The Concise Home Medical Guide

Among the eminent contributors are the following:

R. G. ANDRY, M.A., Ph.D.

MALO BROWN, M.A.

JOCELYN CHAMBERLAIN, M.B., B.S., D.C.H.

GEOFFREY CHAMBERLAIN, M.D., F.R.C.S., M.R.C.O.G.

D. M. B. COLLIER

PETER COOPER, F.P.S.

BARBARA K. HOWELLS, M.B., B.S., D.C.H.

R. F. LAMBERT

MARGARET J. McMAIN, M.C.S.P., S.E.N., O.N.C.

LILIAN M. MORGAN, M.B., B.Ch., N.Sc., D.P.H.

HEATHER RICHARDS

JILL B. ROCK, M.P.S.

LEONARD G. RULE, M.B.E.

E. SILVERMAN, Dip. Soc. Science, Dip. Mental Health

MARY SYLVESTER, M.B., B.S., M.R.C.S., L.R.C.P., D.Obst.R.C.O.G.

D. R. THOMPSON, B.Sc., B.M., B.Ch., D.Obst.R.C.O.G.

Editors:

EDITH J. CONDON and STEPHEN Z. SMITH, M.D.

GROSSET & DUNLAP

Publishers New York

Printed in U. S. A.
ISBN: 0-448-01949-3

1978 PRINTING

CONTENTS

COMMON ACCIDENTS AND EMERGENCIES

Abdominal Injuries

Never give anything to eat or drink to the patient. Cover wound with sterile or freshly laundered material, pad of cotton and firm, but not tight, bandage. If wound runs across the stomach, bend patient's knees and support in this position. Raise head and shoulders, and support them. If wound runs downwards, keep legs straight and do not raise head. These two positions help to draw the two edges of the wound together. Get medical aid at once.

Abrasions

Skin-deep wounds where the protective outer skin has been scraped away or grazed.

Clean the area well with warm soapy water or under running tap to get rid of gravel and dirt. Put plenty of Bacitracin or other non-greasy antiseptic cream on clean dressing, and bandage. Keep the injured part raised to reduce pain and bleeding.

Alcohol

Never give alcohol to injured people unless ordered by a doctor. See also under Intoxication.

Apoplexy

Rupture of a blood vessel in the brain tissue of elderly people causes collapse and unconsciousness with flushed face and noisy breathing. See under Stroke, Apoplectic.

Asphyxia

Suffocation. Where breathing has stopped or there are signs of failure of breathing, begin artificial respiration at once and continue until breathing starts.

The simplest method is mouth-to-mouth or mouth-to-nose breathing into the patient (see p. 22 and illustrations). Head of casualty must be fully tilted backwards to insure clear air. If patient's color does not improve after the first few breaths, look for obstruction in the throat (food, dental plates, vomit, etc.): clear obstruction, tilt head well back and try again. Send for the doctor.

See p. 23 for other methods of artificial respiration.

Berries

Poisonous berries, red, green, or black, are not fatal on the whole to adults but can cause alarming symptoms such as severe vomiting. Get medical aid, try to discover what type of berry has been eaten and, if there are any signs of failure of breathing, start arificial respiration (p. 22). Severe vomiting or diarrhea may cause cramp in the limbs, so give a conscious patient plenty of fluids to which sugar and salt (½ teaspoonful of each to 1 pint) has been added. Never give anything by mouth to an unconscious person.

Bites

Dog. Small punctured wounds with very little bleeding. Cover with dry dressing and get medical aid. Rabies is not likely: a greater danger is from tetanus carried by dog from soil.

Ant, Midge, Bee, Wasp. When bite is on the skin, remove the sting with tweezers or point of a needle sterilized by passing tip through a flame. Apply a weak solution of household ammonia.

A bite near the eye or in the mouth is more dangerous. Apply a solution of bicarbonate of soda (one teaspoonful to a glass of water), or give as a mouth-wash. When sting is in the mouth, get medical aid. (Faintness, pallor, cold skin indicate shock.) In severe cases breathing may fail; apply artificial respiration if this should occur (see p. 22).

Frostbite. See p. 15.

Snake. See p. 17.

Bleeding

Bleeding due to accidents requires immediate action. If severe (gushing or spurting out of the wound) stop flow of blood by firm pressure directly on bleeding point with fingers or thumbs (over a clean pad if at hand). Sit, or preferably lay the patient down to lessen bleeding. Raise and support the bleeding part, unless fractured. Wipe off dirt with clean dressing but never disturb a formed blood clot. Apply dressing, cotton pad, and bandage firmly. Get medical aid.

If glass is in a cut, do not remove it (unless free on surface); raise limb, cover whole wound with a loose dressing and avoid direct pressure on it. Indirect pressure can be used on nearest pressure point (see First Aid, p. 24) to stop blood flow.

For fuller details see First Aid, p. 24. See also under Abdominal Injuries, Cuts, Ear Discharge, Nose Bleeding, Wounds.

Bleeding from internal injuries. Where there is no outside wound, keep patient warm, support in most comfortable position. Give nothing by mouth. Get medical aid. Do not move patient unless it is essential for his immediate safety to do so.

Blisters

From burns and scalds. Do not break blisters. Cover area with sterile dressing or freshly laundered material, apply generous amount of gauze, but bandage lightly. Raise and support a limb. Do not apply lotions, or creams, or butter, etc., in severe cases. Minor everyday small burns and scalds can be treated with suitable non-greasy antiseptic creams.

From chafing or rubbing: treat as for minor burn, p. 14.

Note. If swelling or inflammation persists, get medical advice.

Breath Odor

Acetone odor (smells like nail polish remover) indicates a diabetic who has taken insufficient insulin or omitted an injection; as a result, he may become unconscious and the breath smells of acetone. Immediate medical aid is required. See if patient carries a card or wears a "Medic-Alert" bracelet indicating that he is a diabetic. Call a doctor or get patient to hospital without delay.

Breathing Difficult

Remove any obstruction from the throat. Raise and put a support under head and shoulders, unless fracture of the skull is suspected. See First Aid, p. 21. Get medical help.

Breathing Stopped

Start artificial respiration (p. 22) at once. Send for doctor.

Broken Bones (Fractures)

Act promptly. Treat a swollen sprain as a fracture until the doctor examines it.

(a) Immobilize the whole part (not the small site of fracture) by securing it firmly (not tightly) with bandages over the clothing, after padding between limbs, and with splints (broom handle or umbrella for leg) if necessary, to a sound part of the body to prevent further injury (see First Aid, Figs. 60 and 62). Do not move patient unless essential to his immediate safety to do so, in which case do not attempt this until the part is securely protected against movement (immobilized).

(b) Keep patient warm and at rest. Do not give more than a sip or two of water in case an anesthetic will be given in hospital. Get medical aid.

Fractured skull should not be handled by untrained persons.

For full details regarding first aid for fractures of various bones, see p. 31.

Bruises

Immerse part alternately in hot and cold water. Alternately, apply a cold compress made of a pad of material wrung out in equal parts of alcohol and cold water; when the bruise is near the eyes, use cold water only. If ice is applied it must be in a bag (preferably flannel cloth) or you will 'burn' the patient.

If swelling or pain persists, get medical advice.

Bumps

Treat as for bruises. A hard fall in children may dislocate a joint. If dislocation is present do not attempt to reduce it; support the injured part and get the doctor.

Burns

A six inch burn on a small child will cause immeasurably more injury than one of the same size on an adult. Therefore treatment of burns depends largely upon the surface area injured.

Small burns from electric iron, hot saucepan, etc. Cover burns at once either with a dry sterile dressing, or with an adhesive one to prevent entry of germs; a little antiseptic non-greasy cream may be applied if preferred. Leave dressing in position for about a week unless there is any sign of inflammation, in which case get medical advice. Do not break blisters. If patient seems shocked or frightened, give a warm drink and keep him quiet.

Minor surface burns in adults involving an area smaller than the forearm rarely necessitate a stay in hospital for treatment.

Severe burns from fire or boiling liquid. Do not remove clothing adhering to burned flesh; expert skill is needed, so cover the whole area, including the clothing, with freshly laundered material, a generous pad of cotton, and bandage lightly. Get the patient to hospital as quickly as possible. Keep him warm by covering with a rug but do not use hot water-bottles. Do not give large quantities of fluids to drink, a few sips of water only. For fuller details, see First Aid, p. 35.

Acid burns. Act quickly—remove contaminated clothing. Flood affected part with water. Bathe with solution of two teaspoonfuls of baking soda (bicarbonate of soda) to one pint of water. Then treat as for severe burns.

Alkali burns. Brush off any particles of caustic soda, or caustic oven cleaner, etc., then flood affected part with water. Bathe with solution of vinegar, one part vinegar to one part water. Treat as for severe burns.

Electric burns. Switch off current before touching the patient. Start artificial respiration (p. 22) at once if breathing has stopped. When breathing is restored then treat burns as above under Severe Burns.

Choking

Food in air passage. Pat the patient sharply on the back where the neck meets the shoulders.

Objects, vomit, or blood in the throat. Pass two fingers down the throat and try to remove object. If this fails, put patient on the floor face downwards and pat sharply on the back as above. If this fails after two or three attempts, get a doctor.

If breathing shows signs of failing, start artificial respiration (p. 22).

Cold Injury

See under Frostbite, p. 15.

Colic

(1) From wind or upset stomach, see p. 18.

(2) From food poisoning; get a doctor, keep patient quiet and warm. See Food Poisoning, p. 42.

Concussion

A fall or a blow on the head may cause concussion which can vary from a momentary 'blackout' to stupor or coma. The person often vomits or feels sick while recovering. Partial or complete loss of memory of what happened before the event may be experienced. No injury to the head should be treated lightly—the patient should be kept quiet and, if there has been any loss of consciousness, a doctor's advice should be sought before the patient goes about his normal business.

In cases of stupor or coma, treat as for Unconsciousness, p. 18.

Convulsions

In infants. The body may twitch, the face will be extremely pale or bluish, the breath held, the eyes turned upwards, and a little froth may appear at the mouth. Hold the baby with his head on one side to let the saliva escape. Lay him in crib padded at ends and sides. Apply cool pack to his head and sponge limbs with tepid water. Telephone for the doctor.

Fits. See Epileptic Fits, p. 15; and Diseases of the Nervous System, p. 419.

Coughing

If this comes on suddenly there may be something stuck in the throat: examine for this. Pat patient on the back and give sips of water. Get medical advice if coughing persists.

Cramp

Massage the affected part and apply gentle warmth to painful area. The cramp may be due to loss of fluid through diarrhea, vomiting, or sweating, and it is most important to encourage the person to drink slowly as much as possible of salt water (½ teaspoonful of salt to each pint).

Stomach cramps may be due to food poisoning. See Poisons and Antidotes, p. 42.

Crib Bars

Child's head wedged in. First, reassure the child that no further harm can come. Tell him that while his face is screwed up it is even harder to dislodge his head. Rub the sides of the head and cheeks with oil, grasp the bar on one side and gently try to push the head through. If this does not work, cut the bar above and below the head; use a small saw or even a saw-edged bread knife.

Similar treatment for head stuck between railings, although a metal saw will be required.

Crush Injuries

Treat for shock (p. 21). Treat failure of breathing by giving artificial respiration (p. 22). Get medical aid quickly. Reassure the patient and be careful not to give anything by mouth if internal injuries are suspected.

Cuts

Deep cuts with severe bleeding. Arrest bleeding at once, see p. 13. If cut is long or gaping, take patient to hospital to have it stitched.

Dirty cuts. Brush off loose grit and dirt. Wash under running tap and with swab of cotton dipped in antiseptic to clean wound. Dress cut as on p. 26. If any sign of inflammation see a doctor.

Embedded splinters. Do not remove deeply embedded large splinter of wood, metal, or glass. Take patient to hospital. If needle is broken and embedded, mark with ink the spot where it entered, and take patient to hospital.

Slight clean cuts. Swab with antiseptic, wash off and dab with alcohol; use adhesive dressings from your First Aid box. If wound is painful next day, or shows any sign of inflammation, go to the doctor.

Diabetic Crises

Diabetic Coma. The patient is unconscious, skin dry, breathing like deep sighs, breath smells sweet, pulse fast but weak. Send for doctor immediately, stating signs and symptoms.

Insulin Overdosage. Patient may appear excited or may be unconscious or faint, skin sweaty and pallid, breathing shallow but breath has no special odor. If the patient is able to swallow give him sweets, jam, or a sweet drink. Always test ability to swallow by pouring a teaspoonful of water between the cheek and gums. Call a doctor.

Diarrhea

A sudden attack of diarrhea may denote food poisoning, see Poisons and Antidotes, p. 42. In children it may mean that they have eaten unripe fruit. Always try to find out the history behind an attack. See that fluids are given and if the attack does not disappear quickly, get medical advice.

Dislocations

On no account should any attempt be made to deal with a dislocation other than to make the person as comfortable as possible until hospital treatment is available. Support the joint in the most comfortable position with a sling, with pillows, etc.; avoid jarring or unnecessary movement.

Do not give cups of tea or coffee, only sips of water, as the patient is likely to need an anesthetic when the dislocation is put right: treatment will be delayed if he has eaten or drunk anything.

Dog Bite

See Bites, p.13.

Drowning

Artificial respiration must be started at once if breathing fails. The mouth-to-mouth or mouth-to-nose method (p. 22.) can be started while the casualty is still in the water.

Earache

For mild earache and that associated with the common cold, keep side of face warm (woolen scarf, hot-water bottle). Take a 5-grain aspirin tablet; half for a child of 4 to 8 years. See also Ear, Discharge from.

Ear, Discharge From

If discharge follows an injury, suspect fracture of the base of the skull. Do not move patient. Get a doctor.

If discharge is from some other cause, such as after an attack of measles, see a doctor. Do not clean or dig around.

The doctor will tell you what to do.

Ear, Insect In

Pour a few drops of olive oil or camphorated oil into the ear hole and the insect should float up and can be removed. If insect does not float up or there is anything else in the channel, leave ear alone and get medical advice. Ears can be damaged by unskilled probing.

Electrical Injuries

Switch off current.

See Shock (general), p. 21. If breathing fails start artificial respiration, p. 22.

See Burns, Severe, p. 14 ;35.

In cases of minor shock, reassure the person. Keep him at rest and give warm drinks: warm water containing 1 teaspoonful of bicarbonate of soda to the pint is useful.

Emotional Upset

Can produce primary shock or hysteria, see p. 16. Keep the person warm. Be firm and comforting without giving excessive sympathy. Get a doctor: a sedative may be necessary.

Epileptic Fits

Minor Epilepsy. Pale face, eyes staring, brief period of unconsciousness resembling a fainting attack. Keep patient quiet. Prevent him injuring himself upon objects around.

Major Epilepsy. Patient often has a warning 'aura' (sensation of restlessness, irritability and headache). The fit goes through four stages: (1) sudden loss of consciousness, sometimes preceded by a cry; (2) face flushed and congested, patient rigid; (3) the convulsions start and it is then that the patient may injure himself by violently throwing his arms and legs about, or bite his tongue; (4) the convulsions stop. The patient will be dazed and confused and may act strangely without knowing what he is doing. The duration of the convulsions and the confused state varies.

Treatment. Do not restrain the person; only prevent him from injuring himself or surrounding objects. Place a rolled-up handkerchief, or a spoon handle wrapped in material between his back teeth to prevent the tongue being bitten. Do not leave patient until he is back to normal. For fuller details, see Diseases of the Nervous System, p. 436.

Eye Injuries

Corrosive acids or alkalis in the eye. Wash out with plenty of clean water; a bowlful in which the patient can blink his eye. Get medical aid.

Foreign body embedded in the eyeball: make no attempt to remove it: take patient to the doctor. For grit, dirt, etc., see below.

Bloodshot eyeball or Black eye after an accident may denote a fractured skull. Do not move patient but get medical aid.

Dust, grit, or an eyelash, may cause bloodshot eyeballs. Use recognized eye-wash or make up a solution of salt and boiled (cooled) water, 1 teaspoonful of salt to a glassful of warm boiled water and, using an eye-cup, wash the eyes two or three times a day, taking care either to use two eye-cups, one for each eye, or to clean eye-cup thoroughly for each eye. If this treatment fails within a day, take the patient to a doctor.

Eyes are delicate things and if there is the slightest doubt about the condition—running eye, sticky eyes, etc.—get medical advice. Do not try home remedies and endanger your sight.

Fainting

Feeling giddy, sick; face pale; skin clammy and cold; pulse weak and slow; breathing shallow. Unless the patient has heart trouble, or there is any other reason not to do so, raise the legs higher than the head when laying the person down. Undo tight clothing at neck, chest and waist. Remove garters. Ensure plenty of air. In a crowded vehicle, sit patient on a seat, loosen collar and belt and bend head down between his knees.

If the person does not recover almost immediately, get medical aid. Smelling salts may be given, but do not force the person to take it. If you give smelling salts, test their strength yourself and be sure to apply them with care.

Fatigue

If person faints from fatigue and exhaustion, treat as for fainting and then let him rest, preferably lying down, and keep him warm.

Fireworks, Burns From

See under Burns, p. 14.

Fishbone In The Throat

If the fishbone is stuck in the throat do not try to remove it yourself. You can try giving a piece of dry bread to eat; this may dislodge the bone but, if one or two tries do not succeed, take the patient to a doctor. Keep calm yourself and reassure the sufferer.

Fish Hook In The Skin

If deeply embedded, do not remove it. Take patient to hospital. If superficial, cut line and ease hook through the skin, point first (see First Aid, Fig. 70.).

Fits

See Epileptic Fits, above.

Food Poisoning

Vomiting and diarrhea may be severe. Cramp will indicate that excessive loss of body fluids needs replacing: give plenty of saline solution ($\frac{1}{2}$ teaspoonful salt to 1 pint water) to drink slowly.

Botulism (from infected canned foods) mainly affects vision and produces dry throat, muscular weakness and coldness. Keep patient warm. If symptoms persist, get a doctor.

For fuller details, see Poisons and Antidotes, p. 42.

Fractures

Broken bones must be immobilized immediately by being bandaged firmly to a sound part of the body to prevent further injury (see also Broken Bones, p.13). Treat for shock. Get a doctor. Avoid unnecessary moving as this increases pain. Reassure the patient and remain calm yourself.

For fuller details, see First Aid, p. 31.

Frostbite

After prolonged exposure to cold the ears, hands and feet, nose and face may be affected and the sense of feeling may be lost in the affected parts; the sufferer may not realize he has frostbite. It is most important to remember that on no account must heat be applied nor should you use friction. Do not rub with snow. Take the person into a moderately warm room and cover the affected part.

If exposure has been prolonged, send for medical aid immediately. See also in Vaso-motor Disorders, p. 309.

Gas Poisoning

Turn off the gas, open windows and doors. If the gas tap is not easy to locate, do not waste time hunting for it. Take in two or three deep breaths of fresher air and hold them for as long as possible while dragging the patient out. Crouch low if coal-gas is present since it is lighter than air and rises, but this is not important with gas fumes from gasoline or butane. A second person should have called the nearest doctor.

Treatment. If breathing has ceased apply artificial respiration (p. 22). Keep the patient warm by covering with blankets. Clean the patient's mouth, pull the tongue forward and swab the throat. Oxygen is the best antidote so make sure that you tell the doctor (or the emergency services) that gas poisoning is the cause so that he will bring oxygen or other antidotes with him.

During recovery, the patient may be violent but he should remain in bed for 24 hours. Aspirin and similar drugs should not be taken for the headache.

Sewer fume, car exhaust fume, and smoke poisoning, require treatment as above.

Giddiness

Lay the patient down with the feet raised. Unless there is reason to suppose there is an internal injury, a drink such as tea, coffee, etc. may be given. Recurrent attacks may denote the onset of some illness so see a doctor as soon as possible.

Grazes

See Abrasions, p.13.

Gunshot Wounds

The treatment of gunshot wounds follows the general pattern and rules which apply to any injury associated with severe internal and external bleeding (see p.14; 24). There may be both an entry and an exit wound to treat. The added dangers are (a) the bullet may be lodged in or have damaged an internal organ (lung, kidney, etc.) or may have severed an important blood vessel; or (b) the bullet may have fractured a bone (leg, arm, ribs, etc.). The First Aider must therefore take particular care in handling the patient as these several points must be considered. Treat the wound, or wounds (see p. 18). Treat for shock. Get medical aid at once. Watch for a worsening of the condition such as unconsciousness (see p. 18), or failure of breathing (see p. 22). Treat broken bones (see p. 13; 31).

Headache

Treat with tablets containing aspirin (see Home Medicine Cabinet, p. 56), preferably washed down with milk as this helps to avoid the sick feeling that some people get with these preparations. If the headache persists see a doctor. Children often start one of the infectious diseases with a severe headache.

Heart Attack

There are two common kinds of heart attack. (a) The symptoms of diseases such as coronary disease or angina pectoris are pain, sometimes very severe, over the heart or in the pit of the stomach. The face may be pale or even ashen, and this is due to lack of oxygen in the blood. (b) The second type is where there is chronic heart disease. Symptoms are breathlessness, face a bluish color, the sufferer may collapse suddenly with vomiting or spitting blood, and show all the other signs of shock.

In either case do not move the person unnecessarily. Send for a doctor at once. Support patient in a sitting position but make sure he cannot fall down. Undo tight clothing at neck, waist and chest, remove garters, etc. The patient may carry special tablets to alleviate an attack. Look for them and place one under his tongue. Alternatively, he may carry nitroglycerin tablets.

Hemorrhage

This means bleeding and, if severe, the flow must be stopped at once. If the wound is clean, apply direct pressure to the bleeding point with a pad and bandage; if possible raise the limb. See under Bleeding, p. 14; 24.

Hernia

Hernia is usually referred to as rupture and occurs most frequently in the groin, at the navel, or through the scar of an abdominal wound. Lay the patient down, raise his head and shoulders and support his knees by bending them over a pillow. Get a doctor. Do not attempt to reduce the swelling.

Hiccup

A most effective way of stopping common hiccups is to breathe deeply in and out of a paper bag holding it over the mouth and nose. In some cases it is relieved by taking repeated sips of ice-cold water while the breath is held as long as possible. If the attack persists seek a doctor. In babies, try patting them on the back or give a moistened spoon dipped in sugar to lick.

Household Bleaches Swallowed

Swallowed bleaches (p. 41) produce a choking, burning sensation in the mouth; sometimes vomiting. Detergents cause nausea, stomach discomfort, vomiting. In both cases give milk and copious fluids. Stomach emetic if required (p. 39) and rest in bed.

Hysteria

The temporary condition can usually be dealt with by firm kindness; too much sympathy is bad, but the patient should not be bullied. The more serious form, with body rigid and patient apparently unconscious, convulsions, and falling to the ground, is alarming for the spectator. Treat as for a mild attack but, if patient does not improve, get a doctor who may prescribe a sedative.

Intoxication

It is often helpful to induce vomiting; give stomach emetic (see p. 39) using warm water, in severe cases. Strong black coffee and sugar should then be given.

A smell of alcohol in the breath need not indicate drunkenness; alcohol may have been taken for collapse. If patient is unconscious, treat as for Unconsciousness (p. 18).

Itching

If accompanied by a rash, it may indicate an infectious disease, e.g. chickenpox. Examine the child and report to the doctor. Threadworms (usually in children) often cause itching around the anus particularly at night (see Intestinal Parasites, p.387). Get medical advice to remedy the condition as it can spread quickly among other children.

A sudden skin irritation in a person allergic to certain foods or substances can be relieved by applying an antihistamine cream or ointment, or by taking antihistamine tablets.

Match Poisoning

Give a child milk to drink if match-heads are swallowed.

Nausea

Feeling sick is common, particularly in children. If nausea is due to stuffy atmosphere, ventilate room and take child for a short walk in fresh air; if due to over-tiredness, give a fruit juice or glucose drink and put child to rest; if a preliminary sign of car-sickness, break the journey and let the child walk or get around in the fresh air. Glucose tablets or sweets, and seasickness tablets are often helpful to persons prone to travel-sickness.

Nausea may be due to the onset of infectious diseases: watch for further signs and symptoms such as headache, rise in temperature, listlessness, and if they do not subside within three or four hours, get medical advice.

Nausea in pregnancy, p. 96. See also pp. 39-44.

Needle Embedded In Flesh

If the needle can be easily extracted with a pair of tweezers, do so: if the point has broken off, mark the spot with ink and get the person to hospital as quickly as possible.

Nose Bleeding

Do not be alarmed by what seems to be a great deal of blood. Loosen all tight clothing around the neck and chest, at the waist, remove garters, etc. Seat the person in a current of air and tell him to breathe through the mouth. Pinch the nostrils firmly but do not try to plug the nose. A cold compress applied to the forehead and at the back of the neck may help. Patient must not blow his nose. Reassure children who may be alarmed by a bleeding nose. If bleeding persists, get medical advice.

Nose, Foreign Body In

The person must breathe through the mouth. Do not attempt to remove the object but get medical aid.

Pallor

A shock caused by good or bad news, motion-sickness accompanied by nausea, and vertigo (fear of heights) can all cause excessive paleness of the face. Treat as for Fainting, p. 15, but if pallor persists call in the doctor.

Palpitations

These may occur, particularly in stout or elderly people, after they have had a heavy meal followed by some energetic activity. Palpitations sometimes follow emotional stress and affect persons with heart conditions, In all cases, reassure the sufferers. Make them rest and, if there is any doubt as to the seriousness of the underlying condition, call in the doctor. See Heart Attack, p. 16, and Fainting, p. 15.

Plastic Bags

These must be kept out of reach of children under ten years of age: also out of reach of anyone who has been seriously depressed. If the enveloping bag is placed over the head, either in play or on purpose, a person can die of asphyxia in as little as four minutes. Give artificial respiration (p. 22), if breathing stops.

Poisons

See section on Poisons and Antidotes, p. 39.

Rashes

Diaper rash. Some children have excessively tender skins, and even constant changing does not prevent a painful, red rash. Get your doctor to prescribe a diaper disinfectant and a good ointment. Make sure that the child is kept dry. Use zinc ointment generously. Boil diapers and dry them in the sun. Avoid use of plastic or rubber pants.

Infections. Rashes accompanied by a running nose, signs of a cold or a temperature, may be the onset of an infectious disease. Get the doctor's advice.

Rupture

Common name for abdominal hernia. Sudden swelling, usually in the groin, pain, and sometimes vomiting. For treatment, see Hernia, p. 16.

Scalds

Treat as for Burns, p. 14; 35.

Shivering

Cold. In cold weather it is a natural skin reaction indicating that more covering is needed. Small children and elderly people need extra warmth in cold weather, particularly in the bedroom. Extreme changes in temperature are bad for them and should be avoided.

Fevers. Shivering associated with fevers is a common feature and may be accompanied with a rise in temperature. Guard against the patient getting a chill, keep him warm and maintain an even warm temperature in the room. Get the doctor.

Shock

This condition is present in all cases of accident or emotional upset. Rest, warmth and comforting reassurance are the main essentials of treatment. Warm sweet drinks, sipped, should be given unless there are abdominal injuries, broken bones, or hemorrhage. For fuller details, see First Aid, p. 21.

Snake Bite

In countries where snake-bite poisoning may be deadly, prompt (within two or three minutes) treatment is vital. Tie a ligature on the heart side of the bite: a strong rubber band, firmly applied, is excellent, or strips of clothing tied round the limb can be tightened by twisting with a stick. The ligature must be released for one minute in every twenty to allow arterial blood flow. As the injection of carbolic soap solution provides effective first aid, travellers in snake-infested areas might carry a hypodermic syringe and carbolic or other soap. Shake a piece of carbolic soap the size of a walnut in a cupful of warm water until dissolved, then inject 1 to 2 ml. of the solution under the skin around the bite marks. Get medical aid speedily as patient must receive antivenom serum injections; meanwhile treat for shock. Note type of snake for the doctor to provide the appropriate serum.

Mouth-to-mouth breathing (p. 22) if respiration fails.

Sore Throat

Crush a tablet of aspirin in a glassful of warm water, gargle, and then swallow it. If soreness persists get a doctor. Be sure your child is fully immunized against poliomyelitis, diphtheria, and smallpox: many infectious fevers begin with sore throat.

Splinters

Small easily removed splinters may be treated by easing the point out with a needle boiled in water (5 min.), and then pulling it out with small tweezers. Large deeply embedded splinters should not be disturbed but removed by a doctor or in hospital.

Sprains And Strains

Sprains occur at joints, strains involve muscles: both are painful and rest is usually the best cure. Repeated cold compresses on a sprain may help ease the pain. If a person with a mild ankle sprain must get on his feet, bandage it firmly with a wide Ace bandage over an old stocking. If swelling and pain persist get medical advice, particularly with sprained ankles, in case a small bone may be broken.

Staggering

Alcohol. If due to over-indulgence in alcohol, give patient large quantities of strong black coffee, or tea: if neither is available give plain water or milk to help dilute the alcohol. The smell of alcohol in the breath may mask an illness for which the patient has taken a small drink, so get the facts of the case and inform a doctor if there is any doubt as to the real cause.

Drugs. If overdosage has caused staggering and confusion, retrieve remaining tablets or mixture and get a doctor; if possible tell him what you suspect.

Blows. If due to a blow on the head, keep the person at rest. If there is even the slightest sign of a momentary 'black-out' make him see a doctor.

Sties

Sties are usually caused by an infection in the nose. See a doctor as soon as possible. In the meantime do not allow the person to rub the eye or to wipe the other one with the same piece of material as is used for the infected one. Relieve the irritation or pain by 'spooning', i.e. wrapping a handkerchief around a spoon and dipping it in a bowl of reasonably hot water containing bicarbonate of soda or salt (1 dessertspoonful to 1 pint of water), pressing out excess fluid to the side of the bowl, and applying the 'fomentation' to the eye.

Stings

Insect stings. If the stinger is in the flesh, ease it out with the point of a needle boiled 5 min., then apply the remedy. For bee stings, household ammonia dabbed on usually gives relief (do not use near the eyes). For wasp or ant stings put on olive oil, household ammonia, a saline compress, or baking soda solution (see Bites, p. 13).

Nettle stings can be alarming to very young children, reassure them, and if possible find dock leaves, crush these in your fingers and rub on to the affected area. Calamine lotion or an antihistamine cream may give relief. Some rashes resembling nettle stings may be associated with an allergy or a disease, so if there is no relief from home remedies or there is a rise in temperature, get medical advice.

Stitch

This is a painful spasm of the diaphragm and happens during games of violent exercise. Give sips of water, keep the person quiet, draw up the leg on the side where stitch occurs, apply a warm (not hot) hot-water bottle and rub the affected side gently. Stitch usually indicates that the person is not 'in training' and has over-exerted himself.

Stomach-Ache

Various stomach and intestinal infections cause stomach-ache, sometimes with diarrhea or with vomiting. Keep patient warm, in bed, give fruit juice, and if symptoms persist call in the doctor. Emotional worries and fears may be the cause in young children—try to find the reason and reassure the child. For stomach-ache caused by overeating, a dose of Milk of Magnesia should give relief. In all cases where pain persists get the doctor to check up.

If some foreign body has been swallowed, take the patient to the hospital quickly.

Strangulation

Remove the constriction at the throat. If breathing has failed, start artificial respiration, p. 22, at once. Get medical aid as soon as possible.

Stroke, Apoplectic

Most common in elderly people. Sudden onset is due to the rupture of a diseased blood vessel causing hemorrhage in the brain. The patient is unconscious, with face flushed, pulse slow, and paralysis often on one side. If breathing is noisy, turn him to the three-quarters prone position (see illustration, p. 22) and undo tight clothing. Keep him warm, but do not apply hot-water bottles. Give nothing by mouth. Keep at rest and send for a doctor. If breathing fails, start artificial respiration (p. 22).

Treat as for fracture of the skull (compression). See First Aid, p. 31.

Suffocation

Soft pillows for infants, or plastic bags over the head of a small child may cause suffocation. The face will be blue, showing lack of oxygen in the blood. If breathing has ceased, start artificial respiration (p. 22). Every second counts in getting oxygen into the blood. When breathing recommences, get a doctor. See also Choking, p. 14.

Sunburn

Can be serious; if blistering is severe, get medical aid. If no blistering, make a thin paste of bicarbonate of soda and water, and dab on to affected parts. Antiseptic non-greasy creams, or calamine lotion may give relief, but do not apply butter or grease, and do not break any blisters.

Sunstroke

Often associated with heat stroke symptoms, i.e. vomiting, rise in temperature, cramp. Keep patient in a cool place at rest. For cramp give repeated saline drinks (½ teaspoonful salt to 1 pint of water). Apply cold compress to the head. If symptoms of raised temperature and vomiting persist, get medical attention.

Throat, Objects Lodged In

For easily removed objects, such as a piece of food in the back of the throat, pat patient sharply on the back or remove object with two fingers. If you do not immediately succeed, get a doctor. If breathing fails use artificial respiration (p. 22).

Toothache

The only lasting cure is to see a dentist and have the tooth repaired or extracted; everyone should have regular check-ups. Oil of cloves rubbed on the gum, or aspirin dissolved slowly against the painful tooth sometimes gives temporary relief. See Diseases of Lips and Mouth, p. 357.

Unconsciousness

The most important thing to discover is whether the person is breathing or not. If breathing has failed, start artificial respiration (p. 22). If breathing is satisfactory loosen tight clothing and, unless internal injuries or fractures make it impossible, raise the legs on a cushion or other support, keeping the head low and face turned to one side if the face is pale. If face is flushed and looks congested, or the patient is known to have heart trouble, raise and support the head and shoulders, turn head to one side, and keep the legs low. Get medical aid. See also Fractured Skull, p. 31, Fainting, p. 15, Asphyxia, p. 21, and Epileptic Fits, p. 15.

Varicose Veins

If varicose veins rupture and bleed, immediately raise the bleeding leg. Apply direct pressure over a folded handkerchief on the bleeding point. Apply a bandage below and above the bleeding point firmly enough to stop bleeding. These three bandages must be gently loosened every fifteen minutes. Send for a doctor.

Vomiting

Find out the cause. If a poison has been swallowed, e.g. medicines or tablets left carelessly around, tainted foods, or wayside berries, keep a specimen of the vomit and any pill bottles, etc. for the doctor's information. Send for a doctor.

If overeating has caused vomiting, keep patient at rest. In heart attack vomiting is sometimes present, see p. 16. Guard against and treat for associated shock, p. 21. Get a doctor's advice if the cause is doubtful or if the condition does not respond fairly quickly.

See also Food Poisoning, p. 15, and Nausea, p. 16.

Weedkiller Poisoning

Unless you know the exact substance involved be content with diluting the swallowed poison with large quantities of water or milk: get medical aid quickly. If collapse is due to poison absorbed through the skin, wash the affected areas and remove contaminated clothing. Look out for failure of breathing and apply artificial respiration (not mouth-to-mouth for these poisons), p. 23.

See also under Poisons and Antidotes, p. 44.

Winding

As a result of a blow in the solar plexus (soft part just below the breast bone) the patient may faint or even collapse. Draw up his knees, having laid him down. Keep him quiet. Loosen tight clothing at neck, waist, chest. He should recover within a few minutes. If he does not, get medical aid.

Wounds

Severe wounds with excessive bleeding must be covered, and pressure applied to stop bleeding as soon as possible. See Abdominal Injuries, Bleeding, Cuts; and also Hemorrhage in First Aid section, p. 24. Any inflammation or swelling which persists should be reported to a doctor at once.

FIRST AID

The appalling toll of human life through accidents in the home, on the roads, at work, and on vacation makes an understanding and knowledge of first aid a matter of vital human good-neighborliness when prompt skilled aid not only can save life but prevent an injury becoming worse. In the great majority of accidents, the first person on the scene is the woman from the house nearby. In the home it is the housewife who is faced with giving first aid to the suffocated or scalded baby, or to the elderly person who has slipped on the stairs. There are countless incidents where skilled attention has saved lives. How many more deaths could have been prevented and how much needless suffering avoided if everyone knew the right thing to do!

PRINCIPLES OF FIRST AID

It is true that first aid is ninety per cent common sense and ten per cent knowledge. It is also true that in certain cases, such as when artificial respiration is necessary or severe bleeding has to be stopped or a broken bone 'fixed' so that further injury is not caused, it is the ten per cent knowledge which may make the difference between life and death, and between a good recovery and permanent disablement. It is essential, therefore, that as many people as possible should study the basic principles and be as well versed as possible in both what to do and what not to do.

First aid should be used only for immediate and temporary assistance and at no time should the First Aider attempt to take the place of a doctor. Medical assistance must be obtained with the least possible delay.

The scope of First Aid is:

To determine the nature of the case and to decide on the treatment required—DIAGNOSIS.

To apply these conclusions intelligently, quickly and gently—TREATMENT.

To arrange for the casualty to be removed to shelter—either to his home, to suitable shelter to await further assistance or to hospital—DISPOSAL.

Diagnosis

In order to find out what has happened and the extent of the injuries or the nature of the illness, three points must be considered: (a) History, (b) Symptoms, and (c) Signs.

(a) HISTORY. The story of the accident, or the onset of illness. This may be given by the casualty or by witnesses; items to note would be that the casualty may suffer from a particular disease, the presence of broken chairs, signs of a crash or any other causes which the surroundings may suggest.

(b) SYMPTOMS. These are the sensations felt by the casualty, i.e. pain, numbness, nausea, shivering, etc., which he can tell you about if he is conscious.

(c) SIGNS. Signs are the variations in the condition of the casualty from normal. Extreme pallor which, in conjunction with the history and symptoms, may indicate loss of blood or shock. Congestion perhaps indicating head injury or a stroke. Swelling and deformity indicating a fracture, and bleeding. Signs are probably the most reliable factors in diagnosis, but the combination of the three points should enable the First Aider to weigh up the situation.

Examination of the Casualty

Examination will enlarge on the three points—history, symptoms and signs.

Note the scene, surroundings, and general circumstances of the case, paying special attention to any sources of further danger or injury. If the person is conscious, warn him to lie still and reassure him.

If he is unconscious, immediately find out whether he is breathing or bleeding and take appropriate action (see Asphyxia, p. 21, and Hemorrhage, p. 24). If signs of life appear to be absent, assume he is alive and apply artificial respiration at once.

If he is bleeding, stop it. Arterial bleeding cannot be mistaken as the blood will be bright red and spurting out. A severed important vein is equally dangerous, but the blood will be darker in color and gushing out. It should be remembered that a little blood goes a long way—rather like red paint, so that what appears to be a severe wound may not, on examination, be as bad as it looks, in which case the examination of the patient should be completed before stopping to treat what may be a comparatively minor injury.

Carefully examine the limbs and body for evidence of fractures or wounds, dislocations or other injuries. Fractures and dislocations can be recognized by the limb being in an unnatural position and, if he is conscious, the casualty will complain of pain and loss of power. On no account must a First Aider try to reduce a dislocation and it must be remembered that this is an acutely painful condition (see Dislocations and Sprains, p. 37).

In elderly people, if there is any doubt, suspect and treat for fractures as their bones are brittle and a fracture of the thigh near the hip joint may be difficult to diagnose.

If the casualty has been run over or crushed by a heavy object, suspect and treat for internal injuries (see p. 25; 34).

If his eyes are closed, lift the lids and examine the pupils (see Unconsciousness and Compression of the Brain, p. 18; 31): they may be equal, normal, dilated, or unequal.

In some poisoning cases, burns or stains round the mouth may be the only clue.

In fractures of the base of the skull, blood or fluid may ooze from the ear or nose, or may be swallowed and later vomited.

Treatment

If the cause of the injury is still present, for example if the casualty is in a gas or smoke-filled room, remove him at once. In cases of electric shock turn off the current before attempting to touch him, or make sure you remove him with some non-conducting material (see Electrical Injuries, p. 15).

In cases of asphyxia (failure of breathing, see p. 21) give artificial respiration (p. 22) at once and continue until a doctor states that further efforts are useless. DEATH MUST NEVER BE ASSUMED. Many patients have recovered after hours of treatment.

In cases of severe bleeding apply pressure (see p. 24) at once, a casualty can die in as little as three minutes if bleeding continues.

When a limb is broken it must be immobilized (by being tied, bandaged and perhaps splinted to prevent movement) immediately to prevent a further injury, such as the broken ends being pushed through the skin or into internal organs. A comparatively simple injury could thus be turned into an extremely serious one.

In cases of severe burns and scalds the danger from infection is very great and immediate action must be taken to cover the affected area with sterile or clean material.

Disposal

Having diagnosed *and* treated the condition the next step is disposal. Unless the casualty has been examined by a doctor on the spot or if the accident has happened away from the casualty's home, he must be taken home, to shelter, or to hospital with the least possible delay.

Should the person be required to be moved before an ambulance arrives, the following methods of support and transport may be used with due regard to the injuries suffered.

Support by One Person

Human Crutch. Stand at the patient's side and put one arm around his waist, holding his clothes on his hip; put his arm around your neck and hold his hand with your free hand (Fig. 1). For use when the patient can walk.

Fireman's Lift. Only to be used when the casualty is not too heavy (Fig. 2).

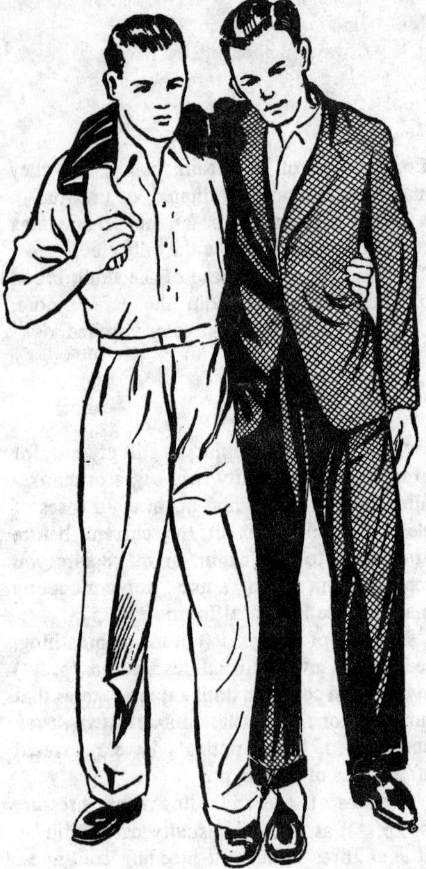

Fig. 1. *HUMAN CRUTCH*

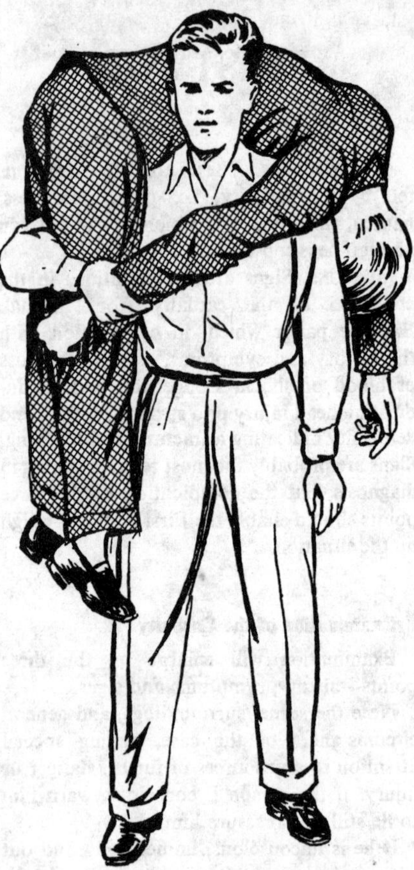

Fig. 2. *FIREMAN'S LIFT*

Cradle Method. If only one helper is present, carefully lift the injured person by passing one arm beneath his knees, and the other arm round his back below his armpits. This method can only be used by a strong assistant for a child or light-weight patient. It cannot be used when there is a spinal injury, a fracture of the leg, or any other serious injury.

Piggyback. If the assistant is strong enough, and if the patient is light in weight and is conscious so that he can hold on, he may be carried on the assistant's back. The assistant should support him under his knees.

Support by Several Persons

Hand Seats. If two or more helpers are available, the patient may be carried by means of hand seats. These are:

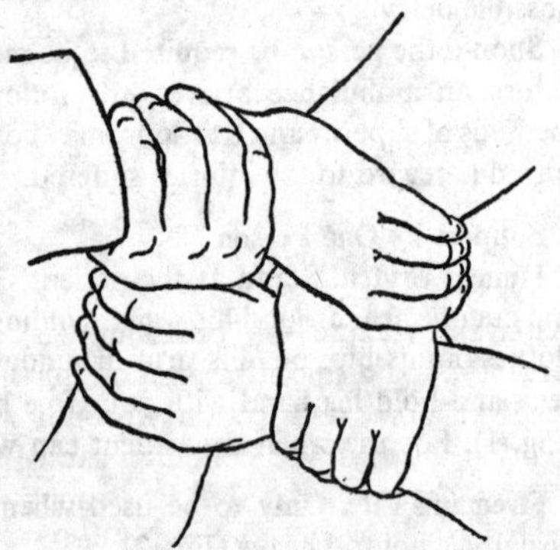

Fig. 3. *GRIP FOR FOUR-HANDED SEAT*

THE FOUR-HANDED SEAT. The patient must help the assistants by using one or both arms to hold round the bearers' necks (Fig. 3).

THE TWO-HANDED SEAT. This is used when the patient cannot use his arms, the patient being supported behind the back by the bearers' two free arms. The bearers' hands should be clasped by hook-grip below the patient (Fig. 4).

In each case the bearers must use cross-over steps when carrying.

Fore and Aft Method. This may be used instead of a hand seat in narrow passages. The hind bearer holds the patient below the armpits and round the body, while the front bearer holds the patient below his knees, walking with his back to the patient's face. The two bearers must then move in step with one another.

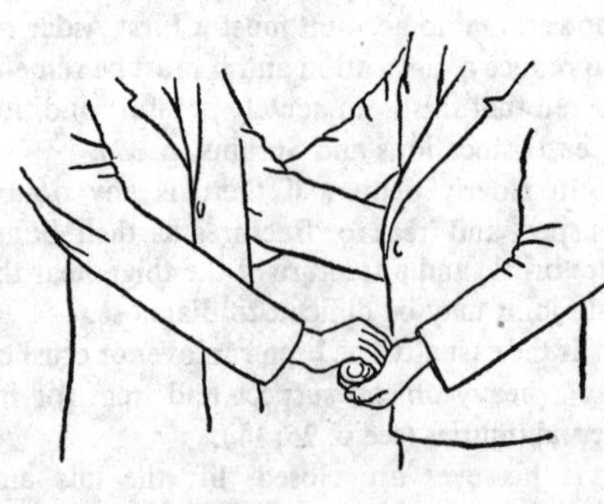

Fig. 4. *GRIP FOR TWO-HANDED SEAT*

An Improvised Stretcher. If no stretcher is available, one may be improvised by turning the sleeves of a long coat inside out, passing a stout pole through each sleeve and then buttoning the coat. A long stretcher may be made by using two coats. The poles will be kept apart if a strip of wood is bound at right angles to the poles at both ends. A door, shutter, or a broad board may also be covered with straw, blankets or wraps to provide an emergency stretcher.

A blanket lift is illustrated on p. 21, Fig. 6. The long edges of a blanket are firmly rolled and then gripped by four bearers, two on each side. This method is mainly used for placing a casualty on a stretcher.

A Bandage Stretcher requires eight triangular bandages arranged as in Fig. 5.

Always test a stretcher before putting a patient upon it. Only carry a stretcher upon the shoulders when going up a hill or stairs.

Whenever possible, avoid lifting a stretcher over obstacles. Keep the stretcher level and steady; carry the patient facing forward, except when going upstairs or up a hill.

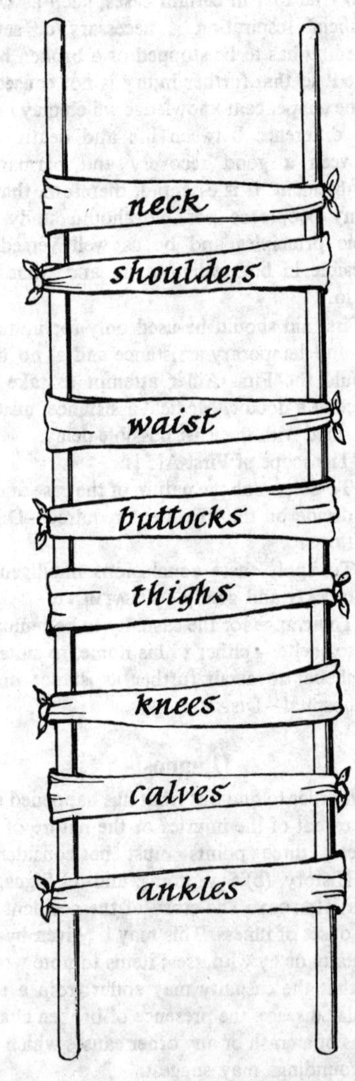

Fig. 5. *BANDAGE STRETCHER*

WHAT TO DO: Summary

1. The saving of life may depend on the quickness with which action is taken.

2. The manner of approach to any injured person and those connected with him should be calm, reassuring and confident. The lessening of anxiety can do much towards reducing the danger of shock, and gaining the confidence of the casualty can help the First Aider to diagnose and treat quickly.

3. Treat failure of breathing, severe bleeding, fractures and shock—in that order.

4. Give artificial respiration at once if breathing has stopped.

5. Stop severe bleeding.

6. Immobilize fractures.

7. Cover wounds and burns with sterile or clean material.

8. Never give alcohol unless ordered by a doctor.

9. Shock is present in all cases of accident or sudden illness.

10. Keep the casualty warm by covering him up but do not apply hot-water bottles. It has been proved that applied heat increases shock, but covering the person reserves his own body heat. Keep him at rest.

11. Improvise dressings and bandages if no equipment is available. Ties, scarves, stockings, etc. will serve as bandages and slings. Clean handkerchiefs, towels, etc. as dressings. Socks, sacking, grass, etc. can be used to pad splints and between fractured limbs. Poles from brooms, umbrellas, tightly rolled newspapers, etc. can be used as splints. Doors, gates, coats, etc. as 'stretchers'.

12. Make use of onlookers to bring help, gather equipment and warn oncoming traffic.

13. (a) Note danger from falling buildings, moving machinery, fire, electric current, poisonous gases, fumes, etc., and guard the casualty against further injury.

(b) If the accident occurs out of doors make sure the casualty is sheltered and not exposed unnecessarily to the weather.

14. Do not allow people to crowd round—give them a job to do.

15. Do not uncover the casualty more than is absolutely necessary.

16. Don't assume that because someone smells of alcohol that he is drunk.

17. Observe any changes in the casualty's color, breathing, pulse (whether it is fast, weak, slow or imperceptible).

18. Never give anything by mouth to an unconscious person or to anyone who will require further hospital treatment. In the first instance you will choke him and in the second, should he require an anesthetic, treatment will be delayed if quantities of fluid have been given.

19. Never give anything by mouth if an internal injury is suspected. If the casualty complains of thirst let him rinse his mouth with water frequently.

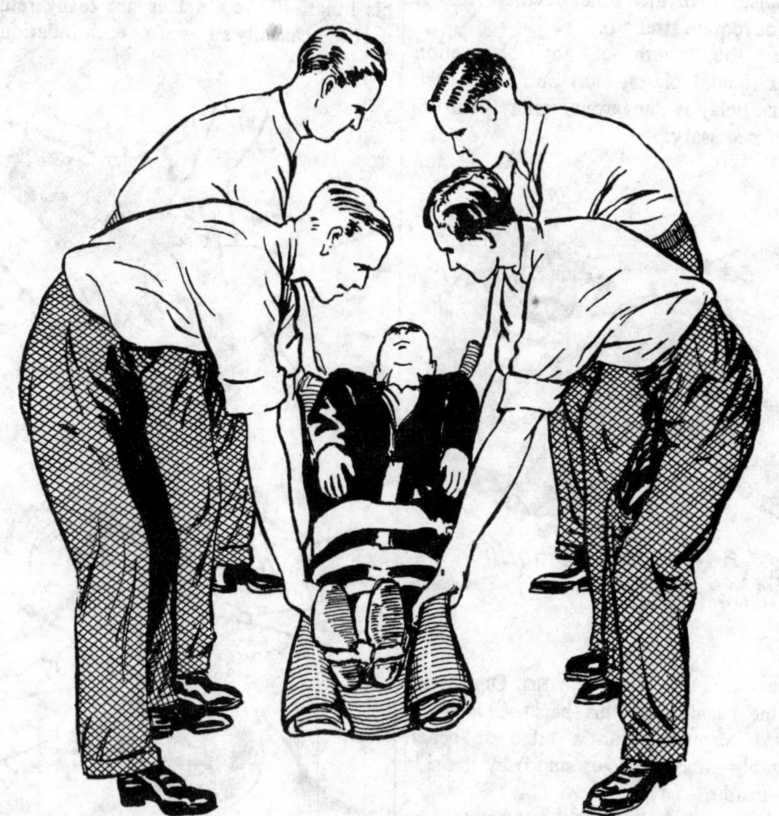

Fig. 6. *BLANKET LIFT*
This is used to lift the casualty on to the stretcher.

20. Remember to remove dental plates from an unconscious person.

21. Always handle injured people as little as possible and with great care and gentleness. Pain increases shock and shock can kill.

22. Never remove deeply embedded splinters or glass.

23. Never break blisters.

24. Leave blood clots on a wound.

25. Loosen tight clothing at neck, chest, waist, and remove garters, etc.

26. When possible give a written report when sending for a doctor. In poison cases every effort should be made to determine the cause so that the doctor can bring any necessary antidote. Save vomit, pill bottles, as these may give a clue to the type of poison.

SHOCK

Shock is present to some degree in all cases of accident or sudden illness. Its severity varies with the extent of the injury and can cause death following severe accidents.

Shock can develop at once or develop later. This delayed development is particularly dangerous as it may go unnoticed, and this is why so much stress is laid on treating and guarding against shock.

Causes. Bleeding, both visible and internal. Burns and fractures, particularly of the femur (thigh), and compound fractures.

General Signs and Symptoms
Faintness and giddiness
Nausea
Pallor
Cold clammy skin
Slow pulse at first which, if shock develops, may become rapid and feeble
Unconsciousness

General Treatment of Shock

Lay the casualty on his back with head low and turned to one side, unless there is a head, abdomen or chest injury, when the head and shoulders should be slightly raised and supported. If he is vomiting or there is danger of any obstruction to breathing, place him in the three-quarters prone position (Fig. 7).

Loosen clothing at neck, chest, waist.

Wrap in blanket, rug, coats, etc.

If he complains of thirst give him sips of water, tea, coffee, etc., unless injuries make this inadvisable (see Hemorrhage, p. 24).

Do not apply friction to limbs; do not apply hot-water bottles.

Keep him quiet and reassured and get medical aid as soon as possible.

ASPHYXIA

Asphyxia (failure of breathing) is an emergency, and artificial respiration must be started at once and continued until the casualty recovers. It is a condition caused by the lungs not getting a sufficient supply of oxygen and if this is not remedied death will occur.

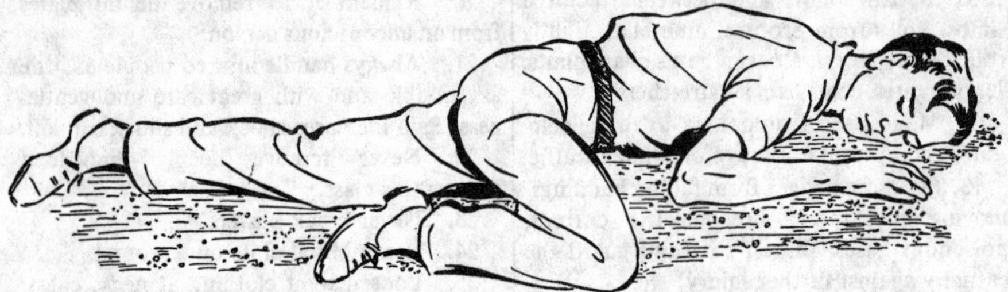

Fig. 7. *THREE-QUARTERS PRONE POSITION*

Causes

1. Drowning when fluid enters the air passages.
2. Poisonous gases, fumes, smoke, motor exhaust, ammonia, certain dry-cleaning fluids, sewer gas, and coal gas.
3. Foreign bodies in the air passages such as food, dental plates, vomited matter; blood in cases of fractured jaws causing choking.
4. Hanging or strangulation causing compression of the windpipe.
5. Swelling of the tissues in the throat caused by burns, scalds, corrosives, stings, or from some diseases of the throat.
6. Injuries to the chest due to accidents in mines, quarries, demolition, etc., or from pressure in crowds.
7. Poisons such as strychnine, cyanide, and morphine, or diseases such as lockjaw (tetanus) and poliomyelitis.
8. Electric shock. Stroke by lightning.

Signs and Symptoms

In the early stages the signs and symptoms are dizziness, shortness of breath, rapid pulse, swelling of the veins of the neck, blueness of cheeks and lips, and congestion of the face. In the later stages breathing is intermittent or absent, pulse slow and irregular, lips, nose, ears, toes and fingers bluish-gray, and there is complete lack of consciousness.

General Rules for Treatment of Asphyxia

1. Remove the casualty from the cause or the cause from the casualty.
2. Make sure there is a free passage of air and remember in unconscious cases there is a constant danger of the tongue falling back and obstructing the air passages if the casualty is lying on his back.
3. Apply artificial respiration immediately —again remembering that if the casualty is not in the correct position the air will not be able to get into the lungs.

Emergency Respiratory Resuscitation (Artificial Respiration)

When a person stops breathing, the blood is deprived of oxygen without which no one can survive for more than eight minutes. It is essential, therefore, to get oxygen into the lungs with the least possible delay. As this action is taken by another person it is called artificial respiration and to stress the urgency it is called Emergency Resuscitation.

There are four methods of artificial respiration in common use for First Aid, and in order of effectiveness they are: (1) Mouth-to-Mouth (or mouth-to-nose) also known as Rescue Breathing, Oral Resuscitation, or the Kiss or Breath of Life; (2) Silvester's; (3) Schafer's; and (4) Holger Neilsen methods.

In some cases the casualty's heart may have stopped beating so that it is necessary to perform external cardiac massage at the same time as artificial respiration, therefore the first two methods are preferred as the casualty is already in the face upwards position.

A change in skin color from blue to pink indicates that the casualty's blood is being oxygenated and that he is responding.

Mouth-to-Mouth Method

Its advantages are that it provides the greatest ventilation to the lungs and can be used more easily and in more difficult circumstances than any other method, and it does not require strength.

Clear the mouth of any obstruction (mucus, dental plates, etc.) but, since each second's delay is dangerous, ignore obstructions if necessary.

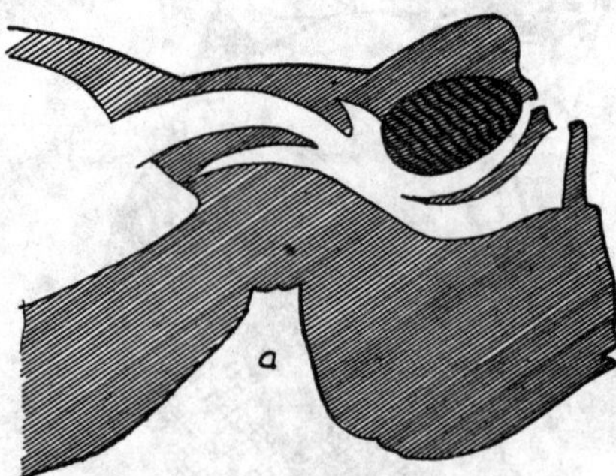

Fig. 8. *MOUTH-TO-MOUTH*

(a) When lower jaw is pushed upwards, the tongue is raised to clear the air passages.

Position of Casualty and Operator. Lay the casualty on his back—in shallow water if drowning, on a table or bench preferably—and kneel (or stand) by the side of his head.

Hold casualty's head in both hands, one hand tilting the head backwards and the other pushing the lower jaw upwards and forwards (Fig. 8b and c).

Fig. 8a illustrates the vital importance of a clear airway. By pressing the head backwards and the lower jaw upwards the front of the casualty's neck is extended and the tongue moves forward leaving the air passage clear.

Inspiration Movement. Open your mouth wide, take in a deep breath and seal your mouth over the casualty's mouth, blocking his nostrils with your cheek (in some cases it may be necessary to pinch his nostrils). Blow into his lungs until his chest rises, then remove your mouth (Fig. 8c). While you are taking another breath the air blown in will be passively exhaled by the casualty.

Repeat six times fairly rapidly, then continue at the rate of ten inflations per minute.

For an infant or young child, seal your lips round both mouth and nose, and blow *gently*. Repeat inflations at the rate of twenty per minute.

Mouth-to-Nose Method

This is a modified method for casualties in a state of spasm whose mouths cannot be opened, or for persons without teeth, or where the operator's mouth is smaller than that of the casualty.

Take up a position by the side of the casualty's head and close his mouth by placing your thumb on his lower lip. After taking in a deep breath seal your lips around his nose without obstructing his nostrils. Blow into his lungs. If the air does not easily return, part the casualty's lips after each inflation.

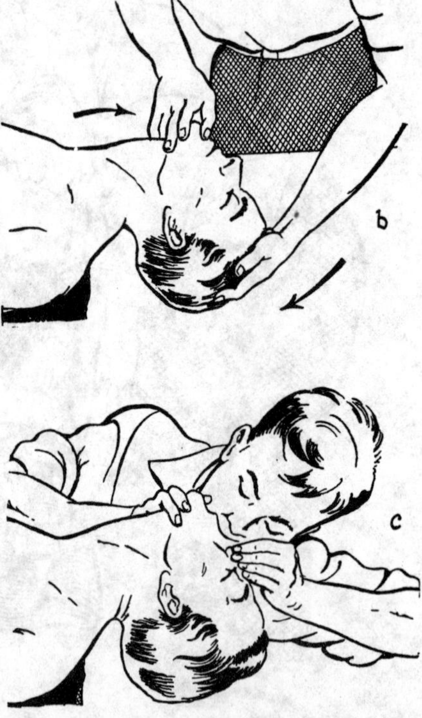

Fig. 8. *MOUTH-TO-MOUTH*

(b) Tilt jaw upwards with right hand. (c) Seal your mouth round the casualty's mouth and pinch his nostrils with left hand.

Silvester Method

Lay the casualty down on his back with a pad (folded jacket or towel, or pillow) under his shoulders so that the head falls backwards.

Kneel at the casualty's head, lean forward and grasp his hands at wrists.

MOVEMENT 1. Cross the hands as in Fig. 9a and press them firmly over the lower chest to force the air out of his lungs. *This will take 2 seconds.*

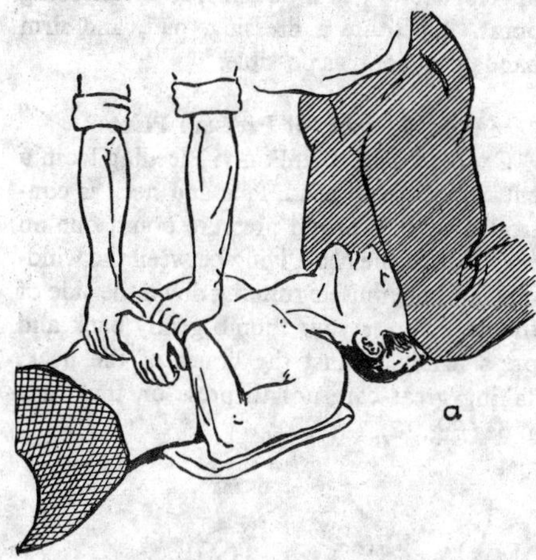

Fig. 9a. *SILVESTER. Movement* 1.

MOVEMENT 2. With a sweeping movement upwards and outwards above the casualty's head, bring the arms as far backwards as you can (Fig. 9b). This releases the pressure and allows air to be drawn into the lungs. *This will take 3 seconds.*

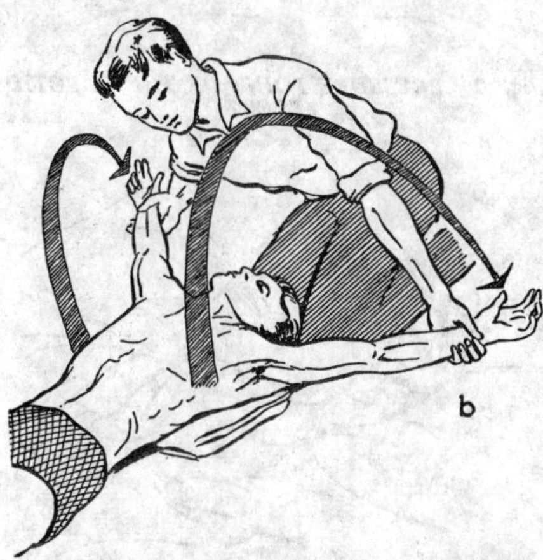

Fig. 9b. *SILVESTER. Movement* 2.

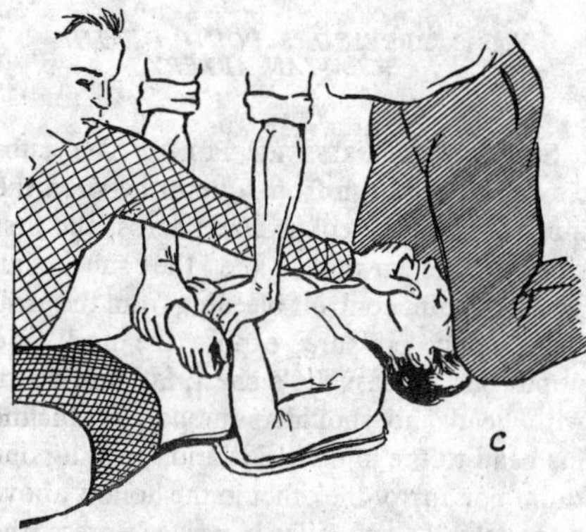

Fig. 9c. *SILVESTER. An assistant can ensure a clear airway for the casualty.*

Repeat these movements rhythmically, 12 times a minute.

Check frequently that the mouth and nose are free from mucus, vomit, or obstruction. Get an assistant to help, if available: he can press casualty's lower jaw (Fig. 9c) to ensure that the jaw is jutting out, and turn the head to one side if necessary.

When natural breathing begins, gradually ease up the rhythmic movements.

Schafer Method

Turn casualty to the face downwards position.

POSITION OF CASUALTY AND OPERATOR. Place casualty's hands one over the other under his forehead, with head slightly turned to one side, if possible, raise hands and head a few inches on folded coat, towel, etc. Kneel on both knees at the casualty's side facing his head and just below his hip joint. Sit back on your heels (as in Fig. 10a) and place your hands on his sides, one on each side of his backbone with your wrists almost touching, thumbs pointing forwards and fingers close together, on his flanks. *Keep elbows straight throughout.*

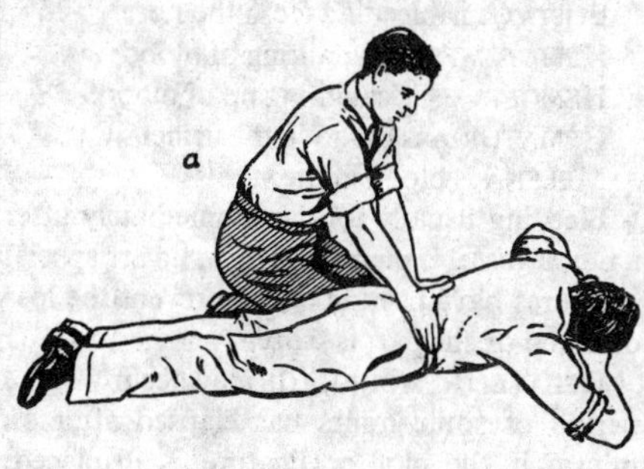

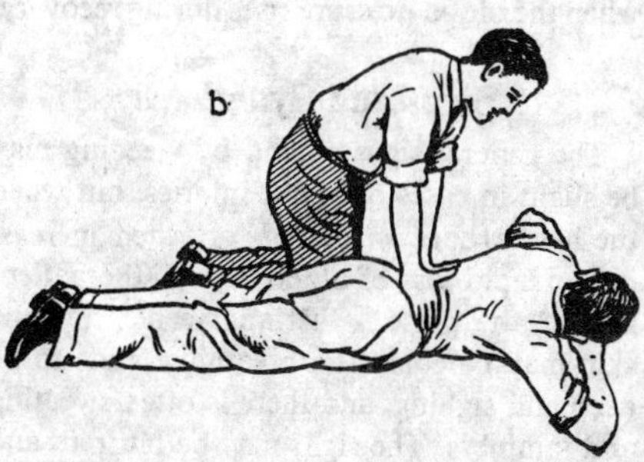

Fig. 10. *SCHAFER.* (a) *Position of casualty and operator.* (b) *Movement* 1.

MOVEMENT 1. Swing slowly forwards, with arms straight, by unbending your knees until your shoulders are vertically above your hands. This causes expiration by compressing the abdominal organs against the ground and on the diaphragm, forcing the air out of the lungs. Count 'One—Two' (2 seconds).

MOVEMENT 2. Swing slowly back on your heels, this relaxes the pressure and induces inspiration. Count 'Three—Four—Five' (3 seconds).

Repeat movements rhythmically about 12 times a minute. At no time bend your arms or 'push', the weight of your body is enough.

Holger Neilsen Method

If the casualty is on his back, turn him so that he is face downwards by crossing his far leg over the near leg. Kneel on the near side by his head. Place his hands above his head. Grasp his far away upper arm with one hand and protect his face with the other and turn him over.

POSITION OF CASUALTY AND OPERATOR Place the casualty's hands, one over the other under his forehead and raise hands and forehead on a folded coat (about four inches in height). His head should be slightly turned to one side. Kneel on one knee six to twelve inches from the top of his head, place the other foot, with heel in line with his elbow. Place your hands on his back over the shoulder blades (Fig. 11a).

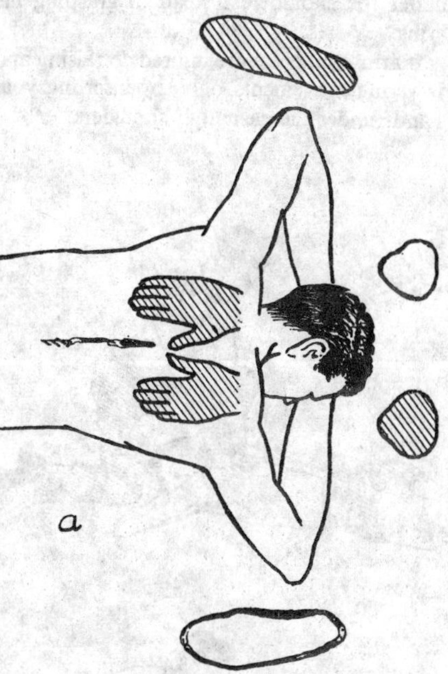

Fig. 11a. *HOLGER NEILSEN Position of casualty and operator.*

MOVEMENT 1. Keeping your arms straight, rock gently forward until your arms are vertical, counting 'One—Two'.

MOVEMENT 2. Rock back, sliding your hands past the casualty's shoulders until they grasp his upper arms near the elbows, counting 'Three'.

MOVEMENT 3. Raise and pull firmly, but not roughly on his arms, counting 'Four—Five', taking care not to draw his hands out of position.

While counting 'Six' replace your hands in the original position and repeat the movements until he commences breathing. The whole operation should take about six seconds and must be carried out regularly and rhythmically. In cold weather cover casualty.

Children. When using Holger Neilsen resuscitation on children the pressure on the shoulder blades should be with the *fingertips only*, and the movements carried out slightly quicker, about twelve complete operations per minute.

For a child under five years of age, the child's arms should be placed straight down his sides. Grasp his shoulders with your thumbs on top and fingers below, and press the shoulder-blades with the thumbs for 2 seconds; then lift the shoulders for 2 seconds. Repeat 15 times per minute. The child may be lying on a table or between the legs of the operator seated on the floor.

The smaller the person, the less the pressure required. All that is required is an amount just sufficient to lightly compress the chest.

Injuries. If there are chest injuries, do arm raising and lowering only, at the rate of about twelve times per minute.

If there are arm injuries, place his arms by his sides and carry out the three movements but raise his chest by inserting your hands under the shoulders instead of grasping his arms.

If arms and chest are injured do raising and lowering movements only, by inserting your hands under the casualty's shoulders.

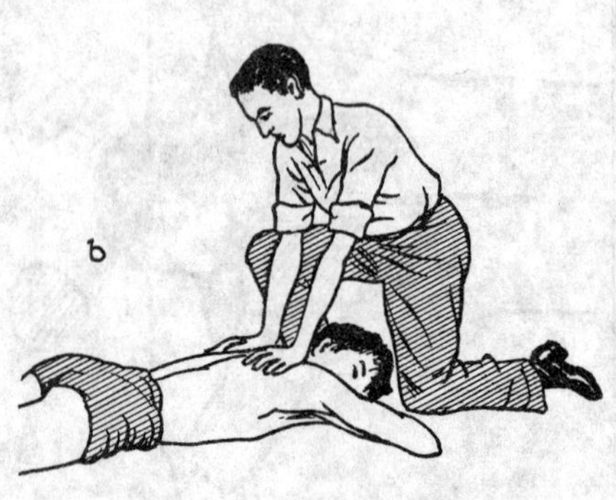

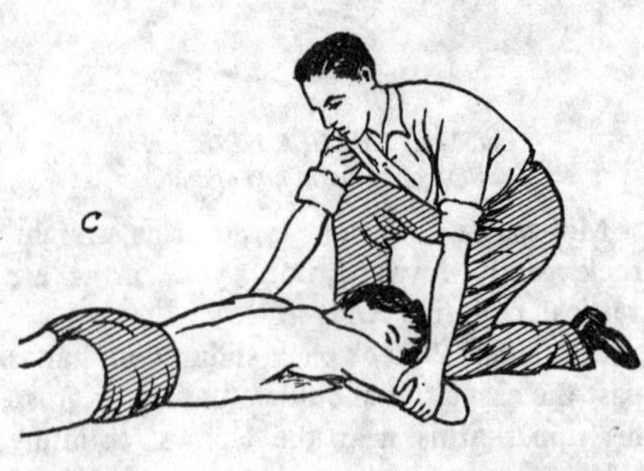

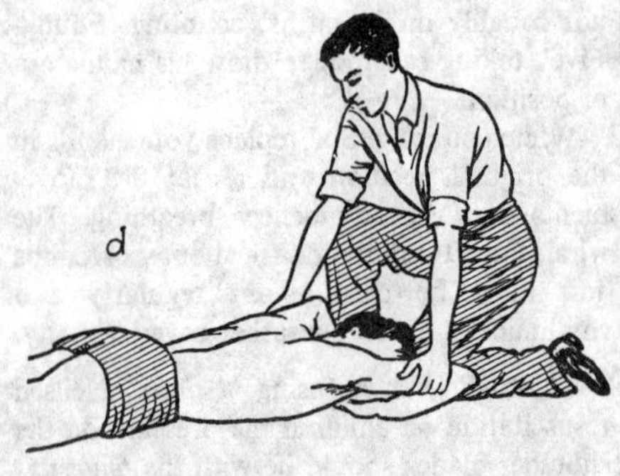

Fig. 11. *HOLGER NEILSEN.* (b) *Movement* 1, (c) *Movement* 2. (d) *Movement* 3.

HEMORRHAGE

Severe bleeding (hemorrhage) must be controlled at once and medical aid obtained with the least possible delay. Bleeding may occur from an artery, vein, or from small capillary blood vessels.

In ARTERIAL BLEEDING, the blood is bright red and spurts out of the vessel in jets corresponding with the pulse beat, and it comes from the cut end of the artery nearer the heart.

In BLEEDING FROM A VEIN the blood is dark or bluish-red, and flows steadily (except in the veins of the neck where it flows faster when the person is breathing out). In venous bleeding the blood issues from the wound on the side further from the heart.

In CAPILLARY BLEEDING, the blood oozes or flows from the surface of the wound, and tends to well up in it.

Bleeding from the surface of the body is called EXTERNAL HEMORRHAGE, while bleeding which takes place inside the body, as in the chest or abdomen, is INTERNAL OR CONCEALED HEMORRHAGE.

Certain names are given to bleeding in different parts of the body.

EPISTAXIS is bleeding from the nose.

HEMATEMESIS is vomiting of blood.

HEMOPTYSIS is coughing up of blood.

HEMATURIA is blood in the urine.

MELENA is blood in the stools.

Bleeding usually follows immediately after a blood vessel is pierced or torn, unless special measures have been taken to prevent the loss of blood or the part is frozen.

DELAYED HEMORRHAGE may occur when a period of some hours has elapsed after an injury, if the clot or ligature is displaced; delayed hemorrhage also often follows shock when the blood pressure rises during recovery.

Signs and Symptoms

The general signs caused by bleeding may be slight in cases of minor injuries, but when the hemorrhage is sudden, or when increasing or rapid loss of blood occurs, the patient is pale, the pulse is fast and feeble, and the skin may be cold. The breathing tends to be deep and sighing, and there is often sweating and faintness. The sight may be blurred, and the patient is restless and thirsty. If the bleeding is not arrested, unconsciousness may follow, with an increasingly fast and feeble pulse.

General Rules for Treatment

1. Lay the casualty down.
2. Raise the injured part, except in the case of a fractured limb.
3. Expose the wound, but do not uncover the casualty unnecessarily.
4. Do not disturb any blood clot which may have formed.
5. Apply pressure: (a) directly on the bleeding point if there is no foreign body or fracture at the site of the wound; (b) indirect pressure on the appropriate pressure point if direct pressure cannot be applied; (c) constrictive bandage.
6. Apply pad and firm bandage over a dressing.
7. Immobilize the injured part.
8. Treat for shock.

Direct Pressure

Apply direct pressure with the thumbs or fingers, over a pad if possible, to the bleeding point. Substitute a dressing, pad, and firm bandage as soon as possible.

Indirect Pressure at Pressure Points

CAROTID PRESSURE POINT. Bleeding from a cut throat, from head, face and neck is controlled by the carotid pressure point, one on each side of the neck, lying between the windpipe and the muscle running down the side of the neck. Press your thumb gently back and press firmly against the bones of the neck, taking great care not to press on the windpipe (Fig. 12).

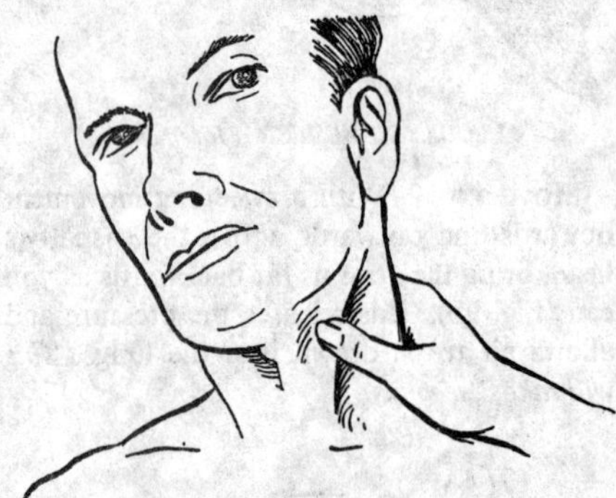

Fig. 12. *PRESSURE POINT OF THE CAROTID ARTERY*

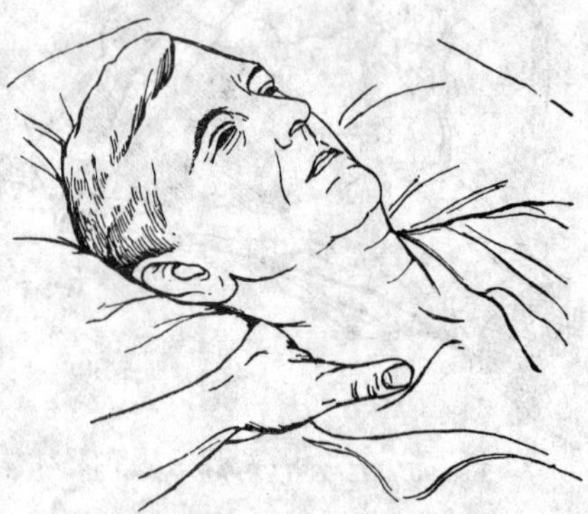

Fig. 13. *PRESSURE POINT OF THE SUBCLAVIAN ARTERY*

SUBCLAVIAN PRESSURE POINT. The subclavian arteries run from a point between the inner ends of the collar-bone, across the first ribs to the armpits, and the subclavian pressure point controls bleeding from the arm.

To apply pressure, expose the neck and upper part of casualty's chest, lay him down with head and shoulders supported. Incline his head to the injured side and, pressing one thumb on top of the other in the hollow above and behind the collar-bone, compress the artery against the first rib (Fig. 13).

Brachial Pressure Point. Bleeding from the arm when this point is nearer than the subclavian pressure point is controlled by the brachial pressure point situated on the inner side of the biceps muscles.

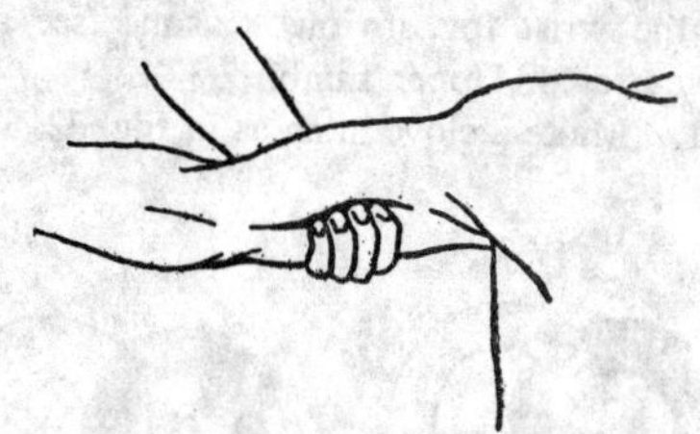

Fig. 14. *PRESSURE POINT OF THE BRACHIAL ARTERY*

Lay the casualty down and compress the artery by passing your fingers under his arm and pressing against the humerus (upper arm bone) (Fig. 14).

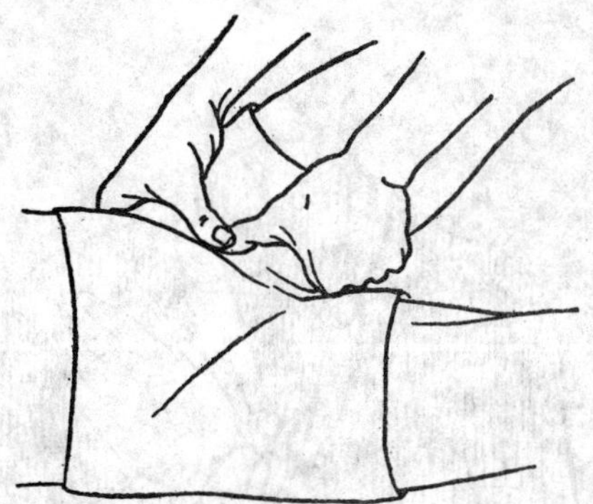

Fig. 15. *PRESSURE POINT OF THE FEMORAL ARTERY*

Femoral Pressure Point. This is situated in the groin and controls bleeding from the leg. Pressure is applied by laying the person down, bending the leg and grasping the thigh with both hands and pressing one thumb over the other at a point in the center of the fold of the groin (Fig. 15).

Constrictive Bandages. Tourniquets are no longer used in general First Aid as they are dangerous in unskilled hands, but constrictive bandages (a narrow fold of bandage, a tie, elastic belt or special rubber bandage, etc.) may be used to maintain pressure for more than a few minutes. It must be tight enough to control the bleeding, but if it is not tight enough it may cause congestion and increase bleeding. When a limb has been amputated a constrictive bandage must be applied at once.

The most effective places at which to apply a constrictive bandage are the middle of the upper arm and the junction of the middle and upper third of the thigh.

If the casualty has to go to hospital a label must be attached to him stating the exact time at which the bandage was applied as it must be released every fifteen minutes. It can be tightened again if necessary. When loosening a constrictive bandage do so gradually, leave it in position so that it can be reapplied should the bleeding start again.

Bleeding from Special Regions

Internal hemorrhage may be visible or invisible. All internal bleeding is serious.

Bleeding from the lungs: Bright red and frothy when coughed up.

Bleeding from the stomach: Vomited, and sometimes looking like coffee grounds.

Bleeding from the bowel: upper bowel—stools will appear black or tarry; lower bowel—blood will appear normal.

Bleeding from the kidneys or bladder: Blood in the urine may give it a smoky or red appearance.

Concealed Internal Hemorrhage

This occurs when there is injury to the liver, spleen or pancreas which have no opening to the outside of the body and the bleeding takes place into the body cavity.

Signs and Symptoms of Internal Hemorrhage. Internal bleeding should always be suspected in crush injuries and immediate medical aid must be obtained. It may be recognized by:

1. Faintness and giddiness, especially if the casualty sits up.
2. Pallor of the face and lips.
3. Cold and clammy skin.
4. Excitability and restlessness.
5. Pulse becoming weaker and more rapid, and perhaps disappearing at the wrist.
6. Breathing becoming labored and hurried; and the casualty may yawn and sigh.
7. Breathing may become distressed ('air hunger'); and the casualty may throw his arms about and call for air.
8. Severe thirst.
9. Unconsciousness.

It will be noted that many of these symptoms apply to cases of severe shock, but air hunger, severe thirst and restlessness are a sure sign that concealed bleeding is continuing.

Treatment. Keep the casualty warm and at rest in the most comfortable position.

Loosen clothing at neck, wrist and chest.

Give nothing by mouth. Relieve thirst by allowing him to *rinse* his mouth.

Remove to hospital as soon as possible.

Attach a note stating that internal hemorrhage is suspected.

Bleeding from the cheek, tongue, gums and tooth socket.

Be careful not to confuse bleeding from these parts with bleeding from the lungs or stomach.

1. Bleeding from the cheek or tongue, if severe, may be stopped by pinching the part between a clean handkerchief, etc. with your finger and thumb.
2. For bleeding from a tooth socket, plug the socket with cotton, place a small rolled-up handkerchief over this and make the casualty bite on it.

Bleeding from the Nose

1. Sit the casualty in a current of air, in front of an open window if not in the depths of winter, with head bent slightly forward.
2. Undo clothing round neck and chest.
3. Tell him to breathe through his mouth.
4. Pinch his nostrils together.
5. Do not let him blow his nose.
6. Do not attempt to plug the nose.

Bleeding from the Ear Channel

This may indicate a fracture of the base of the skull.

1. Lay him down with his head slightly raised.
2. Do not plug the ear.
3. Turn the head slightly to the bleeding side and apply a dry dressing over the ear, and lightly bandage.
4. Get medical aid as quickly as possible. Treat for shock.

Bleeding from the Palm of the Hand

Bleeding from the palm of the hand may be severe and where there is no foreign body or fracture suspected in the wound, apply direct pressure by bending the casualty's fingers over a dressing and small pad (rolled handkerchief) and bandage firmly (Figs. 16 and 17).

Bleeding from Varicose Veins

Bleeding from a burst varicose vein can endanger life if not treated at once.

1. Lay the casualty down and raise the leg as high as possible.
2. Apply a clean pad to the bleeding point.
3. Loosen garter.
4. Keep leg raised.
5. Send for a doctor.
6. Treat for shock.

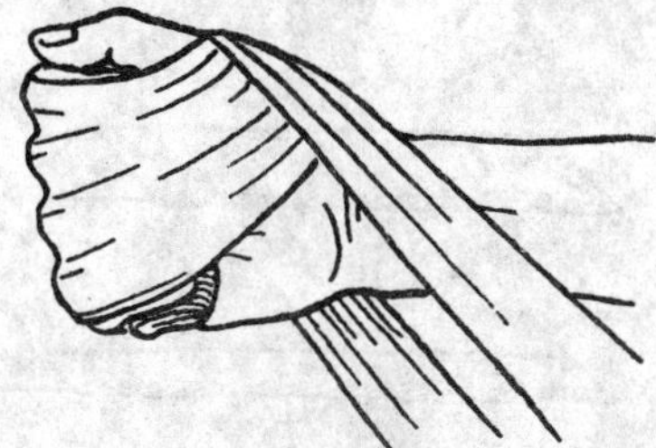

Fig. 16. *APPLICATION OF PAD AND BANDAGE FOR THE HAND*

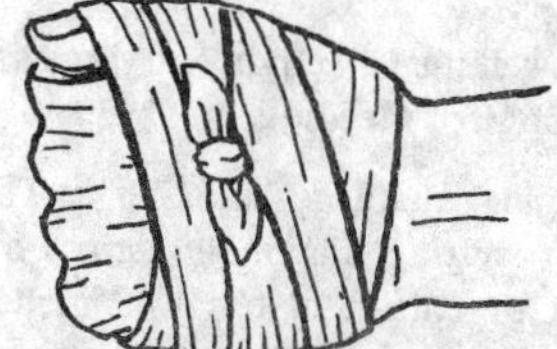

Fig. 17. *BANDAGE TIED OVER THE PAD*

Dressings

Generally speaking, dressings in First Aid are limited to dry sterile dressings because the application of creams, lotions, etc., hampers further treatment. In minor cases, however, certain mild antiseptic creams and lotions may be applied, but great care must be taken to read and follow the manufacturer's printed instructions and to get medical advice at the slightest sign of inflammation or continued swelling.

The purposes of a dressing are to help control bleeding, to prevent infection, and to protect the wound from further injury.

PREPARED STERILE DRESSINGS (gauze): stocked by druggists in various sizes.

A GAUZE DRESSING should be covered with a generous pad of cotton. This also helps to protect the wound from infection and injury.

A COLD COMPRESS (wet dressing) may help to reduce swelling and relieve pain in injuries such as a sprained ankle. A handkerchief, towel, or triangular bandage wrung out in cold water to which an equal part of alcohol may be added, is applied to the affected part and kept wet by dripping on more water. Never apply alcohol solutions to open wounds or to injuries near the eyes.

Bandages

Bandages are used to keep dressings in place and splints in position, to immobilize fractures, to support an injured part, to

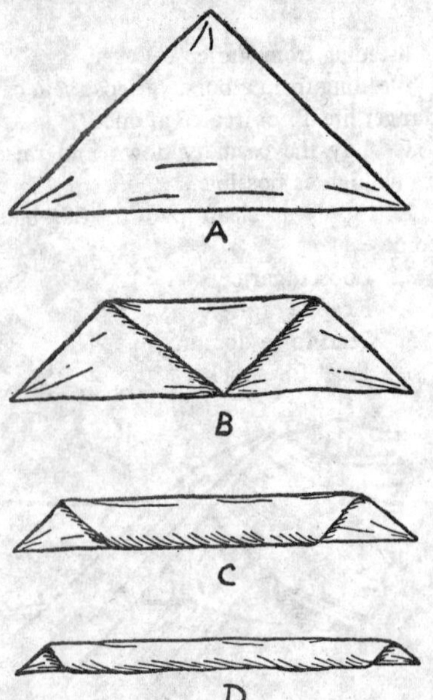

Fig. 18. *TRIANGULAR BANDAGE. A. Bandage spread out. B. Bandage once folded. C. Broad Bandage. D. Narrow bandage.*

reduce swelling, to help in carrying casualties, and to control bleeding.

Triangular Bandages and Slings. These are made by cutting diagonally across a square of linen or cotton material 40 inches wide. They may be used over splints or dressings, or as slings. By folding them into strips of

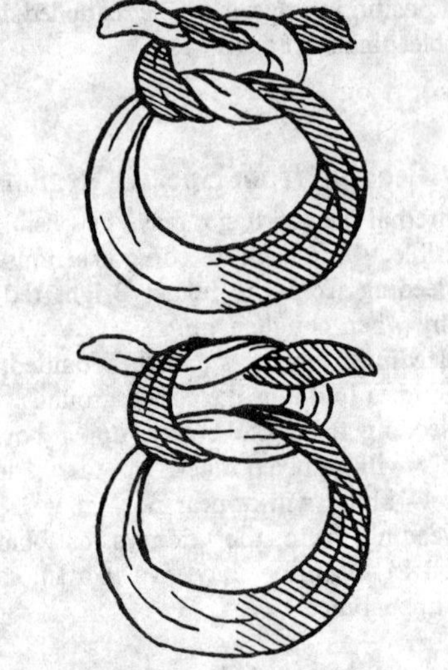

Fig. 19. *KNOTS. The upper granny knot is not used for bandages; the lower reef knot is used for bandages as it does not slip and is easy to untie.*

different widths a broad or narrow bandage may be produced as required (Fig. 18). Reef knots (Fig. 19) are used to secure the ends when the bandage is tied in place.

Improvised bandages may also be made from clean handkerchiefs or other material.

A small arm sling supports the hand and wrist (Fig. 20).

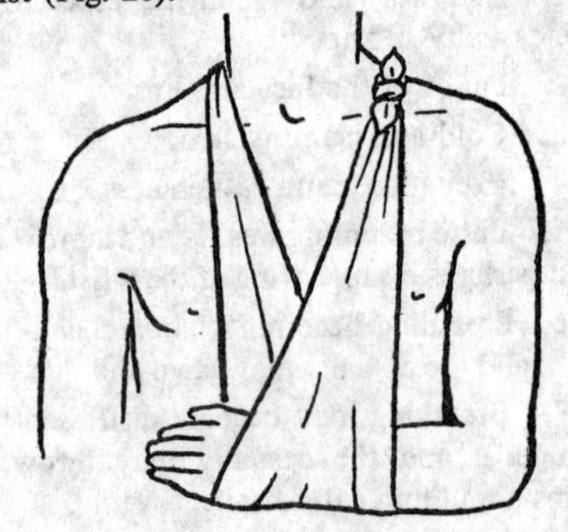

Fig. 20. *SMALL ARM SLING. For fractures of the humerus, or slight injuries to the hand and shoulder.*

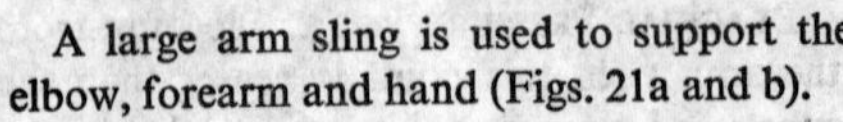

A large arm sling is used to support the elbow, forearm and hand (Figs. 21a and b).

Collar and Cuff Sling. Used in wounds and fractures of the upper limb when the elbow can be bent. It should not be used in fractures of the wrist for obvious reasons (see also Fractures of Upper Limb, p. 33).

1. Make a clove hitch as in Fig. 22.

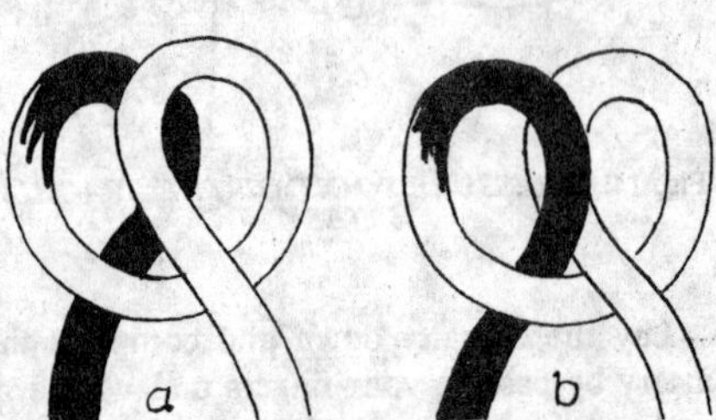

Fig. 22. *CLOVE HITCH.* (a) *Loops to pass over the hand.* (b) *Pass loop 1 behind loop 2.*

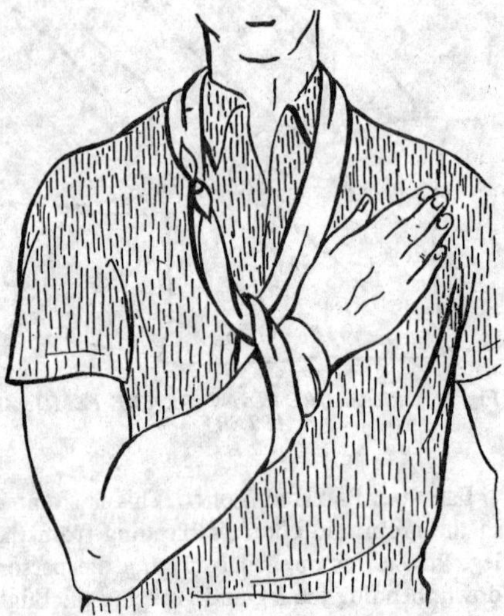

Fig. 23. *COLLAR AND CUFF SLING*

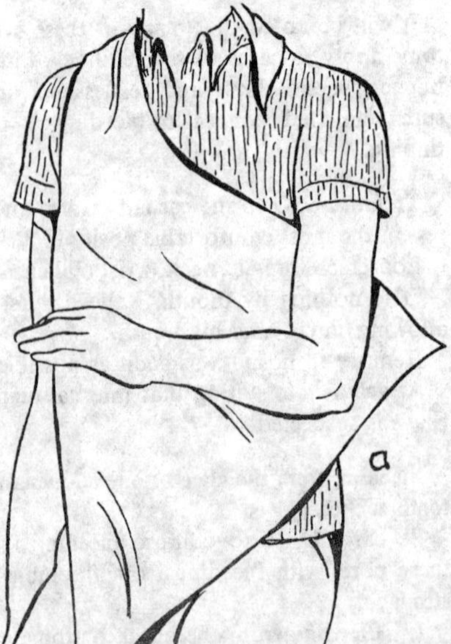

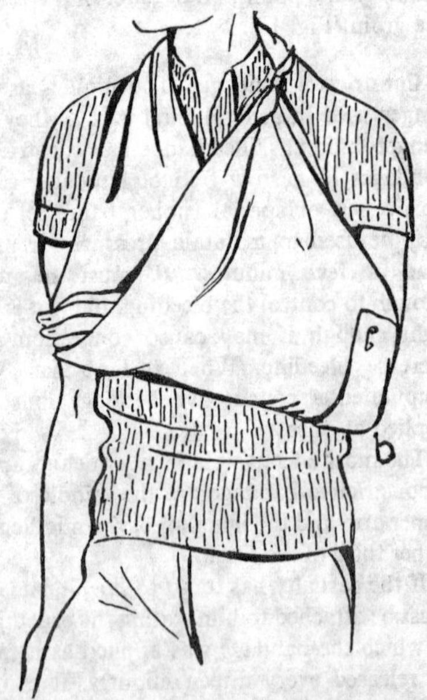

Fig. 21. *LARGE ARM SLING.* (a) *Place triangular bandage as illustrated.* (b) *Tie reef knot in neck hollow and bring point forward at elbow, securing it with a safety pin.*

2. Place casualty's forearm across his chest and slip clove hitch over his hand; tie off so that the fingers of the injured arm just reach his opposite shoulder (Fig. 23).

The Triangular Sling (St. John's Sling). This is used for bleeding from the hand and in fractures of the collar-bone (see Fractures, p. 33).

1. Bend the elbow on the injured side so that the forearm lies across the chest with the fingers reaching the opposite shoulder. Lay the open triangular bandage over the forearm, one end over the hand and the point well beyond the elbow (Fig. 24a).

2. Tuck the base of the bandage well under the hand and forearm, bring the other end round the back and up over the uninjured shoulder (Fig. 24b).

3. Hold the front of the bandage in one hand and tuck the point between the arm and the bandage (Fig. 24b), fold back and secure with a safety-pin (Fig. 24c).

Improvised Slings. Ties, scarves, stockings and belts may be used. If these are not available, then the arm should be left in the sleeve and the sleeve securely pinned to the front of the garment. Alternatively, the hand can be buttoned into the casualty's coat.

Ring Pad. This pad is used to control bleeding from a scalp wound when a fracture at the site of the injury is suspected and pressure on the wound must be avoided (Fig. 25).

Roller Bandages. These are made of woven cotton or some other suitable material, and can be obtained at any drug store in different widths, from 3 to 6 yards long. Crêpe bandages are also useful for support and, being washable, they can be used several times.

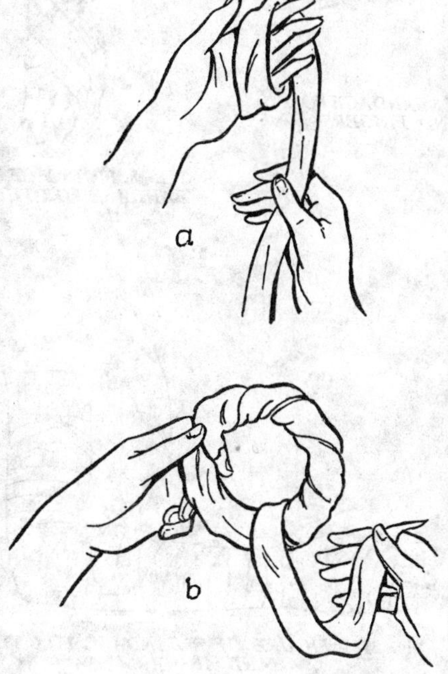

Fig. 25. *RING PAD.* (a) *Wrap one end of narrow bandage around fingers to make a loop.* (b) *Wrap the other end around and around the loop until the ring is completed.*

A bandage 1 inch wide is generally used for the fingers, 2 inches wide for the head and arm, 3 inches for the leg, and 4 to 6 inches for the trunk.

Roller bandages are convenient for use over splints or dressings to keep these in place; they are also used for support of a part, or for pressure to prevent or reduce swelling and bleeding.

Methods of Bandaging. The bandage should be firmly and evenly rolled before use, and the part should be bandaged from below upwards, and from within outwards, each layer of bandage overlapping the layer below. Finally the bandage should be secured by a safety-pin.

The bandage should be neither too tight nor too slack.

1. THE SIMPLE SPIRAL. This form of bandage encircles the part as far as required, and is used on the fingers, wrist, or forearm where it does not easily slip.

2. THE REVERSED SPIRAL is applied with spiral turns so that the bandage is turned downwards over itself at each turn round the limb. This bandage is convenient for use on parts of uneven size, on which a simple spiral does not set properly.

3. A FIGURE OF EIGHT BANDAGE is passed obliquely round the limb, first upwards and then downwards, so that the turns are made in the form of a figure 8.

4. A SPICA BANDAGE is a figure of eight bandage adapted for use on the shoulder, the hip and groin, or the thumb.

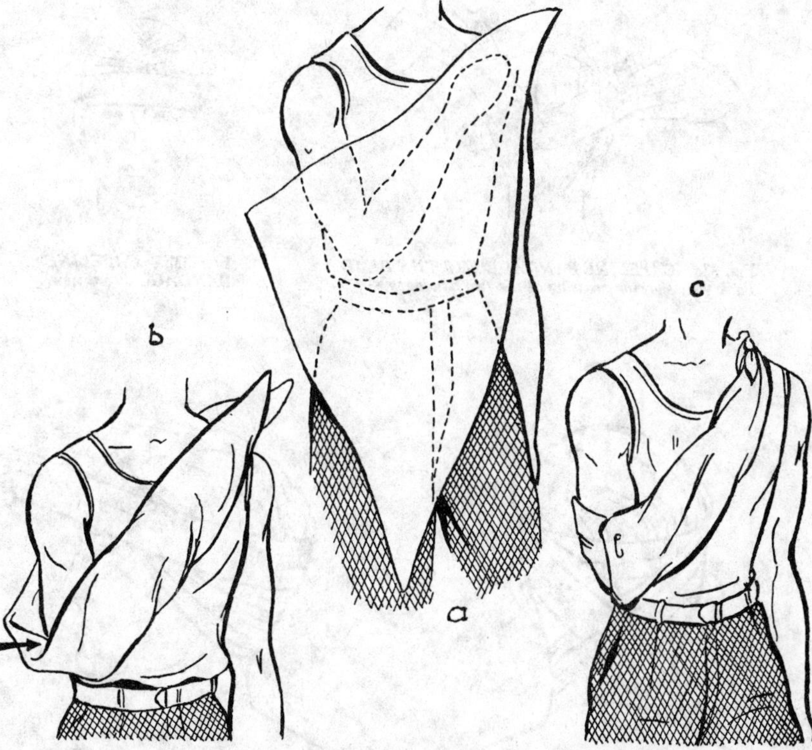

Fig. 24. *TRIANGULAR SLING.* (a) *Place bandage as illustrated.* (b) *Tuck bandage around arm.* (c) *Tie bandage at shoulder and pin at elbow.*

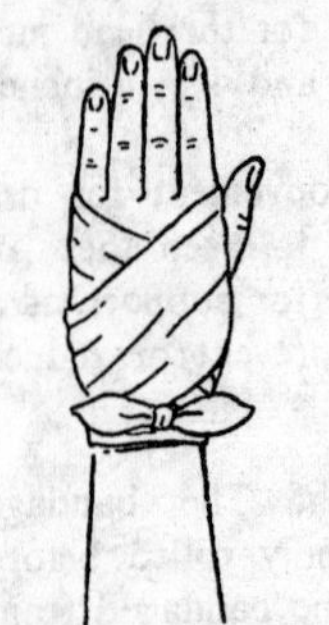

Fig. 26. *HANDKERCHIEF BANDAGE FOR THE HAND.*

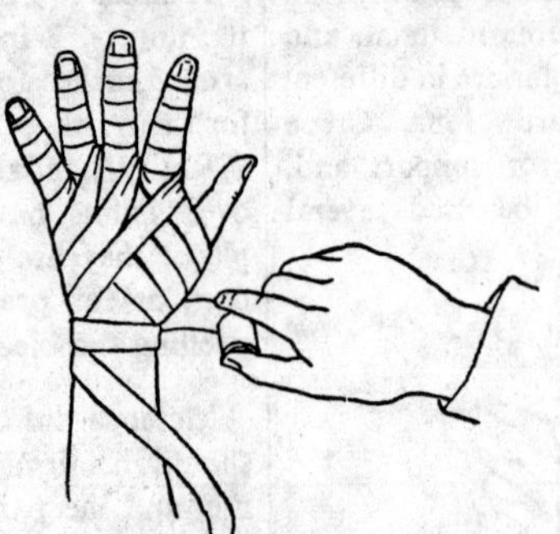

Fig. 27. *FIGURE OF 8 BANDAGE FOR THE HAND AND FINGERS*

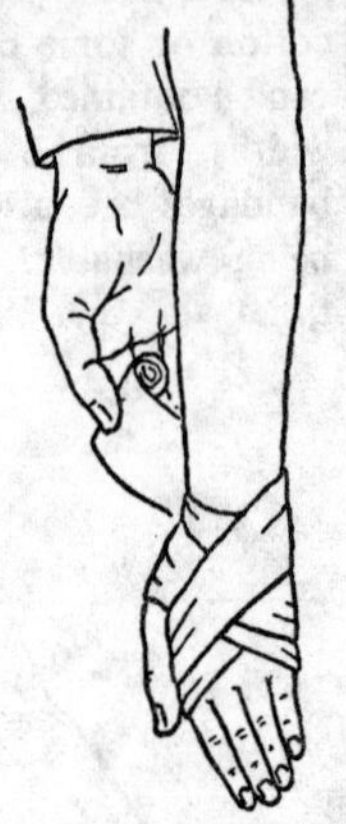

Fig. 28. *FIGURE OF 8 BANDAGE FOR THE HAND.*

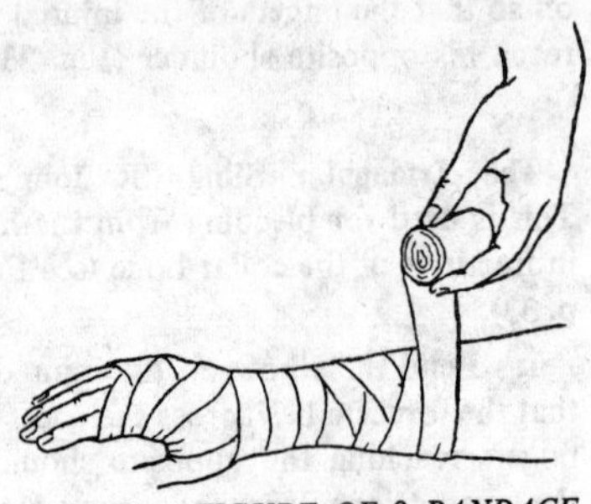

Fig. 29. *FIGURE OF 8 BANDAGE FOR THE WRIST AND FOREARM*

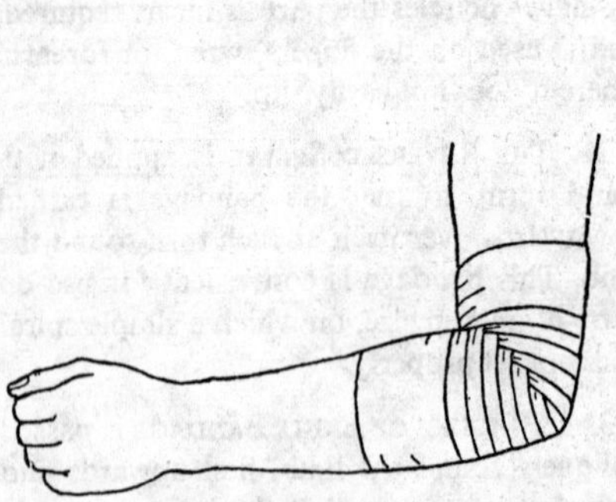

Fig. 30. *FIGURE OF 8 BANDAGE FOR THE ELBOW*

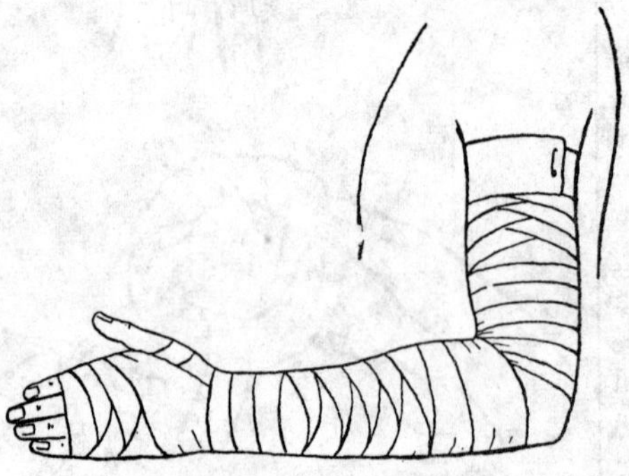

Fig. 31. *FIGURE OF 8 BANDAGE FOR THE HAND AND ARM*

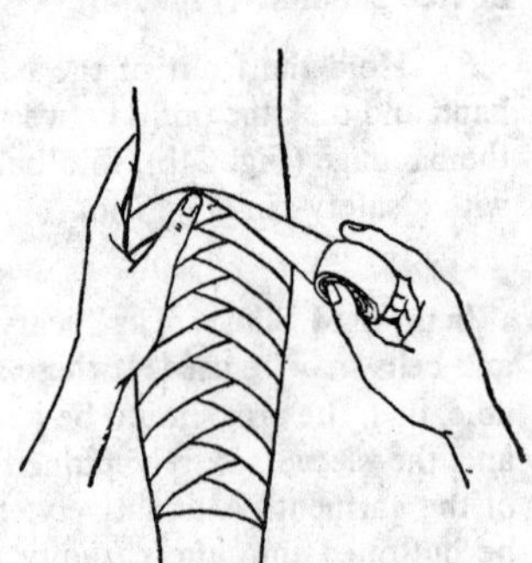

Fig. 32. *FIGURE OF 8 BANDAGE FOR THE LEG*

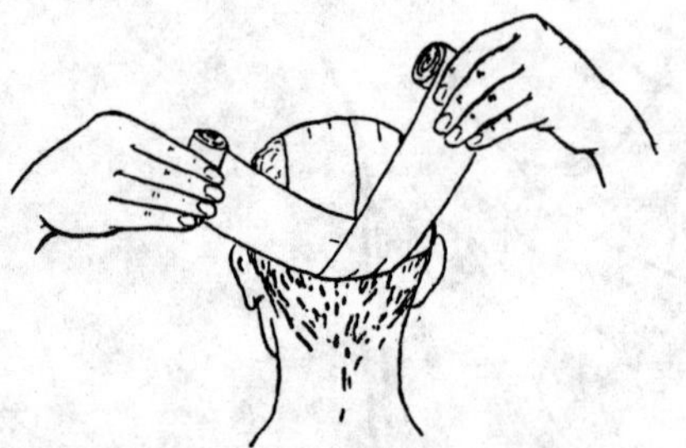

Fig. 33a. *CAPELINE BANDAGE FOR THE HEAD. Back view showing crossing of the two bandages*

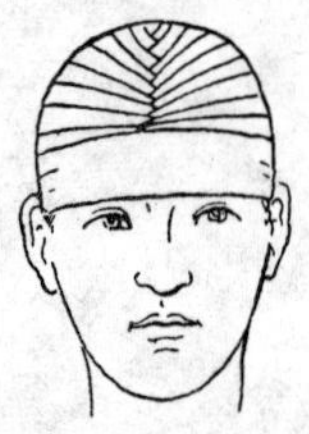

Fig. 33b. *CAPELINE BANDAGE. Front view.*

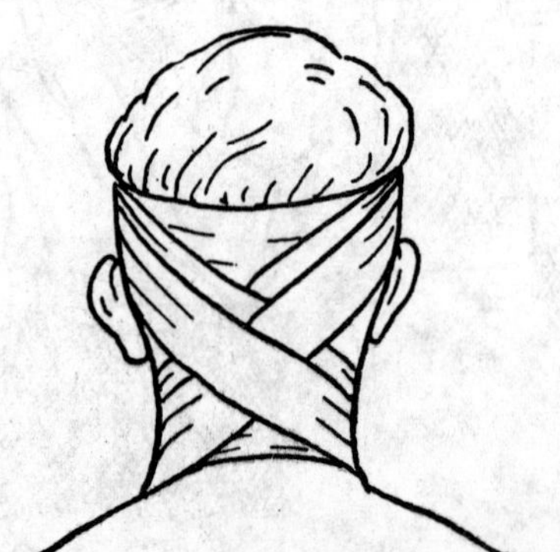

Fig. 34a. *SINGLE ROLLER BANDAGE FOR THE HEAD. Back view*

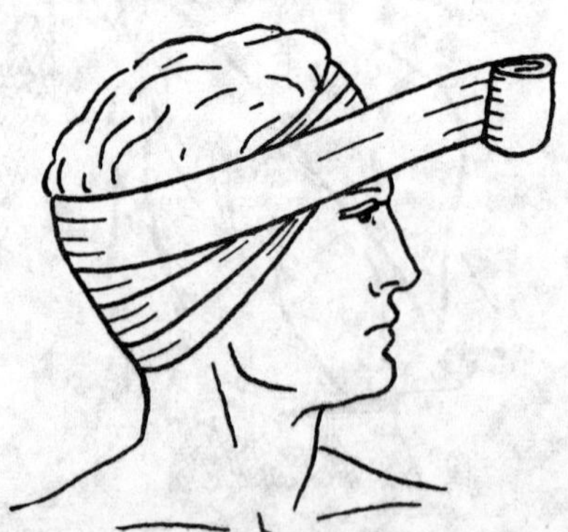

Fig. 34b. *SINGLE ROLLER BANDAGE FOR THE HEAD. Side view*

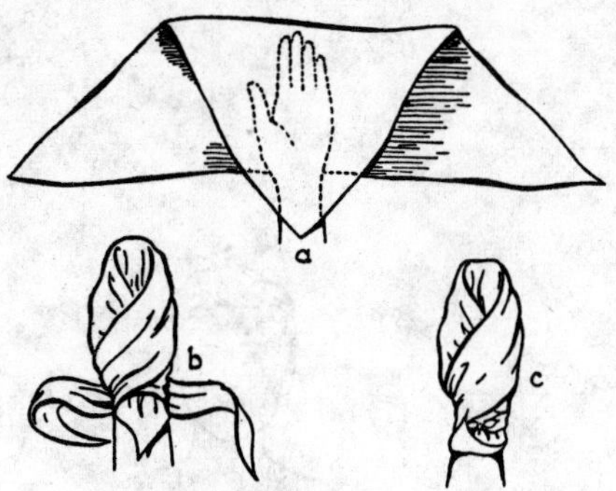

Fig. 35
TRIANGULAR BANDAGE FOR THE HAND

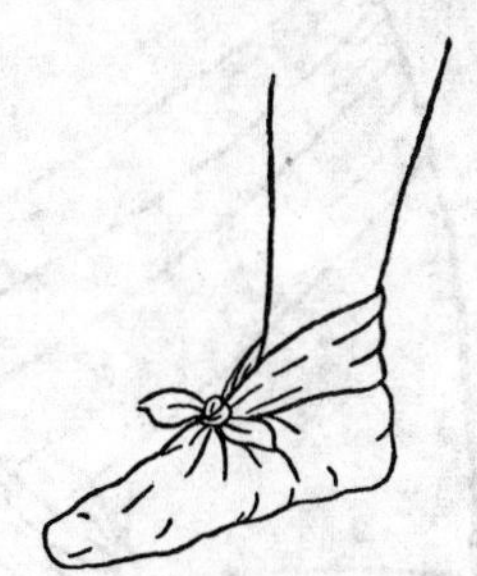

Fig. 36. *TRIANGULAR BANDAGE FOR THE FOOT*

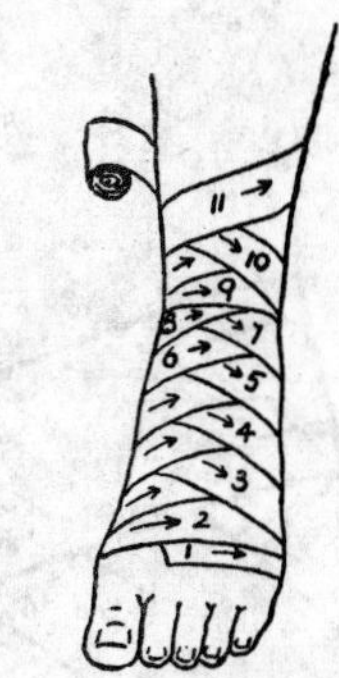

Fig. 37. *FIGURE OF 8 BANDAGE FOR THE FOOT*

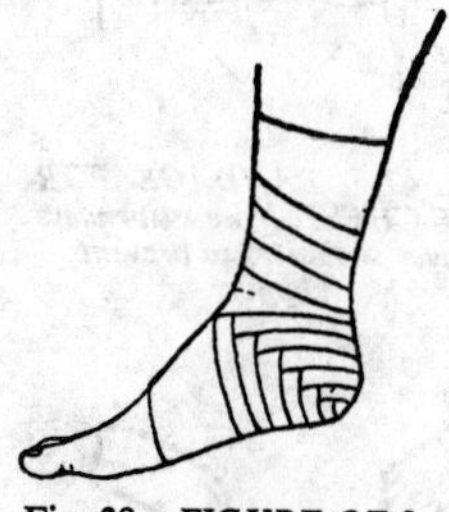

Fig. 38. *FIGURE OF 8 BANDAGE FOR THE HEEL*

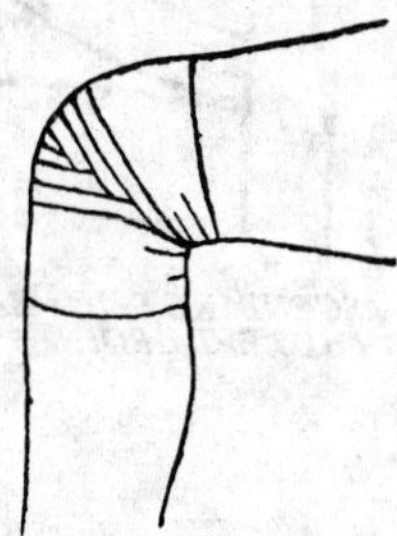

Fig. 39. *FIGURE OF 8 BANDAGE FOR THE KNEE*

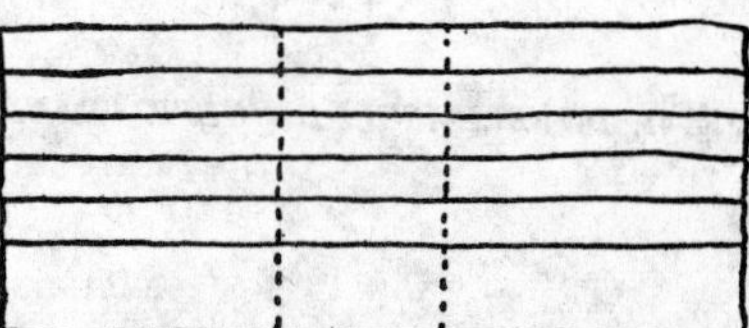

Fig. 40. *MANY-TAILED BANDAGE. Strips sewn together near the center*

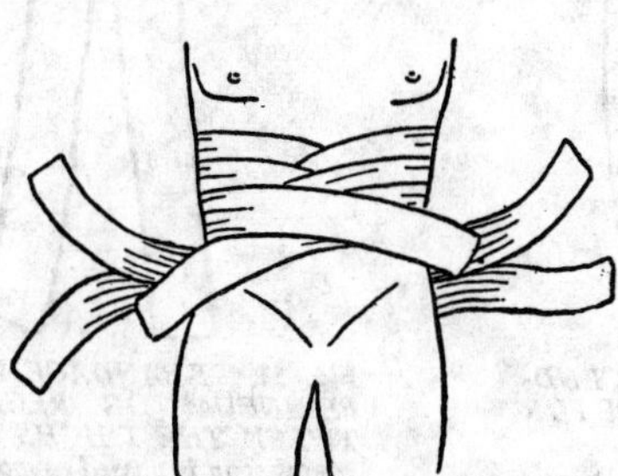

Fig. 41. *MANY-TAILED BANDAGE FOR THE ABDOMEN*

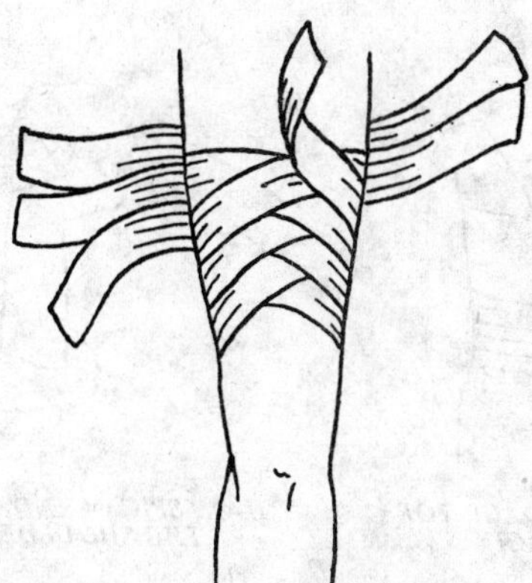

Fig. 42. *MANY-TAILED BANDAGE FOR THE THIGH*

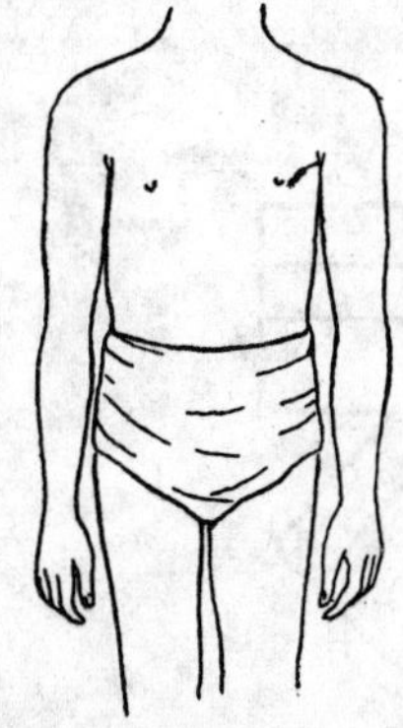

Fig. 43
SWATHE BANDAGE FOR THE ABDOMEN

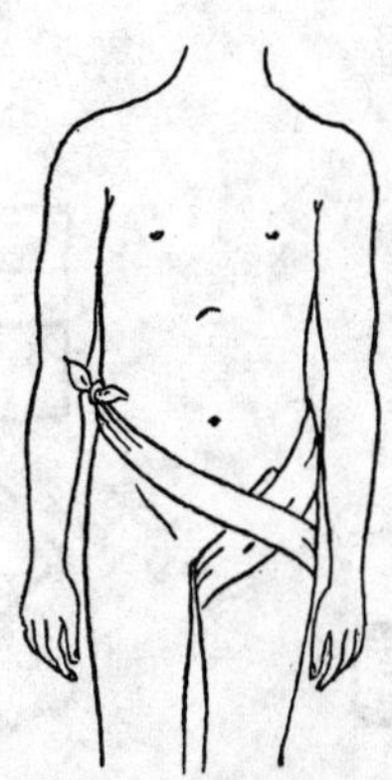

Fig. 44. *BANDAGE FOR THE GROIN*

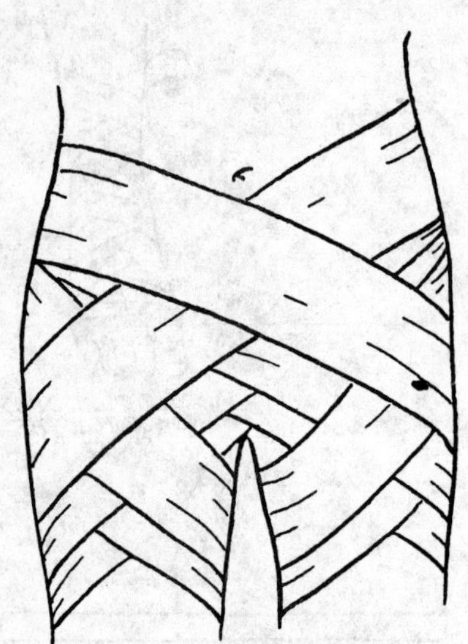

Fig. 45. *DOUBLE ASCENDING SPICA BANDAGE*

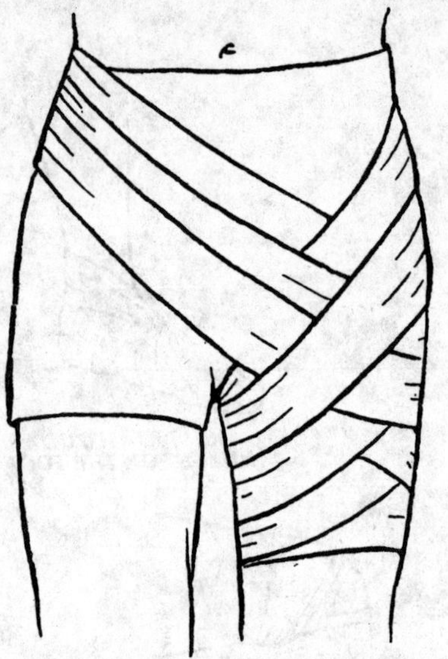

Fig. 46. *SINGLE ASCENDING SPICA BANDAGE FOR THE LEFT GROIN*

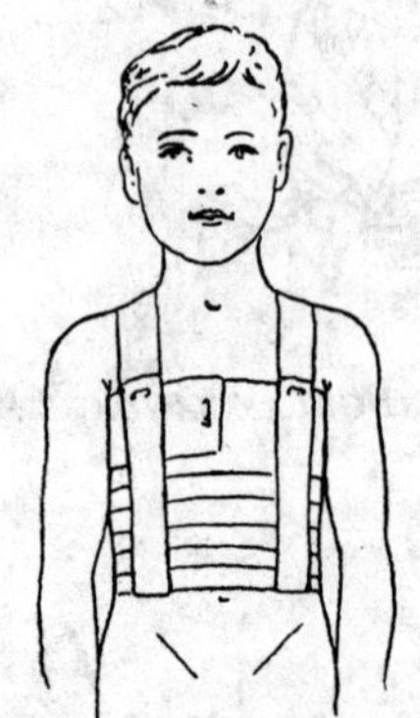

Fig. 47. *BANDAGE FOR THE CHEST. Note suspenders over shoulders to prevent slipping*

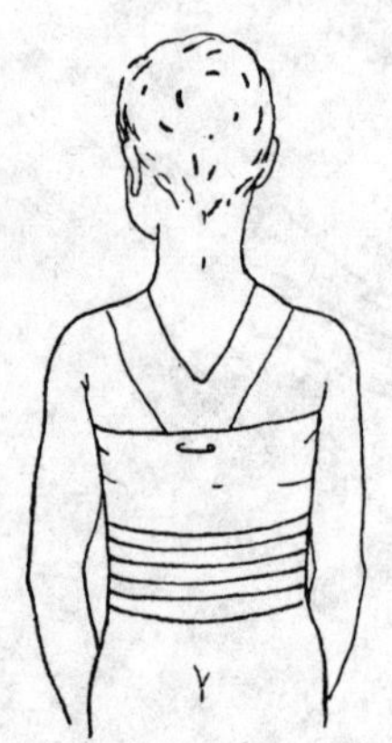

Fig. 48. *BANDAGE FOR THE BACK*

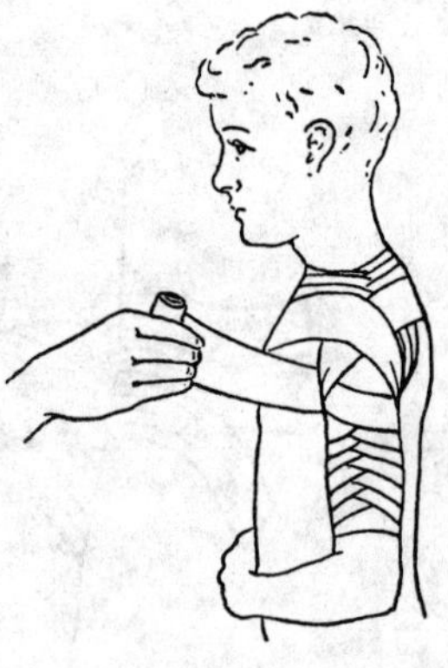

Fig. 49. *SPICA BANDAGE FOR THE SHOULDER*

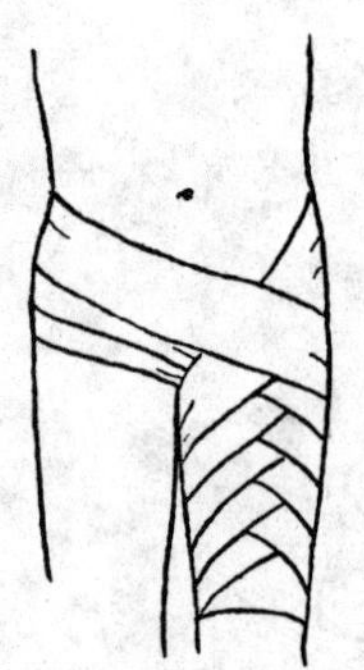

Fig. 50. *SINGLE ASCENDING SPICA BANDAGE FOR THE THIGH*

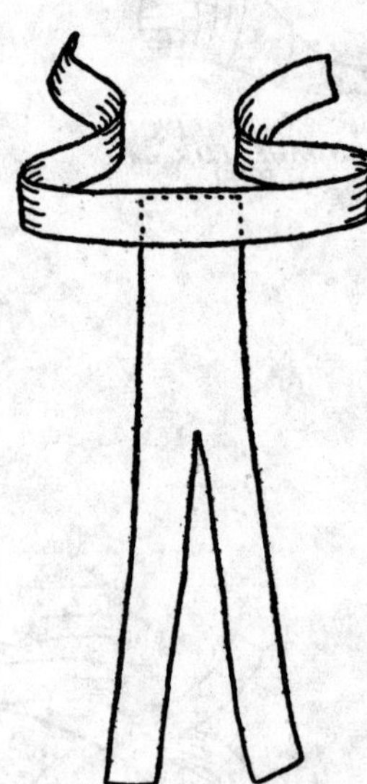

Fig. 51. *T-BANDAGE FOR THE PERINEUM OR REGION BETWEEN THE THIGHS. The horizontal strip is passed round the waist, the vertical strip is carried forward between the patient's legs, and each end is pinned to the horizontal band.*

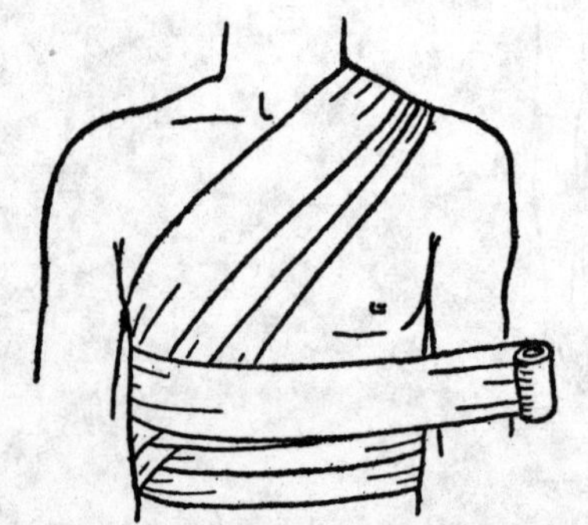

Fig. 52. *BANDAGE FOR THE RIGHT BREAST*

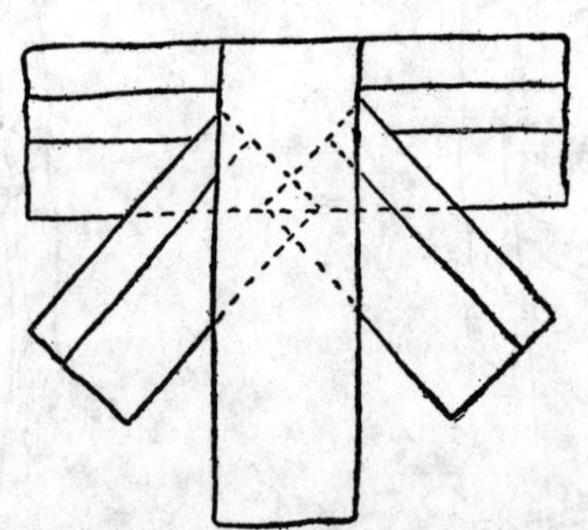

Fig. 53. *DIAGRAM OF MANY-TAILED BANDAGE FOR STUMP OF LIMB*

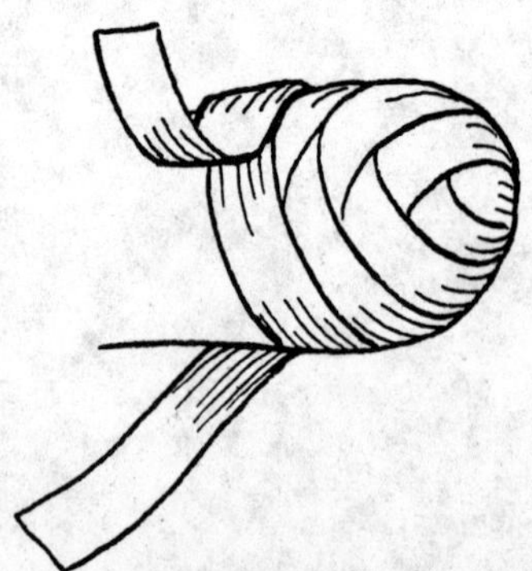

Fig. 54. *MANY-TAILED BANDAGE APPLIED TO STUMP OF LIMB*

FRACTURES

Fractures, the cracks or breaks in bones caused by some form of violence, are due to:

(a) Direct force when the bone breaks or cracks at the site of the injury as the result of a blow, a bullet wound, a crush injury, or a fall.

(b) Indirect force when the bone breaks or cracks at some distance from the site of the injury as in a fractured collar-bone resulting from falling on the outstretched hand.

(c) Muscular force when, for instance, the knee-cap breaks following the violent contraction of the muscles attached to it.

Complications. Fractures may cause injury to joints, arteries, veins, nerves, and vital organs, e.g. a fractured rib may pierce a lung, a fracture of the skull may damage the brain, or a fractured spine may damage the spinal cord, hence the need for immediate immobilization (securing the injured part or limb so that it cannot be further damaged by movement) and for extreme care in handling.

Types of Fracture

SIMPLE OR CLOSED: where there is no wound at the site of the fracture, and no injury to internal organs.

COMPOUND OR OPEN: where there is an external wound leading down to the fracture, such as is caused by bullet wounds, or by the broken ends of the bone protruding through the skin.

COMPLICATED: simple or compound but with other injury resulting from the same accident, from mishandling, or from insufficient immobilization of the injured part.

COMMINUTED: where the bone is broken into several parts.

IMPACTED: where the broken ends are driven into one another.

GREENSTICK: where the bone may crack and bend without breaking completely as in the less brittle bones of children. Also known as an interperiosteal fracture.

DEPRESSED: when the broken part of the skull is driven inwards.

General Signs and Symptoms of Fractures

1. Pain at seat of fracture or near it.
2. Tenderness on gentle pressure on the injured area.
3. Swelling which may make it difficult to diagnose a fracture, so if there is any doubt as to the seriousness of the injury always treat it as for a broken bone.
4. Loss of power, and inability to move the part naturally.
5. Deformity of the limb. Shortening or unnatural position.
6. Irregularity, which may be felt if the fracture is near the skin.
7. Crepitus or bony grating which may be felt or heard.
8. Difference in appearance when compared with uninjured side.
9. Marks on clothing or skin, or the sound of a bone snapping.

General Rules for Treatment

1. Warn the casualty to lie still.
2. Immobilize the part at once. Control hemorrhage (see p. 24).
3. Guard against further injury.
4. Send for medical aid.
5. If necessary remove to shelter.
6. Treat for shock.
7. Never bandage over the site of a fracture.
8. Remember that limbs may continue to swell and that bandages may need adjusting so that they are firm enough to keep the injury immobile but not tight enough to interfere with the circulation.
9. When splints are necessary they must be long enough to immobilize the joint above and below the fracture, and must be padded both for comfort and to ensure that they remain in position.
10. All cases of fracture of the lower limbs must be transported by stretcher.

Fracture of the Skull

Fractures of the skull may occur on the upper part or sides as the result of direct force. Fracture of the base of the skull is generally caused by indirect force as the result of falling on the feet or lower part of the spine, or a blow on the lower jaw.

A skull fracture may injure both the brain and nervous system.

UPPER SKULL. A fracture of the upper skull shows signs of both concussion and compression (see below).

BASE OF SKULL. A fracture of the base of the skull only shows the signs and symptoms of concussion (see below). In addition, blood or fluid may ooze from the ear or nose, or may be swallowed and later vomited. On examining the casualty's eyes it may be seen that one is bloodshot, and later a black eye may develop.

Concussion

This is caused by a blow on the head, a fall from a height on to the feet or buttocks, or a blow on the point of the jaw.

Signs and Symptoms. Varying degree of loss of consciousness, a temporary 'blackout', stupor or coma which may pass into compression without any return to consciousness. Recovery is frequently accompanied by vomiting and a feeling of nausea, and the casualty may suffer a complete loss of memory of the events before and after the injury.

Treatment

1. Clear air passages.
2. If breathing has stopped start artificial respiration.
3. If breathing is not noisy, lay the casualty on his back and slightly raise head and shoulders, turn head to one side and support in this position.
4. If breathing is noisy (bubbling) turn him into the three-quarters prone position as in Fig. 7.
5. Undo tight clothing at neck, chest, and waist.
6. Wrap in blanket or rug but do not apply heat.
7. Never give anything by mouth, neither fluids nor food.
8. On no account leave an unconscious person unattended.
9. When he regains consciousness moisten his lips with water.
10. Look upon all head injuries as extremely serious conditions, even if the period of unconsciousness has been short.
11. Advise the casualty to avoid any physical or mental activity until he has been seen by a doctor.

Compression

This condition is due to actual pressure on the brain, either by the fractured bone pressing on it, or from a blood clot. It may come on after concussion without the casualty regaining consciousness, or may develop later after what seems a period of recovery.

Signs and Symptoms. Although some of the following signs and symptoms may not be immediately apparent, in cases of head injury the danger of compression must not be overlooked.

Unconsciousness. Flushed face. Noisy breathing. Slow pulse. The head may feel hot to the touch. The pupils of the eyes may be unequal in size. There may be paralysis of one side of the body.

Treatment. As for concussion. Get medical aid at once.

Fracture of the Lower Jaw

Caused by direct force and is usually compound since in most cases there is a wound inside the mouth. Fracture of both sides of the jaw is rare.

Signs and Symptoms. Signs or history of injury. Difficulty in speaking. Excessive flow of saliva, usually blood-stained. Pain. Irregularity of the teeth. Crepitus may be felt when the jaw is steadied and supported.

Treatment. Warn casualty not to speak. Make him lean slightly forward. Place the palm of your hand under the jaw and gently press it against the upper jaw. Apply a narrow bandage as in Figs. 55a, b, and c.

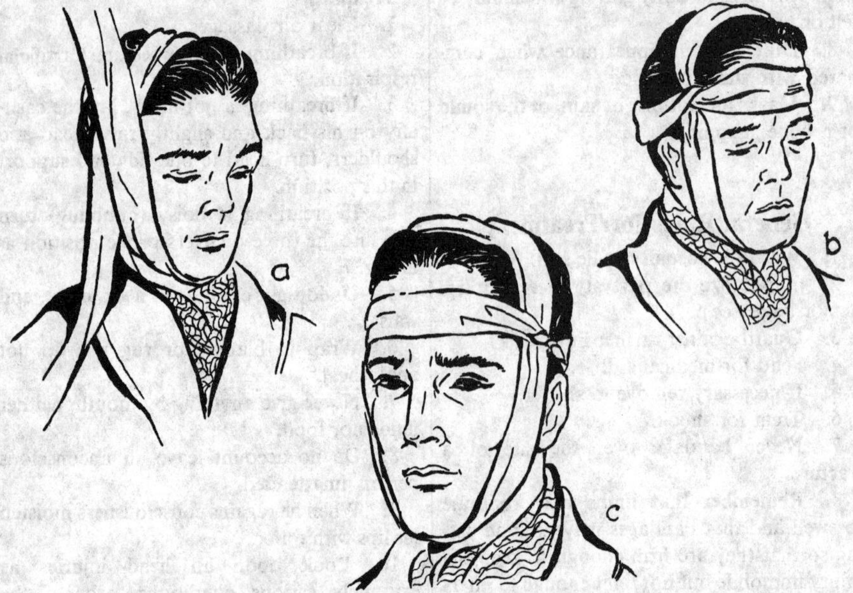

Fig. 55. *FOR FRACTURE OF THE LOWER JAW*

The casualty may want to vomit. Support his jaw with your hand, remove the bandage, turn his head to one side, while continuing to support the jaw. Reapply bandage when vomiting has ceased. Vomiting may have been caused by swallowed blood from a wound in the mouth or of the tongue.

If the fracture is caused by a bullet there may be severe damage and the tongue may slip back and interfere with breathing.

Transport

(a) If he is able to sit up, make him sit with his head held forward.

(b) If he has to be transported by stretcher, which will be necessary if the fracture is comminuted and the wound severe, so long as other injuries allow, place him in a face downwards position with his head projecting over the canvas end of the stretcher. Support his forehead by tying a bandage between the stretcher handles.

Fracture of the Spine

Caused either by direct or indirect violence: by direct violence such as falling across a bar and breaking the spine where it is hit; by indirect violence, such as the neck being broken as the result of a fall on the head.

This is an extremely serious condition and on no account should the person be moved by untrained people unless immediate other danger to life necessitates carrying him to safety. Unskilled handling could result in death or paralysis as the spinal cord can be severed or damaged by the broken and displaced bones.

If the history, signs and symptoms lead you to suspect that the spine may be broken, always treat as such; it is much better to be safe than sorry.

Treatment

1. Immediately warn the person to lie still.
2. If he is unconscious make sure that the air passages are clear.
3. If medical aid is quickly available do no more than keep him warm, and at complete rest.
4. If medical aid is not near at hand or if he has to be moved from possible further injury:

(a) Place pads (newspapers, socks, gloves, scarves, etc.) between his ankles, knees, and thighs.

(b) With great care draw the legs together and tie the ankles by passing a narrow bandage under the ankles, cross it over the instep, and tie off under the soles of the shoes.

(c) Place broad bandages round his knees and thighs. (The thigh bandage should be put in under the knees and gently eased up into position.) Tie off firmly.

(d) Remember that the neck and body should never be bent as this is most liable to damage the spinal cord. Except in cases of fracture of the neck, a casualty with spinal injuries should be carried in the face upward position and extreme care must be taken when placing him on a stretcher.

Transport for spinal injury should only be on a stretcher, and four bearers will be needed because of the great care which must be taken to steady and support the casualty.

Fracture of the Ribs

Cause. Obvious cause as in a crush injury, car accident, etc. or falling in the home and striking the ribs against an object such as the corner of a table.

Signs and Symptoms

1. Pain in the chest at the site of the injury which is increased when a deep breath is taken. The pain is usually sharp.
2. The injured person will breathe in a shallow way to try to avoid the pain.
3. You may be able to feel 'grating' by placing your hand gently over the site of the injury.
4. If internal organs have been damaged the signs and symptoms of internal hemorrhage will be observed and those giving first aid should always keep a close watch for this development (see Internal Hemorrhage, p. 25).
5. An open wound over the site of the fracture may give air direct access to the lungs (sucking wound). The air is sucked in and blown out as the patient breathes. This is a very serious condition.

Treatment for a Simple Fracture of Ribs

Do not remove any clothing except a coat. If bandaging the chest does not give relief, remove bandages and just support the arm on the injured side (Fig. 56).

Treatment for Complicated Fracture of Ribs

1. Do not apply bandages except if there is a sucking wound, in which case apply a dressing and bandage lightly.
2. Support the arm on the injured side.
3. Lay casualty down, raising his head and shoulders; turn him towards the injured side. Support him in this position.
4. Send for medical aid. Complicated fractures of the ribs are stretcher cases.
5. Always treat for shock.

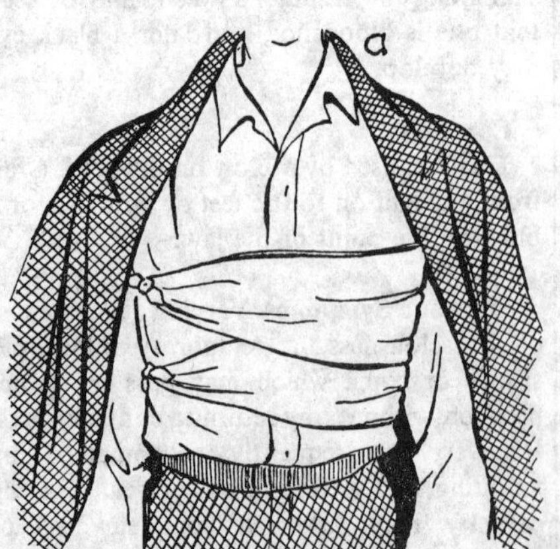

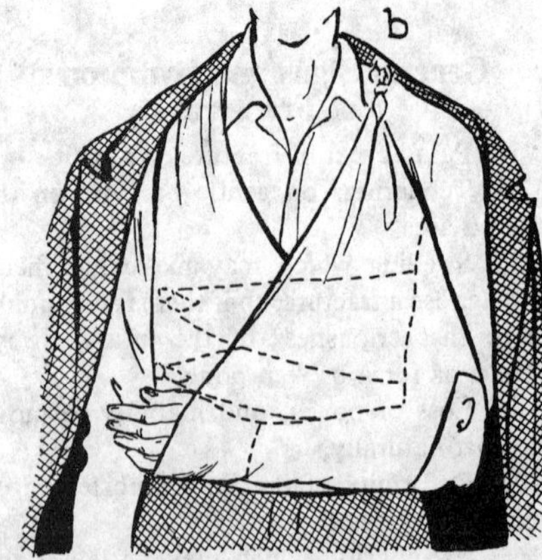

Fig. 56. *FOR SIMPLE FRACTURE OF RIBS.* (a) *Apply two broad bandages round the chest, above and below the injury. Tie bandages on uninjured side.* (b) *Support arm on injured side in a sling.*

Fracture of the Collar-bone

Causes. Falling on the hand with the arm outstretched, or on the point of the shoulder.

Signs and Symptoms. The casualty will usually be supporting the elbow on the injured side, and the arm will be partially helpless. The broken bones can be felt overlapping. Other signs and symptoms of fracture will also be observed.

Treatment

1. Take off coat by removing uninjured arm first.
2. Put a pad from under the armpit reaching to the elbow between the arm and chest (Fig. 57a).
3. Bandage the arm to the side of the chest.
4. Support the injured arm in a triangular sling (see p. 27).
5. Check pulse and loosen bandage if circulation has been impeded.
6. Transport as sitting case unless casualty is suffering from severe shock.

Fracture of the Shoulder Blade

This fracture is usually caused by a crush injury or a severe blow. The general signs and symptoms are apparent and, of course, the history of the accident aids diagnosis.

Treatment

1. Do not remove the jacket.
2. Support the arm on the injured side in a triangular sling (see p. 27).
3. Get medical aid.

Fracture of Upper Limb

If the elbow can be bent without pain or difficulty treat as follows:

1. Do not remove the jacket.
2. Bend the elbow and lay the injured arm across the casualty's chest with fingers touching the opposite shoulder.
3. Apply a collar and cuff sling (see p. 26), except when the wrist is involved.
4. Apply padding between arm and chest, bandage arm to body, first on a level with the top of the shoulder and the second with edge in line with the tip of the elbow.
5. Tie off on the uninjured side (Fig. 58).

If the wrist is involved treat as above but do not apply collar and cuff sling.

If the elbow cannot be bent apply a well-padded splint to the inside of the arm, reaching from the armpit to the fingertips and secure with three bandages, one above the fracture, one below the fracture and one round the wrist.

If both limbs are broken, lay the casualty down, place padding between each arm and the body and secure the arms with three bandages, using the body as a 'splint', the first above the fracture, the second below the fracture and the third round the wrists and thighs, and transport as a stretcher case.

Fractured Forearm splints are only used if the casualty has to be taken a long way or on a rough journey, otherwise the methods already described should suffice.

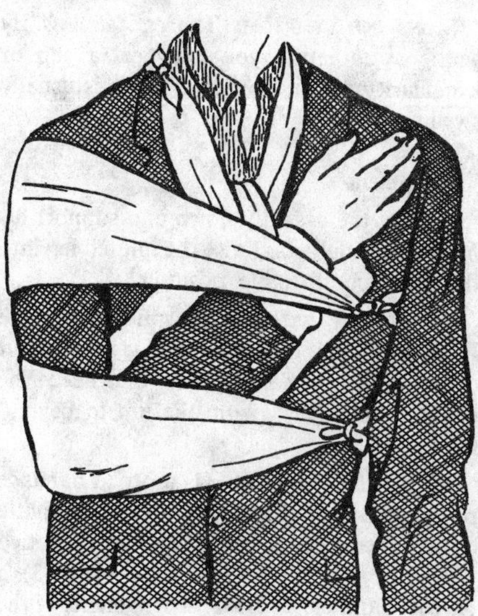

Fig. 58. *FOR FRACTURE OF ARM. Apply a collar and cuff bandage, and then two bandages around body.*

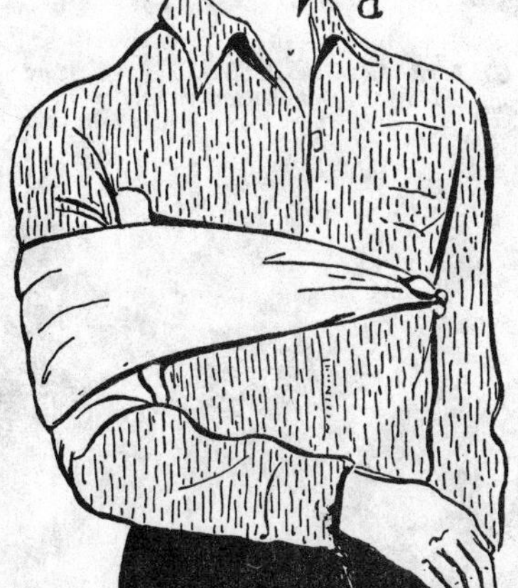

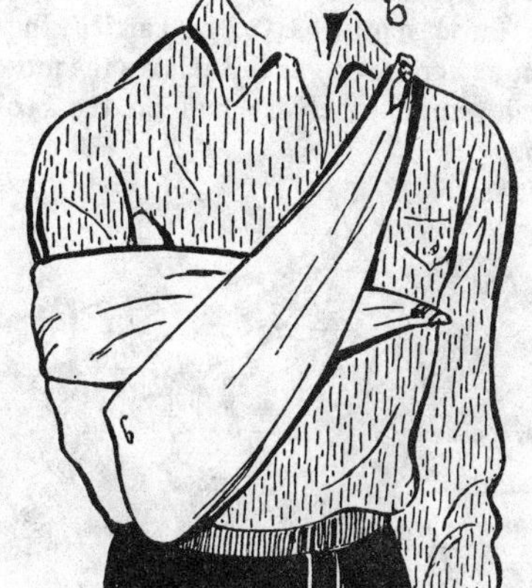

Fig. 57. *FOR FRACTURE OF THE COLLAR-BONE.* (a) *Pad between arm and chest, and bandage arm to chest.* (b) *Support injured arm in a triangular sling.*

Equipment required: two well-padded splints long enough to reach from the elbow to the fingertips, two bandages and one arm sling (see Fig. 56b, p. 32).

Method of Application of Splints

(a) Place the injured forearm at right angles to the upper arm across the chest with the thumb uppermost and the palm turned towards the chest.

(b) Put the splints, one each side of the forearm, from elbow to fingers.

(c) Apply one bandage above the fracture (that is nearest the elbow) and tie off on the outside splint.

(d) Apply a figure of eight bandage round the wrist and hand including the splints.

(e) Place the arm in a broad arm sling.

Fracture of the Pelvis

This is a dangerous condition as it is often associated with some other injury or complication, such as rupture of the bladder. It is usually the result of direct violence, but sometimes a fall on the feet from a height may result in a fractured pelvis.

Signs and Symptoms. Pain, sometimes very severe, in the hips and loins which is increased by movement or coughing. Internal hemorrhage may occur (see p. 25). The casualty may wish to pass water, but will find difficulty or may be unable to do so. If urine is passed it may be dark from the presence of blood.

Treatment. Warn him to lie still, then place him in the position which gives most comfort —for preference on his back with knees straight or slightly bent; if knees are bent, place something like a rolled rug under them to support them.

Warn him that he should try not to pass water.

Apply padding between the legs, particularly between knees and ankles, then tie the ankles and feet together with a figure of eight bandage, by placing the center of the bandage under the ankles, bringing the ends round, crossing the bandage over the instep and tying off under the soles of the feet. Boots and shoes should not be removed unless there is a wound on the foot.

With extreme care ease two broad bandages under his waist and bring them down so that they are under the pelvis, bandages overlapping half their width, and tie off firmly but not tightly (Fig. 59).

Treat for shock. Do not give fluids.

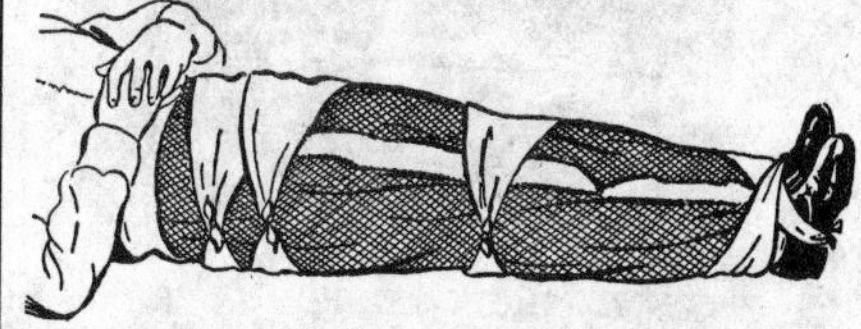

Fig. 59. *FOR PELVIC FRACTURE. Put on bandages in the following order: ankle, pelvis (2), and knees.*

Fractured Thigh (Femur)

A fractured hip is a serious condition, particularly in elderly people, and can be occasioned by comparatively slight causes such as tripping on a rug, and, because the cause seems slight, you may mistake the injury for a badly bruised hip. Fractures of the femur can occur at the upper end (or neck), the center of the shaft, or at the lower end near the knee joint.

Signs and Symptoms. General signs and symptoms such as pain, swelling, loss of power, unnatural position, and shortening. Remember that comparison with the uninjured side can be a reliable basis for diagnosis.

Treatment. If medical aid is readily available, only do enough to make the casualty comfortable, to prevent further injury and to guard against shock, i.e. put pads between his legs and, if his leg can be moved without too much pain, tie the ankles and feet together with a figure of eight bandage (see fractured pelvis).

Tie a broad bandage round both knees.

Tie a broad bandage above the fracture.

Tie a broad bandage below the fracture.

If the leg is too painful to move, warn the casualty to lie still and support and control the movement of the leg by cushions, rolled up rugs, and bags, etc. Reassure him, keep him warm and treat for shock.

FRACTURE OF THE FEMUR WHEN MEDICAL AID IS NOT READILY AVAILABLE OR WHEN THE CASUALTY HAS TO BE CARRIED A LONG DISTANCE OR OVER ROUGH GROUND.

EQUIPMENT. One well-padded splint to reach from crotch to heels.

One or two well-padded splints to reach from armpits to heels.

Eight triangular bandages long enough to go round the body and the splints.

Method

(a) Apply the splint between the limbs reaching from crotch to heels (Fig. 60a).

(b) Tie both ankles together with a figure of eight bandage in 1st position (see fractured pelvis and Fig. 60a).

(c) If one thigh is broken use one splint from the armpit to heels on the injured side; if both thighs are broken, apply splints on both sides.

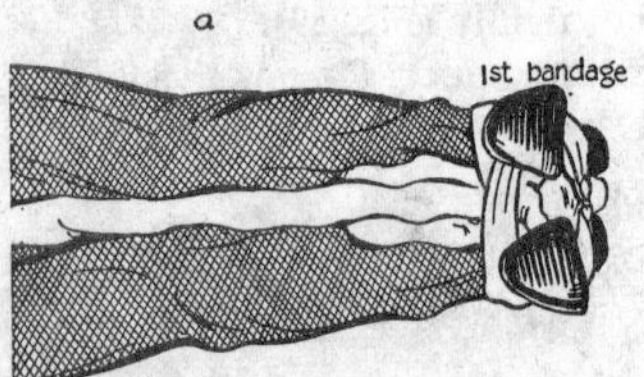

Fig. 60a. *FOR FRACTURED FEMUR. Put padded splints between legs and tie figure of 8 bandage around ankle.*

(d) Place a broad bandage in position 2 under the chest.

(e) Place a broad bandage in position 3 under the hips.

(f) Place a broad bandage in position 4 under both ankles.

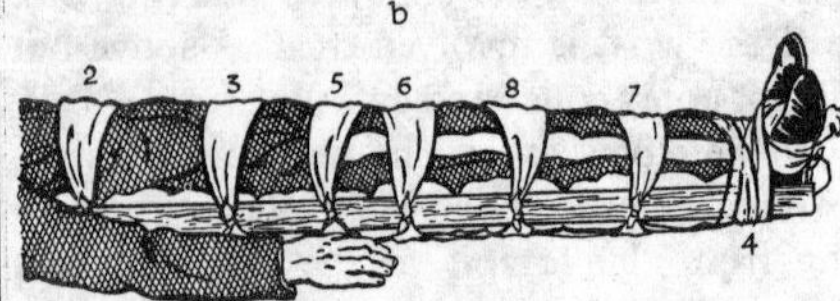

Fig. 60b. *FOR FRACTURED FEMUR. Tie on bandages in sequence marked.*

(g) Place a broad bandage in position 5 under thighs above fracture.

(h) Place a broad bandage in position 6 under thighs below fracture.

(i) Place a broad bandage in position 7 under both calves.

(j) Place a broad bandage in position 8 under both knees.

(k) Tie off bandages so that knots come on the splint (Fig. 60b).

Fracture of the Knee-cap

SIGNS AND SYMPTOMS. The leg is useless. By gentle examination you may feel a gap or irregularity of the knee-cap. There is usually swelling.

Treatment

(a) Lay the casualty down and support his head and shoulders. Raise the injured leg into the most comfortable position.

(b) Place a well-padded splint along the back of the leg, taking particular care to put extra padding under the knee and heel. The splint should reach from the hip to beyond the heel.

(c) Fix the splint with (1) a broad bandage round the splint and thigh, (2) a narrow figure of eight bandage round ankle and foot, tied off under the sole of the shoe, and (3) a narrow bandage to draw the fragments of the broken knee-cap together. Put the center of the bandage above the knee-cap, cross the ends under the knee over the splint and tie off below the knee-cap.

If the casualty has to be carried, the leg must be kept raised as this relaxes the muscles which would otherwise pull on the broken bone.

Fracture of the Leg

If only one leg is broken it is possible, if no splint is available, to tie the injured leg to the uninjured one after padding between the limbs. If both legs are broken, a splint must be used.

1. Place a well-padded splint between the legs.
2. Very gently bring the feet as nearly as possible into line.

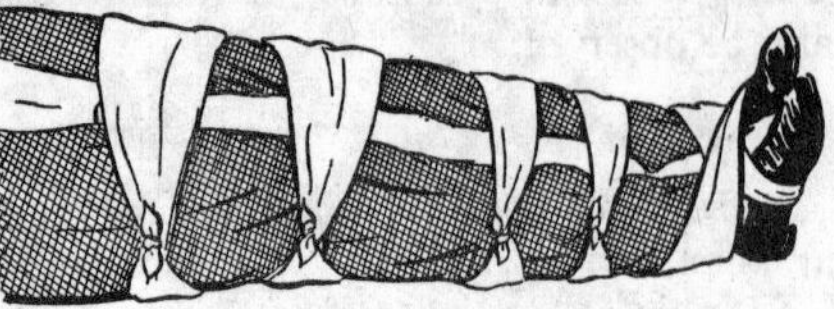

Fig. 62. *FOR FRACTURE OF LEG.*

3. Tie the ankles and feet together with a figure of eight bandage (Fig. 62).
4. Put a broad bandage round both thighs, and one round both knees.
5. Put one bandage round both legs above the fracture, and one round both legs below the fracture.
6. Bandages should be tied on either the uninjured or the less injured leg.

Crushed Foot

If there is no bleeding use the boot or shoe as a splint. Tie a figure of eight bandage round ankle and foot. Raise and support the foot.

If there is a wound, remove boot, shoe, stockings, etc., cutting them off if necessary. Dress the wound.

Apply a padded splint to the sole of the foot, and fix with a figure of eight bandage. Raise and support the foot.

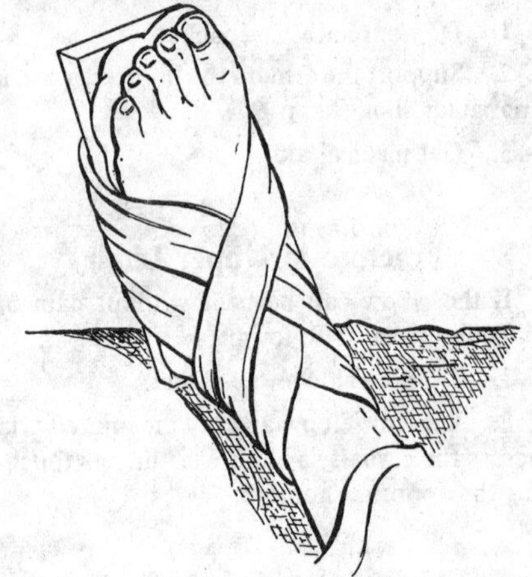

Fig. 63. *FOR CRUSHED FOOT. Tie a figure of 8 bandage round both foot and padded splint.*

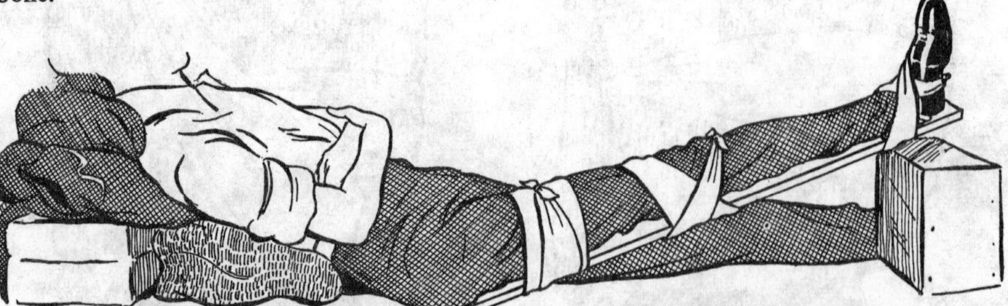

Fig. 61. *FOR FRACTURE OF KNEE-CAP. By raising the leg, the thigh muscles do not pull on the upper fragment of knee-cap. Support the extended leg with a well-padded splint.*

BURNS AND SCALDS

Burns are caused by dry heat such as fire, contact with electricity, friction from machinery, or by strong acids and alkalis.

Scalds are caused by wet heat such as steam, boiling water, or hot fat.

General Signs and Symptoms. Pain. Reddening or blistering of the skin. In severe cases the tissues under the skin may be severely damaged.

The greatest dangers in severe cases of burns and scalds are from shock and infection.

General Rules for Treatment

1. Make sure your hands are clean.
2. Do not apply lotions, creams, etc.
3. Do not remove the patient's clothing.
4. Do not break blisters.
5. Cover the whole area, including the clothing in severe cases, with sterile dressings or freshly laundered material.
6. Bandage lightly. Raise, support, and immobilize the injured part.
7. Treat for shock (see p. 21).
8. In severe cases needing hospital treatment, do not give anything by mouth.
9. In minor cases a non-greasy mild antiseptic cream, or a paste of bicarbonate of soda may be applied. But at any sign of inflammation medical advice must be obtained at once.

SPECIAL CASES. When the face is burnt make a mask out of sterile gauze or clean material, so that the patient can see and breathe, and keep the mask in position with a bandage as for fractured jaw (Fig. 55).

UNORTHODOX TREATMENT. For scalds and minor burns, plunge leg or hand *immediately* into cold water or run tap water on it for at least ten minutes.

Burns from Strong Acids

Treatment

1. Drench the part in water, if possible under a tap.
2. Bathe affected part in an alkaline solution of either baking or washing soda, one teaspoonful to a pint of warm water.
3. Remove contaminated clothing.
4. Apply general rules (above) as suitable.

Burns from Strong Alkalis

Corrosive burns may be caused by alkalis such as strong ammonia, caustic soda, caustic potash, and quicklime.

Treatment

1. If the substance which has caused the burn is powdery or in crystals, brush off as much as possible.
2. Drench with water, under a tap if possible.
3. Bathe the part with an acid solution of equal parts of vinegar and warm water.
4. Remove contaminated clothing.
5. General rules for treatment as applicable.

What to do in Case of Fire

Prevention of Fire

To avoid fire, keep your attic, cupboards and closets clean and as bare as possible, since they are seldom properly ventilated, especially in summer. Rags which may be greasy, or broken toys, or old clothes (the pockets of which may contain matches), may undergo spontaneous combustion, which often takes place at a temperature of 110° F.

Never allow children to play with matches, or to throw burnt matches on the floor.

Use a fireguard where there are children and old people.

House on Fire

If a fire starts, keep your self-control, and smother the fire with a rug or blanket, or throw water on the burning material, not on the flame. If you find you cannot put out the fire yourself, give an alarm. In leaving the room, be sure to *close* the door and windows, because if the room is closed the fire may die out or burn so slowly that it will give time for the firemen to arrive before it spreads to other rooms.

If awakened by the smell of fire at night, do not stop to dress, keep your self-control, wrap a blanket from the bed around you, give the necessary warning to other persons, and then get out of the premises the easiest way you can, closing all doors behind you. Do not go to the floor above the one where the fire is, unless it is imperative to wake others, because heat and smoke ascend.

To escape through passages filled with suffocating smoke, tie a wet handkerchief over the mouth and nose, then crawl on the hands and knees; the smoke rises with the hot air and will be less dense close to the floor. (Fig. 64)

If the whole of the lower part of the house is burning and escape by means of the stairs is cut off, preparations must be made for leaving by the window. If there is no fire escape or ladder, tie all sheets and blankets together by means of reef knots (see Fig. 19, p. 26), which will not slip no matter how much strain is put upon them. Finally, make one end of your improvised fire-escape fast to the bed leg, drop the other end out of the window and, after making sure that it reaches to, or almost to the ground, go down it boldly hand over hand. There is always considerable risk of a dangerous fall resulting from this means of exit, and therefore it should be undertaken only when all other means of escape have failed.

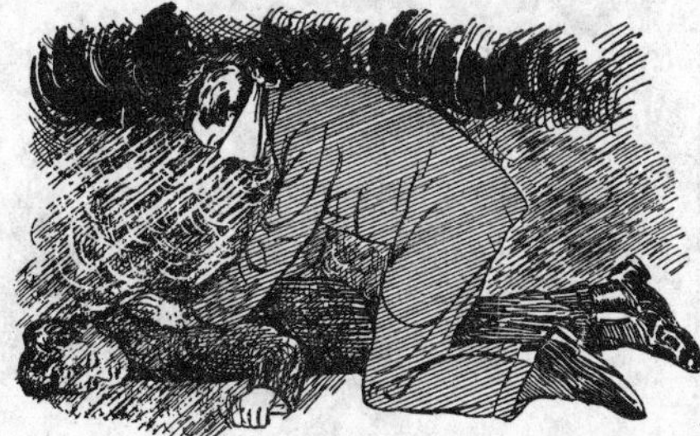

Fig. 64. *HOUSE ON FIRE. Crawl on hands and knees to keep below hot air and smoke.*

Oil Heaters and Lamps

With an overturned oil-lamp there is a sudden and alarming blaze, but if action is taken at once the damage may be confined to the carpet or cloth on which the lamp actually lies. To throw water on the conflagration is useless; burning oil will only be spread over a larger area. The aim should be to absorb the oil and smother the flame, and this should be done by means of some non-inflammable powder such as flour, or sand or earth from the garden.

Clothes on Fire

If the clothes of another person catch fire, approach him by holding up a thick blanket, a rug, or some other thick article to protect yourself against the flames. Wrap it quickly round him and lay him flat down on the ground to put out the flames.

Arrange for immediate hospital treatment, and then wrap the patient in a clean blanket. A little water may be given to the patient if he complains of feeling thirsty while waiting for the ambulance.

If your own clothes catch fire when you are alone, wrap the nearest rug, blanket, thick coat or thick curtain round you, call for help, and roll on the floor to extinguish the flames. Do not rush into the garden or street, because it will make the flames burn faster.

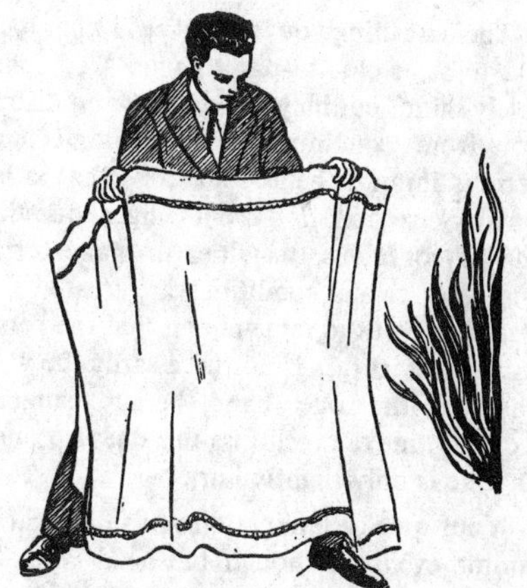

Fig. 65a. *TO EXTINGUISH CLOTHING ON FIRE. Hold blanket, coat or mat in front of oneself and envelop the person so as to smother the flames.*

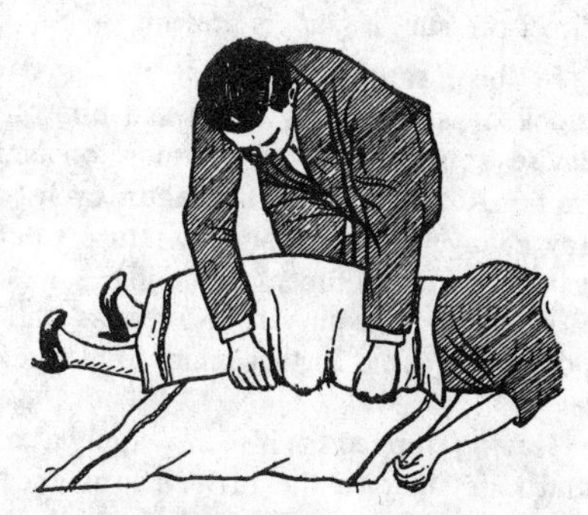

Fig. 65b. *CLOTHING ON FIRE. Push or trip the burning person flat to the floor, wrap closely to prevent air getting to charring clothes.*

A TYPICAL ROAD ACCIDENT

The injuries which one suffers and which can prove fatal are the same whether they happen at home, at work, on the roads—in or out of doors—the only differences being that the additional hazards may vary; equipment may be near at hand or have to be improvised; medical aid and onlookers may be readily available or you may have to cope for some time on your own.

Whatever the scene or whatever the cause or the number of people involved there are golden rules which, if observed, will give the injured the best possible chance of survival and will ensure that they do not suffer as a result of well-meant but harmful attention.

Road accidents tend to be more serious than those which occur in the home, because of the speed with which vehicles travel and the consequent greater damage which results. Complicated fractures and severe bleeding are perhaps the commonest injuries.

In most outdoor accidents more than one person is involved and in order to illustrate how to put the First Aid rules into action, the following imaginary road accident is described.

Collision between motor cycle (injury to the rider, severe head wound and unconsciousness) and automobile (injury to driver, severe arterial hemorrhage of arm and fractured leg, passenger in car shocked but not injured).

The first thing you will notice is what looks like a lot of blood—don't panic. A comparatively minor cut may bleed freely and distract you from examining for more immediately serious injuries, hence the stress that is laid on quick examination and intelligent questioning of conscious casualties to make certain that the serious conditions are treated first. Another point to remember is that the person making most fuss is not necessarily the worst case; on the other hand, because someone does not make much fuss this does not mean that he is only slightly hurt.

Your quick examination will show that the motor cyclist, although the head wound is severe, is not bleeding to death, and although he is unconscious he is breathing. The wound in the driver's arm, however, is serious and must be treated at once (see p. 24) either by direct pressure on a clean wound or by indirect pressure if glass is present.

In the meantime you have reassured the shocked passenger and have sent him off to devise some means of warning oncoming traffic. Return then to the motor cyclist for any change in condition, i.e. return to consciousness or failure of breathing.

Warn the car driver to keep as still as possible to avoid further injury to his broken leg.

Having stopped the bleeding, apply a collar and cuff sling to the driver's arm and set about fixing his leg. Using the unbroken leg as a 'splint', put pads between the legs. Tie the ankles together. Tie both knees together, and put one bandage around both legs above the fracture and one around both legs below the fracture. If there is danger of fire, the casualty should then be removed from the car, but the greatest care must be taken to avoid jarring or unnecessary pain. Have the fire extinguisher—which of course you carry—near at hand. Treat for shock.

So far the motor cyclist has not shown any signs of his condition worsening. There is no blood oozing from his ears or nose, so it would appear that he has not fractured the base of his skull, but he may have a fractured spine so *do not* sit him up; try to treat him without bending his neck or body. Cover him, and treat the wound by using one of the 1 yard packs of sterile gauze over the wound, and a ring pad (see Fig. 25, p. 27) just in case there is a fracture under the wound.

If the accident happens at night turn the headlights of the vehicles on as additional warning to other traffic. Send the passenger for help.

Remember—never move badly injured people unless there is immediate danger, or unless it is raining or snowing heavily.

MISCELLANEOUS INJURIES AND MISHAPS

Bites and Stings

Snake Bites. Venomous snakes are relatively uncommon in the United States, and very few deaths result. The greatest danger in snake bite is from shock, so it is important to reassure the patient and get him to a doctor or hospital as quickly as possible.

If the bite is that of a venomous snake, apply a tourniquet and squeeze or suck out as much venom as possible. See p. 25. The wound from the bite of a nonvenomous snake should be flushed thoroughly and a simple bandage should be applied.

In either case, as soon as first aid has been administered get the patient to a doctor or hospital for further treatment.

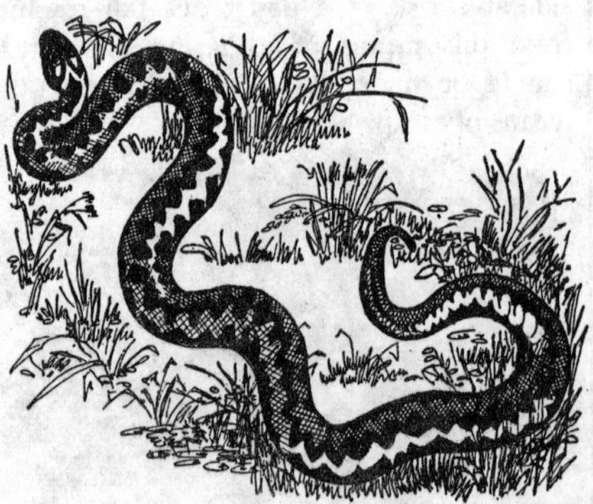

Fig. 66. *VIPER. A venomous snake found all over the world.*

Insect Stings. It is rare for insect stings to endanger life, but they can cause severe pain, swelling and shock.

For treatment, see Bites, p.13, and Stings, p. 17.

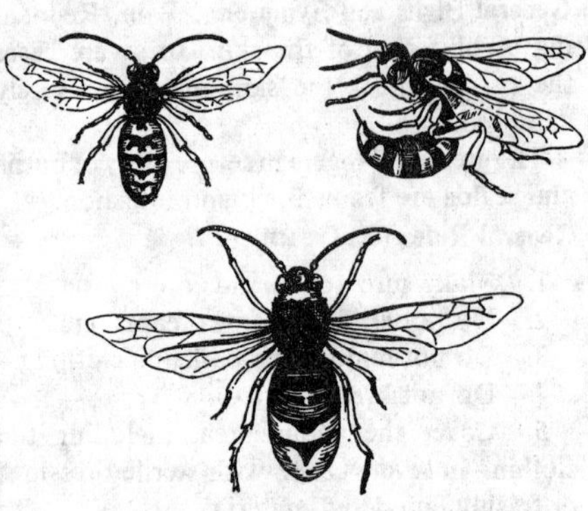

Fig. 67. *WASPS AND HORNET. Top, back and side views of common wasp. Below, the hornet is similar in coloring but larger.*

Jellyfish Stings. The small common jellyfish produces a slight sting and reddening of the skin. A soothing lotion should be dabbed on, or an antihistamine cream applied.

The larger Portuguese Man-of-War jellyfish appears in warm summers around the shores and beaches. Its stings are very painful, and may cause shock, vomiting, and cramp. Remove adherent tentacles. Dab reddened area with a lotion of bicarbonate of soda, apply soap, or cover with an antihistamine cream to relieve the pain. Keep the patient at rest, cover with a rug, and give a warm drink.

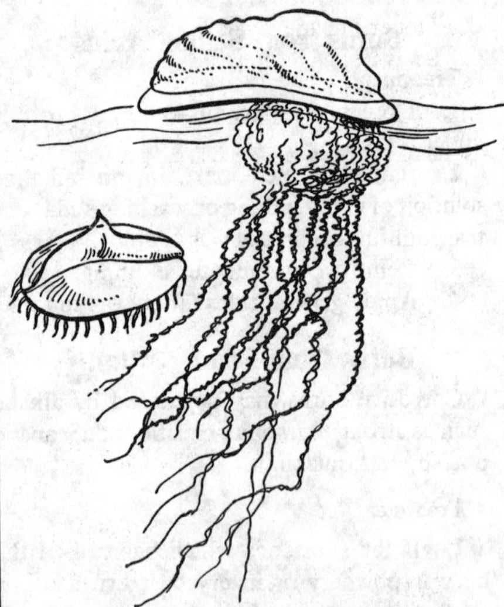

Fig. 68. *JELLYFISH. The small common jellyfish swims just below the surface of the sea. The Portuguese Man-of-War lies partly above the surface with its long tentacles below.*

Nettle Stings. Apply an antihistamine cream, or rub with crushed leaves to ease irritation.

Dislocations and Sprains

These are injuries at a joint. In dislocations the bones at the joint are displaced. In sprains the bones are not displaced, but the ligaments and tissues round the joint are wrenched and torn.

On no account must any attempt be made by a First Aider to reduce a dislocation.

Signs and Symptoms of Dislocations

Severe pain at or near the joint. Inability to move the joint. Deformity: the limb appears misshapen. Swelling usually occurs.

Treatment

1. Get medical aid as soon as possible.
2. Steady and support the limb in the most comfortable position, using padding and bandages.
3. If the jaw is dislocated, remove any dental plates, and support jaw with a bandage.

Signs and Symptoms of Sprains

Pain at the joint. Pain and difficulty of movement of the joint. Swelling and bruising.

Treatment

1. Steady and support injured limb.
2. Expose the joint and apply a wet cold bandage. When wet bandage ceases to give relief, take it off and then reapply it.
3. Severe sprains should be seen by a doctor as sometimes small bones may be fractured.

Eyes: Foreign Body in the Eye

Insects, grit, dust, or an eyelash in the eye may be removed with the corner of a clean damp handkerchief, or, if the object is under the upper lid, the casualty may blink his eye under water. Alternatively, lift the upper lid forward, push the lower lid under it so that the lower lashes sweep the upper lid. Repeat several times; if unsuccessful, get medical aid.

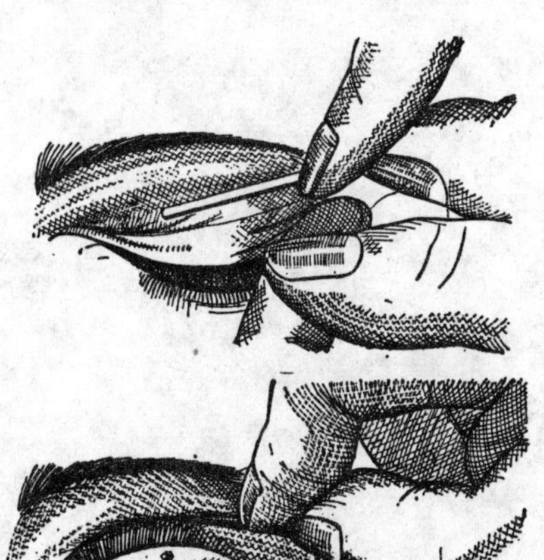

Fig. 69. *TO REMOVE A FOREIGN BODY FROM THE UPPER EYELID.*
(a) *Hold eyelashes firmly with fingers and with other hand lay matchstick (or knitting needle) along upper lid.* (b) *Draw lashes upward to turn lid inside out disclosing foreign body.*

Warn the casualty not to rub his eye.

Never remove any object which is embedded in the eyeball. Apply a soft pad of cotton, secure with a lightly tied bandage and take casualty to hospital.

Fits

The emergency treatment of epileptic fits is dealt with in the section on Common Accidents and Emergencies under the heading Epileptic Fits, p. 15.

Heart Attacks

There are two kinds of heart attack which may have to be dealt with from a first aid point of view.

In the first type there is some interference with the blood supply to the heart, thus preventing the heart from getting enough oxygen; this occurs in such diseases as angina pectoris and coronary diseases. These attacks are usually sudden and may not come on because of exertion. Signs and symptoms are pain over the heart, in the pit of the stomach and down the arm, of an extremely severe nature; and a pale or ashen face.

The other type is due to exertion by patients suffering from chronic heart conditions, the heart being unable to cope with any extra demands made upon it. The signs and symptoms are breathlessness, skin bluish due to lack of oxygen, and sudden collapse, sometimes with vomiting or spitting blood. The casualty will show signs of shock.

Treatment. Do not move the casualty unless really necessary but support him in a sitting position since this causes less strain on the heart. Undo tight clothing around neck and waist.

Send for medical aid at once.

Poisoning

Poisonous substances may be taken into the body (a) through the lungs by breathing in gases, fumes, or smoke; (b) by swallowing; or (c) by injection through snake or dog bite, or by hypodermic syringe.

The greatest danger to life is from asphyxia: see p. 22 for treatment.

General Rules for Treatment

1. Send for medical aid giving, if possible, suspected cause of poisoning.
2. Keep any pill boxes, bottles, etc. which may help the doctor to identify the poison.
3. Keep any vomited matter.
4. If breathing has failed, start artificial respiration (see p. 22) at once.
5. If the patient is unconscious but still breathing, place him face downwards with head turned to one side. Give nothing by mouth.
6. If the patient is conscious and shows no signs of corrosive burning of lips and mouth, make him vomit.
7. If there are signs of burning from corrosive acids or alkalis or strong disinfectants, do not induce vomiting. Give quantities of water, milk, or Milk of Magnesia in water.
8. Artificial respiration must be continued until medical aid is available. Apparent absence of life must not be taken to mean that the casualty will not respond to treatment.

For fuller details on Poisons and Antidotes, see p. 38.

Travel Sickness

Travel sickness can very often be avoided by sensible behavior before and during a journey. Do not eat large, rich or greasy meals, ice-creams, chocolate, or sodas. Dry crackers or chewing gum are much safer. If travelling in your own vehicle, stop at the first signs of sickness in a passenger or in yourself. Give the person who is prone to travel sickness somehting to do; chat with him; play simple games such as car numbers or milestones, estimating the speed of the vehicle by timing milestones and so on.

If you have a favorite remedy, take the tablets in good time and follow the manufacturer's instruction. Pregnant women should not take such tablets if they can manage without them.

If travelling by sea, try to stay on deck in the air but do not watch the horizon.

Needle, Glass or Fish Hook Embedded Under the Skin

Needle or Glass in Flesh

If a needle or a splinter of glass pierces the skin and then breaks so that the embedded portion cannot be seen, at once mark the spot where it entered, keep the part completely at rest (if necessary using a splint or sling), and consult a doctor as soon as possible.

Fish Hook in Hand or Finger

If the hook is deeply embedded treat as for needle above.

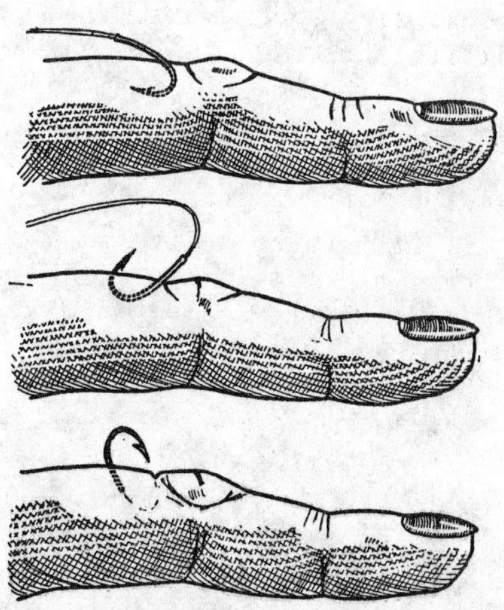

Fig. 70. *REMOVAL OF FISH HOOK. Press barb completely through as illustrated, cut off the dressing of the hook and withdraw the barb.*

If the hook is not too far in the flesh it can be dealt with as follows. Cut the dressing off the hook so that only the metal part remains in; bathe the skin with iodine, and then press on this part and try to force the point out through the skin so that the hook can be pulled out afterwards. If the barb has already pierced through the skin it may be broken or cut off, and the rear of the hook is then extracted. Bathe the wounds with iodine and apply a dry sterile dressing and a bandage. The hand should be kept at rest as much as possible and should not be wetted until healing is complete.

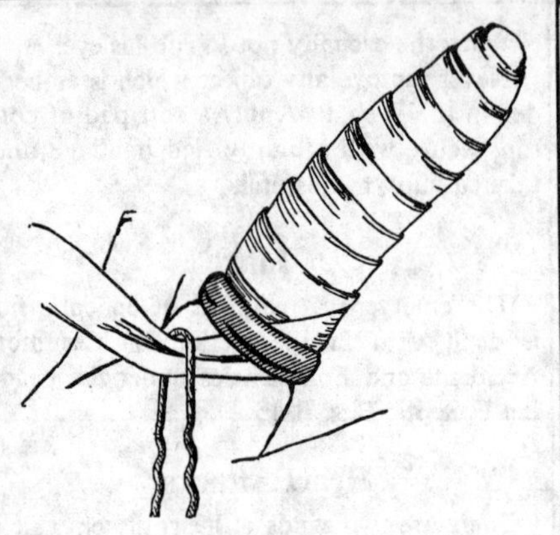

Fig. 71. *RING TIGHT ON FINGER. Wind tape as illustrated and bring free end through with bend of hairpin.*

Ring Tight on Finger

If the condition is recent and temporary, immerse the hand in cold water and rub soap around the ring.

If the finger has swollen, get a length of ordinary tape half an inch or so wide and, beginning at the finger tip, wind it tightly around the finger towards the ring, each turn overlapping as in Fig. 71. This will reduce swelling. Take a hairpin and push the bent end between the ring and finger (palm side) towards the tape. Thread the free end of tape through the hairpin loop and pull the hairpin back. Rub all well with wet soap. Pull firmly on the tape end and as it untwists the ring should move up the finger.

POISONS AND ANTIDOTES

A poison is a substance which damages the body. It has never been defined in law and is classified as 'poison, or other destructive or noxious thing'. Many substances in common use in the house and garden are incredibly dangerous and, when to these are added the contents of the average medicine chest in the house, it can be seen why a knowledge of the commoner poisons and their treatment is of value to the householder, especially if there are young children in the house.

A poison can enter the body by many routes. The two commonest are by swallowing (as with aspirin) and by inhalation (as with gases); other less likely ways are through the skin by absorption (as with compounds containing lead), by injection, or by absorption from the lining of the rectum and vagina.

Treatment depends not only upon knowing what type of poison has been taken or absorbed, but it will be modified by knowing how much has been taken and by which route. Hence any external evidence, such as a half-empty pill box or any pieces of the plant that the child has eaten, should always be left for the doctor to examine.

Great individual variation occurs in the effects of a given poison on different people; some persons have an idiosyncrasy to certain drugs while in those with liver or kidney disease the effects of a certain dose of a poison would be more grave than for a healthy subject. Further, individuals can acquire a tolerance to noxious substances as did de Quincey who, in his biography *The Confessions of an Opium Eater*, describes taking about 300 grains of opium every day with only pleasurable effects, about enough to kill 50 healthy men who were not addicts.

Modes of Poisoning

In the United States poisoning is usually accidental, occasionally suicidal, and rarely homicidal. 'Common things occur commonly' and it is found that 90 per cent of all accidental and suicidal deaths from poisoning are caused by coal gas, lysol, common narcotics (barbiturates and aspirins) or mineral acids in household use.

Certain types of poisons can be grouped by their common mode of action in the body and they may be roughly classified in this way:

(1) CORROSIVE: Strong mineral acids, alkalis and lysol

(2) IRRITANT: Metallic (e.g. arsenic), vegetable (e.g. fungi), or gases (e.g. ammonia fumes)

(3) NARCOTIC: Morphine and barbiturates

(4) CONVULSIVE: Cocaine and strychnine

(5) PARALYTIC: Nicotine

(6) GASEOUS: Irrespirable or harmful if breathed in (e.g. carbon dioxide), or truly poisonous (e.g. hydrocyanic acid)

Many poisons fall into two or more groups, for example phosphorus is both an irritant and a liver poison, and all produce different symptoms.

General Emergency Treatment

Should a person become unwell soon after eating a meal or should he be found in circumstances connecting him with a poison, e.g. unconscious with a box of sleeping pills beside him, or should a child be unduly sleepy after a walk in woods known to contain fungi, then suspect poisoning and act quickly to save life.

(1) **Send for a doctor** and let him know what poison is suspected so that he may bring suitable remedies . . . *or*

Hurry the patient to hospital.

(2) **Treat Respiratory Depression.** Should the poison be domestic gas or exhaust fumes which contain carbon monoxide, remove the patient from the atmosphere and turn off gas taps. The rescuer should stoop low in the room or garage because the light carbon monoxide rises above the air. Ideally, the rescuer should be connected by a rope to someone outside in case he, too, is overcome.

If the patient does not start breathing within 15 to 30 seconds, use artificial respiration (see p. 22) and, if available, oxygen.

Shallow breathing in other cases of poisoning requires prompt clearing of the airway in nose and throat (see p. 22). Dentures and mucus should be removed with the fingers and the patient placed as Fig. 7, p. 21.

(3) **Treat Shock.** Treat the shock that many poisons cause by conserving warmth with blankets (not hot-water bottles); use no drugs but give by mouth only such fluids as may be indicated in that particular type of poisoning.

Meanwhile keep the patient in the head-down position.

(4) **Removing Poisons from the System.** (a) Cyanides are the most dangerous of swallowed poisons because of the speed with which damage is caused. Having rapidly treated the patient for shock and breathing, the first-aider should rush the patient to the nearest hospital Accident Department for specific treatment (see p. 43).

(b) No attempt should be made at home to wash out poisons such as paraffin (kerosene), wood alcohol or furniture polish containing it, and corrosives (p. 40). Vomiting should not be encouraged, especially with swallowed gasoline. Soothing liquids such as milk, castor oil, or mineral oil may be given. For known corrosive acids give chalk in water and for caustic alkalis give vinegar or lemon juice diluted with its own volume of water.

(c) Poisoning by substances other than those in (a) or (b) may require removal of the poison by vomiting or by stomach washout. Although it is better to wait for stomach washout until the patient is in hospital, a simple procedure is given below.

EMETICS. Making the patient vomit up the swallowed poison is not so thorough a procedure as a stomach washout but is used when a washout is not possible. The simplest method is to tickle the back of the tongue and throat.

If this proves ineffective, give an emetic, e.g. mustard, ½ to 1 teaspoonful, in a glass of warm water; or salt, 1 to 2 tablespoonfuls in a glass of warm water; or warm soap solution. *Note.* Do not give an emetic to a patient who is unconscious, who cannot swallow, or who has taken a corrosive poison.

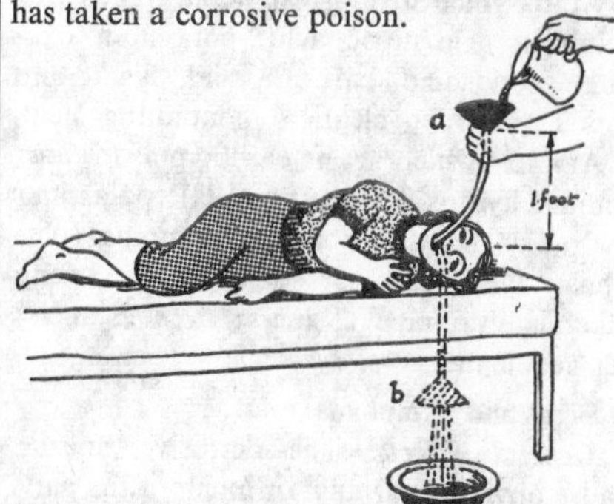

Fig. 1. *STOMACH WASHOUT.* (a) *With patient lying on her side and stomach tube inserted, pour in through the funnel the appropriate solution.* (b) *Lower the funnel and tube as illustrated to allow stomach contents to flow down into bowl on the floor.*

STOMACH WASHOUT. To wash out the stomach with a stomach pump, a long rubber tube is used, about ½ an inch in diameter, and 3 to 4 feet long, passed 16 to 18 inches down the throat. Absence of the syringe bulb makes the use of a fairly long tube necessary so that a syphon action can be attained. The pointed end is lubricated with butter or glycerin and passed into the stomach, an adult requiring about 16 inches of tube to be passed down beyond the teeth. A funnel is fitted into the free outer end, which is then lowered towards the floor over the bowl; fluid from the stomach will flow from the tube, removing the stomach contents which should be saved for inspection. The funnel is then raised and the stomach is washed out by running in 1 pint of soda bicarbonate solution (1 teaspoonful to 1 pint of warm water), or warm water. The patient must be propped in a sitting position with pillows, or may lie on his side if he cannot sit up. False teeth must be removed before the washout is given. The fluid used for the washout should be allowed to flow out and be collected in a bowl. The washout procedure is repeated until the returned fluid is clear.

(5) **Treat Pain.** Many poisons cause pain; ease it with a hot-water bottle to the stomach but *never* give any analgesic such as aspirin. If necessary the doctor may give a correct pain-relieving drug.

Summary. For the first-aider the aims of emergency treatment of poisoning are to keep the patient's airway clear for breathing, treat him for shock, remove what poison you can, and hasten him to the doctor for specific treatments. If no trained person is available then carry on treatment as detailed under each poison but the best place for treating any but the mildest poisonings is in a hospital with skilled care. This applies especially to children for many poisons that children eat exert their effects late and only experienced persons can guard against the dangerous states produced in children.

Corrosive Poisons

ACIDS which are most commonly taken are: sulphuric acid, nitric acid, potassium oxalate, acetic acid, carbolic acid, lysol and metal or toilet cleaners containing acid.

ALKALIS which act as caustic poisons are: sodium hydroxide (caustic soda); potassium hydroxide (caustic potash); ammonia solutions; lye; washing soda; lime; strong alkaline drainpipe cleaners; oven cleaners; carpet cleaners.

Signs and Symptoms

General Effects. The corrosive poisons cause obvious 'burning' or injury of the parts of the body with which they come into contact. Thus in the mouth, throat and stomach swelling, discoloration and erosion are seen. Breathing and speech become difficult and labored, and there is much pain and intense thirst with shock and collapse, and sometimes suffocation. The patient, however, generally remains clear in his mind. He often retches repeatedly and may vomit up blood-stained brown or black material. Convulsions may occur; the skin is pale and cold, or the face may be blue, the eyes sunken, the pulse fast and feeble, and the temperature low.

Characteristic Discoloration and Odor:

SULPHURIC ACID and HYDROCHLORIC ACID both cause gray stains which may go black later, with altered blood.

POTASSIUM OXALATE and OXALIC ACID cause white or brown stains.

NITRIC ACID causes yellow or brown stains.

ACETIC ACID, AMMONIA, CARBOLIC ACID are easily recognized by their odor.

Treatment: (a) Usual

See general rules for treatment, p. 39.

Note. An emetic must *never* be given in corrosive poisoning, nor may a stomach tube be used. An *antidote* must be given to neutralize the poison.

In doubtful cases give copious drinks of cold water or cold milk to dilute the acid in the stomach and decrease its corrosive action.

Treatment: (b) Special

Certain corrosive poisons require special treatment.

CARBOLIC ACID (phenol) and LYSOL differ from other corrosives in that they are quickly absorbed into the bloodstream and general system, causing insensibility. They produce the characteristic signs of corrosive action, and can generally be recognized by the typical odor of the breath. The lips and mouth are white or brown and leathery, and the urine may be green or suppressed. The reflexes may be absent and there is usually stupor. Severe abdominal pain is present just after the poison is swallowed, but passes off later. The abdominal muscles are contracted and hard, and the vomit may be bloodstained and contain fragments of the lining of the stomach; vomiting, however, may be absent. The patient may regain consciousness and apparently improve, and then die from shock some hours later.

Treatment. Alkalis are not given for these poisons. Instead, half a pint of liquid medicinal paraffin is given, or 1 tablespoonful of Epsom or Glauber's salts in ½ pint of milk or water.

It may be possible to introduce a stomach tube with great care, and to wash out the stomach until there is no further odor of carbolic. For the washout, ½ ounce of sodium sulphate or magnesium sulphate in 1 pint of warm water may be used. Milk, or white of egg in water may then be given. Also give stimulants, and keep the patient warm, using artificial respiration if necessary.

If the skin or eyes are injured, bathe the parts with warm castor oil.

POTASSIUM OXALATE and OXALIC ACID. For these poisons egg white or olive oil is the antidote since other alkalis may form poisonous substances.

Irritant Poisons

The common irritant poisons are:

METALLIC COMPOUNDS: The salts of arsenic, various arsenical preparations, copper or antimony, lead, mercury, zinc or tin, and salts of these metals.

IRON SALTS in medicinal tablets.

BLEACHES. Sodium hypochlorite solutions.

FUNGI (p. 42) which contain organic irritant poisons.

IODINE and other corrosives when diluted.

PARAFFIN and GASOLINE

PHOSPHORUS

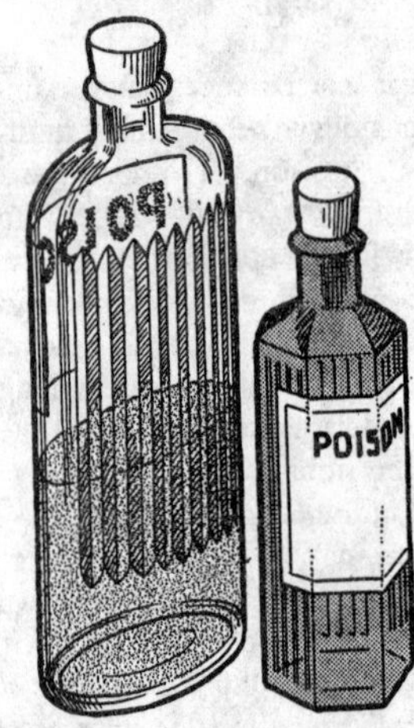

Fig. 2. *TYPICAL POISON BOTTLES. A bottle containing poison must always bear the word POISON.*

Signs and Symptoms

The chief effects of irritant poisons are irritation and inflammation of the parts of the body which come into contact with the substance. The effects are sometimes slower to appear than those which are produced by corrosives.

Vomiting and retching are common, and the vomit may contain blood. Very severe colicky pain and diarrhea develop and, if the patient does not die of shock, the effects caused by absorption of the poison into the system develop later.

General Treatment (Except for Iodine)

An emetic (p. 39) should be given promptly and, after this has taken effect, a purgative must be given. Soothing drinks and general treatment for shock (p. 21) are also required.

Metallic Irritant Poisons

Antimony Compounds. Employed in industry in alloys, foils, safety matches, etc.

Symptoms. In acute poisoning these usually develop in about ¼ to 1 hour, with burning pain, choking, and difficulty in swallowing. There is nausea, continual vomiting and diarrhea, with much pain in the abdomen. The patient has cramps in the legs, and the urine may be suppressed, with delirium, paralysis or coma. When collapse occurs the skin is cold, and the pulse feeble or imperceptible.

Treatment. Vomiting should be encouraged by giving plenty of warm water or, if vomiting is absent, it should be induced by emetics (p. 39). Strong tea may be given and when vomiting subsides give white of egg in water, or milk.

Treat shock by general methods (p. 21).

Arsenic. Much less used than formerly in medicines, some weedkillers, insecticides, and rat poison.

Symptoms. As for Antimony.

Treatment. Stomach washout or an emetic (p. 39) unless patient is in convulsions or unconscious. Keep patient warm in blankets; ice to suck to relieve thirst. Dimercaprolbal is then usually injected to counteract arsenic in the tissues; lost fluids are replaced by 5 per cent glucose in saline given intravenously.

Bleaches. Most household bleaches are 3% to 6% solutions of sodium hypochlorite in water.

Symptoms. When swallowed, they cause intense irritation to mucus linings of the stomach and lungs. Coughing and choking. Severe swelling of the pharynx and larynx but perforation of the stomach rare.

Treatment. Never use acid antidotes. Remove bleach by emetics or by stomach washout (p. 39) using milk of magnesia or milk. Then a purgative. Rest.

Copper Salts. In some fungicides: or from action of acid on copper utensils. See Zinc Salts, below, similar action.

Iodine (Iodine, Iodide salts; and Iodoform)

Symptoms. In acute poisoning iodine causes internal irritation with pain, vomiting, diarrhea and thirst. Strong iodine may also be corrosive. The vomit is yellow, or blue if starchy foods have been taken. The mouth and tongue may be seen to be brown and swollen, and the smell of iodine may be present. Later giddiness, faintness and convulsions may develop.

Treatment. Give starch and water, or cornstarch, and then give sodium bicarbonate, 2 teaspoonfuls in ½ pint of water. If iodine has been taken give starch and water drinks. Then give milk and eggs, milk, or flour boiled with water, or arrowroot.

In chronic iodide poisoning (iodism) there is headache in the forehead, watering of the eyes and nose, salivation, and inflammation of the throat, gums, or air passages. The skin may show a red eruption or acne. The drug must be discontinued.

Iron Salts. Brightly colored, often green, sugar-coated tablets containing ferrous sulphate given to adults for anemia are very dangerous to young children who may eat them like candy.

Symptoms. Pallor, drowsiness, vomiting, blood vomiting, or vomiting of blue-green material, heart irregularity, severe stomach pain and black stools. Forty such tablets have caused death in some cases and the practice of handing out large numbers of such tablets at prenatal clinics make iron tablets one of the commonest causes of poisoning in childhood.

Treatment. If the child has not vomited, induce it (p. 39) although not if the patient is unconscious. Give 1 tablespoonful of bicarbonate of soda in a glass of water to change the sulphate into a less damaging form of iron and induce vomiting again. Keep the shocked (p. 21) patient warm with blankets. In hospital, stomach washouts are repeated, desferrioxamine may be given intravenously, blood transfusion may be needed, and blood salts corrected.

Lead and its Salts (In gasoline additives, some paints and lead lotions)

Symptoms. Acute Lead Poisoning causes dryness and a metallic taste in the mouth, with intense thirst. Colic, constipation and vomiting may be noted, the stools being dark. In severe cases stupor and convulsions develop.

Treatment. Give an emetic (p. 39) and follow with magnesium or sodium sulphate, ½ ounce in ½ pint of water; then give white of egg in water, or milk.

Chronic Cases. Lead poisoning occurs occasionally in painters as an occupational disease but now, by law, paints used for internal decoration and paints used for toys contain no lead. Pallor, colic and constipation are present with 'wrist-drop', mental disturbances, or kidney disease. A blue line is often present round the gums.

Hot water bottles to the abdomen, and enema or a saline purge will relieve the colic.

Further treatment, under medical supervision, will include injections of calcium gluconate and a diet rich in calcium, including milk.

Mercury and its Salts (Corrosive sublimate, perchloride of mercury, white precipitate, red precipitate, vermilion)

Symptoms. In acute poisoning there is a metallic taste, shrivelling of the tongue and salivation, with pain in the abdomen, vomiting and purging. The skin is cold and the pulse rapid and weak. The urine may be suppressed.

Treatment. Give white of egg in water or milk freely, and then give an emetic (p. 39). Keep patient warm and airway clear. Get medical aid. Dimercaprol may be used.

In chronic cases there are anemia and languor, salivation, diarrhea or vomiting, and inflammation of the mouth with a blue 'ine round the gums.

Phosphorous (in matches)

Symptoms. The symptoms of acute poisonng develop in three stages.

(1) Within a few hours there is a taste of garlic, with gastro-intestinal irritation, pain, thirst, abdominal swelling and vomiting of blood. The urine is scanty and may contain blood. The patient may die, or:

(2) Improve for a few days, recover, or:

(3) Develop jaundice, enlarged liver and kidney damage, with prostration, coma, or eventually death.

Treatment. Give an emetic, or repeatedly wash out the stomach (p. 39) using a very weak potassium permanganate solution in lukewarm water. Avoid contamination with the vomitus since phosphorus burns skin and eyes. Subsequent treatment needs close medical care.

Zinc Salts (White vitriol)

Symptoms. The lips and mouth may be seen to be burnt, and there is pain in the throat and abdomen, with difficulty in swallowing. The vomit may contain blood, and convulsions, paralysis or coma may follow.

Treatment. Stomach washout only by skilled person. Give drinks of white of egg and milk, and follow with sodium carbonate, ½ level teaspoonful in warm water. Later give strong tea and demulcent drinks.

Organic Poisons

Aconite

Symptoms. Numbness and tingling of the mouth; nausea and vomiting, pain and breathlessness. Irregular slow weak pulse. Skin cold. Giddiness and unsteady gait. The patient remains lucid.

Treatment. Stomach washout only by a Atropine sulphate, 1 milligram, intravenously by injection. Stimulants, warmth, artificial respiration and friction. The patient must be kept lying down.

Alcohol (acute poisoning)

Symptoms. The breath smells of alcohol. Patient at first excited, violent or dazed. Face flushed, and lips gray or purple. Eyes bloodshot. Pupils often dilated and fixed. Perspiration, giddiness, confusion, later followed by convulsions, stupor or coma. The patient may appear to recover and then die suddenly a few hours later.

Treatment. Stomach washouts or emetic. Ammonium carbonate, ½ gram in a pint of water. Cold showers, and hot coffee if patient can swallow. Artificial respiration and hot water bottles to the limbs. Later warmth and warm wraps. Lay the patient comfortably on a mattress on the floor so he cannot fall and injure himself. Intravenous injections of various stimulants can be used to bring a 'drunk' to a safe state. Pills for sobering up are now on the market but they are not safe or reliable in effect.

Antihistamines

Symptoms. Lethargy and drowsiness, later amnesia and confusion; convulsions occur with severe overdosage. Symptoms are many and vary from patient to patient.

Treatment. Give milk or water. Artificial respiration (p. 22) if needed. Then stomach washout (p. 39) with baking soda (1 teaspoonful to the pint). Convulsions should be controlled with a barbiturate, or paraldehyde. Treat patient in darkened room to avoid stimulation.

Barbiturate Drugs. (e.g. Seconal, phenobarbitol).

Symptoms. Giddiness, confusion, staggering, delirium or coma. Slow stertorous breathing, and blueness of face. Scanty urine. Skin rashes sometimes in phenobarbitol poisoning. Temperature below normal.

Treatment. An emetic or stomach washout (p. 39). Leave 1 pint of hot coffee in stomach, with 30 millilitres castor oil. Apply warmth. Stimulants. Rectal salines. Artificial respiration. Complete recumbency and patient must be sent to hospital.

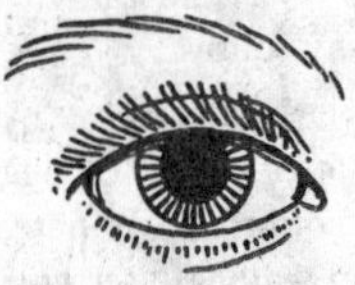

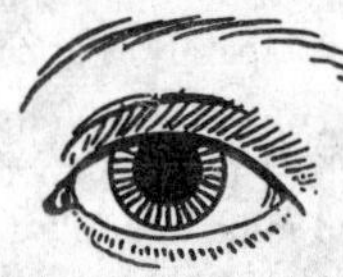

Fig. 3. *DILATED PUPILS IN BELLADONNA POISONING*

Diagram showing the effect of belladonna (deadly nightshade berries; eye drops; liniments) on the eyes of the patient. The black centers of the eyes—the pupils—enlarge far beyond the normal size and the colored rings around them almost vanish. The patient cannot see objects so clearly when the pupils are so widely dilated.

Belladonna; Atropine. In deadly nightshade berries; thorn-apple, eye drops; liniments.

Symptoms. Throat and skin become dry, the urine scanty, or even sometimes suppressed. Skin in most cases flushed, or showing a rash. Fever with rapid pulse and rapid breathing. In the later stages respiration becomes slow. Diarrhea. Pupils much dilated. Delirium.

Treatment. Stomach washout or emetic, p. 39. Wash out the stomach with warm pale pink potassium permanganate solution. Warmth. Stimulants, hot coffee. Artificial respiration if required. Give fluids freely. A short-acting barbiturate to control excitement. Paraldehyde, 10 cc. for delirium.

Camphor

Symptoms. Characteristic odor. Pallor, lividity, vomiting. Excitement and giddiness, with tremor and unsteadiness. Sometimes convulsions. Vomiting and rapid breathing.

Treatment. Copious stomach washouts, p. 39. Purge with 5 to 15 grams of magnesium sulphate in water. Warmth. Artificial respiration. Paraldehyde for convulsions.

Chloral Hydrate

Symptoms. Lividity and coldness of skin, with low temperature. Rapid feeble pulse, and slow breathing. Later coma may follow.

Treatment. Stomach washout or emetic. Warmth, massage, hot coffee. Methylamphetamine under medical direction. Artificial respiration if required. Oxygen.

Cocaine

Symptoms. First, excitement, pallor and dryness of skin, followed by sweating, faintness, and giddiness. Pupils dilated. Pulse and breathing fast. Tremors, convulsions, or mental confusion.

Treatment. If cocaine has been taken by mouth, give stomach washout using potassium permanganate solution. Artificial respiration if necessary. If convulsions occur, barbiturates may be given intravenously.

Dicophane (DDT)

Symptoms. Nausea, excitement, confusion and palpitations.

Treatment. Stomach washout with water. Barbiturates for nervous manifestations, warmth to extremities, stimulants, oxygen and rest in bed.

Digitalis (In heart medicaments. From foxglove)

Symptoms. Headache and languor with abdominal pain, diarrhea and vomiting. Pulse slow and small, with coupled beats. Pupils dilated. Skin cold and sweating. Urine scanty or suppressed. Lethargy or convulsions, delirium or coma.

Treatment. Stomach washout or emetic, p. 39. Copious drinks. Strong coffee. Stimulants. Warmth. Complete recumbency. Quinidine under medical direction.

Food Poisoning

Food poisoning implies acute gastroenteritis occurring within 48 hours after the consumption of tainted or chemically contaminated food or drink, or of poisonous foodstuffs such as toadstools. Foodstuffs infected by bacteria or their toxins provide the commonest type of food poisoning.

Salmonella bacteria (causing 75 per cent of cases) are transferred to food by mice, rats, flies, or by human carriers handling foods. This leads to an infection type of poisoning.

Staphylococcus pyogenes and related organisms produce the toxin type of poisoning. These bacteria are nearly always transferred to food by human beings who carry them on their hands or arms, or in the nose or throat. Less commonly, *Streptococcus* and rarely *Botulinus* are the causative agents, the latter giving rise to a sleeping sickness-like disease.

Infected or exposed food kept in a warm atmosphere is a potent source of danger, especially cooked meat, stews, gravy and soup, milk and milky foods and synthetic cream. Canned foods left open, and eggs, both of which rapidly breed bacteria, may also be dangerous. The danger is increased when prepared or uneaten food is kept for future use without being stored in a cool place or a refrigerator. This is more likely to occur in institutions.

Symptoms. Several members of a household or those who have eaten the same meal are often affected simultaneously. The total dose of the bacterial infection determines the speed of the development of symptoms and their severity; the incubation time indicates the probable cause. Symptoms developing within

(1) ½ hour are probably due to a chemical poison,

(2) 6 hours, a bacterial toxin,

(3) 12 to 48 hours, a salmonella infection.

The symptoms vary considerably in severity, but typically include nausea, vomiting, abdominal pain and diarrhea with colic. In severe cases prostration and collapse occur, due to loss of fluid by the diarrhea.

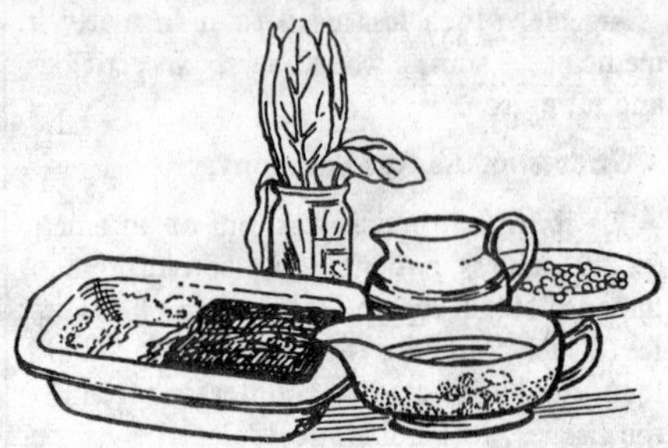

Fig. 4. *FOOD POISONING. Exposed wet foods left unrefrigerated are a source of danger.*

(a) *In cases due to chemicals or toxins* the onset is usually sudden and severe, the patient being collapsed and cold, with a subnormal temperature, but recovery usually follows within 24 hours.

(b) *In the infection type* the onset is later and there may be a rise in temperature, but the illness often lasts for several days. The stools are very loose, watery and foul and sometimes a little blood and mucus are passed.

In all these cases, especially in children, the condition must be diagnosed from acute surgical disorders such as intestinal obstruction. If possible a sample of the vomited material and feces should be sent for laboratory examination.

Treatment. Rest in bed, with warmth, is important and necessary in all cases.

In suspected cases due to chemicals or poisonous foods the stomach should be washed out and the appropriate antidote given as soon as possible.

Warm saline drinks are useful to counteract the loss of fluid, and for 24 to 48 hours only fluids such as tea, broth or fruit drinks are given by mouth. Later a light, very bland diet of milk foods, eggs, steamed fish, jellies, bread and butter, etc. is allowed.

Paragoric is given to control the diarrhea. Codeine may also be prescribed.

In cases of *Salmonella* infection antibiotics are of doubtful value.

The stools should be disinfected with 1:20 carbolic acid, and the nurse must not handle or prepare food until stool tests show absence of infection; this may persist for 14 days or much longer.

The disease is notifiable in the United States. In these cases, sulphonamides and antibiotics are given to prevent secondary infections and aid recovery.

Fungi (Toadstools)

Various poisonous fungi may be eaten accidentally, especially by children. A small quantity, if eaten, will cause intense pain, and death may follow.

The gills of the fungus are always white or creamy-white (in mushrooms they are pink, then brown), and the cup or vulva at the stalk base is a distinctive feature. Found in woods in late summer.

The Fly Agaric (*Amanita muscaria*) is also very poisonous but has a distinctive orange-scarlet cap covered with yellowish raised patches. Found in woods of birch or pine in autumn.

Prompt treatment of the poisoning is vital.

Symptoms. Colic, vomiting, thirst and diarrhea. Excitement passing into coma. Cold skin with slow pulse, and deep stertorous breathing.

Treatment. Stomach washout or emetic, p. 39. Castor oil 1 ounce, or other purgatives. Warmth. Stimulants.

Gases, Poisonous. Coal gas (carbon monoxide); carbon dioxide; marsh gas, sewer gas; hydrogen sulphide; acetylene; chlorine.

Symptoms. Ringing in ears. Nausea and giddiness, with shortness of breath. Lividity and muscular weakness. Rapid pulse becoming imperceptible, with stertor. Convulsions, asphyxia and coma, with dilated fixed pupils. NOTE. The skin is cherry pink in carbon monoxide (coal gas) poisoning.

Treatment. See p. 16. Remove to fresh air at once. Oxygen, or oxygen and carbon dioxide mixture if possible. Artificial respiration. Massage and friction. Warmth.

Hemlock. The poison in the hemlock plant is *coniine* which is similar in effect to nicotine (see below) but it produces more pronounced muscle paralysis.

GELSEMIUM which occurs in yellow jasmine acts similarly and is treated in the same fashion.

Nicotine (as a dust or spray in some pest killers; in tobacco)

Symptoms. Cold sweat, rapid onset of headache, vomiting and abdominal pain; breathing difficult due to paralysis of respiratory muscles; eyesight disturbances; palpitations and dizziness, convulsions and collapse.

Treatment. Stomach washout with dilute potassium permanganate solution, then suspended solution of charcoal. Artificial respiration (important) and oxygen; chloral hydrate for convulsions. Nicotine is fairly rapidly destroyed in the body and the treatment is largely symptomatic.

Opium. Morphine. Nepenthe. Paregoric. Laudanum. Codeine. Diamorphine hydrochloride (heroin), etc.

Symptoms. At first mental excitement, followed by headache and drowsiness. Pupils small or 'pin-point', and face pale or blue, with sweating of skin. Muscular weakness, slow breathing and weak pulse. Later coma and stertor.

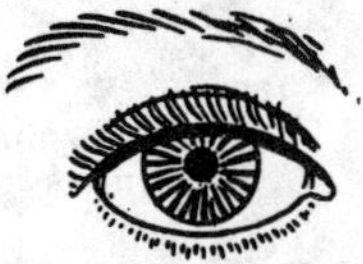
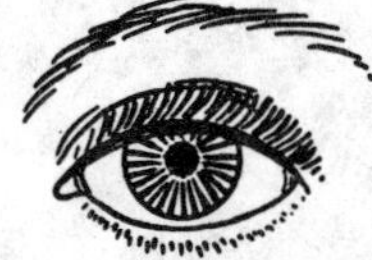

Fig. 5. *CONTRACTED PUPILS IN MORPHINE POISONING*

Diagram showing the effect of morphine, opium, laudanum, and heroin on the eyes of the patient. The black centers—the pupils—of the eyes contract to mere 'pin-points' and the colored rings dominate the eyes. It is similar to the contraction of the pupils seen when a person gazes at the sun on a brilliant summer's day.

Treatment. Stomach washout (p. 39) at once: emetic usually fails to act. Use potassium permanganate solution (1:2000) for repeated washouts. Then leave about ½ pint in stomach.

The stomach should be washed out even when morphine has been taken by hypodermic injection. Douse the face with cold water repeatedly, and attempt to rouse the patient. Nalorphine hydrochloride under medical direction. Supply warmth and give stimulants by mouth or by rectum if patient is unconscious and cannot swallow. Artificial respiration. Keep patient under observation although improvement is noted, in case of relapse. Complete rest in bed. Guard against further self-administration of opium preparations.

Phenacetin (In some headache remedies)

Symptoms. Cyanosis (blueness), vomiting and sweating. There is a red rash in some cases. In severe cases, collapse with feeble irregular pulse, and slow breathing.

Treatment. Water or milk to drink, then emetics (p. 39), stimulants, brandy, warmth to limbs. Smelling salts, artificial respiration (p. 22), complete recumbency.

Prussic Acid (hydrocyanic acid) **and Cyanides**

Symptoms. These poisons act *very* quickly. The breath may smell of bitter almonds, and this sign may be of great value in suggesting the immediate diagnosis and treatment.

Immediately after swallowing there are giddiness, staggering gait and muscular weakness, followed by difficulty in breathing and insensibility. There may be convulsions, and breathing is slow, convulsive and gasping. The patient is profoundly shocked, the skin cold, the eyes fixed with dilated pupils, and the limbs limp. The pulse is imperceptible.

Treatment. URGENT. Artificial respiration must be started immediately, with the patient in the open air. Wash out the stomach, or give an emetic if patient can swallow. Amyl nitrite may, if available, be given by inhalation. If the patient is still alive 2 minutes after ingesting prussic acid, amyl nitrate intravenously may be given.

Salicylates. Aspirin (acetylsalicylic acid), swallowed in quantity, is the major accidental poison to small children. Over 2000 such children are admitted to hospital yearly. Other salicylates are Alka Seltzer; sodium salicylate; oil of wintergreen and methyl salicylate in liniments and ointments.

Symptoms. Nausea and vomiting, ringing in the ears, blurred vision; palpitations and rapid shallow breathing; agitation, delirium or coma. Smell of acetone in the breath.

Treatment. Induce vomiting with fingers or emetic (p. 39) if no convulsions, then delay absorption of the remaining swallowed poison by giving water or milk. If patient unconscious, give nothing by mouth; keep him under warm blankets.

Salicylate poisoning causes complex changes in the body and each case needs individual treatment—hence the need to get medical care urgently. Shock may require oxygen and blood transfusion. Urine and blood need analytical testing to decide upon intravenous fluids. Vitamin K and barbiturates may also be required. In severe poisoning an artificial kidney may be used.

Strychnine. Nux vomica. In some tonics.

Symptoms. Rapid onset of twitching, convulsions; tetanus-like spasms of arms and legs; contraction of facial muscles, head thrown back; eyes staring but consciousness retained.

Treatment. Keep patient warm and in a quiet dark room. Call doctor to give sedatives; then stomach washout with 2 per cent tannic acid. Artificial respiration with oxygen may be necessary.

Tetrachloroethylene (and Carbon Tetrachloride). Used in dry cleaning of clothes.

Symptoms. Vomiting, diarrhea, colic, headache, stupor, and breathing difficulties.

Treatment. Remove the patient into fresh air and apply artificial respiration (p. 22). Stomach washout followed by sodium sulphate (Glauber's salts) 5 grams in a glass of water. If the condition is serious it may be necessary for the hospital to clear the blood with an artificial kidney.

Turpentine. A solvent for paints: in some furniture polishes.

Symptoms. From inhaling vapor or swallowing the liquid: powerful irritation in the lungs or gastro-intestinal tract causing vomiting, excitement, abdominal pain, diarrhea, and painful micturition with urine smelling of violets; characteristic odor in the breath and shallow breathing. Later, convulsions and coma.

Treatment. Remove patient into purer air and ensure absolute rest; move patient by stretcher only and keep him warm with blankets. Emetic (p. 39) if patient conscious. Analgesic, oxygen, etc. only under medical supervision.

Industrial and Agricultural Poisons

Many more people since the war are coming into contact with toxic chemicals in the course of their trade. Excluding the more obvious chemical and pharmaceutical industries, such varying trades and businesses as photography, manufacturing matches, nickel refining, and baking, all have their particular chemicals and poisons which are used for the proper carrying out of their work. To these are added the farmer's increasing use of chemicals on the land and in spraying crops and fruit. Not only are he and his animals at added risk from these chemicals but those who eat his fruit, or drink water that flows through his land, or handle his produce may be affected by the fungicide or pesticide.

Symptoms of Pesticide Poisoning are commonly giddiness, headache, muscle twitching and convulsions. Slow poisoning over a period of time has caused impotence for several months in farm workers using toxic chemicals.

Treatment. Such a poison enters the system by one of three routes. Either it is swallowed, or it is inhaled, or the poison is absorbed from the skin. The immediate treatment is withdrawal of the patient from the source, and removal of as much poison as possible by emetics, by stomach washout (p. 39), by inhalation of oxygen, or by prompt and thorough washing with cold water of all affected areas and removal of contaminated clothing.

Should the poisoning occur in a factory or workshop it is almost certain that the factory First Aid post and the industrial nurse or doctor concerned will be well versed in the management of such poisons as may be met with on the premises.

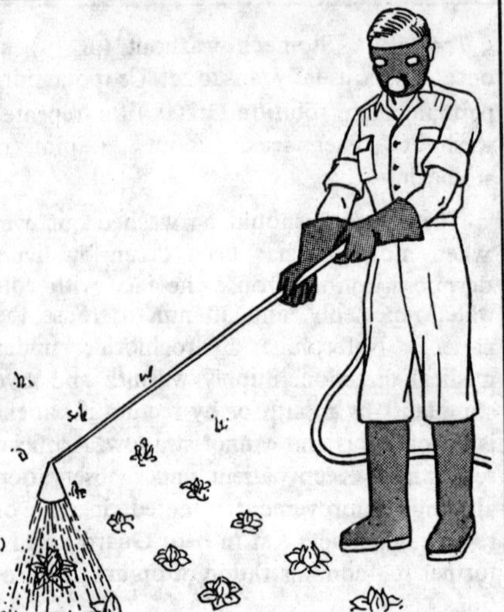

Fig. 6. *SPRAYING A PESTICIDE. To safeguard himself from the dangerous fluids and gases the farm worker should wear protective clothing.*

PESTICIDE. If the accident occurs in the countryside as a result of a pesticide, the doctor might not be familiar with the category of toxic substance used. Hence it is most important to save all vomit and urine for examination. Also, if possible, get the container in which the product was packed and look at the manufacturer's recommendation for treatment since all poisonous agricultural substances should carry these on the label.

The patient should be taken by car to the nearest hospital for special treatment.

Slow poisoning causing impotence is treated with methyltestosterone.

HOME NURSING

Many diseases and ailments can be dealt with at home under the guidance of the patient's doctor or the district nurse, either for the full period of the illness, or after discharge from hospital when the patient still needs special care and nursing. For mothers and those who have to care for sick people in the home there are a number of useful practices which can help to make the patient more comfortable and aid in his recovery.

Behavior of the Nurse. One of the most important things for a person nursing at home to remember is that when a child or adult is ill he will be more sensitive to the behavior and manner of the nurse than at normal times. She must therefore do her best to exercise self-control at all times and be patient, understanding and sympathetic. A good nurse shows willingness and gentleness even in carrying out the most trivial duties. She should try to cultivate a quiet voice and manner and be able to reassure her patient at any hour of the day or night. A good nurse will try to anticipate the needs of her patient.

The doctor must be able to rely on her to carry out his instructions conscientiously and she should give complete loyalty to the doctor and always maintain the patient's confidence in him. She must be able to observe and report to the doctor any changes in the patient's condition and, should an emergency arise, she should remain calm and act with common sense.

Nurse's Dress and Health. In her personal appearance the nurse should be neat and simply dressed. Easily washed clothes are most suitable and low-heeled shoes will prevent tired feet. She should keep herself as clean as possible taking particular care to keep her hands and nails scrupulously clean at all times. Exercise, rest and a well-balanced diet will help to keep her in good health, for this is most essential for nursing.

Outside of the sickroom, mother or nurse must relax and this is where other members of the family can help by taking on some of the many household duties which in the normal course form a mother's daily routine. Any interests—knitting, watching television, visiting the local shops, reading, or a chat with a neighbor—which will reduce strain and anxiety should be encouraged.

Choice and Preparation of Sickroom

Position. Whenever possible the patient should have a separate room; this is essential when nursing infectious diseases. The room should have plenty of light and air and should be located as near as possible to the bathroom.

Furniture. The room should be made easy to clean by clearing out all unnecessary furniture and rugs. Essential requirements are a bed, a table with a washable top or cover for medical and washing equipment, a chest of drawers or cupboard for storage, a bedside table with bell (a cane for tapping will do), an arm-chair and one or two small simple chairs.

Lighting. Whenever possible, the bed should be placed to give the patient a view through the window but care should be taken to keep direct light out of the eyes. At night the main light should be shaded and a bedside lamp is helpful.

Ventilation. Direct drafts on the patient should be avoided. Sash windows give less draft but a screen can be used to protect against draft from casement windows.

Heating and Temperature. If electric or gas heat is used it is advisable to put a shallow bowl of water in the room to keep the air moist. A room thermometer should be kept at the head of the bed to check that the room is kept at an even 70° F as far as possible.

Care of the Sickroom

Everything in the room should be kept as clean as possible. The room should be cleaned every morning after the patient has washed and the bed has been made.

After the room has been cleaned the window can be opened and the room thoroughly aired. Care must be taken to keep the patient warm while this is done. A water-bottle and water for the flowers should be changed daily and any other washable articles, such as fruit bowls, washed. For disinfection of the room after infectious diseases, see p. 49.

The Bed. This should preferably be a single bed raised to an appropriate height to prevent unnecessary stooping and stretching for the home nurse. The bed can be raised on wooden blocks with depressions made to hold the castors or legs.

Bedding. The mattress should be firm but comfortable and several well-filled feather, or rubber-foamed pillows may be needed. For some patients a rubber undersheet and draw sheet may be necessary. Old lengths of sheeting folded to cover worn parts are quite suitable for draw-sheets to cover the rubber sheeting beneath the patient's buttocks. Blankets should preferably be all wool, warm but light, and a lightweight good quality quilt may be used. Electric blankets are best not used but if they are employed now and then to help warm a very chilly patient, the greatest care must be taken to see that there is no direct contact between blanket and patient, and that the blanket is never allowed to get wet, or even damp, or folded or creased. It should never be covered with pillows or heavy bedding when connected to the electric supply or it will conserve too much heat and there will be a risk of fire.

Nylon sheets do not absorb moisture and are not advisable for patients with fever.

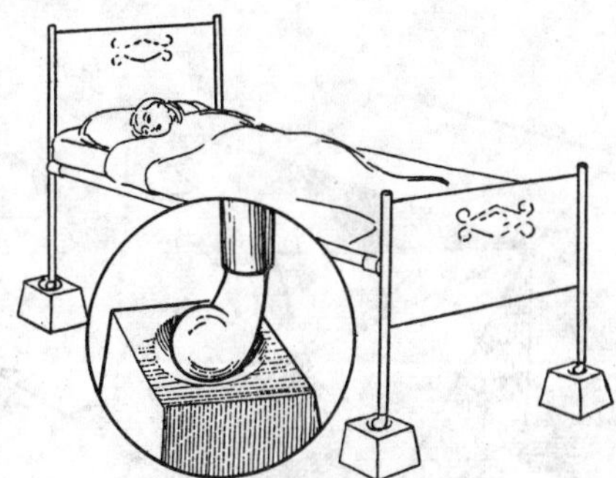

Fig. 1. *BED RAISED ON BLOCKS. This prevents unnecessary stooping for the home nurse.*

Useful Sick Room Equipment

Much of the equipment a patient needs when being nursed at home can be easily improvised.

Backrests. An adequate backrest can be made from a strong cardboard box as illustrated (Fig. 3). Another improvised backrest can be made with a chair (Fig. 2).

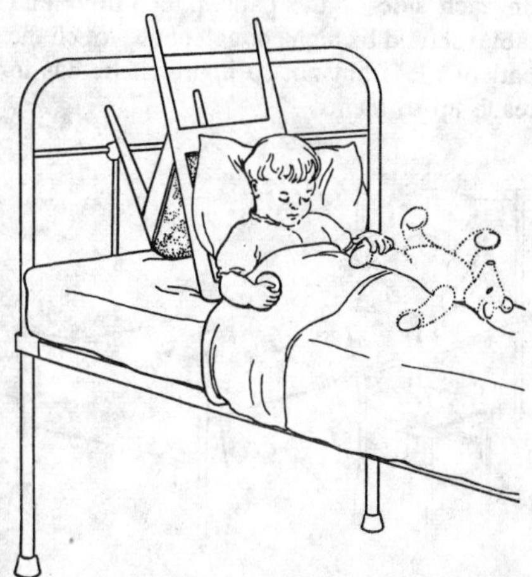

Fig. 2. *IMPROVISED BACKREST USING CHAIR*

HOW TO MAKE A BACK REST FROM A CARDBOARD BOX

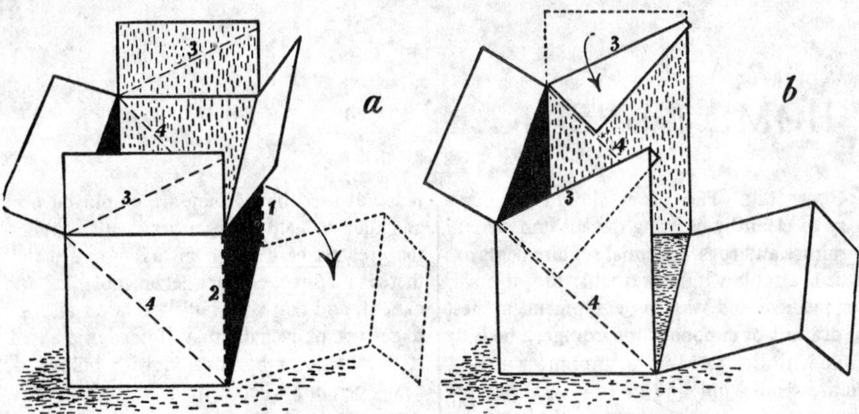

(*a*) With a sharp knife cut down one side at 1 and 2, and open out as shown by arrow points. Score deeply on outside of box at dotted lines 3 and 4.

(*b*) Fold cardboard inwards at both scored lines 3, as indicated by the arrow.

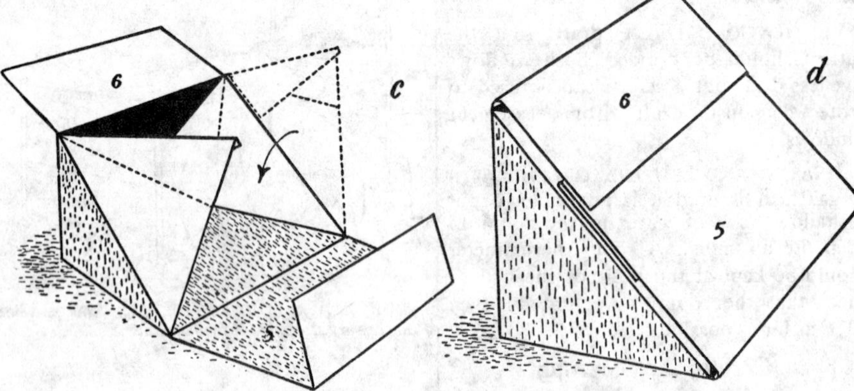

(*c*) Fold cardboard inwards at both scored lines 4, as indicated by arrow.

(*d*) Fold the bottom flap 5 upwards and the short flap 6 over it. The back rest is now ready for a pillow.

Fig. 3.

Bedtable. This can be improvised with a board resting on two chairs (Fig. 4), or by a long wooden box with the two long sides taken out, or by a board rested on two piles of books on each side of the patient. Bed-trays and tables should be high enough not to touch the patient's legs but not so high that he has to reach up to them.

Bedcradles. These are frames over which the bedclothes are placed to keep any weight off an injured or painful part of the body, usually the legs or feet. Bedcradles can be improvised by sawing a hoop in half, crossing the two halves and securing in the center (Fig. 5). Another method is to cut an arch out of a strong cardboard box (Fig. 6).

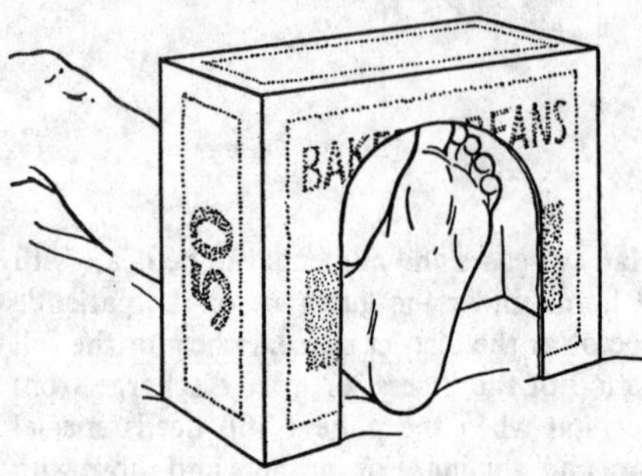

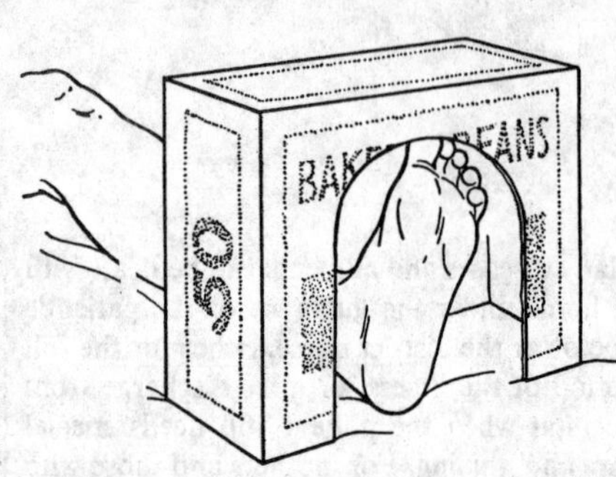

Fig. 6. *FOOTCRADLE. Made from cardboard box*

GENERAL NURSING

Changing Sheets on an Occupied Bed. For making a bed from which the patient cannot be moved, the following routine should be followed.

1. Close the window.
2. Put the clean sheets near the bed.
3. Untuck the bedding all round the mattress.
4. Take off all the blankets except the bottom one (that is just above the patient).
5. Slip the top sheet off from under the bottom blanket which should be tucked round the patient to keep him warm.
6. Remove all pillows except one.
7. Roll the patient to one side of the bed.
8. Fold the used draw-sheet up to and slightly under the patient.
9. Fold back the rubber sheet over the patient's body.
10. Fold back the bottom sheet up to and slightly under the patient.
11. Prepare the clean sheet by folding it down the middle lengthwise and lay the fold along the length of and close to the patient's body. Roll up the top half to the patient's back. Tuck in the bottom half of the sheet.
12. Replace and wipe rubber sheet.
13. The used top sheet can be utilized as a draw-sheet by folding crosswise then lengthwise. Place the second fold close to the patient's body and roll the top half up to the patient. Tuck in bottom half.
14. Roll the patient to the clean half of the bed.
15. Remove soiled draw-sheet and bottom sheet from the other side of the bed.
16. Pull the rolled half of the clean draw-sheet under the patient and fold it back over his body.
17. Pull rubber sheet smooth, wipe it and fold it back over the patient's body.
18. Pull clean bottom sheet under the patient and tuck it in.
19. Put down and tuck in rubber sheet and draw-sheet.
20. Roll patient on his back.
21. Put on clean top sheet, remove the covering blanket and make up the rest of the bedding.

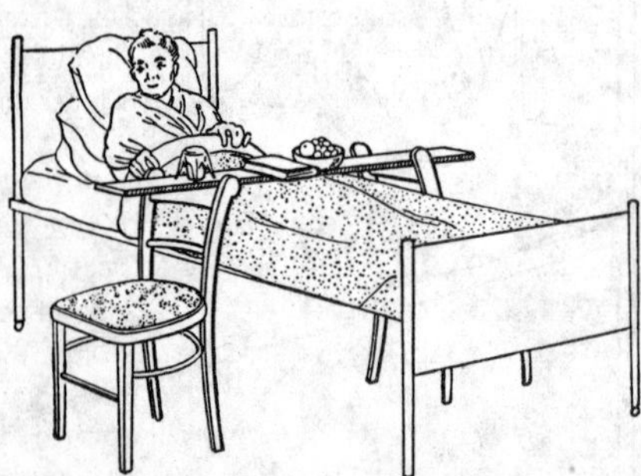

Fig. 4. *BEDTABLE. Improvised bedtable using board with two chairs.*

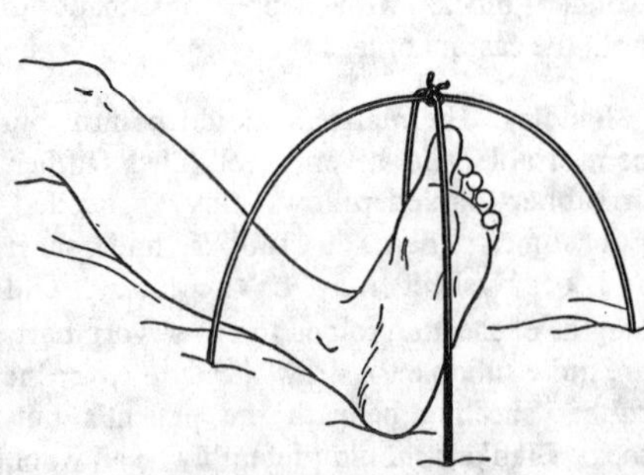

Fig. 5. *FOOTCRADLE. Made from two halves of a hoop.*

Blanket Bath. Close the window and collect all the articles needed for the blanket bath. These will include:

1. Bowl of warm water and jug of hot water to reheat the water if it cools.
2. Soap and two washcloths.
3. Two old blankets.
4. Hot-water bottle if necessary.
5. Talcum powder, surgical or methylated alchohol if necessary.
6. Two towels.
7. Clean pajamas or nightdress.

Untuck the top bedding, take off the top blankets, slip out the top sheet leaving the bottom blanket to keep the patient warm. Cover the patient with an old blanket and remove bottom blanket. Roll the second old blanket under the patient who should then be lying on one blanket and covered by the other. Remove the nightwear. Starting with the face, for which one washcloth should be kept exclusively, wash, dry and, where necessary, powder the patient in front, taking care to expose only a small portion of the body at a time.

Roll the patient first on one side then on the other to wash his back. Make sure the patient is thoroughly dry. Rub pressure areas with skin lotions if necessary and put on clean nightclothes. Brush hair and teeth. Roll the bath blanket from under the patient. Replace sheet and bottom blanket. Remove second bath blanket and replace the rest of the bedding.

Bedpans. The most commonly used bedpan is the type in Fig. 7. If a special type is required the doctor will recommend a suitable one.

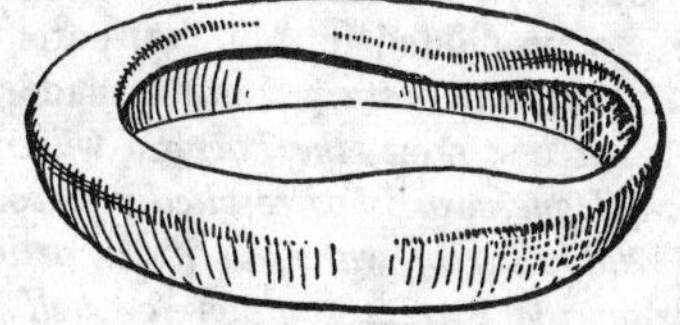

Fig. 7. *BEDPAN*

In cases where a patient is able to sit up in bed quite easily, a bed pan or a strong, fairly shallow household dish is quite satisfactory provided the dish is labelled and kept only for this purpose. A large jar makes a satisfactory urinal. They should be labelled and broken up afterwards.

When giving a bedpan to a patient, the room should be kept warm by closing the window. Warm the bedpan and cover it with a clean cloth. Help the patient on to the bedpan if necessary and leave him alone but stay within call. Remove the bedpan after use and set it on the floor, covering with the cloth, then wipe the patient and take the bedpan out of the room. Inspect the contents of the bedpan for unusual matter such as blood, pus, worms, etc. If anything unusual is present a specimen should be put aside for the doctor to examine. Empty the bedpan and flush the toilet. Clean the bedpan with a brush kept only for this purpose. Rinse under a running tap.

The bedpan should be washed in disinfectant or in a solution of soda and hot water once a day. Urinals and improvised bedpans should be dealt with in the same way. The hands should be washed immediately after cleaning the bedpan, and water should be taken to the patient to enable him to wash his hands also.

Bedsores. When a patient has been confined to bed for a long period, parts, such as the buttocks, heels, shoulder blades and elbows which are under constant pressure, easily become inflamed and tender. Even with the best care the skin on these tender spots may break and a bedsore or ulcer develop. Because of the continuing pressure, such bedsores are often slow to heal so prevention is all-important.

PREVENTION

1. Change the patient's position often.
2. Keep the bed free from wrinkles and crumbs.
3. Put inflated rubber rings, or ring pads under the heels and buttocks; use bedcradles (see Figs. 5 and 6, p. 46) if necessary to carry the weight of bedclothes from sore spots.
4. Always keep the patient clean and dry.
5. Wash the pressure points morning and evening with warm soapy water, drying carefully, and rubbing firmly but gently with topical antibiotic powders.

Some skins respond better to a silicone barrier cream, which is thinly smeared on the pressure areas twice a day for about a week and then once daily. When using a silicone cream only wash the pressure points with warm water about twice a week unless they have become soiled.

6. Ascorbic acid taken in the form of lemon or orange juice every day, or as 50-milligram tablets three times daily will help to keep the skin in good condition. condition.

TREATMENT

If the skin has broken, the following emollient is both healing and soothing:

Castor oil	2 parts
Peru balsam	1 part

Such astringents as burnt alum are sometimes used but for this and other medicaments for chronic bedsores it is best to consult the doctor.

Taking Medicines. Although it seems a simple matter to give a tablet or spoonful of mixture to a sick person, greater benefit is often obtained by strictly following instructions on the label, such as 'Give with plenty of water,' 'Take after a meal,' or 'Rub well in.' The instructions are not mere 'fussiness:' the advised method of using the drug is often as necessary to treatment as the drug itself. Details of why this is so will be found in the Pharmacy section.

Serving Meals. A sick person tends to lose his appetite and it is part of the nurse's job to see that the meals are served as attractively as possible. Only small amounts should be offered at a time and the nurse should coax a reluctant patient without making him feel the food is being forced on him. The tray should be prepared outside of the sickroom. A doubtful appetite can often be cheered by a few small flowers from the garden brought in on the tray. Before serving a meal the patient should be made comfortable and a bedjacket or shawl put round his shoulders. Since sick people tend to become more easily irritated than they would normally, meals should be served as punctually as possible and care should be taken to keep hot meals hot and cold food cold. See also Invalid Cookery, p. 60.

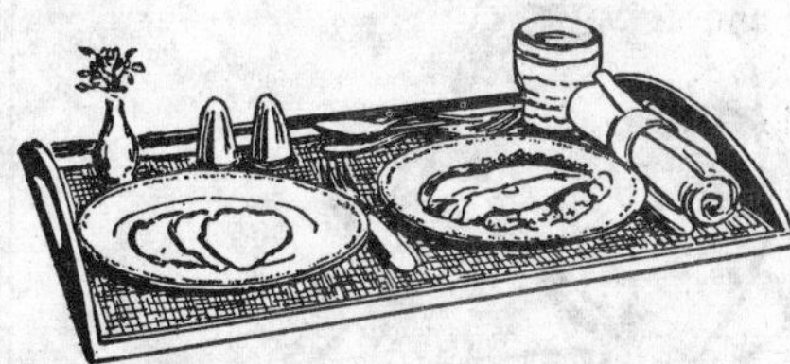

Fig. 8. *MEAL TRAY. Food served attractively can help a doubtful appetite.*

Information for the Doctor

When a patient is cared for at home the mother or nurse is able to observe him constantly. It is therefore often helpful if the nurse can keep some record—temperature, pulse, sleep—of the patient's condition if the doctor wishes her to do so.

Temperature Taking. Temperature charts for daily recording can be bought at the druggists. A note of where the temperature is taken (mouth, armpit, rectum, or groin) should be made as it can vary a little according to the part of the body in which the thermometer is placed.

It is generally the temperature of the mouth which is recorded but the mouth should not be used directly after the patient has taken a hot or cold drink, or after smoking. It should not be used for infants, nor for people whose breathing is difficult, nor for delirious, unconscious or irresponsible patients. The thermometer should not be placed in the groin or armpit if the patient is very thin or has had a hot bath or if a hot-water bottle has been in contact with the area. The temperature of infants, and of adults for whom the usual places are unsuitable, should be taken in the rectum with a round-bulb thermometer.

The thermometer should be shaken down to below 37° C (98° F). This is done by holding the thermometer firmly between the thumb and first two fingers and flicking the wrist sharply several times. Place the bulb of the thermometer under the patient's tongue, or in the groin or armpit. Close the mouth or arm or leg. Leave for not less than three, minutes. Take out the thermometer and write down what the mercury registers. Shake down the mercury, rinse the thermometer under a cold tap, dip in mild disinfectant, rinse again and put it back in the case. When taking the temperature in the rectum, grease the thermometer with vaseline and gently insert the bulb end 1 or 1½ inches into the rectum. Then proceed as before.

BODY HEAT	
Subnormal temperature	95–97° F
Normal temperature	97–99° F
High temperature	100° F upwards

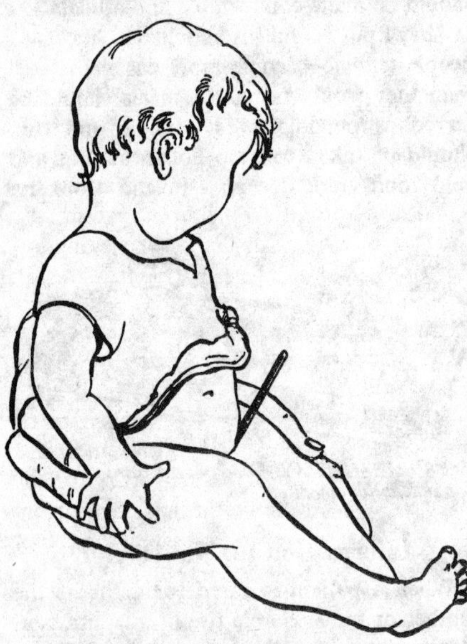

Fig. 9. *TEMPERATURE TAKING. The groin is a suitable place for small children.*

To Take the Pulse. Rest the patient's arm in a relaxed position. Place the tips of two fingers on the patient's wrist at the base of the thumb and count the number of beats in one minute, checking with the second-hand of a watch. Make a note of the result at once.

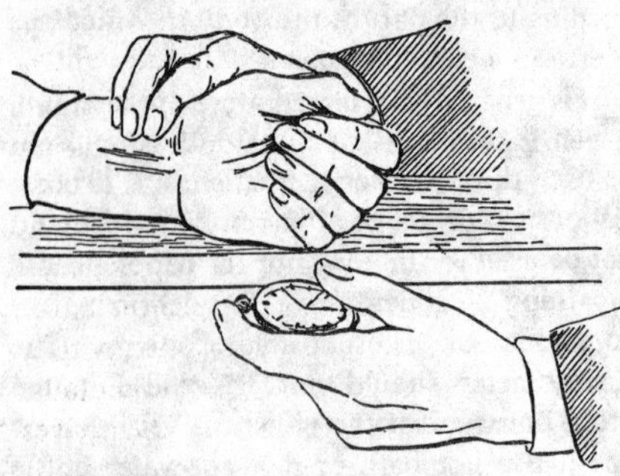

Fig. 10. *TAKING THE PULSE*

The pulse rate becomes slower as a person gets older, except in certain diseases.

PULSE RATES	
Infants	100–140 per minute
Children	90–100 „ „
Adults	60– 90 „ „

General Reports for the Doctor. It is advisable to make a note of the patient's symptoms for each day in order to avoid mistakes. The report, which will vary according to the type of illness, should include such things as:

1. Amount of sleep, food, and liquid taken by the patient.
2. Condition and color of skin, i.e. whether hot or cold, rough or discolored, etc.
3. Observation of urine and stools. (If these do not seem normal a specimen should be kept for the doctor to inspect.)
4. Nausea and vomiting.
5. Coughing, whether dry, spasmodic or with expectoration.
6. Breathing, whether deep, shallow, rapid, noisy, by mouth, etc.
7. Position of the patient's body and his facial expression.
8. Swellings.
9. Pain: if the patient is in pain the location and type of pain, i.e. sharp, spasmodic, mild, etc., should be noted together with the duration of the pain.
10. Dizziness, faintness and chilliness.

NURSING INFECTIOUS DISEASES AT HOME

If a patient with an infectious disease is nursed at home, only the nurse should have direct contact with the patient while he is liable to infect others. The nurse can avoid spreading the disease by taking a number of precautions. Cleanliness is the best protection against the spread of any infection and all the members of the family, especially the mother or home nurse, should be more than usually particular to wash their hands before handling food and after using the toilet. Food should be covered and bins used for soiled dressings or linen should have tightly fitting lids.

Direct sunlight is a good disinfectant so the sickroom should have as much air and sunlight as possible. (In the case of measles, however, the room may be darkened as the eyes become over-sensitive.) Everything possible in the room should be easy to wash. All the dishes, medical equipment, children's toys, and books should be kept apart from those used by the family. Articles which cannot be thoroughly disinfected after the patient recovers may have to be burnt so remember to use only those things which will not be required afterwards. Linen used by an infectious patient should be put in a covered receptacle and disinfected with a suitable disinfectant such as lysol or a carbolic fluid. Instructions on the bottle should be followed implicitly. Rinse the disinfectant out after the stated time, then wash the linen. If it is sent out of the home, the laundry should be informed that it comes from an infectious patient and that it must be disinfected first.

A coverall should be kept on the inside of the sickroom door; it should be put on as the nurse enters and taken off before leaving, and the hands must be washed immediately after attending the patient.

The toilet and bedpan should be disinfected immediately each time the bedpan is emptied. Other waste material from the sickroom, i.e. floor sweepings and tissues should be burnt, or disinfected before discarding.

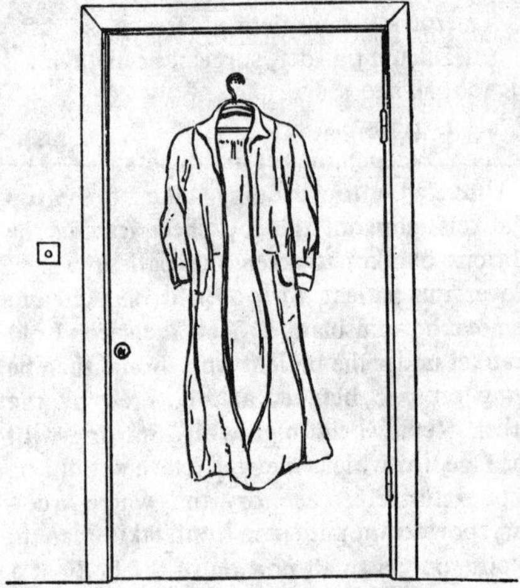

Fig. 11. *SICKROOM COVERALL. Should be kept handy behind the sickroom door.*

Disinfection and Fumigation

The most common methods of disinfection are by heat sterilization and by chemicals. The latter are usually employed in the form of solutions, gases or aerosols (finely divided air spray solutions) and sometimes in powders. Since many of these concentrated chemicals are dangerous, it is most important that the directions given on the labels are strictly followed. Not only is it a question of danger but, if a concentrated substance is required to be diluted in, say, 100 parts of water and the article steeped in the made-up solution for one hour, *the bacteria will not be killed if guesswork has resulted in a solution of 200 parts of water, or if the article remains in the correct solution for half an hour only.*

Fumigation is disinfection by means of fumes or gases.

Disinfection of Skin. Simple washing with soap and water will destroy and remove most contaminating bacteria. If food has to be prepared soon after the nurse has had to handle bedpans, an extra precaution should be taken. The hands should be washed in a medicated soap, preferably one containing hexachlorophane. Hands should not be dried on a towel exposed to the germs of the sickroom; allow the hands to dry in the air, or use paper towels kept in the kitchen or bathroom.

Disinfection of Hair. Ordinary washing with soap or with a medicated shampoo will usually be adequate.

Disinfection of the Mouth and Teeth. For regular use, non-prescription mouth washes are commonly employed for gargling and mouth rinsing.

Disinfection of Nurse's Clothing. During the domestic nursing of infectious diseases, the protective coverings worn in the sickroom require disinfecting and washing apart from the family laundry. Cotton is best soaked overnight in lysol 1 part to 80 parts of water; it is then well rinsed and washed in the usual manner. Woolen material tends to retain this kind of disinfectant even after thorough washing. Prolonged boiling of cotton or linen sheets and towels, and drying in bright sunlight is still an excellent method of disinfection.

Disinfection of Eating Utensils. All china, glassware, and cutlery should be rinsed under a running tap to loosen food particles and then immersed for 10 minutes in a phenolic disinfectant solution such as lysol 1 part in 80 parts of warm water. Each item should be thoroughly rinsed with clear warm water and left to drain; do not wipe with dishtowels which may not be so germ-free as they may appear. Alternatively, after the food particles have been rinsed off, the cups, plates, spoons and other utensils can be boiled (at the boil) for 5 minutes.

Disinfecting Bedpans, etc. Bedpans and urine bottles should always be well rinsed with water before disinfection. Lysol is suitable for disinfecting these articles. Sputum cups (with lids) used in tuberculosis or poliomyelitis need particular care. Alternatively, waxed cartons can be burnt after use as sputum containers.

Disinfection of Bedding. BLANKETS from the beds of persons with an infectious disease are adequately disinfected by immersing overnight in a warm solution (about 105° F) of 160 parts of water to one part of lysol. This long soaking may cause a little matting with some wools.

Infected BED-LINEN and curtains, during the illness, should be put into a covered bucket or tub containing a disinfecting solution and left in it for the recommended time. Rinse out the disinfectant well with plain water before wringing, as many disinfectants are irritating to the skin and are not compatible with the soaps or detergents used in the laundering. A disinfectant solution suitable for linen (cotton, too) is: lysol 8 tablespoonsful to 1 gallon of water (soak for one hour). If lengthy soaking is not desired, the linen can be disinfected by boiling for 5 to 10 minutes in a covered laundry bowl or bucket.

Nursing Sick Children

In general a sick child is cared for in much the same way as an adult but there are certain points of difference. The mother is much the best person a child can have for his home nurse and it is very important in the case of small children.

Particular care should be taken to guard fires and to keep medicines and breakable articles out of the child's reach if these articles have to be kept in the sickroom. If all persuasion fails when trying to give a sick child medicine, a large towel can be wrapped around both arms before giving him a dose by mouth.

Children with chickenpox or other mild illnesses, and convalescents, need plenty to occupy their hands. Toys, books, and so on should be given a few at a time to save exhausting the child and also running out of occupations for him.

Children with whooping-cough need extra comfort and reassurance during severe coughing bouts as they can be very frightening to them.

Children recovering from mild infectious diseases can often be allowed to play outside in the garden (the doctor should first be consulted) before the end of the quarantine provided that they are not allowed contact with other people.

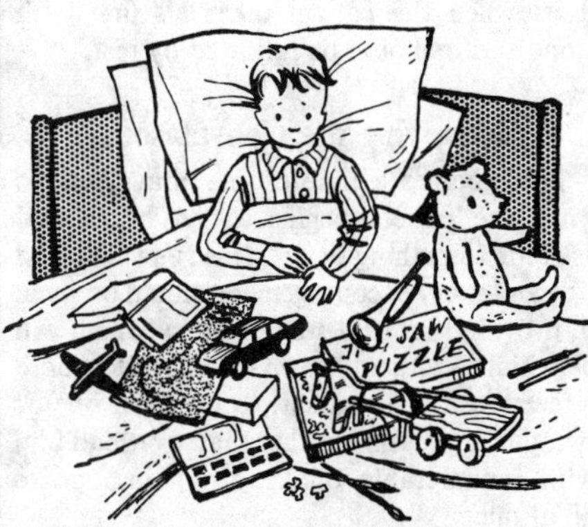

Fig. 12. *TOO MANY TOYS. The convalescent child can only cope with one or two interests at a time.*

CHRONIC SICK AND OLD AGE PATIENTS

Although there are long-term patients among younger people the majority are elderly and in many instances care of the chronic sick and of the aged can be considered together. The attitude of the home nurse towards these people should be particularly sympathetic as many of them are without hope of real recovery. They easily feel neglected and unwanted and a good nurse should, with tact and understanding, try to counteract these feelings by helping to make the most of what they are able to do.

Old people and the chronic sick often have a great desire for independence and this should be encouraged as they can easily fall back into apathy. Handrails, clothes which are easy to get on and off, exercises for the joints, and allowing them to feed themselves (even when this means some mess) will all help old people to do as much as possible for themselves and to retain their interest in life. Some of the best occupations for old people who can get about the house are those which make them feel wanted and of use, e.g. cleaning silver, tidying drawers and boxes, preparing vegetables and arranging flowers. For the chronic sick, activities which have an end-product, e.g. knitting, rug-making, small-loom weaving, play an important part in keeping the patient interested.

Pleasant surroundings are of great importance to persons confined month after month at home. Gay curtains, a pleasant room with a good view from the window, kept fresh and tidy, and with their own personal possessions about will do much to keep up interest and hope. The nurse should also encourage them to take a pride in their personal appearance.

Visitors play a very important part in keeping chronically sick and old people interested in the outside world. Visits should be frequent, regular to avoid disappointment, and of short duration to prevent overtiring. When possible, occasional outside visiting by car should be arranged after consultation with the doctor.

Nursing Relief

Where the burden of long-term home nursing falls on one person it is most important that she should have rest days or a vacation to maintain health, fitness and outside interest. Home helps can be provided from the local authority through the doctor or local visiting nurses' association, while the housewife or nurse is on vacation. In certain cases the doctor may consider it possible to arrange for the patient to go to a convalescent home for a short time.

Old Age Patients

As well as being cheerful, the room for an elderly person should be kept warm and free from drafts at a temperature of 70° F. Small rugs should be removed to avoid possible accidents. A bell should be within easy reach for calling attention.

Beds for old people should be low to allow them to get in and out easily. Care should be taken not to tuck in the bedding too tightly, and plenty of pillows should be provided for sitting up in bed. A firm pillow should be used to support the feet and, if necessary, a bed-cradle used to keep any weight off the feet.

Baths. Old people should bathe regularly. They should be encouraged to use the bathroom, and the bath should be fitted with a rubber slip mat and handrails to prevent falls. It is better to let old people dry themselves and a covered chair should be provided for them to sit on while doing so. Leave the door unlocked and put a bell nearby in case they need to ring for assistance. Drying must be very thorough and powder can also be used.

Hair. Should be washed every two or three weeks and in winter less frequently, as old people chill easily.

A hairdresser should visit the patient every so often to give a trim, and the hair should be brushed daily. A chiropodist should also visit regularly to keep the feet in good condition.

Eyes can be bathed in warm water if they become sore or discharge, and the mouth should be kept clean.

Bladder Control. Old people often lose partial control of the bladder as the muscles become weaker. They must be given every facility to empty the bladder as soon as they feel the need. At night a commode should be within easy reach or they should be offered a bedpan at a regular time every night. Getting up for a short time each day and avoiding liquids at night should help to control this difficulty.

Old people must be carefully watched to see if there is any change in their color, pulse rate, or respiration. Such changes should be reported to the doctor as old folk are liable to chest ailments and the onset of illness in old age is often insidious.

Chronic Sick

The room for a person with a long-term illness must be warmer than usual and draft-proof. The patient will need extra warmth as the circulation becomes sluggish and a bed-jacket and light blanket next to the patient should be provided. Bedsores are most likely in chronic patients so every precaution must be taken (see Bedsores, p. 47). It may be necessary to have special equipment for lifting heavy patients and supporting others who may be disabled. Consult your doctor on the matter. Patients who are bedridden need a constant change of position. Most chronically sick patients are nursed sitting up, whenever possible, to prevent the development of pneumonia. Plenty of supporting pillows will be needed whatever position is used.

Paralyzed limbs need extra support and the doctor may apply light splints. Paralyzed legs should be supported at the feet with sandbags to prevent footdrop. Paralyzed arms should be placed on a pillow and a soft pad placed in the hands to prevent deformity.

Chronic patients who cannot get out of bed will have to use a bedpan, but in less difficult cases a commode or a sanitary chair which can be wheeled to the bathroom and fitted over the toilet should be used. If possible these patients should be bathed in the bathroom once or twice a week. The patient's hair, teeth, and nails should also be kept clean and attended to regularly.

There are a number of aids which can be used for chronic patients who cannot sit up or hold a book, e.g. a frame with mirrors to bring the page into the patient's sight, a projector to reflect the page on the ceiling or a screen, prismatic glasses and automatic page turners. The provision of such aids should be discussed with the doctor. A good handyman may be able to make part of the equipment.

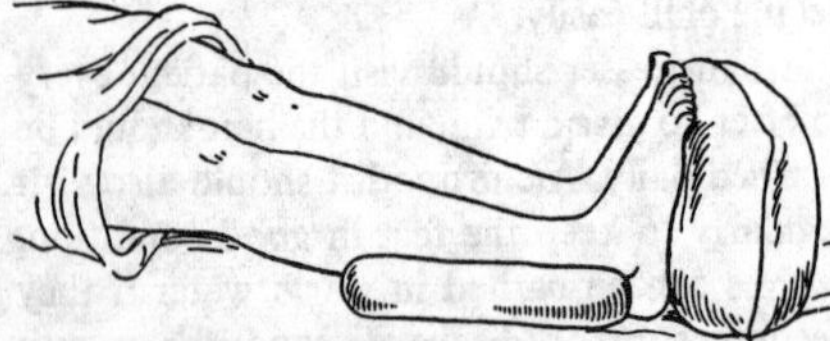

Fig. 13. *SANDBAG SUPPORT. Paralyzed legs should be supported at the feet with sandbags to prevent footdrop.*

CONVALESCENCE

When the worst of an illness is over it is the nurse's job to encourage the patient in every way to become independent and as self-supporting as possible. Praise should be given for every real effort the patient makes.

A convalescent needs just the same careful nursing as the very sick patient and he should not be allowed to exhaust himself by trying to do too much too soon. The nurse should encourage him to exercise his joints and feet as it will be of great help when he begins to get about again. The first time the convalescent is allowed out of bed by the doctor he should be wrapped up warmly and helped to a comfortable chair. The amount of time spent in the chair can be increased daily if the patient does not show over-tiredness. By about the third day he should be able to walk around the room with the help of the nurse and then alone. The amount of time the patient spends out of bed is then increased daily until he is completely recovered. The nurse should be near at hand and ready to assist when the patient takes his first bath alone and it should be followed by rest.

Occupying the Convalescent

There comes a time during convalescence when the patient begins to get bored and asks for something to do. This is a very good sign and every encouragement should be given to provide him with some activity which will help him to forget his own troubles. It is more interesting to the patient to be given one or two things at a time rather than overload him with innumerable books, toys, and games all at once.

The busy housewife or mother is often limited in the time she can spare with the invalid and in the money which she can afford to lay out on extras. Although the radio and television will help to pass some hours, more active pastimes should be included for variety and also for the sense of achievement they can provide. While it is important for the home nurse to encourage the patient to occupy himself and become self-reliant, care must be taken to see that the invalid does not overstrain himself in any way. Whatever activities are decided upon, always talk it over with the family doctor when he calls and get him to state the length of time any activity may be continued, when it may be changed, or when the time may be increased.

Very young children quickly tire of doing one thing and it is necessary for them to have various changes. On the whole, familiar cuddly toys prove the greatest consolation. A few empty cotton spools on a string and tied across the crib so the spools may be pushed backwards and forwards, or a few stones or buttons sealed in a tin which may be rattled will please a very small child.

The under-tens will play happily with educational toys such as building bricks and blocks, various types of peg boards, beads on pegs, giant poppet beads, or plastic screws and nuts. Coloring books and colored pencils or wax crayons give endless pleasure. Bead threading, button sorting, sewing cards, picture lotto, or simple jig-saw puzzles made of cardboard are some of the many possibilities for occupying a child still in bed.

Beads, pegs, etc., for the smaller children must be large.

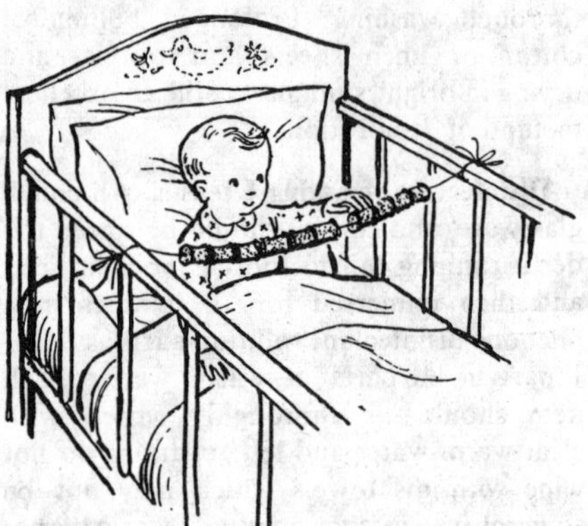

Fig. 14. *THE CONVALESCENT BABY*

Older children, confined to bed or the house for a long time, need not be limited to amusing themselves only. There is no reason why some school lessons cannot be set with the help of the class teacher and with the doctor's permission. Letters to pen-pals, especially if attempted in a foreign language will prove a good exercise.

Learning to use reed pipes or mouth organs will interest many children. Painting and drawing and modeling in clay are good stand-bys and not costly. At Christmas-time cards and calendars could be painted and decorations made for the Christmas tree, and then scrapbooks made with the used Christmas cards later on.

Other suggestions are dish-gardening, paper cut-outs, paper modeling, and weaving, or games such as dominoes, cards, marbles, and solitaire, all of which can be played alone.

Occupation for Adults. The choice is endless. In the early stages of convalescence when quiet pastimes are needed, the radio, television, reading, letter writing, crossword and jig-saw puzzles will generally satisfy. Later, when more activities are undertaken, hobbies are ideal to take up and they may remain as permanent interests. Stamp collecting is one of the most popular hobbies, but match-box collecting, used railway tickets, sea-shells, coins or button collecting may prove equally as absorbing. The family and friends can all help to collect for the patient.

The garden enthusiast may send for gardening catalogues to study or draw plans of his ideal garden. It may be possible to pursue window-box gardening or have a bedside 'cactus garden.'

PAINTING, sketching, drawing, design, draftsmanship or stenciling are well within the scope of bed patients. Light musical instruments such as the flute, harmonica, guitar, or banjo may all be practiced in bed.

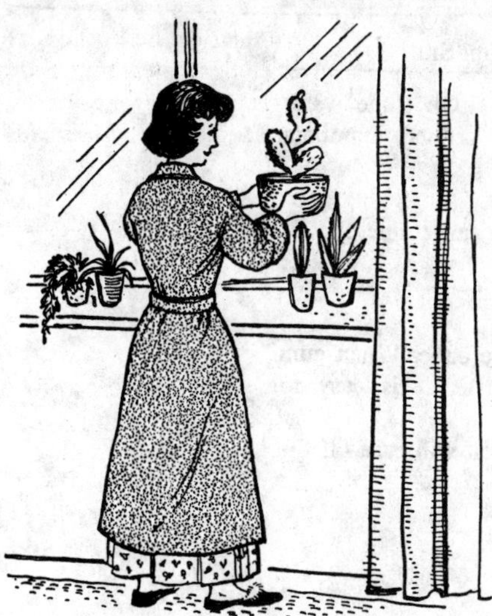

Fig. 15. *THE SICKROOM GARDEN*

MODELING with some of the newer modeling substances need not be a messy job as they self-set to a stone-like hardness and may then be painted.

BOOKS. For those confined to bed but mentally active, this can be a splendid opportunity to study a subject for which there never has been time in the business of general living. A study of a foreign language may later double the enjoyment of a vacation abroad or add to one's qualifications for a new job.

HANDICRAFTS are of special help to those needing some physical activity. Weaving a scarf or table-mats on a small loom is both useful and satisfying. The handyman who is out of bed but about the house could even make his own simple box loom. A simpler type is the card loom—the warp is made by a length of string being threaded up and down through holes in a piece of cardboard or threaded around the serrated ends of the card. The woof is woven in and out across the string and may be of wool, silk, cotton, or even rag.

The housewife sitting up in bed may prefer knitting, crochet, needlework, embroidery or soft toy-making. At such a time she may for once have the leisure to study various cook books or do some of the jobs which invariably seem to get left, such as pasting snapshots in the family album.

Men. Handicrafts which appeal to men are rug-making, basketry, chip carving, puppetry, model-making, leatherwork, or lampshade-making.

Once the convalescent is up and about the family doctor will advise on the possible increase of activities. Some light household chores or various jobs in the garden may be permitted. Using a typewriter or sewing machine, or some carpentry jobs may well be attempted at this stage and the man with a mechanical bent may keep himself busy repairing a radio or clock, or tinkering with the engine of a car or motorcycle.

Older Patients. In the case of the elderly, allow them to do familiar things and at their own pace. Any small job which gives them the idea that they are helping the family gives them a feeling of accomplishment and of being wanted.

When convalescence at home is lengthy, it is often more tedious for the patient than convalescence in hospital or a Home. In the larger establishment there is always something going on—visits from the doctor, routine attentions from the nurses, personal visitors, hot drinks at regular times and so on. At home the patient is left more on his own. To the naturally retiring or bookish types of persons this may be enjoyable but, in general, once the pleasure of being at home has worn off, the convalescent finds that the family has not as much time to spend at the bedside and he is likely to get not only bored but easily irritated.

The various suggestions put forward here for occupying the convalescent can lead to a happier return to health and one less taxing to the patience of the busy housewife or mother who has to care for the invalid.

STAINS AND STICKY SUBSTANCES: HOW TO REMOVE

Bed-linen often becomes stained by the accidental spilling of medicines, cups of tea, or ointments, and a fidgety child or a restless adult convalescing from an illness is very prone to stain and mark his clothes with other substances used for his relaxation and entertainment.

When removing such stains or gummy substances, note the following general points.

Old stains are more difficult to remove than new ones.

Cotton, linen and nylon will safely respond to bleaches or alkaline substances such as ammonia or washing soda, *but* both skin and the cloth must be thoroughly washed with water immediately afterwards.

Wool, silk and rayon, or fabrics partly made of these, will be harmed by alkali and most bleaches.

A useful slow-acting bleach (2 to about 6 hours according to size of stains, cloth, and thickness) is made by putting 1 cupful of hydrogen peroxide solution (20 volumes) into 5 cupfuls of cold water and adding 4 to 6 drops of ammonia solution. Rinse garment well in several waters as soon as the stains are gone.

STAIN	How to Remove from CLOTH	from SKIN
Acriflavine	Treat stain with dilute hydrochloric acid, then wash material in the usual way.	Wash promptly with detergent and hot water. For old stains, soak skin in hot water and rub with lemon juice.
Adhesive tape	Cigarette-lighter fuel will soften the plaster, but remove tape quickly so that softened mass will not spoil fabric.	Squirt lighter fuel over the tape to soften plaster.
Blood	Soak well in cold soft water for 12 hours, rinse in cold water till free of marks; wash in usual way. *or* Soak at once in cold salt water (1 teaspoonful per pint) for about 2 hours. Wash in usual way. *or* If stains are stubborn, soak in borax solution (1 tablespoonful per gallon cold water) for several hours. Wash in cool soapy or detergent water.	

Stain	How to Remove from Cloth	from Skin
Bromine	Dab with sodium hydroxide solution.	Apply Carron Oil (lime water and oil); *or* diluted ammonia solution.
Cellulose lacquer	Rub gently with acetone on cotton wool. *Note:* Acetone will destroy rayon.	Remove with turpentine oil.
Chewing gum	Cover with warm soapy water, then soften with dry-cleaning fluid (carbon tetrachloride).	Chill with ice cube. When gum becomes brittle, it is easy to remove. *or* Cooking oil will ease off the gum.
Cocoa	Sponge with warm borax solution (1 heaped tablespoonful borax per ½ pint warm water).	
Coffee	As for cocoa: repeat till clean. *or* Brush the marks with glycerin, rinse in lukewarm water, press on wrong side with a cool iron. For old stains, soak spots in glycerin, remove most of it with cotton, and apply methylated alcohol.	
Egg (white)	Cover with a solution of warm salt water (1 teaspoonful per ½ pint).	
Egg (yolk)	Wash in soapy water; if stain remains use dry-cleaning fluid.	
Friars' balsam	To remove tackiness from china or glass, wipe over with methylated alcohol.	
Fruit	Pour a stream of boiling water through the cloth, rubbing in borax. Rinse with boiling water. *or* Soak for some minutes in warm borax solution (1 tablespoonful per pint). For old stains on linen, soak the part in whisky. Rinse thoroughly.	
Gentian Violet (Crystal Violet)	Sprinkle a few detergent granules on the stain and rub over with a wet cloth.	
Glue	Use hot water.	
Grease	Silk: apply powdered magnesia on wrong side as soon as possible. Press with a hot iron, having a piece of blotting paper on each surface of grease spot. *or* Use dry-cleaning (carbon tetrachloride) fluid as recommended on label.	
Indelible pencil	Rub with a cotton pad wetted with methylated alcohol.	Easily removed with methylated alcohol.
Ink (ball-point)	Use methylated alcohol. *or* Acetone (but not for rayon). Rub in gently to thin the ink, and wash in usual way.	Remove with either methylated alcohol or acetone.

STAIN	How to Remove from CLOTH	from SKIN
Ink (writing)	Pour milk through the stain several times, then wash in warm water with soap. Bleach in the sun. *or* Wash at once in soapy water. For old or stubborn stains on white cotton or linen: wash, spread stained part over a basin, sprinkle oxalic acid (a poison) on stains, and stream through with the boiling water. Rinse thoroughly in hot water. For silk or wool, wash immediately in usual way; soak stubborn stains in a solution of hydrosulphite of soda (1 teaspoonful per pint of warm water); then wash in usual way.	
Iodine	Ammonia solution will remove iodine stains from most fabrics.	Dab with weak ammonia solution.
Lipstick	Wash in warm soapy water. If some remains, remove with dry-cleaning fluid.	
Milk	Wash in warm, soapy or detergent water. If fabric is still stiff, use dry-cleaning fluid. *or* Rinse in a dilute solution of ammonia. Wash in usual way.	
Nail polish	Amyl acetate or acetone will easily dissolve the varnish (and also rayon!).	
Ointments	As for Grease.	
Proflavine	As for Acriflavine.	
Tea	Immediately cover the stain with salt and leave for a while. Wash in usual way. *or* Soak in boiling water before tea is dry. If stain persists, soak cloth in a hot solution of borax (2 tablespoonsful per gallon) until cool. Colored materials should be well rinsed through the borax solution but not left for a long soaking.	
Tobacco		A mild bleaching solution will remove brown stains. Rinse off well.
Urine	For fresh stains: steep the part in a dilute solution of ammonia for 10 minutes or so, then wash. For old stains: after dampening the stain with dilute hydrochloric acid, repeatedly dab with methylated alcohol. Rinse thoroughly.	
Wine	Make a paste of common salt and water, spread paste over the stain, let it stand for a while, and wash cloth in hot water. Claret stains should have milk poured through them till the color has gone. Wash in usual way. *or* Rinse several times through a hot borax solution (1 tablespoonful borax per pint of water).	

HOME MEDICINE CABINET

FIRST AID BOX

Every home should be equipped with a first aid box containing at least the bare essentials for simple first aid treatment and, as they are used, the supplies should be replaced regularly. Only first aid items should be kept in the box, and they should be clearly labelled, clean, and in neat order so that they are immediately available in an emergency. The box should be kept on a shelf, out of the reach of small children. It should have a well-fitting lid to keep out dust and germs but it should be easy to open, and not locked so that no time is wasted in reaching the contents. Instructions saying what each item is used for should also be kept in the box. A small first aid box, in a dustproof cover, should also be kept in your car.

The following items are suggested for inclusion in a first aid box:

Bandages 1″, 2″, and 3″ gauze
Small package of raw cotton
Sterile gauze squares, separately wrapped
Tin of assorted adhesive dressings
Roll of adhesive tape ½″ or 1″ wide
Several sterile finger dressings
Antiseptic ointment
Box of sodium bicarbonate
Small bottle of calamine lotion
Toothache tincture, or oil of cloves
Small bottle of smelling salts
Boric acid crystals
Nurses' scissors
Clinical thermometer
Tweezers
Eye-bath and sponge
Camel-hair brush in clean container
Package of needles
Box of safety matches
Measuring spoon
Package of safety-pins
Chamois finger sheath

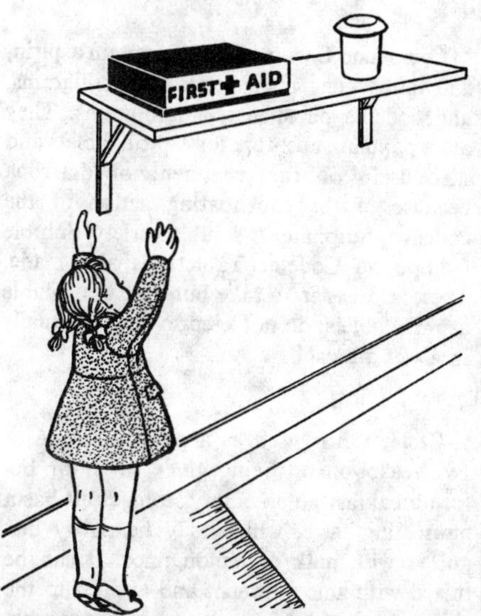

Fig. 1. *FIRST AID BOX. Keep your first aid box on a high shelf out of reach of small children.*

Other items which may usefully be included if space permits but which are not so essential are:

A triangular bandage
Flashlight
Crêpe bandages
Oiled rayon or silk
Table salt
Small tin of mustard

Uses of First Aid Items

Bandages. One-inch bandages are useful for fingers; one-and-a-half and two-inch sizes for hands, wrists and necks; two-and-a-half and three-inch sizes for arms, legs, and ankles, etc. Wider ones are required for body and head bandages. Crêpe bandages are suitable for body bandages and for legs, especially knees and ankles. Adhesive dressing strips are useful for small cuts and abrasions. Adhesive tape may be applied over larger antiseptic dressings to hold them in place. Triangular bandages may prove useful as slings for arm injuries (see also First Aid, pp. 26–30).

Raw Cotton. This is useful for bathing wounds, for hot wet soaks, bathing eyes, in dressings and for retaining heat over plaster dressings and poultices. It is used for applying ointments, liniments, lotions, etc.

Oiled silk or rayon placed over a dressing keeps it moist, or keeps wet soaks hot and moist.

Antiseptic solution is of value for adding to warm water to bathe dirty cuts and abrasions. Antiseptic ointment may then be applied on a dressing to prevent infection in wounds.

Sodium bicarbonate made into a paste with a little water can be applied to insect bites to relieve irritation.

Calamine lotion is a useful cooling lotion for application to bites, rashes, sunburn, etc.

Boric Acid. A solution of the crystals in boiled water (two level teaspoonsful in one pint of water), when cooled to body temperature, makes a soothing lotion to bathe the eyes after removal of foreign particles.

Mustard powder is used as an emetic in cases of poisoning by tablets, poisonous solutions, berries, etc. A tablespoonful is mixed with half a pint of warm water and given to the patient to drink as soon as possible after the poison has been taken.

Common salt in strong solution is also useful as an emergency emetic to make the patient vomit the swallowed poison.

Toothache Tincture, or **oil of cloves,** will relieve the pain of toothache if the gum around the aching tooth is rubbed with a piece of cotton moistened with a few drops of tincture or oil. If there is a cavity in the tooth this should be dried out with cotton and a small plug of cotton soaked in the tincture or oil may be used to fill it.

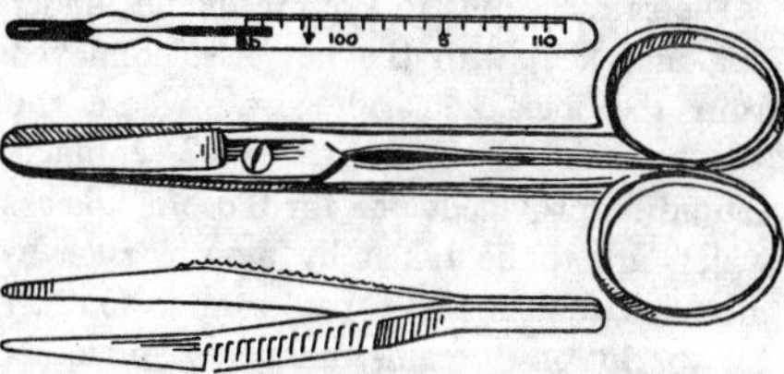

Fig. 2. *FOR THE FIRST AID BOX. Clinical thermometer; nurses' scissors; and tweezers.*

Smelling Salts may be administered in cases of fainting. About twenty drops are given in a wineglassful of water. It should not be given in cases of hemorrhage.

Tweezers with pointed ends are useful for removing splinters, etc. and those with blunt ends for holding swabs to wash wounds. They may be sterilized by being passed through a flame or by boiling for 10 minutes in water.

Needles are useful for removing splinters or grit from wounds. They should be sterilized in the same way as tweezers. If the eye end of the needle is pushed into a cork, the cork may be held in the hand while the needle is passed through a flame. A box of safety **matches** in the first aid box will always provide the means for sterilizing a needle, tweezers, or scissors.

Clinical Thermometer. For mode of usage see Home Nursing, p. 47.

Camel-hair Brush. A small camel-hair brush (kept in a clean container) is useful for removing specks of dirt or insects from the eye.

MEDICINE CABINET

In addition to the first aid items mentioned above, a stock of medicines to cope with minor ailments is an asset in the home. These should be kept in suitable containers in a special cabinet which can be locked.

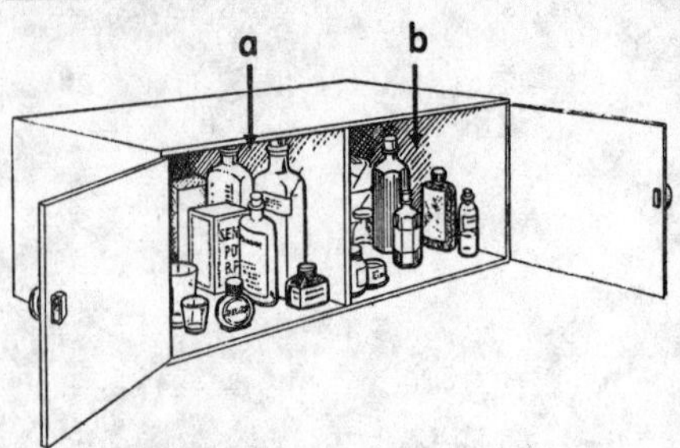

Fig. 3. *MEDICINE CABINET. One section (a) for medicines used internally; and the other (b) for medicines used externally.*

Keeping Medicines Safely

It cannot be too strongly emphasized that all MEDICINES MUST BE KEPT IN A SAFE PLACE. When there are children in the house it becomes doubly important to ensure that nothing is left lying about, no matter how harmless it may seem to be. It is not always realized that many medicinal substances which are quite safe for adults in normal doses can be fatal for children.

The safest way is to keep medicines under lock and key, with the key itself removed from the lock and put away where the children cannot get at it. Two cabinets should be provided: one for those medicines which are to be taken by mouth, such as mixtures, tablets, and capsules, and the other for the lotions, creams, liniments and other preparations which are not for internal use. Having two cabinets will reduce the chance of picking up the wrong bottle. It will also prevent some of the very strong smelling liniments from tainting tablets and capsules. If it is not possible to have two cabinets, then the next best thing is to have one cabinet divided into two sections, one being reserved for the internally used medicines and the other for those used externally.

Some thought should be given to the places where the cabinets are fixed. First, they should be high enough to be out of reach of children. Secondly, they should be in a cool dry room because medicines keep better under these conditions. This is not so important with liniments, lotions, and creams, so that if two separate cabinets are being used, the one holding the external preparations may conveniently be fixed in the bathroom or the kitchen.

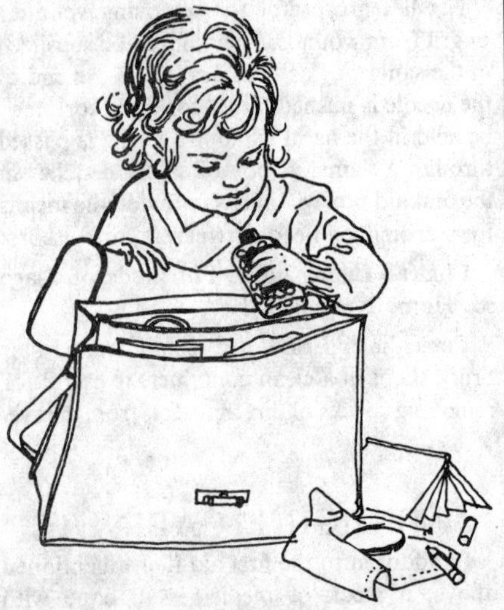

Fig. 4. *MOTHER'S TABLETS. To leave tablets in a handbag easily accessible to small children is careless and dangerous.*

Special precautions should be taken with tablets, capsules, pills, and granules, since some of them closely resemble certain sweets and can be very attractive to children. Besides keeping medicines under lock and key in the cabinet, it is also possible to obtain special tamper-proof containers which are deliberately made difficult for children to open. These containers are also useful if it is the practice to carry a few tablets or capsules in one's pocket or handbag for use in an emergency.

If it is necessary to keep a medicine, for example a cough mixture, beside the bed during the night, be careful to see that it is returned to the medicine cabinet in the morning. If sleeping tablets are left handy for possible use in the night, only one dose should be put out; and this must be returned to the cupboard next day if it is not used.

Medicines Useful in the Home

The following list of useful substances is intended only as a guide; other preparations may be preferred for some purposes, and may be kept instead of those mentioned.

It is more helpful to consider the list in two sections:

A. those which are taken internally; and
B. those which are used externally, either for application to the body or for other purposes;

and, as advised above, the two groups should be stored separately.

Medicines named as essential for the first aid box are marked with an asterisk (*). They are repeated here so that the list for medicine cabinets may be complete in itself, and also because larger quantities may be kept in the cabinet than in the first aid box and so provide a reserve from which the small containers in the box may be refilled. The notes after the lists give some of the uses of the medicines, and the names of some alternative preparations which may be used.

A. MEDICINES FOR INTERNAL USE

- Aspirin Tablets, 300 milligram
- Compound Codeine Tablets
- Castor Oil
- Epsom Salts
- Magnesium Hydroxide Mixture
- *Sodium Bicarbonate
- Soda-mint Tablets
- Throat Lozenges
- Cough Mixture

B. SUBSTANCES AND PREPARATIONS FOR EXTERNAL USE

- *Boric Acid Crystals
- *Calamine Lotion
- Petroleum Jelly; Vaseline
- Witch Hazel
- Hydrogen Peroxide
- Smelling Salts
- Rubbing Alcohol
- Camphorated Oil
- Potassium Permanganate
- Lysol
- Zinc Ointment

A. For Internal Use

Aspirin Tablets, 300 mg. This is the usual strength and adults may take one to three as a dose; young children should have a quarter or half a tablet, depending on their age. The tablets relieve headache, toothache, and other pains. They are also useful for colds and influenza. Many combinations of aspirin with other drugs can be purchased but it is doubtful whether they have any advantage over the plain aspirin tablet for ordinary purposes. Aspirins may irritate the stomach so they should be taken after food, or in milk. Soluble Aspirin Tablets, dissolved in water with effervescence are not so liable to cause stomach upsets but they do not keep as well as the ordinary aspirin tablets. In some people, even small doses of aspirin cause serious reactions. These persons should learn to recognize aspirin under the name ACETYLSALICYLIC ACID, sometimes shortened to AC. ACETYLSAL., since either of these names may be used on the labels of the compound preparations, e.g. Compound Aspirin Tablets (containing aspirin, phenacetin and caffeine), Aspirin and Phenacetin Tablets, Aspirin and Caffeine Tablets, and Compound Codeine Tablets (see below).

Compound Codeine Tablets contain aspirin, 250 milligrams, phenacetin, 250 milligrams, and codeine phosphate, 8 milligrams. They are a popular substitute for aspirin tablets and also useful in the treatment of diarrhea because of the constipating action of the codeine phosphate. A soluble variety, Soluble Compound Codeine Tablets, is also made. These are easier to take but, like the soluble aspirin tablets, do not keep so well, especially in a wet atmosphere.

Caster Oil is used as a purgative, one to two teaspoonsful being given an hour before breakfast on an empty stomach. It has a nauseating taste, which may be partly disguised with milk or lemon juice. It can be mixed with zinc ointment and applied to the skin as an ointment for bedsores or diaper rash.

Epsom Salts (MAGNESIUM SULPHATE) is a rapid and powerful saline purgative; one to four teaspoonsful given in half to one tumblerful of water before breakfast produces evacuation in one to two hours. Wet dressings of magnesium sulphate, an ounce in a quarter of a pint of water, can be applied to boils or carbuncles. **Glauber's Salt** (SODIUM SULPHATE) is an alternative to Epsom salts as a saline purgative and may be taken similarly.

Magnesium Hydroxide Mixture (MILK OF MAGNESIA) relieves indigestion and flatulence and is also mildly laxative. One to four teaspoonsful is the usual dose. Mixed with water it may be used as a mouth-wash to neutralize acid around the teeth. It is also a useful antidote in cases of poisoning by mineral acids.

Sodium Bicarbonate is another handy substance which keeps well and has several uses. A quarter to one teaspoonful taken in a little water neutralizes the acid in the stomach and relieves the pain and distension of indigestion. Alternatively, **Soda-mint Tablets** (which consist of sodium bicarbonate and peppermint oil) may be sucked slowly, or one of the many indigestion lozenges or tablets on the market may be substituted. Sodium bicarbonate dissolves mucus so it is employed in a weak solution (a teaspoonful to a pint) to wash out the mouth and nose; this strength can also be used as an eye lotion, or applied to the skin to relieve itching in urticaria.

Throat Lozenges. It is better to avoid medicated lozenges. All that is necessary is to have a stock of simple pleasant throat lozenges which will keep the throat moist and relieve a slight irritant cough. Cough drops are very suitable but there are many others from which to choose.

Cough Preparations. Many useful preparations are obtainable. Distinguish between those which will stop a cough and those which will encourage expectoration.

B. For External Use

Boric Acid Crystals dissolved in water makes a soothing eye lotion. Boil and cool the water before dissolving the crystals in it. Use about a teaspoonful to half a pint of water. The solution also forms a mildly antiseptic skin lotion but it should never be applied to broken skin.

Calamine Lotion is dabbed on the skin with a wad of cotton to relieve insect bites and stings, heat and diaper rash, sunburn, and itching and redness of the skin.

Petroleum Jelly; Vaseline is obtainable white or yellow, and either is satisfactory as a bland, neutral, and soothing application to sore and chapped skin.

Witch Hazel is a pleasant lotion for small wounds, bruises, and inflamed swellings.

Hydrogen Peroxide. The usual strength is 20-volume. This should be diluted with an equal volume of warm, not hot, water and used as an antiseptic solution to clean cuts and wounds. Somewhat weaker solutions provide useful mouth-washes and gargles, and also remove stains from the teeth.

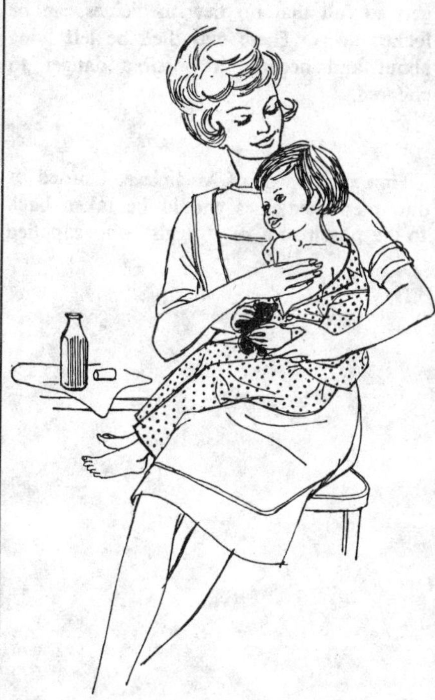

Fig. 5. *WINTER COUGHS. Warmed camphorated oil rubbed on the chest will relieve congestion.*

Rubbing Alcohol is applied to the skin to prevent bedsores. It may also be used as an evaporating lotion to reduce sweating, and to remove sticking plaster from the skin. Cotton soaked in alcohol is used to clean the skin before injections are given.

Camphorated Oil. A little warmed oil rubbed on the chest is helpful in colds to relieve congestion. Vapor rubs are useful alternatives.

Potassium Permanganate dissolved in warm water yields a purple antiseptic solution. For cleaning wounds, 600 milligrams per pint; for a gargle, mouth-wash, or vaginal irrigation, weaker solutions are adequate.

Lysol (*Poison*) is a soapy solution of cresol and is a general antiseptic and disinfectant. A teaspoonful to a pint of water provides an antiseptic lotion. For use as a disinfectant, see Disinfection and Fumigation in the section on Home Nursing, p. 48.

Care of the Medicine Cabinet

Frequent inspection is necessary to check the following points:

(a) That all the medicines and preparations are in stock and in their right place.

(b) That they are all reasonably fresh. Because the period for which medicinal substances may be kept varies with the nature of the substance it is a good idea to write on the labels the date the medicine was bought. Replace stocks which show signs of deterioration.

(c) That the cabinet is clean. Watch especially that drops of the syrupy liquids do not run down the sides of the bottles and contaminate the shelf. Wash all such bottles and the shelf when this happens.

(d) That all containers are clearly marked with the name of the contents and, if possible, with the directions for use. A strip of transparent adhesive cellulose tape over the label will protect it.

Deterioration of Medicines

DO NOT HOARD MEDICINES. It sometimes happens that when a patient has been discharged or when the doctor has changed the treatment, a few doses remain in the bottle of medicine or the box of tablets. *These should be thrown away* unless the doctor advises that they may be kept. There are several reasons why this should be done.

First, medicines do not as a rule keep well. This is particularly true of liquids but it also applies to solid preparations such as tablets and capsules. If they are kept too long, chemical changes take place, with the result that either the medicines lose their activity, becoming too weak to do any good, or they spoil and, if taken, they may upset the whole body system. The time it takes for these changes to occur varies enormously with the type of preparation. Some may keep quite well for a year or more but others may deteriorate in a few weeks. The time also depends on the conditions under which the medicines are kept; a warm damp atmosphere such as in a bathroom usually speeds up the rate of deterioration. It is therefore not possible to give any useful indication of the 'life' of the different sorts of preparations, and the best rule to follow is to take the medicine as directed by the doctor and either throw away what is not wanted, or ask for a further supply when the first has been used up. In this way only fresh medicines will be in use.

The second reason why unused medicines should be discarded is that stocks of drugs provide a real temptation to 'try something first' before going to the doctor. This results in delay in obtaining the correct treatment and may lead to a minor illness developing into a more serious one. It should be remembered that an illness seldom repeats itself exactly in the same patient and is different in another. So a tablet which cleared a headache on one occasion may fail on another, or a cough mixture which was originally prescribed to stop a cough may do damage if subsequently taken to stop a cough which should have been stimulated. Self-treatment is unwise; but the treatment of one patient with the medicine prescribed for another is even more so, and may cause real harm. The opportunities for doing these risky things will be very much less if surplus medicines are not saved up.

If, despite the advice given above, it becomes a habit to hoard medicines it will very soon be discovered that the medicine cabinets are cluttered with boxes and bottles. As a result it will be difficult to find a particular medicine and, if others are there of a similar appearance, there will be the danger of confusing one with another. There will also be a greatly increased likelihood that bottles and boxes will be knocked out of the cabinet and their contents wasted, but possibly the worst result follows when the cabinet gets so full that no new medicines can be locked away. These will then be left lying about and become a possible danger to children.

How to Dispose of Medicines. Unused or unwanted medicines should be taken back to the pharmacist or druggist who supplied them. If this is not possible or convenient, any pharmacist will give advice on the way to get rid of medicines. In the absence of such advice the best method is to pour liquid medicines into a large bucket of water and flush this away down the drain. This procedure is also suitable for solid preparations like tablets and capsules, which usually break up readily if they are allowed to soak in the water. Tablets, etc., may also be burnt but it is not advisable to do this on an open fire; put them in the stove one or two at a time. Do not throw tablets and capsules in the wastebasket or onto a trash pile or anywhere where they may be found by children or animals.

INVALID COOKERY

There are several basic principles which need to be observed by those who have to cater for the feeding of sick and convalescent people.

1. The prime requirement is to see that every item of food or drink purchased and served to the invalid is sound.

2. The protective foods must next be considered. The important thing is to see that they are given in the right amount. This will not be difficult if the diet includes dairy foods, green and root vegetables, citrus and summer fruits, and fish (especially the fat fish). All the vitamins and essential minerals would be included.

3. The requirement third in importance for feeding invalids is the provision of body-building foods—the proteins. These can be provided by meat and fish, although of course some proteins will be given in the dairy foods. Meat is best avoided in the acute early stage of an illness.

4. The provision of calories, largely from the bread group of foods and the sugars, is considered last in catering for invalids since a person lying in bed all day needs to take in far less of these energy producers than a busy active person. In general there is no need for careful assessment of the amount of these foods because the invalid's appetite is a good guide to his requirements. It is really important, however, to see that a patient does not fill himself up with calorie-producing foods at the cost of neglecting to eat the protective and body-building foods. In other words, a patient will not get back on the road to health if he has too high a proportion of cereal, toast, biscuits, ice-cream and bread in his diet.

5. On the question of giving foods containing roughage—the indigestible cellulose part of vegetable matter—to prevent constipation in patients confined to bed, this depends on the nature of the illness. In ulcerative colitis, dysentery, or spastic colon no roughage whatsoever should be given.

The activity of the intestines is reduced in an invalid and it is not to be expected that he will have bowel movements as often as when he was up and about, so there is no need to step up the roughage content. In general, too, roughage increases flatulence and this can make life very uncomfortable for the patient.

The values of the various kinds of foodstuffs—the proteins, vitamins, etc.—are dealt with in detail in the section on Food and Nutrition, p. 65.

Diet in Various Diseases

If a patient is to be nursed at home, the doctor will recommend suitable diets for the specific illness, e.g. gout, or diabetes mellitus. Although dietetic treatment is dealt with in many of the sections on diseases, some brief general notes are given below.

Diet in Fevers

Since febrile patients are usually averse to food but are continually thirsty, milk and milk foods—hot or cold—should form the basis of the diet for the first few days. Fortify the milk with medicinal glucose and cream, and fruit juices with glucose. With the advent of antibiotics and modern therapy, the period of high fever is now much shorter (seldom more than four or five days), and the patients, being less debilitated, may be given jellies, clear soups, eggs and egg custards, and steamed white fish quite early.

Small meals given often are best. The patient should be encouraged to take as much as he can. The early morning drink should be weak coffee or cocoa or a malted milk drink, and this is given again at frequent intervals. In shorter fevers, such as influenza and pneumonia, a more solid diet is given as soon as the fever begins to abate. In typhoid the solids are given quite early in the illness.

BREAKFAST: fine oatmeal or non-bran cereal with sugar and cream, a lightly boiled egg, toast and butter. MID-MORNING SNACK: milk drink and crackers. LUNCH: white fish steamed or broiled with white sauce and puree potatoes; junket or rice pudding to follow. MID-AFTERNOON SNACK: weak tea or a milk drink, and plain cake. EVENING MEAL: lightly cooked egg dish or pureed chicken, milk jelly or ice-cream, toast and butter.

Fruit juice strained from fresh fruits containing vitamin C needs to be given twice daily. Alcohol is permitted to elderly patients (about ½ oz of whisky every 5 hours during the day).

Diet in Stomach Disorders

(a) INFLAMMATION or food poisoning. The stomach must be given time to recover before it can deal with even the mildest of foods: about 24 to 48 hours usually suffices. Warm (boiled) milk can then be sipped in small amounts every two hours. Barley water or glucose may be added. Solids may then be introduced carefully but they must be very digestible (dry toast, plain cake, oatmeal, butter, eggs poached or boiled, chicken, white fish, puréed vegetables, milk puddings, stewed fruit, ripe fruit without skin and pits, barley sugar). Avoid coffee and alcohol.

(b) GASTRIC ULCER. A precise regimen is usually provided by the doctor (see also Diseases of the Digestive System, p. 365) but observe the following general rules.

Spices, condiments, and meat extracts which encourage increased secretion of gastric juice are forbidden. So too are alcohol and tobacco. Roughage is inadvisable.

Milk every two hours neutralizes the excess acids in the stomach. After two weeks or so on a milk and milk-cereal diet, the patient may begin to eat lightly cooked fish and eggs, junket with cream, puréed cauliflower and parsnip, and thin bread and butter. It is important that even these simple meals are unhurried. Meals should be frequent and, if one is delayed, a snack of milk chocolate, plain biscuits or a glass of milk should be taken. Vitamin C in some form must be taken daily.

Diet in Heart Failure

In general, meals should be dry and fluids somewhat restricted. Large meals are likely to strain the heart so the three main meals should be evenly balanced. Full details are given in the treatment of heart failure in the section Diseases of the Heart, p. 300.

Diet in Biliousness

For this upset of the liver the foods are best confined to dry toast, plain biscuits, honey, jam, molasses and golden syrup, and fruit drinks should have glucose added. Avoid alcohol.

Diet in Simple Anemia

Although not all anemias are due to lack of iron, the simple or iron-deficiency form is more easily dealt with if the patient takes foods rich in available iron and also in vitamin C.

For IRON content: liver, kidney, red meat, eggs; green vegetables, spring onions, watercress; black and red currants, raspberries, dried fruits; black molasses.

For VITAMIN C: liver, vegetables as above, new potatoes, brussels sprouts, spinach, turnips, fruits as above, lemons, oranges and tomatoes.

Diet in Common Skin Troubles

Stubborn and frequent outbreaks of boils, pimples and sties are very often alleviated and sometimes cured by a high vitamin diet or a raw food diet.

Wholewheat bread and wholewheat cereal should replace white bread and crackers. For vegetables, any green ones are useful and so are carrots, and potatoes in their jackets. Real lemon juice and blackcurrant juice should be taken sometimes instead of coffee or tea. Soups and stews should have yeast extract added. Bacon, pork, liver and kidney are the most suitable of the meats.

General Notes for the Feeding of Invalids

1. Do not give food if the patient is tired after being bathed or after having injections. Wait until he is comfortable and rested and the room neat before serving meals.
2. Arrange the tray attractively with a clean cloth (changed often) and pretty china. Never leave crumbs or stains from a previous meal.
3. Ensure that hot meals are hot by the time they reach the patient, by warming the plate or serving food in individual dishes direct from the oven. Serve small portions.
4. Ensure that the meal is ready on time. 'Little' things like a delayed mealtime can be a source of irritation and upset the patient; upsets tend to retard recovery.
5. Once the meal is finished remove the tray without delay; sponge the patient's hands and let him rest before seeing visitors.

Planning Meals

Early Stages of Illness

During the first twenty-four hours it is often wise, especially in digestive upsets, to give only water and no food, but this will depend upon the doctor's instructions.

When this stage has passed, boiled milk, or milk and water can be given, or fruit juices with glucose. These can be followed at a later stage by milk puddings, milk soups, dry toast with yeast extract, or jellies.

In Convalescence

Once the patient is beginning to get better a greater variety of foods can be introduced into the diet, but these must be easily digested and meals can be prepared from the following range of foodstuffs:

Bread a day old, or dry toast, oatmeal, plain biscuits.
Milk, sterilized, pasteurized or boiled, or diluted with mineral water or barley water.
Butter
Fish (not shell fish, nor fat fish such as mackerel or herrings).
Eggs, poached, boiled, baked, but not fried.
Meats, lean and lightly cooked. Not pork. These should be introduced last after the patient has safely digested fish and eggs.
Vegetables (puréed): peas, young carrots, beans, cauliflower, spinach, broccoli; avoid the coarser root vegetables such as turnips and parsnips.

Milk puddings
Fresh fruit and stewed fruit

Loss of appetite is common in many illnesses. Therefore, in order to tempt the poor appetite, meals must be made interesting, pleasant and varied, quite apart from the basic nutritional requirements.

Variation in Presentation

Bread can be served as thin slices, fingers, thin sandwiches or toast: alternatives to bread are crackers.

Milk drinks can be varied in flavor: add blackcurrant, raspberry or other fruit juices; coffee or cocoa; sherry or rum.

Texture

Once the patient is off a soft diet it will stimulate his appetite if foods of different texture are served in the same meal, e.g. a soft stew followed by a crisp jam tart. A bland food can be followed by one with a sharp flavor, e.g. steamed fish and baked apple.

Color and Flavor

Much invalid food is white in color, e.g. white fish, milk, milk puddings, and it will stimulate the appetite if color can be introduced. Use colored china, or a colored tray cloth with white china. Colored flavorings in milk may be used and a spoonful of jam can make a white milk pudding look most appetizing, provided jam is allowed in the diet. Parsley cheers the appearance of steamed fish.

Hot or Cold

It helps to stimulate the appetite and provide variety if hot and cold food are served in the same meal or on different occasions during the day, e.g. a hot savory first course can be followed by blancmange, an ice, or fresh fruit; alternatively, a cold meat first course may be followed by a hot, light steamed pudding.

Surprises

Junket can appear much more attractive if served in a small, stemmed glass instead of on a pudding plate.

Try to get a delicacy which the patient has mentioned.

Vary the china used at different meals, if possible, and provide colorful paper napkins which are cheap to buy and attractive to look at.

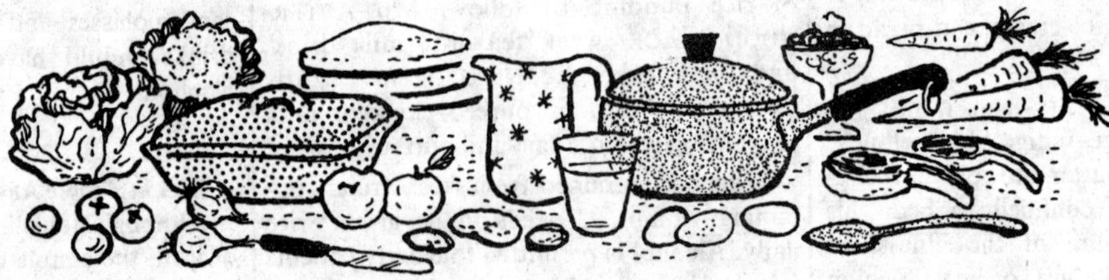

SOME USEFUL RECIPES

Milk Drinks

It is better to drink milk rapidly and if it seems difficult to digest, it can be diluted with water, barley water, or soda water. It does not aid digestion to drink it slowly or to sip it. Pasteurized or cooked milk is easier to digest than raw milk. Some adults find milk constipating, but this is less likely to happen if milk is taken with the food.

Protein Milk

This is produced commercially and can be bought in packages. It is easily prepared and instructions are given on the package.

Milk with Flour

One teaspoonful flour, a little cold water and 1 pint boiling milk. Mix flour with cold water, pour on boiling milk, and boil for three minutes. Grated lemon or orange peel will add a pleasant flavor.

Milk with Meat Extracts

Use the prepared extracts in the proportions stated on the container but use milk instead of water.

Milk with Brandy

One glassful milk, sugar to taste, 1 tablespoonful brandy. Heat milk, sweeten, and add brandy.

Malted Milk

One glassful of milk, or milk and water, 1 tablespoonful of malted milk powder, 1 or 2 teaspoonsful of sugar, small pinch of salt. Mix the powder with a little of the liquid, heat remaining liquid to boiling point and add sugar and pinch of salt. Serve hot or cold.

Milk Punch

¼ pint milk, white of egg (stiffly beaten), 2 tablespoonsful cream, 1 tablespoonful of whisky, brandy or sherry, about 1 teaspoonful confectioner's sugar, 1 teaspoonful of instant coffee powder. Shake all the ingredients together and pour over ice.

Milk and Molasses

½ pint milk, 1 tablespoonful molasses. Bring milk to boil, add molasses, and bring to boil again. Strain and serve hot.

Creamed Soups

Cream of Celery

Four or five sticks celery, ½ cupful boiling water, 1 tablespoonful butter, 1 tablespoonful flour, 1 cupful milk. Cut celery into small pieces and cook in boiling water until tender, then pass all through a strainer. For WHITE SAUCE: melt butter in a saucepan and gradually add flour, then pour in the milk. Cook slowly (stirring) and when the mixture thickens, add the celery purée and blend together.

Cream of Pea

½ cupful of purée made from cooked peas passed through a sieve, 1 tablespoonful each of flour and butter, 1 cupful milk, 1 teaspoonful of sugar, a little salt. Make white sauce with butter, flour and milk (as for Cream of Celery Soup), add purée, sugar and salt. Garnish with finely chopped mint.

Cream of Potato

One large potato washed and sliced, 1 teaspoonful grated onion, boiling water, 1 tablespoonful each of butter and flour, 1 cupful milk, chopped parsley to taste. Simmer potato and grated onion until tender in sufficient boiling water to cover. Make white sauce (as for Cream of Celery Soup). Add potato and ½ cupful potato water, and strain. Reheat, adding chopped parsley.

Cream of Tomato

½ cupful tomatoes (cut up), 1 tablespoonful each of butter and flour, and 1 cupful milk. Stew tomatoes for 5 minutes and strain (a little chopped onion may be cooked with them if liked). Make a white sauce with butter, flour and milk (as for Cream of Celery Soup) and add tomato pulp, a lump of sugar and a little salt. Reheat: if reboiled it may curdle.

Milk Junkets and Puddings

Junket, Plain

½ pint milk, 1 level tablespoonful sugar, rennet as directions on container. Heat milk over low flame until at body temperature (if no thermometer available then test with little finger: about 98°–99° F.). Add rennet and sugar, stir well and put into bowl to set.

Junkets, Various

(a) Add thinly sliced banana, a sprinkle of sugar and squeeze of lemon.

(b) Add coffee extract or powder to milk before adding rennet.

(c) When junket is set, grate nutmeg over and top with whipped cream.

Cornstarch Pudding

½ pint milk, 1 tablespoonful cornstarch, 1 or 2 teaspoonsful sugar (to taste). Mix sugar and cornstarch with a little of the milk. Boil rest of milk then slowly stir into mixture; return this to saucepan and cook until it thickens. Pour into moistened mold to set —or into individual glasses.

This can be varied with different flavors, such as adding a few drops of vanilla extract; or add a little grated lemon peel to the milk while it boils then strain before adding to cornstarch.

Ice-cream

Ice-cream with Evaporated Milk

Can evaporated milk (chilled), 2 oz confectioner's sugar. Beat the milk in a cold bowl until twice its bulk, then add sugar and a flavoring. Beat again until flavoring is thoroughly mixed in, then freeze.

Chocolate Ice-cream

1 cupful thin cream or evaporated milk, ¼ cupful water, 2 drops strong coffee extract, ½ teaspoonful vanilla (if liked), ½ square (½ oz) cooking chocolate, 3 tablespoonsful sugar. Break chocolate into small pieces and melt in the water on a low heat until melted. Stir in other ingredients, and freeze.

NOTE: when ice-cream has been in the refrigerator freezer for about 2 hours remove tray, break up ice-cream with fork and fold in a well-beaten white of egg.

Fruit Beverages

Apple Water

½ lb apples cut into pieces, 2 oz brown sugar, 2 pints boiling water. Pour the boiling water over the apples and sugar and, when cool, put the fruit through a strainer.

Rhubarb water is similar.

Blackcurrant Drink

One tablespoonful blackcurrant jam, squeeze of lemon juice, ½ pint hot water. Pour hot (not boiling) water on the jam in a warmed pitcher, add lemon juice, and leave covered for five minutes. Strain and serve.

Lemonade with Egg White

Strained juice of a lemon, 1 oz sugar, 1 pint boiling water, beaten white of an egg. Dissolve the sugar in boiling water, allow to cool a little then add the lemon juice. Cool, add beaten white of egg.

Strawberry Crush

4 oz ripe strawberries, ½ pint water, squeeze of lemon juice, soda water or lemonade. Hull the strawberries, press them with the water through a sieve and pour on to a little cracked ice in a tumbler. Add squeeze of lemon juice and fill glass with soda water or lemonade.

Egg Dishes

Coddled Eggs

Break an egg into a cup or small dish; pour on boiling water to cover it. Leave for 5 to 8 minutes, drain off water and serve in cup. Very suitable for infants.

Baked Egg

Break an egg into a buttered small dish or cup, season with a little salt and pepper and bake in moderate oven or under a hot grill until set. To make a change, a little cream or milk may be added to this dish; alternatively, sprinkle with a little grated cheese.

Eggs au Plat (quick and easy to do)

Break an egg on to a buttered plate standing on a saucepan of boiling water. Cover with a lid, and leave with water gently boiling until the egg sets.

Egg in Broth

Poach an egg gently until set in a strained veal, chicken, or mutton broth. Lift egg out into a soup plate, cover with the broth, garnish with chopped parsley and serve with thin buttered toast.

Fluffed Egg

Separate the yolk and white of an egg, taking care to keep the yolk whole. Beat the white of the egg until stiff. Put this into a buttered small dish, make a hole in the center and drop in the yolk; add salt and pepper if desired, and a little finely grated cheese. Stand dish in a container with a little water and bake in a moderate oven (350° F) until set (about 10 minutes).

Fish

White fish and poultry appear frequently in an invalid diet because they are easier to digest than red meat, but fat, either naturally in the fish or used in cooking it, is less digestible.

Kedgeree

½ lb cooked (boiled or poached) white fish, 1 oz margarine, 4 oz boiled rice (see p. 62), 1 beaten egg, 1 hard-boiled egg, chopped parsley (and chives if liked). Melt the margarine in saucepan, add the cooked rice, season with salt and pepper as desired, add beaten egg and stir, then add the cooked fish which has been boned and flaked. When this is hot pile on a very hot dish and sprinkle the finely chopped boiled egg over. Garnish with parsley (and chives).

Fish and Egg Pie

½ lb partly cooked fish, 1 hard-boiled egg, ½ pint white sauce (see Cream of Celery Soup, above), breadcrumbs. Flake the fish and put into a glass oven dish, adding salt and pepper as desired. Place slices of hard-boiled egg over fish and pour on white sauce. Sprinkle with breadcrumbs and bake for 20 minutes in a moderate oven. A little grated cheese mixed with the breadcrumbs will add a piquant flavor.

Fish and Tomato

1 lb filleted white fish, seasoned flour (containing a little pepper and salt), ½ lb tomatoes, a little butter, 2 tablespoonsful milk. Wash, dry, and cut fish into neat pieces, dip into flour and put into buttered glass oven dish. Cut the tomatoes into halves and lay a half on each piece of fish, add small pieces of butter and the milk. Cover and bake for half an hour in a slow oven.

Baked Sole

Prepare sole by washing, and trim the fins. Butter an oven dish, lay in the fish and add a squeeze of lemon juice and a little grated onion. Bake in moderate oven for 15 minutes.

Meat

Fresh Ground Beef

1 lb freshly ground stewing steak, 1 small onion, ½ oz dripping or cooking fat, ¼ pint stock or water, 1 tablespoonful flour, a little salt. Heat the fat in a saucepan, add the ground beef and the onion (chopped), stirring with a fork to keep the ground particles from coagulating. When the beef is brown add stock or water and simmer very gently for 1½ hours; add the flour and salt, stir, and simmer for about 10 minutes.

Steamed Chop

Obtain a tender loin chop and put it on a small plate on top of a saucepan of water; cover closely with aluminum foil or another plate, and steam for 30 minutes. Chopped parsley, lemon slices, or a dash of catsup add flavor and color when serving.

Lamb Stew

Cut away surplus fat and dice the meat; put into a casserole, add vegetables as liked, season to taste, cover with water and cook in a slow oven for 1½ hours.

Steamed Steak

1 lb stewing steak cut into even pieces, small carrot, turnip, onion diced, 4 tablespoonsful stock or water, 1 tablespoonful meat or yeast extract, 2 tablespoonsful flour. Roll meat pieces in the flour and put with vegetables, stock and extract into a double boiler, season with pepper and salt and steam for about three hours.

Cheese Dishes

Savory Cheese Custard

4 oz cheese, grated or sliced thinly, small onion partly cooked and chopped finely, 1 egg, ½ pint milk, breadcrumbs. Put cheese in bottom of well-buttered dish, sprinkle the onion and a little pepper over it. Mix yolk with the milk, add pinch of salt, beat egg white until stiff and fold this into the yolk and milk mixture then pour all over the cheese. Allow this to set in a hot oven, sprinkle with breadcrumbs and return to oven for a few minutes to brown.

Cheese Fondue

½ pint hot milk, 4 oz grated cheese, 1 cupful stale breadcrumbs, 1 tablespoonful butter, ½ teaspoonful salt, 3 eggs. Mix all the ingredients together except the eggs. Beat the egg yolks and stir into mixture, then fold in the stiffly beaten whites of the eggs. Put mixture into a well-buttered glass casserole, and bake in moderate oven until set. Fondue should be served immediately.

Cereal Foods

Whole grain cereals—rice, barley, coarse oatmeal—cook according to directions on package.

Barley Water

2 oz pearl barley well washed, thinly peeled rind of a lemon, 1 pint boiling water. Put barley and lemon rind in large bowl and pour on the water. Add sugar as desired, cover, and leave until cold. Strain off the liquor into clean jar.

For thick barley water put the 2 oz pearl barley in 2 pints of cold water, bring to a boil and strain away the water. Add 2 pints fresh cold water (and lemon or orange rind if liked) and simmer slowly for 2 hours. Strain, add lemon juice and sugar if liked, or serve with milk.

To be taken freely in fevers or in inflammations of bladder or kidneys.

Oatmeal

1½ tablespoonsful oatmeal, 1 pint boiling water, pinch of salt. Cook slowly for 2 hours, strain, and add milk or cream. Serve with sugar if the patient wishes it.

Plain Boiled Dry Rice

If accompanied with syrup, jam, cream or milk it will serve as a sweet. Alternatively, it can be served as a side dish to cooked fish or stew, or made into a rissotto (see below) or similar savory dish.

Wash the rice three times. Bring 2 quarts of water to a boil and sprinkle in the rice gradually so as to keep the water bubbling, stir well with a fork. Boil rapidly for a quarter of an hour or so until the grains feel tender when pinched between the fingers, then strain through a colander. Pour boiling water through the rice pile to wash out the gelatinous matter and place for about a quarter of an hour in a medium hot oven to dry the grains.

Rissotto

Cook 4 oz rice as for Plain Boiled Dry Rice, add 1 oz butter or margarine, 2 tablespoonsful tomato puree, 2 oz grated cheese and seasoning to taste. Reheat, put on to hot dish, and sprinkle over with grated cheese.

Creamed Tapioca

Cook 1½ tablespoonsful tapioca, 1 cupful hot milk, pinch salt in double boiler (or in bowl over hot water in saucepan), for 15 minutes. Beat 1½ or 2 tablespoonsful sugar into one egg yolk and stir into the tapioca until it thickens. Lift saucepan from heat and fold in the white of the egg which has been beaten until stiff. This can be served hot or cold, or with stewed apples, prunes or figs for variety.

Flour Foods

Eggless Cake

8 oz flour, 1 teaspoonful bicarbonate of soda, 3 oz butter, 4 oz sugar, ½ lb mixed dried fruit (as liked), a little milk, 1 tablespoonful vinegar. Sift together the flour, bicarbonate of soda and a pinch of salt, rub in the butter and add the sugar and mixed fruit. Stir in enough milk to make a fairly stiff mix, then add the vinegar stirring quickly. Bake in a greased tin in a hot oven (425° F). Nourishing, yet provides a variation in texture from usual fruit cake.

Sponge Cake

2 eggs, sugar and flour each equal in weight to the eggs. Add the sugar to the eggs in a bowl and beat until creamy, sift in flour, pinch of baking powder and small pinch of salt, add 1 teaspoonful of warm water. Bake in a greased baking tin, in hot oven (425° F) for 10 to 15 minutes.

For variation, color the mixture pink with grenadine, or chocolate with a few drops of coffee extract and vanilla flavoring.

Cheese Pastry

4 oz flour, 2 oz margarine, 2 oz grated cheese, 1 large egg, cold water. Season the flour with salt and pepper, rub in the fat, add cheese and egg yolk (not white). Mix to a stiff paste adding water as necessary. Roll out and cut into fingers. Bake until golden brown in a moderate oven.

Vegetable Dishes

Cauliflower au Gratin

Wash cauliflower, break into small pieces, and cook until tender in salted water. Drain. Butter an oven dish, put in the cauliflower pieces, cover with a white sauce (see Cream of Celery Soup, p. 61), sprinkle with grated cheese and buttered breadcrumbs, and bake in a moderate oven until top is brown.

Mixed Vegetables

Any raw vegetables in season can be used and they should be diced or sliced. For each 1 lb of vegetables allow 4 tablespoonsful water and a small pat of margarine, and seasoning. Cook in a saucepan with the lid on tightly and shake often to prevent burning. Serve as soon as vegetables are cooked: overcooking soon spoils the 'fresh' flavor. Garnish with chopped parsley.

Celery

Only good quality fresh celery should be used. Cut away coarse parts and soak for a little while in cold water. Cut into pieces of equal length, put in enough milk and water to cover, season, and cook in saucepan without a lid for about half an hour. Strain. This can be served as a second vegetable or on toast.

Leeks

Remove root and any coarse leaves, wash very well, tie stems together and cook as for celery. Serve with a little butter.

Creamed Turnips

Boil the peeled turnips in salted water (or milk and water) until tender, mash with 1 tablespoonful grated cheese, ½ teaspoonful butter, and a little pepper. Serve hot.

Scalloped Potatoes

Arrange peeled sliced potatoes in thin layers in a buttered baking dish, each layer covered with finely minced onion and seasoned, and dotted with butter. Add a little top milk, cover with breadcrumbs, and bake in moderate oven until cooked.

Celery and Apple Cheese Salad

This is easy to prepare and will add variety to the diet of the convalescent. Chop the celery and apple and mix with grated cheese, add seasoning to taste and a dash of lemon juice.

Cooked Vegetable Salad

Cooked diced carrots, a lesser amount of cooked peas, a few cooked mushrooms. Arrange the vegetables on a dish and serve with mayonnaise separately. This can be varied when other cooked vegetables are available, e.g. cauliflower sprigs, French beans, asparagus.

Fruit Dishes

Stewed Fruit

The best way to prepare a compote of fruit is to cook each fruit separately if possible, mixing them only when about to serve in individual dishes. In this way each fruit maintains its individual flavor and looks more attractive particularly as white fruits, such as apples do not become stained by darker fruit such as blackberries.

Fruit Purée

Place the clean fruit in a saucepan with only enough water to prevent burning. Cook gently until soft. Put through a sieve, add sweetening to taste, and reboil for a few minutes.

Dried Fruit

Apricots, figs, peaches, prunes can be obtained dried and are valuable for the convalescent as they contain useful minerals and vitamins. They can be served raw or cooked after discarding any which are unsound. If served raw they need to be soaked for 24 hours then put through a sieve: honey, milk or cream can then be added. To cook dried fruit soak them overnight, add a piece of lemon peel, bring to the boil and simmer gently until tender. Sweeten to taste and serve either hot or cold.

Loganberry Fluff

½ lb stewed loganberries, juice of 1 orange, 1 egg white beaten until stiff. Add the orange juice to the loganberries, sweeten as desired, fold in the egg white, pile high on small dish and serve.

Blackberries, raspberries or apple purée can also be prepared similarly.

FOOD AND NUTRITION

Anyone whose business it is to provide meals should possess a knowledge of at least the fundamentals of nutrition so that she will know the true value of the food she is providing. The importance in regard to both quantity and quality of an adequate and varied diet for maintaining the body in health is fully recognized today.

In addition, certain diseases can be treated by dietetic measures, and others can be prevented by them.

The science of human nutrition entails the study of food and of the processes of growth, maintenance and repair of the living body dependent on its intake. It answers the questions: what is food composed of? why does man need food? and what does his body do with it?

Food is needed for the following basic purposes:

(a) production of energy (heat, work, etc.);
(b) growth, repair, and reproduction (body building);
(c) provision of substances to regulate the above processes and so maintain health.

THE COMPONENTS OF FOOD

Food components are known as nutrients, and can be divided into the following groups:

1. Carbohydrates provide the body with energy, and may also be converted into fat.
2. Fats provide energy and may also form body fat.
3. Proteins provide material for growth and repair of body tissues. Energy can also be provided, and sometimes conversion to fat occurs.
4. Mineral Substances provide material for growth and repair, and for the regulation of body processes.
5. Vitamins help to regulate the body processes.

Water and oxygen (from the air) are also necessary for life but are not usually considered as nutrients.

Although there are a few foods which contain only one nutrient, most foods contain variable proportions of several different kinds.

Measurement of Nutrient Quantity

Standard units are used to measure the amount of different nutrients. Gram (g.), ounce (oz.), calorie (cal) and international unit (i.u.) are those commonly in use.

The **calorie** is a measure of the energy value of food.

The **international unit** is a measure of vitamin quantity.

Taking into account the composition of different foods and their degrees of absorption by the body it is accepted that:
1 g. of carbohydrate absorbed by and oxidized in the body, produces 4 cal;
1 g. of fat absorbed by and oxidized in the body produces 9 cal;
1 g. of protein absorbed by and oxidized in the body produces 4 cal.

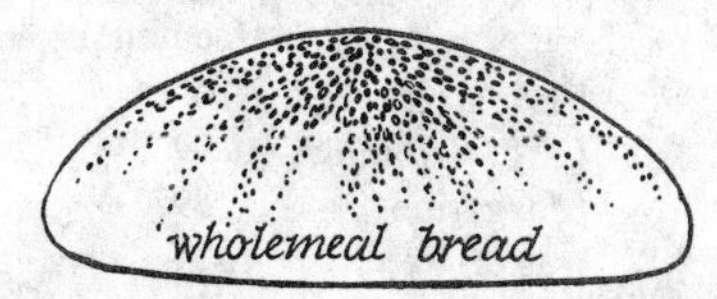

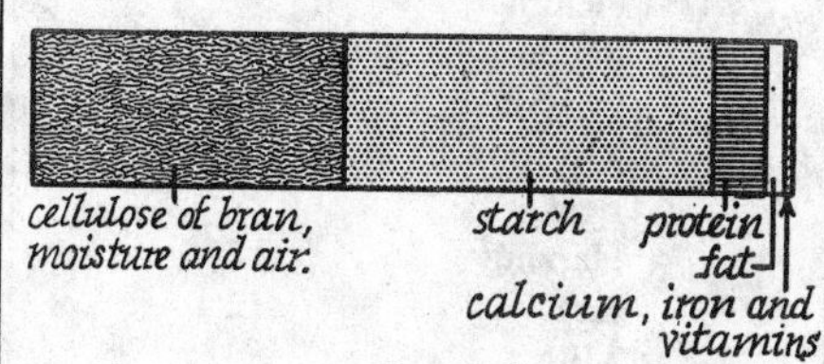

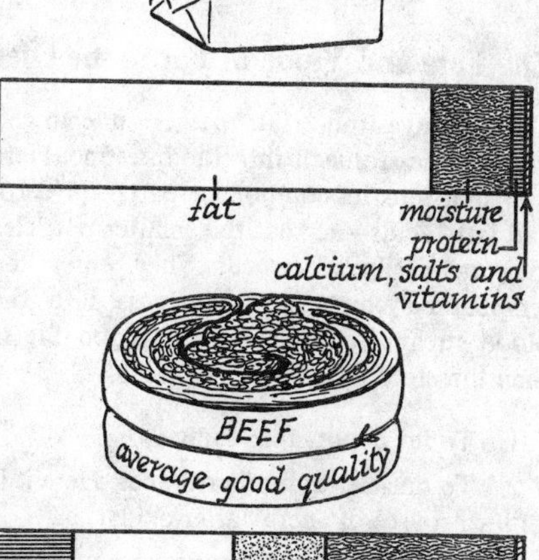

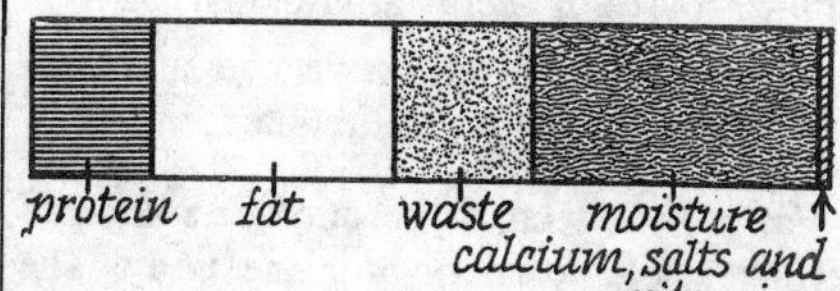

Fig. 1. *BREAD, BUTTER, BEEF. Showing the proportion of carbohydrate, fat, protein, vitamins, etc., in these basic foods.*

CARBOHYDRATES

Carbohydrates are compounds of carbon, hydrogen, and oxygen. They provide most of the energy in almost all human diets. The amount of carbohydrate in the diet varies in different communities. A poor person's diet may contain over 90 per cent carbohydrate, a well-to-do person's 50 per cent. For a normal adult, 55–65 per cent of carbohydrate in the diet is probably a suitable figure.

There are three kinds of carbohydrates:

(a) sugars, which may be monosaccharides or disaccharides;
(b) starches which are polysaccharides;
(c) cellulose which is a polysaccharide.

The diagram below shows very simply the chemical structure of the different carbohydrates:

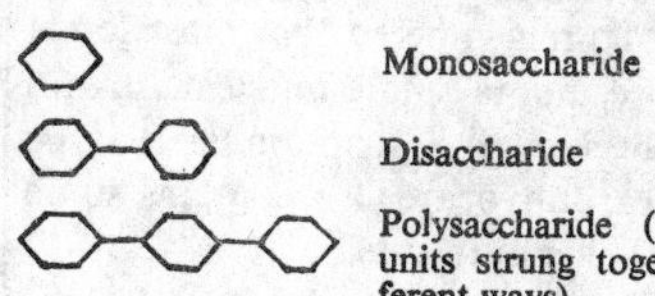

Sugars. Chemically, sugars are the simplest form of carbohydrate.

Glucose. This simple monosaccharide sugar exists naturally in the blood of living animals. It may be made from starch or from a more complex sugar such as sucrose. It plays an important role in the body. It also occurs naturally in plant juices and in fruit.

Fructose. This is another simple sugar and is the sweetest. It forms a part of cane sugar and occurs in plant juices, fruit and honey.

Sucrose. Sucrose is the scientific name for household sugar (cane or beet sugar). It is composed of two simple sugars, glucose and fructose, chemically combined together and is therefore a disaccharide. It occurs naturally in beet and sugar cane, in sweet fruits, and in some root vegetables such as carrots.

Lactose. This sugar is the combination of galactose and glucose. It occurs in all types of milk, including human milk.

Maltose. Chemically, maltose is composed of two glucose molecules. It is formed naturally from starch during the germination of barley, wheat, and other grains.

Starch. This is a polysaccharide made up of combined glucose molecules. Most of the carbohydrate in man's diet occurs as starch. Plants store most of their food as starch, as can be easily observed in cereal grains and the potato. Unripe fruits also contain starch which changes to sugar as they ripen.

The starch is enclosed within granules which cannot be easily digested. Thus flour and potatoes require heating to swell the granules. These then burst and release starch in digestible form.

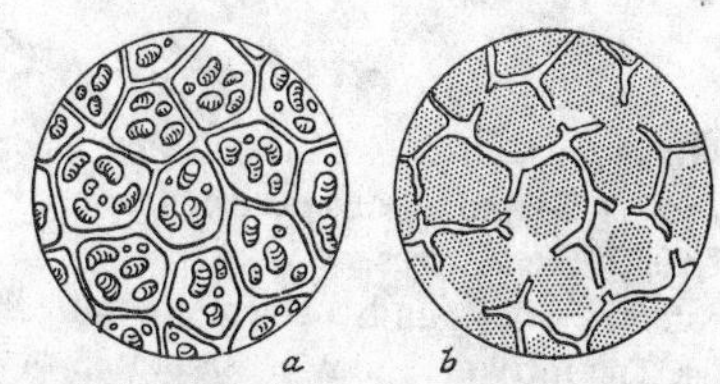

Fig. 2. *POTATO STARCH. (a) Raw starch grains in cells. (b) Cooked gelatinized starch bursts the cell walls.*

Cellulose. Much of the stiffer structure of vegetables and cereal foods is composed of cellulose which forms the cell walls enclosing the starch grains (see Fig. 2). It is only digested to a very small degree in the body, as it is very insoluble. However, it has some value because it gives bulk to the diet.

A chemical product of cellulose—methyl-cellulose—is a material of no food value but which fills the stomach when eaten and gives the effect of 'fulness.' This property may help a person on a reducing diet not to feel hungry.

It should be remembered that most foods contain more than a single nutrient. Bread, for example, as well as containing a large amount of carbohydrate also contains some protein and other nutrients.

Food providing Carbohydrates

FOOD	GRAMS PER OZ
Sugar	28·4
Syrup	20·2
Jam	17·6
White flour	21·2
Oatmeal	18·6
White bread	15·5
Raisins	16·4
Potatoes	4·6
Beans (baked)	4·5
Bananas	4·9
Milk	1·2

The Fate and Value of Carbohydrate in the Diet

Carbohydrates, when eaten, are broken down in the body into glucose which is absorbed into the bloodstream, passed to the cells, and then used. The muscles and other tissues in the body get energy from the oxidation of glucose. The process may be written thus:

Glucose + Oxygen makes Energy + Water + Carbon dioxide

$$C_6H_{12}O_6 + O_2 \quad = \quad \text{Heat and Work} + H_2O + CO_2$$

The glucose that is not used up is stored as glycogen in the liver and muscles. Whenever a meal provides more glucose than the tissues are able to accept, it is converted into fat and deposited in the adipose parts of the body. Excessive storage of fat takes place in obesity.

When there is not enough carbohydrate for the body's needs, protein and fat are utilized butyric acid, which gives butter its flavor, and an unsaturated fatty acid is oleic acid adequate amount of digestible carbohydrate.

FATS

Fats include all fatty materials such as meat fat, butter fat and all oils derived from animal and vegetable sources.

Fats are compounds of glycerol with fatty acids. The fatty acid may be saturated or unsaturated. This simply means that by the addition of hydrogen to its molecule an unsaturated fatty acid will become saturated. An example of a saturated fatty acid is butyric acid, which gives butter its flavor, and an unsaturated fatty acid is oleic acid found in olive oil. Fats are insoluble in water but soluable in liquids such as alcohol, ether, or chloroform (fat solvents).

The main sources of fat in the diet are butter, margarine, meat, and dairy products. Most vegetables and fruit contain very little fat, except nuts and soya products.

Foods providing Fat

FOOD	FAT CONTENT (percentage)
Frying oil	100
Lard, dripping	99
Margarine	89
Butter	84
Peanuts	50
Bacon	46
Cheese	35
Mutton	31
Beef	29
Herring	12
Egg	12
Milk	4

The Fate and Value of Fat in the Diet

After ingestion, fat passes unchanged through the stomach into the intestine. Here it is split into its component parts—glycerol and fatty acids—so that the smaller particles may be easily absorbed. They enter the lymphatic system and then pass into the blood stream. The fate of the blood fat is then threefold.

1. To fat depots for storage.
2. To muscles and other tissues. Here it is a source of energy after oxidation.
3. To the liver for conversion and synthesis into other metabolites.

Fat is thus seen to be another source of readily available energy for the body. The amount of fat consumed in the diet differs in different countries. Many articles of food cooked without fat are not tasty, and the housewife, recognizing this, uses it liberally. Recently, however, there has been some evidence linking excessive fat levels in the blood with coronary artery disease. Some authorities now recommend that middle-aged people leading sedentary lives should cut down on butter, cream, pastries and fried foods.

Very active people, on the other hand, require a high fat intake to supply them with the energy they need. This energy is more readily available from fats than the equivalent weight of carbohydrate, since 1 g. of carbohydrate produces 4 calories, while 1 g. of fat produces 9 calories.

PROTEINS

Proteins are essential components of all living cells, and are necessary for all growth and repair of the human body. Without sufficient protein in his food a child cannot grow.

Proteins are highly complex substances built up of different kinds of amino acids in varying arrangements. The amino acids themselves are less complex compounds of carbon, hydrogen, oxygen and nitrogen—the nitrogen content being their special feature. Some amino acids contain sulphur, and a few contain phosphorus.

Essential Amino Acids. Some amino acids necessary for life can be converted in the body from other amino acids. There are others which are essential to life but which cannot be made in the body; they must therefore be supplied in the diet.

The essential amino acids are:

Isoleucine	Phenylalanine
Leucine	Threonine
Lysine	Tryptophan
Methionine	Valine

Two additional ones for the growing child are:

Arginine	Histidine

There are two sources of dietary protein—animal and vegetable. Plants make their own protein from inorganic materials. Animals cannot do this but use the protein from plants as food. Animal proteins usually contain all the essential amino acids and are often termed first-class proteins. Vegetable proteins may lack one or more, and are called second-class proteins.

ANIMAL PROTEIN	PROTEIN CONTENT (percentage)
Cheese	25
Beef	15
Mutton	13
Egg	12
Milk	3

Meat and fish of all kinds are good sources of protein.

VEGETABLE PROTEIN	PROTEIN CONTENT (percentage)
Peanuts	29
Brown flour	12
White flour	11
Beans (baked)	6

Protein forms part of all living plant cells, and is found in seeds and in green and root vegetables in variable small amounts. Cereals form the most important class of seed foods. The whole grain contains, apart from its large proportion of starch, some useful protein in the embryo and outer layers (bran). When flour is milled, the embryo and parts surrounding (therefore most of the protein) are removed. Thus brown flour contains less protein than the wheat, but more protein than white flour.

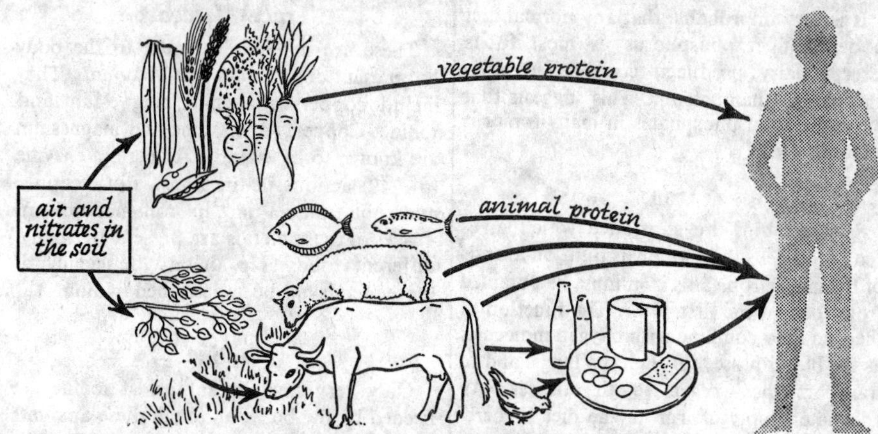

Fig. 3. *SOURCES OF PROTEIN. Plants, using nitrates and other soil nutrients and air, make vegetable proteins. Fish and animals eat plant proteins converting them to animal proteins. Man utilizes both forms.*

The Fate and Value of Protein in the Diet

Proteins are broken down in the gastro-intestinal tract by certain enzymes, with release of amino acids. This takes place partly in the stomach, the process being completed in the small intestine where absorption takes place. It is likely that animal proteins are better absorbed than vegetable proteins—probably because the latter are often in a cellulose covering.

The digested protein passes to the liver where some is built up into new substances or metabolized. The rest passes into the general circulation and then to every tissue in the body. It is then used for:

1. the growth and repair of the body;
2. the production of energy.

As protein is essential for growth, it follows that children and pregnant and nursing women need more than adults who require it for repair and maintenance only. After the above requirements have been fulfilled, any spare protein is used to produce heat and further energy.

The fundamental importance of protein in the diet for growth and repair cannot be overstressed—no other nutrient can be a substitute.

MINERALS

The body contains 19 inorganic mineral substances all of which must come from food. These substances are used for four main purposes:

1. As constituents of bones and teeth (e.g. calcium, phosphorus, and magnesium);
2. As constituents of the varied cells of the body (e.g. iron, phosphorus, sulphur, and potassium);
3. As soluble salts which give to the fluids of the body their composition and their stability, and which are essential for life (e.g. sodium, chloride, and potassium);
4. As agents concerned with release of energy during metabolism (e.g. iron, phosphorus and manganese).

In addition to the substances already mentioned there are a number of other minerals required in very small quantities but which are very essential—notably iodine, copper, and cobalt.

Sodium Chloride

(Common Salt)

All body fluids contain salt, and it is essential for life that the necessary amount should always be accurately maintained. The intake of salt in the diet varies. In general, foods contain relatively little salt. Most of the salt we eat is added at the table or in cooking, or during some stage of preserving or processing the food.

Salt is lost from the body in two ways: in the urine and in the sweat. The loss in the urine is regulated by the kidneys, but there is no control over the amount of sweat loss. However, there is evidence that during adaptation to hot climates, sweat becomes more dilute and so less salt is lost in this way. Extra dietary salt may be needed during this adaptation time, and is necessary when work is done in high temperatures, e.g. by miners in deep pits, by stokers in engine rooms, and by steel workers. If there is a shortage of salt, as for instance in heat exhaustion, a characteristic picture results — muscular cramps, a dry mouth, and mental apathy. There may also be vomiting.

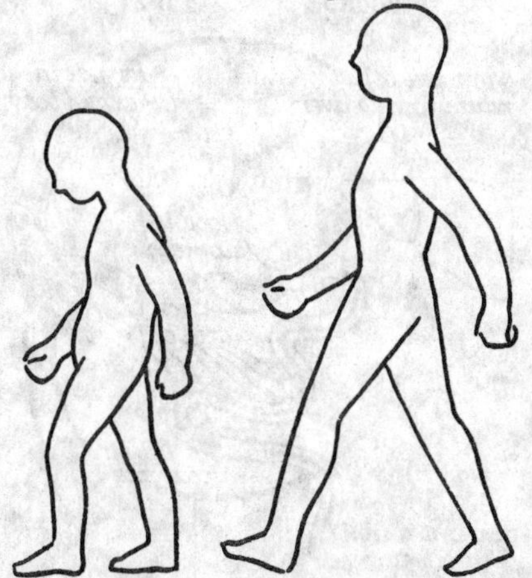

Fig. 4. *THE DIFFERENCE. Without sufficient protein in his food the child cannot grow properly.*

The daily amount of salt needed by an adult is about 4 grams. The average amount eaten daily is about 15 grams. The amount not needed is harmlessly passed out in the urine.

A high salt intake is known to be harmful in congestive cardiac failure, the salt increasing the edema (watery swelling) already present. In this condition a low salt diet is often recommended by the doctor.

Calcium

Calcium has three main functions in the body. It is necessary for:

1. Proper development and growth of bones and teeth;
2. Normal blood clotting;
3. Normal functioning of muscles.

Children need more calcium than adults because there is constant formation of new bones and teeth in childhood. If there is not sufficient calcium in the diet, reduced growth, badly formed teeth, and rickets result.

Expectant and nursing mothers also require extra calcium. The expectant mother is forming the bones of her unborn child, and the lactating mother providing calcium in her milk. If there is insufficient calcium in the diet the mother will draw it from her bone stores, and a condition of osteomalacia in the bones may result.

The main calcium sources are milk, cheese, bread, flour, and green vegetables.

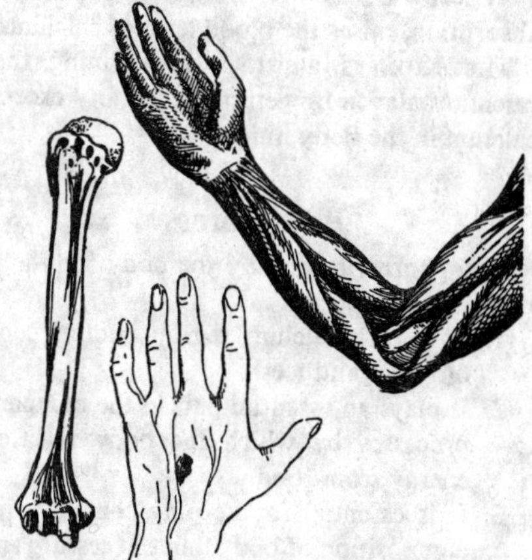

Fig. 5. *CALCIUM is essential for bone growth and development, for blood clotting, and for proper functioning of the muscles.*

Foods providing Calcium

FOOD	MILLIGRAMS PER OZ
Dried skimmed milk	348
Cheese	230
Sardines	113
Liquid milk	34
White bread	29
Herring	28
Egg	17

Absorption of Calcium. There are several factors which are known to influence the absorption of calcium from the intestine into the body. Vitamin D assists the absorption of calcium. Proteins also facilitate this process, probably because the liberated amino acids form soluble calcium salts which are easily absorbed.

Phytic acid and oxalic acid, on the other hand, impede the absorption of calcium. Phytic acid is found in cereal foods such as whole wheat flour and oatmeal, and oxalic acid in rhubarb and spinach. The amounts of these acids in a normal diet, however, are not sufficient to markedly affect calcium absorption.

In certain diseases, e.g. the malabsorption syndrome, fatty acids not absorbed into the body form insoluble 'soaps' with calcium and they are carried (with vitamin D) into the feces. Calcium deficiency results.

Regulation of Calcium Balance. Calcium is stored in bones from which it can be quickly obtained to maintain a constant level in the blood.

Several factors influence the deposition and withdrawal of calcium from the bones. The PARATHYROID GLANDS control the level of blood calcium. Should they become diseased or damaged, the amount of calcium in the blood falls and tetany (muscular spasms) may occur. Rarely, these glands are over-active, the calcium being drawn from the bones and excreted in the urine. Calcium stones may collect in the urinary tract in this condition of hyperparathyroidism.

VITAMIN D, as well as assisting calcium absorption, raises the blood level of calcium.

THE KIDNEYS assist in maintaining the calcium balance by getting rid of any excess calcium in the body fluids.

Phosphorus

Phosphorus is used by the body for three main vital purposes.

1. It is, with calcium, a major constituent of bones and teeth.
2. It plays an essential part in the complex processes by which the body releases energy from food.
3. It is essential for keeping constant the composition of body fluids necessary for the continuance of life.

Thus phosphorus is concerned in the life of all body cells.

Foods providing Phosphorus

FOOD	MILLIGRAMS PER OZ
Cheese	155
Liver	89
Kidney	74
Egg	62
Milk	28
Cabbage	18
Oatmeal	108
Potato	11

It is very improbable that any normal diet is deficient in phosphorus as most foods (except dairy products) contain far more phosphorus than calcium. This suggests that the addition of phosphates in many tonics is unnecessary.

Iron

Hemoglobin, the substance which gives red blood cells their color, is built on a basis of the metal iron. This iron must be obtained from food in the first place. The function of the iron is to combine with oxygen molecules as the blood passes through the lungs, and to transport the oxygen to the tissues. An adequate supply of iron in the diet is therefore essential to health. In fact, a deficiency of iron is a common cause of ill health in many parts of the world.

Once iron is absorbed from food, it is lost only slowly. The red blood cells, which contain the iron, have a life of about sixteen weeks, then the cell breaks up and the released iron is used again. But iron can be lost from the body in two ways: by the excretion of worn cells of the alimentary and urinary tracts and unwanted bile, and when bleeding occurs. Replacement from food is therefore necessary. If not enough iron is eaten in the food then anemia results.

Two points must, however, be observed where the nutritional significance of anemia is concerned.

1. Certain types of anemia may be due to causes other than iron iron deficiency.
2. Once a person becomes anemic he needs larger amounts of iron than can be supplied in food. This is best given as inorganic iron in medicine.

Foods containing Iron

FOOD	MILLIGRAMS PER OZ
Liver, kidney	3·9
Beef	1·1
Eggs	0·9
Mutton	0·6
Raisins	0·5
Peas	0·5
Cabbage	0·3
Potato	0·2

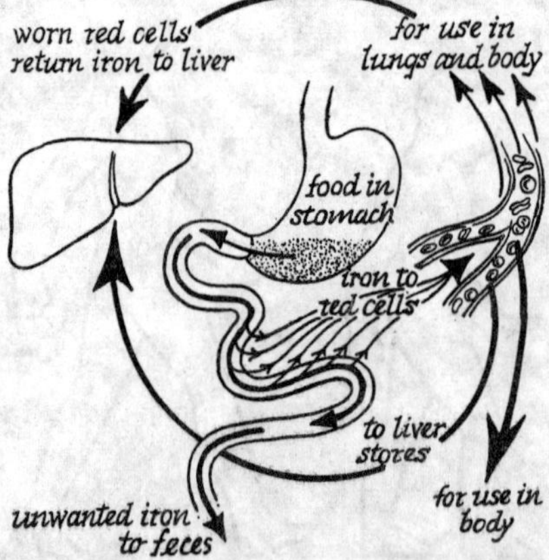

Fig. 6. *IRON. The body wastes but little iron. It re-uses that from worn red blood cells over and over again (see text).*

Trace Elements

These are minerals essential to the body but present only in very small amounts. They include copper, cobalt, zinc, magnesium, and iodine. Copper, cobalt, zinc and magnesium are known to be essential for certain enzyme (p. 249) actions in the body. Both copper and cobalt play a part in iron metabolism. Traces of these metals are present in many different foods. No dietary deficiency of these metals has been described in man.

Iodine

Only very small quantities of iodine are needed by the body, although these amounts are essential. Iodine is concentrated in the thyroid gland and is contained in the thyroid hormone. The activity of this hormone depends on its iodine content.

Foods providing Iodine

- Sea fish and shell fish
- Water
- Vegetables grown where soils contain iodine

The diet becomes deficient in iodine where there is little or no iodine in the soil, as in some parts of Switzerland, America and England. Goiters are likely to result, but they can be prevented by using iodized salt in such areas.

Fluorine

Fluorine is found in bones and teeth, thyroid and skin. The addition of very small amounts of fluorine to drinking water decreases the incidence of dental caries, especially if provided when the teeth of babies

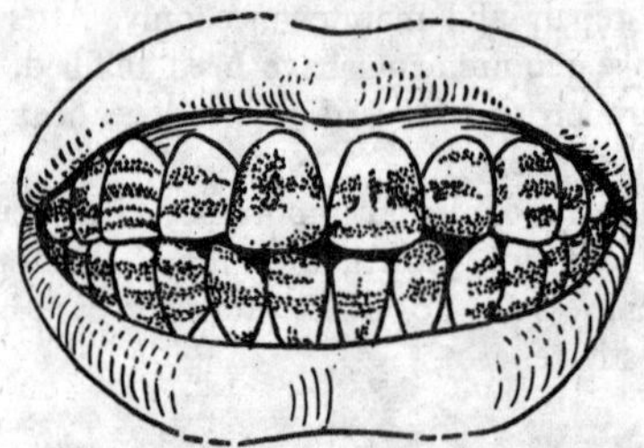

Fig. 7. *FLUORINE MOTTLING. Although minute amounts of fluorine in drinking water strengthen growing children's teeth against caries, even a slight excess will cause permanent mottling of the enamel.*

and young children are developing. As the amount of fluorine in the normal diet is very small, artificial addition to water supplies has been recommended by many dentists.

THE VITAMINS

The vitamins are organic substances essential to the body metabolism. The body cannot make vitamins for itself and so has to obtain them from foodstuffs where they are present in minute amounts.

Certain vitamins are found mainly in fatty foods and are called fat-soluble vitamins, i.e. A, D, E and K. The others are water-soluble vitamins, i.e. the B group and C.

Vitamin A

Vitamin A is found in certain fats and in the fatty parts of foods of animal origin. Some vegetables, e.g. carrots, contain the substance carotene. This is an orange-colored pigment from which animals can make vitamin A. Carotene is thus known as a pro-vitamin or vitamin precursor. Some animals, for example rats, can convert carotene easily into vitamin A. Man is not so efficient in this respect, so vitamin A from animal sources is of more value to him than carotene from vegetable sources. Vitamin A is measured in international units.

Foods containing Vitamin A

ANIMAL SOURCES	INTERNATIONAL UNITS PER OZ
Halibut-liver oil B.P.	850,000
Cod-liver oil (N.H.S.)	20,000
Liver	4,253
Butter	850
Cheese	369
Kidney	284
Eggs	284
Sardines	77
Herrings	43
Milk	32

VEGETABLE SOURCES	INTERNATIONAL UNITS PER OZ
Carrots	5,197c
Spinach	3,686c
Watercress	1,418c
Tomato	851c
Cabbage	255c
Peas	142c

(The letter c indicates that the sole source of vitamin A potency is carotene)

Value of Vitamin A. This vitamin is necessary for the growth of children. It plays a part in the way the eyes perceive light. It also protects surface tissues such as the front of the eyes, and the lining of the respiratory tract, the throat and bronchial tubes.

Vitamin A deficiency results in night blindness and possibly the eye disorders known as xerophthalmia and keratomalacia. Deficiency also causes the skin to be abnormally thickened, giving rise to a condition known as follicular keratosis.

The Vitamin B Group

This group comprises a number of substances often found together in the same foods:

- Thiamine (vitamin B_1, aneurine)
- Riboflavine
- Nicotinic acid (niacin)
- (Cyanocobalamin) vitamin B_{12}
- Pyridoxine
- Pantothenic acid
- Biotin
- Choline
- Paraminobenzoic acid
- Inositol

Thiamine

This substance is unstable at high temperatures so that a large amount may be lost in cooking, canning and processing.

Foods containing Thiamine

FOOD	MILLIGRAMS PER OZ
Dried brewers' yeast	2·75
Pork	0·20
Green peas	0·17
Whole wheat bread	0·12
White bread	0·06
Potato	0·03
Milk	0·01
Sugar	Nil

The function of thiamine is to form a part of the subtle chemistry by means of which a steady and continuous release of energy is obtained from carbohydrates.

Thiamine deficiency results in stunting the growth of children, a special type of neuritis, and in mental changes such as depression and irritability. Extreme deficiency results in the disease of beri-beri (see Deficiency Diseases, p. 398).

Riboflavine

This is a yellow substance possessing a green fluorescence in solution. It is not easily destroyed by heat alone, but is destroyed by heat plus ultraviolet light. Milk should therefore not be left in the sun because in half an hour much of its riboflavine content may be destroyed.

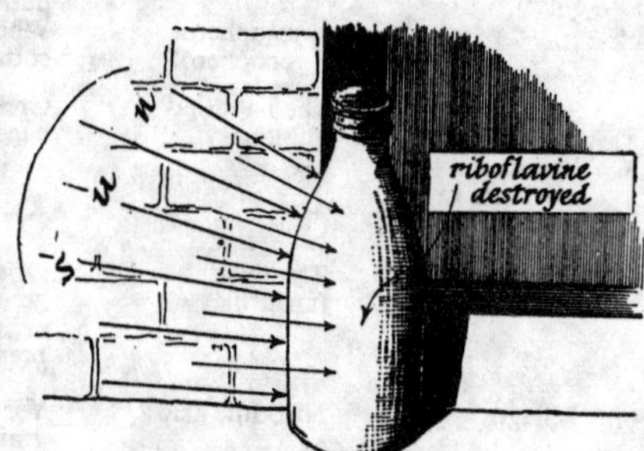

Fig. 8. *DAMAGE BY SUNLIGHT. In half an hour most of the riboflavine content may be destroyed.*

Foods containing Riboflavine

FOOD	MILLIGRAMS PER OZ
Dried brewers' yeast	1·54
Liver	0·85
Meat extract	0·48
Cheese	0·14
Eggs	0·11
Beef	0·07
Milk	0·04

The function of riboflavine is to form a link in the chain of processes through which the body obtains energy from food.

Riboflavine deficiency leads to checking of growth, cracks and sores in the skin and mouth corners, a sore and red tongue (glossitis) and filming of the transparent front of the eye.

Nicotinic Acid

The body converts this substance to its active form—nicotinamide. Nicotinamide can also be formed from one of the amino acids, tryptophan.

Foods containing Nicotinic Acid

FOOD	MILLIGRAMS PER OZ
Meat extract	17·0
Liver, kidney	3·8
Beef	1·3
Bacon	1·1
Wholemeal bread	1·0
Potato	0·3

The function of nicotinic acid is to form another link in the chain of processes through which the body gets energy from food.

Deficiency of nicotinic acid leads to a checking of growth, skin infections, a sore and red tongue (glossitis), and digestive and mental disturbances. Extreme deficiency results in the disease of pellagra, with dementia, dermatitis and severe diarrhea.

Vitamin B_{12}

Unlike other vitamins, vitamin B_{12} contains a metal, cobalt. It is present in milk, meat, eggs, and fish; liver is the richest source. CYANOCOBALAMIN (vitamin B_{12}), and its active form, HYDROXOCOBALAMIN, is involved in the development of red blood cells. It is necessary for growth. Because lack of vitamin B_{12} causes pernicious anemia, hydroxocobalamin (or cyanocobalamin) is used for the treatment of this anemia.

FOLIC ACID. As with vitamin B_{12}, folic acid is essential for the formation and metabolism of normal red blood cells. Without it, the living cell cannot divide. It is present in liver, yeast, leafy green vegetables, and cereals and a mixed diet provides enough for health. But in the extra demands of pregnancy, folic acid is a useful supplement. For this purpose, it is often incorporated with iron in tablets.

The other B vitamins are of biochemical importance, but human deficiences of these have not been reported.

Vitamin C
(Ascorbic Acid)

When planning a diet an adequate supply of vitamin C must be ensured. A diet may be insufficiently provided with this vitamin for two reasons. Firstly, vitamin C occurs almost entirely in vegetable foodstuffs, animal foods contain only very small amounts. Secondly, vitamin C may be easily destroyed by cooking; even if the best methods are used it is difficult not to lose at least half of the total vitamin content of the vegetable or fruit. This destruction is due to the fact that in the vegetable cell there is an enzyme together with the vitamin C. This enzyme is a substance which works with the vitamin in carrying out plant processes. When, however, plant cells are destroyed, either by cooking or by grating, the life of the plant is disrupted and the enzyme destroys the vitamin C. The vitamin content is also lost when plants begin to wilt.

Foods providing Vitamin C

FOOD	MILLIGRAMS PER OZ
Blackcurrants	57
Brussel sprouts (raw)	28
Cauliflower (raw)	20
Cabbage	20
Orange	16
Lemon	14
Grapefruit	11
Potato—new	9
Oct.–Nov.	6
Jan.–Feb.	3
Tomato	7
Apple, plum, pear	1

When seeds, including cereal grains, have sprouted, vitamin C develops in them. When normal sources of vitamin C are unavailable, deficiency can be avoided if dried peas or grains are moistened, allowed to sprout and then eaten in that form. For daily needs eat one orange or a helping of cooked cabbage.

Provided her diet is good the mother's milk provides sufficient vitamin C for her infant. Cows' milk contains a small amount which is, however, easily destroyed in the presence of bright sunlight (as when the bottles are left on a doorstep). It is wise to supplement this source of the vitamin with orange juice or an equivalent (not fruit-flavored cordials) for bottle-fed infants.

Value of Vitamin C. Vitamin C is necessary for the proper formation of the foundation substance that binds together the cells of tissues such as blood capillaries, bone, teeth, and connective tissue. It is also known to play a part in the formation of hemoglobin and in the healing of wounds.

Deficiency of vitamin C leads to checking of growth, susceptibility of the gums and mouth to infection, and slowing of healing of wounds and fractures. Extreme deficiency leads to scurvy with swollen and bleeding gums, and hemorrhage into the skin and elsewhere.

Vitamin D

The body obtains this vitamin from two sources: from food and from sunlight.

Foods containing Vitamin D

FOOD	INTERNATIONAL UNITS PER OZ
Cod-liver oil	2,300
Sardines	280
Herrings	250
Eggs	17
Butter	17
Cheese	4
Milk	0·1–0·7

THE VITAMINS

	Name	*Solubility*	*Associated Deficiency Disease*	*Chemical Name*	*Principal Sources*
	Vitamin A	Fat soluble	Night blindness; Xerophthalmia	Carotene	Halibut-liver oil; cod-liver oil; sheep's liver; butter; spinach; carrot; red-palm oil; apricots; kale.
	„ D	„ „	Rickets	Calciferol	[Reaction of sunlight on human skin]. Halibut-liver oil; cod-liver oil; sardine; herring oil; fortified margarine; egg yolk; butter.
	„ E	„ „	*	α-tocopherol β-tocopherol	Wheat germ; rice germ; yeast; cottonseed oil; green leaves.
	„ K	„ „	Special bleeding disorders, e.g. hemorrhage of newborn or of diseased liver	The naphtha-quinones	Green vegetables, especially cabbage group; tomatoes; egg yolk.
B	„ B_1	Water soluble	Beri-beri	Thiamine (aneurine)	Dried brewers' yeast; cereal germ; meat (esp. pork); fish; eggs; potatoes; peas; wholemael bread; beans; egg yolk.
	P-P	„ „	Pellagra	Nicotinic acid	Yeast; liver; wheat germ; whole grain; meat extracts.
B_2	B_6	„ „	Pellagra in rats	Pyridoxine	Fish (esp. salmon); cereals; molasses; beans and peas; bananas; potatoes.
	G	„ „		Riboflavine	Yeast; kidney; liver; egg white; milk.
	Pantothenic acid		Graying of fur in rats	Pantothenic acid	In all foods, but rich in yeast; liver; egg yolk.
	B_{12}		Pernicious Anemia	Cyanocobalamin	Molds *(Streptomyces)*; liver; kidney; heart; fish; egg yolk.
	„ C	„ „	Scurvy	Ascorbic acid	Blackcurrants; paprika; orange juice; cabbage; spinach; tomatoes.

OTHER VITAMINS

Name	Associated Deficiency Disease	Chemical Name	Principal Sources
Vitamin H (now known to be a B vitamin)	Dermatitis in rats	Biotin	Yeast; liver; raw egg white.
Vitamin P (used in 1937; now identity uncertain)	Fragility of capillaries	Citrin (sometimes confused with hesperidin and rutin)	Lemon peel.

* Despite extensive investigations to date in many parts of the world, there are no convincing results to support the therapeutic usefulness of vitamin E in any disease.

Sunlight acting on the skin can cause the formation of vitamin D in the body itself. Thus, if children receive enough sun on their bodies the amount of vitamin D needed from food is reduced. Similarly, sunlight, acting on certain foods which do not contain vitamin D, can cause its formation.

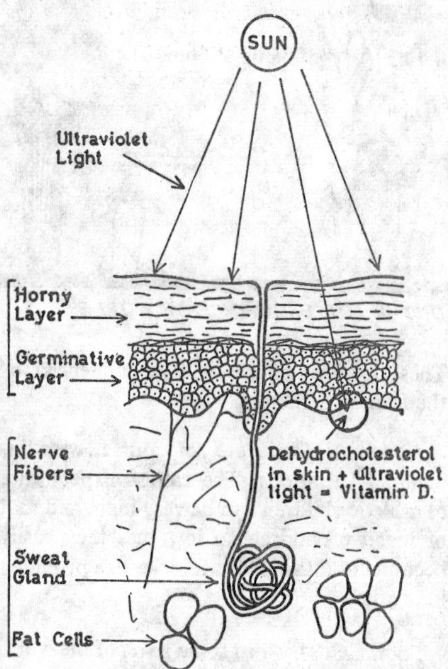

Fig. 9. *SUNLIGHT ON THE SKIN. The ultraviolet rays stimulate the making of vitamin D.*

Value of Vitamin D. This substance is concerned in the laying down of calcium and phosphorus in bones, and in the absorption of calcium into the body. Thus vitamin D is of special importance to infants and children whose bones are growing and developing, and to expectant mothers in whom the bones of a fetus are developing. Adults also require a small amount of the vitamin though not as much as the groups mentioned. Deficiency of vitamin D in the diet may lead to rickets in children and to osteomalacia in adults.

Vitamin E

This is found in milk and wheat germ and in the small amount of fat present in green vegetables. It acts by preventing the oxidation of certain substances in foods. It was thought to play a part in human fertility but there is no conclusive evidence that this is so.

Vitamin K

Vitamin K is found in green plants such as cabbage and green peas and in animal tissues generally. It is essential for normal blood clotting. Deficiency is unlikely in a person eating a well-balanced diet.

WATER AND FLUIDS

Water itself is not regarded as a nutrient as it does not produce any calories, but the need of the body for water is second only to its need for air. Approximately two-thirds of the body weight is made up of water.

The body is continuously balancing the amount of water taken in with the amount excreted.

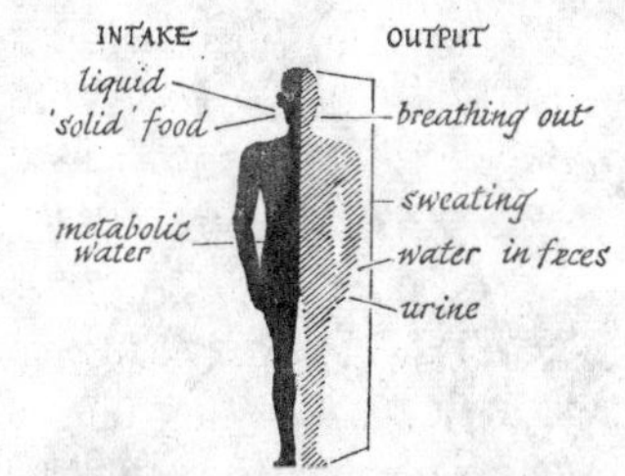

Fig. 10. *WATER INTAKE AND OUTPUT. Solid food is usually damp; metabolic water is released during the chemical breakdown of food.*

In a normal adult doing moderate exercise (either as a job or a sport) the intake and output are approximately equal. If too much is drunk the excess passes out through the kidneys; if too little, a state of dehydration occurs. In a temperate climate at least 1½ pints of water or watery fluid should be drunk daily.

DIGESTION OF FOOD

The foods which are taken into the mouth go through many chemical changes in the various portions of the long digestive tract before they are in a suitable state to be absorbed into the blood, largely through the walls of the small intestine, the unwanted residue being excreted as feces..

The process is described and illustrated in the Physiology section, p. 249.

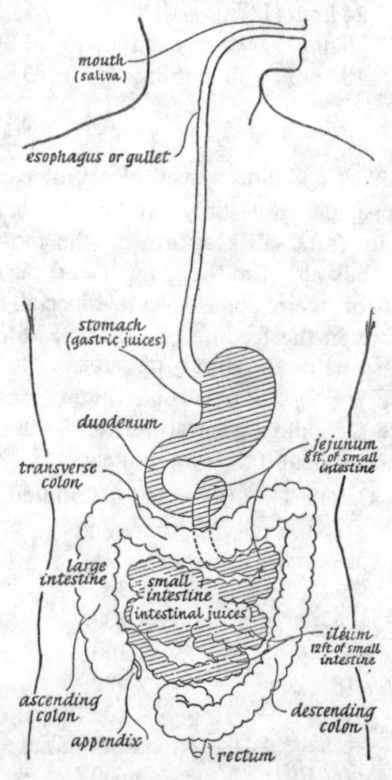

Fig. 11. *THE DIGESTIVE TRACT*

ENERGY AND CALORIES

It has been mentioned earlier that animals get their energy from food and that each of the three nutrients, carbohydrate, fat, and protein can provide this energy. The energy value of food is measured in units of heat known as the large calorie. The average values are as follows:

1 gram of carbohydrate produces 4 cal.
1 gram of fat ” 9 cal.
1 gram of protein ” 4 cal.

(A large cube of white sugar produces about 15 cal).

Energy Value of Some Common Foods

FOOD	CALORIES PER OZ
Cooking fat or lard	253
Butter	211
Cheese	117
Sugar	108
White flour	100
Beef	89
Potato	21
Banana	21
Milk	17
Apple	12
Beer	10
Orange	10
Lettuce	3

The energy produced in the body from food may be utilized in the following ways:

1. In mechanical work (no energy from food is needed for mental work);
2. In growth;
3. In maintaining the body temperature; and
4. In promoting the activity of the vital organs, e.g. the heart beat, breathing, and the circulation of the blood.

Energy for Basal Metabolism

The energy necessary for maintaining body temperature and for the activity of the heart and other vital organs when the body is at rest is called the basal metabolism (see also section on Physiology, p. 249).

The following factors affect the amount of energy expended for basal metabolism:

1. BODY SURFACE. The number of calories needed for basal (as for other) metabolism is proportional to the body surface. The body weight itself can be an accurate enough guide.
2. AGE. The basal metabolic rate is low at birth but rises rapidly to a high level during early childhood. Then it falls to reach the adult level. After the early twenties the energy expenditure decreases regularly till old age is reached.

EFFECT OF MAN'S SIZE AND AGE ON HIS DAILY BASAL METABOLIC CALORIE REQUIREMENT

Person	*Age*	*Height (in.)*	*Weight (lb.)*	*Basal Metabolism*
Schoolboy	18	71	156	1,986
Army Cadet	20	70	150	1,757
Worker	35–39	67	134	1,573
Retired Man	66	67	134	1,431

3. SEX. Women have a lower basal metabolic rate than men owing to their different size and shape, and to the larger proportion of body fat.

4. STATE OF HEALTH. Certain diseases increase or decrease energy requirements: fevers, for example, quicken the metabolic rate.

5. STARVATION. The basal metabolic rate becomes reduced. This serves as an automatic reduction in the body's daily need. Thus the basal metabolic needs of an adequately nourished man amount to 1,550 calories; after a fast of three weeks or more, these needs may be reduced to 1,000 calories. Hence prolonged starvation can reduce the basal metabolism by as much as 30 per cent.

From the above we see that the amount of energy used just to keep the body alive varies from person to person, and is dependent on the factors outlined.

Energy for Everyday Activities

Apart from the energy necessary for basal metabolism, Man needs to use additional energy every time he moves or performs any action. A person who is very active and who has to do strenuous manual work will require more calories than one who may have a sedentary job, or who is lazy.

Below are two lists of the approximate number of calories needed per hour for various activities and occupations.

OCCUPATION	CALORIES PER HOUR
Sleeping	0
Sitting	15
Standing	20
Dressing	33
Walking fast	215
Playing violin	162
Cycling	396
Swimming	576
Skiing uphill	1,015

WORK	CALORIES PER HOUR
Domestic work	
Dishwashing	84
Mopping	210
Bedmaking	456
Sedentary Work	
Writing	20
Typing	30
Tailoring	45
Light Work	
Shoemaking	90
Carpentry	140
Light engineering	140
Very Heavy Work	
Coal mining	320
Woodcutting	380

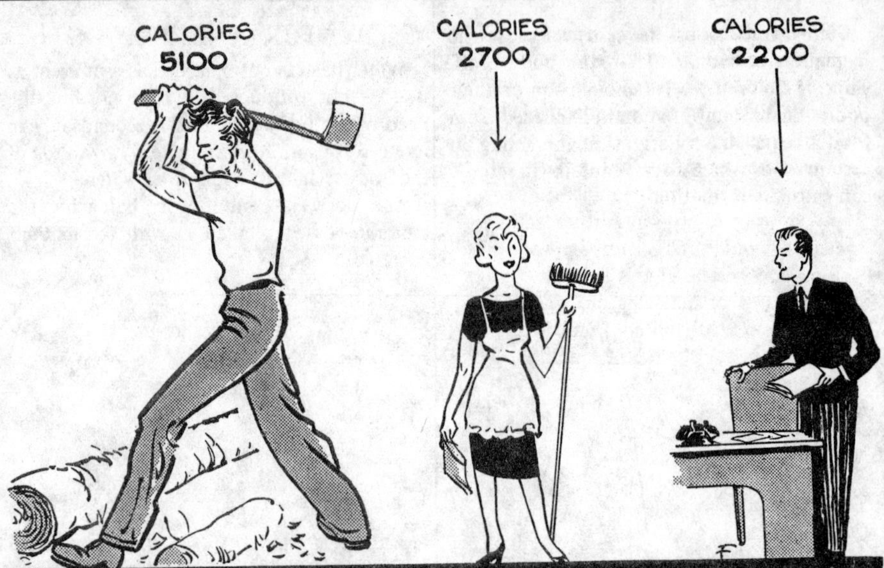

Fig. 12. *THE CALORIE REQUIREMENTS DIFFER FOR EACH TYPE OF WORKER*

We can therefore work out the energy expenditure, and thus the calorie needs of different people performing various activities and doing jobs of work.

	CALORIES PER DAY
Housewife	
24 hours basal	1,500
8 hours everyday activity	360
8 hours working in the home	880
	2,740
Male Clerk	
24 hours basal	1,700
8 hours everyday activity	360
8 hours writing	160
	2,220
Woodcutter	
24 hours basal	1,700
8 hours everyday activity	360
8 hours woodcutting	3,040
	5,100

Children. Children need plenty of calories to provide, not only for their vigorous activity (after all they are on the move all day), but also for the growth and development of their bodies. It is especially important in the feeding of children, however, to ensure that the supply of calories does not come merely from carbohydrate foods because the child's general nutrition will suffer if proteins and fats are too meager.

Calorie Requirements for Children

AGE (in years)	CALORIES PER DAY
1 – 3	1,300
4 – 6	1,700
7 – 9	2,100
10–12	2,500
13–15	3,100 (boys)
	2,600 (girls)
16–19	3,600 (males)
	2,400 (females)

These average figures will be influenced by the following factors.

ACTIVITY. There are, of course, wide individual variations. The caloric expenditure of athletic children can be very high, and that of inactive children so low that they easily become fat if too many calories are provided in the diet.

SOCIAL CUSTOM. In some parts of the world social customs restrict the activities of women, and this may apply from the age of ten or so. On the other hand, in some countries, children are put to work long before growth is complete and their supply of calories should be increased according to the work they do.

GROWTH AND BODY SIZE. The actual weight of the child should *not* be used as a guide. An undersized child may need more calories than one who is well grown and well developed.

CLIMATE. In general, everyone eats less food in a hot climate than in a cold one.

Pregnancy. Extra calories are needed both for the mother herself and for the growth of the fetus and placenta. The mother is heavier and her basal metabolism rises during pregnancy. The extra needs can be covered in two ways—more food and less physical activity. A poor woman with several children will find it difficult to rest—she will have to eat more—whereas a better off woman bearing her first child will be able to cut down her physical activities. On an average, a total of 40,000 extra calories should be allowed for each 9-month pregnancy.

Lactation. The nursing mother obviously needs extra calories otherwise her health and weight will suffer in order to provide milk for her baby. An allowance of 1,000 extra calories per day is recommended for a 6-month lactation.

TOTAL DIETARY NEEDS

Having discussed each separate nutrient and the production of energy from calories we see that for proper health and efficiency different diets must contain adequate amounts of all the nutrients.

The optimum nutritional requirements for different classes of individuals are shown in the following table. No further addition of nutrients would produce any improvement in the general health. If less than the optimum requirements of nutrients are supplied by a diet, an individual will not immediately suffer in health but his efficiency and well-being will be affected.

Search for New Foods

With an ever increasing world population and the threat of world-wide food shortage, the search for new sources of nutrients is essential. A few promising sources are algae, seaweeds, and green leaf proteins.

Chlorella. This is a green alga forming the scum on the surface of ponds. Like all green plants it grows by using the energy of the sun's rays, and can make carbohydrate and protein from carbon dioxide, water, and inorganic nitrogen. Essential nutrients could be extracted from chlorella grown in the laboratory, enabling man to be less dependent on food from the farm and on climatic conditions. But how to make this type of food appetizing has not yet been solved.

Green Leaves and Young Grass. The cow eats grass and turns it into milk. But this is not an efficient process as three-quarters of the protein present in the grass is lost for human use. A process has been devised for extracting protein from leaves and grass in the factory. The product obtained is green, almost tasteless, and has the consistency of crumbly cheese. It could be used as an additive to foodstuffs poor in protein.

Yeasts. By growing certain strains of yeasts in a nutrient such as a molasses solution, large quantities of fat can be produced.

SUMMARY OF DIETARY ALLOWANCES

	Calories	*Protein*	*Calcium*	*Iron*	*Vitamin A and Carotene**	*Thiamine (Aneurine)*	*Vitamin C†*	*Ribo-flavine*	*Nico-tinic Acid*	*Vitamin D*
		G.	*G.*	*Mg.*	*I.U.*	*Mg.*	*Mg.*	*Mg.*	*Mg.*	*I.U.*
Man										
Sedentary	2500	69	0·8	12	5000	1·0	20	1·5	10	—
Moderately active	3000	82	0·8	12	5000	1·2	20	1·8	12	—
Very active	4250	117	0·8	12	5000	1·7	20	2·6	17	—
Woman										
Sedentary	2100	58	0·8	12	5000	0·8	20	1·3	8	—
Moderately active	2500	69	0·8	12	5000	1·0	20	1·5	10	—
Very active	3750	103	0·8	12	5000	1·5	—	2·2	15	—
Pregnancy (latter half)	2750	96	1·5	15	6000	1·1	40	1·6	11	600
Lactation	3000	105	2·0	15	8000	1·2	50	1·8	12	800
Children up to 12 years										
Under 1 year	800	28	1·0	6	3000	0·3	10	0·5	3	800
1–3 years	1300	46	1·0	7	3000	0·5	15	0·8	5	400–800
4–6 years	1600	56	1·0	8	3000	0·6	15	1·0	6	400
7–9 years	1950	68	1·0	10	3000	0·8	20	1·2	8	400
10–12 years	2500	86	1·2	12	3000	1·0	25	1·5	10	400
Children over 12 years										
Girls—13–15 years	2750	96	1·3	15	3000	1·1	30	1·6	11	400
16–20 years	2500	88	1·0	15	5000	1·0	30	1·5	10	400
Boys—13–15 years	3150	110	1·4	15	3000	1·3	30	1·9	13	400
16–20 years	3400	119	1·4	15	5000	1·4	30	2·1	14	400

* Figures are for a mixture of Vitamin A and Carotene.
† There is considerable controversy regarding these figures.

OBESITY, MALNUTRITION, AND OTHER NUTRITIONAL DISORDERS

Food Calories and Obesity

If nutrients are eaten in excess of the calorie output of work, they are converted into body fat. The most fattening foods are those which contain most calories. These are concentrated foods containing little waste and high proportions of carbohydrates and fat, such as pastry, suet pudding, sweet cakes, and sweets.

People become fat because they have large appetites and lead relatively inactive lives. Weight can be lost by eating foods with a lower calorific value, e.g. raw apples instead of apple tart, squash or cauliflower instead of potatoes, and also by increasing regular bodily activity, e.g. walking instead of riding in car or bus (see diseases of Metabolism, p. 391). It is well to remember certain facts about calorie expenditure during exercise. If a man walks for 20 minutes he uses up 70 to 80 calories; if he is thirsty and drinks half a pint of beer, the beer puts back the calories he has used in walking. He should not therefore be surprised if his weight does not change!

Malnutrition

Inadequate amounts of some nutrients in the diet lead to malnutrition, and an inadequate total quantity leads to undernutrition or subnutrition. Starvation is an extreme degree of undernourishment.

The food supply of a country is dependent on social, economic and agricultural factors. In some countries the land and farming development cannot keep pace with the population increase (as in the Far East, Near East and Africa). A state of chronic semi-starvation with episodes of acute famine therefore exists in some parts of these countries. Second to agricultural difficulties is poverty: other factors include lack of cooking facilities, lack of leisure, poor transport, ignorance, inclination and religious customs. Even in Great Britain, some of these factors are the cause of cases of malnutrition that are seen, even today, in old age pensioners living on their own.

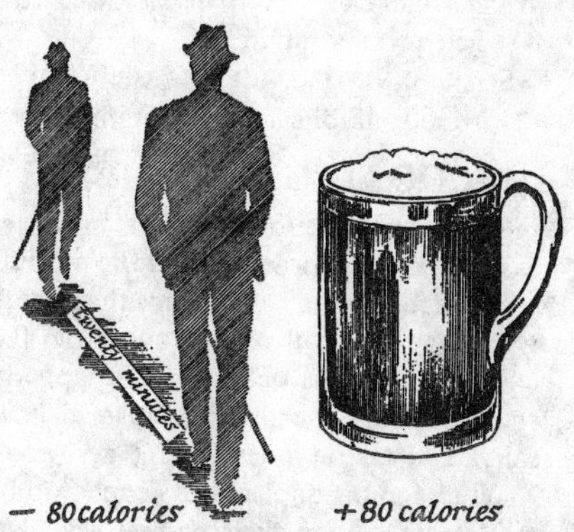

Fig. 13. *LOSS AND GAIN. 80 calories are lost after a short walk; 80 calories are put back in half a pint of beer.*

The diet of the poor in the underdeveloped countries is usually based on one starchy component. Rice is an example. It is noteworthy that if rice is milled much of its vitamin B content (and other nutrient substances) is lost in the portions which are milled off. Beri-beri is very likely to result if this 'refined' rice is used as a basic diet. However, if the unhusked rice is parboiled the vitamin B is fixed into the rice grain and is more difficult to remove at a later stage.

In other tropical diets, the principal food may be cassava or yams. These starches contain very little protein and communities dependent on them are likely to show evidence of protein malnutrition.

Kwashiorkor

This is due to inadequate protein intake. It usually occurs in children after they have been weaned and put on to a diet of starchy soft foods at a time when protein is much needed for growth.

Kwashiorkor is common in Africa as well as Ceylon and India. The disease is characterized by wasting, swelling of the soft tissues of the body (edema), mental apathy, failure to grow, and liver damage (see also Diseases of Young Children, p.516).

Other Nutritional Disorders

Primary disorders of nutrition, or, as they are also called, deficiency diseases, are due to lack of a specific nutritional substance—usually a vitamin or mineral—in the diet. These disorders are dealt with more fully in the section on Deficiency Diseases, p. 397. Systemic diseases in which the body is unable to cope adequately with certain food substances because of a fault in the make-up of the body tissues are known as Diseases of Metabolism, e.g. diabetes mellitus, and are dealt with beginning on page 391.

Deficiency Diseases. The common disorders are:

RICKETS: mainly due to deficiency of calcium in children.

OSTEOMALACIA: an adult form of rickets.

SCURVY: due to deficiency of vitamin C.

BERI-BERI: due to deficiency of vitamin B.

PELLAGRA: due to deficiency of protein and of some vitamin B substances.

KERATOMALACIA: eye disease due to deficiency of vitamin A.

SOME ANEMIAS: due to deficiency of iron; or of folic acid and vitamin C.

COOKING AND MEALS

The process of cooking causes, in almost all cases, a direct improvement in the nutritional value of foods. It also performs the important secondary function of improving the flavor and attractiveness of foods. The appetizing smell of well-cooked food causes a flow of saliva and gastric juice, and the desire to eat.

When food is unpleasant, people will often eat less of it than their bodies need. Nutritional health will suffer if insufficient nutrients are absorbed, and insufficient amounts will certainly be absorbed if too little is eaten.

Cooking Methods

Food can only be cooked by the application of heat in the following ways:

1. Baking, roasting, broiling and grilling require the use of dry heat applied directly to the food.
2. Boiling and steaming require heat applied by means of hot water.
3. Frying calls for the high degree of heat available from hot fat.

Effect of Cooking on Separate Nutrients

1. **Carbohydrate.** In order to be properly absorbed in the digestive tract, starch must be cooked. The starch in uncooked flour, potato, rice or oatmeal, is, as has already been described on p. 65, enclosed in starch granules which are highly resistant to the human digestive juices. When heat is applied in any of the methods of cooking—the baking of flour for bread, the boiling of potatoes, or the frying of a flour batter with fish—the starch granules swell up and burst and the starch itself becomes gelatinized, in which condition it can be completely digested and absorbed.

2. **Protein.** The application of heat to proteins causes coagulation which is most strikingly demonstrated by the change in the white of a boiled egg.

A second effect of heat on many proteins is shrinking. During broiling, for example, a steak shows a pronounced shrinkage due to contraction of the protein of the muscle fibres.

The digestibility of moderately cooked protein is, in general, greater than that of raw protein. For example, the absorption of raw egg is low. Excessive exposure to heat, however, will eventually reduce the nutritive value of protein.

3. **Fat.** Heating fat melts it and, if overheating occurs, the fat becomes charred, producing fatty acids and acrolein.

4. **Mineral Substances**

(a) CALCIUM. The effect of cooking may work both ways on calcium in foods. It is not, however, a factor of any great importance. In the case of milk, for example, heat may cause a slight reduction in the availability of calcium to the body, whereas in cereals the small amount of calcium present may become more available.

An indirect effect of cooking on the amount of calcium in foods is the effect of the calcium in hard cooking water. If greens are boiled in hard water, sufficient calcium may become incorporated in them to double the amount they originally contained.

(b) IRON. In general, cooking tends to increase the ease with which the body can absorb the iron from foods. A second beneficial aspect is the increase in dietary iron due to amounts picked up from cooking water and utensils. On the other hand, there may be certain losses of iron during the cooking of meat if juices containing iron are allowed to escape.

(c) SALT. Salt (sodium chloride) and other soluble mineral substances are lost from foods when they are boiled. This is of little nutritional significance if salt is added during cooking.

5. **Vitamins**

(a) **Vitamin A** and **Vitamin D.** Baking and boiling have no effect on vitamin A or vitamin D but, in frying in a shallow pan, the additional heat plus the free access to air often causes destruction of the vitamin A activity of the fried food.

(b) **Thiamine (Aneurine).** A proportion of the thiamine in foods may be destroyed during cooking for the following reasons:

(i) Although thiamine can stand reasonable degrees of heat, it is destroyed at higher temperatures, e.g. during the baking of biscuits.

(ii) Thiamine is destroyed by baking soda. There is little loss during the baking of yeast buns or bread.

(iii) Since thiamine is soluble in water a proportion is lost in the cooking water during boiling.

(c) **Riboflavine; Nicotinic Acid.** Although these vitamins are susceptible to high degrees of heat and are also soluble in water, losses are small during the ordinary process of cooking. Unusually vigorous treatment, such as, for example, pressure cooking or the 'corning' of beef causes losses of riboflavine and of nicotinic acid.

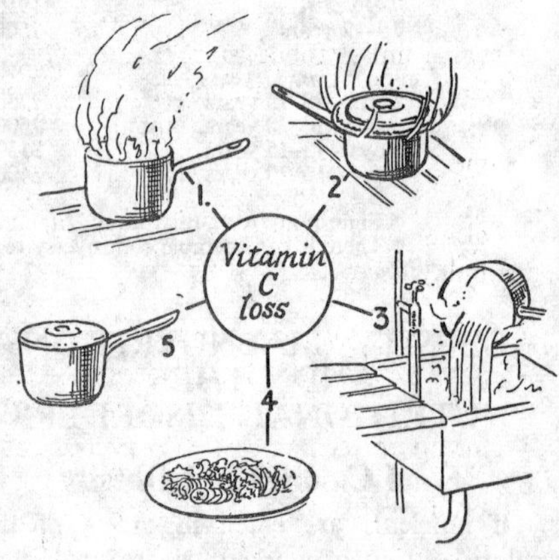

Fig. 14. *VITAMIN C is quickly lost from fruits and vegetables in five ways (see below).*

(d) **Vitamin C.** Cooking is essential to make potatoes, often the most important dietary source of vitamin C, available to the body. But during the cooking a large proportion of the vitamin is destroyed by the heat.

Factors causing loss of vitamin C:

(i) Prolonged heat (long cooking).

(ii) Heat in the presence of air (keeping meals hot).

(iii) Vitamin C is very easily soluble in water (it is lost when cooking liquors are discarded).

(iv) Vitamin C is quickly destroyed by plant enzymes. In the intact leaves or fruits the cell walls protect the vitamin C from the enzymes, but when the green vegetable or fruit is chopped up, the enzyme begins to destroy the vitamin. The enzyme, however, is made inactive by hot water (60°C or above) so that fruits and vegetables placed immediately in boiling water lose the least amount of the vitamin.

(v) Copper in traces from utensils, etc., causes destruction of the vitamin.

METHOD OF COOKING	LOSS OF VITAMIN C
1. Potatoes boiled in their skins	15 per cent
2. Potatoes baked in their skins	20 per cent
3. Potatoes fried	30 per cent
4. Potatoes boiled after peeling	50 per cent

Soup, Stock, and Jellies

Stock is commonly made by boiling meat bones in water but is of almost no nutritional value. The hot water only extracts a small amount of fat and gelatin from the bone marrow and a small quantity of extractives which provide flavor and cause the digestive juices to flow. Stock does, however, provide a certain amount of riboflavine and nicotinic acid.

Stock and Soup cannot be of substantial value unless foods supplying the nutrients—carbohydrates, fats, proteins, minerals or vitamins—are put into them. If, however, meat, vegetables, barley and peas are put into soup it can be of substantial nutritional value although it always remains a comparatively bulky food.

Gelatin, which is a protein, lacks the essential amino acid tryptophan, and contains only minute quantities of some others. The maximum amount of jelly which could be conveniently eaten in one day would be about 1 pint. This would contain about 1 oz of gelatin which would only provide about 110 calories. The nutritional value of jelly, be it calves' foot, aspic, or commercial jellies can thus be said to be negligible. As a pleasant variation to the diet of convalescents, it is useful but the nutrient value then usually depends on the sugar which has been added.

Salads

The loss of about 75 per cent of the vitamin C in green vegetables is almost inevitable during the course of cooking. This loss can be almost completely avoided by eating the vegetables raw in the form of salads. It is, however, important to remember the quantitative aspect of nutrition before recommending the use of salads as a diet.

VEGETABLE	VITAMIN C
1. A convenient serving of lettuce weighs 1 oz and provides	4 mg.
2. A convenient serving of raw cabbage weighs 1 oz and provides	20 mg.
3. A convenient serving of cooked cabbage weighs 6 oz and provides	30 mg.

It can be seen that the consumption of a substantial helping of cooked greens is a better source of vitamin C (and a very much better source of vitamin A) than a serving of raw greens, because the raw vegetable is very much bulkier to eat. Most leafy vegetables are also good sources of riboflavine, carotene, and calcium.

The chief nutritive value of vegetables and fruits in salads is in their supply of carotene (from carrots, endive, etc.) and of vitamin C (from tomatoes, rutabagas, etc.).

Meat Extracts; Yeast Extracts

Meat Extracts provide little nutriment but plenty of flavoring which is useful for stimulating the flow of gastric juice before a meal is eaten. They also contain substantial amounts of nicotinic acid and riboflavine.

Yeast Extracts contain high concentrations of all the B vitamins, and their meaty flavor is very useful in making meals appetizing.

Meals

For everyday purposes a meal can be defined as the amount of food which can be eaten at one sitting and which provides 200 calories or more. There are no fixed rules about the number of meals that should be eaten each day since much depends on the type of work to be done. Experiments have shown that bodily efficiency in general is best maintained on four to six meals during the waking hours rather than two or three. But this does not mean large meals. In fact, United Nations experts state that most American dinners are too heavy for their eaters, whether the dinner is taken at midday or in the evening. In Western countries in general, over-eating is too often a status symbol but it will inevitably damage health.

The amount of nutrients taken at each meal will vary greatly but it is the total daily intake of each nutrient which matters in assessing the health needs of each individual.

Breakfast. As the efficiency of the muscles is lowest in the morning before food is eaten, it is advisable to start the day with a breakfast before going to work. Indeed, better work is done when a cooked breakfast has been eaten. A boiled egg with two slices of bread and butter may be adequate for the office worker, but cereal, eggs and bacon, and several slices of bread and butter and marmalade may be required for the youth or the laborer. All children need a good breakfast before going to school.

Mid-morning Snack. This small meal does not need to provide many calories. Milk or a milk-containing drink, fruit, or a sandwich should suffice, otherwise appetite for the main meal is lessened.

Lunch or Supper. Like the dinner meal, this provides a number of protective foodstuffs, and the proteins, fats, and carbohydrates should all be represented.

Dinner. The main dish should contain a protein, some fat, cooked vegetables or salad, with a sweet course to follow. Soup and coffee are optional, and will partly depend on the season of the year and the amount of fluid consumed for snacks. Protein and carbohydrate should both be eaten at this meal.

[illegible] again at a [illegible] supper had when the previous [illegible] [illegible] [illegible] minutes. There are no fixed rules about the number of meals that should be eaten each day [illegible] each individual [illegible] type of work to be done. Experiments have shown that bodily efficiency is usually better maintained if the food is eaten as six meals during the waking hours rather than two or three. This does not mean more meals, but rather [illegible] between [illegible] [illegible]. American dinner [illegible] to [illegible] [illegible] whether the dinner [illegible] as [illegible] [illegible] every day [illegible] each [illegible] [illegible] is often [illegible] but a pleasant [illegible] healthy.

The amount of nutrients that each meal should [illegible] will vary greatly with the time of day, [illegible] of each meal [illegible] which matters in expressing the [illegible] needs of each individual.

Breakfast. As the majority of the [illegible] [illegible] in the morning before [illegible] [illegible] [illegible] [illegible] the day will [illegible] [illegible] [illegible] [illegible] better [illegible] when [illegible] breakfast [illegible] [illegible]. A [illegible] egg [illegible] slices of bread and butter may be adequate for [illegible] [illegible] butter [illegible] [illegible] [illegible] of bread and butter [illegible] [illegible] [illegible] [illegible] [illegible] [illegible] [illegible] [illegible] [illegible] before going to school.

Mid-morning snack. This [illegible] [illegible] to provide [illegible] [illegible]. Milk or a [illegible] drink [illegible] or a sandwich [illegible] [illegible] [illegible] [illegible] and [illegible] [illegible].

Lunch or [illegible]. [illegible] this provides a quantity of protein [illegible] [illegible] [illegible] [illegible] [illegible] [illegible] [illegible] for [illegible].

Dinner. [illegible] dish should contain protein [illegible] vegetables [illegible] [illegible] [illegible] [illegible] [illegible] [illegible] [illegible] [illegible] and [illegible] [illegible] [illegible] year and [illegible] [illegible] of [illegible] [illegible] [illegible] [illegible] concentrate [illegible] both be [illegible] at [illegible] [illegible].

[illegible] [illegible] to [illegible] and [illegible] [illegible] [illegible] [illegible] [illegible] [illegible] [illegible] [illegible] [illegible] [illegible] [illegible] added.

[illegible]

The [illegible] of [illegible] [illegible] [illegible] [illegible] [illegible] [illegible] [illegible] [illegible] during the course of cooking [illegible] [illegible] [illegible] [illegible] [illegible] [illegible] vegetables [illegible] [illegible] [illegible] form of [illegible] [illegible] however [illegible] [illegible] the [illegible] [illegible] [illegible] [illegible] [illegible] [illegible] a diet.

[illegible]	[illegible]
[illegible] [illegible] [illegible] [illegible] [illegible]	[illegible]
[illegible] [illegible] [illegible] [illegible]	[illegible]
[illegible] [illegible] [illegible] [illegible]	[illegible]
[illegible] [illegible] [illegible] [illegible]	[illegible]
[illegible] [illegible]	60 mg

[illegible] [illegible] [illegible] the consumption of [illegible].

The [illegible] value of vegetables are [illegible] [illegible] [illegible] [illegible] [illegible] [illegible] [illegible] [illegible] [illegible] [illegible].

[illegible] [illegible] and [illegible]

[illegible] [illegible] [illegible] [illegible] [illegible] [illegible] [illegible] [illegible] [illegible] [illegible] [illegible] [illegible] [illegible] [illegible] [illegible] [illegible] [illegible].

[illegible] [illegible] contain [illegible] [illegible] [illegible] [illegible] [illegible] [illegible] [illegible].

[illegible]

[illegible] [illegible] [illegible] [illegible] [illegible] [illegible] [illegible].

[illegible] vitamin C is quickly destroyed by [illegible] [illegible] in the later stages of [illegible] in boiling water [illegible] [illegible] least amount of [illegible].

[illegible] copper [illegible] [illegible] from utensils [illegible] causes destruction of the vitamin.

[illegible] [illegible] cooking	[illegible] of vitamin C
1. [illegible] [illegible] [illegible]	[illegible] per cent
2. Potatoes baked in their skins	[illegible] per cent
3. [illegible] [illegible]	30 per cent
4. Potatoes [illegible] after peeling	[illegible] per cent

[illegible], [illegible] and Jellies

[illegible] [illegible] [illegible] [illegible] [illegible] [illegible] bones in water [illegible] almost no [illegible] value. [illegible] [illegible] water only [illegible] a small amount of [illegible] [illegible] from the [illegible] marrow and a small quantity of [illegible] which [illegible] [illegible] [illegible] [illegible] [illegible] [illegible] [illegible] [illegible] [illegible] [illegible] [illegible] [illegible] of [illegible] and [illegible].

[illegible] nutritional value [illegible] [illegible] [illegible] [illegible] [illegible].

HEALTH AND HYGIENE

The family that is healthy gains much more enjoyment and satisfaction from life than the one in which its members are ailing, at cross purposes with one another, and ignorant of how to keep fit and sociable. The health of a community depends largely on the mothers, and to a lesser degree on the fathers, since the doctors, hospitals and various medical services deal mainly with those whose health has deteriorated, and those who are sick and incapacitated.

The vast majority of people are born healthy and this good health needs constantly to be maintained against weather, infecting organisms, accidents, bad feeding customs, dirt, food shortages, and foolish traditions. In the battle for health the housewife is sometimes at a loss as to what is the best way to deal with a situation. She cannot always trust old domestic customs because more scientific knowledge has shown that better health can be maintained by newer methods, and for her family's sake she must learn them and how to apply them.

FOOD HYGIENE

The finest food in the world, selected with the greatest care to provide the family with a balanced diet of proteins, fats, carbohydrates, vitamins and mineral salts can easily be ruined for human consumption by careless and unhygienic storage and preparation. Living creatures and plants are naturally able to ward off and combat many of the innumerable bacteria and micro-organisms in the air and water around them, but non-living foodstuffs cannot do this and soon become contaminated unless they are protected in one way or another.

There are five main points to consider in keeping foods in good condition:

1. General cleanliness;
2. Moisture;
3. Time;
4. Temperature;
5. Foods particularly vulnerable to bacterial contamination.

If these points are all known and taken into consideration, the likelihood of food poisoning will be greatly reduced. Although it is almost impossible to have food entirely free from micro-organisms (some are not destroyed even after prolonged cooking), it is essential to keep contamination to a minimum.

The danger can be realized more clearly when it is known that a single micro-organism, in favorable conditions such as moisture and warmth, can multiply to 2,000,000 in about seven hours. It is clear then that the sooner fresh food is cooked and eaten the more wholesome it will be.

Favorable conditions for the multiplication of bacteria are temperatures around 98° F (that is about normal body temperature), unclean food, unclean surfaces used for preparing and storing food, powdered and dehydrated foods to which water (or moisture from damp storage) has been added, and other highly susceptible foods (see p. 146). It should be noted that foods which have been left on a shelf or cupboard for a few days and become infected with *Salmonella*, *Staphylococci* or *Clostridium botulinum* usually appear to be quite sound, but they are a potential danger. The bacteria *Salmonella*, of which there are some 150 varieties, is the most common food contaminant (see also p. 42).

The Kitchen

As the kitchen is the main center of food preparation, considerable thought and planning should go into its design and layout. Most modern kitchens have easily cleaned surfaces throughout, with constant hot water, sound floors, and walls in good condition. All of these things are essential for good food hygiene. Many kitchens are still far from being ideal but, with the variety of new materials now available, any kitchen however antiquated can be made easier to keep clean with hard plastic surfacings, stainless steel, with good quality paints, and with vinyl and other composition floorings.

Floors. Ideally these should be hard, easily cleaned and vermin-proof. Wooden floors absorb water, are dusty and can harbor vermin: they should therefore be covered. Linoleum, though cheap, will not wear so well as vinyl floor coverings, slate tiles or some of the new composition tiles which make attractive easy-to-clean surfaces.

Walls. These should also have easily washed, hard surfaces. Eggshell paint or tiles in conjunction with an absorbent ceiling preparation (to counteract condensation) probably give the most satisfactory results available today. If paint is used it should be frequently renewed. Paints containing granulated cork help to minimize condensation but if it is very bad a steam extractor may be needed.

Equipment. Sinks and draining boards should be made of porcelain, stainless steel, fiberglass, or smooth plastic materials. Wooden draining boards can carry infection even after thorough cleansing.

Table tops and other working tops in the kitchen should be covered with enamel, a hard plastic or some other easily cleaned, nonporous material. Shelves should preferably be made of glass, metal, tile, or other non-

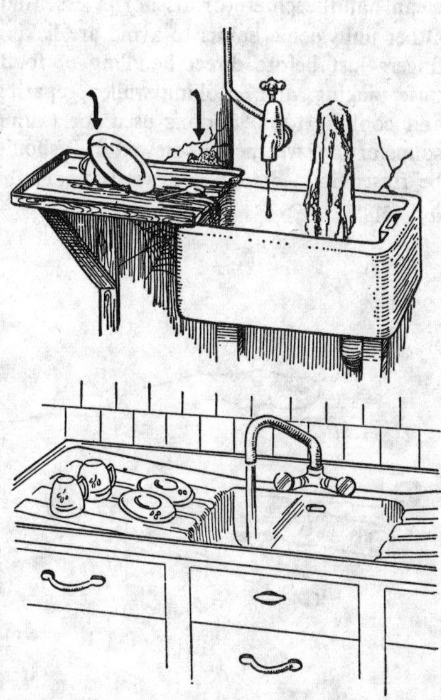

Fig. 1. *KITCHEN SINKS. Above, the neglected sink, the wooden draining board, cracked dishes and broken walls all offer a harbor for germs. Below, the hygienic draining board, uncracked cups and tiled walls offer no attraction to germs.*

porous material. Wooden shelves can be made more hygienic with an application of hard gloss paint. Stoves, saucepans and smaller equipment should all be kept clean—particularly in the corners—and in good repair.

Trash cans should have well-fitting covers and should be kept outside the kitchen, and should be kept disinfected and in good repair.

Water which has been used for scrubbing floors or for rinsing soiled diapers should not be emptied into the kitchen sink.

Washing Up. Cutlery and dishes should always be thoroughly washed after use, with a good detergent and hot water. Dish cloths should be changed frequently although rinsing with clean hot water and drying on a rack may be preferred to drying dishes with towels.

Remember to rinse out milk bottles. Avoid using chipped and cracked dishes; bacteria can lurk for a long time in cracks. Dishcloths and mops should be boiled and renewed regularly. Particular care should be taken when washing bottles, dishes and cutlery used by babies and by children already ill; sick-room cups, spoons, etc., are best washed separately.

Personal Hygiene. A high standard of personal hygiene is essential for people preparing food. Hands should always be washed before handling food, particularly after using the toilet and after using a handkerchief.

Finger nails should be kept clean and aprons changed frequently. If a person is suffering from an infection, particularly of the nose or chest or of the bowels, she should handle food as little as possible and take extra care when it is necessary to do so. Coughing and sneezing into the hands should be avoided and a clean handkerchief (or tissue) is essential. Other unhygienic habits to avoid are licking fingers just before direct handling of food, nose picking, and smoking while preparing and cooking food. Spoons used for tasting soups or the sweetness of stewed fruit should be rinsed immediately afterwards under the hot tap.

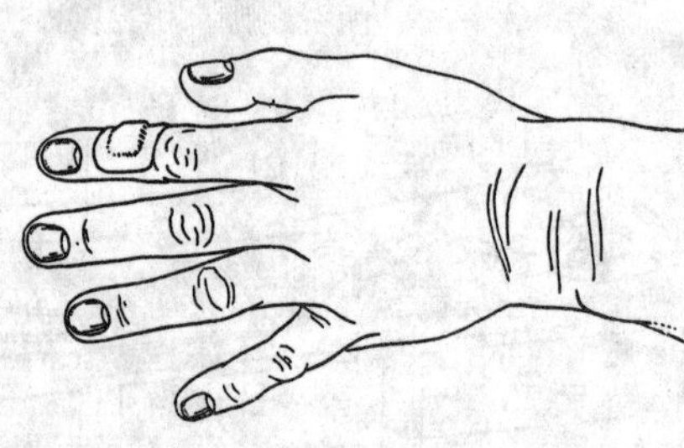

Fig. 2. *PERSONAL HYGIENE. Food handlers should cover cuts and sores with a waterproof dressing.*

Cuts and sores on the hands or fingers should be covered immediately with a waterproof dressing.

Fresh vs. Stale Foods

Buying Food. Food should be bought selectively for its freshness to the eye and nose. It is particularly important to recognize freshness in meat and fish and the sensible mother will teach her daughter (and son) when they are shopping to notice the difference in appearance of fresh and stale foods.

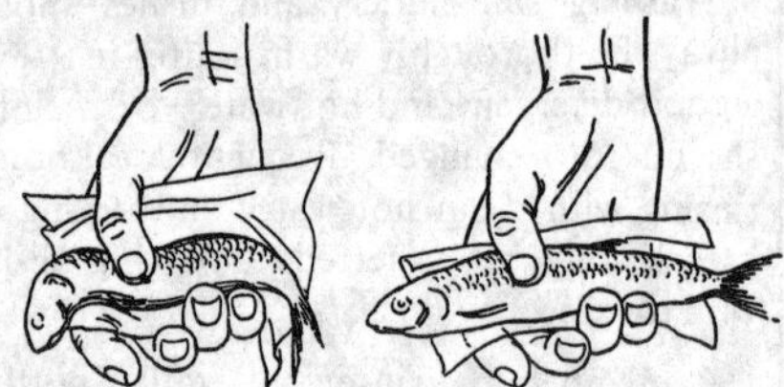

Fig. 3. *FISH, STALE AND FRESH. Avoid the flabby fish and choose the firm one.*

The housewife should shop in stores where the food, premises and attendants are clean. Where unhygienic conditions and practices exist the housewife should draw the attention of the management to them. Animals should be kept under control if they must be taken into food stores. Always make sure that food is wrapped in clean paper—particularly fish, meat, cakes, etc.—or in sound containers; provide a clean shopping bag for purchases.

Cooking. In the interests of food hygiene, food should be handled as little as possible before cooking. It should be cleaned and cooked thoroughly and for health's sake it should be eaten immediately, particularly the foods which are more likely to cause food poisoning (see p. 42). Pre-cooked food which is stored needs thorough recooking, not just heating up.

Gravies, soups, and sauces should be freshly made just before they are eaten. Fried, broiled and grilled foods should be cooked on both sides to safeguard against any bacteria not being destroyed. Roasting temperatures are generally high and the temperature charts which are usually supplied with cookers should be followed.

Frozen eggs should only be used for baking at high temperatures such as are used for sponge cake or pastry. If reconstituted dried eggs are cooked lightly (scrambled eggs, omelettes) they must be eaten immediately. If milk dishes are to be eaten cold they should be stored in a refrigerator. Food should never be left to 'keep warm' in or on a warm stove for long periods.

Foods Susceptible to Contamination. There are certain kinds of food which are particularly liable to contamination. Extra precautions can be taken to prevent them from becoming potential sources of food poisoning. One of the most important precautions is never to store such foods in a warm room or cupboard. Other precautions are dealt with under 'Cooking,' above.

MEAT. Bacteria, particularly *Salmonella* and *Clostridium welchii*, multiply rapidly in 'made up' dishes such as pies, sausages, and pressed beef, so these foods should be eaten fresh.

EGGS. Dried egg powder, frozen eggs and duck eggs are highly susceptible to *Salmonella* contamination although egg powder does not become vulnerable until it is mixed with water, and frozen eggs until they are thawed.

GRAVIES, SOUPS AND SAUCES. These 'wet' foodstuffs are particularly susceptible if made some days before being eaten. The time interval allows the *Salmonella* organism to multiply rapidly.

MILK AND MILK DISHES. Milk is a highly perishable commodity and milk dishes, i.e. custards, puddings, and cream (real or synthetic) are all prone to infection by *Salmonella.*

UNCOOKED FOODS. Salads, watercress, and shellfish need special care when being cleaned and prepared as they are possible sources of typhoid and paratyphoid fevers and of diseases caused by worms. Typhoid bacteria thrive in polluted waters.

FROZEN FOODS. These are liable to rapid deterioration once they have begun to thaw. They should never be refrozen after being taken out of a deep freeze.

GELATIN. Gelatin should be heated to near boiling point before use as it is prone to carry infection.

Food Storage

As far as is practicable, food should be bought immediately before it is prepared and eaten. Food that is stored should be put in suitable containers and cupboards where food pests cannot reach it. Except for a few dry substances such as white sugar and salt, food should not be stored in a warm room. Storerooms should be kept free from waste food and paper, both of which encourage pests, and also free from damp which encourages mold growth (mold is not harmful in itself but will spoil food). Bread, flour, cakes, etc. should be kept in covered tins or bins.

Stores of foodstuffs should be checked regularly for signs of deterioration and anything of doubtful quality thrown out, e.g. 'blown' cans, fermented bottled fruit, and dry foods infested with weevils. Canned food should be eaten as soon as possible after opening

'Blown' cans show a swelling, usually at the ends, which indicates that there is imperfect sealing and that the contents are contaminated by a micro-organism which is producing a gas. Dented cans are not necessarily contaminated though the risk of a minute break is greater than with undamaged tins. Test a dented can by covering it with water in a bowl. If bubbles of air come up, then the contents are contaminated.

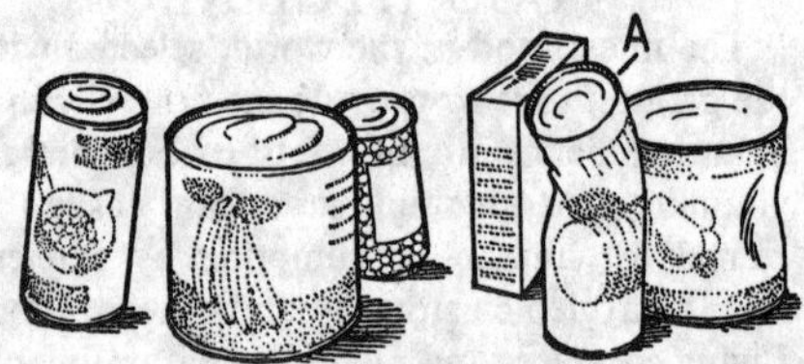

Fig. 4. *'BLOWN' AND DENTED CANS. The first three cans show a swelling which indicates imperfect sealing and possibly contaminated contents. Can A is dented, but not blown, but it may have a crack through which air can contaminate its contents.*

Storing in a Refrigerator. All the more perishable foods, such as milk and milk dishes, meat, fish, and cooked left-overs, should be stored in the refrigerator. The following simple storage rules will ensure that food is kept as fresh as possible.

1. Never overfill a refrigerator but allow room for air to circulate.

2. Do not place really hot food into the refrigerator as it raises the inside temperature causing condensation and consequent deterioration of all the food within. Allow hot food to cool as rapidly as possible in a suitable place before storing it.

3. The refrigerator must be cleaned and defrosted regularly to prevent tainting and to ensure that the correct temperature is maintained.

4. Never put food that may be 'off' in the refrigerator because freezing will not make it fresh again and it may contaminate the rest of the contents. Low temperatures prevent the multiplication of bacteria but do not kill them.

5. Metal and glass containers should be placed at the bottom of the refrigerator as condensation forms on them and may drip on to food below.

Food Pests

Houseflies. These are very common pests, especially during the warmer months. They are dangerous as they breed and feed in dirty places, e.g. animal excrement and decaying animal and vegetable matter which contain billions of bacteria. They will then enter houses and shops contaminating food in two ways: by walking over it with bacteria-laden feet and by secreting a digestive juice on the food—this juice often contains bacteria.

CONTROL. Flies can be kept out of store rooms by covering the window with wire 30-mesh screen. Keep food covered or in fly-proof cupboards. Refuse should be kept covered and bins emptied often.

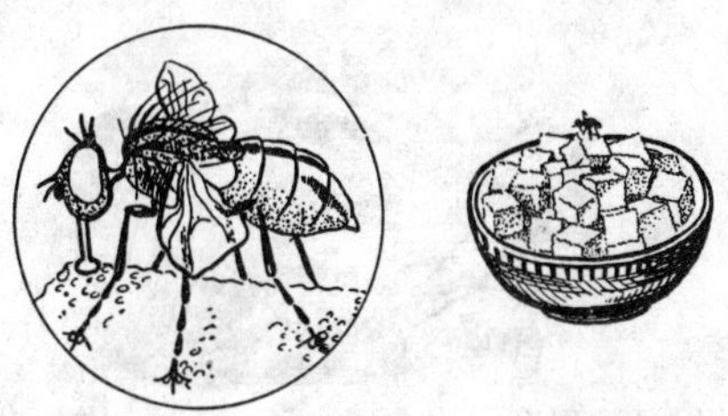

Fig. 5. *HOUSEFLY. Sugar being contaminated by the housefly.*

Commercial fly sprays are sprayed in the room as a fine mist and have an immediate effect on the flies. Care must be taken, however, not to spray food (the shopkeeper will tell you which sprays are safe to use with food about).

Bluebottles. The blowflies are normally outdoor species which breed on the bodies of dead animals and insects. This powerful attraction towards the smell of flesh will often cause them to enter houses, particularly where meat or fish is lying.

If meat containing blowfly maggots is eaten, it may cause diarrhea but there is no likelihood of the maggots surviving in the alimentary canal.

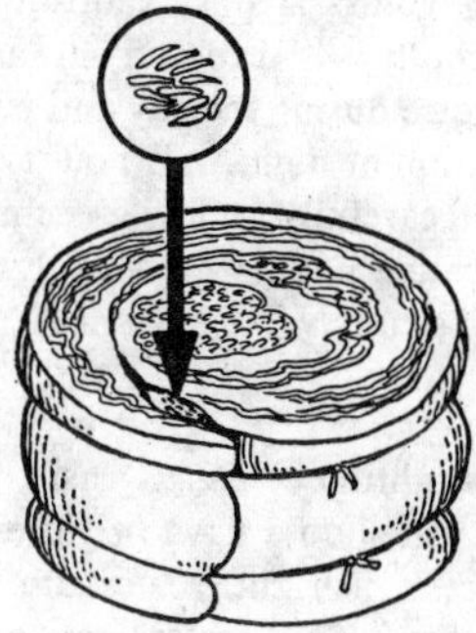

Fig. 6. *BLUEBOTTLE EGGS. These are usually laid in crevices of exposed meat.*

CONTROL. As for House-flies, above.

Cockroaches. These insects can contaminate food. They are nocturnal in habit and live in cracks and crevices in floors and walls, particularly where there is warmth.

CONTROL. An insect spray should be sprayed or sprinkled into cracks and crevices. Food should be protected with covers. Cracks should be repaired.

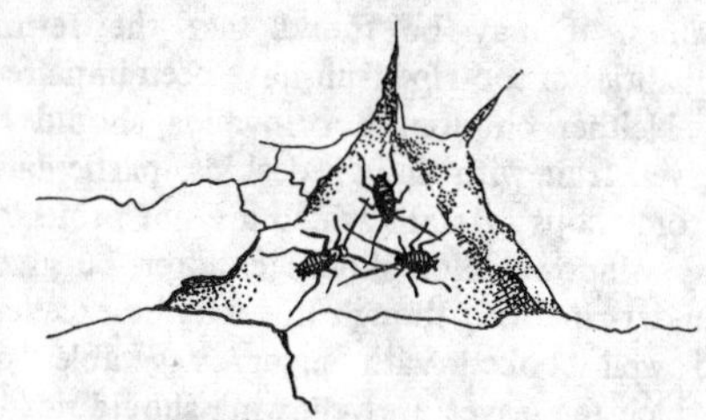

Fig. 7. *COCKROACHES. These insects live in cracks in walls and floors.*

Ants. Both garden ants and house ants can carry germs from place to place although they are more of a nuisance than a danger. The garden ants generally nest in the soil under stones and the house ants in warm buildings, i.e. kitchens, centrally heated dwellings, behind plaster, or under the floors or foundations.

CONTROL. Leave no crumbs around. The nests of garden ants can be destroyed with boiling water. Commercial ant-killing powders should not be used near food stores nor left accessible to children or pets.

Wasps. These are a nuisance in late summer and are attracted by sweet things and fruit. They can contaminate food.

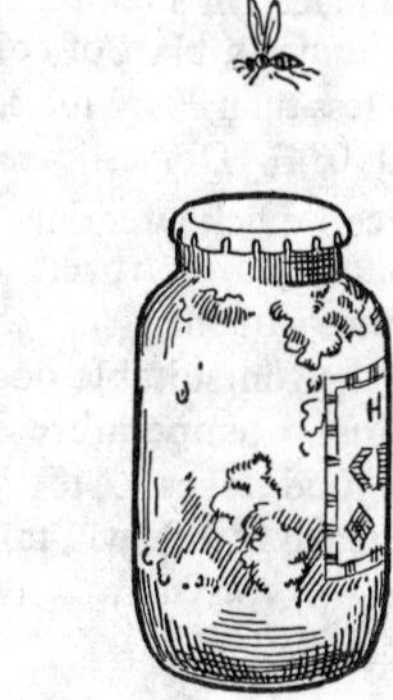

Fig. 8. *WASPS. Keep sweet things covered, particularly in late autumn.*

CONTROL. Keep jams and other sweet things covered. The nest can be destroyed by careful burning at dusk when most of the wasps have returned for the night.

Mites. These minute insects are about one-fiftieth of an inch in length and are detected by a grayish dust around the food. They attack flour, pudding mixes, pearl barley, dried fruit, jam, and cakes. They are generally found when food has been stored for long periods particularly in warm, moist, badly ventilated places.

CONTROL. As the amounts of susceptible foods stored in ordinary households are small the infested foods are best thrown out.

Biscuit Beetles. These beetles live on foods such as spices and biscuits. The adult beetle is about one-tenth of an inch long and is generally seen when an outbreak is well in progress. The larva and grubs can penetrate packages of foods.

CONTROL. Insecticides in the form of dusts, sprays and smokes should be used in the pantry after removal of open food stores.

Grain Weevils. They will attack grain foods such as rice, barley and macaroni. The weevil is about one-tenth of an inch long and the eggs are laid in the surface of the grain. Infested food may become hot and musty.

CONTROL. Store grain foods in temperatures below 55° F. In farmhouses, or places where large quantities of whole grain are kept, the grain can be mixed with insecticidal dust, or fumigated.

Silver Fish. These wingless insects are harmless from the point of view of contaminating foods. They like the dark and are found mainly in older houses. They may damage book bindings if left undisturbed.

Rats. It is not unusual for rats to infest houses in over-crowded cities and they may be a nuisance in farmhouses and in dwellings near grain warehouses. Rats can gnaw through almost anything from concrete and water pipes to food and clothing. They spread *Salmonella* food poisoning and can carry other specific diseases like plague. Because they are creatures of habit their paths can easily be traced.

CONTROL. Buildings should be kept in good repair. Rubbish and waste food must not be left in open containers. Traps should be set at right angles to the rats' run. Poisoned animals will generally die in inaccessible places and poison bait can be dangerous to children or pets in the house. As rats are suspicious animals, unpoisoned bait (preferably cereals) should be left for a few nights before adding poison to allay their fears. Dead rats should be handled with gloves, and hands washed after using poisoned bait.

Mice. Mice are a fairly common pest in houses—particularly older ones. They can contaminate and destroy food, woodwork and fabrics.

CONTROL. Stop up holes. Keep food in containers. Keep rooms free from crumbs and waste food. Mice can be poisoned in the same way as rats. They are easy to trap; cheese and breadcrumbs are the best bait.

COOKING FOR HEALTH

The food we eat serves two purposes, in children it provides the material whereby the body may grow and, in both children and adults, the food substances are utilized by the body to replace the cells and tissues worn out by the constant processes of breathing, moving about, working with muscle and brain, as well as the thousand and one activities of being alive.

It is important therefore, that those who are concerned with providing meals should have some simple basic knowledge of food values and of their nutritive qualities. A detailed account of these qualities will be found in the section on Nutrition, but here we are concerned with the practical aspects whereby the housewife can provide meals to keep her family in good health.

In planning meals it is obvious to anyone that men, or women, doing heavy manual work, particularly in the open air, require more muscle-replacing foods (proteins) and energy-giving foods (carbohydrates and fats) than sedentary office workers, who will be better served with more fruit in their diet.

Food Nutrients

Carbohydrates provide the body with energy; fats provide energy too, but can also encourage accumulation of fat in the body.

Proteins provide material for growth and repair of body tissues, and they also can provide some energy.

Mineral salts, in small amounts, provide vital material to aid growth and repair, as well as for the regulation of the body processes. Vitamins are essential to certain body processes.

Very few foods contain only one nutrient; most are a mixture and thus the value of a particular foodstuff may depend as much on the amount of the food usually eaten, as upon the quantity of the essential substance in it. For example, potatoes are more valuable than parsley because, although the latter contains more vitamin C reckoned on a 'weight for weight' basis, potatoes are eaten in greater quantity than parsley.

Shopping

The first business of the housewife in feeding her family will be buying the food. If she is fortunate enough to have a garden, fruit and vegetables can be home grown.

Vegetables and Fruit

Freshly gathered vegetables contain more vitamins, particularly vitamin C, than when bought from a shop where they are not always as fresh as they might be.

Although today most people are better educated about the nutritional value of food many younger housewives do not know what to look for to ensure that they are getting

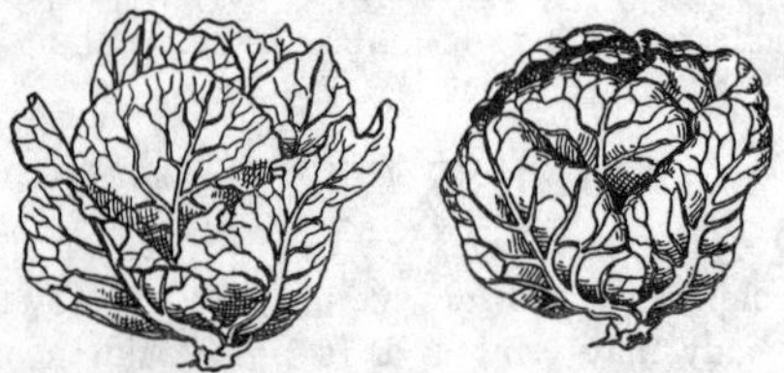

Fig. 9. *CABBAGE. The leaves of a fresh cabbage stand briskly upward while the leaf tips of the wilted cabbage flop inwards.*

quality, freshness and the best value for money. Two important points, the most expensive foods are not necessarily the most nourishing, but on the other hand a food bargain may not always be as good as it appears at first sight. This is particularly true of fruit and vegetables. Over-ripe fruit, for instance, although offered at bargain price is often rotten at the core and much of it will need to be discarded. Even for jams and jellies, it may be found that the setting qualities of too-ripe fruit have been impaired.

Neither children nor invalids should be given fruit with damaged skins, particularly from shops or stalls which are not protected by windows. Nor should children be given under-ripe fruit though this may be excellent if well cooked with sugar. Vegetables on which the leaves are yellowing should not be purchased. Lettuce, from which the roots have been cut should be examined, as it is one of the tricks of the trade among less reputable grocers to trim the outer leaves away, exposing quite a good-looking heart which will, within a short time, have lost all its crispness. Spinach particularly, though rich in mineral salts, is extremely perishable. Look to see that all leaves are fresh and green and not interspersed with sodden ones which rot with amazing rapidity. It is often better to buy some well-known brand of frozen vegetables because the peas, sprouts, etc. will have been gathered at the height of their perfection. It is probably in vegetables that the housewives have derived the greatest benefit from deep freezing.

QUICK FREEZING of foods means that the freshly picked fruit or vegetables, or the fresh fish or meat, is placed in a temperature below −20° F, often under a blast of cold air. The food freezes in less than 30 minutes. After that it is stored at 0° F. Domestic refrigerators cannot produce 'quick freezing,' but can safely store packages of frozen foods in a deep freeze compartment.

DEEP FREEZING in suitable domestic appliances requires a temperature of 0° F to −10° F. The food takes 6 to 7 hours to freeze, but to reach 0° F it will take 15 to 24 hours. Color, flavor, and vitamins are retained by this method.

Meat

In shops selling meat, there is a growing trend, in response to public demand, to display joints of meat already cut and priced —'Buying by the Unit' rather than by the pound.

Beef. When buying shin beef, or knuckle of veal for invalid broths, remember that gristle makes the broth gell better. Close-grained meat is always tougher and is generally used for stewing, for cooking in a casserole, or for boiling. For roasting and broiling, use the best meat which is interlaced with minute veins of fat. It is only when the animal is getting old that this fat gives place to gristle and sinew. With beef, too light red a color means that the animal is immature; and if it is rather coarse-grained and dry looking, it is cow beef, from which most of the nutriment has been taken by long milk production and calving.

Lamb. Good quality lamb is pale-fleshed with a pinky tinge. Bones, after cooking, are white and if splintered the center marrow is pink, and this whitens as the animal ages. The modern dislike of fat meat has resulted in a demand for excessively lean meat, often at the expense of quality.

Poultry

Poultry today is comparatively one of the least expensive of meats. Chicken is easily digested and therefore plays an important part in feeding the sick. A 'broiler' is a chicken which is grown and fattened to maturity in a very short period. Since it has never, like the old barnyard bird, had to scratch for a living, it is free of gristle and tough sinew. At 7 to 10 weeks old, these birds are processed, killed, eviscerated, trussed, wrapped in special vacuum film and deep frozen. Throughout all these processes the broilers are handled in the most hygienic way.

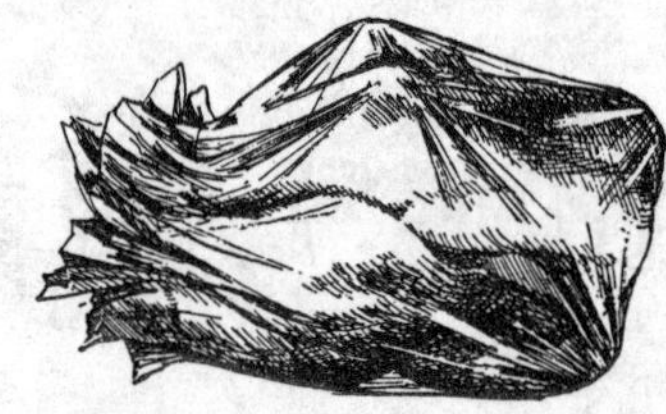

Fig. 10. *QUICK FROZEN POULTRY. Undo film covering at vent end to allow escape of moisture or the flesh will turn sour.*

Quick frozen poultry should be sold from a frozen food cabinet and thawed out at home by being kept at room temperature. The film covering should be undone at one end to allow moisture to escape and to prevent condensation within the bag, for this tends to 'sour' the flesh.

Housewives should be wary of shopkeepers who sell oven-ready poultry from an unrefrigerated counter. Frozen food will not keep in good condition in an ordinary domestic refrigerator for more than 72 hours. The latest refrigerators have a special drawer for frozen foods. Never, in any circumstances, should an attempt be made to refreeze foods that have thawed out.

Be on guard against shops where oven-ready poultry is exposed to an ordinary temperature during the day and put back into refrigeration at night. All poultry should be examined carefully for any greening round the vent because poultry, if slightly 'off,' does not smell strongly like meat or fish.

Fish

The condition of fish is easily recognized. All wet fish should have bright eyes, and on really fresh fish the scales are bright and shimmering. The scales are a protective armor against bacteria, which is why fish such as mackerel (which has no scales) needs to be eaten in a really fresh condition. Freshly caught mackerel is stiff, with a slight upward curve of the tail.

The flesh of fish is as useful a source of animal protein as that of meat. The fat, unlike that of meat, provides vitamins A and D in the diet. The proportion of this fat differs widely in different kinds of fish: fat fish (herring, mackerel, salmon and eel) contain five to eighteen per cent of fat; white fish (cod, haddock, sole, whiting, flounder, etc.) contain less than two per cent.

It is interesting to note that cod and halibut, whose livers are so rich in oil, have a fat-free flesh. They are therefore always better served with a creamy sauce.

Cod, which some people find dull, can be made really tasty. For example 1 lb. cod, the cheaper large fillets are excellent, should be cut into squares, browned slightly in olive oil, placed in a fireproof glass or earthenware casserole, with a cup of cooked rice and four or five sliced medium-sized tomatoes, after rubbing the dish with a clove of garlic. Pepper and salt to season. A tablespoonful of chopped parsley, a pinch of dill seed, marjoram or mixed herbs, a small quantity of sliced gherkin or pimento can be added according to taste. Then the casserole is put in the oven (without a cover) until the fish is soft and flaky. Serve with creamy mashed potato.

Children usually enjoy eating a dish with so much color, although they may complain about eating pale steamed cod.

Fat Fish. It is important that housewives know when fat fish, such as herrings, are in season. Fat fish are in poor condition after spawning and, by law, some kinds are not allowed to be exposed for sale during this period.

Fish of which the bones are eaten provide a source of calcium and phosphorus: the group includes herring, sardines and sprats. Many people neglect cheap and nourishing sprats because they smell somewhat strongly when being cooked, or they are 'fatty.'

FISH IN SEASON

January
Cod, Flounder, Haddock (fresh and smoked), Halibut, Skate, Sole.

February
Cod, Eel, Flounder, Haddock, Halibut, Oysters, Skate, Sprats, Sole.

March
Cod, Flounder, Haddock, Halibut, Herring, Rainbow Trout, Salmon, Skate, Sole, Sprats.

April
As for March, with the addition of Salmon Trout.

May
Cod, Crabs, Flounder, Halibut, Herring, Lobster, Mackeral, Mullet, Smelts, Sole, Whiting.

June
As for May; Crabs and Lobster are more plentiful.

July
As for May with the addition of Hake, Pike, Prawns, Salmon Trout, Shrimp.

August
As for July.

September
As for the previous summer months with the addition of Bass and Oysters.

October
Cod, Flounder, Haddock, Hake, Halibut, Herring, Oysters, Scallops, Sole, Whiting.

November
As for October; supply of Lobster depends on the weather.

December
As for October.

Cooking Equipment

The importance of planning and cleanliness in the kitchen is dealt with under kitchen hygiene, p. 77, but here we need to consider the choice of cooking equipment which will best serve the family needs.

Basic Utensils

Pots, pans, and kitchen tools used for food preparation and cooking should be of good quality and chosen carefully. While it is most attractive to have all the pots, pans and kitchen gadgets to fit in with a color scheme, the young housewife should not be too much influenced by a desire to possess a kitchen that appears to have everything. It is much more important to have a few well-chosen utensils which serve their purpose adequately and which can be kept clean easily. It is almost impossible for a really busy woman to keep a large conglomeration of utensils clean in a small kitchen.

Saucepans. Six saucepans, two large, two medium and two small are needed for cooking a normal varied diet One person living alone could manage with four. Aluminum pans are the easiest to keep clean and are satisfactory for all cooking. The discoloration oi aluminum from water boiling in it has no injurious effects and may be removed by boiling water to which a little cream of tartar has been added.

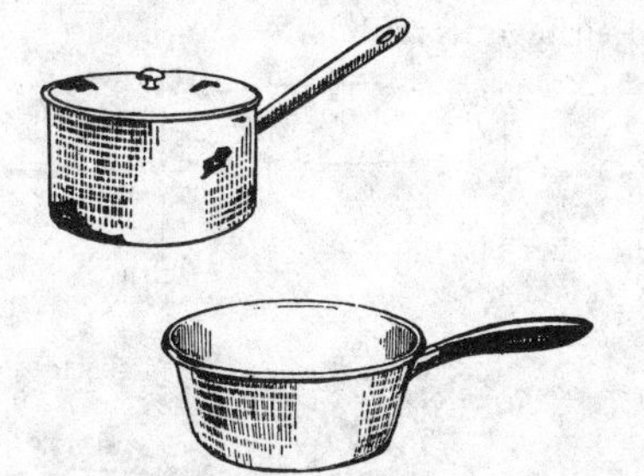

Fig. 11. *SAUCEPANS. Once enamelware has become chipped it will readily chip further and the chips may get into the food. A modern aluminum saucepan with heatproof handle is a better buy.*

If enamel is used, buy a good brand that will not chip. Chipped enamelware should never be used; once the surface is broken it will chip further and it is difficult to keep the damaged surface clean and wholesome. It is best to use aluminum pans or fireproof glass cookware. A double-boiler is used for making boiled egg custard, lemon or orange pudding, etc. A shallow frying pan should have a heavy base to prevent burning; iron is better than aluminum. An egg poacher, though not essential, is most useful, particularly for invalid cookery; none of the egg is wasted and its symetrical shape makes it look attractive. A roasting pan, two baking pans and at least one cooky sheet will be required.

Bowls and Casseroles. Three casseroles and two pie plates will be needed in every kitchen. Fireproof ovenware is being used more and more because it has so many advantages. It is so easy to keep clean and the food can be served as well as cooked in it. A large earthenware mixing bowl and a rolling pin are also required. An enamel-topped table that is kept spotlessly clean makes an excellent substitute for a pastry board and saves storage space. A pointed gravy strainer can also be used as a flour dredger. The pastry brush should be kept spotlessly clean and discarded immediately it begins to shed hairs. An electric food mixer and egg beater saves a lot of work, but it is expensive for a small household. A small hand-operated egg beater, which can be used as a food mixer, is a very inexpensive and useful gadget.

Sieves, Mincers and Gadgets. A Mouli® grater saves a lot of trouble. It has three small circular grates, the finest with holes hardly larger than a big pin point. All kinds of purées can be made with it or cream soups strained. It is ideal for invalid cookery or for baby's purees. There is a similar device, with four cutters for slicing and shredding vegetables and fruit, or cutting potato for chips.

A good grinder is extremely useful though more expensive; and much time and mess is saved by having adequate small gadgets such as a fish scaler, enamel or stainless steel soup ladle, potato peeler, apple corer, corkscrew, can opener, kitchen scissors, and food chopper.

A set of paring and carving knives with a knife sharpener is essential.

Aluminum Foil. Cooking in aluminum foil is economical, and it can be put to a number of uses. Different vegetables can be boiled in the same saucepan, by twisting them up in separate squares of the foil which is grease- and moisture-proof.

For roasting, the meat or poultry is wrapped in it with the necessary amount of fat and, in this way, all the natural juices are preserved. It is particularly good for meat that might be a little tough, but slightly longer cooking time should be allowed. Cover steamed puddings with foil and there is no need to tie down, and no fear of water penetrating. For roast meat or any food that is required to be crisp outside, it is not suitable, or else the foil should be removed just before cooking is completed and the heat increased for browning.

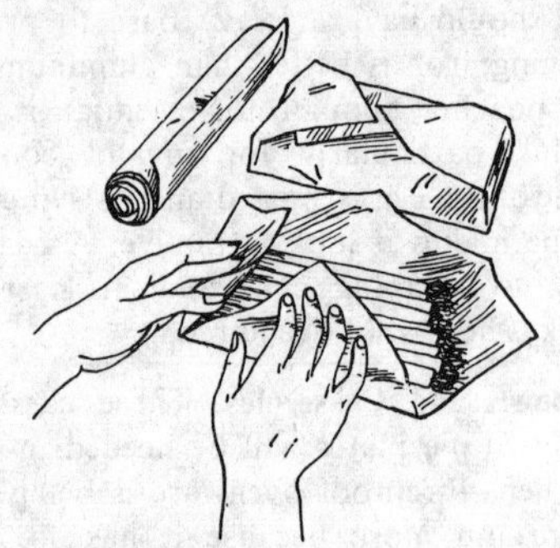

Fig. 12. *ALUMINUM FOIL. Has many domestic uses, particularly for storage of green vegetables and in cooking meats.*

Aluminum foil is excellent to wrap up green vegetables before putting them in a refrigerator. Washed, drained, and wrapped in foil, lettuce will keep crisp and fresh for a week in a refrigerator, as well as free from contamination.

Pressure Cookers

Pressure cookery has become popular during recent years, chiefly because of the economy in fuel and time. In this type of cooking it is possible to cook at temperatures above the normal boiling point of 212° F. It is a valuable method of cooking foods that usually require long slow cooking, such as the cheaper cuts of meat, meat soups, stews, and root vegetables.

There are a number of pressure cookers on the market and in each case the instructions given by the manufacturers should be followed with care. The cooker should never be filled too full, not more than two-thirds for solid foods and about half for fluids or cereals. Times given on the chart should be followed, but allow for slight variation in thickness of some meats or poultry.

Pressure should always be allowed to drop to normal before any attempt is made to open the pan. Either reduce the pressure immediately by allowing cold water to run over the side or, in the case of items such as stewed fruit, milk puddings, etc., allow the pan to cool slowly at room temperature.

After use, the cooker must be well washed and put aside, with the lid off.

Types of Cooking Stoves

Circumstances, rather than preference, often control one's type of fuel and method of cooking. Open coal ranges are seldom used today, except in the remoter parts of the countryside. Electricity is gaining in popularity because of its cleanliness, but gas holds its own for various reasons, one being that there is no fear of supply failures. Oil-burning stoves are used in country areas where other fuels are not easily available.

The latest cookers, either using gas or electricity, often have ovens with thermostatic control, enabling cooking time to be set in advance. If a complete meal is put in the oven, make sure tnat all the items require the same cooking time. The foodstuffs which need slower cooking, such as milk puddings, are placed on the lower shelves, but root vegetables such as carrots are sometimes found to be hard when the poultry or meat is cooked; brief preliminary par-boiling is a remedy. For cooking on solid electric or other flat plates, utensils must have heavy machined bases to ensure quick transference of heat to the center of the saucepan and to eliminate waste of heat. For non-solid plates (coiled electric rings or gas jets) thinner pans can be used.

Washing Greasy Pots and Pans

Easy cleaning of cooking utensils depends on the methods employed. Greasy meat pans are best simmered in water to which soda or some detergent has been added. Aluminium pans need only hot soapy water without soda, or else a detergent: for the inside a nylon pad suffices, though a small amount of mild abrasive may be needed to remove traces of starchy food. Pads of steel wool are best for the outside. Earthenware casseroles, glass ovenware and enamel dishes are easier to wash in hot soapy or detergent water, if they are first soaked in cold water. Frying and omelet pans, after the fat has been poured off, should be well rubbed with a pad of absorbent paper and a little salt. Omelet pans need not be washed unless any particles have stuck to the surface, but store them upside down against dust. Pans or dishes used to cook or serve fish should be soaked immediately in cold water to remove the odor.

When boiling green vegetables that have a strong smell (cabbage, broccoli or sprouts) place a small piece of stale bread on the top of the lid where the steam emerges; it will absorb the steam and diffuse the smell.

Turning Scraps to Good Account

Unnecessary wastage in cooking should be avoided, though of course there must be unusable refuse such as outer leaves of vegetables and peelings (that is unless you are a countrywoman and keep a pig or your children have pet rabbits).

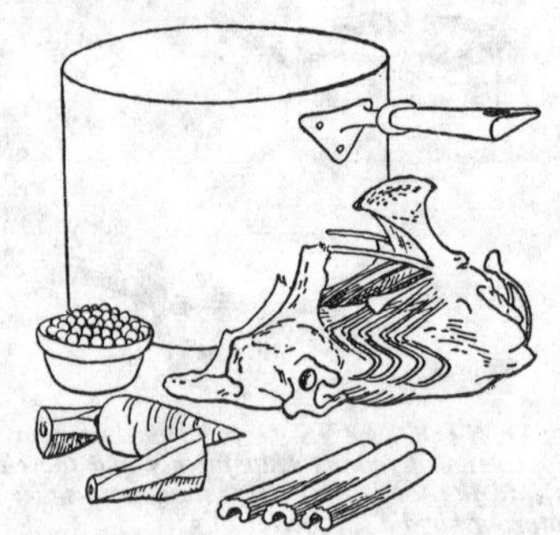

Fig. 13. *FOR THE STOCK POT*

Bones, carcasses of poultry, celery tops left over, cooked root vegetables, can all be utilized to make stock for soup. If the stock from such left-overs is not sufficiently flavored, it should be strained, left to cool, skimmed of fat and cooked for twenty minutes with the addition of one of the well-known dehydrated soups which are on the market. The quantity used should be in accordance with the quantity and quality of the stock.

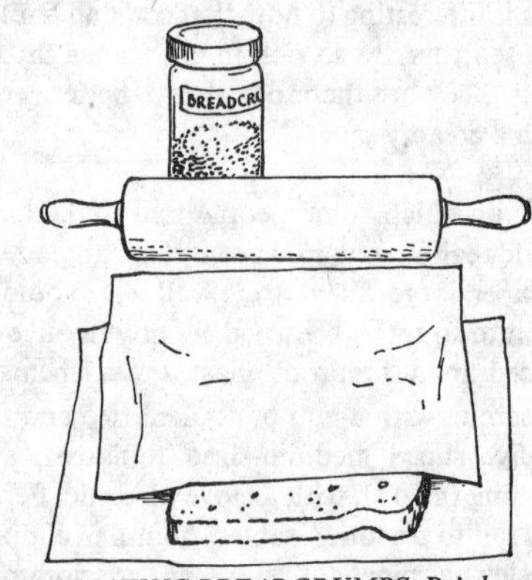

Fig. 14. *MAKING BREADCRUMBS. Dried crusts, or baked stale bread (covered with a napkin to prevent pieces flying about), crushed with a rolling pin makes useful crumbs for coating fish, apple charlotte, etc.*

Careless housewives waste bread more than any other food, which is totally unnecessary. First, never cut into a new loaf until the one in hand is finished. Save stale white bread for making bread pudding, adding to steamed puddings, etc.; but of course, throw away any that may have become moldy and scald the bread box out. Fingers of stale bread or crusts can be left in an open tin in the oven until they are crisp. Young children love to nibble them and these homely rusks are useful for the teething baby. The dried crusts can also be crushed with a rolling-pin. Stored in tins, or jars, thay have many uses—for coating fish before frying, for making Apple Charlotte, or for sprinkling on a large variety of different dishes.

Cooking for One

Cooking for one is sometimes a difficult problem. Women who live alone or whose husbands are often away may suffer slightly from lack of adequate nourishment because it 'hardly seems worth while bothering about this or that for only one person.' Broiled foods are ideal, entailing the minimum of work. There are, too, many excellent canned foods sold today which can be combined with fresh foods to make quickly prepared meals.

Fillets of any kind of white fish need the minimum of preparation; a pat of butter (or margarine) on an enamel plate, a light dusting of flour, pepper and salt. Cook skin side first, turn, add a little more butter, sprinkle with finely chopped, fresh parsley and a squeeze of lemon juice. If preferred, a dash of essence of anchovy or Worchestershire sauce. Breakfast bacon thinly sliced is easily grilled on a plate with a sliced tomato and left-over potatoes rolled into tiny balls; when ready sprinkle with parsley.

Mushrooms too, peeled and sliced if large, will cook nicely under a broiler. Smoked fish should be scalded before broiling. Chops and steaks retain flavor and juices better when broiled. Omelets with a variety of fillings are ideal when cooking for one. Cheese is invaluable for toasting and for making Welsh rarebits. Cheese and eggs are first-class body building foods. With a cheese omelet, accompanied by a small package of frozen spinach or a mixed salad followed by fruit, you have an ideal lunch for one.

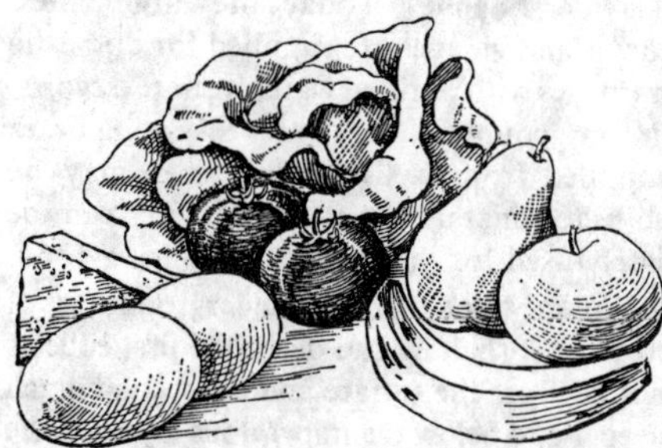

Fig. 15. *LUNCH FOR ONE. For those who live alone such foods as these are quick to prepare yet provide a good balance for the diet.*

Stews for one are not as good as casseroled meats. A dinner that can be put into any oven and left unattended is a casserole of meat (cut into pieces) and vegetables, well-scrubbed potatoes in their jackets, milk pudding or baked custard, and baked apples.

Cooking—Its Values

Many a busy mother must have asked herself whether it is really necessary for her family's health that she prepares and bakes and boils and stews day in and day out. Wouldn't meals of raw foodstuffs do? or perhaps canned foods? Let us see what we gain by cooking our food.

Advantages of Cooking

1. First of all there's the matter of flavor and tastiness. We are all born with sensitive taste buds on our tongues, and sensitive receptors for appetizing (or other) smells in the lining of our noses. Even the smallest baby purses his lips and rolls his first drop of orange juice or cod-liver oil around his mouth to get the flavor of the strange new substance.

Cooking improves the flavor of many of our foods and it brings out new and pleasant flavors in others. What a delightful fruity tang cooked apricots have compared with raw ones! Natural sole provokes no desire but what a pleasure it is to eat it well cooked! An attractive flavor stimulates the appetite and sets the digestive juices flowing.

2. Cooking makes meats, poultry, fish and eggs—the main protein foods—easier to digest. Meats which are lightly cooked are more digestible than well-done or overcooked meats, and even the latter are easier to digest than raw meat. Cheese also contains a fair amount of protein but it toughens when cooked and is then less digestible.

3. Cooking starchy foods such as rice, wheat, oats and potatoes is most essential since raw starch is almost incapable of digestion in the human alimentary tract. The heat of cooking splits the starch granules and gelatinizes them and in this form the human digestive juices can utilize them.

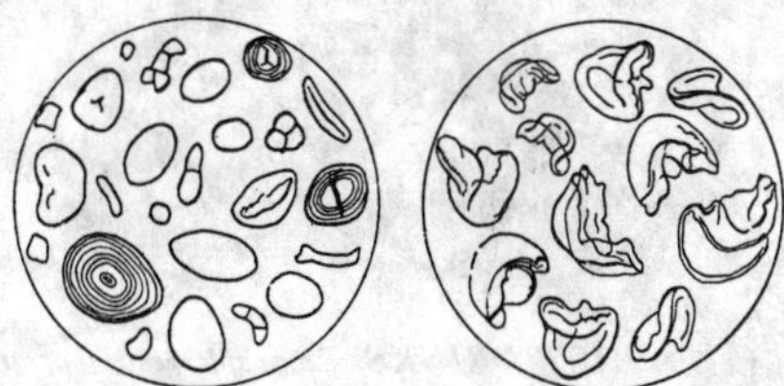

Fig. 16. *STARCH GRANULES. (a) Indigestible granules of raw wheat starch. (b) After boiling, the granules break, the starch becomes gelatinized, and is then easy to digest.*

Cane sugar, on the other hand, although it belongs to the carbohydrate class of foodstuffs, is not much changed by cooking. Yet even it, when cooked with acid fruits such as blackcurrants, gooseberries, apricots, and strawberries undergoes a chemical change, turning it partly into glucose and fructose which are more digestible than the original sugar.

4. Cooking softens and ruptures the 'roughage' or cellulose of vegetables and fruits. Although the fibrous cellulose of these foodstuffs is incapable of being utilized by the human digestive system, the softening up by cooking enables it to pass through the stomach and intestines with less irritation than the raw form. This is more important for babies, invalids, those with a delicate digestive tract, and for old people than for sturdy normal persons.

5. Most bacteria and other microorganisms affecting foodstuffs are killed by heat so that cooking serves to prevent infections. It is recommended that slow cooking of meat (joints) at low temperatures overnight (or for 17 hours) should not be done because the temperature inside the joint seldom rises above 150° F and there may be some germs (*Salmonella* and *Clostridium*) left unkilled. Ordinary cooking temperatures will kill them all.

Milk is pasteurized before being sold and although the pasteurizing temperature is well below boiling point it is sufficient to render the milk safe for consumption.

6. Parasites in meat are killed by cooking and although today the healthiness of animals used for meat is of a high standard, and the inspection of slaughter houses is strict, occasional outbreaks of worm infestation —especially from pork—have occurred.

Disadvantages of Cooking Food

1. Boiling vegetables in water certainly draws out of them some of their potassium and magnesium salts, but fortunately it has little effect on the more important calcium and iron content. The potassium and magnesium salts are easily replaced in the average mixed diet.

2. Cooking removes the important vitamin C (ascorbic acid) from any food but it has practically no effect on the other vitamins. Cabbage or sprouts lose about two-thirds of their vitamin C during cooking, so it is advisable to cook them quickly and serve them promptly. It is very easy to replace the daily requirement of vitamin C by taking fresh lemon, orange or tomato juice, or blackcurrant syrup.

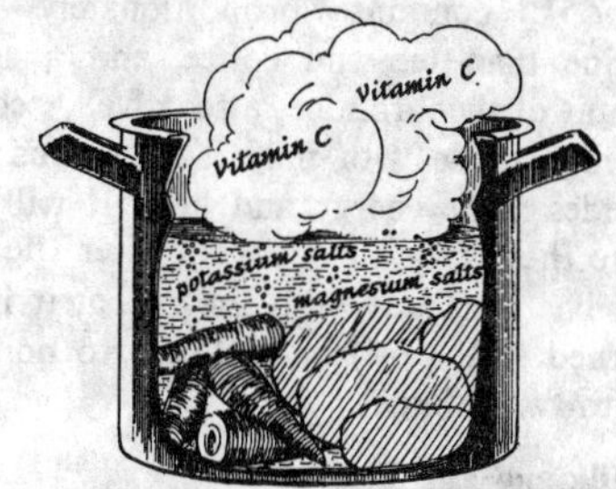

Fig. 17. *VITAMINS AND SALTS. Cooking drives off vitamin C and draws out magnesium and potassium.*

3. Fat which is allowed to become intensely hot develops a substance known as acrolein which is very irritating to the digestive system, so there is particular need for greater care when frying than in other forms of cooking.

BEVERAGES

Apart from quenching one's thirst, some beverages can be a useful source of vitamins and minerals and others, particularly milk, supply enough nourishment to be considered as food.

Tea, Coffee, and Cocoa

TEA contains caffeine, tannic acid and a volatile oil. The caffeine stimulates the nervous system and heart; it promotes the passage of urine and relieves fatigue. Tannic acid is injurious to the mucus membrane lining the stomach and intestines, but there is less tannic acid in freshly made tea than in tea which has been allowed to stand; the addition of milk to tea also inactivates the tannic acid and is therefore beneficial. Tea should never be drunk very strong, nor after it has stood for more than five minutes in contact with the tea leaves; after this the tea should be poured into another warmed vessel. The fragrance of tea is due to very small amounts of essential oils in the leaves.

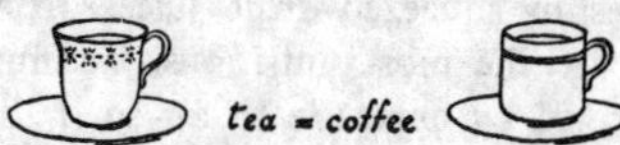

Fig. 18. *TEA AND COFFEE. The average cup of tea contains about the same amount of stimulant as the average cup of coffee.*

COFFEE contains about the same quantity of caffeine and tannic acid as tea, but is more expensive. The tannic acid in tea and coffee delays the digestion of food, especially of meat and proteins, and should not be taken with dinner or supper, especially by persons suffering from dyspepsia, as is a common habit. Both tea and coffee are unsuitable beverages for children, as they are too stimulating for the nerves and brain.

The drinking of 'instant' coffee has become very popular. Instant powders are made of extract of pure coffee and there is as much stimulating caffeine in a cup of instant coffee as in one made directly from the ground beans. The difference as a beverage lies mainly in the flavor.

COCOA contains proportionately less caffeine than tea and coffee, and a small amount of theobromine, a sedative. A cocoa beverage made with milk is nutritious and provides some energy and heat. It will improve the flavor of cocoa if, after the hot milk has been added to the cocoa, it is all returned to the pan and allowed to boil for one to two minutes.

Milk and Egg Drinks

Beverages made from milk or egg, or both, are very nourishing and rich in body-building foods. They are excellent for children and invalids. It is important to remember, however, that milk alone is not a completely adequate diet, except for infants.

Many children and adults do not like the flavor of plain milk and the following recipes are some pleasant ways of disguising it.

MILK DRINKS

½ pt. milk — flavoring to taste
2 teasp. sugar — (fruit or vanilla)

Fruit flavors are best. Mix well and serve cold.

MILK SHAKES

Use a rotary mixer: it is quite cheap and gives the shake a professional look.

one or two ripe bananas — 1 teasp. chocolate powder
½ pt. milk — few drops vanilla flavoring

Sieve bananas and add chocolate powder. Mix well. Add milk (and vanilla if used). Mix well again, using rotary mixer in last stage when fruit has become very liquid.

Any soft fruit is suitable for this recipe.

EGG NOG

1 fresh egg — few grains salt
1–2 teasp. sugar — flavoring to taste
½ pt. hot or cold milk — (fruit, sherry, or wine)

Beat egg and sugar together very thoroughly and then pour on the milk. Add flavoring.

Fruit Drinks

Freshly squeezed fruit juices from ripe fruit are the most nutritious. Vitamin C is destroyed by exposure to air so if the fruit has to be squeezed some time before serving it should be kept in an airtight container, in the refrigerator if possible. It is better to take fruit juices one flavor at a time; orange juice and lemon juice for instance neutralize each other so that you do not get the flavor of either.

Canned fruit juices retain their vitamin C content to a large extent and may even be better than juice from inferior fresh fruit. Any 'tinny' taste can be eliminated by allowing the juice to stand in a jug for 15 minutes or so before using. It helps to improve the flavor by mixing a little fresh juice with the canned juice.

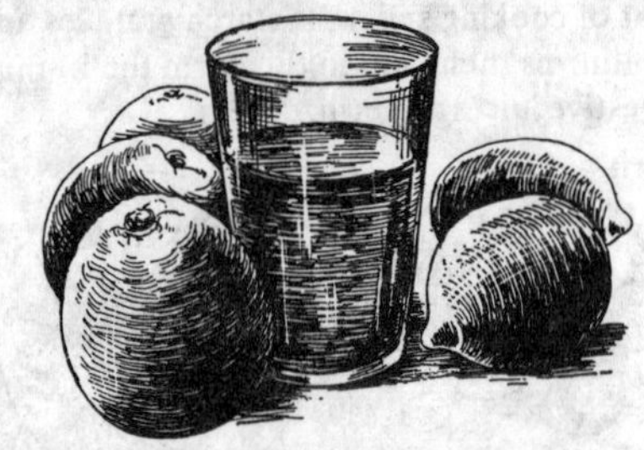

Fig. 19. *FRUIT DRINKS. Enjoyable iced, hot, or cold.*

Hot fruit juice, particularly lemon or blackcurrant, is good for relieving colds, but the water added to the fruit juice should be just below boiling point.

LEMONADE

4 lemons — 2 pts. boiling water (= 4 cupsful)
4 oz. sugar (= ½ cupful)

Peel lemons thinly, put rind and sugar into a jug. Pour on the boiling water and stir until sugar dissolves. Leave to get cold, then strain and add the lemon juice.

ORANGEADE

3 small oranges — 2 pts boiling water
2 tablesp. sugar — (= 4 breakfastcupsful)

Make in the same way as lemonade, above, using the orange rind grated.

Alcoholic Drinks

Alcoholic beverages appear to be stimulating because they relax mental awareness and release inhibitions. They are also temporarily warming since they cause dilatation of the skin blood vessels. If taken in small amount alcohol stimulates the flow of digestive juices and so helps to digest a meal, but if taken in a large quantity it hampers digestion.

BEER made from malted barley and flavored with hops. According to the type of beer or stout, it has an alcohol content of about 5 to 8 per cent as well as digestible sugars, so that it could be considered as a food. One pint of good ale contains almost the same amount of carbohydrates as 1¼ ounces of bread.

WINES. White and red wines, suitable for taking with meals, have become increasingly popular. It is usual to serve red wine with stronger meats and a white wine with fish or with light meat like veal. The average alcohol content of wines is about 16 per cent.

HOT PUNCH is warming and refreshing in the winter and is said to be good for colds. Rum punch is an old drink, but a cheaper wine punch contains:

1 bottle cheap red wine
½ pint water
juice of two oranges
tablesp. sugar
grating of nutmeg

Mix all the ingredients, including skins of oranges, in a saucepan and heat until very hot, but be careful not to allow it to boil. Serve immediately. It should be drunk as hot as possible.

WATER

Water is even more essential to man's existence than food. It is therefore of prime importance in any country or community to ensure that water supplies are plentiful and that the water is clean and wholesome.

Water Supplies. Today the large cities, towns and villages are supplied for domestic purposes with purified water from reservoirs. in the country this water is sometimes supplied from wells. Rain water may be collected in tanks and, if boiled, can be safely used for drinking or preparing food.

Water which collects underground is of two types, shallow and deep: the first collects not far from the surface and the second much deeper and below the impervious layers in the soil. The shallow water is soft and comes to the surface in springs. It is an unreliable source as it can easily be contaminated and when the rainfall is low the flow becomes lower and may disappear. It can be tapped with a shallow well. The deep water layers are relatively pure as they are filtered through hard layers in the soil. This water collects calcium and magnesium salts and is therefore hard. It may come to the surface as a natural spring or can be tapped for deep artesian wells. All wells providing water for human consumption must be properly constructed and lined and must be at least 100 feet away from any source of contamination. Waste water must not be allowed to seep back into the well.

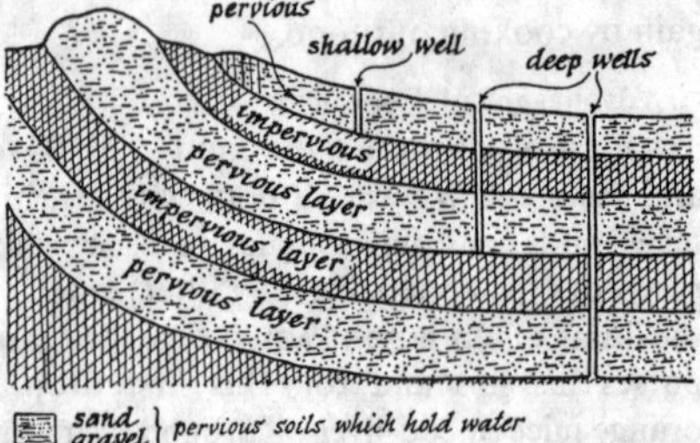

Fig. 20. *WATER SUPPLIES. How both shallow and deep water is tapped at various layers.*

Rivers also supply a large amount of water to towns and cities but this has to undergo thorough purification. Pollution from trade waste, detergents, and sewage has to be rendered relatively harmless before it can be disposed of in rivers.

Properties of Water. Pure water consists of two elements chemically combined. Each water molecule is made up of two hydrogen (H) atoms linked to one atom of oxygen (O) and can be expressed by the chemical formula: H_2O. However, since water is a great solvent it often dissolves and contains in solution many impurities some of which are good for health and some are harmful.

Good water is without odor, is perfectly clear; when poured from one vessel to another it should form air air bubbles. Boiled and distilled waters have a vapid flat taste, owing to the absence of carbon dioxide gas and atmospheric air which are driven off by boiling and distilling. A hundred cubic inches of good river water contain about 1½ parts of carbon dioxide and 1¼ parts of air.

Carbon dioxide gives to mineral or soda water its brisk and pungent taste; without this gas and atmospheric air, water is insipid and not palatable as a beverage. Hence if it is boiled or distilled for purification a large surface of it should be exposed to the air so that it may reabsorb from the atmosphere the gases it has lost, and may regain its taste.

Types of Water

Hard water contains sulphates and bicarbonates of calcium and magnesium and is uneconomical compared with soft water. It is poor for washing woolens, hair and skin, and necessitates the use of larger quantities of soap to produce lather; it leaves scum in sinks, baths and plumbing pipes, furs kettles and water heating apparatus making them less efficient, and if boilers are not regularly cleaned they may burst. Certain types of hard water, such as those containing more than 600 milligrams of calcium salts per gallon, may cause indigestion and diarrhea to persons with a delicate digestive system.

TREATMENT. A combination of lime and soda will soften hard water. Boiling hard water deposits the bicarbonates of calcium and magnesium as fur and is a satisfactory method for softening small quantities. Lime is used for softening larger amounts of this type of water. Sulphates of magnesium and calcium can be removed by adding soda.

Soft Water. Surface water and rain contain no mineral salts and are therefore 'soft' to the touch. Rain falling in industrial areas, however, is full of impurities, e.g. soot and acids, and must be purified before reaching the consumer. Soft water does not fur kettles and pipes but over a long period it may dissolve the metal of the pipes, especially lead. For all domestic purposes, however, it is much more economical than hard water.

Healthful 'Impurities.' In the course of passing through various earths and rocks, water usually contains small quantities of certain minerals valuable to health. Iodine is absolutely necessary for the efficient functioning of the thyroid gland. In areas where water is poor in this vital mineral, some of the local inhabitants are likely to develop goiter and, if it is completely lacking, the children develop so meagerly that they are cretins, stunted and imbecile. Since medical science has in this century discovered the cause of cretinism, it is now an easy matter to prevent it by adding iodine to the local water supplies, or by using iodized tablet salt.

Minute quantities of fluorine in water are helpful in safeguarding dental decay if fluorinated water is taken by young children while the teeth are developing. Too strong a fluorination, however, can cause mottling of the enamel.

Hard water, despite its many drawbacks, is better for bone and teeth formation than soft water.

Diseases Transmitted by Water

Unclean water is an easy medium for transmitting several diseases. The water may be contaminated through leaking pipes or badly made wells, or more directly by infected animals, birds, or vegetable refuse. Infected people bathing in rivers or reservoirs can pollute the water with the micro-organisms of disease.

Some of the disorders transmitted by water are:

1. Intestinal worms
2. Diarrhea and stomach upsets
3. Athlete's foot
4. Poliomyelitis
5. Typhoid and Paratyphoid
6. Dysentery and Cholera.

Most of these diseases can be transmitted when contaminated water is taken by mouth. In the case of athlete's foot, the skin fungus is usually picked up from the damp floor of a communal bath house or swimming pool. Water-borne cholera, a scourge of India, has recently been brought under control by inoculating hundreds of thousands of pilgrims before their ritual purification in the Holy River Ganges.

Do not consume water from open ponds: water in running brooks is usually safe. Do not bathe when suffering from colds, body discharges, or skin infections: you are more likely to infect other people who share the swimming pool than do harm to yourself. Keep bathing suits and towels washed and clean, not merely dried off after use. Use the toilet before swimming.

Ice can be as easily infected as water or food by handling with dirty fingers, and disease organisms frequently survive in it. Children should therefore never be allowed to suck ice from ponds or rivers. Even ice made in the refrigerator at home should always be made from tap water.

BATHING AND CLEANLINESS

The seven million pores of the skin should be kept clean to preserve health. When bathing is neglected, and the undergarments are not changed sufficiently often, perspiration accumulates and dries upon the skin with the oily matter secreted by the oil-glands and with the dead scales of the skin.

The regular use of soap and warm water ensures a healthy and clean condition of the skin.A warm bath should be taken frequently, preferably immediately before retiring to bed, since this reduces the risk of subsequent chills. In young and healthy persons a cold bath or shower may be beneficial in the mornings and is invigorating, but should not be taken by aged or debilitated persons, or by those with heart disease or high blood pressure.

Cold Bathing. Water applied to the skin at a temperature below 24° C (75° F) is called a cold bath. For persons with the constitutional energy to bear it, it is a very powerful tonic; it stimulates the skin circulation and the tone of the muscles.

REACTION. The first effect of the application of cold water to the skin is the sudden contraction of all its vessels, and the return of the blood to the internal organs. The nervous system, feeling the shock, causes the heart to contract with more energy and pump the blood back with new force to the surface areas. This rushing of the blood back to the skin is called a reaction and, when it occurs rapidly, it is evidence that the system is in a condition to be benefited by the cold bath.

When this does not take place, and the skin looks pale and is covered with 'goose flesh,' and chilliness is felt after bathing, then the bath has been too cold or too prolonged, or the bather has too little reactionary power for this form of bath. The latter conclusion should not be accepted until cold water has been tried with various modifications, such as (1) beginning with tepid water and gradually lowering the water temperature; (2) bathing for a time, at least, in a warm room; or (3) beginning the practice in warm weather, and applying the water at first with a sponge from which most of the water has been pressed out. With some or all of these precautions, most persons may learn to use the cold bath. It should always be followed by brisk rubbing with a coarse towel.

The Sponge Bath. For persons who are feeble, only a part of the body should be exposed at a time and this part, having been quickly sponged and wiped dry, should be covered, and another part exposed and treated in a like manner. In this way all parts of the body may successively be subjected to the bracing influence of water and friction, with little risk of an injurious shock. The only requirements for carrying out this simple plan of bathing are a sponge, a basin of warm water and two towels.

The Shower. The shock to the skin and nervous system produced by a shower of cold or cool water is much greater than that from sponging. Besides the sudden application of coldness there is the stimulation of the skin by the fall of the water droplets. Shower baths are excellent for those who are robust and full of vitality, but are unsuitable for invalids and delicate persons.

The Warm Bath. A temperate bath ranges from 75° to 85° F; a tepid bath from 85° to 95°; a warm bath from 95° to 98°; a hot bath from 98° to 105°. A warm bath is of the same temperature as the surface of the body, and produces no shock. To those who are past middle age, the warm bath taken for half an hour twice a week is beneficial. It is a mistake to suppose that the warm bath is weakening; it has a soothing and tranquilizing effect. It renders the pulse a little slower and the breathing more even. If the temperature of the bath is above 98°, the pulse rate is quickened.

The temperature of the warm bath, as of the cold, should be made to range up and down according to the vigor of the system and the circulation of the individual. The aged and the infirm, whose hands and feet are habitually cold, require the bath temperature to be well up towards the point of body temperature. The pulse should not be made to beat faster by it, nor should sensations of heat or fullness be induced about the temples and face.

Turkish, Russian, and Sauna Baths

The Russian bath is essentially a steam bath while both the Turkish and the Finnish Sauna are taken in dry heat to produce copious sweating. They are all invigorating but should be taken with caution by the elderly, by those with high blood pressure, or by fatigued or debilitated persons.

The Russian Bath. In the center of the building is an open space where one undresses. Around this space are doors opening into small rooms filled with vapor. In the center of each room is a series of steps leading nearly to the ceiling. The bather lies on the lowest of these steps and then gradually ascends to higher and hotter ones. The first sensation is that of suffocation, and breathing is difficult, but soon perspiration bursts through the pores and breathing becomes easy and agreeable. The steps vary in heat from 96° to 110° F, and in earlier times the temperature ranged very much higher than this. Bath attendants then flog the bather with birch twigs or coarse towels, lather him well with soap and, after the soap is rinsed off, rub him down and put him under a shower of ice-cold water. The shock is great, but the sensation is pleasant after a few moments. In the past, the bather was made to rush out steaming hot and roll in the snow. For those with a tendency to heart disease, palpitation, vertigo, or blood pressure, the vapor bath should be indulged in with great caution or not at all.

The Turkish Bath differs from the Russian bath in that the atmosphere is dry. The bather first enters the 'frigidarium' or cooling room where he undresses, and passes into the 'tepidarium' or warm room, the temperature of which ranges from 110° to 140° F. The heat induces a gentle perspiration and prepares the system for exposure to a still higher temperature. This is attained in the 'calidarium,' the temperature of which varies from 140° to 200° F. In this room the bather undergoes the operation of kneading or shampooing by attendants. To get the full benefit of a Turkish bath this process should never be omitted, the attendant's hands alone being the sole means of friction. After the sweating, shampooing and soaping, the bather passes into the 'lavatorium' or wash room. Here he begins with a warm shower-bath, the water gradually being changed to cool, and then to cold. This not only washes off perspiration and soap, but also closes the pores and causes a vigorous reaction. The bather then returns to the cooling room where he lounges, wrapped in a sheet, to await the secondary perspiration.

The Turkish bath is one of the most invigorating and refreshing health institutions we have. It is devoid of danger to almost all in average health, if used in moderation. Fear is often expressed about passing from the hot-air room to the cold-water bath but there is no danger in passing into cold water while in a state of profuse perspiration. Adverse changes are brought about through the nervous system of the skin; when this is raised above the normal temperature cold water causes less shock.

Sauna Baths. The sauna baths of Finland are essentially the sweating type. The small, enclosed, compact bath-house (the sauna) is lined with birchwood which gives out a pleasing, mildly pungent aroma due to the heat of the stove in one corner. In Finland the stove is heated with wood logs and the smoke can sometimes be a nuisance but in modern city saunas, electricity does the heating. On slatted wooden shelves, which make the room look like a large airing cupboard, the bather lies in a dry heat of 80° to 100° C (178° to 212° F). The stone or granite-block floor is dampened occasionally by the attendant to give quick humidity, and before long the bather is sweating freely.

A quick warm shower is then taken in the adjoining room, mild towelling, and back to the sweating-room for about 15 minutes. Then a cold shower is taken and the sweating repeated. Three or four showers are taken and finally the bather has a plunge into a cold bath. He dries off and lies down to rest for about a quarter of an hour. The attendant then gives light massage and this is followed by a final relaxed rest for fifteen minutes.

General Rules for Bathing

Certain precautions must always be taken before indulging in any bath. Never take a bath on an empty stomach, as did the Romans, nor immediately after meals, nor should a bath be taken when one is very weary or exhausted.

Warm baths simply relax and cleanse. After all other baths, whether hot air, vapor, or sea bathing, a good glow of the skin should follow.

Elderly people should use warm baths and mild Turkish baths. Cold bathing chills an older person's skin too much and depresses the nervous system. Cold sponge-bathing is a useful adjunct to other health measures in the young and middle-aged, often being a good preventive against catching cold.

Sea-bathing should not be indulged in by the very old or young, by those whose circulation is feeble, or by persons who have heart disease, chronic lung disorders, arteriosclerosis, Bright's disease, or those who are debilitated. A full reaction and a good glow must ensue, and not too much time be spent in the water. No hesitancy should be harbored about plunging in at once, as less heat is thus lost from the body.

SLEEP

During sleep the body is in a state halfway between consciousness and unconsciousness. While conscious, the body responds actively to signals from the brain. During sleep the activity of the whole body is slowed down but remains responsive to the brain, unlike unconsciousness when the brain ceases to respond to stimuli from the skin, eye, and other sensory organs.

Most human beings spend a third of their lives sleeping but the amount of sleep they require varies among individuals, the need for sleep becoming less as a person grows older. It has been thought that eight hours' sleep was the right amount for all adults but people vary in their requirements which average between six and nine hours a night.

The mechanism which sends us to sleep is not fully understood but is generally thought to be brought about by the activity of a 'sleep center' in the brain. Relaxation has a great deal to do with going to sleep. Generally a person is unlikely to go to sleep unless he is both mentally and physically relaxed. But if he is involved in a monotonous activity, such as driving long distances on straight roads. he may fall asleep despite the tension he is under.

Functions of Sleep. One of the most important functions of sleep is to re-store energy in the body. The number of calories used during sleep is about half those required during wakefulness. Sleep, however, does not appear to be solely governed by fatigue since many people who suffer from insomnia can become exhausted without falling asleep and some of those who have slept much of the day can still sleep at night.

It is believed that sleep may play an important part in the growth of skin tissues, by permitting the skin cells to utilize their own glycogen instead of giving it up (via the bloodstream) to the other body tissues as happens during the normal activities of wakefulness. Sleep is certainly one of the most important healing agents known to medicine.

Sleep reduces the activity of the body. Breathing becomes more regular, the heart beats more slowly and blood pressure falls.

Less oxygen is taken in and more carbon dioxide given off. The kidneys work more slowly and the blood becomes more dilute. In old people, however, the kidneys often lose the power to lessen activity during the night.

Types of Sleep. There are two types of sleep, 'light' sleep and 'deep' sleep. The average adult generally falls quickly into a deep sleep which gradually changes to light sleep about 3 or 4 a.m. Sleep then becomes deep again until about 6 a.m. when it gradually becomes lighter until the person finally wakes up. The activities of the body are at their lowest during the phases of deep sleep. It is believed that dreaming only occurs during light sleep.

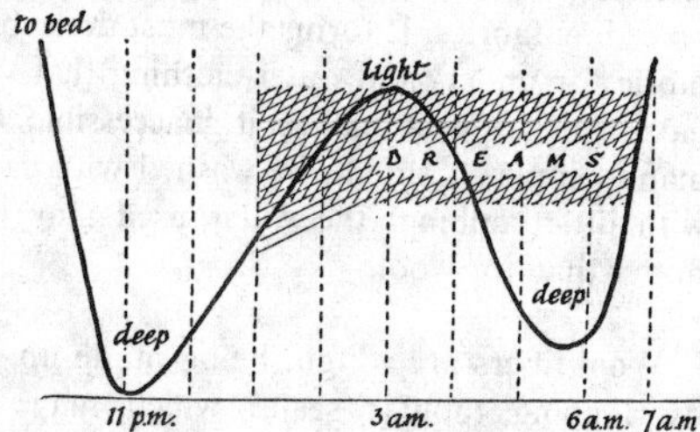

Fig. 21. *SLEEP GRAPH. Diagram showing periods of deep and light sleep.*

Relaxation

Relaxation of both mind and body is the best preparation for sleep. Lying down in a horizontal position relaxes the muscles, reduces the load on the heart and other organs, brings down the blood pressure and dilutes the blood.

It is thought that the most suitable position for sleep is on the side (left or right) with the body supported by the overlying knee and the top forearm resting on the mattress. Most people change their position a number of times during sleep, even the quietest sleepers are said to change as many as twenty times during the night. These movements probably prevent the body from becoming stiff by keeping the distribution of the body weight even.

The body remains sensitive to heat and cold during sleep so it is important that bedding

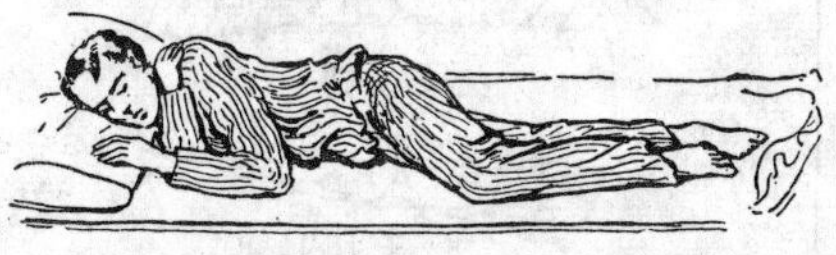

Fig. 22. *AN EXCELLENT POSITION FOR COMFORTABLE SLEEP*

should be warm and light for maximum relaxation.

Closing the eyes, particularly in darkness, relaxes the eye muscles and stops them sending messages to the brain. If one continues to send mental pictures to the brain this will prevent the onset of sleep, so it is important to relax the mind as well as the body. The ears appear to take longer to relax and to cease sending messages to the brain and remain more receptive during sleep than the eyes. Therefore loud or unfamiliar noises may keep people awake.

To get the maximum value from a short sleep during the day people should lie down in bed in a darkened room with the door closed.

How to Relax. Full relaxation is a complete negation of effort. 'Trying to relax' implies some mental effort. You do not 'try,' you give in and yield up your awareness, your worry, your bodily erectness and muscular tension.

It is therefore necessary to lie down in a quiet room comfortably, and with a warm light covering. Even if your mind is full of worries and plans when you first lie down, begin to 'unlock' your muscles. Begin with one arm: sense and tense each upper arm muscle and then let it go quite limp, then the muscles in the lower arm, the palm, the fingers. Do the same with the muscles of the other arm. One by one 'unlock' the muscles of one leg, then of the other. Then your face: you will be surprised at first to find how many small but important face and neck muscles are taut and strained. The forehead, the eye muscles around the lids, the eyes themselves, the cheek, the muscles around the mouth, even the ears—one by one let them yield.

These limp muscles offer no resistance to stretching. The relaxed body and limbs have the semblance of a rag doll. The nerves to and from these muscles convey no messages.

The art of full relaxation is not learned at one attempt but everyone is capable of learning it. At each time of relaxation you will find yourself 'unlocking' still other muscles with an increasing sense of relaxation and slipping away from the cares of everyday bustle.

Children and Sleep

Children require a greater amount of sleep than adults but their individual needs differ greatly. Most babies and very young children sleep during part of the day but will refuse a daytime nap when they no longer require it. Children generally take the right amount of sleep for their personal requirements though emotional difficulties may prevent their getting it (see also Child Care, p. 116). It is quite normal for small children to wake early in the morning.

Preparing for Sleep. Children must be reasonably tired before they can sleep but not overtired as this may keep them awake. The room should be darkened in summer if the child has difficulty in getting off to sleep. Adjust the bedding to make certain that the child does not become too hot or cold and, if he is worried by the dark, provide a night-light so that his fear will not keep him alert.

Parents should not work themselves into a state of worry if a child does not go to sleep immediately on being put to bed as this worry may be communicated to him. A friendly routine at bedtime with a song or story is an excellent preparation for the child before sleep.

Insomnia

Many people suffer from insomnia. Except in rare cases this is not a disease; it is more often caused by psychological difficulties rather than by physical disabilities. Over-excitement, worry, shock and nervous tension, as well as indigestion, are all common causes of insomnia. People suffering from chronic insomnia and those who find difficulty in sleeping because of pain or illness can be helped by sleeping drugs. These will be prescribed by the doctor and the doses should be strictly observed as overdosage can be dangerous. Barbiturates should never be taken with alcohol. Sleeping pills are usually prescribed for short periods only as they can be habit-forming and will not then cure the insomnia. In really difficult cases a visit to a psychiatrist may be of more use than pills.

The important thing for those who suffer from insomnia is to learn to relax and not to worry about the amount of sleep they are not getting.

Aids to Sleep

1. Make sure you are neither too hot nor too cold.
2. Tossing and turning will not help sleep; find as comfortable a position as possible, and relax.
3. Relax the muscles deliberately by tensing them first and feeling them relax, one by one.
4. Follow a relaxing routine before going to sleep. A hot bath is often helpful. Avoid working until the last moment.
5. Reading in bed and counting sheep are stimulating to many people and do not help relaxation.
6. Make sure the room is quite dark and there are no avoidable noises. The ears can be plugged with cotton if necessary.
7. If in need of extra sleep go to bed earlier, relax, and avoid worrying.
8. Hunger causes contractions of the stomach. If hungry before going to bed have a small snack; a big meal before bedtime may retard sleep. Hot milk or hot milk beverages are particularly helpful for aged persons who cannot get off to sleep easily.

Beds and Bedding

The quality of the beds, mattresses, and bedclothes often affects sleep. When we are very tired we may rest even upon a board, but sleep will generally be more sound as well as more refreshing if the bed be somewhat yielding. Forms of bedding which have become popular are the inner spring and rubber foam mattresses.

Rubber foam mattresses should be of the thicker kind—five inches or more in depth—because this gives more firmness to the natural springiness of rubber.

Inner spring mattresses vary considerably in the number and type of springs they contain and in the durability of the padding material in them. It is better for sound refreshing sleep in a healthy posture to purchase as good quality a mattress as possible. A sagging bed in which one sleeps with an unnatural curvature of the spine is harmful, especially to persons prone to backache, lumbago, or other rheumatic affections.

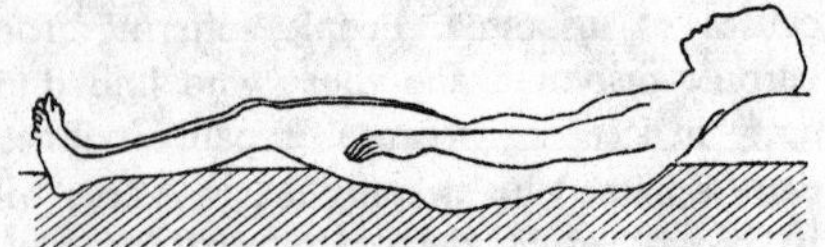

Fig. 23. *A SAGGING BED. This causes an unnatural curvature of the spine.*

Bedding. In hot weather linen sheets are preferable to cotton and are used by those who have ample means, but cotton ones are very suitable for general use, and in winter, preferable. Cotton ones are best, particularly the flannelette ones, for those who suffer from rheumatism. Heaviness in a blanket usually indicates that it is not made entirely of wool and such a blanket will provide less warmth than cellular ones which are light and have the additional good quality of being porous. We should sleep under as few clothes as possible consistent with comfort.

The practice of sleeping with the face entirely covered with bedclothes is very unhealthy and is particularly dangerous for old people. It compels one to breathe the same air several times.

One pillow, neither too hard nor too soft, is adequate to retain a good sleeping posture. For older people, particularly those with bronchitis or heart disease, several pillows will be needed as they sleep better in a slightly sitting position.

CLOTHING

The clothes we wear are intended, or should be intended, to fulfil three purposes; to maintain warmth in winter, coolness in summer, and health at all times. The atmosphere which surrounds us conducts away the heat which comes to the surface of our bodies. In summer or in tropical countries the atmosphere, when very hot, may impart heat instead of conducting it, while in winter we require the protection from the cold afforded by our clothing.

Clothes have no power to manufacture or to impart heat. They only retain and keep in contact with our bodies the warmth generated within us. A good clothing material should (1) retain the natural warmth of the body; (2) absorb perspiration; and (3) be washable, light and durable.

The color of clothing is also of some practical importance. Dark colors absorb the light and heat of the sun's rays much more than lighter ones and, since colors which absorb heat are also good radiators, the dark colors have the highest radiating power.

White reflects heat and rays of light, and is a bad absorber and bad radiator of heat. White garments are therefore cooler to wear in tropical sunlight.

Excessive clothing hampers movement, and makes the skin clammy and less able to react to changes of temperature. Loose clothes are warmer than tight-fitting ones since they retain a layer of warmed air near the body. Heavy clothing is not necessarily warm clothing.

Types of Fabric

The materials in general use for clothes are cotton, linen, silk, artificial silk, wool, nylon and other fabrics produced from man-made fibers, leather, and fur. Today many clothes are made of a mixture of these materials and it is always wise to look at the label or inquire from the shop assistant about the composition of these mixed fabrics. This is important both from the point of view of washing or dry cleaning the garments and of considering whether the cloth will be a bad conductor of body heat (a warm material) or a good conductor (a cool material).

The following list of fabrics is arranged in the order of capacity to retain heat and moisture, and, in reverse, it gives the order of capacity to conduct heat away and permit evaporation of moisture:

Plastics, Nylon, Fur, Leather, Wool, Silk, Rayon (Artificial Silk), Cotton, Linen.

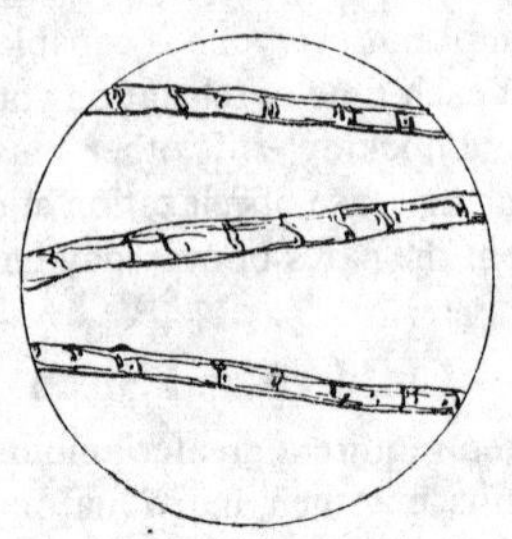

Fig. 24. *LINEN FIBERS*

Linen is woven from the plant fibers made from flax. It takes up moisture which evaporates and so cools the skin, and it conducts heat rapidly away from the body and therefore always feels cool to the touch. It has other qualities which compensate in some measure for this cooling effect; its fibers, for instance, are round and pliable which makes linen cloth smooth and soft and nonirritating.

Cotton—also a plant fiber—is somewhat warmer than linen because it is not such a good conductor of heat. The perfection to which its manufacture has been carried makes it a rival of linen in softness and pliability. It does not absorb as much moisture as linen, and therefore better retains its powers as a non-conductor. The fibers of cotton are not round and smooth like those of linen, but are flat and spiral with sharp edges; modern methods of manufacture, however, have produced fabrics which cannot affect the most delicate skins. The cellular weave used for some cotton underwear provides minute traps for the warm air from the body surface, and thus counteracts the cooling quality of smooth close-woven cotton cloth.

Linen is better than cotton for binding up wounds where there is tenderness of the surface.

FLANNELETTE is made of cotton and, being fleecy, is warmer than smooth cottons, but unless specially treated it is easily inflammable.

Silk, like linen, has a round fiber which is even softer and smaller. It absorbs less moisture than cotton, and in its power of retaining warmth it is superior to both the preceding fabrics. It forms the most desirable fabric for under- and outer-clothing that we have, but its cost makes it inaccessible to many people. It should be washed with care with little rubbing; the water used may be hotter than for wool.

Wool fibers are rough, being made up of overlapping tubular scales which may be highly irritating to some skins. Wool fiber contains a natural fat so that it does not absorb moisture readily and it holds much air among its twisted fibers, the air acting as a poor heat conductor. For infants or adults with delicate skins, or for persons with eczema, woollen underwear should not be worn next to the skin, but it may be worn over a linen or cotton undergarment. Being a good non-conductor, it will in this way preserve the warmth of the body without irritating the skin.

In cold climates wool is one of the best materials of which clothes can be made. In all cold and temperate regions, it may be worn by most people in the form of thick or thin garments nearly all the year round.

If washed with very hot water or bleaching substances, wool shrinks and becomes harsh because the fat is removed from the fibers.

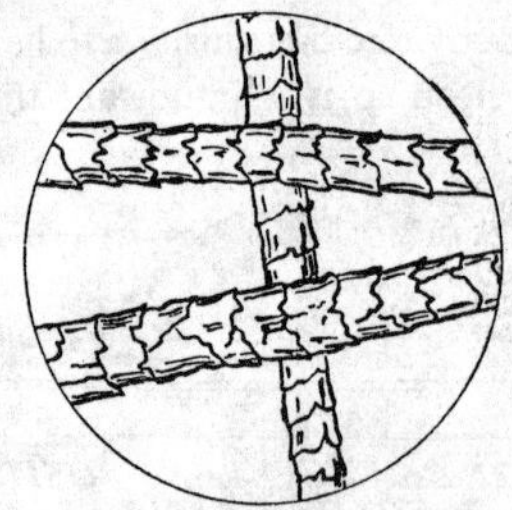

Fig. 25. *WOOL FIBERS*

Therefore it should be washed in warm soft water with good soap or soap flakes (less preferably a gentle detergent), dried away from strong heat and ironed with a damp cloth.

Artificial Silk or Rayon materials are made from the cellulose of plants and trees and the fibres are not so strong as those of silk. It does not absorb much moisture, and because it rapidly conducts heat away it is a cool fabric. Although extensively used for underwear, it is mostly 'woven' in a lacy or a knit form so that air is trapped in the spaces and less heat is conducted away.

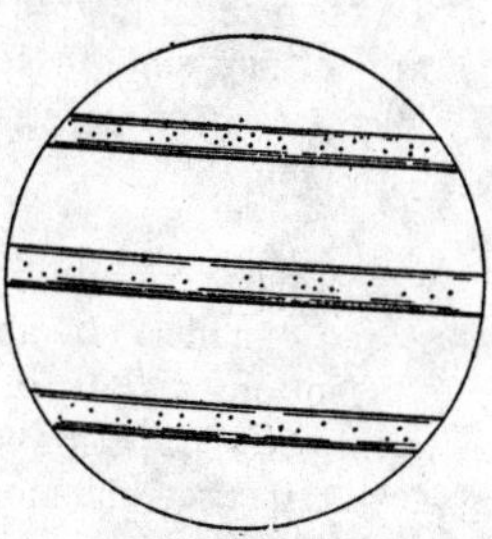

Fig.26 *NYLON FIBERS*

Nylon, and the newer synthetic fibers are increasing in popularity because they are quick drying and need little ironing. Their long, smooth, solid fibers do not absorb moisture but when they are cut short, spun like wool, and knitted, the interstices permit some of the moisture to pass through.

Nylon is difficult to ignite; it melts but does not flare.

Leather and Fur provide the warmest of clothing. They are windproof and therefore very suitable for really cold climates or severe winters.

Rubber. Rubber garments worn next to the skin hinder the evaporation of sweat and are unhealthy. Shoes made of this material soon cause the feet to become clammy and damp, since the perspiration cannot escape through the rubber. Such shoes, if worn in the open air, should be taken off immediately on entering the house.

Shoes

Shoes should fit correctly and be neither too large nor too tight, since either misfit will cause corns. Tight shoes also give rise to bunions and ingrown toe nails. High heels are not advisable, especially when the wearer is required to do much standing or walking; the heels should be low and broad to permit a steady balance and correct posture, especially during childhood and pregnancy.

Shoes are generally preferable to boots, because they allow freer movement of the ankle joints.

SOME PRACTICAL CONSIDERATIONS ON HAVING A FAMILY

Plans Before Marriage

During courtship the young couple who are planning to marry are provided with a chance to get to know one another and discuss in much intimate detail their hopes and desires, their likes and dislikes—in fact their general attitude to life. This gives them an opportunity, if they so wish, to change their minds before taking the final step of marriage. In this exchange of confidences, the subject of having a family is most important for it sets the shape of their whole future. The great majority want to have a family.

Hereditary Factors

In a few cases some doubt may arise about the desirability of having children because of a physical defect in one of the potential parents or in his or her family. In such cases the young couple should consult the family doctor. Epilepsy is a disorder which seems to be inherited in some families and it is advisable for persons from such a family not to have children. Where epilepsy occurs as a solitary instance in a family, the affected person married to a normal person is no more likely to produce an epileptic child than two normal people. A person with muscular dystrophy or a related muscular disorder carries within himself (or herself) a factor causing defective muscular development. Although this factor is not a dominant one, nor is it very common, the mating of two people each with such a factor greatly increases the likelihood of their producing an infant with muscular dystrophy.

Mental disorders and mental deficiency vary greatly in their causative factors. In manic-depressive psychoses and in schizophrenia, the disorder occurs more frequently in families with the trait than in ordinary families. In the case of mongoloids there seems, as far as recent investigations are concerned, to be some familial defect in the genetic make-up, but how it arises is not yet clear.

Tuberculosis is not inherited as a congenital fault, although some people of slender build are more prone to the infection. It is due to infection of part or many parts of the body with tuberculosis bacteria. If the mother is infected, the disease could, of course, be passed on to the baby if the mother nurses it herself.

Deformities such as harelip and cleft palate, spina bifida, and clubfoot are due to malformations during the development of the infant and the chances of one of these anomalies happening are small. Blood group differences in the two potential parents are no bar to the production of healthy children now that medical science can cope with the occasional complication due to the Rhesus factor (see Physiology, p.240).

If one of an engaged couple knows that there is no likelihood of his (or her) being able to have a child, or that it is inadvisable because of the risk of passing on some defect, it is wiser that this should be made known to the other *before* marriage, and perhaps discussed with the family doctor, who may advise on adopting a child.

Budgeting for Baby

In general, the longer the engagement, the more ready are the couple to set up house, home and family once they are married. Again, if there is little money, the young woman may remain at work for a while to help set up the home, deferring the question of starting a family until a certain sum has been earned. It is much better for the future harmony of the marriage that these items are planned in outline early rather than that they should be left to chance.

Career versus Baby

There are many women who have special gifts and training and who feel that they should make use of their capacities outside the home circle. For career women who marry and have children, too, the fitting in of the dual role may mean many sacrifices, and careful planning of both work and family routines. The important matter from the family point of view is that the baby (or babies) is provided with a really good nurse or mother-substitute (see also Child Care, p.118), and the parents must be prepared to accept the natural situation in which the infant is likely to become more attached to his nurse than to his actual mother. Such matters as these must be conscientiously thought over, discussed by both the prospective parents, and carefully planned so that the young child will not be deprived of loving attention in his vital early years.

Many young mothers today, realizing how important the first four or five years are to a small child, forgo their careers for those years and go back to their professions or special work once the child reaches school age.

For mothers who wish to earn a little extra money or be partly occupied with a job out of the home, the difficulty is not so intense, though planning for a first-class mother-substitute is equally important.

Control of Pregnancy

We are concerned here with the creation of a harmonious family life centered around the producing and raising of children. The mechanical and chemical means of controlling pregnancy are, specifically, the concern of the family physician, the obstetrician and gynecologist, and family planning clinics. For those who wish to practice birth control it is best to do so under the professional guidance available.

During the menstrual cycle there are periods of maximum and minimum fertility. Look at the figure below. For five days before ovulation (the day the ovum or egg passes out of the ovary on its way to the womb) and for three days after this, conception is most likely. The ovum is only capable of being fertilized for one to two days: sperm cells can probably live for about five days in the uterus or Fallopian tubes but, as the precise time of their viability is not known, it is safest to allow an extra day or two without inter-

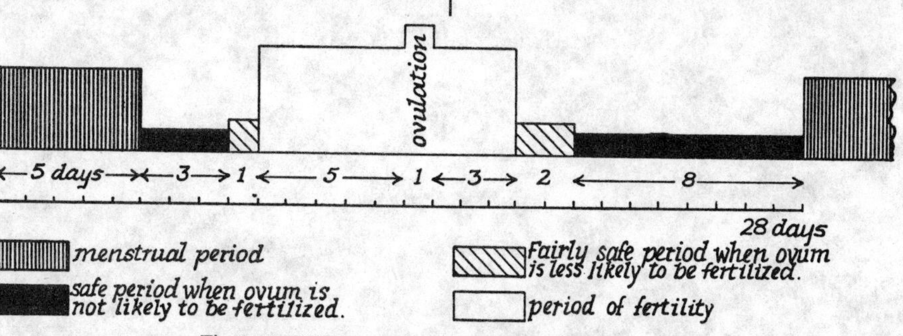

Fig. 1. *A TWENTY-EIGHT DAY MENSTRUAL CYCLE*

course. Menstruation normally occurs 14 days after ovulation.

The 'Safe' Period. The great difficulty with this method of control is that there is so much variability in menstrual cycles. Not only is it that some women have cycles lasting only 24 days and others perhaps 34 days but some women vary greatly from one period to the next. With such great individual irregularity it is impossible to predict an identical or regular safe period for all women. Even for a woman whose menstrual cycle is a regular 28 days, it is essential for her to keep a detailed diary (and preferably charts) of the menstrual dates for at least six months, and make adjustments for the longer and shorter cycles when calculating the 'safe' days. It is surprising how much irregularity is often noted. Casual mental calculations, of course, do away with all 'safety.'

For the 28-day woman, the ovulation day occurs on the fourteenth day after menstruation began. Her fertile period will then be from the ninth to the seventeenth days inclusive, and for the remainder of the cycle she should be reasonably safe. To be on the safer side, however, it is wisest to refrain from intercourse for a day or two on each side of the fertile period.

After childbirth or a miscarriage the cycles may modify in pattern so that the Safe Period needs to be calculated afresh.

Fertility Problems

Not every young couple who sets up home with the intent to have a family is able to produce babies. There are many possible reasons for this inability to have children and, if the years go by and children do not come, the obvious course is to seek medical opinion and examination.

In the early months of married life it may be just shyness, or ignorance of how the body works and is formed, which leads to inadequate intercourse. Read the first part of the section on Functional Changes and Diseases of Women for details of how the woman's body functions.

If marital relations are satisfactory but no child has arrived, a reversal of the 'safe period' (see above) may be utilized. Fig. 1 indicates a period of high fertility in a woman five days before, during ovulation day, and three days after it. The maximum fertility, as far as is known, is on the day prior to ovulation and the ovulation day itself (14 days before the next period in a 28-day cycle). Intercourse on those two days is more likely to result in pregnancy than at any other time.

Fitness to Conceive. Only about 2 per cent of women who seek medical advice about their infertility, have a medical condition which would make pregnancy inadvisable. Pulmonary tuberculosis, for instance, should be cured before a woman has a baby because she runs a serious risk of high blood pressure and an extension of the disease after childbirth; pregnancy should not be undertaken by women with chronic kidney disease.

Infertility due to abnormalities in structure of the child-producing organs is dealt with in Sterility in the section on Functional Changes and Diseases of Women. These anomalies can only be assessed by careful medical examination of either or both prospective parents.

Families in Early and Late Marriages

The tendency for earlier marriage, the couple still being in their teens, poses a problem, especially for those with smaller incomes, of having a baby or a family without adequate housing or household goods to accommodate the new family group.

Living with In-Laws. If economic circumstances make it necessary for a young couple to share a house with parents, the first essential is to come to an agreement at the outset for each pair largely to lead their own private or independent lives. The young couple must have at least one room in which they can be completely private and invite their friends (or the parents) when they wish. If this separation is firmly established at the beginning much heartache and bitterness is saved later on. It will not be long before the young people consider the question of having a baby.

It is a great anxiety to bring up children decently in shared houses. The poor infant is usually unduly checked and scolded so as to prevent his disturbing the rest of the household. The young mother is increasingly fearful that the baby may be resented if he cries and that her ideas of child care are being well criticized. Great forbearance and much genuine affection between the old and the young are necessary for such an arrangement.

Late Marriages. For mature people who marry later in life the matter of having a child or family, before the wife's capacity for child-bearing has become reduced, is often a point of serious concern. Much depends upon the age of the woman. Fertility in women decreases in many cases after the age of twenty-eight although there are the exceptional women who bear two or three children after marrying later than forty years of age.

If a family is desired and a pregnancy is not begun in the first year of marriage do not delay seeking medical help and advice. The ovulation days of maximum fertility should be chosen for intercourse (see p. 91).

PREGNANCY AND CHILDBIRTH

A child is conceived at the moment of union of a sperm cell with an ovum (or egg cell) within the mother's body. Each cell brings half of the necessary characters and when they fuse a new being has begun his existence, and thereafter for the woman the whole pattern of her life will be modified by the responsibilities of her mothering role.

Conception

How is a woman made aware of the fact that she has conceived and is pregnant? Since women generally menstruate every 28 days, the failure to menstruate at the expected time will make a married woman suspect that conception has taken place. Once the fertilized cell has become implanted on the wall of the womb it busily divides and grows, utilizing the mother's blood as its source of nourishment. Menstruation normally ceases when the womb is supplying this nourishment to the immature growing fetus.

The woman may seek confirmation from her doctor who can test her urine for chemical substances only produced when she is pregnant—chiefly chorionic gonadotrophin. There are a number of proprietary test substances available in prepared packs. The test itself can be completed in quite a short time, usually in about two hours, and the woman can be informed of positive or negative results the same day.

The woman may perhaps wait for two months before seeking confirmation, but by then she may be aware of other changes in her body which adapts itself to the needs of the developing fetus. The breasts swell and the ring of skin around the nipples becomes brownish; nausea may be noticed in the mornings; there may be tingling as the breast tissue modifies for production of milk.

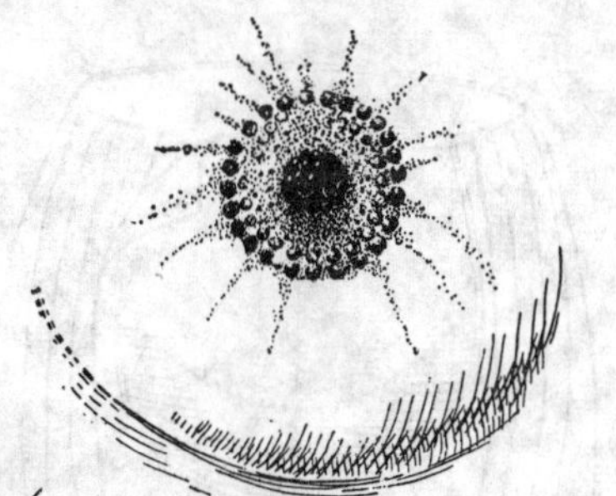

Fig. 1. *A SIGN OF PREGNANCY. An early indication is the aura of brownish coloration around the nipples.*

In a few cases, however, menstruation continues for two or three months when conception has occurred. A single missed period does not necessarily indicate pregnancy—it occasionally occurs in anemia or illness, as well as early in the menopause (see p. 144, and Functional Changes and Diseases of Women).

Estimation of the Date of Birth. If a woman's periods are normally regular and cease soon after conception, the date of expected birth can be fairly accurately calculated, although the precise date will depend on the date conception occurred. The common duration of pregnancy is nine months, 40 weeks, or 280 days. Conception is most likely to occur within 9 to 16 days from the first day of the preceding menstruation; the birth date, however, is reckoned to be nine months plus seven days from the first day of the last period seen.

Quickening. Movements of the baby within the womb are generally felt after about four months and may be an indication of the stage of pregnancy. Quickening is the first slight fluttering or knocking of the fetus within the womb, and this becomes stronger and more definite as the baby grows bigger.

CONDITIONS AFFECTING THE FETUS

In the single small fertilized cell in which the child's life begins lie all the genetic factors and elements which decide the qualities he inherits from his parents and ancestors. These characteristics are contained in the chromosomes and genes (see Physiology), and their various combinations may result in many millions of different personality patterns, so that no two babies are exactly alike, even so-called 'identical twins.' The developing fetus grows by continuous cell division, until there are finally over twenty billion cells. In the very early stage of development these are alike, but differentiation takes place as the various parts of the body such as the brain, bones, muscles, eyes and so forth are formed; and since each of these different structures is formed at different times, the conditions and stresses affecting the mother at different times during her pregnancy are likely to affect the development of different parts of the fetus.

Apart from actual mechanical injuries, any effect on the infant's development after about four weeks following conception occurs mainly through the mother's bloodstream, which carries food and oxygen to the fetus and removes waste products.

Drugs or toxic substances may therefore have some action on the baby; such substances may be nicotine (from tobacco smoking), alcohol, sedative drugs like the barbiturates, aspirin, and many other medical substances which affect the oxygen supply. A pregnant woman often loses the wish to smoke, but in any case it is better to give it up altogether. If this is impossible, the number of cigarettes smoked should be reduced to three or four daily. Smoking leads to constriction of the uterine vessels and so reduces the supply of food to the fetus. Alcohol, also, should only be taken in strict moderation, if at all.

The effect of drugs on the infant's development has been only too tragically observed with the use of thalidomide given as a sedative to mothers in early pregnancy during 1959–1962. The drug passed via the placental blood and damaged the immature limb buds and other parts of the fetus. Although thalidomide is now prohibited, some other drugs are not above suspicion. It is wiser to take more rest for minor discomforts in early pregnancy, rather than take drugs unnecessarily.

Nutrition during pregnancy is also important; the diet must be ample, well-balanced, and supplemented by vitamins, calcium, and iron. A balanced diet will help to prevent pregnancy disorders in the mother and imperfections in development of the baby. The baby, however, generally gets sufficient nourishment even at the mother's expense.

Some gain in the mother's weight is bound to occur in pregnancy and is normally from half to one pound per week. If there is more gain than this, the mother should ask her doctor to prescribe a suitable diet. Fat-forming foods such as cakes and pastries, puddings, cereals, biscuits, sweets, and sugar should be limited, fruit being eaten instead. If the gain in weight is still too much, a low-salt or salt-free diet may be recommended by the doctor.

Certain diseases in the mother can also affect the development of the fetus. German measles during the first four months of pregnancy can cause deafness and malformations in the infant. Syphilis can infect the fetus; gonorrhea may cause infection of the eyes at birth with subsequent blindness. Inadequate nutrition may be provided by mothers suffering from wasting diseases such as tuberculosis or diabetes mellitus. For further details see Disorders of Pregnancy.

It can be seen therefore that protection from toxic substances, an adequate diet and the maintenance of the mother's good health and happiness play a very important part in a baby's prenatal development.

Various fanciful stories and old wives' tales of supposed harmful influences on prenatal growth should be dismissed as coincidences and superstitious beliefs, but it is probably true that constant anxiety, or fear, may lead to chemical changes in the mother's blood which would affect the child's nervous system, giving rise to irritability and nervousness in the newborn child.

Long high-altitude flights, especially in the early months of pregnancy or near full term, are inadvisable because of the risk of oxygen lack in the blood which can occur in non-pressurized aircraft; sickness in bad weather and bumpy flights; fatigue and the difficulty of movement in a confined space, particularly for the legs; and the risk in using the seat belt in the later months of the pregnancy.

Effect on the Mother

Emotional Instability. The expectant mother should try to maintain a happy and serene state of mind, avoiding as far as possible all unnecessary worry and emotional upsets throughout her pregnancy. It is common, however, during these months for a woman to find she cries more readily than usual, or is easily irritated, or upset by quite small things. This increase in sensitivity is quite normal, and the husband should do his best to make daily life as smooth and trouble-free for her as possible.

Marital Intercourse During Pregnancy. The advisability of intercourse during pregnancy often causes some anxiety. It is safest if this is given up during the first twelve weeks because during this time the implantation of the fetus is taking place in the womb and should proceed without risk of disturbance. If intercourse does take place, it must be avoided at the times the menstrual periods would ordinarily be due, since in women who are prone to miscarriage it is most likely to occur at these dates.

As the abdomen increases in size after the third month, it is best to adopt the side-to-side position during intercourse, which is more comfortable and safer, since it prevents pressure on the womb. After the eighth month, it is also best to refrain from intercourse, as it may lead to premature labor. The husband should be particularly considerate to his wife during the whole of her pregnancy, and not make undue demands upon her.

PERSONAL CARE

Some women fear that pregnancy will spoil their looks and attractiveness but this need not happen if an expectant mother takes care of herself and pays attention to certain aspects of health and beauty care.

Skin and Hair. A daily warm bath helps to keep the skin healthy, and the use of a coarse towel afterwards is good for the circulation. Sunbathing, with carefully graduated exposure so that the skin does not burn or redden, is good for general health, but the head and eyes should be protected from direct sunlight.

The Skin and Complexion may need extra nourishment if they become dry; a good skin food should be used regularly each night and a protective non-drying foundation cream applied during the day.

Hair, Hands and Nails should also be given regular careful attention, so that a generally well-groomed and well-cared for appearance is kept right through the nine months.

Teeth. Care of the teeth is very important at this time, and foods with a high calcium content—milk, cheese, cauliflowers, etc.—should be eaten so that the mother's blood does not 'borrow' calcium from her teeth for the bony structure of the fetus.

Feet. To prevent flat foot due to the extra weight-bearing, shoes must be chosen to allow correct posture while standing and walking. Shoes with too high or pointed heels are unsafe for balance and throw the whole spine and pelvis out of position, so that the abdominal muscles tend to sag, and the pelvis and spinal ligaments and muscles become strained and fatigued. The flat types of casual shoes, or slippers (with non-slip sole) can be attractive as well as comfortable, and are made in variety of styles and colors.

Daily Barefoot Exercises for the feet are very helpful. Here are two simple but useful ones.

(1) Rise slowly on tiptoe with the arms extended sideways for balance: sink slowly. Repeat 15 to 20 times.

(2) Stand with the feet slightly apart and roll feet outwards, to stand on outer edge of soles; curl the toes firmly under the foot. Return to normal standing position. Repeat 15 to 20 times.

Abdomen. The muscles of the abdominal wall become stretched during pregnancy as the womb increases in size, and the skin also undergoes changes. Light massage of the abdomen with olive oil or a good skin lotion should be carried out daily to keep the skin supple, the skin being rolled between the fingers in folds; this should do much to prevent the appearance of the white lines or stria often seen in the later months of pregnancy.

Breasts. The nipples vary in different women, and may be large or small or, in a few cases, may be inverted into the breast. The size and shape of a mother's nipples are of great importance in breast feeding. The nipples should be pulled out daily during pregnancy—in the bath is a good time—and gently massaged with oil or skin food to prepare them for suckling (see also p. 100). If one or both nipples are actually inverted, the doctor should be consulted about the possibility of breast feeding.

Clothes for the Expectant Mother

Maternity clothes can be comfortable, gay and attractive, and an expectant mother should continue to study her appearance and look fresh and charming throughout her pregnancy. For the first twelve weeks ordinary clothes can be worn, but these will later become too tight, and will be uncomfortable and unsuitable. All tight clothes must be put aside. The brassière should give good support without any constriction and should be adjustable to allow for the increasing size of the breasts. Corsets and tight girdles are, of course, not to be worn; a good adjustable maternity belt has no constriction at the top, but provides some support below. Tight elastic in knickers and garters must not be worn as they predispose to varicose veins.

Maternity clothes, such as two-piece dresses or 'separates' with adjustable skirts and loose tops, pinafore dresses, or loosely fitting dresses without belts provide a variety of suitable styles for indoor wear; coats should be loose and easy to slip on and off.

With a little care and not too much expense, the expectant mother need not feel in the least dowdy, and can, if necessary, often continue in a job until the seventh or eighth month without embarrassment.

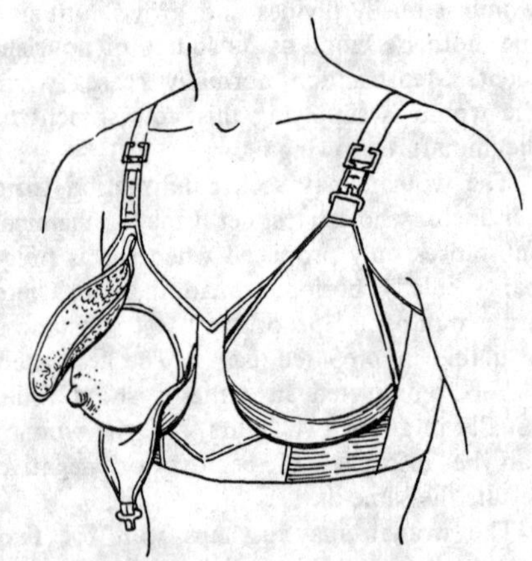

Fig. 2. *MATERNITY AND NURSING BRASSIERE. The drop cups have a hook and eye adjustment. The illustration also shows a pad in place for absorbing milk secreted in early lactation.*

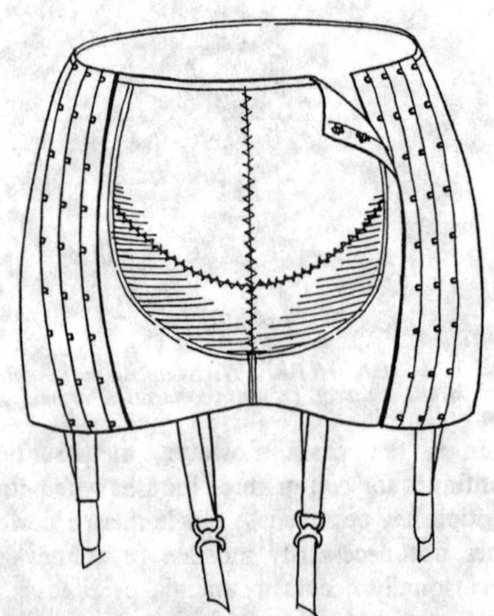

Fig. 3. *MATERNITY BELT. The net elastic front comfortably supports the enlarging abdomen and the rows of stepped hook fastenings allow for expansion.*

PRENATAL CARE AT THE CLINIC

No young wife today need let her happiness in having her first baby be marred by alarmist neighbor's talk or fearsome descriptions of childbirth. When her pregnancy is confirmed by her doctor's examination, he will then arrange for her to have prenatal care either by a doctor with special experience of obstetrics, or at a local clinic, or at a hospital prenatal clinic. At many of these clinics classes are held where the mothers can discuss their problems and where they are given full explanations of the birth process. They will also be taught about the importance of relaxation and how to relax and how to keep fit.

Regular medical supervision from the second or third month is always necessary to prevent any complications either during pregnancy or labor, and to minimize possible risks for both mother and child.

Examinations

At the first visit to the prenatal clinic the expectant mother is asked about her general health. The urine is tested to ensure that the kidneys are working normally and that sugar or albumen is not being passed. The heart, lungs, teeth, and abdomen are examined, and the weight is recorded. Visits are generally made monthly, and then every two weeks for the last two or three months. The blood pressure and urine are tested at each visit.

The measurements of the mother's pelvis are made to decide whether the birth of the baby is likely to be straightforward at full term. In cases where the hip girdle and pelvis are small, labor may have to be induced early, since a small baby makes delivery easier.

The abdomen is examined by the doctor to determine the size of the womb as pregnancy advances. After the third month the womb rises above the pubis, or bony front rim of the pelvic girdle. Later the position of the baby can be felt. A baby is normally delivered head first, and in the later weeks of pregnancy the head should be down in the pelvis. In some cases the baby does not turn, and remains head uppermost or lies transversely across the abdomen; the doctor then often attempts to turn the baby by manipulation. If this does not succeed the baby may then be born in the 'breech' position, i.e. buttocks first.

Twins. If the mother is carrying twins these may be felt by the doctor when he examines the abdomen; the womb will be rather larger and heavier than when there is a single fetus, and the abdomen is often more prominent. The presence of twins can be confirmed by X-ray examination, and two fetal hearts may be heard by the doctor in the seventh month or later. Extra care is needed during a twin pregnancy. The mother needs to rest more and must be careful to avoid prolonged standing or fatigue. Her blood pressure must be taken very regularly, and a supporting belt with shoulder straps may be advisable to help the abdominal muscles.

Iron Tablets. If the expectant mother is found to be anemic (from deficiency of iron) she is given iron tablets or pills to take throughout pregnancy; the pills are generally supplied to most pregnant women to prevent anemia.

Prenatal Exercises and Fresh Air

A daily walk in the fresh air should be taken to stimulate the muscles and circulation and help keep all the organs of the body healthy. Nowadays many prenatal clinics advise special exercise to make labor easier and to help breast feeding. Giving birth to a child involves considerable muscular work, and the body must be prepared and trained.

Breathing Exercises

These are important because the enlarging uterus tends to compress the other abdominal organs and lungs a little, and it is then easier to breathe shallowly, using only the upper part of the lungs. The amount of oxygen supplied to the blood is lessened just when more is needed to supply both mother and fetus. Breathing exercises should be practiced daily in front of an open window, or better still in the garden.

Stand with the feet about 18 inches apart. Rise on tiptoe, lifting the arms sideways to shoulder level, and breathing in slowly and deeply. Then lower the arms and heels, breathing out fully. Repeat this about ten times.

Prenatal Exercises

1. Stand upright and hold the back of a firm chair. Rise on tiptoe and tense all the muscles of the body. Descend to a squatting position with the knees widely separated. Lean back, with weight on the heels, bend the head forward and arch the back; straighten the legs, and return to the erect standing position. These movements exercise the pelvic ligaments and muscles.

2. Sit on a rug; bend the legs with the knees outwards and the soles of the feet together. Hold the ankles, with the forearms between the knees; with the elbows push the knees down and outwards to stretch and mobilize the pelvic joints.

3. Kneel on a rug and rest the forearms and forehead on the floor. Extend (hollow) and then arch the spine slowly but firmly, to mobilize the spine and relieve backache.

4. Sit on the front half of a firm chair with the legs apart. Place the hands on the insides of the knees and push them outwards, rocking forwards with the back hollowed, and then backwards with the back rounded and knees relaxed.

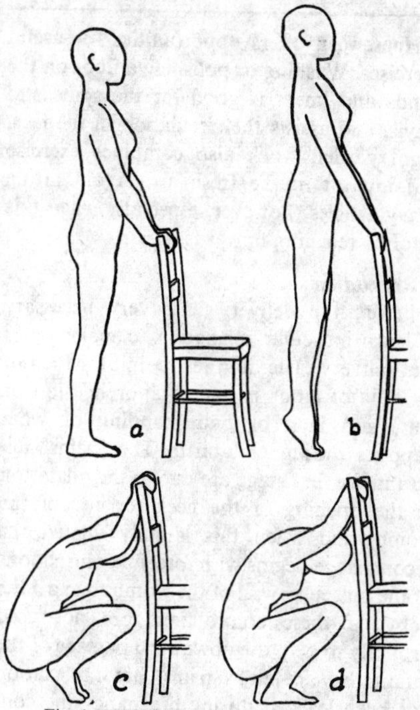

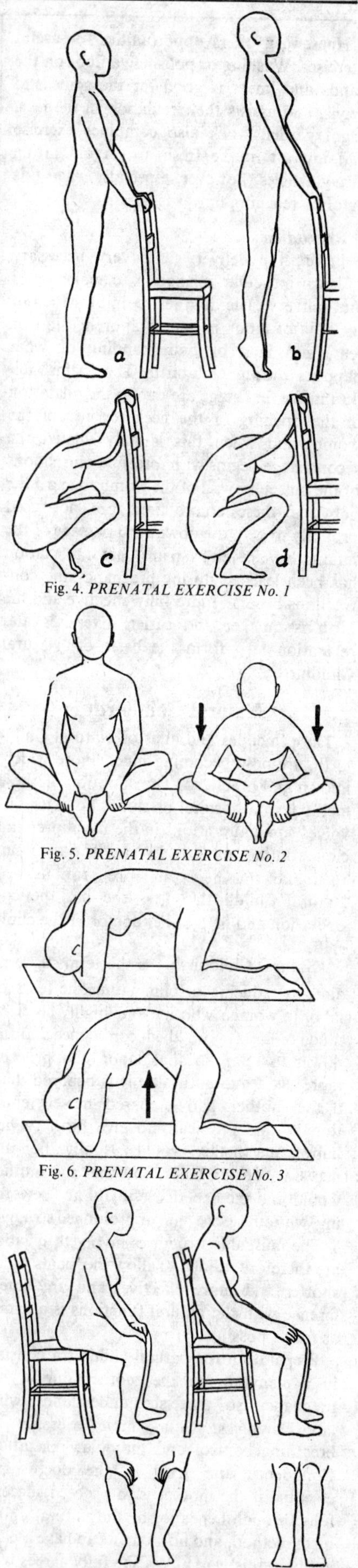

Fig. 4. *PRENATAL EXERCISE No. 1*

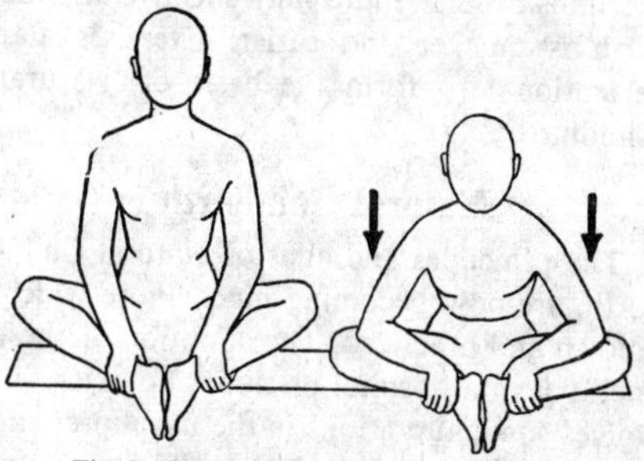
Fig. 5. *PRENATAL EXERCISE No. 2*

Fig. 6. *PRENATAL EXERCISE No. 3*

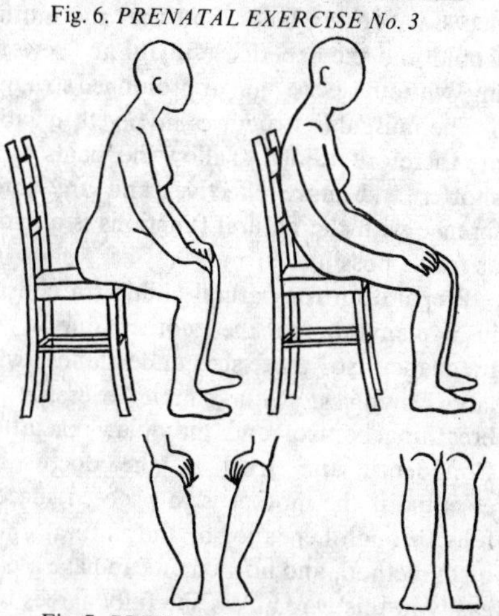
Fig. 7. *PRENATAL EXERCISE No. 4*

Housework offers opportunities for useful exercises. Washing or polishing a floor on the hands and knees is good for the spine and pelvis, and assists the circulation in the legs. Light garden work also combines exercise and interest in the fresh air. Avoid lifting heavy articles, however, especially when this involves reaching upwards.

Relaxation

Before the delivery it is very necessary to learn muscular relaxation to make labor and delivery easier and less painful. Much of the pain of labor is due to apprehension or fear, and lack of understanding of what happens during childbirth. The 'pains' felt during the first stage are due to the dilatation of the opening of the neck (cervix) of the womb, and when this is fully dilated the second stage begins with forceful contractions of the muscular wall of the womb to expel the baby. If these contractions are not used properly to help the downward passage of the infant, they are felt as 'pains,' but if relaxation has been learned during pregnancy the contractions become more fully effective and the birth is quicker and easier. Exercises and relaxation also form the basis of 'Natural Childbirth.'

Natural Childbirth

The principles and aims of Natural Childbirth, are now becoming much more widely known and practiced. The adoption of these methods in a hospital or clinic, however, involves some alterations in the usual prenatal clinic routine, and it is not easy for a woman to make the necessary preparations for Natural Childbirth unless she has the cooperation and help of her doctor or the clinic staff.

'Natural Childbirth,' as the term suggests, aims at reducing or eliminating the fears of labor in women who live our highly civilized mode of life. It gives them confidence and the power to relax so that labor can proceed more easily and naturally. It is believed that, if the mother had prepared herself emotionally and physically to give birth to her baby, anesthetics would usually be unnecessary during labor, and that the mother would find the experience joyful and rewarding, without severe pain or prolonged struggle.

The muscular structures involved in labor are therefore trained to allow the 'pains' to be shorter and more effective, and any interference with the natural functions is avoided as far as possible.

Preparation for natural childbirth consists in explanation to the mother during her pregnancy so that she understands what labor involves, with simple exercises in breathing control and muscular relaxation. Confidence and trust in the doctor are essential if the mother is to proceed successfully through her labor by the natural childbirth method, and no woman can have a baby easily in this way unless she fully agrees with the aims and principles. The husband should also approve and agree, and is welcomed if he wishes to be present at the birth.

The baby is not put in a separate room from his mother, as is common in many hospitals, but stays in a cot by the bed so that she can 'mother' him and feel contented by his nearness.

AILMENTS AND DISORDERS

Occurring During Pregnancy

Morning Sickness. This is common and occurs mainly in the first three months. A feeling of sickness may, however, be felt at other times of the day, or in the evenings, and may persist up to six or seven months, varying from slight nausea to quite distressing retching and vomiting. Eating a dry biscuit or a lump of sugar will generally help. Meals should be eaten as dry as possible, with drinks between meals. Rich or fried foods should be avoided, as well as fatigue and worry.

Constipation. Drink plenty of water and take reasonable regular exercise. Fruit, dried fruits, orange juice, salads and vegetables may be taken plentifully. All-Bran is helpful. Piles are likely to develop during pregnancy if the bowels are constipated and there is much straining, so it is important to adjust the diet and keep the bowels regular. Never take castor oil or strong purgatives.

Frequency of Passing Water. This is a very common complaint, due to the pressure of the enlarging womb. If it disturbs sleep at night, do not drink any fluids after two hours before bedtime. Take more water in the mornings and during the day.

Varicose Veins (See also Diseases of the Heart). These distended veins are painful and tend to develop in some women during the later half of pregnancy. Walking exercise is very useful, but avoid prolonged standing as much as possible; whenever resting during the day, lie down and raise the legs horizontally on a comfortable support. If the legs swell, or varicose veins begin to appear, use an elastic stocking, and never wear any tight clothing or garters.

Cramp. Cramp often occurs during the night, and may be partly due to lack of calcium and partly to pressure from the enlarged womb. Take plenty of milk, cheese, and green vegetables, and tell the doctor who may prescribe calcium tablets. A glass of water with half a teaspoonful of salt taken at night is sometimes useful.

Toxemia. Headache (with or without vomiting) after the first three months, or blurring or any disorder of sight, or swelling of the face or hands, should be reported to a doctor immediately, as such signs may indicate toxemia. For fuller details see Disorders of Pregnancy.

Vaginal Discharge. If this is profuse it may cause discomfort, with irritation and soreness of the vaginal opening, and perhaps smarting on passing water. The common vaginal discharge is known as leucorrhea or 'whites', and consists of a mucoid non-inflammatory fluid; if the discharge is yellow or thick, the doctor should be consulted at once, and a thorough examination made. For leucorrhea warm vaginal douches of soda bicarbonate or salt and water (1 teaspoonful to 1 pint of warm water) may be used twice a week, and constipation must be avoided.

Hemorrhage. Bleeding from the vagina may indicate threatened miscarriage. The patient should go to bed at once and a doctor be sent for immediately. For the causes, diagnosis and treatment, see Disorders of Pregnancy.

Miscarriage. Although the great majority of women go through the nine months of pregnancy without any threat of miscarriage, certain sensible precautions are advisable.

1. Do not let yourself get overtired.
2. Never undertake heavy lifting jobs, or work involving straining, pushing heavy fúrniture, or stretching upwards.
3. Be extra careful at the times menstrual periods would be due, and avoid marital intercourse at these times.
4. Do not take prolonged or heavy exercise such as heavy gardening, or long journeys by bus, train, or car.
5. Avoid chills, emotional upsets, risks of falls, undue strain or anxiety of any kind, sea journeys, influenzal infection any situations with risk of injury crowds, crowded vehicles, competitive sporting events, etc.
6. Wear sensible shoes with broad heels to reduce the risk of falls.
7. Never take strong purgatives during pregnancy.
8. Make regular visits to the doctor or clinic.

THE CONFINEMENT

Apart from the baby's own necessities such as the crib, bedding, bath, toilet articles and clothing (see Layette, p. 110), the mother wi need nightdresses opening down the front fo breast-feeding, and maternity brassières.

Time for Delivery

Labor may take place at any time from the seventh month onwards. If the birt occurs between the 28th and 38th week that is more than 2 weeks before full term (40 weeks), it is said to be premature. Premature babies may be born alive, but the greater the prematurity the smaller the bab will be, and the more care it will need t survive and thrive. Premature labor may b due to various causes such as shock or a fa accidents or injury, placenta previa, toxemi or acute fever; or it may be deliberate induced by the doctor, in some cases, if t mother's measurements are small, or f other health reasons.

Attendant. When labor is thought to have begun the midwife or the hospital doctor should be at once informed, by telephone, and details given as to the 'pains,' show of water or blood, and any other points of useful information (see Stages of Labor).

Hospital and Transport. If transport is to be by car, arrangements must be made in advance. Clean towels should be placed on the seat, with cushions for comfort and to reduce jolting. A blanket should be laid over the mother, who should keep her feet and legs up on the seat and relax as comfortably as possible. A bowl or bedpan should be taken in case urine needs to be passed or the water breaks and a warm water bottle in cold weather. An experienced woman attendant should be present during the journey.

Presence of the Husband. Nowadays some young husbands feel they should share the experience of childbirth with their wives by being present during labor; this is especially the case where the wife has prepared for the delivery by Natural Childbirth methods, in which it is thought to be important for a husband to watch the birth. The husband can give the wife moral as well as physical support and encouragement. Some women may not like the idea of their husbands seeing them during labor, but others feel the shared experience makes the marriage bond closer, and that the husband's presence is natural and a great help, especially during a first labor in which the first stage is more likely to last several hours.

A number of hospitals now make arrangements for the father to be with his wife during labor, and, even if he does not watch the last stages and the actual birth, his presence during the first stage is generally a great comfort to the wife, and helps to reduce the husband's anxiety during a separation often lasting some hours.

The Stages of Labor

Labor takes place in three separate stages.

In the FIRST STAGE the mouth of the womb dilates, with regular and intermittent contractions of the womb giving 'pains' of a colicky type; these gradually increase in frequency and strength, and usually last one or two minutes, with 10- to 15-minute intervals. The passing of mucus, known as a 'show,' continues, and it may become tinged with blood. The bag of water in which the baby lies enclosed in the womb may break early, but more generally this does not occur until the second stage. When the neck of the womb is fully dilated and open, the second stage begins. In a first delivery the first stage may last up to 18 hours or more, and unless the water breaks early the mother may sit up and move about the room during this time.

THE SECOND STAGE. The mother must now lie down, with the nurse in attendance. The pains have a bearing-down character and are stronger than in the first stage. The mother is encouraged to use these pains to push the baby down the birth canal, and to rest and relax between them. The second stage ends with the birth of the child; in first deliveries it lasts two hours or more, but in subsequent labors may be very short indeed, and the baby may be born without much warning.

THE THIRD STAGE is shorter and easier, and follows a rest of ½ hour up to 2 hours; it ends in passing the 'afterbirth' or placenta. After this the mother can rest and sleep.

Birth Positions of the Baby

Delivery of the baby may take place by various presentations. Normally the head presents and is delivered first, with the occiput (or back of the head) toward the front of the mother's body, the soft skull bones being molded in the birth canal to prevent injury. If the face is in front labor is likely to be longer. When the baby has not turned head downwards at full term it may be born as a breech (or buttocks) presentation, or if the mother's pelvic measurements are small and delivery is likely to be difficult, the doctor may advise a Caesarean operation (see Disorders of Pregnancy). Today the course of most labors is foreseen, and plans for delivery are made accordingly.

After Delivery

Bleeding (Post-partum Hemorrhage). Some loss of blood after passage of the afterbirth always occurs, but the womb should normally contract and prevent severe bleeding. If the afterbirth is slow in being passed, or some portion is retained, the womb may remain relaxed and distended and severe bleeding follow. In these cases the womb is massaged by the doctor's hand, through the abdominal wall, to compress it and assist contraction. Occasionally the placenta needs to be removed by hand, and this of course must be done with strict surgical asepsis.

If labor is normal and there is no tear or other complication, the mother will be allowed to sit up and get out of bed during the lying-in period, to lessen the likelihood of 'white leg,' or phlebitis in the leg.

Vaginal Discharge. This will continue for up to two or more weeks, gradually changing from red to brown after seven days, and finally becoming white. If, after two weeks, the discharge seems profuse or smells unpleasant, the doctor should be informed.

Diet. For 24 to 36 hours after labor the diet should be light, with milk, fruit, semi-solids, and cereals. After this period the mother must be given a good varied diet for her own recuperation and to provide the supply of breast milk.

After Pains. These are normally felt for up to about two weeks, and are a sign that the womb is contracting down to regain its normal size and to expel the 'lochia' or secretions after the birth.

THE NEWBORN BABY

When the baby has been delivered the doctor sees that it begins to breathe naturally and that its color is good. Generally the child soon lets out a shrill cry, but sometimes it may be necessary to slap it gently on the back, or to draw off mucus from its throat by means of suction through a soft rubber catheter, the child being held head slightly downwards to allow drainage. Babies who are born in partial asphyxia look white or bluish, because the breathing and pulse are poor.

Tying the Cord. When the baby is breathing properly (usually within two or three minutes) the navel cord is tied securely by the nurse in two places, about two inches from the naval, with sterile ligatures; the cord is then cut with sterilized scissors between the two tied places.

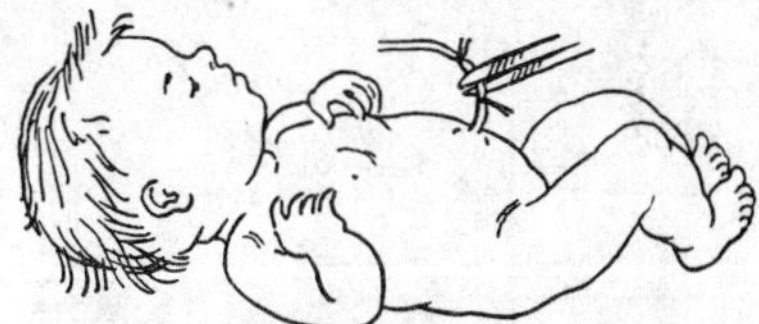

Fig. 8. *CUTTING THE NAVEL CORD*

The Eyes are generally treated with silver nitrate (2 per cent) solution, or penicillin, to counteract any infection from the birth canal.

Washing. After a normal birth the baby is washed gently and dressed by the nurse The body is often covered with a greasy substance called vernix caseosa, which is removed by rubbing gently with olive oil before bathing.

The cord must not be wetted, and is covered with a sterile gauze pad dressing.

LYING-IN PERIOD

The first twenty-four hours after delivery are a resting period for both mother and baby. When the mother has held her baby in her arms and shared her joy with her husband, she will feel that the nine months of waiting and the labor have brought their full reward. In some hospitals the babies are kept in a separate room, except at feeding times, but at home the mother will probably like to have the crib near her own bed. Then she can see the nurse bathe the baby, change diapers and learn the details of baby care. If she is in hospital, before she leaves the nurse will tell her how to bathe and diaper and dress and how to handle her baby.

The lying-in period generally lasts for about ten days if the birth was straightforward, although the mother may leave hospital earlier to rest at home.

The Breasts. During the first three or four days the breasts do not form milk, which is preceded by a watery fluid called colostrum. The baby is generally held to the breast about six hours after birth and thereafter three or four times a day until the milk comes in. At first the breasts may feel rather tight and tender, but if the baby sucks well this should soon pass off. If it does not, the nurse in charge should be told, as it is important to avoid congestion and engorgement of the milk ducts (see Baby Care, p. 100).

Postnatal Exercises

These are important to help the womb return to its normal size and position, and to strengthen the abdominal muscles which have been stretched for four or five months, as well as the spinal and pelvic ligaments which have borne the extra weight and strain.

After delivery, if there is no tear, the mother should lie on her stomach during the afternoon rest in the lying-in period, to help the womb return to its normal position in the pelvis. In some cases it tends to turn backwards as it sinks down and become 'retroverted' (see Diseases of Women).

The following exercises are simple to do, but most effective in helping to restore good muscle tone.

1. While lying on stomach with head turned sideways, stretch the arms straight forward, raise the head and look forward, and press the legs together to contract the buttocks and abdominal muscles. Relax and then repeat several times.
2. Repeat these movements lying on the back. Breathe in during the contractions, and out during relaxation.
3. Lie on the back, with tne legs and arms straight. Draw the knees upwards, with the feet resting on the bed. Slide the palms of the hands under the buttocks and lift them from the bed, pressing the thigh muscles together, and contracting the abdomen and buttocks. Lie back on the bed, rest, and then repeat.
4. Kneel on the bed on hands and knees with the feet together and hands about 12 inches apart. Arch the back, bend the head down, contract the abdomen, the buttocks and thigh muscles. Bend the knees until the buttocks are resting on the heels and the forehead lies on the bed. Relax the elbows and remain so for 2 or 3 minutes.

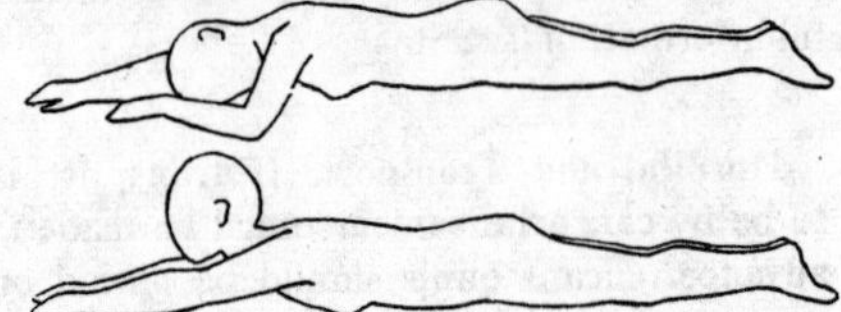

Fig. 9. *POSTNATAL EXERCISE No. 1*

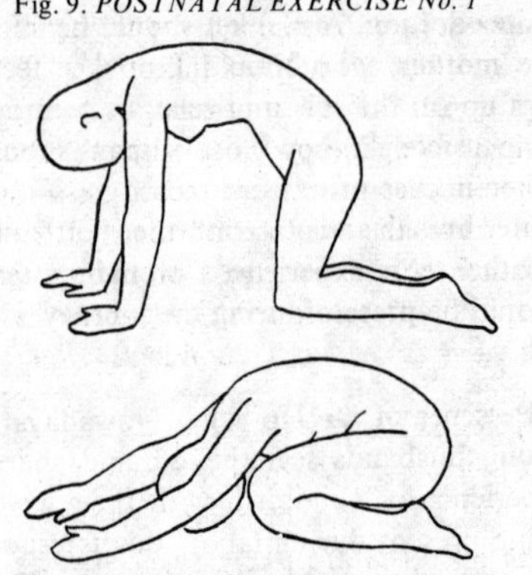

Fig. 10. *POSTNATAL EXERCISE No. 4*

BABY CARE

In baby care, the first essential is for the parents to have a happy confidence that they are doing the best for their child. This instinctive care from kindly parents is most important to the helpless infant. It is a fundamental part of all mothering—a quality so difficult to define by those who study human behavior, yet so natural to all good parents who have the welfare of their children at heart. Even the youngest of babies quickly gains a sense of security when handled lovingly, gently, and confidently, talked to and smiled at and fed happily when he needs it.

Of course there are innumerable details which have to be learned by parents about looking after and bringing up babies, and some mistakes are likely to be made in the process; most thoughtful parents, however, can overcome or avoid many of the common pitfalls.

As far as the outward physical signs are concerned a healthy baby is making good progress when he shows:

An average steady gain in weight each month;

Readiness for each feeding, and good appetite;

Peaceful sleeping periods;

Normal stools, with regular bowel actions;

Firm muscles, healthy smooth skin, pink cheeks and rosy lips;

Bright eyes and active movements of limbs;

General contentment and normal steps in progress; and

Teething without much disturbance.

THE NEWBORN BABY

The Skin. A newborn baby may at first sight be rather a disappointment to his parents. The skin of the body and face is often red, and the face may be wrinkled or puffy—especially around the eyes. The baby's body may be covered with rather downy hair, which comes off after about a week.

Small red mottled spots are quite common, especially on the back of the neck, between the eyes, and on the upper eyelids; these gradually disappear without treatment. Small 'port wine' and 'strawberry' marks often fade in a year or two though larger ones may require surgery.

Up to 50 per cent of negro babies have 'blue spots' (concentration of pigment) which could be mistaken for bruises but they fade within a few months.

The Baby's Head. The size and shape of the newborn baby's head should be carefully noted by the doctor, and also the grooves and the spaces called fontanelles between the bones of the skull. At birth the average circumference of the head is 13 to 14 inches.

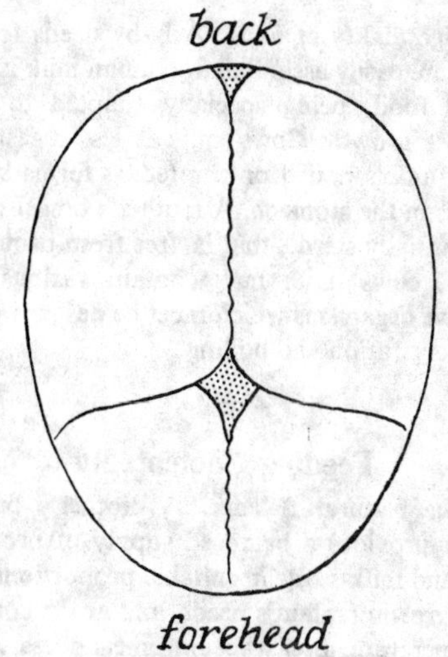

Fig. 1. *FONTANELLES. The space between the back skull bones is almost closed at birth although the front fontanelle usually takes twelve to eighteen months to close.*

The shape of the head varies in different races, and in some babies the skull is not symmetrical, but this is not usually important, and generally becomes less noticeable when the hair grows and as the child grows older.

The fontanelle above the frontal bones generally closes between twelve and eighteen months after birth. The fontanelle above the occipital bones is generally almost closed when the baby is born at full term.

The Scalp. At birth the baby usually has a soft growth of down (lanugo), or there may be thick dark hair on the scalp; this will be shed and by six months the new hair should be making good growth. At birth a swelling is sometimes seen on the top of the skull; this is due to pressure during labor and to edema, but it disappears within a few days.

The Eyes. For a short while after birth a baby cannot 'see' clearly objects or people around him. He is aware of light and dark and of moving shapes before he can see faces or focus on objects in the room. When he is a month old his eyes should follow a moving light and at two months he can see objects fairly well.

A newborn baby often squints during the first few weeks of life, but this generally disappears as his powers of vision develop. In some babies the squint is more apparent than real, particularly if the eyes are set close together. If by the age of three months the baby's eyes are not straight most of the time he is awake, a doctor's advice should be sought.

The Abdomen. When an infant is quite young the abdomen is normally rounded and this fulness continues until he is three or four years old, but at five years the muscles are stronger and the abdominal wall is firmer and flatter. If the abdomen is abnormally large a doctor should be consulted.

The Umbilical Cord. The cord is usually cut about two inches from the baby's abdomen; the stump must be kept dry and aseptic until it separates from the navel, which usually occurs after about a week from birth. In many cases the baby is not bathed in a bath until the cord is off so as to avoid wetting and infection; he is sponged on the nurse's lap instead. If the cord does become wet it should be dried with alcohol. An antiseptic powder may be used if there is any discharge, but, if there is any redness or sign of inflammation around the navel, a doctor should see it at once.

Occasionally a small protuberance or hernia, up to the size of a small cherry, persists in the navel. This commonly disappears in time and it is not usually necessary to apply adhesive strapping support which makes the skin sore.

Premature Infants

All babies weighing less than five and a half pounds at birth need special care and, if the infant weighs under four pounds, such attention is best given in hospital. Otherwise care may be undertaken at home if facilities are adequate and a good nurse is in attendance.

FEEDING. This may present problems, since the baby's stomach is small and his powers of sucking and swallowing are often feeble. The infant requires 3 ounces of fluid and 60 to 75 calories per pound of body weight during each 24 hours. At first a very small baby may need to be fed every hour; breast milk should be given whenever possible. As the baby gains weight the intervals between the feeds are increased. Tube feeding may be necessary if the baby cannot suck or swallow, while a dropper is used when the baby can swallow, but cannot suck.

FEEDING INFANTS AND YOUNG CHILDREN

Correct feeding is one of the most important contributions to health and normal growth in early life, and certain basic needs must be met.

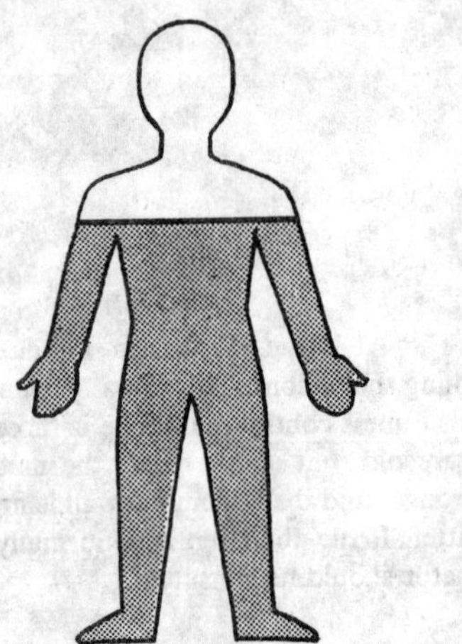

Fig. 2. *BODY FLUIDS form* 70 *per cent of the body weight.*

Fluids. Water is the essential medium for all the processes taking place in the body, and the body fluids form about 70 per cent of the body weight. Lack of water or fluids from insufficient intake, or from excess loss as in vomiting, sweating or diarrhea can seriously affect a baby's health in a very short time. The minimum amount needed by a full-term baby is 2½ ounces per pound of body weight per day, and premature babies require rather more. In feverish disorders, diarrhea, and after vomiting the intake must also be increased.

Calories. When foods are absorbed during digestion they provide fuel for oxidation, to give out heat and energy and for growth. The unit of heat is called a calorie.

Human milk	20 calories per fluid ounce	
Cows' milk (raw)	20 ,, ,, ,, ,,	
Reconstituted full cream dried milk	20 ,, ,, ,, ,,	
Reconstituted half cream dried milk	16 ,, ,, ,, ,,	
Unsweetened full cream condensed milk	50 ,, ,, ,,	
Sugar	15 ,, ,,	4 Grams (level teaspoonful)
Cereals	12 ,, ,,	

From the age of two weeks to six months a baby needs about 50 calories per pound of body weight per day, while a premature baby needs 65 or more calories (see also Useful Feeding Data, p. 101).

Protein, Fats, and Carbohydrates

PROTEIN foods, found in milk, fish, egg white, meat, cheese, peas and beans, are essential for growth and repair in the body, and about 1 gram of protein per pound of body weight is required daily, i.e., a 13-lb. baby needs nearly half an ounce (13 grams) of protein a day.

CARBOHYDRATES (sugars and starchy foods) and FATS provide body heat and energy, and about 1½ grams per pound of body weight are required daily.

MINERAL SALTS of calcium, phosphorus and iron are important for the bones and blood, while small amounts of iodine, sodium, potassium, magnesium and sulphur are also needed.

VITAMINS are accessory food substances which are essential in maintaining growth and health (see Food and Nutrition, p. 65).

Digestibility of Food. A baby needs foods that are easily assimilated. Human milk is the ideal food, being specially adapted to the baby's growth. Cows' milk is less digestible and, unless boiled or citrated, it forms large curds in the stomach. A mother's breast milk is normally sterile, that is, free from bacteria, while cows' milk may contain various infective organisms which must be destroyed by pasteurization and boiling.

Feeding Contentedly

The Natural Balance. A mother's breast milk provides a balanced supply of protein, fat and milk-sugar in suitable proportions for the growing infant's needs, and at the correct temperature. Breast feeding means less work for the mother and less expense. A breast-fed baby seldom suffers from constipation.

Oral Phase

The close natural contact of a mother and infant during breast feeding gives the mother a deep satisfaction and gives the child the feeling of love, protection and security. Babies, whether breast- or bottle-fed, who receive the stimulus of gentle 'mothering' during the feeding period will respond more happily than those who are only dutifully fed as a routine.

The main interest in the young infant's life are the events which center about his mouth —his powerful instinct to suck, the flow of warm milk which satisfies his hunger, and the intimate mouth-play through which he expresses his sense of contentment and happiness. This early and important stage is known to psychologists as the 'oral phase' in life and it leaves a deep and lasting impress on the personality (see Adolescence, p. 127; and Formation of Personality, at the beginning of Psychiatric Disorders).

Scientific tests have recently shown that very young babies thrive better and develop a better sense of security if held mainly on the left arm near the mother's heart-beat.

The Diet of the Mother before childbirth affects the subsequent supply of breast milk and she should have extra milk, cheese, vitamins, and iron tablets.

Breast Feeding

Care of the Breasts

Most mothers today want to breast feed their babies if possible, and success depends to some extent on the preparation and care of the breasts during the pregnancy. They should be washed with soap and water every day and the breast tissue gently squeezed towards the nipple; often a few drops of milky fluid can be expressed in this way. Engorgement and obstruction of the ducts when the milk comes in about three days after the child is born is unlikely after regular preparation. If it does occur, it can be eased by early massage and expression of the milk by hand.

If the nipples are small or depressed, they should be pulled out daily during pregnancy and a little lanolin rubbed in.

CRACKED NIPPLE. It is often advisable to stop nursing from the affected side for one or two days to allow the nipple to heal. To empty the breast, express the milk by hand three to four times during the day. Alternatively, a nipple shield may be used during suckling. Keep the nipple clean and dry; if inflammation occurs, consult a doctor at once.

ENGORGED BREASTS. It may be necessary when the breasts are tight to express some of the milk before the baby can feed, because he will not be able to take hold of sufficient breast tissue to suck. This engorgement sometimes occurs towards the end of the first week and may last about three days.

Baby's First Feeding

Some twelve hours after birth, the baby should be put to suck for about a minute at each breast. The breast will only yield a thin watery fluid, colostrum. Most babies 'play' at the nipple at this first introduction and no mother need worry if the baby does not suck vigorously. The baby should be put to the breast again after six and twelve hours. On the second day he should be suckled three-hourly, increasing from one to three minutes at each breast, and on the fifth to tenth days increasing from four to eight or nine minutes at each breast. Night feedings may be omitted if the infant is asleep.

The time taken for feedings varies with different babies and at different ages. Between the third and fifth days the mother's milk secretion is usually well established.

The nipple should be bathed and guided into the baby's mouth, being held between the first and second fingers. See that the baby's nose is not pressed against the breast, or he cannot breathe. He should be given each breast each time, the first breast being well emptied before changing over. The opposite breast should be used first at alternate feedings. As the baby becomes stronger he may take all he needs in two to three minutes.

If the baby tends to chew on a nipple, take him off the breast for a few moments and then let him begin suckling again. Restless or thirsty babies may be soothed with extra drinks of warm boiled water between meals.

BREAST MILK SUPPLY. The mother's milk supply often falls somewhat when she gets up and about after her delivery. This reduction may be only temporary. She should persevere with breast feeding, ease up on housework and take a rest with her feet up each afternoon. A drink of cold water before a feeding is often helpful.

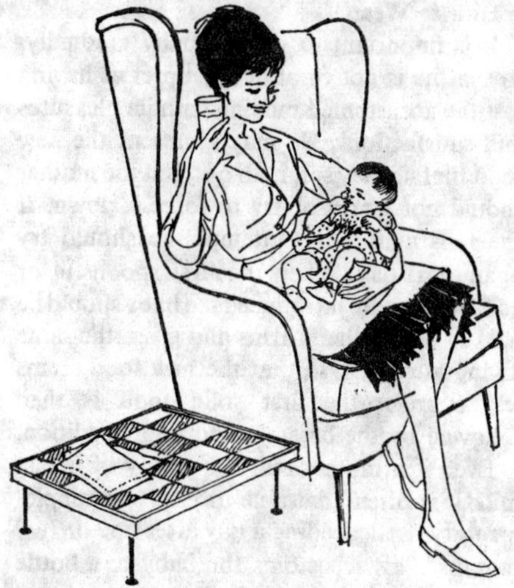

Fig. 3. *BEFORE BREAST FEEDING drink a glass of cold water, or milk.*

Complementary and Supplementary Feeding

Complementary Feeding

Sometimes the breast milk is insufficient and the baby does not gain weight adequately. When the gain is unsatisfactory over a period of two or more weeks a complementary bottle feeding may be recommended immediately after the breast feeding, at one or more times during the day (see Useful Feeding Data). Often at the 2 p.m. or 6 p.m. feeding the baby needs the extra bottle because mother is tired after the morning's work, or an outing, and the breast supply has become reduced.

Supplementary Feeding

A supplementary feeding is a bottle given *instead of* a breast feeding.This is often more convenient than complementary feeding and saves time. On the other hand, emptying the breasts at regular three- or four-hour intervals does help to keep the breasts active.

Test-weighing

Before deciding on supplementary or complementary feeds, the baby is often test-weighed before and after each feeding for three or more successive feedings, to find the amount of breast milk he has taken and how much more he requires. A ten-pound baby, for instance, needs at least 25 ounces a day (5 ounces for each of his five 4-hourly feeds). If test-weighing shows that he only gets 3 ounces of breast milk at one feeding he requires 2 further ounces in a complementary feeding.

Bottle Feeding

Cows' milk does not contain the correct balance of protein, fat and carbohydrate for a baby's growth, and has to be modified to make it more digestible. It must also be sterilized to prevent possible infection from diseases such as tuberculosis, scarlet fever, typhoid and paratyphoid fevers, and diphtheria.

For infants, cows' milk is used in three main forms: fresh liquid, dried, or evaporated.

Cows' MILK must *always* be boiled for a baby's feed. It is also safer to scald or boil pasteurized milk for about 3 minutes when it is to be given to a baby under a year old, or preferably two years. It is particularly important that the milk should be boiled in the following circumstances:

1. In hot climates, or in hot weather if there is no refrigerator.
2. If the infant has diarrhea, or looseness of the bowels.
3. During periods away from home, or when traveling.
4. During epidemics of diphtheria, typhoid fever, or poliomyelitis.

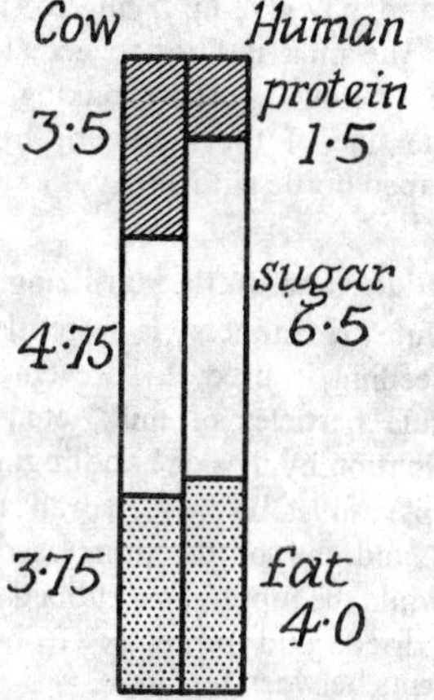

Fig. 4. *HUMAN vs COWS' MILK. Note the differing proportions of protein, sugar, and fat.*

DRIED MILK FOODS are sterile and keep for several months in unopened tins, and are convenient during periods of travel, on holiday, or in tropical climates. They are also more easily digested than liquid fresh cows' milk, and are easily prepared for use in the right dilution by adding boiled water. Most dried milks contain added vitamins and iron.

EVAPORATED MILK (unsweetened) is cows' milk evaporated to one-third of the original volume, and is prepared for infant feeding by adding boiled water and sugar to make a mixture of correct strength. Condensed milk is a sweetened form, but, when diluted, it is unsuitable for routine feeds as it contains insufficient protein or fat for normal babies. It may be useful as a temporary measure for sick infants who have some difficulty in digesting fats or protein.

Useful Feeding Data

FEEDING TIMES. The baby may be fed every three hours until he weighs 9 lbs. and then is gradually changed over to feeds every 4 hours; or he may be fed 4-hourly from the beginning.

Feedings are commonly given at:

6 a.m.	9 a.m.	Noon	4 p.m.	7 p.m.	10 p.m.
or,	6 a.m.	10 a.m.	2 p.m.	6 p.m.	10 p.m.

For the first five weeks or so, some babies need to be fed at night—somewhere about 2 a.m., but after the sixth week the baby should sleep from 10:30 p.m. until 5 or 6 a.m.

BABY'S WEIGHT DETERMINES QUANTITY. A normal baby gains about 1 ounce per day for the first one hundred days after the first ten days of life, then about ½ ounce a day until the end of the first year.

A baby needs 2½ ounces of fluid, and 50 calories per pound of body weight per day. For example, a baby weighing 12 lb requires at least $12 \times 2\frac{1}{2} = 30$ ounces of fluid, and $12 \times 50 = 600$ calories per day.

Breast milk normally provides 20 calories per fluid ounce. Liquid cows' milk also provides 20 calories per fluid ounce, but has more protein and less sugar than human milk; therefore cows' milk should be diluted and sugar added when given in place of breast milk to babies under nine months.

In premature or underweight babies the amount required is calculated on the normal or expected weight according to age, not on the actual weight.

DRIED MILK may be 'full cream' or 'half cream.' Some babies can digest a full cream milk mixture from birth. Half cream milk food is usually given during the first few weeks of life, and also for delicate babies under a doctor's supervision—although babies kept too long on half cream may be underfed.

SUGAR must be added to feedings made from liquid cows' milk, full cream dried milk, and unsweetened evaporated milk because these milks do not contain as much sugar as human milk.

Feedings during First Four Weeks

Cows' MILK MIXTURE, for 24 hours:

Boiled milk	10 to 20 fluid ounces
Boiled water	10 to 15 fluid ounces
Sucrose (Cane sugar)	7 level teaspoonsful

FOR HUMANIZED DRIED MILK give 2½ level level measures of milk powder mixed with 2½ ounces of boiled water for every pound of body weight. Do not add sugar.

Give 2½ ounces of mixture daily for each pound of body weight. A 7-lb. baby therefore needs 7 x 2½ = 17½ ounces daily. Divide into five feedings (every four hours) = 3½ ounces per feeding. Some babies may require more than the average quantity and this should be allowed if the infant appears to be hungry.

Feedings after First Four Weeks

Cows' MILK. Give a mixture of two-thirds cows' milk, one-third water and 2 level dessertspoonsful of sugar to the pint. For 30 ounces of mixture for the day's feedings use:

Boiled milk	20 fluid ounces
Boiled water	10 fluid ounces
Sugar	3 level dessertspoonsful

When the baby is old enough to have 6 or more ounces of milk mixture at each feeding the mixture may gradually be made stronger, so that at nine or ten months he is given undiluted cows' milk. If the baby seems hungry after a bottle feeding and cries, he may be given a little more of the mixture; if he does not finish some of his feeding do not try to force him and do *not* keep the remainder for his next feeding.

Dried Milk Mixtures:

Full cream milk powder (unless otherwise instructed)	**2 level measures**
Boiled water	**2½ ounces**
Cane sugar	**½ teaspoonful**

For the daily allowance, make up at least 2½ ounces of this mixture for every pound of body weight.

Temperature of the Feedings

Test the temperature of the mixture by shaking out a few drops on the inside of the wrist or on the back of the hand. If the milk mixture is too hot it will hurt the baby's mouth and even injure his stomach; if it is cold it is indigestible and may give him colic. The milk should be heated to 98.4°F, body temperature. It should never be over 100°. The bottle should be kept warm during a feeding by wrapping it in a piece of flannel and, while the baby is bringing up gas, the bottle should be put in a pan of hot water.

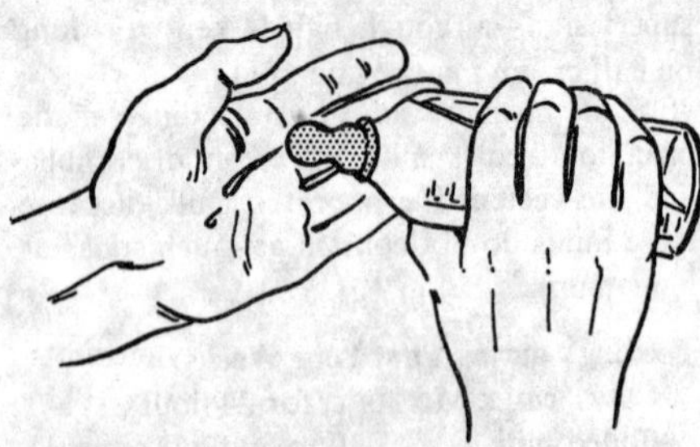

Fig. 5. ***TESTING TEMPERATURE. Test the temperature of the milk mixture by shaking a few drops on the wrist, or the back of the hand.***

Equipment for Bottle Feeding

A large saucepan to sterilize the bottles
2 or more bottles
Bowl or large heat-proof measuring pitcher, with fork or mixer
Teaspoon to measure sugar. Dessertspoon
Sugar in covered container
Hot boiled water
2-4 Nipples. Saucer or small bowl
Small glass or plastic bowl or saucer to cover niples
Salt (for cleaning nipples after use)
Bottle brush
A glass or earthenware bowl (capacity 2 to 3 pints)
A washable tray
Bowl (for hot water to keep bottle warm during feeding)

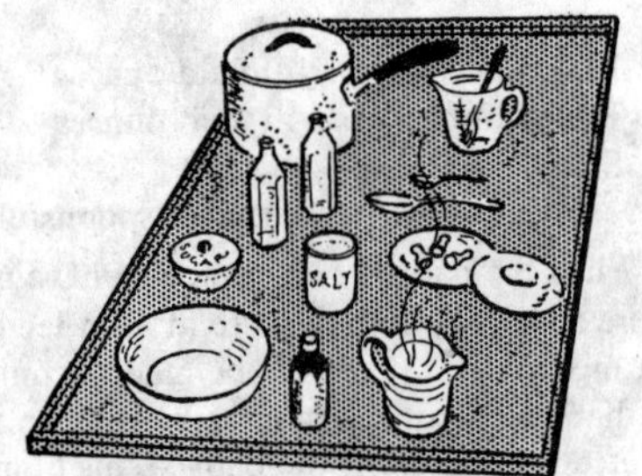

Fig. 6. *EQUIPMENT FOR BOTTLE FEEDING*

Nipples

The milk must not flow too fast; one drop per second when the bottle is held down is the right rate. If the hole in the nipple is too small, enlarge it with a red-hot sewing needle. Do not use a nipple which is old and soft as the flow may be too fast.

A baby needs to suck to give his jaws and muscles exercise. A newly born baby (and up to the age of about 8 weeks) cannot suck so strongly, so a three-holed nipple is generally used. If the bottle has no valve, it may be necessary to withdraw the nipple from the baby's lips every now and then to allow air to enter the bottle as the milk is sucked out.

A feeble or a premature baby may not grasp the need to release the nipple from time to time and may give up trying to suck when he finds the milk is hard to get. This difficulty may be overcome by making an air inlet in the side of the nipple or by using a boat-shaped bottle with a valve.

Cleanliness and Bottle Sterilizing

Absolute cleanliness is essential, when bottle feeding is used, to prevent infection from stale particles of milk, etc., or from contamination by flies or handling; the bottle and nipples must be washed well after each feeding, and the bottles immersed in cold water, while the nipples are rubbed with salt, rinsed, dried, and protected from contact with germs between feeding.

Sterilize the bottle, nipples and valves each day by covering with cold water in a saucepan and boiling for about five minutes.

WEANING

Weaning, or 'mixed feeding' as it is called today, consists in gradually changing the baby's diet from liquid milk to solid foods, although the term is sometimes used to describe the change from breast feeding to bottle or cup feeding. When the baby is between three and five months old, or when he weighs fifteen pounds, he needs more food and calories, for growth and increasing activity, **than milk alone can provide. Although he cannot chew food until he is about six months old, the additional food can be provided in soups, in strained or sieved foods, purées, jellies, and in milk puddings.**

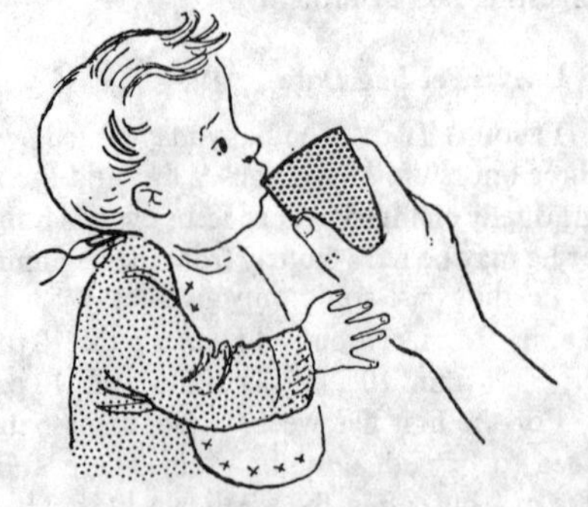

Fig. 7. *A NEW ADVENTURE. A drink from a cup*

How to Wean

It is important to wean a baby gradually, so that he is not emotionally upset at having lost the accustomed nursing with its pleasures and satisfactions. He may so resent the new food that he may spit it all out, but the mother should not worry or try to force it down. If she fails at the first attempt she should try again next day. When the first spoonsful or cup feedings are introduced the baby should be **held in the mother's arms and given the same loving attention, so that the new food seems less strange; the first solid food is then followed by the breast or bottle in addition.**

Even if a mother still has plenty of breast milk it is often advisable to give one supple- mentary bottle feeding a day after one or two **months. This accustoms the baby to a bottle and also makes breast feeding less arduous for the mother.**

Some babies of about four months will take their first sips of orange juice or fluid from a cup quite happily, while others may not be ready and may not find swallowing and breathing easy at first. The later the baby is first introduced to a drink from a cup the more he will probably resent it, and many babies find a bottle at bedtime much more soothing for their last feeding.

A bottle-fed baby often dislikes a cup more than a breast-fed child, but as soon as he begins to use a cup fairly well the bottle feedings may gradually be cut down one by one, the last (about 10 p.m.) being retained longest.

Weaning from the breast should not be started during a hot spell, when the baby is cutting a tooth, or is in any way out of sorts, and it must never be done suddenly. A mother should aim at breast feeding a baby for seven or eight months, and some babies may then change easily over to a cup without using a bottle. Give one feeding a day of milk or dried milk mixture instead of one breast feeding, for 4 or 5 days; then give two bottle or cup feedings, and miss two breast feedings for another 4 or 5 days, and so on, the weaning being gradual and taking from at least two, and sometimes up to five, weeks.

Solids

When the baby is three or four months old a little soup or vegetable broth may be given once a day; this may be a powdered or canned **baby soup, or fresh home-prepared broth, a** little being given just before 2 p.m. feeding, **and the amount increased gradually. The other solids, such as cereals, egg, fish, strained fruits, strained vegetables, and milk puddings, are then introduced gradually. Only one solid should be introduced at a time, to allow the** baby to get used to a new flavor.

Rusks. **When a baby is about five months old, a hard rusk should be given before the** 10 a.m. and the 6 p.m. feedings. **He will soon learn to hold it, but should never be left alone while chewing it in case he chokes. The exercise helps his jaws to develop and keeps his**

PLAN FOR WEANING

	6 a.m.	10 a.m.	2 p.m.	6 p.m.	10 p.m.
Breast feedings	Breast feed	Breast feed	Breast feed	Breast feed	Breast feed
Stage 1	”	”	”	Milk mixture	”
” 2	”	Milk mixture	”	”	”
” 3	”	”	Milk mixture	”	”
” 4	”	”	”	”	Milk mixture in bottle
” 5	Milk mixture	”	”	”	Milk mixture in bottle

Each stage takes about one week but may vary if the child is a slow feeder or unwell.

gums healthy. Rusks may be made by baking fingers of stale bread about ½-inch thick in the oven until golden brown, and they should then be kept in an airtight container. Never dip these rusks in milk or soup, or pieces will break off and the baby may choke.

Feeding Himself

A baby soon likes to hold a spoon and make efforts to feed himself, and he should be encouraged to try although he is sure to be messy at first! He will often manage some feeding quite well by twelve months, but it may be about eighteen months or two years before he can manage by himself. If he plays with his food, throwing it about, or squeezing it in his hands, it should be moved from his reach, and the mother should continue the feeding with a spoon. When he can sit up alone, it is better for him to have a suitable chair than to sit on his mother's lap.

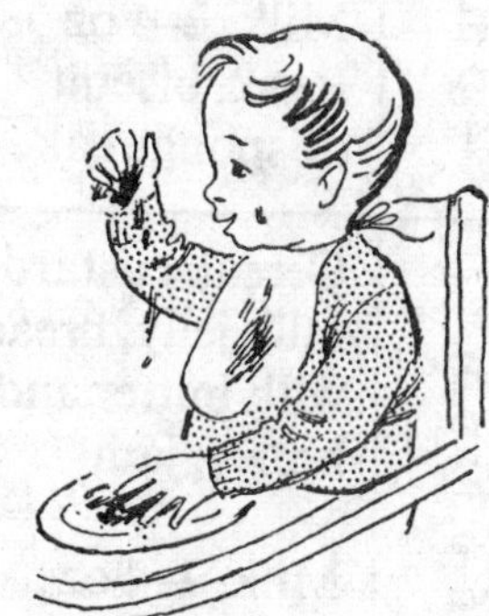

Fig. 8. *GETTING THE FEEL OF HIS FOOD*

Feeding Problems and Difficulties

Some babies on occasion want to be fed up to thirty minutes before the usual three or four hours are up, especially in the early days after birth before regular feeding times have become a habit, or because the mother's breast milk varies in amount at different times of the day, and the previous feeding may have been smaller than usual.

Demand or Schedule

The mother, particularly the young mother with her first baby, is faced with a dilemma. Shall she yield to the baby's demands and feed him whenever he is hungry or shall she keep him on a schedule? The normal baby by the time he is about three weeks old and has been fed on demand is *averaging* four hours between feedings anyway—sometimes he will wait five hours, sometimes he gets hungrier after three.

To allow a baby to lie and scream when he is hungry gives him a sense of insecurity and loneliness which may cause signs of tension later on; on the other hand feeding him when he cries and seems fretful will lead to indigestion and loose bowels as well as taking up more of the mother's time and energies. A little boiled water may soothe him if he is just thirsty, or he may settle down if the diaper is changed. A mother generally soon learns to distinguish between the cries of real hunger and of discomfort and, even if on some days one or more feedings are given early, the mother should aim at regular feeding times within a few weeks when a good supply of breast milk is established, or the bottle feeding requirement has been balanced.

Air Swallowing

The feed-in-a-hurry baby who swallows a good deal of air is apt to get colic and have screaming attacks; the mother should control milk flow by holding the nipple between the first and second fingers. In other cases some article in the mother's diet may cause colic in the baby. If air swallowing occurs with bottle-fed babies the nipple of the bottle should be checked for a proper rate of flow (one drop in 1 to 2 seconds).

Overfeeding

Overfeeding is much less common than underfeeding, but may occur if the supply of breast milk is ample. The baby's digestion becomes upset and, although at first the gain in weight is more rapid than usual, this is followed by no gain, or even a loss.

Signs

1. Three or more bowel movements a day; the stools are first soft, bulky, pale, later becoming greenish and watery.

2. Throwing up part of the feeding, and sometimes vomiting between feedings.

3. Irritability, crying, restlessness, and attacks of colic.

When a breast-fed baby is overfed he may be given one or two tablespoonsful of warm boiled water just before the feeding, and the feeding time cut by about a minute, or he may be fed from one breast only at each feeding. The weekly gain in weight should average about 8 ounces up to three months, but it may be more some weeks and less in others.

Underfeeding

This is much more common, especially in breast-fed babies, when the mother gets up after the delivery and her milk supply may be temporarily reduced. She should not give up, however, during this phase, as generally the supply becomes sufficient if the baby is sucking well.

Signs

1. Fretful crying before, between, and sometimes after the feeding.

2. Small gain in weight, or some loss.

3. Constipation with hard small dark stools.

4. Gas and colic

5. Wakefulness at night or early morning.

Sometimes, however, the underfed baby does not cry a lot and lies rather quietly, sleeping a good deal; but weekly weighings or frequent test-weighing after feedings will show that this gain is insufficient.

Failure of Breast Feeding

Breast feeding may be unsuccessful for various reasons:

1. The baby's birth may be premature, and he may suck feebly and not obtain sufficient milk.

2. Hare lip or cleft palate may make feeding difficult, or there may be so much regurgitation that the baby swallows insufficient amounts of milk.

3. The mother's nipples may be small and the baby a non-vigorous sucker.

4. The mother's milk supply may be delayed in coming in, may be insufficient or may fail for various reasons. She may be worried about the baby's progress, or she may wish to give up breast feeding and fail to persevere in the attempt.

To Increase the Breast Supply

1. The breast must be emptied at each feed; if the baby does not take all the milk, the mother must express the remainder by hand.

2. The mother must get plenty of sleep, and rest as much as possible in the afternoons.

3. Drink a glass of milk, fruit juice, or water a quarter of an hour before each feeding.

A SCHEME FOR MIXED FEEDING

	3–4 months	4–6 months	6–7 months		7–9 months
Early a.m.	Breast feed or Bottle feed	Breast feed or Bottle feed	Breast feed or Bottle feed		Orange or fruit juice to drink on waking
9–10 a.m.	Cereal: (oats, wheat, etc.) 1 teaspoonful mixed smoothly with 2 oz boiled cows' milk Breast feed or Bottle feed	Cereal: up to ½ cupful Rusk or crust with honey Breast feed or Bottle feed	Cereal: ½ cupful Rusk or crust with honey or seedless jam Milk drink from cup	7.30–8 a.m.	Cereal: ½ cupful Coddled egg, or egg yolk. Bacon, tomatoes, fish roes etc. Milk drink
1–2 p.m.	Soup or broth, 1–2 oz: add sieved or strained vegetables (carrot, cauliflower, etc.) Breast feed or Bottle feed	Soup, ½ cupful with sieved vegetables. Add coddled egg, flaked fish, or lean minced meat. Custard or milk pudding, with sieved apple or prunes Water, boiled and cooled, to drink	Soup, ½ cupful with sieved vegetables. Add egg, flaked steamed fish or lean minced meat or chicken, etc. Custard or milk pudding, with sieved apple or prunes Water, boiled and cooled, to drink	10.30 a.m.	Milk drink
				Noon	Mashed potato, sieved vegetables. Minced meat, fish liver, rabbit, chicken, etc. Fruit and milk pudding. Stewed apple, plum; mashed banana, prunes, etc.
4 p.m.	Orange or blackcurrant juice	Orange or blackcurrant juice	Orange or blackcurrant juice	4 p.m.	Milk, 2–4 oz Rusk, biscuit or sponge cake
5–6.p.m.	Cereal: 1 teaspoonful mixed with 2 oz boiled cows' milk Breast feed or Bottle feed	Cereal: ½ cupful Bread and honey Breast feed or Bottle feed, or 4 oz milk from cup	Cereal: ½ cupful Bread and honey or seedless jam Breast feed or Bottle feed or 4 oz milk from cup	6–6.30 p.m.	Cereal, custard, milk jelly, bread with butter and honey, jam Milk, 2–4 oz
10–11 p.m.	Breast feed or Bottle feed if baby is awake. Discontinue if baby sleeps all night	Breast feed or Bottle feed if baby is awake. Discontinue if baby sleeps all night	Milk feed as at 6 p.m. if baby is awake. Discontinue if baby sleeps all night	10 p.m.	Milk if child wakes. May be given in a bottle

Vary the cereals, stewed fruits and milk puddings, soups and solid foods

4. Use hot and cold sponging for the breasts (hot sponging for 1 to 2 minutes, followed by cold water for a few seconds). Continue this for 5 to 10 minutes, once or twice a day, one or two hours after the previous feeding.

In some cases the milk comes in too quickly and the breasts become engorged, with subsequent reduction in the supply. If supplementary feedings are given in the first few days breast feeding may be more difficult to establish, so it is better to give boiled water, or sugar and water, until breast feeding begins, normally about the third day.

Bottle Feeding Difficulties

Some babies may find certain ingredients difficult to digest, and if upsets occur the doctor's advice should be sought. The protein casein in milk may lead to colic and constipation and the milk may need to be modified by diluting it with water, or by acidification with lactic acid. If there is difficulty in digesting fat the child is pale, fretful and usually thin and highly strung; the bowels are loose, pale and sometimes contain slimy mucus and there is abdominal pain and often sickness. Starch is the other ingredient about which there may be difficulty and starch indigestion may develop when cereals are introduced during weaning, with abnormal fermentation in the bowel. This could lead to rickets through interference with absorption of vitamin D, and the cereal should be introduced in small amounts.

Loss of Appetite and Poor Appetite

A young baby's appetite may vary somewhat from day to day; an attack of gas, crying, overtiredness, or a hot spell in summer may send him 'off his food' for a day or two.

Colds, eruption of a tooth, or more serious illnesses also lead to early loss of appetite, but a raised temperature and other signs of illness will indicate something amiss, and a doctor will be needed to decide the cause if the baby does not take two or three meals with his usual appetite. Meanwhile give fruit juice drinks or water. In a toddler, loss of appetite may sometimes be due to emotional disturbances, or to the home environment, the child becoming tense and anxious as a result of parental mismanagement or quarrels, or of jealousy of a brother or sister, usually younger than himself.

PERVERTED APPETITE (pica) is sometimes seen in children over two years of age, when the child eats soil, plaster, coal, or other odd substances; this may be due to irritation from threadworms, or to some mental or emotional disorder, in which latter case he may also suffer from nightmares, habit tics, or sleep-walking. If the condition persists, a children's specialist may be needed to decide the underlying causes.

Variety at Mealtimes

Children's meals should be varied to avoid monotony, and should be served attractively in gay bowls, mugs and dishes. If a baby or young child eats less at one meal or during one day he will generally make up for it sooner or later, and it is wiser to allow him to choose the type and amount he requires, without too rigid insistence on each food item. Some children need from 40 to 45 calories for each pound of body weight, while others maintain good health on only 30 calories. As long as the gain in weight is fairly steady and the child is in good health, has regular bowel movements, and takes a reasonable quantity of milk, protein foods, vitamins and other necessary foodstuffs, the mother should not worry unduly as to how the daily menus are composed, especially over short periods.

A small child should not, however, be offered several choices of food if he refuses the meal supplied, or he will soon develop fads and fancies, and make mealtimes a tiring and anxious business. A variety of foods, of course, is advisable, especially of cereals, strained vegetables and milk puddings; these should be smooth, and the cereals and puddings may be flavored with jam, blackcurrant syrup or stewed fruit when the child is learning to feed himself with a spoon. Small first portions, with second helpings, are better than large portions especially after any illness.

BABY'S BOWEL MOVEMENTS

For the first two or three days after birth the stools are blackish-green, rather sticky, and are called 'meconium;' they gradually become brown, and then orange-yellow, as feeding becomes established.

Breast-fed babies vary considerably in the number of daily stools. To begin with there may be a movement after nearly every feeding, but after three or four weeks there may be only one each day, and some healthy contented breast-fed babies may have bowel movements only every two or even three days. This does not indicate constipation, provided that the stools are soft, orange, and fairly smooth.

The bottle-fed baby's stools are more solid and yellow or brownish, and he has fewer movements than a breast-fed infant. If the stools should be darker, more formed than normal, the feeding may need to be increased or light brown sugar used instead of white sugar. Sometimes the baby may need extra drinks of boiled water in hot weather, or a little extra fruit juice, or sieved prunes.

Loose green stools, with diarrhea, may be a sign of serious infection and a doctor should be consulted early (see also Diseases of Children). If the stools are green or very curdy, without being frequent, some adjustment of the feeding may be necessary, especially when mixed feeding has begun. Prune puree causes the stools to be darker than normal. Some babies pass rather green stools fairly regularly, without any other signs of upset, and the mother need not worry if the baby is gaining weight and is contented.

Laxatives and purgatives should not be given without medical advice. Laxatives are habit-forming if given too often and tend to make the bowel lazy. Purgatives, which are much stronger, may make constipation worse, and it is dangerous to give a dose to a child with abdominal pain before he is seen by a doctor. The pain may be due to appendicitis or obstruction of the bowel.

Enemas and infant suppositories are used in specific cases of illness by a doctor, but otherwise are best avoided except under medical instruction.

BATHING

A baby should be given a daily bath, in normal circumstances, and this should be given before a feeding, in a warm room without drafts. Soap, towels, powder, diapers and clean clothes should be put within easy reach beforehand. The bath is usually given before the 10 a.m. feeding up to about four or six months. Then it may be more conveniently changed to 5:30 p.m. For bathing, the main requirements are:

Bath on stand, or bowl on table
Mild toilet soap
Large towel and waterproof sheet for lap
Baby's towels (warm in cold weather)
Cotton (clean or sterile)
Chair without arms
Diaper pail
Safety-pins. Powder. Zinc cream or ointment. Lanolin. Toilet tray
Diapers. Clean clothes
Clean facecloth (gauze or soft linen)
Small sponge
Soft brush, and comb
Water for bath, about 100° F (tested with elbow or bath thermometer) for babies up to about 6 to 8 weeks; then gradually reduce to 80° F. *Always* put cold water in first.

A Sponge Bath

If the baby is on your lap, wrap his body in a warm towel.

First the eyes are swabbed with clean moist cotton, wiping from the nose to the outer side. Clean the baby's face with water without soap; the cloth may be used around the finger to clean the ears, but do not let any water run in. If there is mucus in the nose a small twist of cotton (not on a stick) can be used to clear the openings of the nostrils, but do not push the cotton up.

The scalp should be washed every day for the first four to six weeks with a little soap on the hand, and then well rinsed. Dry the face and scalp gently. After a month or so, a shampoo three times a week should be sufficient. 'Cradle cap' is a greasy scaly crust that forms on some babies' heads; to remove it, rub on some olive oil or vaseline overnight and shampoo the scalp in the morning. This will need to be repeated several times.

When washing the infant's body, attend to the folds of skin in the neck, armpits, groin, and genital areas; also wash between the fingers, toes and buttocks. Rinse off all the soap carefully and dry thoroughly by patting all over, then powder lightly so that the powder does not cake in the folds; lanolin may be used in these parts to prevent chafing. Zinc ointment or cream can be used on the buttocks when they are sore, as an added protection. If the skin is dry, a baby oil preparation can be used instead of powder. Never let the baby breathe in any powder.

Some doctors today advocate no-soap cleansing of infants up to two weeks.

A Tub Bath

A baby should enjoy his daily bath, and care must be taken when he is first put into a bath to see that he is not frightened. Put him in slowly, letting him feel comfortably supported; a towel laid in the bath helps to prevent slipping. It is sometimes easier to wash the head, face and neck before lowering him into the water. As the baby becomes a little older he will enjoy his bathtime and should be encouraged to kick and splash for exercise (see also p. 108). After about four months the family bath may be used.

In boy babies, if the foreskin of the penis retracts easily, this should be done daily in the bath to wash off any accumulated secretion and the foreskin must always be pushed back to cover the glans or tip afterwards.

The muslin facecloth should be boiled frequently. The finger and toe nails should be kept short and cut straight across to prevent accidental scratching.

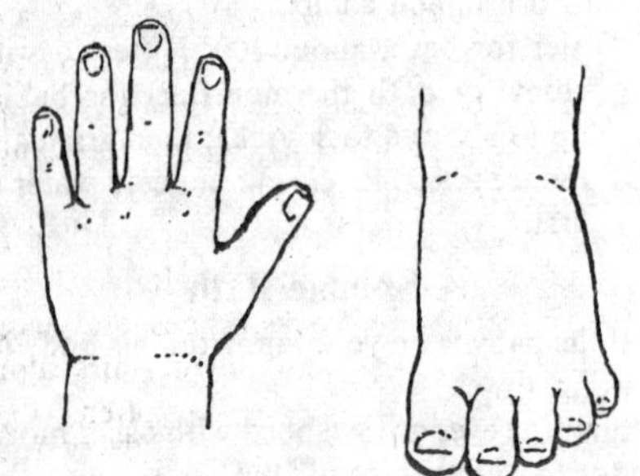

Fig. 9. *NAILS should be cut straight across and kept short.*

CRYING

For the first year or more, a baby's only way of expressing himself is by crying. In the first weeks of life he has two instinctive fears, of loud noises and of falling, but he also feels discomfort or pain, hunger, thirst and loneliness, and he cries to attract attention or for comfort. A mother soon learns to distinguish her baby's different cries, although at first they all sound alike. If he is hungry a baby cries loudly but, if he is not fed at once, crying makes him more unhappy and he will learn not to cry too long before a feeding is due, unless he is really underfed, or the last feeding was insufficient. Now that 'on demand' feeding is more common, a baby is less likely to be kept to strictly timed feeding schedules and the mother does not have to worry about slight irregularities before the routine feeding times have become established.

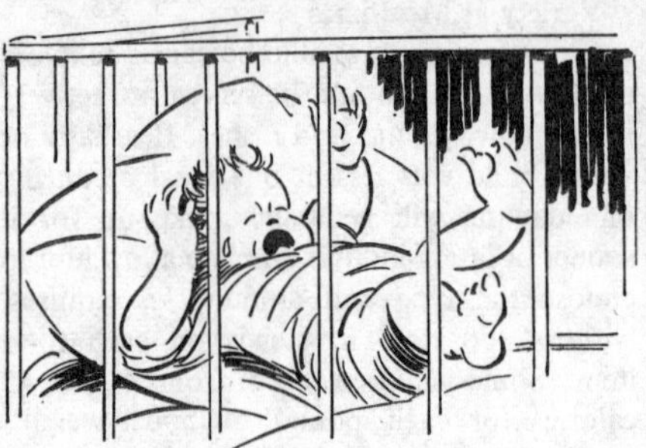

Fig. 10. *FRANTIC CRYING is bad for the baby.*

Colic or gas may cause pain soon after a feeding, or the baby may have a wet or soiled diaper and need changing, or he may just feel lonely.

When a baby is teething he is very likely to be fretful and irritable, and needs more 'mothering.' Prolonged or constant crying with no attention is bad for the baby who feels lonely and unhappy; sometimes just a drink of boiled water and a change of position may be sufficient to quiet him. Most babies, however, will probably cry for up to ten minutes a day without the mother needing to worry, and it is not necessary to pick him up every time he whimpers a little. If he is carried or rocked for too long periods he may get insufficient sleep and become too insistent on being nursed.

COLIC

When a baby cries or screams soon after a feeding, this may be due to colic, which is commonest during the first three or four months. The pain is due to 'cramp,' or irregular bowel movements with spasm along the intestinal wall. The baby draws up his arms and legs, and his face is red from the pain and discomfort. Some babies tend to have attacks of colic in the afternoons, or after the 6 p.m. feeding. Usually the gas has not been brought up after the last feeding, or perhaps the baby may have swallowed too much air, or he may be tired or cold, or need 'mothering.' Certain foods may cause colic in some cases, or the food given may be too cold, too slow, or too much. It is best not to wean the infant or change the bottle feeding without a doctor's advice. Sometimes certain items of food in the mother's diet may lead to occasional colic in a breast-fed infant.

When a baby has gas or colic, the mother should pick him up and hold him against her shoulder and pat his back or rock him gently; she may also try laying him on his stomach across her knees and rubbing his back. Changing his position will help him to pass gas, and a drink of warmed boiled water may also assist. Colic is not serious although it is often a great worry to the mother, but she will generally find the baby is gaining weight and is otherwise healthy. A doctor may advise other treatment when colic is severe—perhaps a warm enema, a pacifier, a warm bottle (well protected) in the carriage or crib, an anti-colic nipple with bulbous tip for the feeding bottle, or medicine to relieve bad attacks.

TEETHING

An infant or young child is often fretful or 'off his food' and may have a slight 'cold' with a runny nose and rather loose stools for a few days when a tooth is coming through the gum. These are common signs of teething and are not serious. If such signs occur after the age of five months the mother should look in the baby's mouth to see if the gum overlying a tooth is red and swollen; if there is much dribbling and normal temperature, an erupting tooth is probably the cause. Aspirin is not recommended for infants under one year of age but 1¼ to 2½ grains may be used for children of one to five years if the tablets are crushed in milk and given no more than three times in a day. The baby should be given hard objects to bite on, such as a bone teething ring or plastic spoon handle.

If the baby is constipated, small doses of milk of magnesia may be given, with (a mixture of the above) may be given, with extra drinks of boiled water or fruit juice during the day. A doctor should be called if there is any fever, bronchitis, or diarrhea with green stools.

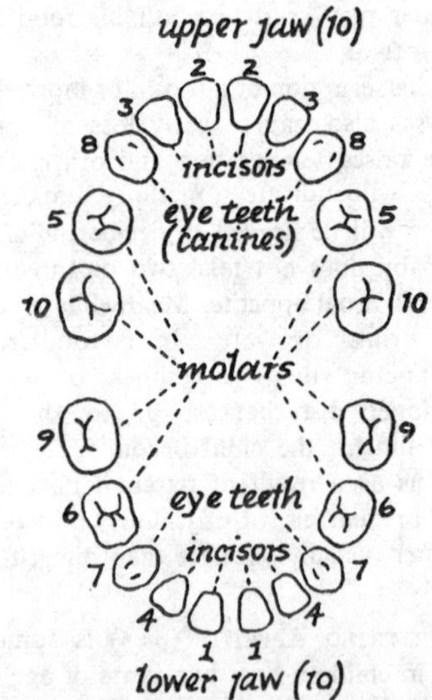

Fig. 11. *MILK TEETH. Diagram to show average order of appearance of temporary teeth.*

Eruption of Teeth

The actual ages at which the different teeth appear are very variable, and parents should not worry if any of the teeth are rather late in erupting when there are no other signs of backwardness in growth.

TEMPORARY TEETH	APPEAR (age in months)	SHED (age in years)
Two lower central incisors	5–6	6–7
Two upper central incisors	6–12	7–8
Two upper lateral incisors	8–13	8–9
Two lower lateral incisors	7–14	7–8
Lower first molars	10–16	10–11
Upper first molars	12–17	10–12
Canines	12–22	9–11
Upper and lower second molars	20–30	10–13

PERMANENT TEETH	APPEAR (age in years)
Upper first molars	6–7
Lower first molars	6–7
Lower central incisors	6–7
Upper central incisors	7–8
Lower lateral incisors	7–8
Upper lateral incisors	8–9
Lower canines	9–11
Upper first premolars	10–11
Lower first premolars	10–12
Upper second premolars	10–12
Upper canines	11–12
Lower second premolars	11–13
Upper and lower second molars	12–14
Upper and lower third molars (wisdom teeth)	17–25

As a child nears the age of two he wants to copy everything his mother and father do. This is a good time to provide him with a small toothbrush of his own. He will only make a casual job of it but he will enjoy doing it and find it less of a duty than if he begins later on.

VACCINATION AND IMMUNIZATION

Every young child should be immunized against diphtheria, pertussis (whooping-cough), poliomyelitis, smallpox and tetanus. A short interval follows each injection before immunity develops, so it is important for immunization to be carried out before a child may be exposed to any risk of infection.

Diphtheria immunization is perhaps the most important for children under one year of age in whom the mortality rate from this disease can be high. Although outbreaks of diphtheria are rare now that immunization is widespread, the risk of infection still remains.

Pertussis (whooping cough). **Vaccination** should also be given early as this disease can be most distressing and dangerous for small babies.

Poliomyelitis Vaccine. This is quite simple to take—just a few drops on a piece of sugar—but is most effective against a potentially crippling disease.

Smallpox Vaccination, by inoculation into a scratch made on the skin, produces immunity for several years. Primary vaccination is best carried out at thirteen to fifteen months and revaccination some four to five years later.

Tetanus Vaccine. It is important that tetanus vaccine should be given to infants and children because everyone who is injured and gets dirt in the wound runs the risk of contracting tetanus (or lockjaw).

Measles Vaccination is newer. It may not always prevent a child from catching measles but it will be a milder form without complications.

Other Infections. In certain circumstances, as when living or traveling abroad, typhoid immunization may be advisable after the first year of age. In the case of yellow fever, vaccination should be postponed, when possible, until the infant is at least nine months old. It must not be given at the same time as vaccination against smallpox.

Parents should keep a clear record of all these procedures in case the child is moved to another area, or care of another doctor.

GROWTH AND DEVELOPMENT

Although average rates of growth and phases of child development are recognized, **individual babies rarely make exactly the same progress. Most mothers like to feel that** their baby is more advanced, but it should be realized that, although the first two teeth may be a little late in appearing, several may then be cut at once. Some babies are more active than others and gain weight less quickly than **a more placid though heavier child. The active baby will crawl a month or more before the less lively infant. Some children never crawl but go straight to standing and then taking a few steps, and walking. Heavy babies may not walk alone until they are fifteen months or more, and, if their progress is good in other ways, the mother should not be concerned.**

For the first year or more a baby may use both hands equally before he begins to show right- or left-handedness. Encourage him to use his right hand for a spoon or rattle, but let him use whichever he wants. If he seems to prefer using his left hand, do not prevent him, as prevention will confuse him and may lead to stammer or difficulties in talking, and to later difficulties in writing and reading.

Some Milestones in a Baby's Development

AGE	
4 weeks	Baby can turn head to one side, and sometimes lifts it for a moment. Watches a dangling toy held in front of his eyes, and follows it a little way.
6 weeks	Smiles when suitably encouraged.
8 weeks	Takes hands to mouth. Watches a dangling toy move from side to side. Makes vocal sounds.
12 weeks	Lying on stomach he can lift his head and shoulders with support from forearms. When held up, he can hold his head fairly steady. Tries to grasp a toy held within reach. Recognizes mother. Turns head in direction of sounds.

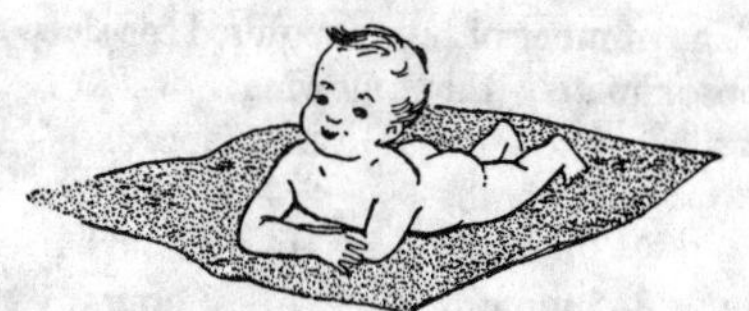

Fig. 12. *AT TWELVE WEEKS. Lifts head and shoulders.*

16 weeks	Head steadier when he is held upright. Recognizes breast or feeding bottle. Laughs aloud.
20 weeks	Ticklish. Can hold a bottle.
24 weeks	Rolls from prone (front down) to supine position (on back)
32 weeks	Bites on a rusk or crust.
36 weeks	Begins to crawl. Can sit steady. Sometimes stands with support. Understands 'No.' Imitates sounds.
40 weeks	Begins to crawl. May try to take steps when supported by hands Plays pat-a-cake, bye-bye, etc Says some syllables such as Da, Ta

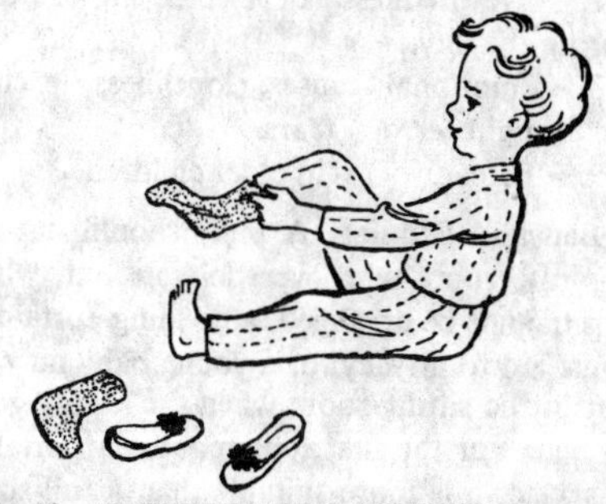

Fig. 13. *AT TWENTY-TWO MONTHS. He puts on socks and shoes.*

44 weeks	Understands several phrases. Plays give-and-take game. Puts one object inside another.
48 weeks	Walks with support. Waves bye-bye.
52 weeks	Walks with one hand held. May crawl on hands and feet. May say two words. Offers toy when asked.
15 to 18 months	May control urine during daytime. Crawls upstairs. Feeds himself and holds cup without help. Takes off shoes and socks. Points to parts of body when asked. Points to objects in pictures when shown. Temper tantrums may begin.
21 to 24 months	May put three words together in a sentence. Takes off simple clothes. Puts on socks, shoes and pants. Goes up and down stairs alone. Runs without falling often.
2½ years	Goes on simple errands in room or house. Knows full name.
2½ to 3 years	May be 'dry' at night. Jumps with both feet.

SLEEP

Hours of Sleep. The young baby needs a great deal of sleep to allow the digestive processes to proceed and for physical growth to take place, but the actual number of hours varies with each child. The newly born baby sleeps for a number of short periods during the day and longer at night. The hours are gradually reduced until the baby sleeps for about 13 to 16 hours at twelve months.

The number of hours required for sleep are approximately the following:

AGE	TIME (approx.)
1–2 months	14–20 hours
2–3 months	14–18 hours
3–5 months	14–17 hours
6 months	14–16 hours
1 year	13–16 hours
2 years	13–15 hours
3 years	13–14 hours

Sleeplessness may be due to a variety of causes, such as:

1. The baby is too hot or too cold.
2. Poor ventilation in the bedroom, or too much light.
3. Hunger, thirst, gas, colic, or indigestion; or constipation.
4. Noise and disturbance.
5. Colds, coughs, feverish complaints: teething.
6. Discomfort. Wet diapers.
7. Overtiredness, or insufficient exercise during the day.
8. Emotional causes: loneliness, excitement, night terrors, fears.
9. Threadworms in older children.

Bed and Bedding. A baby should have a separate room whenever possible but, when this cannot be arranged, a dividing curtain is some aid to privacy; or a young baby may be put in the sitting-room when the family goes to bed. For the first four months a portable basket crib is more suitable than a full-sized bed. The mattress should be firm and covered with rubberized or plastic sheeting. A pillow is not necessary for a young baby, but if used later it must never be soft; a flat pad is recommended for safety, since a tiny infant is unable to turn himself away from a smothering fold of a soft yielding pillow. A washable sleeping-bag is useful in cold weather for a toddler, particularly if the bedclothes are likely to be kicked off.

Settling Down. When a baby is put to bed he needs to learn that his mother cannot keep on picking him up to play with him and, providing he is comfortable and is given a little mothering and reassurance, he should soon drop off if left to settle down quietly. A warm bath given before the six o'clock feeding instead of in the morning often helps to make the baby sleepy and ready to drop off quietly. A soft piece of muslin for a young baby or a soft toy for an older child to cuddle is also a help in settling him down. Sedatives or soothing syrups should never be given except on a doctor's advice.

TOILET TRAINING

This is a subject about which mothers often become very anxious. Some mothers claim that their babies were clean by twelve months and this may well have been so, but most babies are not 'trained' by this age and it does not mean that they are less intelligent.

A baby's control of his bowel and bladder movements depends upon the co-ordination of certain muscles and nerves and this only develops slowly. At first his reaction to nature's demands is purely automatic and his ability to exercise control does not normally begin to develop until he is ten months old.

A young baby's bowel movements, however, are often regular and there is no reason why a mother should not take advantage of this regularity. She can often anticipate his needs and watch for signs of action, such as straining with reddening of the face, and try to use the pot in time. It is important to remember however that the 'potty' should be warmed so that it is not associated with discomfort and that the baby should not sit on it for more than five minutes. But success at this time is a matter of luck rather than training in the proper sense.

It may seem odd to think of the processes of evacuation as pleasurable, but to a baby they are because they are associated with his most primitive urges. Training to be clean is his first lesson and he may resent it.

It is commonsense, and not weakness, to avoid clashes of will and to deal with the situation in a matter-of-fact unemotional way. It is now realized that too strict or insistent a 'training' in a baby's first year is unwise. If he soils himself or behaves well, do not make a fuss. A calm word of praise or blame is enough, and above all avoid emotional appeals such as 'do it for Mummy.'

If the baby takes a dislike to the pot do not scold or smack since this will upset him and cause him to be tense and obstinate. Put the pot away and reintroduce it again in two to three weeks. This means going back to diapers which means more work, but it is quicker in the long run. Such setbacks are common but are only phases and, if treated calmly, will pass.

A year-old baby may find training difficult, but by eighteen months will be responding, and may ask for 'potty' in his own way or even bring it himself. At about two years of age, training becomes simpler, most of the resistances have gone and the toddlers are often proud of their successes.

A child continues to wet at night for some time after he has learned clean habits during the day. Many toddlers are dry most nights between the ages of two and three years, except when teething. A mother who allows her child to learn clean habits when he is old enough to understand, and who does not worry or scold about 'accidents' before he is three years old is less likely to have behavior problems.

SUNSHINE AND FRESH AIR

Every baby needs plenty of fresh air and sunlight. The best time of day is early morning when the sun's rays do not burn easily. The ultraviolet light rays help to develop vitamin D in the skin, this vitamin being essential for healthy growth of the bones and teeth. Ultraviolet rays are also present in reflected atmospheric light in open places. It is not wise to let a very young baby lie exposed for more than a short time to direct sunshine; the baby carriage should then be put in a shaded place, facing away from the direct glare. A canopy is advisable on hot sunny days.

In the house, good ventilation helps to prevent infection, poor appetite and listlessness; lack of fresh air encourages flabby muscles and poor circulation. Fires of all kinds, except electric fires, burn up the oxygen in the air, so it is especially important to have heated rooms well aired and windows kept partly open day and night.

The bedroom should be at least 12 feet by 9 feet, and the window should have an area of 2 square feet open to the outside air; a large opening admits less draft than a smaller aperture.

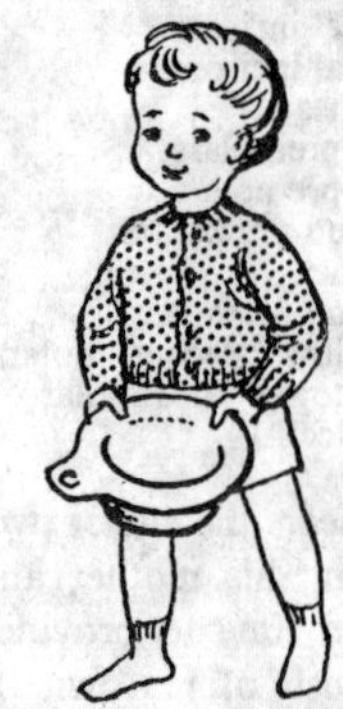

Fig. 14. *AT EIGHTEEN MONTHS he will bring it himself.*

On fine warm days, toddlers and older children can be allowed to play in a bathing-suit, or shirt and pants, with a covering for the head and back of neck in hot weather. On colder but bright days a child can get the benefit of sunshine by playing near an open guarded window where the sunlight comes in, instead of spending the day in a dull room.

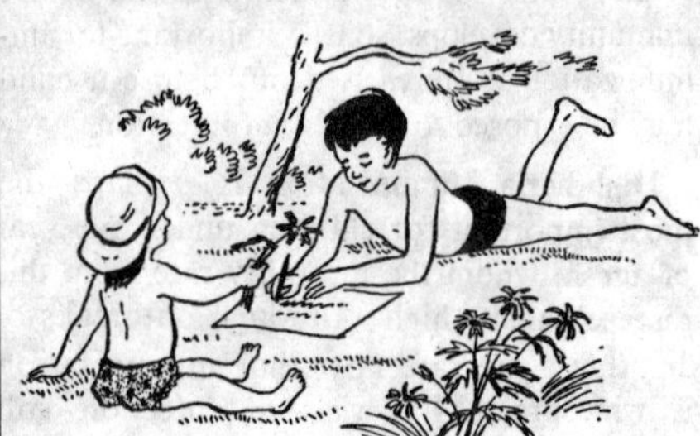

Fig. 15. *IN THE GARDEN for fresh air and sunshine.*

EXERCISE

Even quite young babies need exercise, and regular daily periods should be allowed from three to four weeks after birth to develop firm healthy muscles and bones, and to encourage a good circulation of the blood; exercise also helps to prevent constipation and undue fatness, flat feet, bow legs and a weak spine.

AGE 3 TO 4 WEEKS. The baby should lie undressed on his mother's lap in a warm place and out of a draft; a suitable time is before the bath. He can be encouraged to kick and stretch his back and limbs for a few minutes, and the arms, feet and legs may be gently massaged, directing the pressure upwards towards the body. He should also have his diaper removed and be allowed to kick for a little while before each feeding.

AGE 3 MONTHS. Put a folded towel or blanket on the floor or on a large table and let the baby lie flat; let him kick and move his arms and legs freely. Then turn him to lie on his stomach, massage his back and help him to hold up his head. He will gradually begin to try to roll or turn, or pull himself up a little way when holding on to your fingers.

AGE 4 TO 5 MONTHS. When undressing the baby for bed, hold him round the body under the armpits, and help him to bounce and jump on your lap, as well as letting him kick on a rug on the floor. In the garden on a fine day, he will also enjoy lying on a rug to kick and exercise his limb and trunk muscles.

A TODDLER should be allowed to walk barefooted for a little while each day to strengthen his feet muscles. Be sure the floor is free from splinters and not slippery.

PLAY

As the baby grows he has longer periods awake during the day, and will sometimes like to be near his mother (and other people) so that he can see and hear her, and have some of her attention; he can enjoy her company without needing constant nursing.

Remember that a baby from about six months onwards will soon want to put everything he touches or holds in his mouth and he should only be given safe rattles, teething rings, toys and strong plastic dolls. Painted, celluloid, or brittle plastic toys and sharp objects, or things that break easily or can be pulled to bits are dangerous.

A play pen is very useful and should be put away from drafts; in it a child may learn to pull himself up and support himself standing. Soon, however, he will want more freedom to explore around the room, and should not be kept in the pen for too long at a time, though a variety of playthings may help to keep him occupied while his mother is busy with housework.

An open fireplace must always be enclosed by a safe fire screen. Matches, breakable objects, and sharp pointed things such as knives and knitting needles must always be kept well out of reach.

Toys and Playthings. Simple toys and playthings are much the best for young children; they are less easily broken and are available in more variety. The child learns to use his imagination when playing with bricks or simple wooden toys and ordinary household or kitchen objects, empty boxes, wooden pegs, plastic bowls and so on. He also learns to use his hands to build and balance his playthings and make things fit, later copying his mother in her different kinds of work.

When a child is allowed to help and imitate his mother by using a brush and pan or a duster, and is given small errands and jobs to do, it is easy to gain his confidence and affection and he is more easily 'managed.' He should never be interrupted too suddenly in any occupation, but quietly warned that it is time for an outing, or the next meal, etc., which should be suggested as a happy alternative rather than as a necessary item in routine.

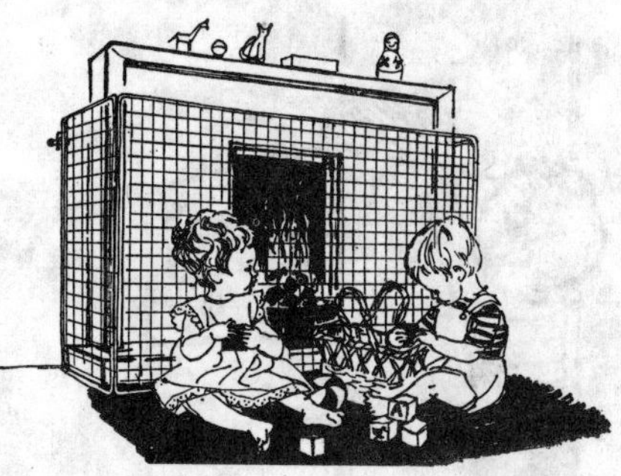

Fig. 16. *SAFE. Children can play freely when the fire screen is firmly fixed.*

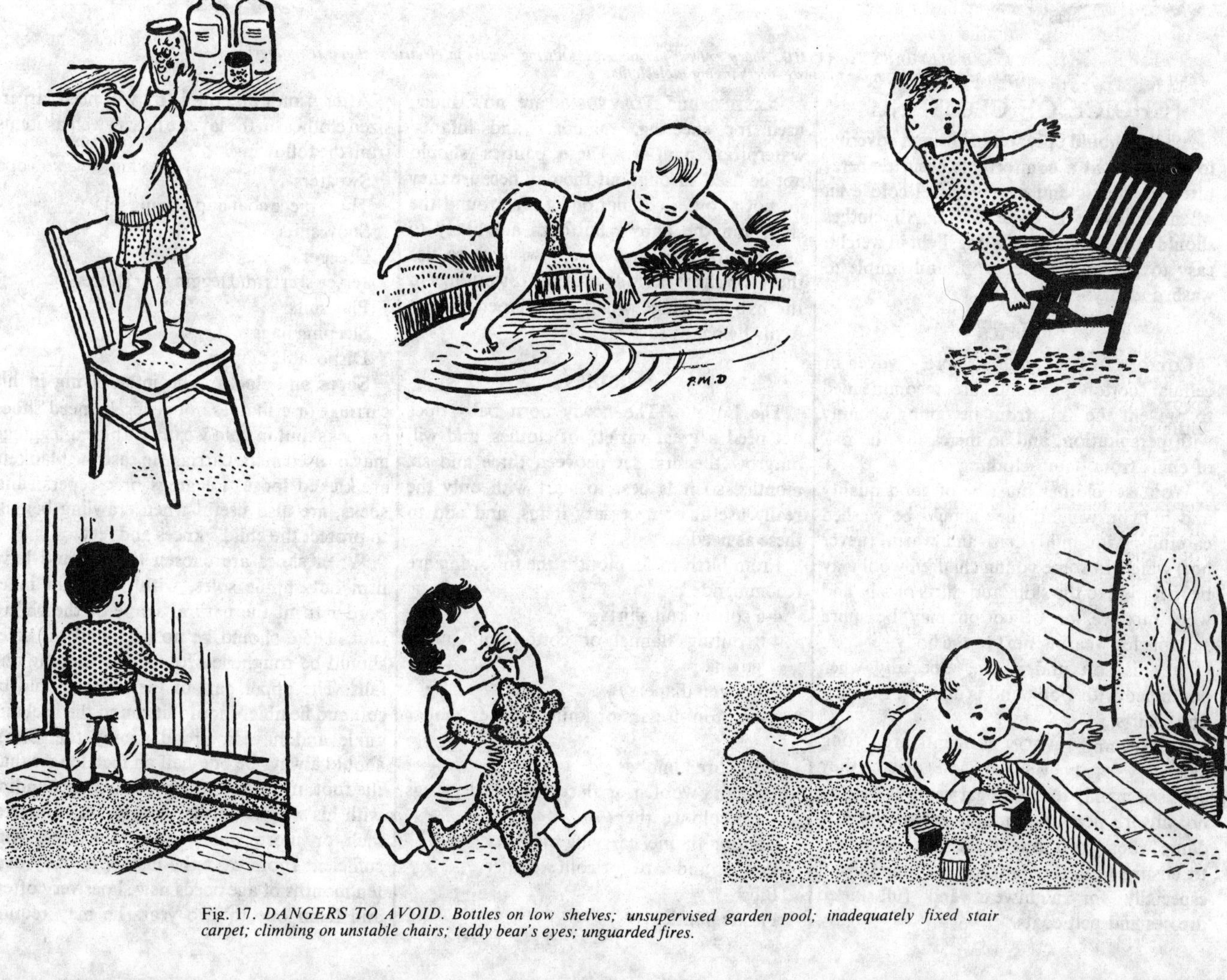

Fig. 17. *DANGERS TO AVOID. Bottles on low shelves; unsupervised garden pool; inadequately fixed stair carpet; climbing on unstable chairs; teddy bear's eyes; unguarded fires.*

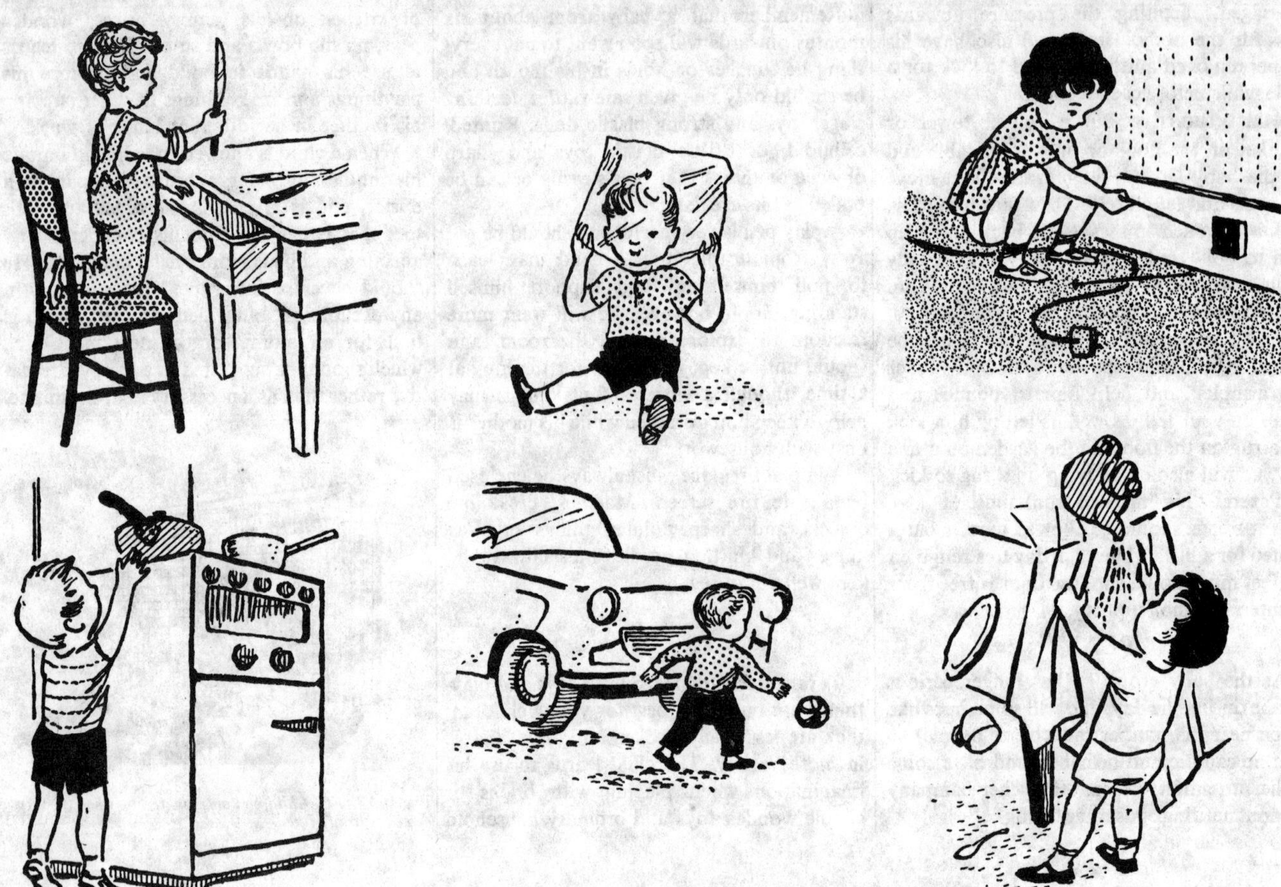

Fig. 18. *DANGERS TO AVOID. Sharp knives; plastic bags; knitting needles in electric sockets; tempting saucepan handles; balls in the roadway; overhanging tablecloths.*

CHOICE OF CLOTHING

A baby should only wear sufficient covering to keep him at a comfortable even temperature. His hands and feet may feel cold even when his body is quite warm. All clothes should be loose, non-irritating, light in weight, easy to put on and take off, and simple to wash and dry.

Fabrics

COTTON. In hot weather, loosely woven or cellular cotton garments are recommended to prevent the skin from becoming clammy with perspiration, and so increasing the risk of chills from damp clothing.

WOOLEN clothes must be of good quality and light in weight; they should be washed carefully with mild soap and warm (never hot) water. In some young children wool may be irritating to the skin, and shirts of silk and wool mixture, or of cotton may be more suitable for wearing next to the body.

SILK is soft and warm, especially when combined with wool, and is useful for dresses and shirts.

RAYON and NYLON garments are strong and very easily washed and dried; they are used mainly for outer garments as they do not absorb perspiration and so become very damp when worn next to the skin. Be careful to ensure that the fabrics are flameproof, especially for nightwear and full-skirted dresses and petticoats.

PLASTICS and POLYTHENE are now much used for sheeting, raincoats and infants' waterproof panties. These panties should not be used throughout the day because they do not allow a circulation of air around the skin, and the baby's buttocks are likely to become irritated and sore; it is best to use them for short periods only, as for outings in the baby carriage when the diaper cannot easily be changed.

Clothes

The Layette. The newly born baby does not need a great variety of clothes, and will outgrow the first set between three and six months, so it is best to start with only the really useful or necessary items, and add to these as needed.

From birth to six months the following are recommended:

- 4-6 cotton knit shirts
- 4-6 outing flannel or cotton knit night gowns
- 4-6 dozen diapers
- 3-4 cotton dresses or knitted jersey diaper sets
- 3 or more kimonas
- 2-3 pairs woolen or fleecy cotton leggings for cold weather
- 2 outing flannel carrying blankets
- Booties and caps for cold weather
- Bibs
- Plastic panties

After 6 months, the baby will need larger-sized clothes on the layette list, as well as items from the following:

- Sweaters
- Three piece coat and legging sets
- Snow suits
- Creepers
- Jersey shirts and leggings or shorts
- Play suits
- Sleeping bags
- Disposable diapers

Shoes and Socks. The infant lying in his carriage or crib does not generally need shoes or socks, but in cold weather knitted leggings may be used in the carriage in case the blankets are kicked loose. Leggings or creepers, and socks, are also useful when crawling begins, to protect the child's knees and feet.

When shoes are chosen they should have firm but supple soles, with a straight inner border to fit the natural shape of the child's foot. There should be no heel, and the soles should be roughened to prevent slipping and falls. The upper part of the shoes should be soft and flexible, should fit round the heel and ankle and have a broad roomy toe. Shoes should always be one-half an inch longer than the foot, measured when the child is standing with his weight on the foot, and one-quarter inch or more wider across the toes, with sufficient room over the instep. A baby over ten months of age needs new shoes very often, and from one to two years he may require them every two or three months to prevent cramping and distortion of the toes, or pressure spots where the skin may become red or thickened.

Sandals are practical and comfortable for indoor wear up to school age, as well as for outdoor wear in fine warm weather.

Care must be taken to ensure that socks are large enough since too short a sock can cause nearly as much damage in cramping the toes as too short a shoe.

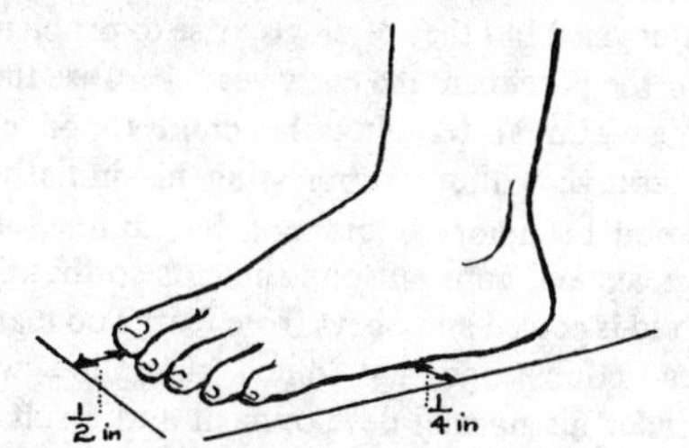

Fig. 19. *FOOTWEAR. When measuring the child's foot to get the size for new shoes, add the extra measures as shown.*

HABIT PROBLEMS

Some habit problems such as thumb-sucking, nail-biting and bed-wetting are often difficult to overcome. In the beginning the young child behaves as he does because he just follows his inclination, but sometimes the behavior becomes a habit because the parents appear worried and concerned, and this makes the child feel the center of attention. In other cases there may be some underlying tension or emotional disturbance, with a sense of insecurity.

Thumb-sucking

Sucking is a very strong instinct and one of the main pleasures of infancy. A baby will often resort to thumb-sucking when he is tired or hungry and this can become a habit which may persist for months or years, and any attempt to interfere will make him cross and unhappy. He should be given plenty of 'mothering' and when he is going to sleep he can be given a soft diaper or soft toy to cuddle. Most children, even if they still suck their thumbs in their bed at night, grow out of the habit at the latest by about five years of age.

A Pacifier. In a few cases persistent thumb-sucking may push the baby's front teeth forward and the lower teeth backward, but this does not affect the position of the permanent teeth which start to erupt at six years of age. A pacifier (or 'dummy') is less likely to displace the teeth and is sometimes recommended to prevent thumb-sucking or to soothe a baby who has attacks of colic. Some doctors and parents, however, consider 'dummies' to be unhygienic as they may well be if used carelessly. A baby who has a pacifier is often ready to give it up from between the age of six months and two years, while most babies who suck their thumbs go on much longer. A pacifier must always be kept absolutely clean.

Head Banging and Rocking

A baby may develop the habit of banging his head against the crib rail and thoroughly alarm his mother. The habit is not dangerous, but the sides and end of the crib can be padded, and if he rocks or shakes the crib, a carpet underneath nailed to the floor will reduce the noise. The habit may help to relieve tension, and sometimes extra mothering will make the baby more relaxed at bedtime so that he drops off to sleep more easily.

Breath Holding

Some babies show anger or resentment by holding their breaths when they cry until they go blue in the face. This naturally frightens the mother but she should try not to show her alarm because it is the baby's way of trying to get what he wants, and he will repeat the trick if he feels it is successful. Meanwhile she should try to distract him so that he forgets about the frustration. It is best to try to calm such a child in a good-natured way, and to help him get over his crossness quietly; a little crying will not hurt him, but if he is smacked or scolded sharply he will feel angrier than before and probably behave more unreasonably.

Nail-biting

This should be treated like thumb-sucking and the parents should not scold. The habit is usually due to some kind of tension, and occurs when a child is excited, worried, tired or lonely. The child often does not realize that he is doing it, and the mother and father should consider whether there is some emotional strain that can be put right—too much correction, interference or scolding, or bullying from older children may have started the habit, or a lack of interesting occupation. As a girl gets older she can be encouraged to keep her hands nice, and a little lanolin will help to prevent brittleness and tearing of the nails.

Occasional bouts of nail-biting may be due to overexcitement or overtiredness and a quieter routine should be arranged.

Bed-wetting (see Child Care, p. 125).

Masturbation

Masturbation, or 'self-abuse' as it sometimes used to be called, is very common among infants and quite young toddlers, and often causes unnecessary worry to the parents. From the age of two years it is often noticed that the child is interested in exploring different parts of his body, and losing interest in the earlier pleasures of thumb-sucking. The pleasurable and soothing sensation of handling or rubbing the genital parts is comforting to a child when he feels uncertain, insecure, shy, or just lonely. The mother should treat the matter casually and kindly, and make sure that he has a sufficient variety of interesting playthings and occupations, and the companionship of children of his own age to prevent boredom or loneliness.

At one time masturbation was looked upon as a disgraceful and dangerous indulgence, and it was even taught that it might lead to insanity, but it is now regarded as a natural solace or pleasure sometimes indulged in almost unconsciously by many children. The chief associated risk lies in the feeling of guilt or anxiety it may give rise to if the parents appear to be shocked or unduly concerned.

Masturbation in early childhood is not sexual in the adult sense and the child should never be punished or scolded for it, since he may later find it difficult to regard sex in adult life naturally and without feelings of fear and guilt.

A young child's clothing, especially the diapers and overalls, should always be comfortable, loose and non-irritating. Masturbation should always be differentiated from local irritation, worms, a tight foreskin or inflammation of the penis. To prevent loneliness in bed or during resting periods, a soft toy should be allowed in the crib or carriage for the child to cuddle.

GROWING UP

A baby's characteristics and temperament begin to form even before birth; the mother's health and outlook during pregnancy, her environment and state of mind all contribute towards the health and happiness of the baby after he is born. Even in the early months the baby enjoys his 'walks' in the walker the mothering at feeding times, the play and exercise during bathing, and he needs an atmosphere of quiet calm love and a regular daily routine with no feeling of worry, fuss or inattention to his needs.

Later, he must be able to trust his mother, and feel confidence in her decisions so that it is easy for him to do as she wishes. He begins to develop ideas and a will of his own and to assert himself—going through the stage of 'negativism,' when he likes to say 'no' to his mother and refuses to co-operate. This is a normal though trying phase, but by wanting to assert his will he is learning how to hold his own.

He also becomes much more observant, and wants to explore rooms, corners, and objects, 'getting into everything' and keeping his mother constantly on the watch for fear of danger or accidents. Overprotection by the parents at this stage will make the child timid, although the risks of serious accidents must be minimized by precautions and common sense.

Management should be positive rather than negative. A child will often resent an order not to pull the cat's tail; instead he can be told to let the cat have a nice sleep. The parents should avoid saying 'don't' and should interfere as little as possible. As a baby becomes a toddler he needs to explore and experiment, and he should not be continually told what he may not do, or punished because his mother is alarmed or annoyed; instead he should be given a reasonably safe place to play in, with suitable playthings and a sound chance to develop and use his increasing activity without damage to himself or the home.

Consistency of Parental Control

Mothers and fathers must aim at consistency, not alternating between indulgence and strict discipline, above all gaining their children's confidence and trust by firm but kindly authority. More children are probably spoiled by lack of love and understanding than from lack of actual discipline. When a baby or young child is ill he usually gets extra attentions and favors, and sometimes it is difficult to return to ordinary routine and control; this must be done by gentleness with firmness, as recovery and convalescence proceed.

Temper Tantrums

All young children become emotionally upset at some time and lose their tempers because they cannot have or do just what they want. A child may show he is angry by violent screaming, by lying on the floor, kicking, trying to hurt other people and breaking things, by throwing himself about, or sulking and refusing to co-operate or do as he is asked. These outbursts are likely to occur from the age of one year onwards and express the child's rage and helplessness, as he becomes more aware of himself as an individual and of his own desires. Sometimes such emotional upsets affect the child himself so that he becomes ill, or flings himself about and injures himself. The actual tantrum may be the final outcome of a series of frustrating situations or restrictions of which the parents have been unaware. After the age of two and a half years, anger is less likely to be shown against routine restrictions, but occasional conflict with parents, relatives or anyone in charge of them becomes more apparent and is part of the growing-up process and learning to live with others. A healthy child who feels secure and happy and who is not overtired can face up to a fair amount of frustration, but violent surges of emotion, disappointment, or anger can lead to a feeling of panic in a small child because he does not know how to deal with them.

If the mother or father always give in to a child's insistent demands or outbursts of temper to avoid 'scenes', outbursts may become a habit. The parents should remain as quietly patient as possible, and reassuring, and do nothing to increase the child's rage; even if he appears likely to harm himself by banging his head on the floor he will not really injure himself. When he begins to calm down, some distraction and comfort may be offered. He should not be scolded when the tantrum is over, what he needs is reassurance. It is often possible after a time to anticipate the sort of situations which cause these upsets and to avoid them

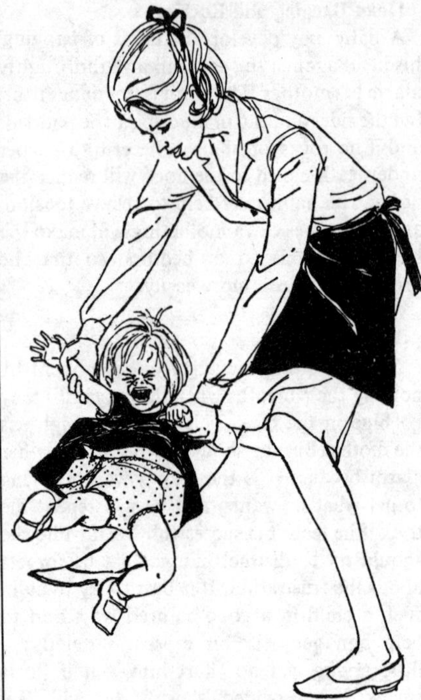

Fig. 20. *TEMPER TANTRUMS*

Tension in Infancy and Early Childhood

A mother may ask why her child appears to be 'highly strung,' with nervous habits, irritability, or minor symptoms of anxiety. It is not often easy to find a single cause at once, but any event or circumstance which upsets a child and causes anxiety of some kind may give rise to a state of tension. Any sense of insecurity even in the earliest days after birth will lead to fretfulness and anxiety, and it is important for a young baby to have an adequate time for suckling, this being one of the strongest instinctive pleasures in a newborn child.

The development of a child's character is affected by the relationships and behavior of the people around him, especially those in closest contact, such as his parents and later his teachers. If he feels accepted and approved, and not too much is demanded of him, he learns to adjust himself to people and situations without strain or anxiety. Children who do not feel accepted, and who are lonely, timid, or emotionally disturbed in other ways become anxious, irritable and 'tense' with signs of stress in their habits, temperament and behavior.

Spoiling

Parents who 'give in' to a child easily, so that he comes to think he can have or do what he wants if he cries or makes enough fuss, soon have a 'spoiled' child whom it is very difficult to manage or train. He will also expect to get his own way with other children and later on with relatives and teachers, and will become aggressive, non-co-operative and a poor 'mixer' socially. A parent may be too indulgent or too strict because of similar treatment in his or her own upbringing, or a mother may want to go to the opposite extreme and avoid the mistakes of her own parents. Spoiling may sometimes be a substitute for love, when a parent does not wholeheartedly accept a child.

The Aggressive Child

A healthy child has a great deal of physical energy, curiosity, tenacity and determination. These qualities are valuable and necessary in later years but they often give rise to problems for the parents in the early years because they must aim at teaching the child to be co-operative without suppressing his initiative. Good behavior should not be attained by threats and constant punishments so that the child is cowed and obeys from fear. Too many restrictions and too much discipline will hinder his normal development and result in lack of self-reliance and will-power, or in resentment and lack of co-operation with ordinary regulations and with authorities in general.

A small child has a short memory and he is too young to understand the reasons for many of his parents' cautions and prohibitions which are needed for an ordinary well-planned routine and home life. Patience is needed to help him to conform; some frustration is inevitable, and a very determined child will find more difficulty in yielding to parental wishes than one with a more placid or docile temperament. A determined child easily becomes aggressive when confronted with authoritative orders or threats, but may not always show it by immediate outbursts. If he is afraid to show anger he may become destructive with his toys instead, or may bully other small children.

A young child's aggressive acts and behavior are often triggered off by causes outside of himself or his own control, and parents should try to make it easier for him to behave reasonably without too strict management or retribution and humiliation.

The spoiled child is also often aggressive but this is because he has become too accustomed to getting his own way by self-assertion (see also p. 118).

First-born and Youngest Children

The position of a child in any family influences his character and personality. The first-born presents certain problems because his parents have little or no previous experience to fall back on and are concerned and anxious about management and training, and make mistakes more easily.

The youngest child may get the least attention from his parents, or he may be rather overindulged because he is the baby. As he grows he may be handed over to his brothers or sisters a good deal of the time and get less mothering, but is not likely to be lonely unless there is much difference in age between the children.

EMERGENCIES

When to call a Doctor

1. If the child's temperature is over 101° F, or if he appears ill with a lower temperature. The younger the child, the more necessary it is to avoid delay.
2. If the breathing is affected, if the lips are blue, or there is laryngitis, hoarseness, or harshness of voice.
3. If there appears to be pain or tenderness in any part, especially in the abdomen (when not apparently due to colic).
4. For vomiting (apart from ordinary 'throwing up' in infants) or vomiting with diarrhea.
5. If poisoning is suspected.
6. If a dislocation, fracture, spinal or head injury, concussion, or abdominal injury is suspected.
7. If bleeding cannot be controlled.
8. If a child appears abnormally drowsy, is semiconscious, or has convulsions.
9. If a child becomes delirious.
10. If earache is suspected, if the ear discharges, or there is swelling behind the ear in the mastoid region.
11. For foreign bodies in the nose, or ears, or if some solid object is swallowed or becomes lodged in the throat.
12. If a child cannot pass water.
13. If a stoppage of the bowel is suspected, or there is severe constipation.
14. For generalized or spreading rashes (apart from eczema and diaper rash).
15. In cases of burns with blisters, or scalds.
16. For blood in the stools or in vomited material.
17. For injuries or infections of the eye.
18. For more serious lacerations and cuts, especially those contaminated by dirt. For injuries associated with shock.

CHILD CARE

All parents wish that their children will grow into contented and well-adjusted adults. It is during infancy and the early years of childhood that the seeds of the child's future character are sown, and the type of adult that he will later become depends largely on the influences at work during this early period. The physical well-being of the child is, of course, important—but far more important is a happy family life with a home background of harmony and content.

The family unit of Father, Mother and Child is the backbone of the home. Guidance of the children is a joint responsibility of both mother and father. The child who is given love and security by both parents is a child who will grow up with few complexes, fears and anxieties, and who will later be able to do the same for his own children.

It follows then, that in a home where the parents are constantly quarrelling or on bad terms with one another, or in a split home where there has been divorce or separation, this important love and security cannot be adequately given. From a very early age the child can sense tension in the home, and will become tense himself. When his loyalties are divided between father and mother he becomes confused, and the results will be far-reaching, affecting his later personality.

GENERAL MANAGEMENT

Feeding of Young Children

The mother who fusses and worries too much about what and how her child is eating is laying the foundation for battles at mealtimes and for food fads in the years to come. It is comforting to realize that experiments in the feeding needs of children have shown that, provided the child is offered a suitable variety of food, he will naturally select a balanced diet for himself, and will never starve.

However, a knowledge of the basic foodstuffs essential to a growing child is necessary information for the mother, and there are certain points which will help to ensure that the child is feeding as well as possible. If he is to eat well he must have a healthy appetite. Such an appetite is encouraged through sensible general management as to fresh air and exercise, eating and sleeping.

Three meals a day of a varied diet that is also well balanced should be given and, what is very important, the child should have no snacks between meals. The manner in which food is offered is also important, as will be seen in the section on Poor Appetite. Forcing a child to eat some sort of food, that he obviously cannot bear the sight of, will stop him from eating even the things he enjoys.

Types of Foodstuff. A child's diet will principally contain protein, carbohydrate, and fat, with vitamins, mineral salts, and water.

PROTEINS. These are the body builders. Together with the much smaller quantities of mineral salts and vitamins they are essential for tissue building and growth. Children require relatively more of this type of food than adults. Proteins are mainly obtained from animal sources such as meat, fish, eggs, cheese and milk. They are also contained in soya flour and the pulse vegetables, e.g. peas and beans. For further details see section on Food and Nutrition, p. 65.

CARBOHYDRATES are the sugars and starches. With the fats they provide the balance of the calories the child needs (added to the calories from proteins). They provide energy, act as fuel for the combustion of fat and may be converted into and stored as fat. Rice, bread, honey, potatoes and breakfast cereals are typical carbohydrate foods.

There is a common tendency to overfeed a child with starchy foods, particularly with cakes, cookies, bread and sweets. As most children have a 'sweet tooth,' it is so easy at times to keep them quiet by giving in to constant demands for more cookies and sweets. If your child must have something to chew between meals—give her an apple.

FATS provide the fuel store in the body. Cooked fat is more indigestible than uncooked fat, so provide easily digested fats such as those found in butter, egg yolk, and milk. Peanut butter, although a useful source of vegetable fat, does not suit all children.

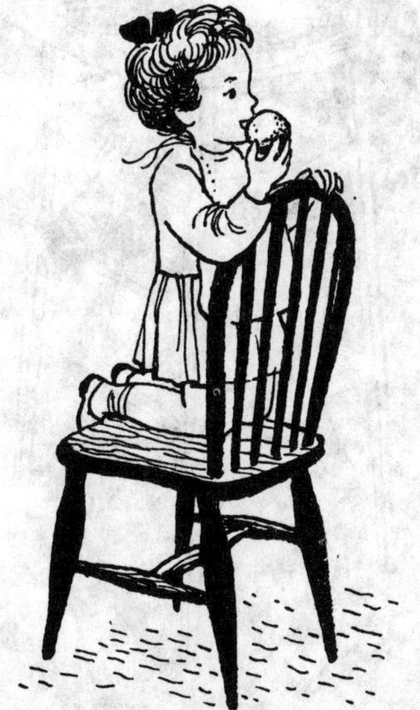

Fig. 1. *GIVE HER AN APPLE*

VITAMINS are chemical substances present in small amounts in certain fresh foods, and some (vitamin C) are easily destroyed by prolonged cooking. They are essential for the proper growth and development of bones and other tissues in the body, and also increase the resistance to various diseases.

VITAMIN C occurs in oranges, grapefruit, lemons, blackcurrants, tomatoes, potatoes and apples.

VITAMIN D is found in milk and certain oils, and is also formed naturally in the skin when the sun's rays shine on it. In winter, a child needs extra vitamin D in the form of cod-liver or halibut-liver oil, or the synthetic equivalent in tablets.

Severe lack of vitamin C in the diet leads to scurvy, and lack of vitamin D to rickets.

MINERAL SALTS. Although these are only found in minute quantities in foodstuffs, they are essential for tissue building. The most important are iron, calcium, phosphorus and iodine. Iron keeps the blood 'rich' and prevents certain forms of anemia. Calcium and phosphorus help to make strong bones, and iodine keeps the thyroid gland going. Good sources of iron are liver, egg yolk and leafy vegetables. The best source of calcium is milk.

MILK is an essential part of a child's diet. It contains water, protein, carbohydrate, fat, vitamins, calcium and other mineral salts. Up to seven years of age one pint per day (at the most 1½ pints) in various forms, is quite sufficient. More than this amount will lead to a poor appetite for other food. Excessive amounts also lead to constipation—so beware of forcing too much milk upon your child.

WATER. Although water has no food value, a child needs to drink it during the day, especially in hot climates. The body needs water for carrying out the vital functions, and it is essential for digestion and elimination of waste products. Sufficient water in the diet tends to prevent constipation.

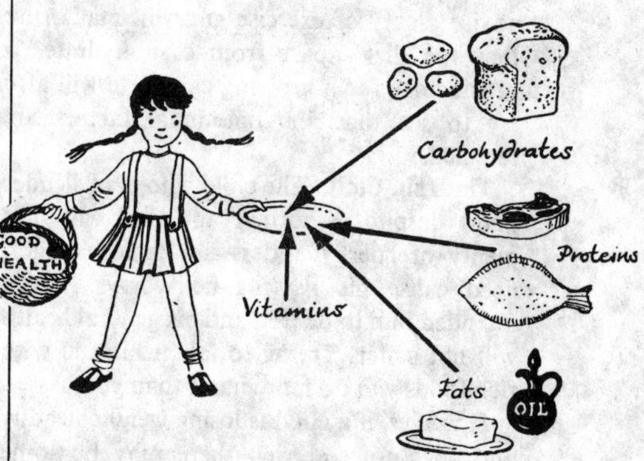

Fig. 2. *FOR GOOD HEALTH give her a balanced diet*

Appetite Problems

The Fat Child. If a child is grossly overweight, the doctor who has examined him and excluded any glandular cause (which is very rare), will probably advise a modified type of diet and plenty of exercise. We are not considering here the natural plumpness that occurs in many children before puberty, but the truly obese boy or girl. This type of child may have an inherited large appetite, especially for starchy foods. One of his parents may be very fat. In another obese child the cause of his fatness may be that he is subconsciously unhappy and eats to compensate for it, but many cases of obesity are difficult to explain.

Whatever the cause, excess weight is not healthy. The child is made miserable by his weight when other children tease him. The fat child is a natural target for ridicule, and who would not be demoralized when cries of 'fatty' and 'pudge' are constant reminders of one's size? Such a child is also more prone to succumb to diseases such as recurrent bronchitis. With increased weight the arches of the feet tend to flatten and painful feet result. This, together with his weight, makes the child less active, and exercise becomes a burden until it is abandoned.

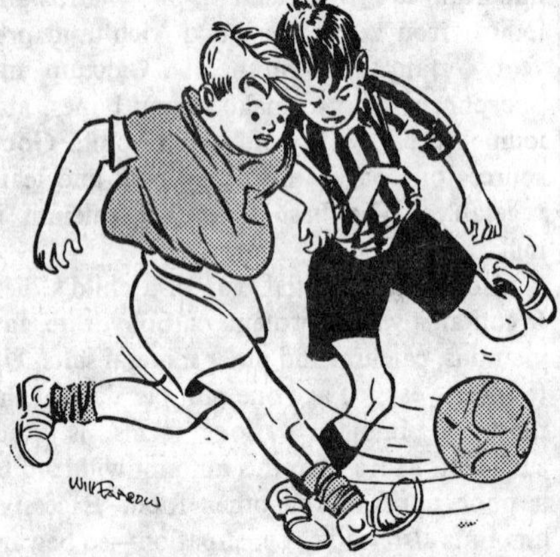

Fig. 3. *THE FAT CHILD needs exercise too.*

Cutting down drastically on starchy foods will make him lose weight, but great patience and perseverance are needed on the mother's part to succeed in doing this. A great incentive to the child is to have a pair of scales and watch his own weight records.

Get the help of your doctor and the results will be well worth it all. The doctor will also advise plenty of exercise and will make sure that the diet, apart from carbohydrate, is satisfactory for a growing child. He will also try to see that any emotional factors are rectified.

The Thin Child. The child who is of slender build despite a normal appetite, who has plenty of energy and is not losing weight, need cause his parents no worry. Nature intended him to be thin and his general health will not suffer. Trying to fatten him up with rich foods will do more harm than good.

However, if a child is losing weight steadily and does not feel well there may be some physical or emotional cause for it, and a check up by your doctor is necessary.

Poor Appetite and Food Fads. When a child is ill it is usual for him to go off his food for a few days. As long as he is having plenty to drink all will be well, and once he is better he will eat as well as ever.

But the well child who has a poor appetite is another problem, and this is probably due to mismanagement and overanxiety on the mother's part. Perhaps he is having too much milk; or sweets and cookies and snacks are being eaten between meals. These will fill him up so that he doesn't feel hungry at mealtime. Maybe he is offered his meals in the wrong way. If his plate is overfilled he will be put off by the mountain of food to be eaten, however tasty it is. It is better to serve small helpings so that he will ask for more.

If the child senses that his mother is worried because he is not eating, if she is always coaxing or bribing him or making him eat, then he soon finds that here is a way to be 'top dog.' Meals become a miserable ordeal for the mother with the victory going to the child. So adopt a relaxed attitude at mealtimes but offer nothing between meals. If he won't eat, don't make him. You know he will never starve so you must not mind if at some meals he hardly eats a thing. You will soon have a hungry child, learning to enjoy his food.

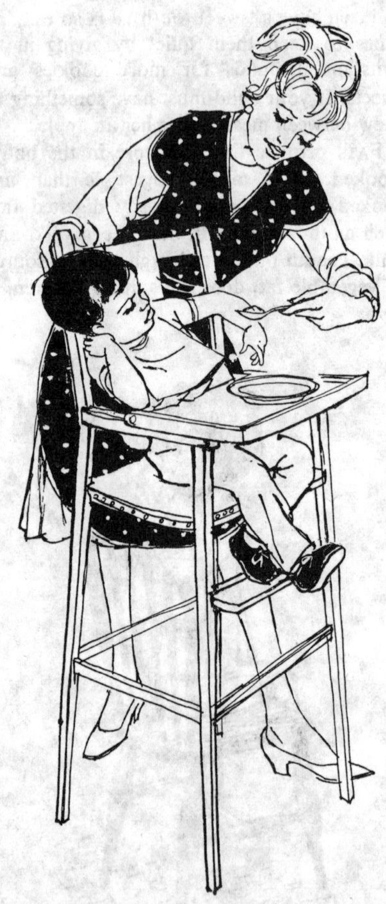

Fig. 4. *MEALTIME PROBLEM. Do not fuss if he will not eat.*

Constipation. A faulty diet is one of the most frequent causes of constipation in the otherwise healthy child. To correct it, increase the roughage in the diet with such foods as fresh fruit (apples, bananas, etc.), prunes, vegetables, and bran cereals. Make sure that the child is getting plenty of water, especially in summertime, otherwise the stools are likely to be dry and crumbly. If laxatives have to be used, milk of magnesia, or a fig syrup is safe, but the giving of laxatives should never become a habit.

Other factors may contribute to constipation. A school child may find that he is too rushed to give proper attention to his bowels. A younger child may have been mismanaged at the toddler stage with failure to institute regular habits. Occasionally there may be more severe emotional reasons present. The child who is ill in bed will nearly always be temporarily constipated but this is nothing to worry about. As soon as he is better it should right itself when diet and activity return to normal.

If the child complains of pain on passing a stool, he must be seen by a doctor. There may be a small tear of the back passage. The pain would cause fear of having movements and lead to constipation—the constipated stool thereby making the tear worse. If the child feels unwell and the constipation is long standing or associated with acute symptoms, a doctor must be consulted, as constipation also occurs in various organic conditions.

Sleep

A child should sleep in a room separate from his parents and in his own bed. The bed and mattress should be firm with one flat pillow and light but warm coverings. The room must always be well aired.

The amount of sleep needed varies from child to child and decreases as he gets older.

AVERAGE SLEEP TIME	
At 2 years	12 hours at night
	1 hour or so in the day
At 5 years	11–13 hours
At 8 years	10–11 hours
At 12 years	10 hours

Variations in sleep requirements, however, are common and normal. Up to the age of four or so, it is advisable to carry on with a midday rest in bed even if the child does not go to sleep at this time. As well as giving the child a rest it will give the mother an hour or so to relax and put her feet up.

To encourage a child to sleep well at night make sure that he is happy during the day and getting plenty of fresh air and exercise. Establish a nightly routine and a regular bedtime.

Sleep Problems such as waking at night, poor sleep, and nightmares often occur in infancy and childhood. They usually indicate that the child is under some emotional strain or that his sleep régime is not being handled properly. Being sent to bed should never be used as a punishment, for this will associate bed and unpleasantness in the child's mind.

If too much fuss is made over a child who stays awake or keeps on waking then it may encourage him to try to keep awake to get further attention. It is a great temptation, on some occasions, for parents to take a child into their bed but such a habit, once started, is very difficult to break and is best not begun under any circumstances.

Excitement at bedtime will also discourage sleep. Fathers coming home shortly before young children are due to go to bed should curb their very natural desire to romp with them. A quiet little game or a story, and a helping hand to mother to put them to bed is more helpful for everyone.

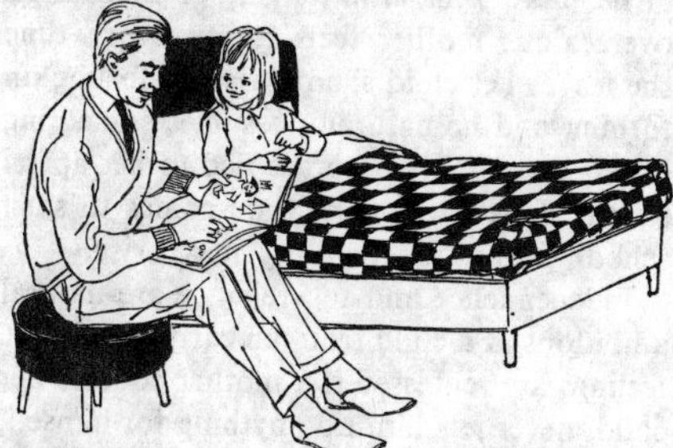

Fig. 5. *BEDTIME. A story from father is better than a late romp just before going to sleep.*

With a serious sleep problem the best plan is to consult your doctor before the situation gets out of hand. He will check up on any possible physical cause such as earache, toothache, or a blocked nose and will advise what to do. He may in some cases prescribe a safe sedative.

Clothing

Simple clothing which will wash well, wear well, and needs a minimum of ironing is the ideal. It must be comfortable to allow freedom of movement, with easy fastenings for dressing and undressing.

A not-too-short shirt with pants, of cotton or wool, perhaps combined with nylon, or other synthetic fiber, are excellent for underwear. These materials, especially in a cellular weave, allow evaporation and are efficient insulators against heat loss or gain. The old maxim 'wool next to the skin' may be conveniently forgotten these days. Wool itself is occasionally irritating to sensitive skins and may not always wash well, especially if frequent laundering is necessary. Nightdresses, pajamas and other types of clothing can be bought in non-inflammable materials. Mothers would be wise to make sure of getting this type of nightwear and so prevent a possible tragedy.

In hot climates and in the summertime clothing must serve the purposes of protecting the body from excessive heat and permitting the body to lose its heat easily. Thus clothing in general should be lightweight, ideally of cotton materials and white or light colored to reflect the sun's rays. It should be loosely fitting.

Children who are used to the sun and heat will derive great benefit from *controlled exposure* to the sun, and a healthy tan all over is evidence of good health in the normal child.

Children traveling from a temperate to a tropical or semi-tropical climate must be very carefully acclimatized before full exposure to the sun is allowed.

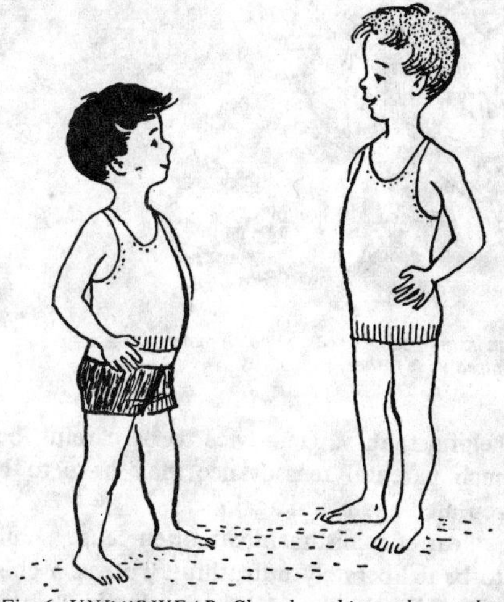

Fig. 6. *UNDERWEAR. Shrunken shirt and pants leave a dangerous gap. Let the shirt fully cover the body.*

Shoes. Great care should be taken when choosing shoes for a child. Much adult foot discomfort may arise from badly-fitting shoes and cramping socks in childhood. Shoes must be comfortable and of the correct size and fitting. The soles should be firm and non-slipping. The heels should fit snugly and the toe should be broad, allowing plenty of room.

Many makes of shoe are manufactured in broad, medium and narrow fittings. Make sure you go to a shoe store where there is an experienced children's fitter who will measure your child's foot and advise on the best type of shoe. Since the shape of children's feet vary, even in the same family, do not pass on shoes from an older to a younger child.

Personal Hygiene

General Cleanliness. The habits which a child learns during the formative years will remain with him for life. It is better for the mother to supervise washing during the child's early years and to see that he is reasonably clean. However, since a child will inevitably get dirty at play, too much insistence on cleanliness will spoil his fun and may lead to frustrations on both sides.

The nightly bath which he had in babyhood should be continued. A firm habit should be made of washing the hands after going to the toilet and before meals. Paper towels should be available to children.

Teeth. From the time a child is two years old he should be cleaning his teeth regularly after meals. Usually he enjoys doing it as he takes pride in copying what his mother does. The teeth should be brushed vertically from the gums, and not across the mouth.

Dental visits should be started when the child is three years old, and continued regularly every six months. Dentists recommend that the first few visits should be for noting how the teeth are developing and not necessarily for treatment. When the mother has her teeth cleaned, the child should accompany her for part of the visit. The child gets used to the dentist in this way, and these visits may prevent scenes later on.

While the mother was carrying her child she was making sure of a good foundation for his teeth by drinking plenty of milk and taking extra vitamins and calcium. Make sure that this excellent beginning is followed up by preventing tooth decay during the childhood years.

The exact cause of dental caries is not yet known, but research has shown that too much sugar and to a lesser extent starches, especially between meals, will cause particles to stick between the teeth and encourage decay. Eating hard fruit such as apples, particularly after a meal, is good for the teeth as this has a cleansing action.

In the United States and Canada a minute amount of fluoride is added to the water supply in a number of towns, as it has been shown that this substance may prevent cavities in the teeth if taken in the drinking water early in childhood.

Care of the Hair and Nails. From an early age try to make hair washing and nail cutting a pleasant pastime instead of an ordeal. Hair should be washed about once a week, and it is a good plan to use a special child's shampoo which does not make the eyes smart. Make a habit of washing the brushes and combs at the same time—they should be kept scrupulously clean. As for the nails, keep them cut short since they are much easier to keep clean that way.

Toilet Training. By the time he is about two and a half years old the average child is usually dry during the day and 'toilet trained.' A regular time of going to the toilet is a habit to be encouraged early in life. It is not a good thing to accustom the young child always to use the same pot or toilet. Later on, when he starts school or goes away on holiday you may find that the child refuses to open his bowels in strange surroundings.

Around the age of two and a half he should be encouraged to pull his own pants down and up, and gradually over the next year he will be learning to attend completely to himself. Later, teach your child to wipe himself properly and, of course, always to wash his hands after going to the toilet.

Pride in Appearance. Boys, as well as girls, will benefit when they grow up if they are taught to take a pride in their appearance in childhood. Too much fuss over clothing is unnecessary since it may lead to a vain and fastidious child. But with suitable parental example a young boy and girl will enjoy

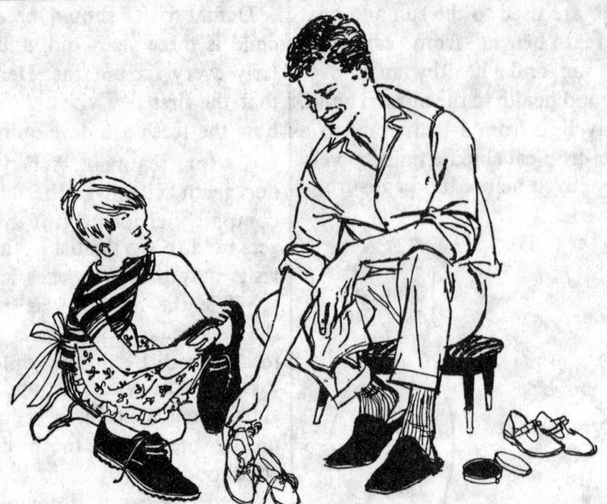

Fig. 7. *SHOES TO CLEAN. Jobs which have to be done can be much more fun when they are shared with father.*

keeping their clothes and themselves clean and neat. When father cleans his shoes, for example, his son should be encouraged to join in, while the daughter will notice the care and pride which mother takes over her clothes and appearance and will be only too keen to do likewise.

ENVIRONMENT

Security. The enormous value to the child of a happy home life has already been mentioned, and cannot be too strongly emphasized. Most young people who come before Juvenile Courts have been found to have an unsatisfactory home background which has lacked love and security. This has resulted in producing an unstable and dissatisfied individual—the juvenile delinquent.

As a parent you will wish to give your child the best possible security, and want him to look to you for friendship as well as for love and comfort. You naturally expect him to bring his troubles to you and to confide in you, and he will do this all his life if you listen patiently and enter into his own special world.

Never make light of a child's fears. What may seem rather silly to you may assume disproportionate images in his mind. Children of all ages may fear storms, lightning, deep water, pain, darkness, insects and animals and many other things, including quarrels between parents. These situations create tension and the child may react by having nightmares, by bed-wetting, thumb-sucking, or cruelty to pets, or he may get on badly with his friends. Such things are only temporary if, deep down, the child feels that his parents understand and will protect him. But if such habits continue the doctor should be consulted.

Explanations about lightning or pain or barking animals, which add to a child's knowledge of the world about him, will help him to keep fears at bay and he will begin to see how normal these things really are. It is better to try to build up a child's self-confidence and his belief in his ability to deal with his problems. When a child hesitates, an attitude of 'You can do it' is much more helpful than vague advice to be careful, but such parental reassurance may have to be repeated again and again.

Fear of punishment can often cause a child to be deliberately untruthful. To ask a child 'Who did this?' or 'Did you do this?' in an extremely angry voice may cause him to deny his guilt stubbornly. It is not always easy for parents to refrain from asking hasty and impulsive questions when they are irritated and upset but a kindly approach will help the child to tell the truth more willingly.

Father and mother should agree on their methods of handling their children, and any discussions or arguments on this point should be arranged well out of earshot of the child. It is terrifying for a child of any age to hear his parents quarrelling or losing their tempers with each other. Arguments occasionally must take place, and repressing them leads to other troubles, but tempers should never be lost when the children are around.

Routine. Up to the age of five years a definite routine in each day enhances the child's sense of security. If changes are to be made they must be made gradually, the child being warned beforehand and the mother at hand to reassure until the child is used to the new situation.

Discipline. Firmness with tolerance must be a basic attitude of the mother and father, and through the parents' firmness the child will learn obedience.

The toddler age—up to three and a half—is probably the most difficult to manage. One minute the child is a delightful and appealing little person, the next, he is screaming 'No' (his favorite word) and refusing to obey. He is passing through successive stages of personality development with varying behavior patterns which are often puzzling to his parents (see also Baby Care, p. 111).

Losing one's temper and forcing obedience is not the way out. No parent wishes to break a child's spirit. On the other hand it gives a child a sense of insecurity if you insist one minute on a certain thing being done, and then, when the child refuses, you give in to keep the peace.

What then is the way to handle him? From the beginning parents must make up their minds, and tactfully make it clear to the child, what are the situations where he has no, or little, freedom of choice, such as going to bed, getting up, times for meals and for coming home, and washing hands before meals and after going to the toilet. On other occasions, a compromise between his will and yours, made in a confident and pleasant manner, or an alternative distraction, will usually be effective.

Many conscientious and sensitive mothers tend to be overprotective in their effort to shield the child from various harms. But overprotection and spoiling will not help him to develop independence. A child cannot have his mother with him every minute of the day, or have every material longing granted. If an overzealous mother feels guilty every time she leaves her child she passes this feeling on to him, and he naturally assumes something is very wrong. He becomes tied to her apron strings. Later, when the time comes to start school, separation troubles may arise.

Independence and self-reliance are natural ambitions in a child from an early age. These feelings are repressed if a mother coddles her child, never lets him do anything for himself, and spends her whole time entertaining him. Self-reliance is encouraged, on the other hand, if the child is allowed to help around the house and to fend for himself as much as possible.

As the child grows older he should be allowed more freedom. The junior school child will become much more venturesome and this should be encouraged. He should be given some opportunity to take part in family councils and discussions. When planning outings let the child make his suggestions and take them into consideration. In these ways each child is made to feel a useful member of the family unit.

When you need to reprove your child, which will sometimes be necessary however well you manage him, never threaten him with the bogy-man or the policeman. Such threats have very harmful effects on a young child's mind. Your child should be taught that a policeman is his friend and is always ready to help him.

The Working Mother. There is no doubt that up till the age of five years there can be nothing to equal a mother's full-time care. However, in certain situations a mother, for one reason or another, decides to carry on working. She may have to work if she is a widow or her husband does not earn enough. If she is a professional woman she may find full-time housework intolerable and may decide that it is more beneficial to her child and herself to be a contented working mother, than a discontented housewife. Probably the best solution under the circumstances is part-time work, when the mother can spend some part of the day with her child. Whatever the reason for a mother working she cannot do so happily unless she has a suitable person to look after her child. A grandmother or relative at home, provided there is complete agreement on management, is the most suitable person. Otherwise, careful selection of a substitute must be made.

Once the child goes to school, arrangements are easier. It is important, however, for the mother to try to arrange her working hours so as to be at home when the child returns because mother's absence can often cause anxiety and insecurity in the child.

The Child's Room. Whenever possible a playroom or den, which is the children's very own, is an excellent arrangement. If this is not feasible a corner of the living-room, designated as theirs, is an adequate substitute. This is the children's own little world, and here they should be allowed to do much as they please, and not be nagged to keep it neat the whole time. The fact that such a room or place

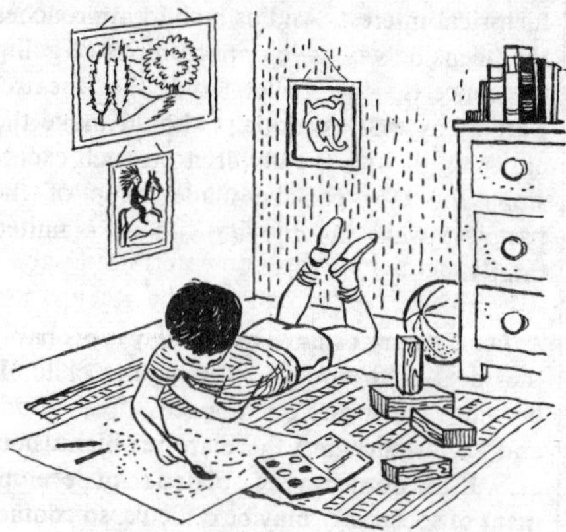

Fig. 8. *A CORNER OF HIS OWN*

belongs to the children is a great incentive to them in keeping their belongings well organized and putting them away at the end of the day.

Sometimes an eight- to ten-year-old child will want to leave certain toys such as trains, cars, etc. in position for continuation of play next day and it is a good thing to allow this if at all possible. Where this is not suitable, due to shortage of space, a frank explanation to the child will help to avoid upsets.

Let him have a say in how his playroom or bedroom is decorated and let him arrange it himself. He will do so with eagerness and concentration. Provide some chairs and boxes of a suitable size, a low table and a blackboard. Have plenty of cupboard space or storing boxes where his treasures and belongings can be stowed away. Choose an easily cleaned and non-staining floor covering so that paint-water, for example, can be spilled without too much anguish on your part. A plastic type of tile is probably ideal, although similar materials such as linoleum will do just as well.

Safety in the Home. Most accidents in the home are preventable.

Fires must *always* be guarded, and boiling water must never be left unattended. All medicines, disinfectants, poisons, and tablets should be locked well out of reach of children —especially now that some dangerous tablets not only look attractive to a child and resemble sweets, but also taste nice. Poisonous or inflammable liquids should never be stored in empty bottles with old labels left on. Steep stairs should have gates, floors under carpets or rugs should not be highly polished.

Above all, remember, prevention of an accident in your home is your responsibility.

Sex Information

Sex and the Young Child. The theory that ideas and attitudes acquired early in childhood go on to color adult life is now widely accepted by modern thinkers. The way, therefore, that parents handle the approach of their children to sex, from the earliest age, is especially important.

From as young as two and a half to three years of age the child will be conscious of a difference between the sexes, and will begin to ask questions. An unembarrassed and uninhibited attitude on the parents' part when answering questions of this kind will foster the same sort of attitude in their children when they grow up.

Questions should not be turned aside with a blush, and the old gooseberry bush or stork story is no substitute for a cheerful explanation. If frank and candid answers are given, then there will be little danger of the child getting distorted information from others, who may put untrue, twisted, and ugly ideas into the young child's mind.

Do not let fear of what other people will think of your methods interfere with the foundation of normal attitudes in your child. Occasionally you will find that grandparents or older relatives believe that sex is a taboo subject, not fit for a young child, but they are confusing coarse adult sexiness with the child's simple desire for information.

The right vocabulary should be used for the various body parts. If the mother is pregnant it will be a good opportunity to tell the young child that the baby is growing inside. As the child grows older he will want to know how the baby started. He can be told that baby grows from a seed or egg already in the mother—later the father's part is simply explained, and in this way the child accepts the whole process as quite natural.

Some parents may be afraid that their children are getting this type of knowledge too early. Children can only absorb knowledge at the level at which their understanding has reached. They are usually satisfied with simple straightforward answers and will usually be able to trust their parents if told that they will understand more fully when they are older. This sort of truth never hurts if it is given in the right way, and the child is more secure if he feels he knows the truth.

Preparing for Puberty

Before adolescence both the young girl and boy should have explained to them the changes that are going to take place (see Functional Changes in Women). It is a great shock to a young girl to have her first menstrual period without knowing what it is and why she has it, or for a boy to have a night emission and sex dreams without being aware that all boys have this same problem to contend with.

It is important to avoid children feeling that there is anything dangerous or wicked about sex. Such ideas may affect their whole attitude to love and marriage later on, and may lay the foundations of fear of childbirth and failure in marriage. The child is not naturally embarrassed by sex, unless parental or outside influence has led him to feel that way. He should accept it as a natural part of life.

Bearing in mind this frank advocacy of informing the young and growing child about sex, it must be remembered that the child will grow up as a member of a conventional society and must therefore be taught certain standards and habits of self-control, and encouraged to conform to the general pattern of the world he will live his adult life in. That is to say, an element of privacy and modesty should be gradually introduced as the child mixes more and more with groups outside his home.

It is how the parents get on together, and their attitudes to the social code and religious teachings which will have the greatest effect on the moral standards of the child in later life.

Fresh Air, Sunshine, and Exercise

In winter, as well as summer, it is of great benefit to a child to be out in the fresh air daily. It is sometimes tempting to stay indoors in a nice, warm atmosphere, but fresh air is invaluable. Even when the weather is cold, running around in the open air will give the child the exercise he naturally needs, will encourage a healthy appetite and bring color to his cheeks.

In the summer, sunbathing should be encouraged. Whenever possible allow the child to strip and run around and play with the sun shining directly on his body. But sunbathing should be done cautiously—a short period of two to five minutes at first, and gradually increasing the time. It should never be overdone to the extent of sunburn.

As has been mentioned, vitamin D is formed in the skin by the direct action of the sun, and that is one of the reasons why exposure to it is so beneficial. But there are some children, particularly fair children, whose skins are abnormally sensitive to the sun, and exposure can cause burning, allergic reactions, and much discomfort for them. Such children should be well protected when they go out in the sun, especially by the sea. There are several useful sun-protecting creams and lotions on the market and they should be used liberally on sensitive skins.

Vacations. Getting away for a vacation each year is something to which the whole family looks forward. The mother who has been tied to her home for the whole year deserves some time away from household chores. Father will get a chance to relax and the child will also enjoy the novelty and change.

The seashore, particularly in an uncrowded area, is certainly the ideal place to choose when children are small. The freedom of the sands and water, especially for apartment dwellers, cannot be rivalled, and sea air is the healthiest atmosphere to be found.

With the younger child, problems over vacations may arise. A timid two-year-old may be extremely upset by a sudden change in routine and environment, and in such a case the best plan is to put the trip off for a few months, or, if father's plans cânnot be altered, to make the best of a vacation at home for that year. The journey itself must not be too long, unless the child is a seasoned traveler.

As the children grow older there is much to be said for parents and children taking their vacation, or some part of it, away from each other. This arrangement certainly means that mother and father have each other to themselves, and can relax completely. But sound arrangements for the children must be made —otherwise neither party will benefit. Boys and girls who are Scouts will probably thoroughly enjoy a camping vacation. A visit to school friends or relatives is a good alternative.

If you are going to a hotel or boardinghouse, make really sure that it has facilities for putting up children, and that children will be genuinely welcome. There is nothing worse than having to keep children unnaturally quiet and controlled while on vacation, just as they are longing to let themselves go.

The City Child. Living in an apartment without the use of a garden has its problems and disadvantages, but the city child has many compensatory advantages. Great ingenuity may be needed to create in an apartment the atmosphere of space and freedom which a child needs. Plenty of built-in cupboards and orderly habits on the part of the parents will make things easier.

Fresh air and outings are more necessary to the child who is cooped up in a small apartment than for those with gardens around the house. Shopping expeditions, where the child has to hold onto mother's hand and beware of traffic, are not sufficient to provide for his needs. Make as much use as possible of parks and open spaces around the locality; there the child can run about, shout, jump and generally 'let off steam.' Most parks have recreation areas with swings, slides and sand boxes. Playing on these, as well as being great fun for the child, also gives him an opportunity for exercise and the company of other children.

At weekends, trips to the country, though they need some effort on the part of parents, are well worth while and provide a stimulating change of environment particularly for school age children.

From a very early age a city child must be made traffic-conscious. Safety rules should always be practiced by the mother, and the child will copy. If pedestrian crossings are always used, if the child is taught to look both ways and then back to the oncoming cars, if his parents never step into the road from behind a stationary car, then these actions will become automatic in the child's mind too. A child who has been well trained in this way will allow you to have peace of mind whenever he is out on the streets by himself later on.

Because of the imperfect social world in which we live, there is another lesson which must be taught to children. This is never to speak to, or take sweets from strangers, or to accept lifts in cars, however friendly such an offer may appear. Instill this teaching from an early age and as the child gets older you can explain the reason. Tell him 'a stranger may want to take you away from home and may hurt you.'

A city provides for a child, as he grows older, many fascinating places to visit. These will widen his interests, increase his general knowledge and lay the foundations for an active, cultured and inquiring mind. In a big city, the zoo will probably be the place to choose for a first outing. Later, he will enjoy going to museums, art galleries, and places of historical interest. And as a child approaches the 'teens he will have opportunities of going to concerts, the ballet, and the theatre. Fathers as well as mothers should make the effort to go with the children on such excursions for they can be made some of the happiest ways of enjoying life as a united family.

The Country Child. The country is probably the ideal environment for a young child. It provides clean air, open spaces, fresh foods and less traffic—but there are problems here also. If the house is very isolated then development of sociability may be difficult, so contact with other families in which there are young children should be arranged whenever possible.

When settling in a remote district, make sure you know how to get hold of a doctor or other medical aid. However healthy a family may be, accidents in isolated places do happen, and the sooner expert help can be obtained, the better. Sanitation may be somewhat

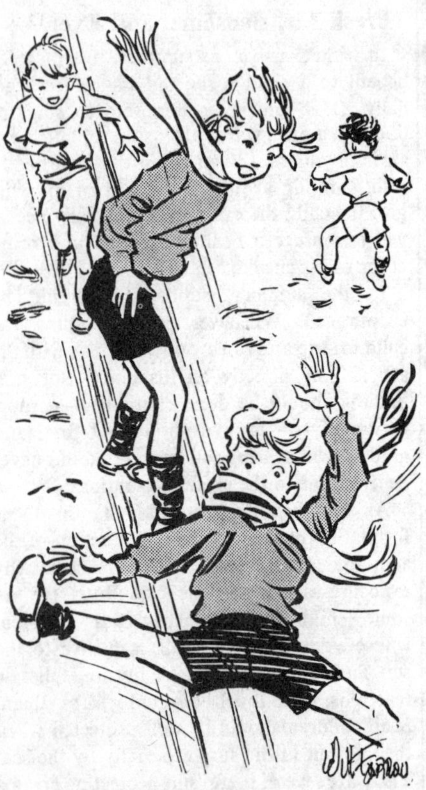

Fig. 9. *CITY CHILDREN. Let them make use of parks and open spaces where they can let off steam.*

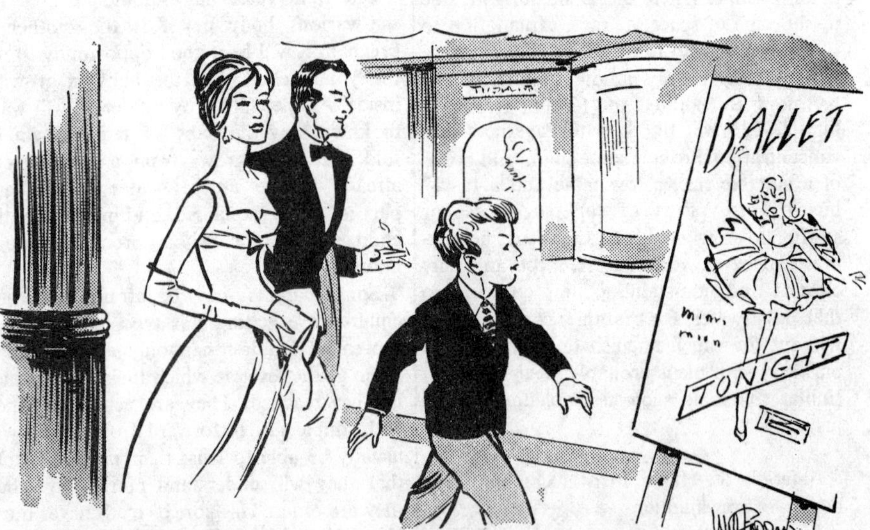

Fig. 10. *FAMILY EXCURSION. A visit to the ballet is one of the advantages of living in the city.*

primitive in remoter areas so that great care must be taken to ensure cleanliness, especially when the children are very young. Non-flush toilets need regular cleaning and disinfecting, and rubbish should be placed well away from the house.

Today, with the radio and television in many homes there is not much fear of country children lagging behind their town cousins. Books of every kind will stimulate the children's outside interest, and trips to the nearest towns will show them how other people live.

RECREATION

Play. The child at play is not just a child keeping himself amused while his mother gets on with her household tasks. No—it is the means by which he learns and experiments and finds out what life is about, and in this way he prepares himself for life. Play materials stimulate his thought and imagination. They teach him co-ordination of hand and eye, and develop his natural aptitudes.

Play also serves as a release for the emotions. A child may play out his fears in make-believe games, he also expresses his feelings for people through play. It develops the child's skills and is a serious and essential part of his growth to adulthood.

When a child is absorbed in some activity, try not to cut it off sharply if it is time to do something else. The passage of time has little meaning to a child at play although it has only too much to a busy mother. It is better to warn him, for instance, that it will be time for bed soon, and let him finish what he is doing first. We all know how frustrating it is to be suddenly interrupted while in the middle of some vital project.

A mother who understands what play is about is better able to provide the child with the materials he requires for his development.

Play Equipment. In general, toys and play materials should be simple. They should be constructive and promote thought and experiment. Flimsy cheap toys and too many toys defeat their own purpose and lead to carelessness and frustrations. Select play materials which are suitable to the age of the child. For example, the older boy enjoys making toys either for himself or for younger brothers and sisters. A handyman father can often encourage and show him how to use tools properly. A building set for a nine-year-old will keep him joyfully occupied for hours, while a four-year-old will tinker with it but not understand it properly and will soon lose interest.

For two- to six-year-olds provide facilities for playing with sand and water, ideally out of doors, but indoors too if possible. Of course there is bound to be some mess so make provisions for this beforehand. The pre-school child loves to imitate his mother, so give him an apron, a cloth, a small dustpan and brush and you will be finding yourself enjoying housework with him, even though it will take twice as long and the results may not be perfect.

Some of the different types of play material are listed below:

EXERCISE TOYS:
- Ball
- Tricycle
- Rocking horse
- Baby walker
- Wheelbarrow

'LEARNING' TOYS:
- Picture books
- Drawing paper, colored (sticky back) paper
- Crayons and pencils
- Blunt scissors
- Blackboard attached to wall
- Colored blocks, and construction toys
- Tools (hammer, nails, saw, wood)
- Plasticine

OBJECTS OF AFFECTION:
- Dolls
- Teddy-bear
- Soft toys
- Doll's clothing
- Bed for the doll

'MAKE-BELIEVE' TOYS:
- Farmyard animals
- Cars, tractors, etc.
- Old boxes, cotton spools, ribbon
- Telephone
- Clothes for dressing up

The Garden. If you have a garden much of the child's time will be spent out of the house when the weather allows. Some types of basic play equipment in the garden will allow a child to get the maximum enjoyment and exercise out of doors. A swing and a slide are great fun and provide good exercise. An outdoor sandpit with bucket and shovel and containers will aways keep a young person busy. Some sort of wading pool will be appreciated in hot weather—either a permanent concrete pool or the inflatable type, where a child can paddle and splash to his heart's content. Even a large tub or bowl of water can be enjoyed by the smaller children.

Hobbies. From the age of about eight or so most children develop some sort of hobby which they take up with great enthusiasm. Usually, as the child grows older and his interests change, so does the hobby—sometimes with remarkable rapidity and regularity. It may be stamp collecting or watching trains, knitting, needlework, or making a scrapbook, or some other fascinating pastime.

However short-lived it may be, encourage each enterprise and, what is more important, show genuine interest. Remember that a hobby is usually the personal choice of the child. It is something he is passionately interested in, a venture of his very own of which he is very proud, and over which he will take the greatest care and pains. It is, in fact, an extension of play as discussed earlier on. But no parent should be upset when he or she has entered thoroughly into the spirit of some scheme to find it suddenly dropped and something else embarked upon. This is a natural sequence of events, especially in the younger child.

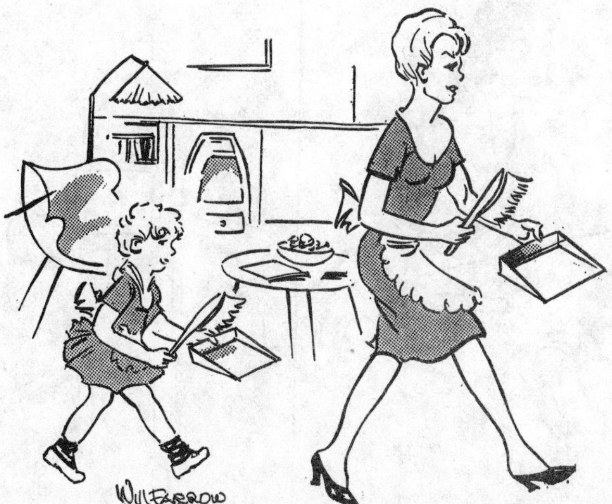

Fig. 11. *COPYING MOTHER. The younger child loves to 'help' with dustpan and brush.*

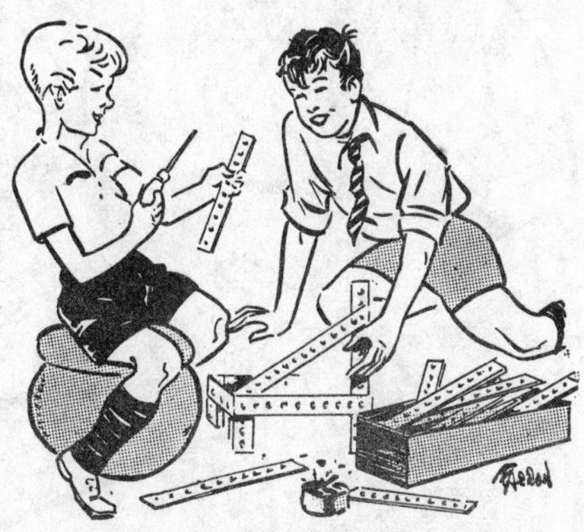

Fig. 12. *CONSTRUCTIVE TOYS*

Group Activities and Games

Being with other children should start from an early age and continue throughout childhood. Co-operation, sociability and initiative, 'give and take,' and tolerance; all these necessary qualities are developed through the contact of a child with others of his own age.

At two years old the child enjoys another's company but co-operative play is not yet developed. He plays alone although he may keep a wary eye on what his companion is doing. By the time he is three he will be starting to play with another child, and at five will enjoy group play.

From this age till around ten or so, make-believe games of Doctors, Mothers and Fathers, and Cops and Robbers are greatly enjoyed and should not be discouraged. In this sort of play children are finding an outlet for emotions which cannot come to the surface in other ways. It is a sort of safety-valve which, if curbed, may result in aggression or delinquency in later life.

Running and skipping games such as Hide-and-Seek, Hopscotch, and Tag are other favorites at this age. Suitable surroundings should be provided for these games. City children should be taught to use recreation grounds, special playgrounds or play streets; playing in traffic-ridden streets should be forbidden.

Organized games such as football, soft ball or hockey further allow scope for exercise and expenditure of energy. They teach a child to take orders and to lead. A spirit of competition and fair play is developed through them.

Family games can be enjoyed by parents and children alike. Here, with the whole family taking part the family gathering is encouraged and the give and take in family life is fostered. Such evening entertainments, when homework is over, are a companionable alternative to sitting in silence glued to a television set.

Children's Organizations. From the age of seven a child can become a Cub or Brownie, later on a Scout, or join one of the Red Cross or other responsible youth organizations. This type of semi-official club for youngsters is admirable in organizing supervised group activities. The people in charge are specially trained, and meetings are held in properly equipped premises. Outings and camps are organized, and competitive games and tests as well as other activities teach loyalty and team spirit.

The tests and badges for which the child works are a real incentive to learning in an enjoyable way. Energies and daring, which under other circumstances might be put to mischievous use, are harnessed and directed into meaningful channels.

Books, TV, and Music

Books. A child enjoys picture books from an early age. He loves seeing drawings of familiar objects again and again. From two and a half he is clamoring for stories, first about himself and the things around him; later, interest grows in the outside world and far away places. As soon as he can read by himself he should be encouraged to do so, but he will still enjoy and benefit from being read aloud to.

Reading has innumerable values for the child. Through it his knowledge is increased and imagination stimulated, and he acquires a thirst for yet further knowledge and experience.

A careful selection of suitable books must be made, not only the right book for the right age, but also to suit the individual child. An oversensitive young child, for example, may be terrified by the story of Red Riding Hood, whereas another may not be affected at all. Horror Comics are quite unsuitable for children; they have nothing comic about them and deal mainly with gangsters and sex, being produced for illiterate adults who are not interested in good literature.

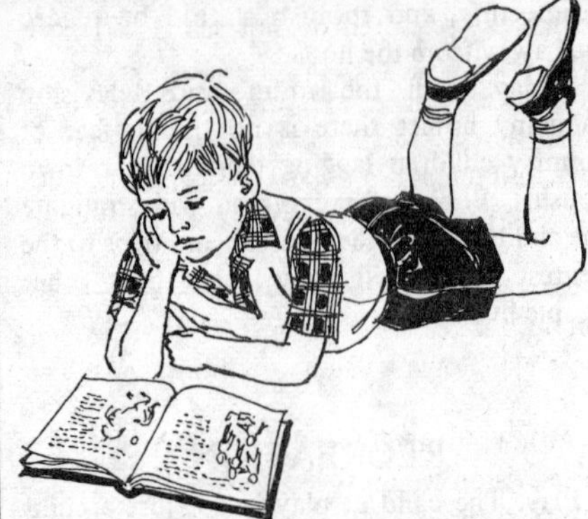

Fig. 14. *THE MAGIC OF BOOKS*

On the other hand there are many illustrated magazines, genuine fun comics and better quality paper-back books which are suitable for children, including such well-loved classics as *Wind in the Willows*, *Treasure Island*, and *Alice in Wonderland*.

Children's libraries are most useful for the voracious reader, and librarians are only too willing to help with the choice of books.

Television. Parents are sometimes very worried about the effects that television viewing may have on their children. If certain rules are laid down in the household then a happy medium between overviewing and never switching on the set can be achieved. There is no doubt that overviewing is definitely harmful to the child. Never start the habit of viewing at mealtime, however tempting this may be. The child cannot be expected to eat his meal properly if his attention is continuously being distracted.

For older boys and girls, set homework must always be finished each day, and parents should never be taken in by such pleas as, 'I can concentrate better with the television on.' Make sure, however, that children are not skimping their work to watch a favorite program.

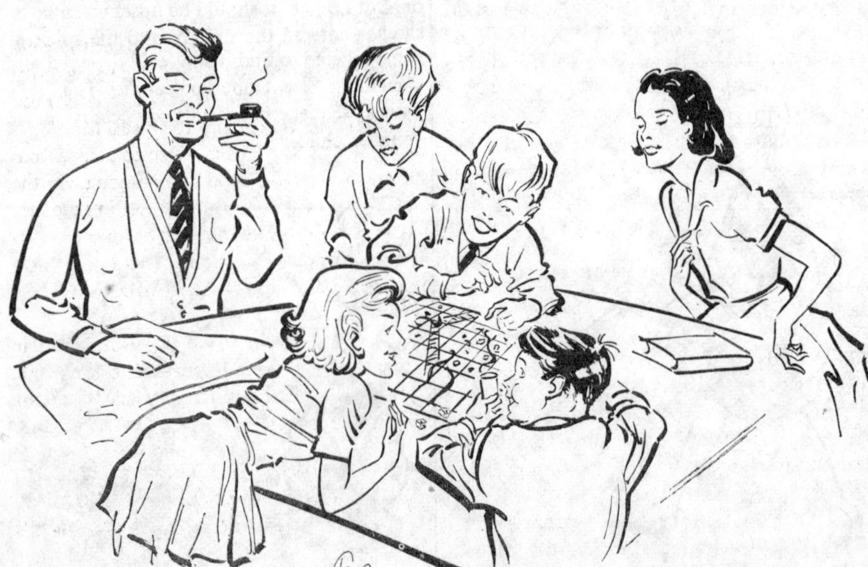

Fig. 13. *GAMES help to foster sociability within the family circle.*

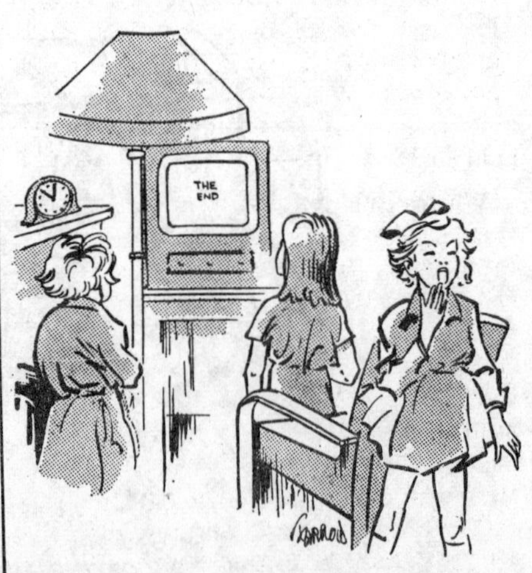

Fig. 15. *TELEVISION TIREDNESS*

The effects of watching violence, brutality and immorality portrayed in programs meant for adult viewing may be harmful to the child, and it is the parents' responsibility to see that children do not see such scenes. Fortunately these programs are usually late in the evening, and announcements often warn that a specific play or documentary is not suitable for children. Certainly, late evening viewing which will interfere with bedtime is a habit that must never be started. Teachers sometimes justly complain that children are too tired to concentrate on school class-work owing to late evening viewing the night before.

Although much is said about the dangers of television we must see the whole matter in perspective. There are many shows suitable and meant for children, and no harm arises from adventure stories and many of the Westerns. In fact, selective viewing can be of definite value both in educating and broadening the child's mind and in stimulating his imagination. It can bring into his home much that is going on in the world which he would never be able to experience otherwise. The selecting is largely the parents' responsibility.

Radio and Music. From an early age most children respond eagerly and readily to music. The radio provides a child with a never-ending source of all types of music, and he soon begins to build in himself a sense of rhythm and musical appreciation. In the preschool age he loves jumping up and down in time to it, exercising his muscles as well as his musical sense.

If the family does not own a phonograph, inexpensive children's phonographs are available. There are a large variety of children's records which introduce the listener to the instruments of the orchestra and the stories told in classical music.

Pets

Some sort of pet, whether it be a cat, a dog, or a rabbit, is an asset to the home with young children. Certainly where the child is the only one or separated from his brothers and sisters by some years, a pet may provide an excellent outlet for affection and companionship. The whole subject of choosing and keeping domestic pets is dealt with in some detail in the section, 'The Household Pet.'

When a child is used to being with animals from an early age he acquires familiarity with them and is taught not to be afraid. If the child looks after his pet by himself he develops a sense of responsibility and he will not be cruel to animals. He will become familiar with all sides of animal life—feeding, mating, birth, and suckling of the young. Watching these events will help him to assimilate knowledge of reproduction quite naturally.

Overfriendly overtures to strange dogs and cats, however, need to be discouraged as they might end in disaster.

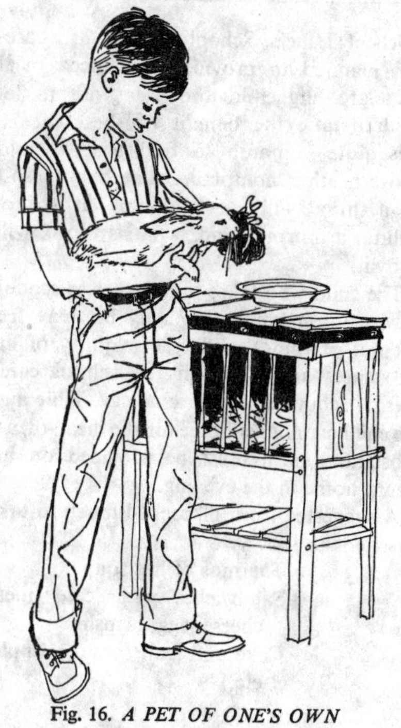

Fig. 16. *A PET OF ONE'S OWN*

SCHOOL

The Nursery School. At a certain age most children benefit by attending a nursery school for a few hours each day. The morning is the time usually chosen. Nursery school is by no means essential but it does provide many real advantages for the child. The best age to start is around three years old. A few children will be ready at two and a half, but a timid shy child may react very badly to being placed in such a school at too early an age.

Care must be taken over the introduction of the child to the nursery school, and the management of the first few days. This applies especially to children who are not used to being away from their mothers. The child must never feel that he is being pushed out of the way for the morning, with his mother breathing a big sigh of relief once he has gone. It is not wise for a young child to start nursery school on the arrival of another baby, as this is likely to give rise to feelings of great resentment and may produce scenes either at home or during school hours. A sensible plan is for the mother to take the child to the nursery school and show him around and watch the other children playing for a few days before leaving him to cope on his own.

Nursery school has special value for the only child, for the child who seldom comes into contact with other children, and for the city child living in a small apartment.

Make sure that the nursery school has been approved by the local health authority. There are rigid regulations concerning the size of the premises, the lighting and heating arrangements, the amount of garden space and the toilet facilities. These regulations are for the child's benefit—so beware of non-approved nurseries as they usually fall well below the required minimum standard.

Sociability is, of course, one of the principal advantages a child will stand to gain. It is essential for a child to mix with others of his own age, essential for building his character and for helping him to adjust to the realities of life. It is also a preparation for that great day when he is five and goes to the 'big school.' Children who have attended nursery school usually adapt themselves much better to the primary school than those who have not.

Most nursery schools have trained teachers, and the children take part in many fascinating activities which they would otherwise be unable to do. There is freedom and space for group dancing, games, and acting. There are specially designed apparatus and toys available, paints and clay, and bars for climbing—things which it may not be possible to have at home.

The mother, too, may get some precious hours to herself, while the child is learning to be independent and widening his horizons.

Primary School

First Days. Starting school is indeed a great step in every child's life. The first few days and weeks are most important, and every mother wishes this period to pass smoothly and without too much upset on either side.

Most children are eager to start school and this attitude is encouraged if the mother prepares her child wisely for the great day. The right idea about school should be built up in a child's mind—that it is a happy and interesting place, where every child goes to learn more about books, drawings, and numbers, and where there are games to play, songs to sing and things to make. Children with older brothers and sisters will look forward to being 'grown up' and joining them in the many interesting activities which they have already heard about. Most under-fives will have watched schoolchildren on the playground, and in the afternoon seen them coming home from school.

However well-prepared and eager the child is, the first days must inevitably be a great strain. The school building and the classroom are unfamiliar and he has to sit still for longer than he is used to. There are strange faces and strange noises and bells keep ringing. So the child needs extra love and care during the first few days. The mother must be prepared to listen with great attention to his doings and adventures and admire the 'work' he brings home to show her.

All children want to be the same as their schoolmates and it is important to them not to be dressed differently, and to have the right equipment.

Parent-Teacher Relationship. The teacher is an all-important figure in a schoolchild's life, and the sort of person she is, and her methods, will play a large part in keeping him happy and well-adjusted at school.

There should therefore be an open and free contact between parents and teacher. Parents should make full use of any Parent-Teacher Association that may be attached to their child's particular school. It is important to go to the meetings of such an Association since there one learns about school policies and projects, and is able to discuss any parental problems. Mothers and fathers should be prepared to confide their child's problems in the teacher, and the teacher will reciprocate by sharing the child's difficulties with his parents.

Never criticize the school or teacher in front of the child, and do not sympathize with his grievances too readily without first looking into the circumstances. It is important that the mother should encourage as happy a relationship between teacher and child as possible, but this cannot be achieved if the mother constantly takes the child's side about minor grievances and puts the blame on the teacher.

A good school will ensure that not only is there liaison between parents and teacher but between the teacher and the school doctor, and the family doctor if necessary. Such a relationship is especially valuable if the child is having difficulties with work or seems to be unhappy at school.

Slowness at School. If a child seems unnaturally slow or behind the others the cause may be a physical one—perhaps he has a slight degree of deafness or his eyesight needs attention. One type of hearing trouble is high-frequency deafness in which the hearing for high notes is defective, whereas other sounds are heard normally. If such disabilities are not recognized early both the parent and the child will go through much unnecessary suffering.

There are some children who are naturally slow and will never be particularly good at lessons. The future happiness for such a child depends entirely on his parents. They must never expect too much, and if they are disappointed they must not show it in front of him. It is not his fault. A child usually wants to please his parents and he is doing his best not to be a failure in their eyes. A slow child should be given every encouragement—praise him for trying and accept him for what he is.

It is not unusual to find that a child who is not good at lessons will have some other aptitude. Whatever it is—cleverness with his hands, a love of animals, a musical sensibility —it should be encouraged and allowed to flourish. It will serve as compensation for both child and parent. Children who are driven beyond their capacities are bound to suffer emotionally, and their characters will be adversely affected. In extreme cases they may resort to cheating in an effort to secure a good place in class, or they may give up the unequal struggle, become apathetic, and stop trying at all.

School Lunch. School lunches are carefully planned to provide a balanced meal for a growing child and it is wise to let children take the benefit of these meals. It is quite common to find that a child whose mother complains that he 'doesn't eat a thing' will eat his lunch at school without a murmur and, what is more, will enjoy it.

The child who takes sandwiches to school, however nourishing they may be, may feel left out of things when the majority of his classmates are eating in the school cafeteria. If school lunches are not available and the child cannot get home for the meal, then a substantial meal must be provided on his return home in the evening.

A suggested form of packed lunch to take to school is:

Thermos of hot soup
Sandwiches with cold meat cheese, egg, or fish
Cake and fruit (orange, apple, etc.)

Minor Infections. At the start of each new term some mothers are very distressed when their children immediately go down with colds, coughs, and sore throats. Between the ages of five and seven such troubles are very common. They are often inevitable as the child is exposed to many germs with which he has not been in contact during the holidays. As he grows older a partial immunity is built up and the time lost from school becomes less.

When there is a school epidemic of one of the childhood infectious diseases such as measles, chickenpox, mumps, or German measles, the child who has not had the disease is the most likely to succumb, but if he is in normal health it is just as well that the childhood diseases are finished with at an early school age. At this time the school work he misses is far more easily made up than at the later time of examinations. German measles present a special problem. The most dangerous time for a woman to contact German measles is in the first three months of pregnancy, because this disease may have an effect on the unborn child. Therefore it is often advised that mothers of little girls should make sure that their daughters *do* catch German measles in childhood to prevent any likelihood of trouble in child-bearing years. Some really keen mothers organize 'German measles parties' to make absolutely sure that their girls catch this minor infection at a time when it is comparatively harmless.

Boarding School. Some parents may consider sending their child to boarding school, but there are certain types of children who will not be happy away from home. This applies to those boys and girls who are very sensitive and especially devoted to their home. They will find great difficulty in adjusting themselves, and although they may appear happy enough their emotional development may be hindered.

When the home life is unsatisfactory through divorce or illness, or if the parents have to go abroad, the sending of a child to boarding school may be inevitable.

In other cases there are valid medical reasons for sending certain children to a boarding school—many asthmatic children, for example, are completely free from attacks during a school term.

Special Schools

It is very reassuring to parents of a child with a disability, that there are good facilities for his education in the form of Special Schools. Such schools are part of the public school systems or are privately endowed. The staff in these schools, as well as having a true vocation for this type of work, have received special training for teaching the blind or the deaf and children with learning disabilities, emotional problems and physical handicaps.

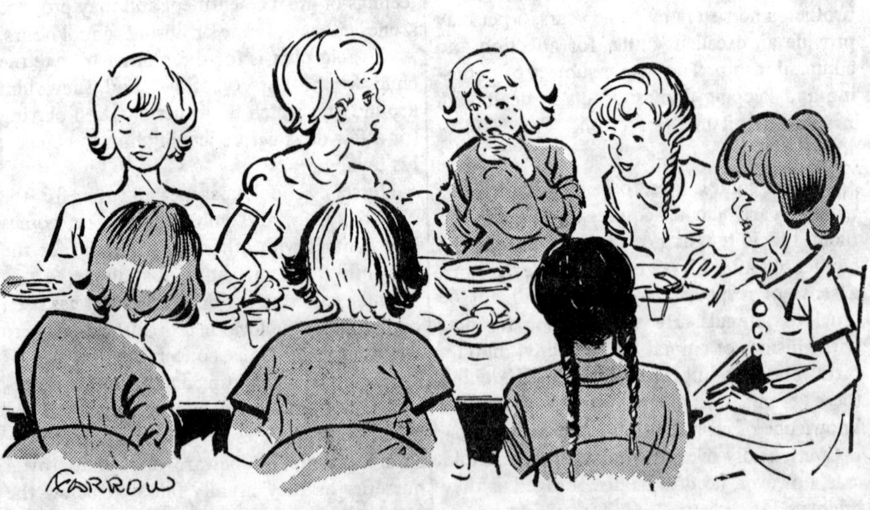

Fig. 17. *GERMAN MEASLES PARTY*

Medical Care

The Family Doctor. The family doctor or pediatrician should be chosen with some care. It is best to go on a neighbor's recommendation rather than haphazardly signing on with the nearest doctor, although how near he is will affect the choice to some extent.

The good doctor and the wise parent are able to carry on a friendly and useful relationship.

Much depends on the approach of the parent to the doctor—and as the health of the child is partly in his hands it is wise to be considerate in seeking his help. Find out the times of his office hours and try never to be late for an appointment. Many people are annoyed if they are not allowed in after hours. These hours have to be strictly adhered to, otherwise a busy doctor will never have time to start on his rounds. If you need a home visit, telephone in the morning before 10 a.m. (except in emergencies). This will greatly help the doctor in planning his day.

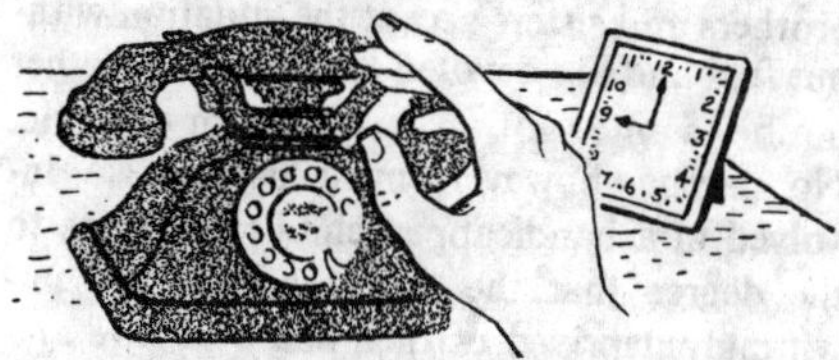

Fig. 18. *THE DOCTOR'S VISIT. Telephone him before 10 a.m. if you need him to come to your home.*

If you are genuinely worried about your child confide the full trouble to your doctor and you will find that he will always try to help and reassure you. Never be afraid that he will think you foolish—after all he is there to help you and he realizes that small matters may grow out of proportion in a worried mother's mind. On the other hand, too much fuss over minor ailments will encourage your doctor to regard you as a person who makes much ado about nothing.

Clinics. Public clinics are established in urban areas to give the same medical care as the family physician.

Inoculations. By the age of two years children should be completely immunized against diphtheria, whooping-cough, tetanus (lockjaw), and poliomyelitis. They should also have been vaccinated against smallpox. For further details, see Baby Care, p. 107. Booster doses against diphtheria are given before school entry at five years of age and again at eleven years.

SPECIAL PROBLEMS OF CHILDHOOD

Jealousy of the New Baby

The arrival of a new baby in the family is bound to have its effects on the other children. It is especially liable to create a problem when the baby is the second child and the first is under five years old. Jealousy is a reaction which is to be expected. It is a very natural reaction which springs from a basic feeling of fear—fear that the new baby is to take the child's place, that the love and security he has will be lost, and that his happiness is threatened.

A sensible parent will prepare the way before the baby is born. A few weeks or perhaps months beforehand the child should be told that a baby is on the way. This will give him time to get used to the idea gradually. If any changes have to take place to accommodate the new baby they should be made before the infant is born. The child may need to be moved into another room, for instance, or into a bed from a crib.

If the mother is having the baby in hospital, the person remaining in charge of a young child at home must be someone familiar.

The return home from the hospital is also important. It is probably better for the mother to greet the child without the baby there, and then to introduce the new arrival. Not too much fuss should be made over the baby, and if visitors come to see him they should be tactfully persuaded to pay some attention to the others before admiring the new infant. Encourage the child to help with the baby as much as possible. He will feel very important fetching clean diapers or the baby powder, or being allowed to mind the baby while mother is out of the room.

It is natural for the child to want to be more a baby himself at times—do not ridicule this and give him extra love and cuddling at such a time. Appeal to him as 'grown up' and able to do so many things that a little baby cannot.

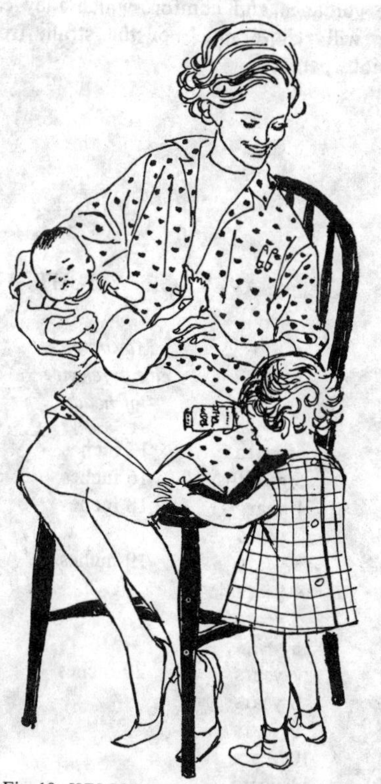

Fig. 19. *HELPING WITH THE NEW BABY*

It is a good idea to give the child a doll with all the baby accessories so that he can copy what mother is doing. He can give the doll a bottle while baby is feeding, dress and undress and bathe the doll, and in this way will not feel left out of things.

If the child is about to go to a nursery school, this should be established some weeks before the expected birth, so that he does not feel pushed out of the home and rejected by his mother on account of the new baby.

The main thing to keep in mind is that jealousy is a natural feeling at such a time. The child finds it very difficult to understand that the mother can love both baby *and* him, and this love, which is his main security, seems in danger of being lost. Jealousy must be dealt with sympathetically and effectively and never suppressed. If the feeling is submerged in the child by punishment or other means, then it may show itself in other more subtle ways such as bed-wetting or tantrums. The feelings themselves may be carried through into adult life.

Bed-wetting

A child usually becomes dry at night between the ages of three and four and a half. Bed-wetting beyond that time usually causes much anxiety, annoyance and extra work for the mother, and must also cause discomfort and guilt in the child.

A knowledge of some of the theories of bed-wetting, and the fact that in most cases it can be successfully cured with the help of your doctor, will do much to encourage the mother who is faced with this difficulty.

There are really three different kinds of bed-wetting. The first is rare and is usually associated with other symptoms. The cause is some physical disease of the urinary or nervous systems. Bed-wetting of this kind can be easily identified by the family doctor's examination, with or without hospital consultation.

The second is where, once a child has become dry for some time, he reverts, after a varying interval, to wetting the bed. In such a case there is usually some emotional factor responsible, such as the arrival of a new baby, a severe illness, separation of the parents, or moving to a strange neighborhood.

The third is where the child has never been dry, and continues wetting the bed most nights. In these cases the exact cause is not fully understood, but a plausible explanation is that it is to some extent hereditary. The brain of the deeply sleeping child is not able to get messages from the bladder to suppress the urge to pass water, or to awaken the child so that he will get up and pass it.

The treatment is different for each type of bed-wetting. Where it is mild, with minor emotional factors, the mother will be able to deal with it by herself with some simple advice from her doctor. Contrary to popular belief, restricting fluids at bedtime will not be of much use; the child will only imagine himself to be more thirsty than he actually is, and a battle over drinking at bedtime may result. Some authorities advocate lifting the bed-wetter out of bed to pass water at about 10 p.m. but this has also been found to be ineffectual since it is often difficult to get the child back to sleep again. Moreover, if the child is not fully awakened to empty his bladder, then the reflex of wetting while asleep is only encouraged.

Nothing is ever gained by scolding or punishing a bed-wetter. The five-year-old will only become more tense and rebellious and the older child is usually ashamed of the weakness already. He is not doing it on purpose, and he is only too keen to wake up in a dry bed. He needs reassurance and help with whatever situation appears to have started the trouble. The keeping of a chart with dry nights marked in, and wet ones left blank will, in a number of cases, be an incentive to co-operation on the part of the older child. The doctor may prescribe some tablets or a mixture to be taken while this régime is being followed.

The persistent form of bed-wetting responds in some children to treatment with an apparatus known as the electric alarm or 'buzzer.' This should only be used on the advice of the family doctor, who will refer you to a hospital or clinic where such an apparatus may be obtained. Each child is first investigated to discover whether or not this form of treatment will be suitable. The device works by waking the child, by means of a bell, soon after he has begun to pass water, and in this way teaches his brain to recognize messages from his bladder which are now fortified by sounds from the bell. This is only suitable for children who are old enough and willing to co-operate.

Test investigations so far have shown that this type of treatment does not have a bad effect on the child's emotional development.

The Only Child

The upbringing of an only child or a baby that comes many years after his brother or sisters is somewhat different from that of a child in a family group. The parents may be able to do more for him; he will probably have more toys, better clothes and more attention. The fact that he gets more consideration from his parents gives him an added self-assurance which may be useful in later life, provided it is not associated with selfishness or aggressiveness. He will also be more in the company of adults and more easily gain information and new experiences, perhaps from being taken about more.

It is often implied that an only child because he has more things and more attention is also a 'spoiled' child, always wanting his own way and getting others to do what he wants. Spoiling, however, is seldom the child's fault. Parents who let their child have his own way when it is likely to be harmful to him are shirking their responsibilities or being selfish.

Some parents of an only child feel that he is a tie which interferes with their pleasures and outings, and that he has to be taken with them unless he can be handed over to relations or friends. If this happens too often it can lead to a feeling of rejection and insecurity in the child, and create problems.

Wise parents will find other children for an only child to mix with so that he has friends of his own age. In this he has somewhat of an advantage in that he can probably vary these friends according to choice and not be constantly in the company of older or younger brothers or sisters.

Nursery schools can provide company, occupation and interest for the only child of three or four years of age, before he is old enough for primary school. In later childhood, visits to friends, and farm or camping holidays will provide young companionship, although this may not quite compensate for the happy shared life of a large family.

The Handicapped Child at Home

The attitude of the family towards the physically handicapped child will be the most important factor in determining what sort of person he grows up to be. It is easy to give advice, but difficult indeed for parents to adjust themselves emotionally and to accept the situation. It is natural at first for them to have feelings of rejection and guilt about a handicapped child, but today there are many organizations, societies and clubs which have a sympathetic attitude and a practical understanding of the handicapped child's problems. The guidance and comfort which they can give will relieve much of the strain from anxious parents.

Let the family doctor advise you from the start. He will be able to recommend the best way to manage, and will refer you to specialists if necessary. He will tell you what to do about education and will sort out any problems and queries—however trivial they may seem.

At home the aim of the whole family will be to treat a child with a handicap as naturally as possible, as a normal person in fact. This natural attitude will ensure that the child grows up without self-consciousness and in a happy frame of mind. If a lot of fuss is made, and if the mother makes the very natural mistake of being overprotective, the child will be made to feel 'different' from an early age.

Stares and whispers from strangers are incidents that cannot, unfortunately, be avoided. They must be faced resolutely, accepted, and ignored. Pity is also harmful—the child will be far happier without it.

The attitude of the parents communicates itself to the other children in the family. Fortunately, it usually happens that the brothers and sisters accept the situation without fuss and are devoted to the child whether he be a mongol, a cripple, or spastic. No parent, however, must become so involved in a handicapped child's problems to the degree that the other children are unwittingly deprived of their share of love and attention.

Occasionally, if the handicapped child is the first-born, the parents will determine not to have any more children, but to devote themselves to this only child. Such a policy will only do more harm than good both to the parents and the child, as such a child benefits enormously from the companionship and the give and take of family life where there are several children.

AVERAGE WEIGHT AND HEIGHT IN CHILDHOOD

Age	*Maximum circumference of head*	*Average weight*	*Average height*
at birth	13 inches	7 lb	20 inches
6 months	16 inches		
1 year	18 inches	22(19–24) lb	29(28–30) inches
2 years		28 lb	33 inches
3 years	19 inches	33 lb	37 inches
4 years		37 lb	40 inches
5 years		41(37–46) lb	42 inches
6 years		45 lb	44 inches
7 years	20 inches	49 lb	46 inches
8 years		55 lb	48 inches
9 years		61 lb	50 inches
10 years		67 lb	52 inches
11 years		73 lb	54 inches
12 years	21 inches	79 lb	56 inches

THE ADOLESCENT STAGE

I
HOW PERSONALITY IS DEVELOPED

The adolescent, being neither child nor mature adult, is very vulnerable, but has both rights and duties, a fact which is often overlooked by some righteous adults who are inclined to deplore the frivolity of youth which they themselves have forgotten.

Years of psychological research has helped people to gain more understanding of human relationships, but during the last few decades there has been a shift in approach to such studies as adolescence. Let us look at some of these theories before dealing with the practical problems presented in everyday life. Modern 'mental hygienists,' and especially the psychologists among them, now tend to treat such human topics by 'explaining' how behavior develops and how it can be controlled. They endeavor to do what all scientists are aiming at, that is to predict behavior, given a particular set of circumstances.

It must be remembered that as yet no unified theory of psychology has emerged, and various theories exist side by side. The topic will be discussed from the point of view of (a) psycho-analysis, and (b) social psychology. These two are viewed by some experts as antagonistic to each other and by others as complementary.

The psycho-analyst is inclined to view the problems of adolescence as having very deep roots which go back into babyhood and childhood. They consider that the majority of adolescent problems have a good chance of being solved fairly easily and quickly, no matter how complex they may seem at the time, provided that the first seven years or so of the youth's life has been satisfactory from a psychological point of view. To put it in another way, most analysts take the view that it is the 'unsoundness' of child-family relationships during the first few years of his life which is at the bottom of a youngster's disturbed behavior in adolescence, and not so much the particular stresses and strains during the adolescent period itself. A delinquent adolescent therefore is thought to have yielded to adolescent temptation not so much because of his present bad company and his lust for money but because, more basically, his very early home background has been such as to leave him with unsatisfied needs. This makes him badly want to 'take' things, as if he could thereby in a symbolical way 'take' the love of his parents which, unconsciously, he feels to have been withheld from him in his very early childhood. Adolescent problems are said to be in the main merely an extension of those of babyhood.

Freud and Psycho-analytical Theory of Early Childhood

Freud, the father of psycho-analysis, starts his theory of character formation by saying that all people are essentially governed by two opposing forces or instincts: the life-force (Libido) which is referred to in general as the need for love, and the destructive-force (Thanator) which is more commonly referred to as the death wish. Most Freudians have come to base their theory on that of the Libido only. According to this, Freud suggests that human beings have surging through them from birth a fundamental need to love and be loved. This need for love—libido—is said to be neither good nor bad but merely the very force of which life itself is made. According to this theory, if this need is not satisfied early one must expect an unbalanced personality pattern to emerge in childhood. It will show itself more during adolescence and adult life when pressure in the environment produces breakdowns just as pressure applied to a cracked cup will break it.

Freud held that the moment a child is born the libido seeks fulfilment and, if fulfilled, this helps to produce the kind of personality which makes for a stable baby, a stable adolescent, and a stable adult.

Oral Phase

First of all the libido strives to find its natural goal and outlet in what is known as the 'oral phase,' which means the stage in the baby's life when he gains his main satisfactions from the use of his mouth, chiefly by sucking. Freudians therefore stress the importance of the way in which breast feeding—and bottle feeding too—is carried out. Satisfactory emotional experiences at that time should help the baby towards the building up of a secure personality. Conversely, insecure emotional experiences suffered by a child during breast feeding may lead to an insecure personality pattern which can be observed even in babyhood but which will become only fully apparent later, particularly during adolescence, when the complexities of life may produce breakdowns in those whose initial emotional experiences have been faulty.

The oral stage, therefore, is seen by Freud as sensualized and high charged emotionally. It requires great skill and insight on the part of the breast feeding mother in the handling of the infant (see Breast Feeding, p. 100). Hence, in this theory, great emphasis is placed on the necessity of making each mother aware of her vital responsibility in helping her baby at this early stage. Good mothering in the first few months of the infant's life is simply the mother's ability to allow a baby to feel deeply secure. Provided that this first stage of the oral phase is successfully carried out, further experiences await the baby and will affect its character development.

Sooner or later the baby must learn to tolerate frustrations, within reason. It must not always expect to have its milk supplied on demand but only at given times and under appropriate circumstances. Inability to learn this, it is thought, could sow the seeds of later temper tantrums or ill-directed teenage aggressiveness when frustrations arise in adolescence. Hence, it is felt by Freudians that a child, if wrongly handled during the oral stage, can develop oral-greed instead of oral-need, and thus in later life develop into the kind of person who is forever neurotically greedy and demanding, and usually unable to wait patiently for the things he wants.

Anal Phase

Not only waiting, but also the ability to give has to be learned in babyhood. It is at this stage that Freud introduces his concept of the anal phase as the logical successor to the oral phase, one which he believed must also be dealt with satisfactorily. This phase is associated with excretory functions. Everyone is aware of the problems which arise when attempting to train a child to gain control of bladder and bowels. According to Freud the baby at this time experiences emotional feelings for practically the first time in his existence (see Toilet Training, p. 108). The baby is thought to have to learn (among several things) how to control his aggressiveness. The emotional experience of freely giving love to the mother, which is said to accompany physical production of excreta by the baby, is thought to be capable of turning quickly into hate and anger towards the mother during the later stages of the anal phase. Thwarted love of the toddler expresses itself by the angry withholding of waste products, thus subtly forcing the mother once more to supply the full measure of love which the baby feels has been withheld from him. Far-fetched as all this may seem, psycho-analysts claim that many cases of stress seen in children and adolescents are reversions to babyish forms of constipation or diarrhea, and severe difficulties of this sort have their roots in the anal phase.

Oedipus Complex and Electra Complex

According to Freud, the next stage in the child's development which is important and has far-reaching effects upon personality development in the Oedipus complex in boys and the Electra complex in girls, which are explained in the 'Role of Father.' The psychoanalysts believe that, unless these phases are resolved satisfactorily, difficulties will occur in adolescence when the young girl or boy is becoming interested in the opposite sex and seeking a marriage partner.

Latency and Adolescence

Freudians point out that once these three phases have been worked through, the child undergoes for about seven years before puberty a period of 'latency' when he deals with life in a less emotional way. This occurs roughly durin the junior high school age when the child is normally inclined to attend to school matters rather than to sensual ones.

Once puberty and adolescence is reached, however, the earlier forgotten emotional pangs of the development stages are thought to reawaken. Psycho-analysts believe, therefore, that the problems of the adolescent stage are not merely the results of difficult situations in which an adolescent finds himself, but are basically the result of much deeper and fundamental difficulties.

Id, Ego, and Super Ego

There are several other aspects of the Freudian theory which require brief mention in order to fill out the picture of personality formation. Freud considered that there are three layers of consciousness. The deepest and most inaccessible and by far the largest layer is the Unconscious (also termed the Id). The second layer is the Ego, which is mostly conscious, and is responsible for one's ability to say to oneself: This is 'I' or my 'Ego', and which is unique and different from the Ego of other people. Lastly, there is the Super Ego which can be considered as one's ability or moral capacity to distinguish between right and wrong and between accepting or rejecting the values of one's parents and society. The

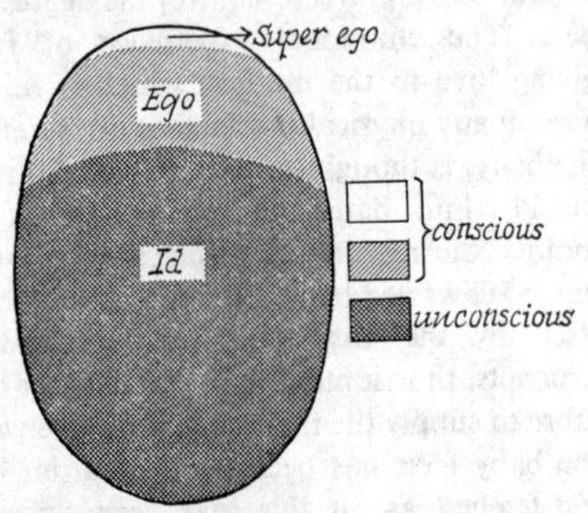

Fig. 1. *LAYERS OF CONSCIOUSNESS. An indication of the proportions of the conscious and the unconscious.*

powerful, more primitive, and hidden instincts of the Id seek to influence the Ego, while the Super Ego acts as a censor and a brake upon such actions. For example: Id says 'I *want* to do this,' Ego says, 'Very well I shall do this,' Super Ego then says 'This is wrong—my parents or society *would not approve* of my doing this.' If the Super Ego is normal or of sufficient strength then its censorship upon such actions will be effective.

Between the Unconscious and the Conscious there is said to exist an intermediary stage of 'pre-consciousness' (all too familiar in the morning when the alarm clock has gone off and one is not quite certain as to whether one is consciously aware of the fact or still unconsciously dreaming about it).

According to Freud, good mental health, especially in adolescence, is related to the extent to which a person can recognize consciously what he is up against and deal with normal conflict situations in a rational manner. The converse is the irrational and unconscious behavior of some adolescents under stress which seems to make them 'rebels without a cause.' They rebel against authority (father, teacher, an employer, or a code of conduct) not so much because authority is directly frustrating them, but because authority recalls, unconsciously, the earlier non-resolved emotional conflicts of childhood in relation to mother and father.

According to this theory then, the extremely maladjusted adolescent requires psycho-analytical treatment to enable him to bring the repressed and unconscious memories of his childhood difficulties into consciousness. Once this is done he will stop being anti-social and adopt a mature and adult pattern of behavior.

Freud held that psycho-analytical treatment was only very rarely required; in most cases life itself acted as the most efficient of all masters. Adolescence is a necessary schooling stage through which all individuals have to pass if they wish to graduate ultimately to full adulthood and maturity. He further held that no individual can fully attain maturity. Life is one long struggle with oneself to overcome aspects of one's childhood and adolescence.

Social Psychologists' Viewpoint

Some social psychologists agree and others disagree with all or some aspects of Freudian theory. Most of them tend to approach the study of the adolescent from a slightly different angle which need not necessarily conflict with psycho-analytical views.

They see the adolescent as a person who is caught between two worlds since he no longer belongs to the world of the child nor as yet to that of the adult. He is therefore seen as a frustrated person who has at times no clear goals or, if he has, he often knows that he has very little chance of achieving them quickly. Often the adolescent does not yet know what he really wants or what he ought to want. When he was a child he knew that playing cops and robbers in an imaginary world transformed his average life into one of thrills and excitement. He knows vaguely that he can no longer play like a child, but what is he to do instead in order to have his average existence transformed once more into a life of thrills? The door to delinquency or to brooding may thus lie open.

The educator's job, therefore, is to provide the adolescent with new goals, to inspire him, and to help him achieve these goals. When childish play no longer satisfies the youth, a wise educator may open up a new world of wonder for him by introducing him further into the realms of skills and crafts, and of the arts—to music, to literature and painting.

Wise parents and educators should also help the adolescent to understand worthwhile human relationships and to adapt himself to the needs of society and his family. He may have no clear concept of how to set about making himself agreeable to others or to behave in a socially acceptable way. In another era, much of this was handled by the Church. Nowadays, while the Church is still keeping an eye on tasks like these, it is the parents and teachers who more than ever before need patience and wisdom to steer the adolescent through his turbulent years, especially with the emergence of sex as a part of his life. This is not always easy to do in an environment which brings sex to the adolescent's notice nearly every minute of the day, on cinema and TV screens and in magazines. None of this need present any lasting difficulty to an adolescent who feels secure owing to the fact that he has been prepared for it by his parents. If insecure or unprepared, however, much unnecessary conflict can develop which may take years to resolve.

Facing the Adult World

As he leaves school the adolescent faces the problems of the world of adult work. During his last years at school he may have idealized his future world of work. How different and frustrating it may turn out to be after the first six months in a factory, in an office, or at a university! Yet, with the guiding advice of a loving adult ready to explain and teach him to adjust himself to these new experiences, how interesting the adult working world can be!

As the youth enters his new world, he also begins to find that he is physically more capable. He can run a mile without puffing and can play sports without tiring easily. His whole physical and social horizon is being daily widened, and every new and exciting experience demands new adjustments until through gradual repetition they become habitual—and eventually adulthood is achieved.

New friendships are made at this stage of life which often require different handling from the earlier and more naïve ones made at school. The jealousy of a co-worker, often older, can damage the idealism of an adolescent who is just emerging from a more innocent childhood. Conversely, the enthusiasm of an elder may set a shining example for the rest of the young man's life. Adolescence is an age of trial and error, of extremes, and of ups and downs until gradually a more balanced view of life is learned.

Guiding the Adolescent

At the present time it appears that a balanced view is emerging which stresses the need for supporting the adolescent without robbing him of his individuality. Guidance requires some knowledge of basic psychology combined with commonsense on the part of parents and educators. It is not enough for parents to deplore the standards of behavior of some adolescents; they need to start to study and learn the reasons why some adolescents behave in a particular fashion. Only then will parents and educators be better equipped to deal effectively with youth's problems and, better still, to help prevent serious problems from arising. We make the plea for more and more adults to spare some time to read some of the innumerable books on the subject and to make an effort to understand and guide young people. In so doing the adult can do much for adolescents in laying a sound foundation for the development of mature adult behavior in later life when our society needs sound adjustment.

II
THE PRACTICAL DIFFICULTIES OF GROWING UP

The adolescent child is undergoing continuous change. Almost overnight he has to leave the protected sheltered existence of home and school and begin to shoulder some of the responsibilities of adult working life. At the same time changes are taking place in his body, in his strength and in his mental powers, and all these he has to learn to control. Frequently his emotional reactions to ordinary everyday problems cause confusion to himself, his parents and the people with whom he comes into contact. He crams into a few years a great deal of experience and comes under influences both good and bad which may have a profound effect upon his adult life.

It is the parent, or the adult in charge, who has the main influence upon adolescent development. The young person is not mature enough to have an objective view about himself. It has become fashionable in some quarters to regard adolescents as young adults but this is very misleading and can even be dangerous when it leads to thrusting responsibilities upon a young person before he is sufficiently mature to deal with them. His self-control is not well established and while he is discovering what his capabilities are he gains some protection from the manner of his early upbringing as well as from the restrictions and limitations imposed by his family. But such restrictions must be imposed with care and consideration for his growing need for independence.

Adolescence has been described as a time when the growing individual becomes aware of adult problems and it lasts until he or she has come to terms with the adult realities. The challenges which every adolescent has to face are:

1. Learning to act independently without leaning too much on his parents and friends;
2. achieving a natural and relaxed relationship with the opposite sex;
3. deciding upon, and preparing himself for, his future profession or occupation; and
4. learning the responsibilities of citizenship.

HEALTH AND BODY CHANGES

Physical Changes

Physical changes are a fundamental aspect of adolescence. The sex glands come into operation altering the physical appearance and mental make-up of the young boy or girl. Between the ages of eleven and twelve years, there is a rapid acceleration until the peak is reached at roughly fifteen years of age. A gradual slowing down in the process then takes places until, at about eighteen years of age, adolescence in the narrow physical sense is complete. Many children in their later school years are ready for adult physical expression.

There is considerable variation in this development which tends to show earlier in girls than in boys. It is rare for adolescent traits to appear before the age of ten years. Some children may show little sign of physical change until they are fourteen years or even older and may appear younger than their age group. There is no cause for anxiety as this in no way affects general intelligence and they usually catch up later on.

Changes in Girls. The girl's breasts develop, hair begins to grow under the arms and around the labial area and the hips broaden (see also Functional Changes of Women). The girl is often self-conscious about these changes and may be embarrassed when she thinks that others may notice. Menstruation will begin about this time and it is extremely important that the girl is prepared for this by her mother. The first monthly period can be a very frightening experience for a young girl unless she knows what will happen and why. Menstruation should never be referred to as 'the curse' or 'being unwell' but more positively linked with future satisfactions in bearing children. Periods are often irregular at first; many girls have no pain associated with menstruation but may feel a little tired and lax. It is, however, always better for the girl to be active even from the onset, since activity promotes a better flowing away of the discharges; young girls may need reassurance on the matter.

Changes in Boys. A boy's voice begins to deepen, hair begins to show on his face, around his genitals and under his arms, and there is enlargement of the sex organs. The emission of fertile semen will begin at this time and is associated with a more frequent and stronger erection of the penis which indicates that a boy is now capable of procreating. Emission usually occurs for the first time during sleep and it should be explained to the boy that this fluid contains sperms which, when joined to the ovum produced in woman, would lead to conception of a baby, and it has no other function than this. A boy may feel when he first has this experience, that he may lose his strength; he will need the assurance that this outflowing will cause him no harm.

He may feel embarrassed, even humiliated by his inability to control these bodily reactions at first and he will need reassurance from his parents. If he has no knowledge and has only heard vague or misleading rumors he is likely to be frightened or anxious. Just as a mother prepares a girl for menstruation so the father should explain these matters to his son. If he finds this difficult he can enlist the help and co-operation of the doctor or club leader to explain this perfectly normal stage of development. Parental silence can lead a boy to believe he is ill, or has done something wrong.

UNDESCENDED TESTES. It occasionally happens that one or both testes have not descended into the scrotum and it is easy for this condition to be overlooked in a young boy unless a specific examination has been carried out. Not infrequently it is only discovered when pubertal changes draw attention to that part of the body. An undescended testis cannot produce sperms although one normal testis alone is capable of doing so. A doctor should be consulted and treatment for this carried out early in puberty. In some cases injection of hormones will correct the defect; other cases may require surgical treatment.

Masturbation. During the period when the sexual urge is crystallizing and the young boy is experiencing nocturnal emissions, masturbation is very common. Few normal adolescents have had no experience of it. For the majority it only occurs occasionally and they grow out of it.

Although masturbation is common and does not have dire physical effects it is a bad habit because it tends to stop the development of mature emotional relationships, and adolescents should be helped to overcome it. This is not easy and will require effort on the part of the young boy or girl who will probably be worried about it. Explanations made quietly and wisely by a trusted adult about the developing physical urges helps, and the young people should be encouraged to take part in activities and interests to absorb their energy. The continuation of this habit is more common in boys and girls who have not enough to occupy them.

Emotional Changes

Sudden unexpected changes in mood are common in adolescents and are, as a rule, due to the physical changes which are taking place: excitement and delight can quickly change to tears and anger.

The adolescent finds it difficult to adapt himself to other people's personalities because of his inexperience; he becomes impatient and intolerant. He will sometimes appear hostile and tactless and usually resents criticism. These reactions are a cover for his own uncertainty even though he may appear outwardly confident. The more importance he attaches to the criticism, the more resentful he may appear. He often reacts very strongly to parental criticism because he feels the criticism is unfair and he has not been allowed to give his reasons and express his point of view. If the situation continues until

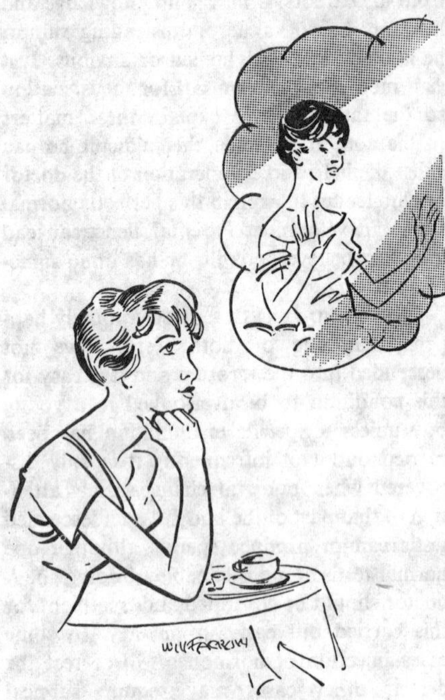

Fig. 2. *DAY-DREAMING*

he feels completely disapproved of, he may cease to make an effort to co-operate.

Parents and other adults dealing with such 'growing-up pains' should praise effort as well as success. It can be pointed out to the young person that it is not wise or necessary to reveal all his feelings in society. He may think it is 'dishonest' not to 'speak his mind' but it can be explained that to speak impulsively may cause unnecessary unhappiness to others, and also he may not always know the full facts of a situation.

Day-dreaming is another common characteristic of adolescence. The young girl's dream of becoming a great actress may never be realized but she gains enormous pleasure from the dream. No harm is done providing she does not at the same time withdraw completely from coping with everyday life.

The borderline between normal adolescent behavior and serious emotional problems is a narrow one, and temporary outbursts of bad behavior are not serious, although exasperating to deal with. Harassed parents sometimes exaggerate the psychological difficulties of adolescence but, if a young person is continuously anxious about everyday problems or his behavior seems likely to get him into trouble with teachers, employers, or the police, then he needs extra help from parents or doctors, or both, as soon as possible.

General Care

Food Needs. Because adolescents are growing fast they need plenty of good food. A boy between thirteen and fifteen years will need at least as much food as a moderately active man, and a girl, during the years when she is growing fast, will need as much food as an active woman. Providing there is no tendency to become grossly overweight no limit should be put on the amount an adolescent eats. Meals should be regular and a balanced diet should include vegetables, fruit, milk and whole grain cereals; body-building protein —in meat, fish, eggs, cheese—is essential at this time. Encouragement to take a hearty breakfast is wise.

Dieting. Girls very often become plump in their early teens, and need the reassurance of knowing that this 'puppy fat' will go away later on. In spite of such reassurance they may wish to diet. Indiscriminate dieting at any age is never wise and the taking of tablets, except under medical advice, may affect health and development. A girl may cut out such valuable foods as milk, potatoes and bread in the mistaken belief that they cause the overweight. It is wiser to help to arrange a more balanced diet (see section on Nutrition, p. 65) and to see that the girl has plenty of exercise. In extreme cases a doctor should be consulted.

Fatigue and Rest. Adequate sleep is essential to adolescents and they should be encouraged to have 8 to 10 hours most nights. Their leisure activities usually take a great amount of energy.

Bodily growth at this time may proceed smoothly or in sudden spurts. The old phrase 'outgrown his strength' has a sound medical basis; sudden gains in weight and height cause physical and mental fatigue and the young person may at times be better left to sit quietly with a book, or not be nagged if he finds it difficult to rouse himself in the mornings.

Parents often become exasperated with teenagers who seem to have boundless energy for their own activities but are 'too tired' when asked to do something for others. In many cases this can be quite genuine because they put a great amount of energy into their activities, and fatigue can be forgotten while something exciting is going on, only to be felt later.

Smoking. Lung and lip cancer and its association with smoking have quite ousted the earlier concept of the peaceful solace given by the fragrant weed of tobacco. In countries the world over, social-minded persons are endeavoring to stop or at least modify this widespread habit. Naturally enough, they want to prevent the formation of the habit which usually begins in youth. What makes an adolescent boy (or girl) start smoking? It makes him feel bold and manly (or the girl, sophisticated) to copy a habit which he associates with being a full grown adult. Basically, it is the adults who need to change such a concept by setting a new example of not smoking. It is a big problem for parents everywhere.

Young people today have and earn good money and raising the price of cigarettes and tobacco will not be an effective deterrent. Warning of the dangers of smoking to health is only likely to be of use if coupled with a good example.

Alcohol. Many families have definite ideas on this subject and forbid teenagers to have alcoholic drinks. It is clearly best for them to have no alcohol, but this is often not achieved and some parents may decide to lay down moderate rules to lessen the likelihood of 'forbidden adventures.' If an adolescent drinks excessively then there is something wrong and advice should be sought from a doctor or responsible person. Reliable investigations have shown, however, that in spite of newspaper reports adolescents on the whole drink far less alcohol than soft drinks and coffee.

Ailments and Illnesses

There are few serious physical illnesses occurring specifically in adolescence but there are a number of ailments to which young people appear prone.

Skin Problems. Many adolescents have a tendency to develop pimples and blackheads on the face, back and chest. This can be unsightly and cause them a great deal of embarrassment. Blackheads are due to dirt and dust settling on excess fatty secretion of the pores. Regular cleansing of the skin with good soap, really hot water and brisk towel drying will usually keep blackheads from forming. They are more common in boys than girls and make their appearance at fifteen or sixteen years of age and often do not clear up until nineteen or twenty years, or even later.

For the more deep-seated condition of acne, see Skin Diseases.

Dental Decay. Grave disquiet has been expressed at the number of children and adolescents who have needed dental treatment or who had mouths full of decayed teeth. This is a real danger to health and, when dental treatment is required, it should be sought as soon as possible. Young people should be encouraged to make six-monthly visits for dental inspection.

Earache, particularly of the middle ear, should never be neglected or ignored. Merely to give the sufferer an aspirin and send him to bed, although this may give temporary relief, is quite inadequate: the doctor should be consulted. Hearing is too valuable to be lost on the threshold of adult life (see Ear, Nose and Throat Diseases).

Sore Throats, Tonsillitis and Catarrhal Infections are relatively common in young girls. Smoking can make this condition worse.

Those who are rather susceptible to these complaints should stay at home at the first sign of the trouble and remain in an even temperature for 24 to 48 hours; this is often more effective than doses of medicines. It is important to keep warm, and although light clothing is suitable in a heated house, school or office, a warm coat for cold winters is a worthwhile investment for outdoor wear.

Tuberculosis. This is one of the few serious illnesses which can be a special danger to the adolescent and during the late teens. Tuberculosis is no longer as prevalent as it was over twenty years ago but it has by no means been eradicated. Medical preventive measures are explained fully in Chest Diseases. The ordinary safeguards for the young person are to avoid overcrowded and badly ventilated rooms, etc., whenever possible, and to get plenty of fresh air and good food.

Venereal Diseases. Although a recent report on Adolescence found that in a number of treatment centers as many as one in five of the patients were teenagers, much more investigation is required as this increase in venereal diseases by no means proves that there is a general rise in promiscuity among adolescents. It is a serious responsibility for all parents and those in charge of groups of adolescents to see that their young people do not run the risk of infection. It can be pointed out to them that the incidence of these diseases is negligible except from sexual intercourse especially of a casual nature.

If gonorrhea or syphilis is contracted, early treatment is essential to avoid the dangerous consequences of these diseases. For fuller details, see section on Venereal Diseases.

Physical Appearance

Today adolescents tend to be taller, heavier and healthier than their parents or grandparents were at the same age. Some of their facial features—noses, chins and mouths—will change before they settle into the proportions they will have in adult life and young persons are often self-conscious about it. They may not mention this awareness of self-change to their parents and it is obviously not wise for parents to remark unnecessarily about it. On the other hand parents often become exasperated when the young person spends hours before the mirror, and may mistakenly think that praise will only make the boy or girl more vain, but a young person can gain a lot of reassurance if his or her good features are approved.

Awkwardness. In early adolescence a boy or girl often blushes, 'falls over his own feet,' and drops things. This may be partly due to rapid and uneven growth but is mainly associated with a new self-awareness and usually happens when he is self-conscious or thinks he is being watched. Such awkwardness rarely shows itself in a setting where a youth is not self-conscious, as in sports. He will usually grow out of this difficulty and little can be done about it in the meantime. It is wiser not to draw attention to it.

Posture. Correct posture is something which many adolescents need help to maintain. Round shoulders are common in girls between the ages of eleven and fifteen. They are very self-conscious about their developing figures and may go about with round shoulders and bent backs in order to try to hide their busts. This is just a phase from which they will recover but it helps if they are not teased about it and are encouraged by their mothers to wear pretty clothes. Exercises, swimming and games will also help.

The main difficulty in overcoming round shoulders is that hunching of the back easily becomes a habit. Mothers may have constantly to remind and encourage their daughters to 'stand up' or 'straighten' their backs long after the self-conscious stage has passed. It is better not to allow the girl to get overtired, for this can make the habit worse.

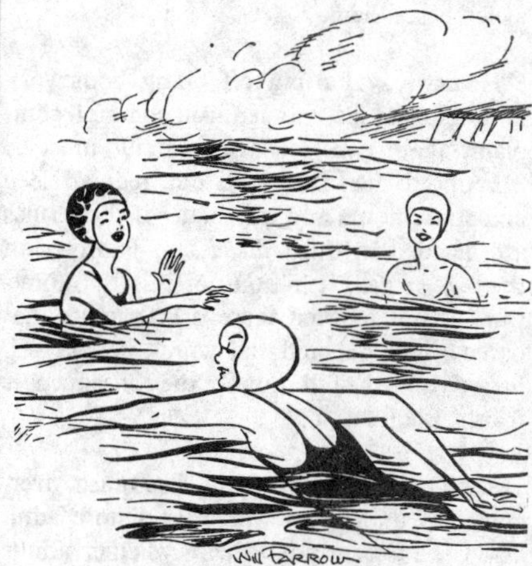

Fig. 3. *SWIMMING EXERCISE. For fast growing adolescents swimming is one of the finest forms of exercise.*

Clothes. Choice of clothes is very much an individual matter. Adolescents have very definite ideas what styles in clothes they want and are often influenced by the latest and exaggerated fashion and it is better that there should be some give and take on both sides of the family. The final decision must rest with the parents where clothes are considered totally unsuitable, but this is best done by tactfully suggesting alternatives. At this time young people are developing their own taste and need helpful advice on colors and cut, on how to dress to suit one's own shape and style, and not merely to follow the latest exaggerated fashion.

Adolescents and Sex Instruction

Many parents have difficulty in deciding what to tell their children about sexual relationships, fearing that knowledge may lead to experimentation without realizing the possible consequences. On the other hand, there are dangers in leaving growing children in ignorance in the modern world where young people mix freely with each other and sex is constantly brought to their attention in movies, on television and in newspapers. Ignorance is not the same as innocence. If a young person is taught to respect sex as a part of life he is less likely to run wild and is helped to accept sexual maturity as a normal part of growing up.

Ideally, sex instruction should be given by parents and it is less of a shock to the adolescent if this has been given gradually throughout childhood. For parents who find it difficult or 'don't know how to start' there are many excellent books and pamphlets. It is often easier, when both parents and young person have read the book, for questions to be invited. (See also the beginning of Functional Changes of Women.)

ADOLESCENTS AT HOME

Some young people manage to get through their adolescence with a minimum of upset and difficulty but for most adolescents it is a time of strain which requires careful handling by the family. It is between the ages of twelve and sixteen years that adolescents can be most difficult in the home. They begin to demand independence and to be considered grown up and resent being treated as children. They take themselves very seriously and want to think and act for themselves. They are often so wrapped up in themselves that they are impervious to the feelings of others, and do not realize how difficult it is for their family to cope with their moodiness and lack of tact and co-operation. Because they are so unsure of themselves they do not know whether they are behaving normally for their age and whether they are right or wrong. They usually want everything at once and when this is not possible they feel that the family is trying to keep them down and does not understand them. This can lead to continuous arguments about trivial matters such as early bedtime, going out, punctuality, neatness in appearance and in the home, and adolescent girls are frequently resentful when asked to help with housework. They are often extremely critical if they consider that older children in the family are getting more freedom and responsibility. At the same time they are often 'bossy' towards their younger brothers and sisters who in turn resent it and may tease and make fun of them.

When there are no difficulties teenagers seem to make some. Even under the mildest parental guidance, they seem to need to demonstrate their ability to make decisions and they will do this often in trivial ways such as wearing unsuitable clothes, grumbling about food or the places to which their parents wish them to go.

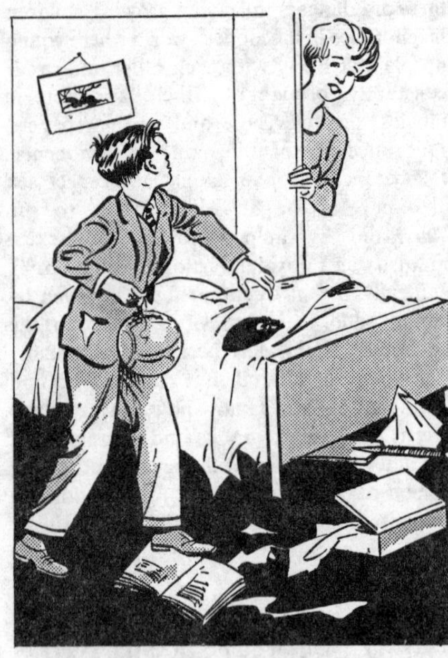

Fig. 4. *THE DISORDERED ROOM*

Youths like to take risks, and go in for rough sports and fast driving. Some risks are necessary to help to train their judgment, but many of them have no real sense of danger and will ride on a motor bicycle without wearing a crash helmet, or speed at 80 or 90 m.p.h. under unsuitable conditions. For such youngsters, restrictions have to be imposed in their own interests. Whenever possible, however, a restriction should be coupled with a privilege.

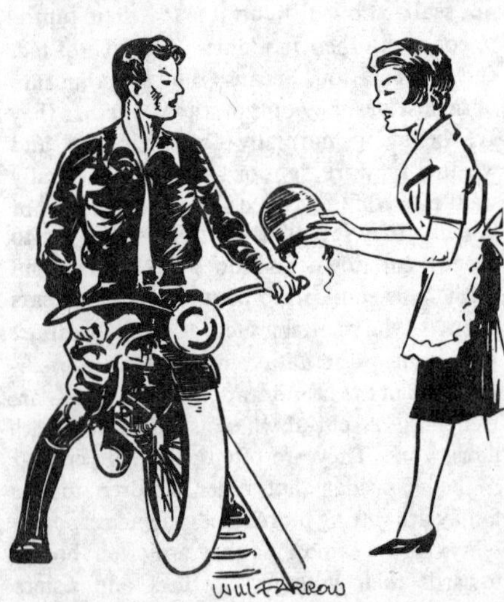

Fig. 5. *ADVENTURE—WITH SAFETY*

Parental Control

Wise parents realize that underneath the rebelliousness their teenagers not only need guidance but want it. They genuinely prefer to have some rules for living, some standards by which they can measure their growth as adults. They expect their parents to disagree with them sometimes, and need to have limits set for them. They can take a certain amount of strictness, providing they are sure that their parents love them. It is best to give adolescents reasons why they cannot go to certain places and stay out late, such as 'I don't want you to go there because they drink too much and are badly behaved,' or 'You must be home early to get enough rest and sleep, and it is not wise for a young girl to be out too late.'

Hitting or smacking an adolescent offends his growing sense of dignity and makes him very resentful. Parents frequently become exasperated if they feel their authority is being flouted, but it is wiser to wait until everyone has cooled down and discuss the matter calmly. Some compromise between teenager and parents is always possible in this way.

Time spent in giving adolescents the opportunity to 'air their views' is well worth while. They frequently express their opinions forcibly but this should not be dismissed as 'back talk' and 'cheekiness.' Discussion helps to train them to be reasonable and to straighten out the thousand and one problems which beset them.

Homework. Putting off doing homework until the very last moment is a common complaint against the teenager. Parents must be firm about rules for nights out, regular sleep and study hours and it is better if these rules are decided in quiet discussion jointly with the boy or girl. If in spite of this the homework is not finished there is little more that parents can do, and the young person will have to take the full brunt of the consequences from school.

The Over-confident Youth. The brash, over-confident adolescent will often ignore adult advice and seem not to care whether adults approve of him or not. In reality, however, he desperately needs to be approved of and, in spite of his antisocial attitude, he needs a great deal of patient acceptance and goodwill before his behavior will improve.

Change in Parental Role

Parents of adolescents often feel in need of sympathy themselves. Quite suddenly their pleasant, reasonably amiable child changes into a tactless person who is both rude and selfish at times and difficult to cope with without loss of patience. They realize that their child is inexperienced in dealing with the complicated situations which will arise, and may run into difficulties without their help. This brings about a conflict between the wish to protect the child and the wish to see him stand on his own feet. Even the most understanding of parents may find that their earlier intimate relationship with their child lessens at this time and that he has some difficulty in discussing problems with them.

In some cases, parents may find that their growing child's views and opinions are contrary to their own but they have to come to terms with such a situation and possibly accept the difference if it is made in all sincerity.

The following suggestions should help parents, or adults in charge, to maintain a mutually valuable relationship with their young people.

1. Maintain an atmosphere of affection and confidence in the home.
2. Acknowledge the importance of teenage problems particularly boy/girl relationships and try to work them out by mutual discussion.
3. Tactfully guide the young people towards realizing their own capabilities as well as their limitations.
4. When a firm stand on controls and rules of behavior is necessary give a reasonable explanation.
5. Be willing to compromise whenever possible.

ADOLESCENT FRIENDSHIPS

Friendship plays an important part in the life of the adolescent. The more casual relationships of earlier years are no longer enough, and friends must be able to share new feelings and experiences. Girls in particular usually tell their innermost secrets to their chosen friends and much of what they discuss seems trivial to adults. Boys on the whole do not seem to need such an intimate relationship with their friends as girls. They will want to be away from home much more: girls often visit their friends' homes while boys seem to prefer to roam around with their pals.

The maturity with which an adolescent adjusts socially to new and wider friendships will depend considerably upon the stage of development he had reached in childhood. If he has had sound attachments earlier to his parents and felt loved and secure, his new friendships will be of the same quality. An adolescent who finds it difficult to break away from strong emotional attachments to his parents will not be able to live a full satisfactory life in the wider social world—emotionally he is still a small child. Learning to live apart from the parental sphere and enter a new one is an important part of growing up in the late teens. Parents have to learn this as well as their sons and daughters.

Crushes. Teenage girls in particular develop 'crushes' on teachers, relatives, older friends or a member of the opposite sex. This is quite normal and they are almost always innocent associations. They usually pass as the girl gets older and becomes ready to establish a more lasting love relationship.

Cliques and Groups. Many of the doubts of adolescence are discussed and resolved in cliques and groups. They think up codes of behavior of their own and these fads spread like wildfire only to be replaced almost immediately by another. Most of these fads are quite harmless and are left behind as the young person becomes mature. Many parents worry unduly if their teenage child becomes involved with a group in case the chances of his getting into serious mischief are greater (see also Leisure, p. 134, and Delinquency, p. 136).

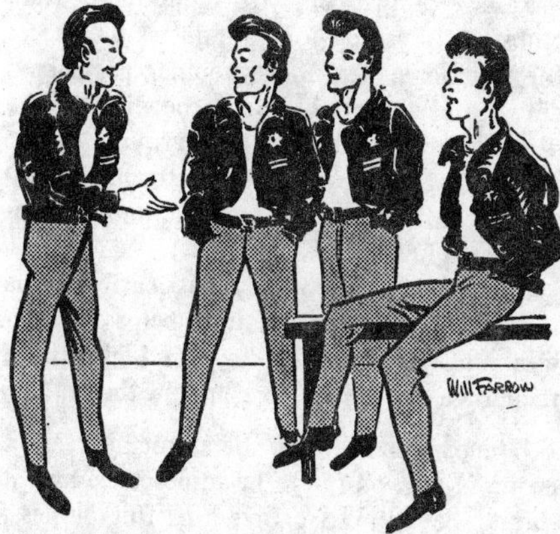

Fig. 6. *CLIQUES AND GROUPS. Being like the rest of the gang is common in the 'teens.*

Undesirable Friendships. Few parents find they approve of all the friends their teenage sons and daughters choose, but young persons are usually very loyal to their friends and too much criticism can make them cling to them unduly. It is rather important to recognize this characteristic since misunderstanding can lead to a real rift. For instance, if a mother finds something wrong with all her daughter's friends and says they are bad mannered, careless or shy, the girl may take to meeting her friends outside. In this way a mother will quickly lose her influence over her daughter for she will not be sure who her friends are or where the girl goes to meet them. In other cases a mother of a teenage girl who states flatly and dogmatically, 'You are not to go around with Betty. I do not like her and will not allow it,' may well encourage the most normal teenager to see her friend behind her mother's back.

Friendships are easily made and rapidly broken at this time and young people usually discover their own mistakes in time. If a friendship which parents think undesirable continues, it is best to get to know the other young person at first-hand by inviting him or her to the house. If the parents then feel certain that harm may come from the friendship they should discuss the matter frankly with their own boy or girl. They will be in a much stronger position with their first-hand knowledge rather than dismissing the friend because of rumors; and this should appeal to the teenagers' sense of fair play. There are bound to be protests and arguments about 'rights to choose one's own friends,' but an unheated and fair explanation from the parents will usually suffice once the young person has calmed down, and he can 'save face' among his friends by blaming his parents.

Friendships with the Opposite Sex

Courtship, marriage and parenthood are just around the corner for adolescents. Before they can settle happily in marriage they have to learn how to get on with persons of the opposite sex. Parents often worry because there is a gap in time between sexual maturity and the time young people are ready to marry, but if a young person has always been encouraged to develop a sense of personal responsibility and respect for others and has been helped to adjust to earlier sexual strivings, his relationships at this time will usually be wholesome.

In spite of the fact that boy–girl friendships provide some of the happiest times in the teenager's life they can also cause much unhappiness. Few teenage boys and girls escape some disappointments and many tend to dramatize the situation. When parents are discussing these setbacks with their teenage children it often provides the opportunity to explain that most adolescents feel shy and nervous and unsure of what to do when they first start going out with persons of the opposite sex. They need the reassurance of knowing that these feelings will become manageable in time. If parents assure them that they know they will not do the foolish things some young people do, it can lead to a discussion of behavior when out on a 'date.' It can be pointed out to them that they have much greater freedom to associate with members of the opposite sex than exists in many other countries and with this goes the responsibility to behave sensibly and wisely.

THE LATE DEVELOPER. Some adolescents who are slower in maturing or extremely shy may not show any interest in the opposite sex until they are seventeen, eighteen or even twenty years of age, and consider interest in the opposite sex as silly. In itself there is nothing wrong with this providing the young person does not become a misfit. A girl may find the girls she has known moving away from her as their interests differ, and, unless she can find a friend of her own kind, she may feel rather isolated. If that happens parents should try to give her special encouragement to make acquaintances and reassure her that in time she will 'catch up.'

Parental Attitudes to Friends

Supervision should be neither too strict nor too lax. An overprotected young person may run amok or be painfully shy when he or she finally gets away. The teenager who has always been encouraged to develop self-confidence and a sense of responsibility and allowed to go out providing her parents know where she is going rarely lets herself or her parents down. Neither boys nor girls deviate a great deal from the pattern set for them in childhood.

At some time or other most parents have to say 'no' to their teenage children. There is certain to be resentment, accusations of unfairness, and so on, but, if young people are persistently staying out late or becoming reckless, parents need to be firm. How this is done is important and if the young people are told in a friendly, reasonable way they are more likely to accept the discipline.

Listening sympathetically to teenagers' problems gives parents and teachers a good opportunity to influence boy–girl relationships. Adolescents will often be very open one day, then secretive the next, about their feelings. It is better not to force the issue when this happens but leave the way open for a talk some other time. When they ask questions it helps them to form their own ideas if parents suggest alternatives with such phrases as: 'Have you thought of this?' 'What would your friend think?'

Bringing Friends Home. Home is the best place for young people to meet each other and it avoids a great deal of irresponsible behavior, but giggling and the sound of noisy records can often get on the nerves of other members of the family. Some reasonable limits have to be set and adolescents are not always unreasonable providing they have enough opportunity to 'let off steam.'

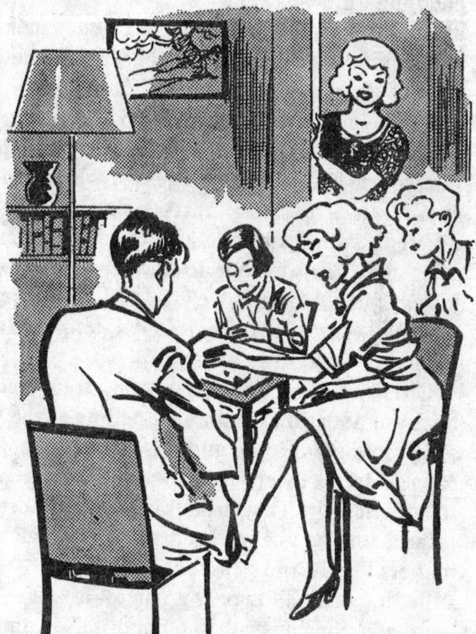

Fig. 7. *BRINGING FRIENDS HOME*

When parties are held parents should always be somewhere around as, although they would not admit it, teenagers are more likely to be cautious when parents are somewhere near. It is better to suggest group activities and games which will keep the party going and may discourage couples vanishing into dark corners.

Dating. It is only too easy for a teenager to get the impression from television, newspapers, magazines, and poster advertisements for commercial products that the most desirable thing in life is to be attractive to the opposite sex. It is not surprising therefore that attention from boys and admiration from girls is sought after and is thought to be the most important part of being grown up.

Many young people nowadays want to be allowed to go out with the opposite sex as young as fifteen years of age and many parents wonder what is the proper age to start. This is very much an individual matter and there is little doubt, with adolescents maturing earlier than even one generation back, that 'dating' does take place earlier and presents a problem. If parents genuinely think that their daughter is too young they should discuss the matter with her showing that they appreciate her feelings, explaining that she is just a little too young yet, and that it is possible sometimes to want to do things before one is ready. Assure her that as soon as she is ready for boy friends you will not prevent it. If, in spite of this explanation, she is insistent, make some compromise such as allowing occasional meetings in your house, and so prevent possible meetings without your knowledge.

Petting. The disturbing aspect of boy–girl relationships from the parents' point of view is the custom of petting. How best can they help their teenage children to develop a realistic attitude towards it and learn to control their sexual feelings? Kissing and cuddling are natural ways of showing affection for the opposite sex but such expression of feeling has to be kept within bounds. It has to be explained quite frankly, but in a non-hostile manner, that constant prolonged petting can lead to pre-marital intercourse and possible pregnancy which can spoil their lives. Different people can take different amounts of sexual stimulation. It is often hard for someone to know when he is losing control of his feelings and therefore partners must always be considerate of each other.

Girls are often reassured to be told that boys are not as insistent about petting as they sometimes seem to be and it is not necessary to yield to all their requests in order to keep their friendship. They usually have much more respect for the girl who refuses to treat such matters lightly and irresponsibly.

Petting after all is only a part of establishing a relationship with the opposite sex and in order to establish a lasting friendship or prepare for marriage young people must know much more about each other. Although kisses and caresses are signs of affection for a person, it is belittling to behave in this way with casual acquaintances. Some young people may get the idea that practice in love-making will help them to establish satisfactory relations in marriage but they need to know from their parents that this is not so and that the guilt and tension so produced often has the opposite effect.

Parents can help to keep petting within reasonable limits by encouraging teenagers to take part in group activities and avoiding leaving young couples alone too long.

Courtship and Marriage. It seems to parents that not long after their adolescent child has started going out with someone of the opposite sex he or she becomes attached to one in particular and the object of such a relationship is usually matrimony. Most young people have a number of boy or girl friends with whom for a time they have a steady, reasonably intimate relationship. This is normal and healthy for it is only by experience that they will come to know the sort of person with whom they are likely to be happy in marriage. Parents may fear that prolonged close friendships may result in marriage before the couple are prepared. It is better to encourage the young persons to discuss their friends and what they mean to them and it is in frank reasonable discussions of this nature that parents can influence their children to adopt a responsible attitude to marriage and all that it entails.

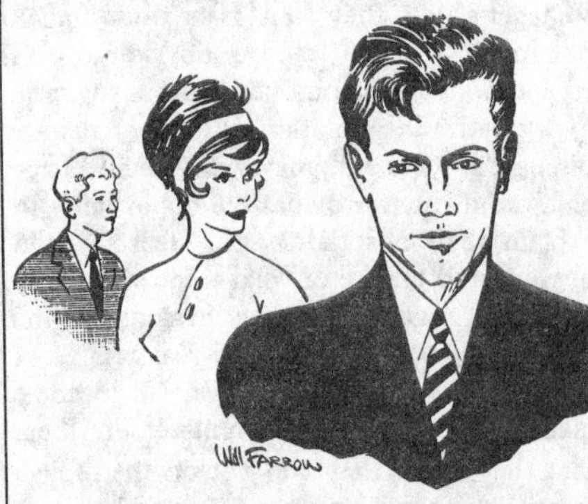

Fig. 8. *INFATUATION for the smart looking young man may often be mistaken for love.*

Adolescents, particularly girls, can mistake infatuation for love and it is not easy for parents to help them to see the difference while they feel so intensely. Open opposition to a boy may only cause a girl to stand up for him. When an opportunity presents itself, wise parents will encourage the young girl to weigh up the boy's good and poor points, and assess them in relation to her own personality and to what sort of marriage and future she wants.

The marriage rate among adolescent girls today is high: one in four is married before she is nineteen years and one in two before she reaches twenty-one. Quite a number of girls have matured considerably by their late teens but girls who marry so early are bound to need a great deal of advice, and in many cases practical help, during the early years of the marriage.

Use of Leisure Time

Adolescents whose parents have a genuine interest in how they spend their leisure are much less likely to wander off at a loose end and land themselves into difficulties.

Clubs. Society would be the poorer without the adventurousness of youth but the high-spirited youth often needs his leisure organized for him. This can be done in an efficient youth club which can utilize his energy, aggressiveness and need to make friends.

Youth club leaders offer a variety of interests—sport, hobbies, crafts and the arts—and, in order to provide for all interests, a single club may have to offer facilities for swimming, football, baseball, judo, wrestling, boxing, running, body building, gymnastics and indoor games in sport alone. Such activities when combined with a congenial job can go a long way towards helping a youth in the give and take of the world outside his home and in building a balanced attitude to life.

Some young people frown upon separate clubs for boys and for girls unless they meet for functions. The most popular are mixed clubs, and these will vary according to the neighborhood and class background of the members. Many prefer an informal atmosphere with dancing and music, and are not interested in hobbies.

Interest in a club may flag easily if the members become bored and it helps to maintain interest when the boys and girls have their own committee to help run the club.

Groups. Wanting to be a member of a group is a strong urge in adolescence and it should be allowed expression. But aimless, unorganized, group activity can quickly degenerate into mischievous behavior since each may tempt the other into taking risks. It takes a very strong-minded youth to withstand the 'dares' of his gang. It is part of the parents' responsibility, however, to keep a watchful eye upon their son's companions and the groups he joins with. If these seem unsatisfactory, discuss the possible consequences with the boy and encourage him to think for himself that it is childish rather than manly to do things just because he is dared.

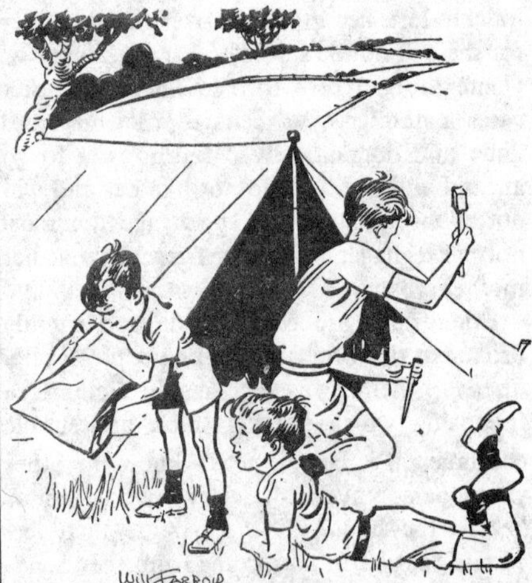

Fig. 10. *CAMPING. Their first vacation without Mom or Dad.*

Vacations away from Family. Adolescents often ask to be allowed to take a vacation away from the family. A mother may be hurt to realize that her young son or daughter does not wish to spend this time with his parents and brothers and sisters, but to force a

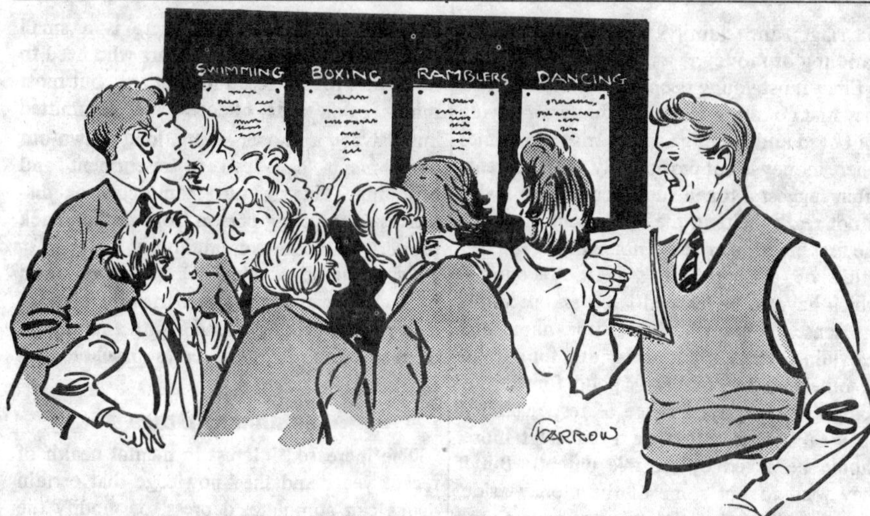

Fig. 9. *YOUTH CLUBS. A keen and active youth club leader may offer a great variety of interests to his young members.*

teenager in this matter may only spoil everyone's vacation. It is best to recognize this adventurous wish to do something on one's own and, providing there is proper supervision, to allow the boy or girl to go.

ADOLESCENTS AT SCHOOL

Examinations, tests, and reports assume enormous importance in the schoolchild's life, and often worry him a great deal. A reasonable amount of anxiety is normal in children, particularly if they set themselves high standards, and some children manage very well in spite of it. Many boys and girls, however, can become overanxious, particularly if parents have stressed the importance of the examination too strongly, and such children will need a great deal of reassurance. Some counterbalance is necessary to develop self-reliance and a sense of responsibility—encourage them to do things in the house or garden which it is known they can do well or, if they are in the late teens, allow them to join a club. Perhaps they can be allowed more time to relax with their friends, even if this means cutting down the number of hours for study. In the long run it will usually prove wiser because the really anxious child will not absorb knowledge even though he is studying his books, but he may come back refreshed after a period away from them.

Last Year at School

As young people are maturing more quickly they need to be taught extra subjects which are stimulating, particularly for children who are not intellectual. There is a need for education for adult life at this time and it should include such subjects as budgeting and family planning as well as discussions on spiritual and moral issues. Parents and teachers need to encourage young people's interest in varied leisure activities such as music, painting, nature study, photography and sports.

Many children feel frustrated in their last year at school. They feel grown up and bored by the restrictions of their school life. Parents can help to relieve this boredom and create a sense of responsibility by gradually allowing extra privileges, such as staying up later, staying out later occasionally, and sharing family visitors.

Wanting to Leave School. A desire to leave school before the school course is completed may be due to failure or lack of interest in school work, or the child may be emotionally upset. Sometimes the situation can be eased if there is an alteration in some of the subjects studied or the youngster is given a little extra encouragement from a member of the school staff, and in this the Principal can usually help. If the school work is really beyond a child's capacity then it is better to allow him to take some other more suitable course of study or training. To force such a young person to stay on at school may only increase his sense of failure.

Higher Education

Usually by the time a child is fifteen years the Principal will have a good idea of the child's intellectual capabilities and can give advice about future training. If entrance to college is contemplated certain compulsory subjects have to be studied. Training for some professions is long, arduous and expensive.

GOING OUT TO WORK

Choice of Occupation

Few decisions are more important to a young person than the choice of a job or career. The enjoyment or satisfaction he will get from his work will be partly determined by the kind of home background he has, partly by his own natural interest in the job, and partly by the attitude of his new adult workmates or colleagues. Choosing the right or a suitable job early enough will usually prevent frustration and aimless drifting from job to job. The young person must be allowed to make his own choice but he needs to be presented with various alternatives from parents, relatives, or employment exchanges. Although some children know from a very early age what they want to do in the future, most have no understanding of the problems involved or of the importance of planning ahead. A young person is usually very flexible and, given the opportunity, can succeed in a variety of jobs but he will do best in the field which interests him most and which uses his best abilities and aptitudes and where he is able to learn the skills without great difficulty.

Parents have to help the adolescent to take a realistic view of himself. Many young people know what they like and have a pretty good idea of the sort of things they might be able to do, but some have mistaken ideas of their own talents and many others can be encouraged by parents and other interested adults to do much better than they think. An adolescent may choose a particular occupation because it is the only one he knows much about, and it helps if he is able to talk it over with people doing a variety of jobs, such as relatives, friends or neighbors.

Girls' Attitude to Work. Most young girls plan to marry sooner or later and bring up a family. But although a young woman may not consider her work to be of prime importance

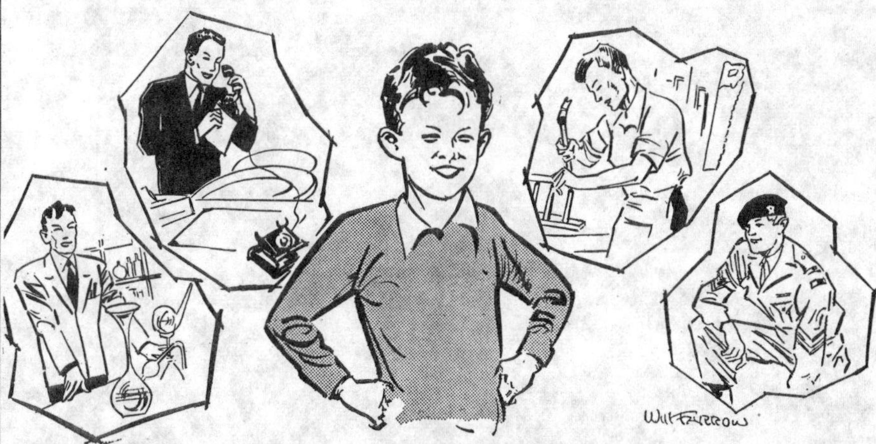

Fig. 11. *WHAT SHALL HE BE? It is wonderful to be fifteen and have the whole world to choose from.*

she should still choose carefully. It may be five or ten years before she marries and satisfaction in her work can affect her attitude to life and marriage. The discipline of full-time work can be a help when planning a home. Even after marriage she may of necessity have to work for some time, and many women become lonely and return to work once their children are growing up. Some skill and capacity to hold down a job is then invaluable.

Reactions to Work

Starting work is rarely easy. During his last term at school the youth will eagerly look forward to being free and independent with money of his own. Where there is good morale in the place where he works he tends to react very well. He is usually anxious to succeed and to be approved of. There are times when he will need sympathetic understanding from his parents to be able to adjust to his world of work, particularly when he becomes unduly discouraged by normal setbacks which are quite new to him or when he feels resentful about 'taking orders.'

Tolerance and restraint on the part of older people towards the youngsters they work with is extremely important. Today young people start work at a later stage in adolescence than their fathers and they have been stimulated to look for opportunities and to be more critical of accepted standards. When young people are outspoken and sometimes tactless, this can cause difficulties, but the young person will settle down more quickly if handled in a firm, reasonable manner, and this may often mean 'not noticing' every sign of aggressiveness or immaturity.

Earning and Spending

Some young people are able to earn considerably high wages before they have learned to exercise self-restraint, and parents of adolescents between the ages of fifteen and eighteen will need to exercise some control over the money they possess. Young people naturally want exciting clothes and amusements but they also have to learn to save for the future, when the responsibilities of marriage and family necessitate careful handling of money.

Since most young people live at home when they first go out to work, the matter of paying for board and lodging usually arises. In homes where money is not particularly short, parents often suggest a token sum each week but this is not really helping the adolescent at all. In the first place he or she is not learning the real value of money and domestic economy, which have to be learned later, and secondly the sense of contributing to the home and providing extras, if not necessities, for parents or others in the family is good for the developing youngster's sense of responsibility. So a fair contribution, or even a bit more, should be asked by sensible parents. But if they wish to put some of the money aside, without telling the adolescent of course, and use it later to help set up house for the young person on marriage, or for some other special purpose, the bonds of family affection will be strengthened when the inevitable break with home arises.

DELINQUENCY AND PUNISHMENTS

When newspapers seem to make a point of giving sensational reports of juvenile delinquency it is not surprising that parents of teenagers become alarmed at any sign of misbehavior. It is necessary, however, to distinguish between youthful mischief and delinquency. Most young people at some time associate with undesirable people, stay out late or dare each other to do wrong things for the fun of it and then grow out of this stage. It is not one particular incident, but continuous antisocial behavior on the part of a young person, which constitutes real delinquency.

Although there has been an increase in juvenile delinquency all over the world, what is considered to be delinquent behavior differs from country to country and from generation to generation.

Dealing with Delinquency. Indignation at violence is understandable and this frequently leads to a demand for severe punishments for all delinquents. Certainly there is a small minority of dangerous offenders who need to be dealt with in closed institutions, but most minor adolescent offences are committed impulsively, and over-severe, long drawn-out punishments can lead to resentment and brooding. This in turn can delay or discourage the young person from settling back properly into the community.

Of inestimable value is a good probation officer who can offer a stable friendly relationship with the young offender with a minimum of restriction. In some cases psychological treatment is required.

Youth and Drugs

The increased interest in mental health of recent years and the knowledge that certain drugs can stimulate, depress, or modify the state of mind has led to much publicity on the subject. A number of young people particularly, with a desire to experiment, to alleviate boredom, or to burn the candle at both ends are intrigued to take drugs without their knowing fully the long-term effects the drugs will have on the human brain and body. Medical research cannot as yet supply all the answers although investigations are being carried out in a number of countries. Enthusiastic pleading to permit freely the use of marijuana, for instance, is no substitute for tested facts.

Since in the next decade the number of psychotropic drugs is certain to increase, knowledge of their effects, of their value or harmfulness, and of their ability to produce addiction should become available. The human brain is a most delicate organ and once harmed it cannot be repaired like a cut finger. Valuable as LSD or amphetamine may be to the psychiatrist in treating his patients or as morphine is for cancer pain, to treat these drugs as new toys is both a personal and social abuse.

Fortunately, it is but a small minority who become involved in drug-taking and it is well known that most of them are of somewhat unstable personality.

See pp. 590, 593, 594.

WOMAN AS WIFE AND MOTHER

The great importance of happy family life in the successful upbringing of children is widely recognized in the world today, and more interest is taken in family welfare than ever before. Doctors, nurses, clinics and social workers have been studying the essential needs of the family as a whole, the expectant mother, and the infant and child from before his arrival at birth until the end of his school years and emergence into the adult community.

A Mother's Different Roles

Bringing up a child to be a healthy, happy and mature adult is a responsible undertaking, and it is the mother who normally plays the most important part in a child's early life. Moreover, she has more than one role to play. In the family circle she is also the wife with her husband's health and comfort to study and she may help him in his work; she is the housekeeper in charge of the house and home; and she exists as an individual in her own right, with her own friends, interests and activities which should not be continually submerged by the demands of family life. Later she may become a grandmother on whom the younger generation leans and to whom they turn for advice and help. In addition she may also work outside her home to help the family income, or because she enjoys the interest of independent work or a career.

At different periods of her life, certain of a woman's roles become more dominant. This is particularly so when she is carrying a child and during the breast feeding months.

FAMILY ADJUSTMENTS TO THE PREGNANT MOTHER

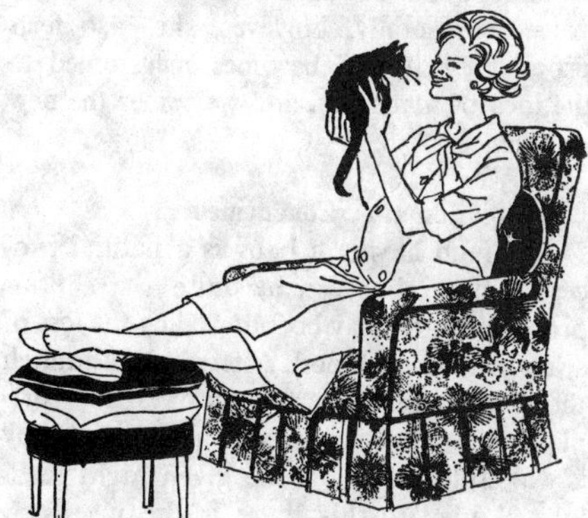

Fig. 1. *FEET UP whenever possible during pregnancy.*

The expectant mother will usually regard her pregnancy as a happy time of preparation for the arrival of the new baby, and will prepare her family for the inclusion of a new member. Since the arrival of a baby generally makes changes in the family's mode of life, each member should be prepared to make some adjustments in the household routine. The father and the older brothers and sisters should demand rather less of the mother's time and be ready to help and share in the general domestic activities.

Husband and Father

The knowledge that his wife is pregnant may cause a husband to feel proud and confident, or he may be rather reluctant to face the prospect of becoming a parent and sharing his wife with the newcomer in the home. In general, however, he adjusts himself to the situation as his wife's pregnancy advances.

A wife needs extra affection and consideration during the rather long waiting period of pregnancy and her husband can help her in many ways to avoid overtiredness, depression and the minor ailments of pregnancy. He can see that she has sufficient rest, and he can share some of the routine duties in the home such as shopping on Saturdays, helping more with the preparation of meals at weekends, playing with the older children in the family or taking them on outings, and helping in the preparations for the new baby, especially if a nursery has to be planned or repainted.

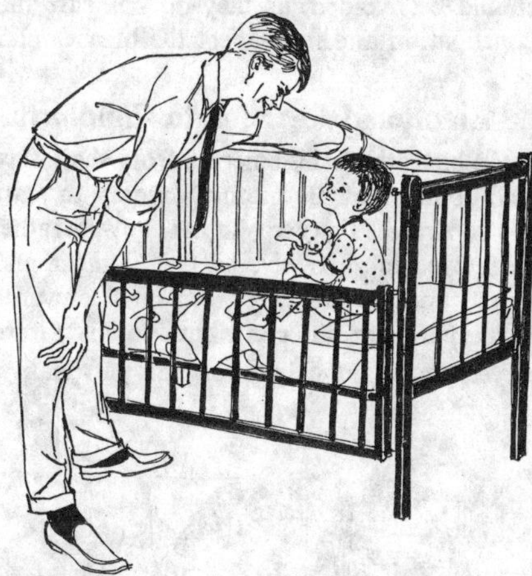

Fig. 2. *BEDTIME. Get the toddler used to a routine with father before the new baby arrives.*

Although the arrival of a first baby confers the status of father on the husband, his own views on this may vary widely. A father often has a less instinctive feeling of parenthood than the mother. He may regard the care of children, especially of a young baby, as a woman's job and that to appear too enthustastic about the infant is unmanly. Once he has helped care for the child and handled him he will find that his own interest and pleasure grows. Father's early practical interest in his young baby will be rewarded by the child's acceptance and confidence, which later develops into love and happiness in his father's company.

The example which a father sets to older children—between five and twelve years of age particularly—in showing consideration and care for his pregnant wife is most important in forming the pattern of behavior of these children to their own marriage relationships later in life.

Brothers and Sisters

A young first child, being the sole object of his parents' interest and affection, may easily feel that his own importance is suddenly diminished when a second baby arrives. His sense of security and happiness are threatened, and the rival to his parents' affection may be bitterly resented unless the way has been carefully prepared before the newcomer arrives.

The parents can prevent jealousy by telling a young only child, some weeks before the expected date, of the hoped-for arrival of a brother or sister so that he gets used to the idea by degrees. Any preparations which change the child's own ways of life, such as removal to a new bed or bedroom, should be made well in advance so that he does not feel he is giving up anything to the newcomer. (See also Jealousy of New Baby, in Child Care, p. 125.)

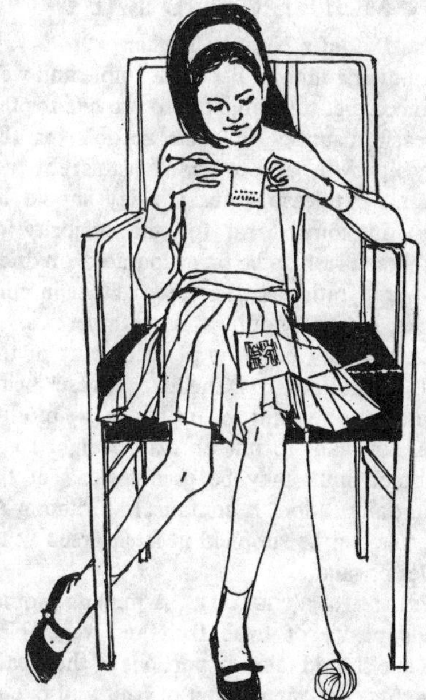

Fig. 3. *BIG SISTER helps by knitting bootees for the new baby.*

If there is a child under three years of age in a family of older children, they and the father should give the youngest one extra attention and companionship before the baby comes, so that he has some substitute for the loss of some of his mother's interest and love when she has to give up more time to the newcomer. They can also take turns bathing him and putting him to bed, to accustom him to a new routine in advance.

Children over eight or ten years of age can be encouraged to take a positive share in running the home and helping with the various chores, according to their age and ability. A girl will often be pleased and proud to help her mother prepare the family meals sometimes, setting the table, and by taking over the cooking or preparation of a simple meal in the evening or at weekends, especially if she is allowed to help choose the food items. A girl often enjoys being shown how to make some of the small garments needed for a new baby, such as small knitted vests or bootees.

Boys and girls can often help with the shopping, and a boy may be willing to help with the dishes, gardening, keeping his own room neat, helping his father clean the car or do decorating jobs around the house, if he knows it will give his mother the opportunity for extra or the necessary rest. The mother should always express her thanks and gratitude for special help given by her family.

Grandmothers

Grandmothers, even if they do not live in the family home, like to be asked to 'baby sit' sometimes, and to help make baby clothes for which the mother of a family may find she has little time. A grandmother or elderly woman friend of the family who is handy with a needle is an invaluable aide to a busy mother, particularly when she is pregnant or has a young baby.

MOTHER AND BABY

The Diet of a Nursing Mother

A nursing mother needs an ample and well balanced diet to enable her to provide for the increasing supply of milk needed for the baby's growth, and to guard against fatigue.

MILK. At least a quart a day should be taken in some form for the majority of mothers. Fresh milk or evaporated or dried milk preparations can be used, either in milk drinks, soups, puddings, or with cereals.

Cheese may take the place of part of the milk, 2 ounces of Cheddar cheese being equal to one pint of milk. If a mother does not want to put on extra weight some skimmed milk may be used instead of the fresh daily ration. It contains less vitamin A, but this can be supplied in fresh green vegetables or salads.

FRUIT AND VEGETABLES. A nursing mother needs plenty of fresh fruit and vegetables, and she should take six portions of these each day. At least one portion of fruit and one of vegetables should be eaten raw. Oranges, grapefruit, lemons, tomatoes, potatoes and green and root vegetables are always available.

MEAT, FISH AND POULTRY. Two good portions of these protein foods daily are advised, lean cuts of meat and liver being recommended.

EGGS. One or more eggs each day should be included, an omelette or other egg dish being interchangeable with one of the meat dishes.

BREAD AND CEREALS. Brown bread (whole wheat) or enriched loaves or cereals or flour products should be taken three times a day to provide energy and calories.

BUTTER AND MARGARINE are easily digested fats and provide vitamins A and D.

WATER AND FLUID DRINKS. A nursing mother needs plenty of water which may be taken as fruit juices, weak tea, and soups. A drink of cold water taken a quarter of an hour before breast feeding is often found helpful.

VITAMINS AND IRON. Mothers are often given combined preparations of vitamins to guard against possible shortage. Iron tablets are also prescribed, but great care must be taken to prevent these being eaten as 'sweets' by young children, who may in this way take a fatal dose. They should always be kept locked up.

Constipation

After a confinement constipation is often a common complaint, especially during breast feeding. It may prove troublesome for many weeks, particularly if piles have developed during pregnancy. A diet containing plenty of fluids and perhaps some bran added to a cereal dish, should help to produce regular action of the bowels. Exercises to restore the abdominal muscles (see illustrations, p. 98) and a daily walk are beneficial. Laxatives should be avoided, as they do not cure the constipation and may affect the breast milk.

Emotional Reaction to Childbirth

At birth the baby emerges from the safety and comfort of his mother's womb to start his separate existence; he can now breathe, he moves more freely, he feels hunger and thirst, and he can cry; from birth onwards his experiences all contribute to his future development and help to form his personality.

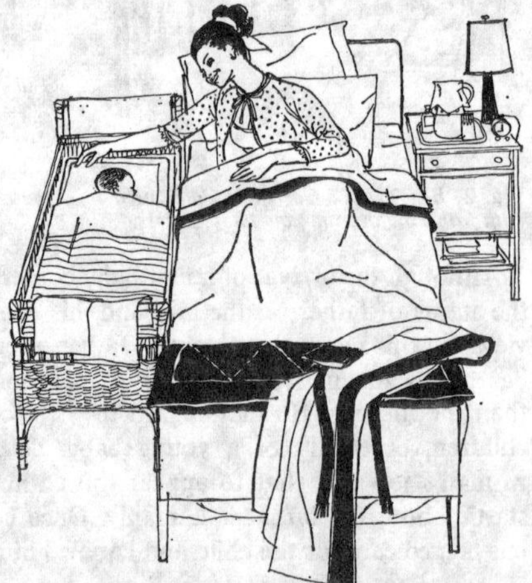

Fig. 4. *NEARNESS is important for both mother and infant during the lying-in period.*

His mother's attitude towards him from birth onwards is therefore very important. If she has been afraid of labor and delivery, this may have added to its difficulty, making the actual birth prolonged, with an increased risk of physical injury to the baby. It may also influence the mother's feelings towards the baby, so that she does not feel the natural spontaneous joy and love a mother should feel towards her child.

Separation of Mother and Baby

In many hospitals the baby is often kept away from the mother, sometimes in a different room, except at feeding times; this is unnatural and, although it may lessen the risk of infection and give the mother more rest, it may also make her feel she is not playing her proper part in being able to comfort him when he cries, or knowing when he seems hungry. Today, therefore, it is becoming more common for the baby to be left near the mother, where she can see and hear him, and where he will not be lonely or left crying for indefinite periods. She can hold him and cuddle him after his feeds until he is ready to drop peacefully asleep, the contact being satisfying to both, and giving him the sense of love and security that is so essential for his contentment, and for the happiness of the relationship of mother and child.

Depression during Pregnancy

Many mothers, even among the best, complain of some degree of depression during pregnancy or after the birth of the baby, and in a few cases this depression is quite severe. The mother blames herself for not feeling more wholeheartedly maternal and adds a sense of guilt to her despondency and low spirits. If the mother realizes how common this is, and that it will wear off as she grows to understand and love her baby, she is less likely to feel perturbed.

It is true that a first pregnancy ends the more carefree days of early marriage, with a limitation of social or other recreations, and even if a woman has really wanted a child during pregnancy she may begin to have certain doubts about the responsibilities involved. Generally, however, she also feels proud as well, and becomes accustomed to the idea of maternity, and welcomes the new experience.

Depression after Confinement

Although having a baby is a natural process, a first labor can be quite a strenuous proceeding and may be followed by the loss of a fair amount of blood. Afterwards, although the new mother rests for ten days to a fortnight, her nights may be disturbed if the baby is wakeful and has to be given night feedings. Added to this there is the necessary adjustment to a new routine, fitting in the time for the feeding and care of the baby and for the extra washing which has to be combined with the usual housework and family duties.

If a mother is breast feeding her baby she needs a rest during the afternoon. In many cases, when she begins to take up her usual domestic work, she finds that the milk supply is not so plentiful as when she was resting in bed; this of course adds to her worries, especially if the baby appears fretful or hungry, and does not gain weight so well. A nurse will often be able to help a mother to plan her day, so that she does not try to get through quite so much household cleaning or heavy work for at least the first month after the confinement. If the milk supply does diminish during the third or fourth week it is not always easy to re-establish it at th right level.

If a mother realizes that depression is not unusual at this time she will worry less and not blame herself. Then she soon begins to enjoy the feeding, bathing and mothering sessions as she gains experience and confidence in handling the new baby. In quite a number of cases a mother's natural love for the child only develops gradually after the birth, as she takes him into her own care and feels his dependence on her, and can enjoy watching him grow and develop.

The husband may sometimes feel rather neglected as the wife takes on the role of mother, but he should not let moodiness or displeasure thoughtlessly upset her, and she in her turn should encourage him to play his part as a father and share with her a natural pride and interest in their baby.

Enjoy your Baby

Many mothers say they enjoy looking after the second baby more than the first. This is generally because they are now more experienced, and are less apprehensive. They do not worry so much about a punctilious routine and keeping to hard and fast rules of management, and know better how to deal with crying, feeding and nursery care, so that there is more time to enjoy the baby and play with him, giving him the interest and love he needs.

Crying may be due to many things, including discomfort from wet diapers, hunger, gas or colic, tiredness, fretfulness, or just boredom. He may need company and want to feel his mother is near. To be held in her arms and rocked for a little while does not 'spoil' a baby, as long as the mother is sensible about it.

As the baby gets older he will not always want to be put in the baby carriage out of the mother's apparent sight, and may be happier near the window; but for his sleeping periods a young baby needs a quiet place where he can drop off easily without noise or disturbance.

Every baby is a different individual, with differing needs and temperament, and a mother should accept him and love him for himself, whatever his apparent shortcomings so that he becomes confident and happy in the security of his family circle, developing the worthwhile attributes of his own particular personality as he grows.

Help in the Home

When a mother begins to get up and about after her confinement, it usually means a sudden return to full domestic duties, with the added work of looking after the new baby; if she is breast feeding him, this is an extra drain on her time and energies. A husband should do all he can to help her and be understanding and patient, giving her extra affection and encouragement, as well as practical assistance.

Visitors should be kept to a reasonable minimum for the first few weeks, and be asked to come at suitable times to fit in with the baby's feeding. If extra domestic help can be arranged for the first month or two, this will give the mother a better chance of regaining her strength, keeping her breast milk sufficient to supply the baby's growing needs, and helping her to enjoy her baby as well as getting the necessary afternoon rest. Even part-time help two or three times a week for the heavier cleaning will be well worth while.

Practical measures for reducing the effort required in running the household with a new baby include a washing machine and automatic drier, electrical aids in the kitchen, and the simplification of routine and cooking for a few weeks. Diaper washing can be kept to a minimum by using disposable paper diapers, or by putting one inside a cotton square before the bowel action is expected. A baby laundry service can be a great help although of course it involves extra expense.

After a complicated labor or Caesarean section home help may be a real necessity for one or two months after the birth. The eased routine and postponement of heavy housework will allow the mother's abdominal wall to regain its normal strength and supporting function. If the muscles of the abdomen and vagina remain stretched and sagging, the internal organs drop and the pelvic ligaments supporting the womb become permanently lax; this will lead to general visceroptosis and perhaps downward displacement of the womb with troublesome frequency in passing urine, which may necessitate a subsequent surgical operation.

The Housebound Young Mother

The early marriage trend among young people today means that about seventy per cent of young women and over fifty per cent of men marry before they are twenty-five. In most cases the first baby arrives within a year or two, and others may follow fairly quickly.

The young mother is tied to her home and children, and both she and her husband have to plan their leisure and recreations accordingly. Even with a car, long or late outings or weekends away from home cannot easily be undertaken with a young baby. Television, radio, gardening, sewing and knitting, household do-it-yourself jobs and so forth take the place of movies, dancing, theaters, concerts,

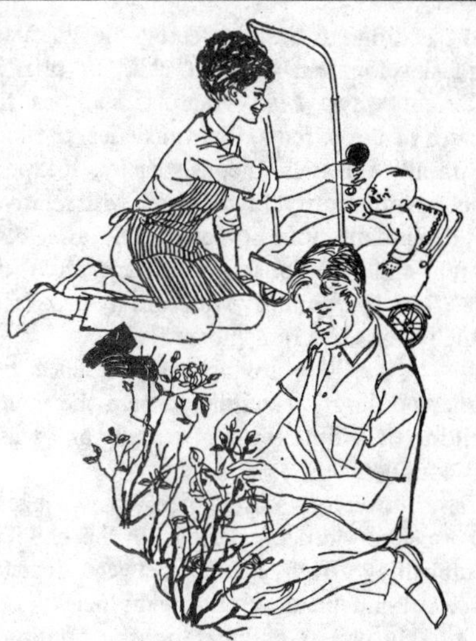

Fig. 5. *SHARED INTERESTS enrich family life.*

visits to neighbors and all-day outdoor excursions or sport.

This adjustment to parenthood may come comparatively suddenly, although the young mother will need to curtail her activities to some extent during her pregnancy. In giving up her job or career, she will have lost many of her contacts and interests outside the home.

Having a new baby is an adventure for a woman. In the role of mother, life revolves around the care of the child and his growing needs. In the early days after childbirth many young mothers leave their homes only for very short periods for household shopping, doctor's visits, and short calls on friends or nearby relatives.

A woman should not be less of a wife when she becomes a mother but should show her husband that motherhood has enlarged her understanding and sympathies as much as, or even more than, before the baby's arrival. This companionship is most important to the young wife who may find that being almost completely tied to the house can lead to frustrations, boredom and loneliness, however much she may love her baby. Shared interests in books, music, gardening, house decorating or politics, begun in the early years of marriage, continued perhaps in lesser degree during the housebound period, will make a foundation for happiness together in the later years when the children may leave home. Parents who lose interest in each other are apt to become unduly possessive with the children.

MOTHER AND YOUNG CHILDREN

Early Relationships

The general behavior and relationship of parents, and especially of the mother, in the early stages of a child's life are among the most important influences on his development. In every family the parents' behavior, patterns and attitudes tend to change and vary at different times, affecting the character and development of each child in turn in different ways. Many factors, such as the health of the parents, their anxieties, tensions or family quarrels, inconsistencies, inexperience or immaturity, involvement with relatives or dependants and so forth, may affect the parent-child relationship at any age, and there are four particularly important principles which should be remembered.

1. A mother's loving care, patience and understanding is essential to help the young child to develop a sense of security and trustful confidence.

2. Between two and three years of age is an especially crucial period for the child in establishing a right balance between dependence and independence of the mother.

3. The parent–child relationship continues to change as the child grows; for the first six months after birth the mother plays the biggest part in providing for the infant's needs; then the baby gradually begins to develop the need for increasing independence and from this stage onwards over-mothering and over-protection must be avoided. It is important for a mother to understand the stages of personality development, and to be able to make corresponding adjustments in her own behavior at the right times.

4. The parents' personalities, relationship and behavior, and the atmosphere in the home are associated with similar trends of behavior and personality traits in the children.

Mothering

Very early after birth a baby begins to form a definite relationship with his parents and senses their approval or disapproval, and acceptance or rejection. When a mother loves and is pleased with her baby she conveys her feelings by fondling, talking and smiling with her endearments, and he will feel this tenderness and acceptance, and gradually become responsive to her affection.

The influence of the mother has such a profound effect on a child that he learns to see the world through her eyes. Her attitudes and opinions will be reflected in his behavior and beliefs until many years later when he begins to learn to form his own ideas and standards of conduct. He will probably also pass on his own childhood experiences to his children.

When a mother does not feel the normal love for her child in the early months, he has no one else to turn to, and feels rejected; this affects his sense of security and he becomes tense, anxious and emotionally starved and disturbed, so that in later life he will be incapable of forming satisfactory friendships or deep relationships with other people because he has not learned love and acceptance in very early childhood.

After the first early years the child comes under other influences from other relatives, adults, and children, at school, at play, and in the characters he meets in books, stories, on television, or in history, and if the mother is wise she leaves him open to these new experiences. Through them he gains contact and understanding of the world outside the home, and learns to make his own judgments and how to take his place in life.

Favoritism and Intolerance

A mother and father should not decide too firmly in advance whether they would like a boy or girl, in case they are disappointed and feel they cannot make the necessary adjustment; but generally the arrival of the child, whatever its sex, brings its own happiness, and the baby is loved for itself. Some mothers may feel that they do not love all their children quite equally and blame themselves for this difference; but since each child is different, especially in ease of management, this discrepancy is often more imagined than real. A good mother is equally devoted to all her family, but when occasions of stress and strain arise and she feels irritated or impatient, she may blame her own reactions unnecessarily. Children are human beings, and cannot be perfect or easy to cope with, and impatience with certain behavior or characteristics is very common for either parent. Since we cannot choose our children, our main aim must be to help them make the best of themselves and to develop their best qualities to the full, strengthening them and helping them to overcome weaknesses as far as possible.

The Management of Young Children

Discipline. The real art and foundation of management in the training of a child, however young, is by example and later by leadership. An overanxious or a bad-tempered mother will have a nervous or difficult child. For most parents management is a question of finding the right balance between strictness and permissiveness, and the majority of mothers and fathers do manage to find this fairly soon by experience and commonsense.

When the parents are affectionate and sensible, the degree of authority or indulgence matters less than when the mother or the father is harsh or weak in their attitude to enforcement of discipline. Different generations of parents have held different views on obedience and respect for authority but it is now realized that while children should be able to respect their parents and understand their views so that they co-operate more readily, more difficulties and problems are caused by lack of love than by lack of firm discipline and punishment.

Nowadays children tend to be less often 'spoiled' or really difficult in their early years since parents are more anxious to know what is needed in care and training.

Compromise. Forty years ago much more rigid views were held about infant feeding; the food had to be supplied in stated quantities at stated intervals 'by the clock' regardless of the particular baby's physical needs, his activities, size and rate of growth, and digestive powers. Today, feeding by self-demand is agreed to be a more natural and sensible method, and much more flexible feeding times are recommended from birth onwards. In the same way mothers are now encouraged to give their babies more comforting, fondling and love from the beginning, which has had happier results for both mothers and babies.

If, however, either of the parents has had a strict upbringing, it may be difficult for her (or him) to approve and allow more latitude to the children for fear of 'spoiling' or worse consequences. Most parents manage to work out a reasonable compromise but not always before mistakes have been made. The parents must have confidence in their own judgment and be able to be firm about matters affecting a child's health and safety, such as proper bedtimes, hygienic toilet habits, washing the hands before and after meals and after using the toilet, decent manners in eating, and fitting a child into the life of the family as a whole, so that he becomes a useful, happy and well-adjusted member.

Contrarily, a mother who has rebelled against her own unduly strict upbringing is likely to be more indulgent to her own child and may carry this rather too far before she realizes that the child is getting out of hand. In other cases a mother may continually give in to a child's demands because it is the easiest thing to do at the time and saves a 'scene,' but the child soon learns how to get what it wants and will begin to cry, scream, stamp or throw himself down for any little whim, because this has worked on previous occasions.

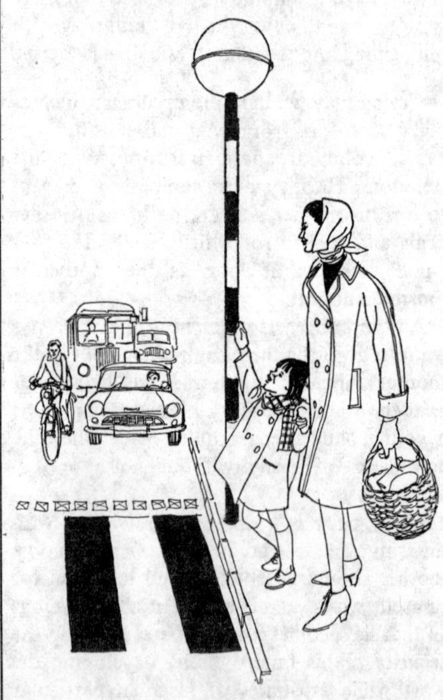

Fig. 6. *SAFETY RULES are necessary for city children.*

It is only fair to a child to teach it that 'no' means 'no' and not 'perhaps' or giving in if the child makes a nuisance of himself. Reasonable strictness, with firmness and helpful 'reminders' rather than nagging or peremptory tones will generally achieve the best results and co-operation. The child should feel that his parents are kind and fair and reasonable, and that he in his turn is approved by them.

Until a child is old enough to be trusted to do certain risky things safely, however, such as play in the street or cross a road, light the gas and so forth, it is better to have strict rules against them, and to take the necessary precautions. At the same time the child should be taught why taboos are necessary for the time being. Later on he can be taught the right way to do such things safely.

Punishment. The main reasons for naughtiness, be it actual disobedience or mischief of some sort, are curiosity, the desire to experiment, increasing physical energies and ability, and other natural processes which cannot and should not be too firmly suppressed; but the mother may be alarmed or upset, and vent her own feelings on to the child by slapping or punishing him. All parents have moments of anger, but forbearance and patience will give better results. Punishment may also be the expression of the mother's own uncertainty, anger, and the need to impose her will to establish her sense of superiority. The wise and mature mother anticipates and perceives her child's motives and reactions more easily, and finds the child easy to manage because she has the right approach and has his welfare truly at heart. Good sense, patience, reasonableness and good-natured cheerfulness are the best means of guidance and training.

It is also most important that mother and father work together and uphold each other, setting suitable standards of behavior. The mother should not ask the father to deal out punishments for minor disobedience because she does not like to exert her own authority; this is unfair and creates in the child's mind the idea of the father as someone to be feared, instead of someone who is strong and just and kind, and the protector of the family.

Over-protection and Possessiveness

A mother needs to be loving, cheerful and confident, so that the child feels secure and accepted in the family group. An over-protective mother, however, will encourage over-dependence in the child. An apparently over-devoted mother may be subconsciously resentful toward the child; such a mother needs constructive advice, not merely criticism. In other cases, a woman may have lost a child previously, or she may be trying to fulfil some emotional lack in her own life, centering her entire interest and ambition on her child.

Such mothers must be helped to realize that although the child does need care and devotion he also needs to grow up, and this means allowing him to develop confidence in himself and his own abilities and to achieve independence mentally and physically as well. This is necessarily a gradual process, with perhaps temporary setbacks or even returns to infantile states such as nightmares, a sense of insecurity when a new baby arrives, bed-wetting in the older child, or fearfulness of the new life at school. The mother's firm but comforting attitude towards a child's fears is his greatest help toward overcoming them. In some cases the allaying of fears needs to be done fairly quickly, as in getting used to a nursery school or sleeping in his own bed, but if he is scared of animals or of trying new skills such as getting on his first bicycle, these activities can be allowed to wait until he is ready to try them out.

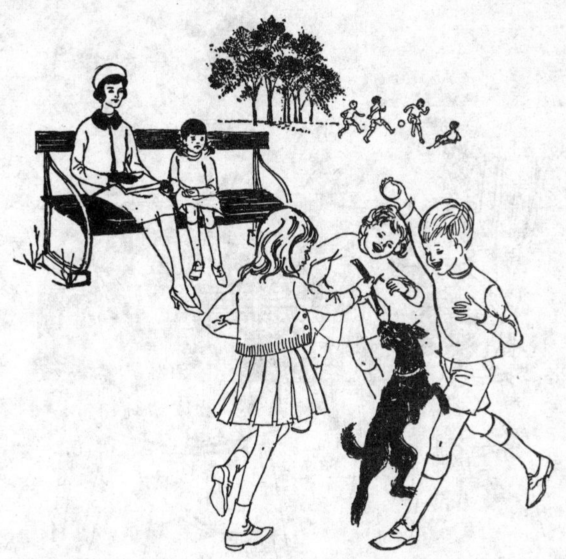

Fig. 7. *THE OVER-PROTECTED CHILD. How much fun and companionship she misses when she is not encouraged to play with other children!*

Affection with Equability

The mother's attitude which will be most helpful to the child is one of loving acceptance, kindness, cheerfulness and helpful training towards independence. Children whose mothers are affectionate and equable in their relationship are generally confident, responsive to affection, and outgoing in their own attitude to life and to the world around. A good parent combines patience, understanding and reasonable firmness, giving the child sufficient freedom to develop its own interests without excessive criticism, interference or continual supervision.

Managing Without a Father

Absent Father. If a husband is away from home for prolonged periods, the mother should try to keep him supplied with details of a baby's progress and development to stimulate his interest and affection. Not only can she send information as to gain in weight, teeth, walking, talking and physical progress, but she should describe his character and behavior, personality, temperament (placid, determined, wilful, co-operative and so forth) and report his day-to-day behavior, comments, questions and activities so that the father has some picture of his child as an individual. He can thus take a personal interest in his development, and not feel he may come home to find his offspring a comparatively unimagined stranger. He will also to some extent be able to share the mother's family problems during his absence. The mother should also talk to her child about his father and plan with the child how they will enjoy having him come home to share and help in their activities.

Where there is no father, or after divorce or separation, bringing up children can be a much more difficult and perplexing job. Then the mother's courage, patience, unselfcentered devotion, cheerfulness and good sense are all-important. She is bound to feel lonely, discouraged and uncertain at times. To help her through her difficult phases and to face up to problems as they arise, she should keep in touch with friends, other married couples with children, and although looking after a home and young children may appear to be a full-time occupation she will be wise if she finds some outside recreations to provide some change of scene and adult interest, which will help to reduce domestic worries and irritations to a more normal level, and enable her to view them in truer proportion.

A boy growing up solely in the care of his mother should be encouraged to play with other boys when he is over two years of age, so that he can develop his masculine interests and traits and learn how to hold his own and mix with boys easily, in preparation for the school days ahead, and to prevent 'mother-fixation.'

A mother must also avoid over-protection and undue possessiveness and it is best to begin to 'share' her children at an early age.

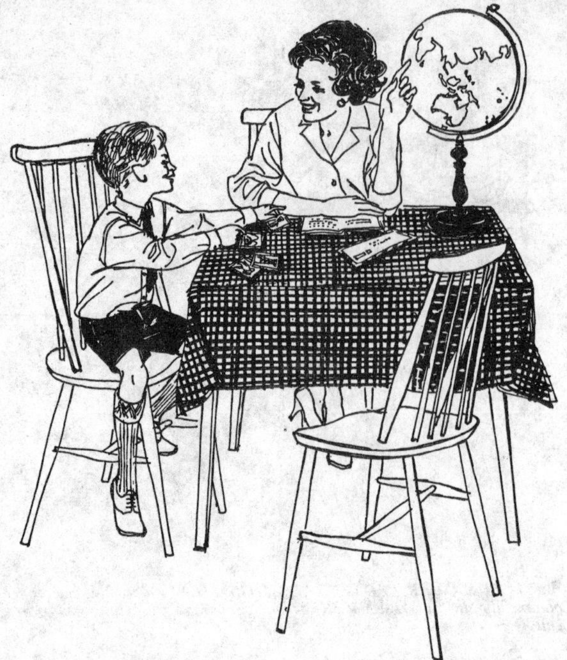

Fig. 8. *WORLDS AWAY. Father may be in a distant land but he is well remembered at home.*

An over-anxious mother in sole charge of a child may be so cautious or fearful all day long, continually warning or preventing him from doing what he wants that he in turn becomes timorous and unventuresome, with no initiative or self-confidence, or else rebellious and difficult to manage.

Divorce. The effects of divorce on the children, especially a young child, are necessarily different in different cases. Where there has been considerable friction and tension, the children may suffer less after the separation than in the disturbed emotional atmosphere of an unhappy home. In either case the child's sense of security is likely to be upset to a varying degree.

When the divorce or separation does occur, it must be explained to the children that each parent still belongs to them, and they should continue to see both when this can be arranged; they should also be told that neither of the parents is entirely to blame, so that the children do not take sides and lose their affection and trust in either.

If the mother has the custody of the children, as often happens, each child should see the father at as regular intervals as possible, without sudden cancellations or arbitrary postponements which cannot be explained to the children. Criticisms and interrogations after such visits must be avoided, since they may make the child distrustful of each parent and increase his sense of insecurity by undermining his loyalty and affections.

Young Children's Questions

At first girls often talk more and say more words than boys of the same age, but after six years of age this becomes less apparent. A four-year-old child says 'kill' and 'die' without meaning permanent death but merely to put out of action someone who has caused annoyance, and a mother should not be unduly alarmed at such remarks.

From one-tenth to one-fifth of a child's conversation in the first five years often consists of questions relating to all that goes on around him, and his constant use of 'why' expresses his growing and natural curiosity. When a child asks questions about God or Heaven a non-religious mother should say 'no one really knows' rather than make evasive replies or pretend indifference.

Since it is by means of conversation that a child listens to words and learns to talk clearly and correctly, and adds to his stock of knowledge and store of words, his mother should find time to talk and explain things to him however small he is and should tell and read him stories from the age of two years onwards. Children, of course, often continue to ask questions and prolong conversation to get attention from their parents, as well as to obtain reassurance or information.

Working Mother

Work Outside the Home. In some families a mother has to work outside the home to contribute to the family income. This may be really necessary where the husband and wife have separated, where the husband is an invalid, or where the family finances have become really insufficient for its needs. A few mothers feel the need of a career and may be able to provide a good substitute to look after the children. Every mother, however, should understand that for young children security and love, as well as physical care, are absolutely essential to happy and healthy development, and that for every child his mother is the natural source of love, attention, care and security. The younger the child, the more he depends on his mother for satisfaction of all his various and increasing needs.

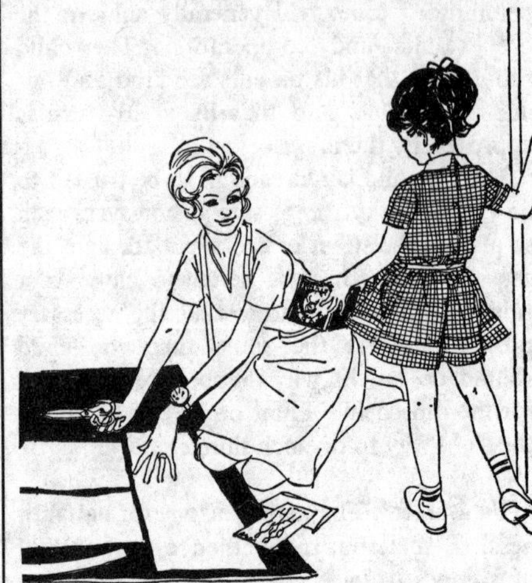

Fig. 9. *EARNING AT HOME prevents separation of mother and family.*

If a mother realizes how vital her own presence and care are to a baby or young child, she will feel more rewarded and gain more fulfilment if she devotes herself to her family, at any rate in the early years.

A mother should also remember that when she does undertake regular work outside her own home, even part-time, the double duty may lead to much strain and fatigue, thus reducing her capacity to play her own part adequately in her family circle. The benefit of increased income may be outweighed by exhaustion and neglect on the part of the mother, and by loneliness, unhappiness, and insecurity for the children.

Enjoyment of one's children requires relaxation and tranquillity, with an understanding that can only be gained by sharing their daily life and growing years.

Day Nurseries can seldom provide enough attention, interest and love for every child, especially babies under one year, and there is always more chance of infections such as colds, sore throats and diarrhea. Where the mother is compelled to work, even for part of the day, it is better to find a relative, or perhaps a friend, or another mother to look after the child and give him individual, reliable and affectionate care, especially for the first twelve months.

After eighteen months or two years the companionship of one or two other children helps him to learn independence, self-confidence and the art of sharing. After the age of three a small nursery school or day nursery may prove satisfactory for part of each day if the staff is adequate and experienced. If a child feels sure of his parents' love and has a basic sense of security he will probably settle down after three or four days without much emotional upset.

Mother Substitute or Nurse. In choosing any helper, such as a friend or nurse, a mother should look for kindness, reliability and sense, some experience, cleanliness and cheerful good nature, as well as ensuring that the helper is not likely to be neglectful or over-severe. The mother must also have confidence in a nurse, and not dispute her decisions or authority unfairly in the child's presence or let herself become jealous over the child's affection for, or dependence on, the 'mother substitute.'

The Baby Sitter

In these days there is usually little or no domestic help with the children, especially in the evenings when the wife would sometimes like to go out with her husband. This problem can be eased by the employment of a 'baby sitter' who will come to the house and take over the care of the child or children while the parents have their outing. When looking out for a suitable person to undertake this responsibility it is wise to obtain good and reliable references or to have some personal knowledge of the sitter, who must be honest, kind to the children, intelligent and generally trustworthy. She should be asked to arrive in good time before the mother's departure, and be given certain instructions.

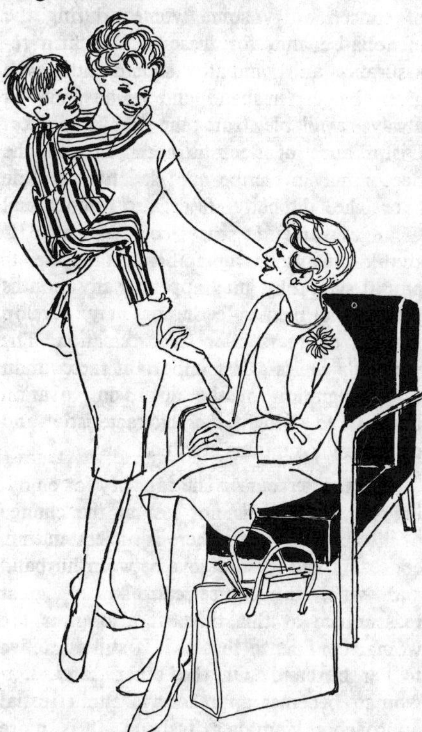

Fig. 10. *THE BABY SITTER. The child and baby sitter should be introduced beforehand.*

1. The telephone number of the mother or of some chosen responsible adult who will be on call.
2. The telephone number of the family doctor.
3. Instructions on feeding (times, food quantities, etc.) and toilet routines.
4. How to handle the baby when he cries. Each baby varies in response to unaccustomed handling.
5. Where towels, diapers, etc. are kept.

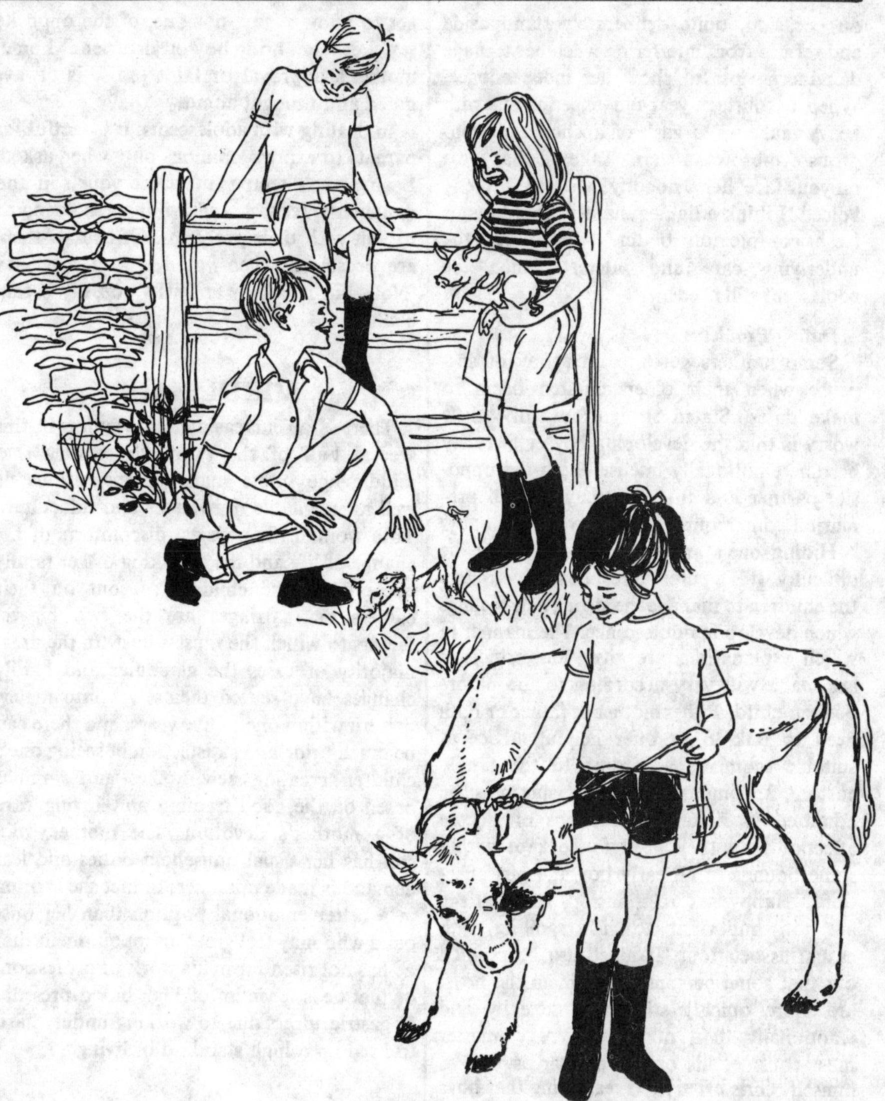

Fig. 11. *FAMILY HOLIDAY ON THE FARM*

6. Instructions as to ventilation, heating and night light, etc.

It is best of course if a baby of over four or five months of age knows the sitter but in any case he should see her before the mother goes out. The sitter should have had some experience in handling babies and feeding, especially giving bottles. No sitter should take charge of a baby if she has a cold, sore throat, or other similar infection, or has been in contact with an infectious fever of childhood.

Family Vacations

After the arrival of one or more babies, the husband and wife generally find that the question of a vacation becomes more of a problem, both financially and because they have to consider the baby's needs away from home. Motoring or boating, for example, are unsuitable, and may not provide the necessary washing facilities or quiet atmosphere for a young baby. A visit to relatives may be arranged, but often the wife finds she has as many chores to do as in her own home.

Renting a bungalow or cottage or a visit to a friendly farmhouse where paying guests are welcome and children not objected to, may prove a solution, especially if a bungalow or cottage is shared with friends so that the duties may be divided. This may also give children of two years onwards companionship and playmates. Some hotels and holiday camps make special provision for young children, including care at mealtimes and in the evenings, but these services may prove too expensive for many families. The new motels are less expensive than hotels, are more free and easy, and provide fairly good washing and cooking facilities and often restaurants for main meals, some having space for the children to play in the adjoining grounds.

COPING WITH TEENAGERS

The mother of adolescent children should wean herself stage by stage from the close mothering care needed for younger children. This effort should be made quite consciously —not merely be allowed to happen. She must on occasion, quite deliberately stand aside and refrain from interfering when her teenage daughter wants to show her independence. When a fourteen-year-old experiments with heavy make-up, a gash of lipstick and wondrous eye-brows, a stern 'Take off that mess on your face' helps nobody, whereas a quietly voiced 'I think a lighter shade might suit your fresh complexion better,' will imply the underlying care and interest which the adolescent still needs.

Dating Problems

Some mothers get into an agony of suspense when their older children begin to make dates. Stated straightforwardly, their worry is that the developing boy or girl may become emotionally intense about the opposite partner and that this may lead to premarital intercourse and even a baby.

Hiding one's anxiety will never solve the difficulty. It is a parental responsibility to help the children to manage the strong new feelings which develop in adolescence. The manner in which explanations are given and criticisms are made will vary according to the nature of each child. Either mother or father or both need to talk to or offer helpful advice at suitable moments according to the family custom. Kissing and some caressing must be admitted as natural expressions of sincere affection, but they need to be kept within some bounds in all early boy and girl affections. Happy sex relationships in marriage are too important to risk spoiling with casual associations. It must also be pointed out that some persons, more often the boys, are more quickly stimulated sexually and emotionally than others are. A youngster must consider his or her partner as well as himself. Girls often need reassuring that boys are not always as insistent about petting as they may appear to be.

Side by side with such direct advice, it is in the adolescents' own interests to encourage their group activities—clubs, sports, hiking, amateur theatricals—where the young people get to know many, not one, of the opposite sex. Let them bring boy or girl friends home; mother's approval or faint praise is always noted and thought about.

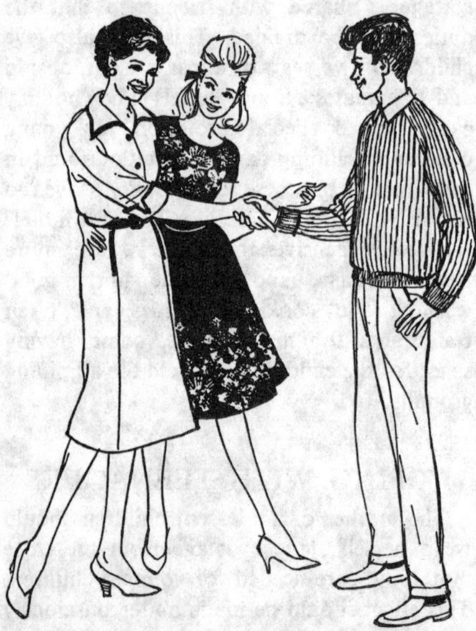

Fig. 12. *INTRODUCING THE BOY FRIEND*

In dealing with adolescents, it is tactful for parents to express opinions only when asked. Losing one's temper may lose your son and daughter's respect and willingness to come to you with their problems. Of course, there are occasions when you feel you must sav 'No'—but it is how and why you say it that counts.

MIDDLE AGE

There is an increasing appreciation in this second half of the twentieth century that middle age offers many compensations as well as inevitable drawbacks and difficulties. To a woman the physical discomforts of the change of life and the shrinking of her family circle when the children set out on their careers or marriages are the two biggest factors to which she must adjust. In the great majority of cases the glandular and bodily changes have settled themselves into a new pattern within one to five years, and there can be much pride and satisfaction in seeing one's children creating new homes and families based on the good training and loving care of a mother's devotion. The mother, too, still has her usual household duties and less demand is made upon her. In fact she is often in a better emotional position than her husband who may feel great disappointment that he has not risen far in his work or profession, or that he is a victim of high blood pressure or gastric ulcers due to working unduly hard to keep up a high standard of living.

The Change of Life

In the majority of middle-aged women the irregular and scantier menstrual periods and final cessation of menstruation takes place with little or no discomfort or upsets. In others there may be difficulties of varying degree. To some the very fact that their child-bearing period is over is a source of depression, yet, looked at sensibly, nature has made a very sound provision that women do not exhaust their bodies by bearing children in their less vigorous years. It is an interesting fact that over the last fifty years or so the average age at which menstruation ceases has become later so that many more women have the menopause at about the age of 52.

Although it is normal in the early stages of 'the change' to miss periods for one, two, or three months, medical advice should be sought if there is any irregular bleeding or blood-stained discharge *between* the period dates as this may indicate a uterine disorder which may be serious and need early treatment.

Flushes. The most common complaint is that of hot flushes. Very few women avoid this although it varies greatly in intensity. There is usually a sudden feeling of heat (or cold) and some flushing, particularly of the face. It feels much worse to the sufferer than it appears to the onlooker who may not even be aware of it. In severe cases it is accompanied by excessive sweating—this is more likely to occur when the woman is tired out, or sometimes during the night with consequent disturbance of sleep. The flushes are caused by glandular changes which temporarily upset the balance of the blood circulation (see also under Physiology). Since any glandular disturbance of the body is liable to cause emotional reactions, it is not surprising that many women at this stage have outbursts of excitability, over-activity, exaggeration of small grievances, brooding over imagined slights and feeling misunderstood. It can be a trying time for husbands and children as well as for the woman herself. Only patience, loving sympathy and an understanding of what is happening can help the situation. If a woman realizes that her emotional menopausal symptoms are getting out of hand she should see her doctor since these symptoms can be greatly relieved by estrogen preparations taken in small tablet form.

Fears and Insomnia. Fears of insanity or of cancer worry some women during the menopause and, for these dreads, firm reassurance and sympathy should always be given by the husband and friends, and is always available from the family doctor. Disturbance of sleep is common and the doctor may prescribe mild sedatives to tide over the difficulty (see also Functional Changes and Diseases of Women). It should always be remembered that menopausal symptoms may appear many months before the menses cease or may develop months or years after their cessation. The woman's age is a less important factor than the recognition of the decreasing ovarian activity to which the characteristic and disturbing symptoms are due.

Sexual Intercourse. The capacity for enjoying sexual union is not lost at the change of life. In fact, where there is understanding, consistent and trusting love between husband and wife, intercourse can be of great reassurance at this time. It also gives the woman confidence that she is still attractive to her husband. On the other hand, if a woman becomes apprehensive about sexual approaches from her husband, it is more often due to his lack of loving sympathy in the everyday business of living together since this can create a sense of apartness instead of unity in the marriage.

In the early stages of the menopause, when a wife first misses one or two menstrual periods, she may wonder whether she is pregnant or not, particularly if she has been neglectful in using contraceptives. A pregnancy can occur at this time but the chances are small compared with those of women in their twenties. If in doubt consult your doctor who can arrange for a pregnancy test.

Contraception should not be dispensed with until two years have elapsed since the last menstrual period.

Fresh Interests

The life pattern of women the world over is, in the age-long natural course of events, divided into two phases—the fertile period and the non-fertile. In Europe, the U.S.A. and other highly developed countries the number of healthy, active women who survive for long years into the second period is high compared with those in India, for instance. Historically speaking this aspect of affairs is comparatively new and it is obvious to sociologists, politicians and to these women themselves that there must be new thinking on the subject of planning our society to accommodate the energy, intelligence and skills of this large section of the community.

It has been suggested by eminent sociologists that women might take up their outside-the-home careers and jobs in the late forties. Because of the indisputable fact that they live longer than men they could continue in these careers or jobs for some years longer than men. Shorter hours or part-time jobs might be planned for those less physically strong. In the Second World War innumerable women in their forties and fifties showed that they were perfectly able to learn new crafts, trades and professions with speed and accuracy.

What do they gain? The obvious first factor is more to spend—theater tickets, better vacations, better clothes for figures not quite so youthful, entertaining friends, helping with expenses of grandchildren, or pursuing a hobby put aside because of lack of time or money during the time of child-rearing. And in the pursuit of these varied activities boredom is lost and interest gained, social horizons are widened, and life is lived more fully.

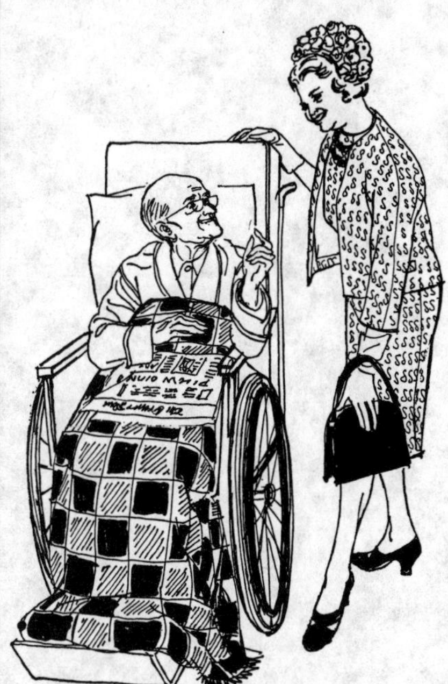

Fig. 13. *A VISIT. A kindly and worthwhile service to those who are lonely and incapacitated.*

For those who prefer the quieter life at home the greater freedom from family duties offers an opportunity for activities of a more individual kind. How many books have you wanted to read and not had time to sit down and enjoy? Perhaps you are a keen gardener and can create a beautiful garden. Or make your own clothes—and some for the grandchildren, or for the local bazaar. If you want to give a quiet service, there are so many lonely and partly incapacitated old people whose lives would be brightened by a visitor.

Renewed Marriage Relationship

As the children grow up, marry and leave home, the dependence of wife and husband on each other rapidly increases. Those who have been good friends and contented lovers throughout the years will find little difficulty in rediscovering the pleasure of doing things together and for each other. The wise wife will go half-way to meeting her husband's interests and hobbies even if they are not primarily her own, and the reverse is also true. The outward signs of affection which have often been laid aside when the children kept the parents, and the mother particularly, busy, need to be renewed to sweeten the fresh relationship.

Many middle-aged husbands need reassurance and love intensely at this stage of life and those who find happy sexual intercourse with their wives will not look for it outside of their homes. A wifely kindness is very important in this as well as in the daily details of living. Infidelity on the part of the husband is usually the culminating point of a number of earlier frustrations, maladjustments and incompatibilities. The loss of good looks, disablements or ill health which may make their appearance around middle age can draw couples closer together with the love, unselfishness and tenderness which may be revealed.

FATHER AND THE FAMILY

I

IMPORTANCE OF FATHER'S ROLE

The most primitive family unit of mammalian life, as far as is known, consists of the mother and her child. Through the drama of childbirth the immediate and close connection between the mother and her child can be understood, even by the most primitive of people It is only in relatively recent times of mankind's evolution that the importance of the role of the father has been recognized in connection with the basic unit of mother and child. Among some primitive Australian aborigines, for instance, the part a male played in begetting children has only recently been understood. Sexual intercourse was in no way thought to be related to conception or to the event of childbirth taking place after so long a period as nine months.

Biologically speaking, there is some justification for the past over-emphasis of the mother as the chief source and donor of life. As one goes lower in the animal world there is plenty of evidence to support the view that while the fertilization by a male often seems necessary, though not always in some species, the complex burden of child rearing is carried out by the mother without the need for a subtle interplay between male and female. Female fish, for instance, after having been fertilized, need never see the corresponding male fish again and do not require him psychologically to stand by in constant support until the young fish are born, nor thereafter. This is not the case with birds, who are placed higher by scientists, for male birds help their females considerably in nest building and in feeding their young. When we come to Man we find further progress in this direction, since in advanced civilizations and individuals it is increasingly appreciated just how important a role a father plays as a basic member of a family unit.

Even today the importance of the father's role is either often underplayed, misunderstood, or simply ignored. Very recently a few books on fathers have appeared, but not enough to establish the idea that the father is a necessary and vital counterpart to the mother in relation to their child. This is all the more surprising if one remembers that to the Victorians 'father' was regarded as something of a bogey-man. Today many American males are said to be content to leave not only the burden of child bearing but also that of child rearing to their wives. In contrast, the anthropologists tell a fascinating tale about the Arapesh tribe in New Guinea where the traditional Western roles of mother and father seem rather blurred in that both the mothers and fathers take it upon themselves quite arbitrarily as to which of them at what time is to do this or that with the child in order to help it become a mature adult.

The Father in Western Society

In our Western society, despite differences in class or community, a more or less uniform pattern of the roles of mother and father in relation to their children can be seen. Mothers are thought to be the primary agents, especially with young children and girls, and fathers are considered as secondary agents whose specific influence on their children is thought to become important only in the later part of a child's, especially a boy's, life.

This current and traditional picture in our civilization seems to be reflected in many phases of life and is emphasized by aspects of psycho-analytical theory. So many books today give advice to mothers on how to be truly motherly by ensuring that no unavoidable separations of mother and infant occur during the first few years of a child's life, but there still seems a great need for informed books to encourage the development of adequate and appropriate mother and child relationships.

There now seems to be an equally great and emerging need for the recognition of the importance of the father's role in child rearing. It is exciting to think that this new movement offers to parents, teachers and others a chance to help forward a neglected human relationship which should improve the modern child's growth to maturity.

The subject is here examined from several points of view, before dealing with the more practical aspects and problems in part II.

1. The role of the father as understood through psycho-analytical theory.
2. The role of the father as understood through non-psycho-analytical theory.
3. The role of the father in specific relationships, e.g. in different class structures; delinquency; boy or girl associations, etc.

The Oedipus Complex

Psycho-analytical theory has a great deal to say about the importance of the role of the father from the point of view of character development of boys and girls. (Further remarks about the theory can also be found in the section on Adolescence, p. 127.) The theory revolves around the concept of the famous Freudian Oedipus complex. The idea is that at about the age of five, boys and girls begin to recognize their own masculinity or femininity. This recognition, in boys, is said to come about through their incestuous feelings towards their mother, and the boys' subsequent feelings of rivalry towards their father. According to this theory, the feeling of rivalry is said to be accompanied by the fear that the father in his omnipotence is capable of de-masculinizing the little boy. This imagined drama gives rise to the need to allay fear and to resolve this Oedipus complex. This resolution is said to come about, in most cases quite naturally, by the boy's recognition that the best way of overcoming his mixed feelings towards his father is not to want to fight him (or through him authority in general), but to identify himself with him, to become a 'chip off the old block.' In this way the boy's aggression and anxiety are thought to become socialized, appropriately channelled, and reasonably resolved. If all this proceeds according to plan, father–son relationships are said to become good and wholesome, easily and naturally. If on the other hand this identification with the father is not made by the little boy, then, not only are father–son relationships said to be strained, but, the boy is likely to adopt a continuously rebellious attitude towards authority and father-like figures, e.g. teachers.

The task of fathers therefore, according to this theory, is to recognize this whole principle and to act in their relationship with their sons accordingly. To deal wisely with the natural aggressiveness which boys are said to express against them, fathers require great patience and imaginative wisdom in dealing with their young sons. This does not mean that fathers should refrain from curbing boys' aggressiveness when necessary, but it does mean that when fathers train or punish their sons this must be done through love and with an understanding of the inevitability of the Oedipal situation and its eventual resolution. The role for the wise father to adopt, according to this theory, is one of assisting his young son to pass naturally through the conflicts of the Oedipal situation. He needs, too, to keep reinforcing the resolved Oedipal situation throughout the boy's later development in life. In practical terms, this means that the father should set a consistently good example of masculinity to his son.

The Electra Complex

The role of the father in his relationship with his small daughter is said to be similar though not identical with that played in relation to his son. The little girl is also said to be going through an equivalent of the Oedipal phase, known as the Electra complex. The difference between her and her brother's problem is that in her case she is said to have romantic wishes not towards her mother but towards her father, and that this needs a natural and ultimate resolution. The father's task, according to this theory, is first to understand the force of her feelings for him and then to channel them gradually and patiently in such a way that she will ultimately wish to identify herself once more with the mother whom her father loves. Through this identification with her mother the little girl is said to be enabled to become truly feminine, a state of affairs which requires gentle reinforcing throughout the girl's development.

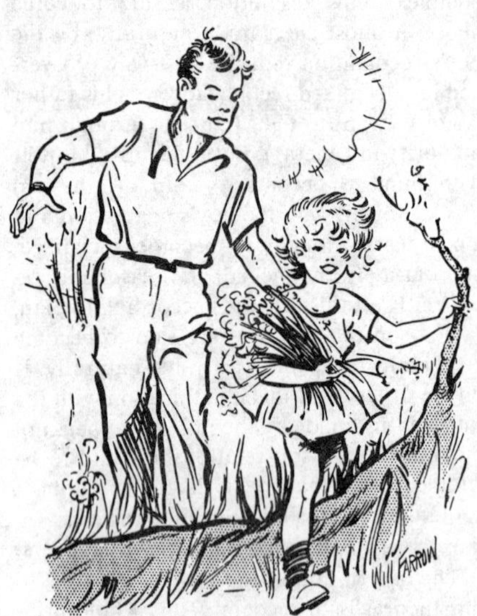

Fig. 1. *A HAPPY FATHER–DAUGHTER RELATIONSHIP*

The role of the father in all this, therefore, is not to overstimulate or spoil the girl by giving in too much to her romantic feelings towards him. At the same time he needs to bring about a warm relationship between himself and his daughter which should enable her in later life to seek out the right sort of male partner in her life who will have some aspects of her father's personality. Such a partner would be visualized by her not as a person against whom to rebel but as a person through whom perfect unity of opposites can be achieved.

Setting a Good Example

As mentioned earlier, there are theories other than the psycho-analytical one which help to throw light on father-child relationships. In social psychology very little, if any, emphasis is placed on the alleged Edipal relationships between fathers and their children, especially those allegedly taking place around the fifth year of life. Instead, the emphasis is placed on the concept that parent-child relationships develop naturally step by step, from birth to adulthood. Great attention, therefore, must be paid to each step. This involves the application of what is technically known as aspects of learning theory. In its development, every young creature, including the human child, makes stepwise progress when it is ready and has the capacity to absorb and learn new behavioral patterns or rules. As each step is reached, the parents should take advantage of it to emphasize, constantly repeat, and impress the new bit of learning upon the receptive body and mind of the child, e.g. teaching him to use a saw, or to give up a chair to a tired person.

By observing these 'rules,' the father is to ensure that his 'good' image is absorbed by his children and that this is consistently reinforced over the years with regular frequency. Moodiness on the part of the father (or mother), or inconsistencies in upbringing (ranging from over-indulgence one minute to over-punishment the next) are considered to be harmful to the growing child. The role which ought to be played by the father, therefore, according to the theory of social psychology, is to set a consistently good example and to instill worthwhile precepts in order to stimulate the right kind of growth in his child, be it a boy or a girl.

Social Variation

It may appear as though the assumption has been made that it is fairly easy for fathers to set a good example, and that such behavior is more or less uniform throughout society. This is, of course, not so. In father–child relationship, different patterns emerge according to the family, class, circumstances, or country, etc. For example, father–son relationships in working class families differ in some respects from those of non-working class families. Talk of, or resort to, various degrees of violence and aggression—'I'll hit you if you do it again'—and swearing, are alleged to be more common among working class families than non-working class ones, and find expression and specific reinforcement via father–son relationships. The picture of a healthy, vigorous and to some extent over-aggressive (working class) father is alleged to be a reassuring and often appropriate one for the boy to emulate since the lad has to learn to hold up his head among his peer group. In contrast, non-working class fathers, with their more subtly hidden forms of agression and violence, are said to set an example for their boys which is more complex to follow, especially in an environment which places less and less emphasis on violence in interpersonal relationships, and where working class and non-working class customs (or mores) intermix owing to 'class emancipation.'

Fathers and Working Mothers

It appears also that subtle changes of mores in all classes have appeared since the general emancipation of women. Mothers, who once were stamped as inferior by a world largely dominated by males, were regarded by children as weak and fathers as all-powerful. Todav, in some families, fathers become more 'powerless' in relation to wage-earning mothers, and this situation can, in extreme cases, lead to delinquency as a boy's protest against a seemingly weak father. Often, of course, delinquency is encouraged by a situation at the opposite extreme, where a father, far from being too weak, is considered by the boy or girl to be too aggressive and lacking in understanding. In such cases there is a great need on the part of fathers to convey a better image of themselves to their children at the deepest level. The children then have a feeling of being loved by the father just as much as by the mother, and they are prepared to be dealt with by fathers in a fair, constant and self-assured way. How can this be achieved by fathers, however, if they are no longer self-assured of their masculinity and robbed of their self-confidence by those wives who are over-emancipated and bossy? Wage-earning wives who assert too much authority in the home may also have this demasculinizing effect upon the father. How also can fathers impart feelings of self-assurance to their children, and thus give guidance, in societies where religious and ethical value systems are undergoing a series of changes? The vague threats of wars or of economic insecurity make their mark on people in industrialized communities, where individuals tend to become increasingly isolated (i.e. de-socialized) and correspondingly more lonely, insecure, and therefore more aggressive or neurotic.

Know Thyself

The answer to much of this seems to lie in the simple little phrases of 'Know thyself' and 'Know the truth and the truth shall make ye free.' Self-knowledge, and understanding of how the human mind and personality develop is, thanks to books on the subject, easier to gain today than it was only one generation ago. The road to self-knowledge can never be easy nor quick but requires patience and hard work through reading and listening, thinking and discussion with other like-minded people who are interested in spreading good 'mental health' throughout communities in an endeavor to make the world a better and happier place for all to live in. Fathers and mothers might therefore take it upon themselves to study their own roles in relation to their children very carefully. This should enable parents and children to respond with the right amount of interflow of love and responsibility to one another and to society at large.

II

FATHER IN THE HOME

How may the foregoing theoretical considerations be applied by the ordinary father in his home setting? Family responsibilities are now increasingly shared and rarely is father the traditional tyrant. Modern families are smaller and father takes some share in looking after the baby or helps wash the dishes with no loss of prestige. But he is still the head of the family with special responsibilities, and he should gain the love and respect of his family by behaving as a responsible and trustworthy male parent.

All children copy the behavior of their parents and if mother and father are thoughtful and considerate their children will develop similar characteristics. Good manners are best learned by example; saying 'please' and 'thank you' and not interrupting conversations are absorbed by the child within the home. Father and mother need to support each other without being unfair to their children. Bickering and arguments in front of children are far more nerve racking for the bewildered youngsters than many parents realize. Differences of opinion and even open disagreements will arise, but these must be settled privately by the parents without the children being present.

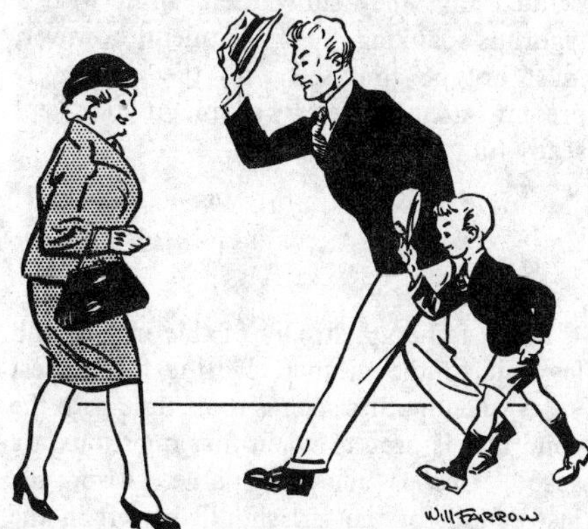

Fig. 2. *GOOD MANNERS are best taught by example.*

Father as Husband

Father's attitude to his wife, and mother of his children, is extremely important, not only for her well-being, but also for the influence this has upon the children and the general atmosphere in the home. However much she may love her family, a mother can become bored with always being tied to the house. Father can sit in sometimes while she goes to see a friend or to an evening class. He can bring interests home and read and discuss events from newspapers and books with her; suggest outings together and help to make arrangements for a sitter; plan, with the children, birthday surprises for her. It is not difficult to think of many such little pleasures which mean a great deal to the mother, and set a good example for boys as to how a husband should treat a wife.

When his wife is pregnant a little extra consideration is important. This does not mean treating her as an invalid. Most normal healthy women are very well during pregnancy, but they can tire easily and to be able to rest more often than usual and to be relieved of a little of the 'running about' can make all the difference between reasonable good humor and anxious irritability. When the new baby arrives it means extra work for the mother, certainly in the early stages, and father may well suffer by not having meals ready on time, etc. Tolerance, and even some help, are more likely to help her to re-establish her routine than too much criticism. He can help too with the other child, or children, who may not take too kindly to the advent of the new baby, by giving them extra attention or, on occasion, taking a turn with the newcomer so that his wife may give the other children more attention.

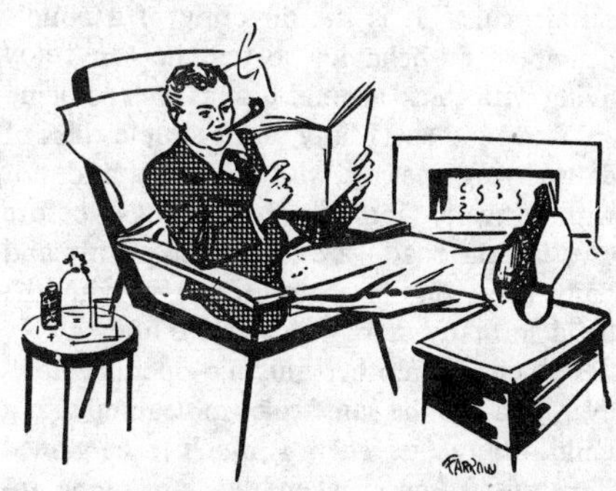

Fig. 3. *FATHER'S TURN to sit while mother goes out for the evening.*

Here, perhaps, a plea should be made for consideration for father when he is tired because of his work. Older children should be told that father's overtime is to buy them a new coat, or provide the money for a holiday. Wife and children must respect strains that may result, and be tolerant.

Father and the Under-fives

Most fathers are restricted in the time they are able to spend with their children and may only have the opportunity at weekends or on holidays, unless they arrive home in time in the evenings for a bedtime game or story and a goodnight kiss. These games and stories can be a great source of joy to the child and, even though father may feel tired, the effort is well worth while because children seem to grow up so quickly when father has only the weekends at home. If the child wants to play when father comes home try to ensure that the game is not too boisterous as this will cause overexcitement and may delay him settling down to sleep.

The Baby and the toddler until about the age of two finds it difficult to cope with the attentions and instructions of more than one person at a time. Trying to divide his affection bewilders him and is more likely to lead to tension and tears. In general he will maintain a more affectionate attachment to his mother while obeying father.

At Three. At about three he will like doing things in a special way. He likes a set routine and will become upset if this is varied. He will begin to enjoy bedtime stories, particularly from father, and will find it difficult to understand if he is disappointed.

At Four. When a child is four he is beginning to become independent and less easy to please. He is able to enlarge his world to include his mother and father at the same time. He can move about quicker, has a great deal more energy and is high spirited. He has a more controlled use of his hands and can do little jobs about the house or help father in the tool shed. He may even be trusted with blunt scissors. Father and mother must be consistent in their attitude towards him: if father says he can cut pictures out of a magazine, it is damaging to the child's security for mother to take it away. Even at this early age a child knows quite well that he will get his own way if he plays one parent off against the other. This usually leads to dissension and should therefore be avoided. There can be no joy if parents disagree.

Father's Importance to the Older Child

Father's influence upon a child now becomes more positive. He can allow the child to 'help Daddy' even if only for short periods, not merely to 'give mother a rest' but so that he and the child get to know each other. He can take him to visit some place of interest or to a football or baseball game. From about the age of seven years he can teach the child to use tools.

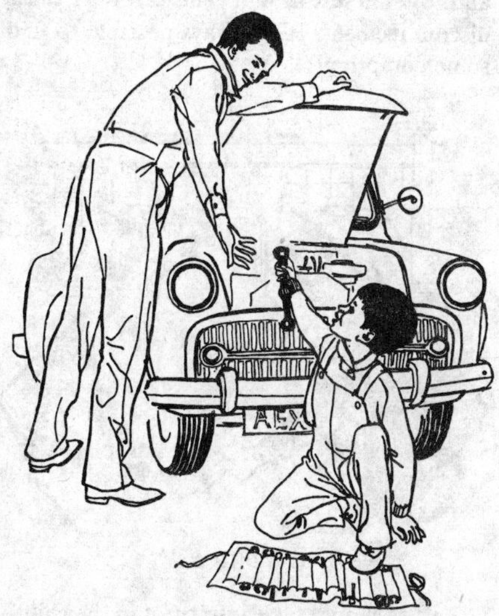

Fig. 4. *IN THE GARAGE. Learning to be handy with tools like father.*

As we have seen in the first part of this section, p. 147, father has a particular and somewhat different role towards his son and his daughter. Sons, in particular, come in for possible 'spoiling' from their mother, and they are the main sufferers from what psychologists call 'mother-fixation'. It is often hard for a mother to realize how dangerous and selfish such over-possessiveness can be, but father can counterbalance this by having a more relaxed, less emotional relationship with his son. Girls, on the other hand, may fare rather badly if there are boys in the family who are being spoiled by mother, so that love and understanding from her father becomes very important to the growing girl. A little knowledge and thought can help to avoid emotional pitfalls.

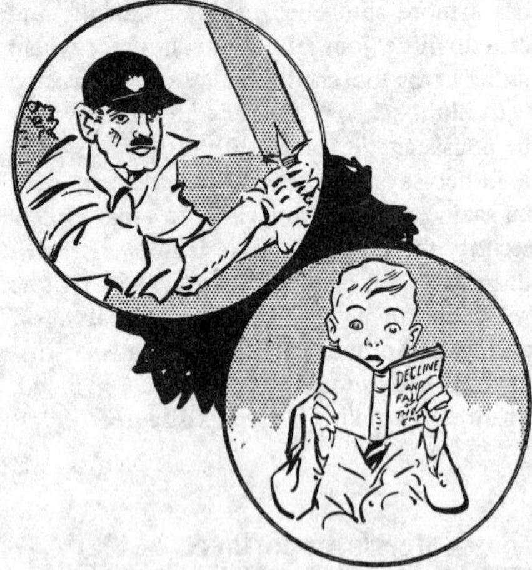

Fig. 5. *FATHER AND SON may have opposing tastes.*

If father is to share interests with his children it is obviously easier if they have something in common, but it may happen that a child, particularly a boy, shows no enthusiasm for the things his father likes. He may prefer intellectual pursuits and have no inclination for sport, or vice versa. This cannot be helped and father must not show too much disappointment, or blame his child and lose interest in him. This can only cause discouragement. It is always possible to find some compromise.

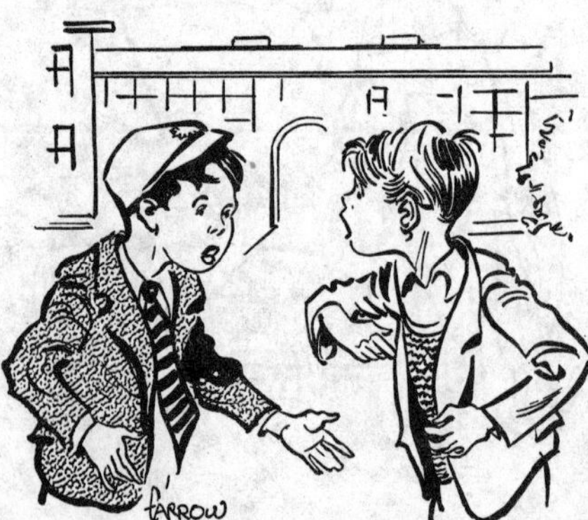

Fig. 6. *'MY DAD SAYS . . .'*

Father should take an interest in the child's school for it occupies a great deal of a child's life, and he should give encouragement providing it is not overstressed and makes the child anxious and nervous. School and its interests are often regarded as mother's province, but father should play his part and attend parent–teacher meetings and school concerts too, whenever possible.

No one who has heard remarks in playgrounds, parks or streets, such as 'I'll ask my Dad' or 'My Dad says' can doubt his importance to a school child.

Constructive Discipline

Firm, but gentle, handling is essential for children. Obedience must be founded on respect. If a child is driven to obey and has his 'spirit broken' by harsh, dictatorial methods he will cease to have any affection for his parents and may become deceitful and disliked.

The word discipline is often misused. It is not primarily concerned with punishment but is a manner of training and learning with certain rules. It is the directing of a child's activities and behavior so that he can enjoy living with those around him as well as being enjoyed by them. Many of the simple rules of daily living—eating with a spoon and not with fingers, looking both ways before crossing the road—are taught frequently and daily by a mother because she is with the child so many more of his active hours.

Father and mother must co-operate, however, and use the same rules in dealing with a child of any age. There is much to be gained if parents discuss, when they are alone together, incidents in the child's behavior from their two points of view. Not only will father become more fully acquainted with his children's joys, failures and successes but mother's anxieties and frets about the children can often be put into a calmer and more objective perspective by father. How much more constructive and worthwhile will discipline then be when parents discard the older method of mother's demanding that father punish the child for some act of disobedience, the rights and wrongs of which neither parent really sorted out!

Punishment

Many of the troublesome actions of small children are not done purposely and do not need punishment. On the other hand, a child who wilfully disobeys a rule or a clear request needs some form of correction to improve his behavior. Angry words from father, if used rarely, are often sufficient punishment for most children for they will make an impression on them and the misdemeanor is not likely to be repeated. Disapproval, in itself, is often enough for some children to feel cut off from parental love; such children are easily encouraged by the assurance that mother or father knows they can do better.

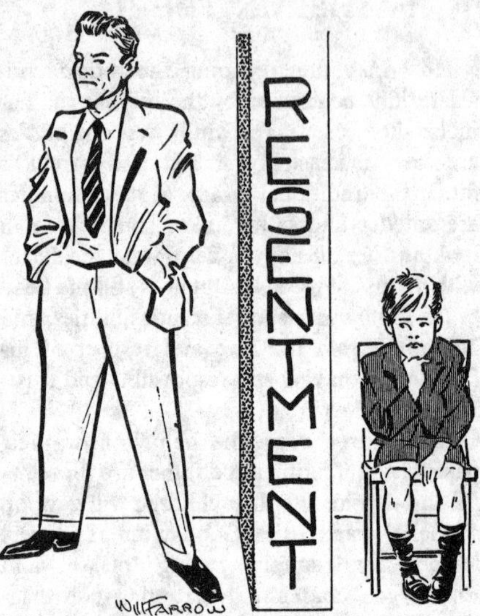

Fig. 7. *HARSH TREATMENT from father may create a wall of resentment between child and parent.*

Spanking, yelling and slapping are all rather unsatisfactory because, in making the child afraid, they arouse resentment which can grow into a tough barrier between child and parent. Of course there are the odd occasions when father and mother become so exasperated that they show their upset with a vigorous spanking. Such treatment, however, must not be confused with the cold ever-present threat implied by a cane or stick kept ready for 'naughty children.'

Sex Instruction

Many fathers fight shy of this matter and leave it to the mother. During the earliest years when mother spends most time with the child and is around when first questions are asked, this is understandable. Also, sex instruction for the girl should be left in the main to the mother. But with the growing schoolboy, father should help. Not merely facts but attitudes are being imparted. If father has established a good relationship with his son, the matter should not be too difficult. Boys should be told the complete facts of life when they reach puberty, which usually comes later in a boy than in a girl. In modern life when young people mix freely it is essential not to leave them in ignorance. It is true they may 'find out' but it is not good for a child to discover these important facts as a result of childish confidences, often garbled and frequently frightening, making the whole subject rather cheap and nasty. An open, healthy, but serious attitude on the part of the parent is likely to breed in the child a respect for himself and his girl friend, and strengthen him to avoid pitfalls. If father finds the subject particularly difficult to deal with, there are many good books published to assist the diffident parent; they can be given to the child to read at his leisure and he should be invited to discuss them afterwards if he wishes.

In some schools, the teachers deal with the subject of sex, and a father who finds it difficult to discuss the matter with his son might ask the teacher for his assistance.

Careers

Helping a child to decide upon future work may sometimes be difficult. Older children are frequently undecided and their ideas are slow to mature. They need help, and boys in particular need the help of their fathers. Advice and discussion should be handled carefully and tactfully to avoid pushing the child into something he does not want to do. The subject is dealt with in Adolescence, p. 135.

GRANDPARENTS AND THE ELDERLY

The Role of Grandparents

When a mother and father have seen their own family grow up and develop into happy and responsible individuals, and though they are often still carrying on with their own work and interests, it usually comes as a joyous experience when grandchildren are born. It can bring with it new experiences and new vigor. Good grandparents can often be a great help to young parents who may feel much more secure knowing that grandparents are there to be consulted if necessary. They may be able to give practical help. If parents have to be away, it is usually much better for the child to be left in the care of grandparents than of strangers.

To be successful grandparents, however, often calls for considerable ingenuity and wisdom. Some daughters or daughters-in-law may look upon a grandmother's counsel as always or necessarily out-of-date, or resent asking advice when they wish to feel independent. If the grandmother attempts to thrust information and precepts upon the mother, disagreements and tensions are likely to follow, especially over a first grandchild. Generally, however, grandparents are wise enough not to interfere unduly, even if new child-rearing methods do cause them considerable surprise and some anxiety. Frank discussions on whys and wherefores between the young parents and the older generation are usually the best solution. The baby is the mother's responsibility and she has the mother's right to make decisions and decide methods of routine and management, but she should give reasonable reassurance to allay any anxiety the grandmother may feel. If a grandmother guards against interference she is more likely to be consulted or have her opinion asked when occasion arises.

Domineering Grandparents

A few parents never let their children attain real independence, and rule even their adult lives to a varying extent, sometimes in mistaken kindness or through possessiveness. When the first grandchild arrives, the son or daughter may find it difficult to steer clear of apparently well-meaning advice. Grandparents should never attempt to play the part of parents unless, of course, they are in sole charge of the child. Any kind of criticism of the parents by the grandparents in front of the child must be avoided, since it is likely to undermine or alienate the child's sense of trust and security, and lead to possible conflict and tension which the child will soon come to share.

The young parents should be willing to listen to the grandparents' advice, but should also be prepared to take their own stand in making decisions and, above all, not to get angry or resentful. Suppressed anger in the parents and heated arguments with the grandmother are often a sign of timidity or submission that has been controlled and repressed over a long period, and finally breaks out. A more mature way of dealing with criticism and interference is for the young mother and father to show a quiet assurance that they are doing the best for the child according to their own views, by explaining what these views are, and by handling the child with self-confidence. This will usually carry more weight, and should lead to an easier relationship between the two generations. If it fails, consultation with the family doctor should help to ease the difficult and unhappy situation, and also give assurance to the grandmother, who may be genuinely anxious as to the parents' adequacy and the advisability of their methods.

The Child in Grandparents' Care

When a baby or older child is left in the grandparents' care, some compromises may be necessary for general management, but happiness and confidence, suitable and regular meals, the requisite amount of rest and sleep, and attention to regular bowel actions are the main requirements, after safeguards have been made against accidents. A grandparent can often give a small child a very happy form of companionship, and usually has more leisure than the busy mother or father, so that more time can be given to play and storytelling. A grandmother or grandfather thus becomes a dearly loved companion and enjoys the child's affection and interests wholeheartedly without feeling too much responsibility about 'spoiling' or general management.

THE ELDERLY

A great deal of thought continues to be given to possible ways of making life more pleasurable and useful to the elderly. Medical, social, and psychological factors all play their part but the most important factor is to ensure that elderly persons remain integrated in the general life of the community as far as possible and do not become isolated and lonely. Attempts are made when planning new homes for the over-sixties, or when altering the existing buildings, to make them as homely as possible and to avoid an institutional atmosphere.

The strengths and weaknesses of elderly people who continue in employment are being assessed and it is often found that their slowness is balanced by their reliability and experience.

The study of the diseases and minor ailments which occur in old age has greatly extended as a branch of medicine, and geriatric units which study and deal with the health and problems of the elderly have increased in number in the last few years with a consequent lessening of many of the worst effects of such illnesses.

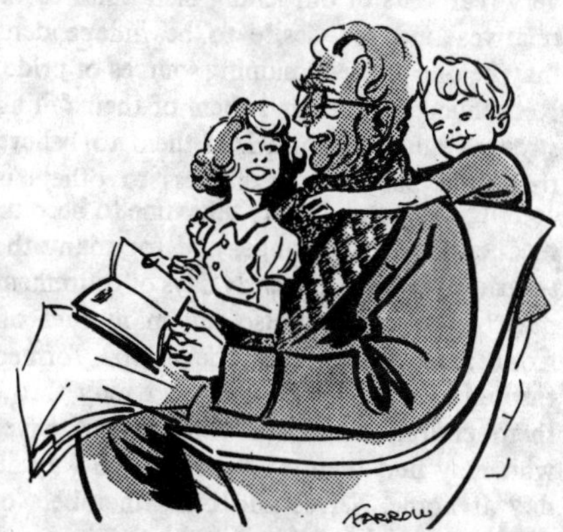

Fig. 1. *GRANDFATHER often has more leisure to become a dearly loved companion.*

The exact nature of the bodily processes of ageing is still not known, but certain disabilities and slowing-down processes arise and are known. All old people do not experience all these effects and there is no specific age at which they occur. The tissues of the body become less sensitive resulting in the slowness and a certain clumsiness sometimes observed; the bones become more brittle and easily fracture. The mind seems to become less alert.

To be happy in life is the desire of everyone and this is no less so in old age. It is important for older people to come to terms with their reduced capacities, and relatives, friends, and everyone coming into contact with them can help by arranging their surroundings so that no undue suffering is caused by possible infirmities. A little thought and consideration can often prevent accidents and illnesses and so enable older people to gain as much satisfaction as possible from the abilities which remain.

Retirement

Men. Retirement can be a tremendous blow, particularly to men, and can have repercussions in all aspects of life, affecting their happiness and security. Often their main interest, and certainly their main activity, has centered around their work and perhaps sporting activities. At retirement these may come to a sudden and complete stoppage. A man's pride frequently lies in his strength and skill in work and in his leisure activities. In many cases work helps to maintain health and a standard of living which is almost certain to diminish at retirement. When there has been this emphasis upon work, some form of occupation in the future may be essential. Some may delay retirement as long as possible believing that their authority and prestige will be weakened by relinquishing a good post. Others may take on a different or less responsible job with a smaller salary. This is not necessarily a tragedy, for a less exacting job is not so exhausting and the quieter home life preferred by older people makes less demands upon the purse.

Older people are not always as unwanted as they sometimes make out. They may have very real fears of burdening their children or relatives and the desire to be independent may be one of the remaining sources of pride. Retirement may remind them of their failing strength and skill, and lead them to believe that their period of usefulness to others is coming to an end. It may take time to become reconciled to the change, and for many the transition stage of the early days of retirement may be the worst. It also cuts many men off from associations and friendships formed through, or at, their work, and may throw them entirely upon the company of wives who may find them aimlessly in the way all day at home. Wives and other members of the family need to be particularly tolerant and considerate during this stage of readjustment.

Women who have been out to work, in contrast to men, rarely find retirement produces such drastic changes in their way of life. If married, they have mainly thought of their job as supplementing the family income and perhaps a way of meeting others, but not, as with men, as their main source of prestige and association. Their satisfactions come largely from their home and family. A housewife's duties continue much the same after retirement.

A wife's role in the household is an important one and much of what she does can affect the retired man. He may be around the house a great deal of the time and frequently may wish to be in the same room as her for company. This often leads to frustrations and alterations in her household routine. She should, if possible, draw her husband into a few of the household duties even though he may be slower and may not do them exactly as she would wish. To complain or grumble at the man only increases the tension and can be a source of unhappiness.

Employment for the Elderly

Planning for retirement is not only wise, it is really essential and should begin well before retiring age.

Preparing for Retirement. For those who have been for years in a steady job and have a pension to rely on, plans should be made for living on a reduced income. The upkeep of one's present house or apartment may be too high once a full wage or decent salary goes. Will you retire to the country or take a smaller house? Will you share with a relative of your own age group or divide your accommodation with a son or daughter? If you are fit and healthy will you continue to work at some minor job, and what is available for you? Such matters as these should be planned and discussed even five to ten years before retiring so that you can begin the change-over before the sharp break comes. The break will be far less sharp if a change of house is already made, a less exacting job fixed up, or a useful hobby begun which can be turned to profitable account when one has more time to give to it. Successful hobbies which have been taken up by those nearing retirement age include dog-breeding, poultry keeping, house painting and minor repairs, gardening, auditing for local shopkeepers, and, more specifically for women, knitting, bead making, dress-making, part-time clerical or typing work.

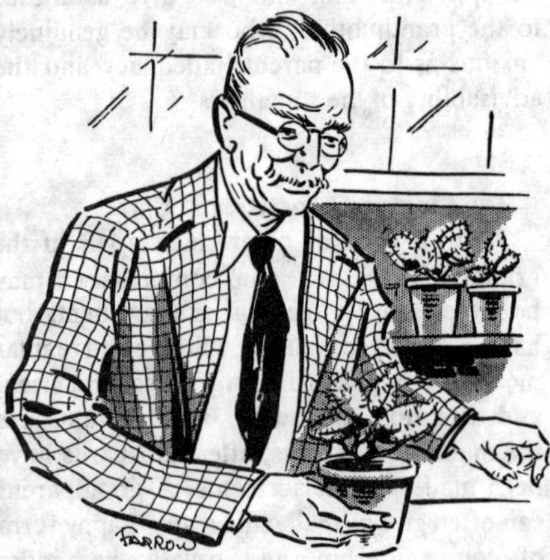

Fig. 2. *SUCCESSFUL HOBBIES may be turned to profitable account on retirement.*

Jobs for the Over-Sixties. Because an increasing number of people in their sixties today are still fairly active and healthy, a considerable amount of research and thought is being given to finding ways and means of providing whole or part-time jobs for those who wish to continue at work. Some employers will allow people to continue working after retirement age if they wish, but this may mean different work with less responsibility.

For men, new work after retirement is often part-time or spasmodic, and is frequently unskilled, e.g. a night-watchman's job, taking small deliveries for a grocer or florist, and odd gardening jobs. Some firms in the larger cities provide materials for light work to be done at home.

Women on the whole fare much better than men and find it easier to obtain work after retirement. Single women, too, seem to find work or leisure time activities when they retire.

But whatever the work, so long as it gives the person a sense of usefulness, it has fulfilled its purpose. Earnings from such work may be small but can be a source of pride and joy to the recipient. In addition, the carefulness and accuracy with which an older person tackles a job is well appreciated by those who employ them.

Sheltered Workshops. There are a few workshops for the elderly. Here the work is carried out under 'sheltered' conditions and is paid for at a piece rate. These are pioneering experiments, but may well be extended in the future. Such workshops and clubs have shown that tasks which are not too complicated, and within the intellectual and physical scope of the individuals concerned, can be learned by people of 70 years and over, although it may take them longer to learn the job. In some sheltered workshops and clubs, craftwork of good quality is produced by people who only learned to use the tools and materials when over the age of 60 years.

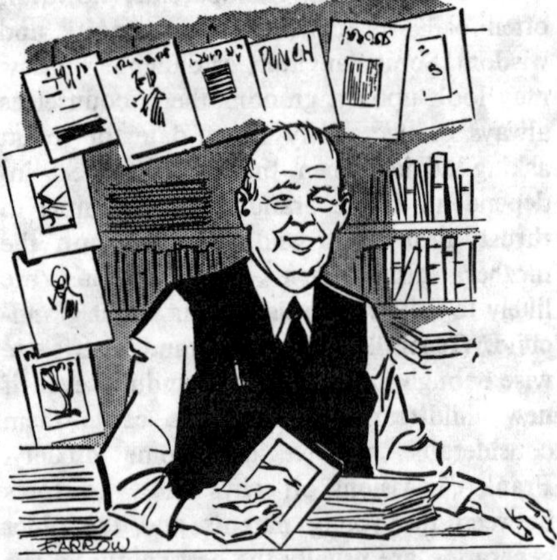

Fig. 3. *A PART-TIME JOB in the late sixties helps to eke out a small pension.*

Mental Adjustment

Complaints of grumpiness, selfishness, and a tendency to interfere are sometimes levelled against elderly people but these attitudes are often due to their feeling of uselessness and being unwanted rather than to any natural irritability. It does not help them at all when younger people think they 'have done their bit' and should sit peacefully in the corner with nothing to do. Such 'peace' can easily lead to complete idleness, which, once established as a habit, is very difficult to break. This in turn only increases their feeling of being unwanted. The more an elderly person can be persuaded to do, the better, and this will produce a corresponding increase in his or her self-respect and in maintaining good health. Provided the work is not beyond the physical and mental capacities of older people, the occupations given them should not be the most menial ones, but those suited to their past experience or adaptability—gardening, embroidery, book-keeping, brass and silver polishing, etc.

It is better if they have some set routine or a household job which is regarded as their province and responsibility. The care of young children is especially suited to them since the very young and the old have a number of similarities, for example, both like repetition and both are unhurried in their activities. Further, the elderly have time to spare.

Another way of overcoming the unwanted feeling and of giving pleasure at the same time is to have a family pet which is dependent upon the elderly person for care.

Although elderly people will seldom openly admit to a feeling of uselessness it can often be a cause of considerable unhappiness for them. This is shown by worry over minor details, in particular over money, and by compulsively repeating small meaningless acts. Their 'pottering' and 'fussing' around is often an attempt to prove that they are still useful.

They will often try to blame their 'uselessness' on others and so gain some relief from their frustration. It may be kinder on occasion not to point out their mistakes. They are frequently aware of their own shortcomings and too much should not be asked of them. They should be asked to do one thing at a time as too many requests at once may cause them to become anxious and confused.

Loneliness is not just a question of living or being alone. A person can be lonely when living in a family or group, if his interests are totally different and he is not invited to participate in family or group life. On the other hand, a person actually living alone but in constant contact with friends and relatives can be much less lonely. Old people may find 'modern' attitudes different from the way they were brought up and therefore difficult for them.

The best way to prevent or combat loneliness is by social contact and companionship, and clubs play an excellent part in this. In most areas there are Over Sixties clubs, Golden Age groups, or clubs organized by churches. Some old people are reluctant to go to clubs but, once encouraged and helped to go, they enjoy them. Visitors for the elderly give great pleasure and it is important not to disappoint them once a promise has been made. A view from a window on to the street can be a great source of interest and pleasure for those who cannot walk far.

Boredom in the elderly is not necessarily due to lack of work as to lack of something to work *for*, lack of some real goal. And this cannot be alleviated by repetitive, perhaps meaningless, tasks. Taking an interest in life involves the will to work and the need to work for someone or with some end in view. Elderly people may become discouraged just 'pottering' in the garden, but will take new interest if they grow vegetables or flowers for a Flower Show. Financial reward may be important, as even a few dollars gives a feeling of achievement. Events of special interest should be within the bounds of possibility and not too far ahead, such as planning for Christmas or looking for birthday presents. Also, it is a good thing (even if the advice is not always taken) to ask 'what do you think?' It gives the older members a feeling of being part of the family.

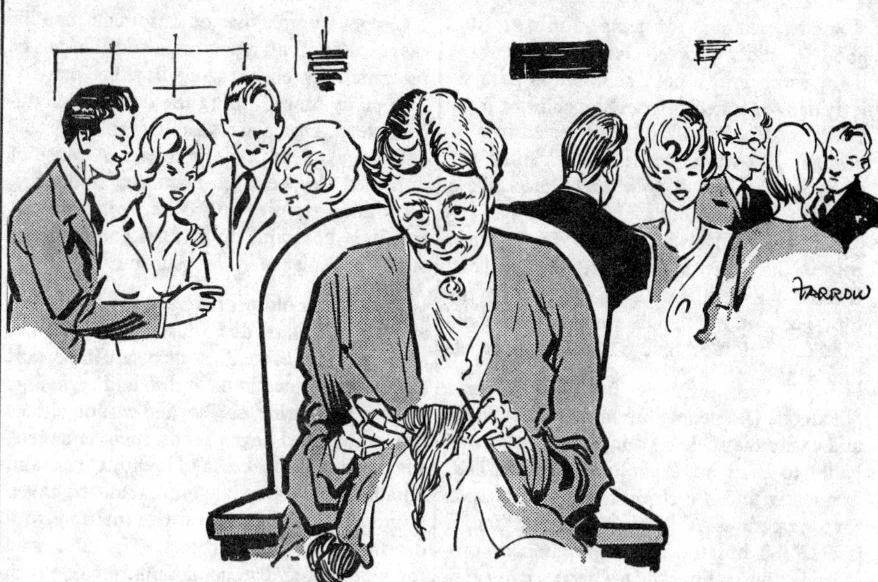

Fig. 4. *LONELINESS. One may live surrounded by family and their friends yet feel quite alone if they do not invite participation.*

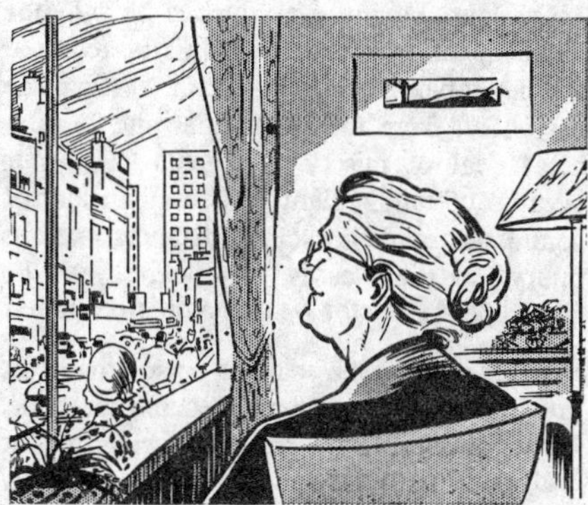

Fig. 5. *A WINDOW ON THE STREET is a great source of interest and pleasure to housebound persons*

The Family Group. Probably the most important link for old people is their contact with relatives. Neighborliness and friendliness are important and give much pleasure, but it is the feeling of being a member of a large family group (cousins, nieces, nephews, friends and friends' relatives) which gives the most joy. In these connections old people may find enough to interest and occupy them from day to day, and to give them a sense of security.

General Care of the Elderly and Old

Personality does not change in old age, but becomes more clearly defined. For instance, a cheerful person remains cheerful and the sociable remains sociable and they retain their sense of humor. A great many remain fit and active, to a greater or lesser degree, for most of their lives—their interests and activities are the keynote of this—but thought and care is often needed to prevent deterioration in others. Such consideration devolves mainly upon the relatives since about 97 per cent of all elderly people are living outside of institutions. Some understanding of their physical needs helps to make life pleasant for all in the household.

Comfort. The elderly feel the cold more acutely because the circulation of their blood is slower and because they are unable to move about quickly and easily and so create warmth for themselves; this may result in numbness and fumbling. They are also particularly vulnerable to drafts. In spring and autumn they may need to have a fire when other members of the family do not feel such need.

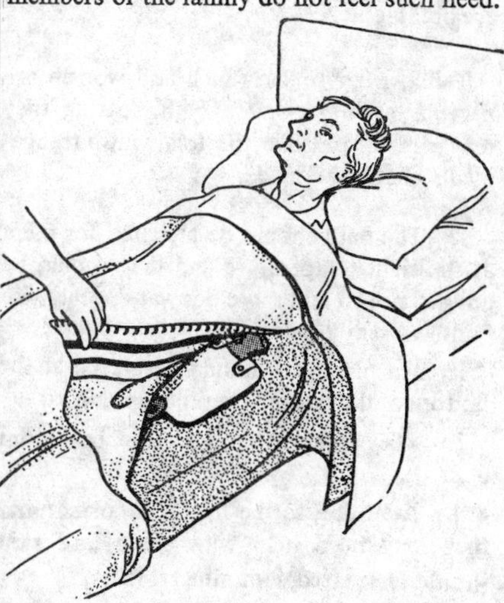

Fig. 6. *HOT-WATER BOTTLE is best placed between the blankets for an older person.*

Sudden changes of temperature are not good for older people. Going from a warm living-room into a cold bedroom is particularly bad for sufferers from bronchitis or from heart trouble. Beware of unprotected fires or heaters. Hot-water bottles are essential for their comfort but it is wiser to place these between the blankets as hands and feet become less sensitive with age and may be burnt before the sufferer is aware of the heat. Electric blankets should be placed *over* the top sheet, and a member of the household should switch it off before the old person gets into bed.

Fatigue. Old people tire much more quickly and easily than when younger and may react badly to loud noises or bright lights. They frequently find it a strain to watch television for long periods. A certain amount of exercise is essential but too much exercise, or prolonged conversations, or tea parties can cause them to tire quickly.

It is a mistake, however, to treat them as children merely because they become confused or simple; they will certainly resent it because they retain their awareness of what is going on around them and can usually find a reason for what they are doing.

Clothing. Elderly people have their own ideas about the type of clothes they want to wear and they frequently wear too much. Air should be able to circulate around the body, and heavy clothing may prevent circulation. The most suitable clothing is loose fitting, light, and warm. Dresses and shirts which unbutton completely like a coat are easily managed. Stockings and socks should be chosen and washed with care; if they are too tight they can impede the circulation and cause numb cold feet.

Feet can lose their shape and support if slippers are worn continuously and older people should be encouraged to wear proper shoes for some of the time. If tying laces is a problem, expanding laces which allow the foot to be pushed into the shoes are obtainable.

Toilet. Many elderly men and women are nervous about taking a bath, fearing they may slip. If possible the following arrangements should be made:

1. The bath should be prepared for them at the right temperature and they should be advised not to add more hot water, otherwise faintness may occur.

2. An old towel should be placed at the bottom of the bath to prevent slipping.

3. They should not lock the bathroom door.

4. Attention to the feet is important and they may need help with this. Hard skin should be treated with mineral jelly.

5. A brisk rub down following a bath helps the circulation, and a rest is advisable afterwards, preferably on the bed.

Sleep. Complaints of insomnia can be exaggerated in all age groups and this can be prevented by encouraging daytime activity. Too many 'naps' during the day spoil night-time sleep. Drugs and sleeping tablets should only be given on doctor's orders. A cause of disturbed sleep can be nocturnal frequency, a common occurrence in the over-seventies, and it is advisable to have a commode or other convenience in the bedroom.

Diet. Many old people have good appetites and an adequate diet must contain all the essential types of food. Proteins are important and are contained in meat, fish and eggs. Fats (butter, margarine, cheese) and carbohydrates (the starch and sugar foods such as sweets, sugar, chocolates, cereals, bread, cakes, and potatoes) are essential, but should be taken in moderation since excess can interfere with digestion and may lead to obesity. The need for vitamins and mineral salts remains high and the best sources of these are fresh fruit and vegetables (although they are contained in some other foods too). Calcium is particularly important in the elderly because their bones become more brittle; it can be obtained from milk, cheese, tinned fish, and in some degree from green vegetables. Two pints of fluid daily should be taken whenever possible.

Physical Handicaps

Physical handicaps can hamper the elderly a great deal, but the health services today can do much to help ease their difficulties (see also p. 179 and p. 185).

Eyesight. Failing eyesight can be a major handicap and all too often this is accepted as inevitable. It can result in cutting the person off from many activities and cause a great deal of misery. Accidents can occur because of failing sight and result in loss of confidence and in some instances serious injury. In most cases, however, it can be remedied if a doctor or optician is consulted.

Deafness. This may cause a person to retreat into a world of his own and become apathetic. He soon gives up the strain of trying to hear and, in turn, family and friends may tire of trying to communicate with him. It is not always necessary to shout, but if the speaker stands so that the deaf person can see his mouth, and speaks clearly, it is surprising how well the deaf person can follow the conversation. Deafness may sometimes be caused by wax in the ears, and this can be remedied by the doctor. If, on the other hand, it is due to a more serious defect the doctor may recommend a hearing aid.

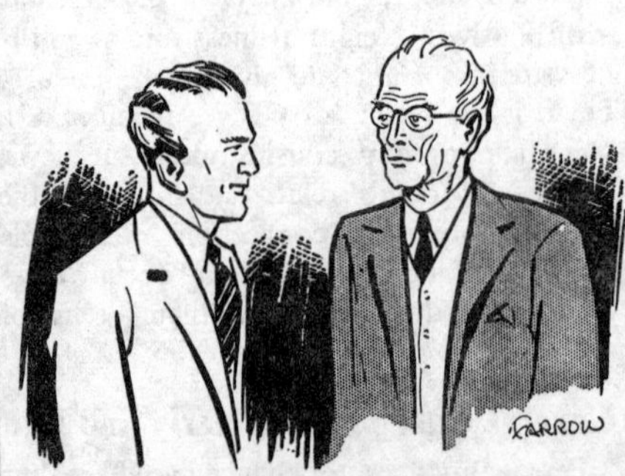

Fig. 7. *HELP THE DEAF PERSON by standing so that he can watch your lip movements.*

Dentures. Properly fitting dentures can make a great deal of difference to health and comfort. Gums may shrink causing the dentures to fit badly and be discarded. Too often this leads to inadequately chewed food, or requests for mashed, soft or 'slop' food. In turn this can cause indigestion and constipation.

Elderly people can be very resistant to adopting such aids. They frequently become rather set and rigid in their ways and cannot be bothered to make the necessary effort. If they can be tactfully persuaded, and perhaps accompanied for fittings, they will gain a great deal and avoid much misery.

Minor Ailments and Diseases

Weaknesses and disabilities which begin to be more noticeable in old age may be of recent onset or may have their origin in the past. A new symptom may cause further fears of dependence and result in instabilities and difficulties, and, although old people need to be shown sympathy, it is twice as useful when sympathy is combined with a cheerful spirit and practical help.

Digestive Disorders

INDIGESTION is common and it is often found that the person has suffered from this trouble earlier in life. Special diets are only useful if taken regularly and they may present difficulties about cooking or be beyond the purse. Dentures should be checked to ensure that food is being chewed properly and if necessary the doctor should be consulted.

CONSTIPATION is a common complaint but may become worse as increasing age leads to a more sedentary life. Practical points, such as ensuring that the toilet is easily accessible, the seat high enough and, if necessary, a handrail fitted on the wall, should be attended to. The doctor's advice should be taken about suitable drugs since too liberal a use of medications can produce diarrhea and be weakening.

There is a popular belief that eggs, milk and cheese should be avoided as they cause constipation, but these are very valuable foodstuffs for elderly people. Add fruit, particularly prunes, vegetables, brown bread and cereals to the diet of constipated persons, bearing in mind that an over-indulgence in fruit and vegetables may cause diarrhea. It may help to give a glass of hot water first thing in the morning to flush the system. If constipation persists the doctor's opinion should be sought.

Urinary Difficulties

FREQUENCY OR PAIN on passing water is common and may be due to a variety of causes. It may help to minimize night-time disturbance if little is drunk after 6 p.m., but the total daily intake should not be reduced. Urinary accidents are less likely to occur if the person has interests and occupations which keep him busy. If the condition persists consult the doctor.

Blood Circulation

Although many old people suffer from high blood pressure it may show few symptoms and in such cases it is often better for the sufferer not to know he has it. A quiet life, relaxation, and gentle exercise form the best régime, unless the doctor orders otherwise.

VARICOSE VEINS must be treated at whatever age they may occur and the treatment course may be prolonged. Slight abrasions in this condition can easily lead to ulcers. Bandaging under medical supervision and the use of elastic stockings may be essential.

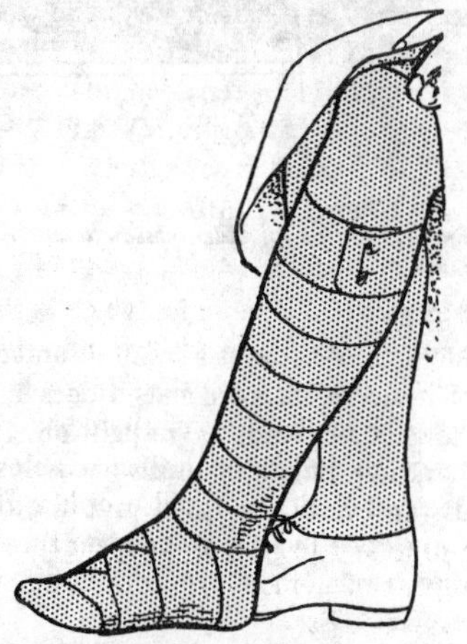

Fig. 8. *VARICOSE VEINS may need to be supported with bandages to enable the patient to live a more active life.*

Skin Disorders

SWEAT RASHES may occur where two skin surfaces meet, such as under the breast or in the groin, and may result in a shiny, cracked, red surface. Suitable clothing which is non-irritant (cotton, or wool-mixture fabrics) should be worn where this is likely to occur, and the skin surface should be cleaned and treated with a baby talcum powder or with zinc and castor oil ointment.

PRURITUS, OR ITCHING, is unpleasant and troublesome. The doctor should be consulted for treatment, and it is advisable to reduce the amount of detergent, bath salts, or soap used in washing. Frequent applications of ointment may be necessary.

FINGER- AND TOE-NAILS must be kept short and clean. As they often become rather horny in old age, they are best cut directly after a bath when the nail is softened. A watch should be kept when new shoes are worn as they may rub. Foot infections, causing inflammation or cracks in the skin between the toes, must be watched and cleared up completely with medicated powders or ointments. No one can be active if suffering 'from their feet.'

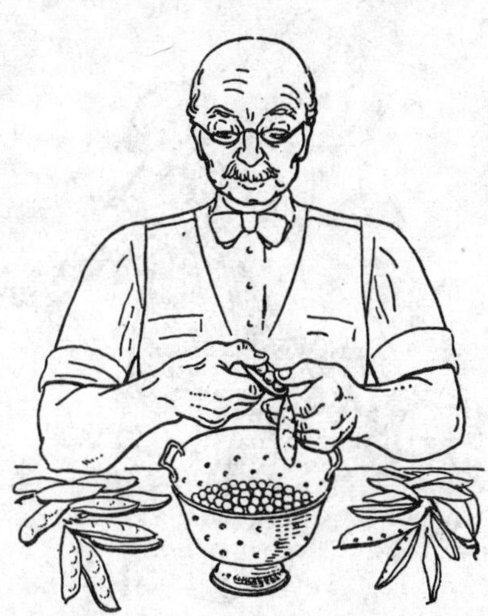

Fig. 9. *RHEUMATIC HANDS may be kept mobile by the mild exercise provided by homely jobs.*

Rheumatic Diseases

If a person has an acute, inflammatory and painful attack of rheumatism, rest in a firm and warm bed is essential. But in old people with one of the rheumatic diseases, the condition is often comparatively quiescent and chronic, and activities within the capacities of stiffened legs and fingers are very helpful in preventing further stiffening. Winding wool, dusting, shelling peas, writing letters, tidying up, and straightening drawers are homely jobs which help mobility without causing undue strain. Clinic treatment and exercise can be arranged through the patient's doctor.

Bronchitis

Chronic bronchitis can cause great suffering, and men suffer from it twice as frequently as women. Every effort should be made to prevent colds or chills which may lead to a bronchial affection. Each attack progressively weakens the tissues of the lungs, but careful nursing can improve the condition, and many bronchitic subjects learn to take sensible care of themselves. Patients should avoid changes of temperature, going out of doors in damp weather, and smoking—the latter should be given up completely; avoid being visited by persons with head colds. Breathing exercises can be most beneficial (see p. 196).

Strokes

These are the most feared of all the disorders of old age. They are caused by rupture of a blood vessel in the brain, and may vary in duration, severity and after-affects (for fuller details see Diseases of Old Age).

Accidents

Last, but not least as a cause of illness and disability in the elderly, is accidents. A recent survey revealed that 74 per cent of the fatal falls in the home involved old people over 75 years old.

Unexpected attacks of giddiness and loss of balance may be caused by sudden changes in posture. A sudden rush by a child or adult past an old person who is unsteady on his feet may easily cause him to lose his balance, and fall. In a household where there are people of varying ages the younger people should be made aware of these natural difficulties which come with old age and be prepared to go about the house more carefully when grandmother is around. Old people should be encouraged to sit down before bending to tie shoe laces and, where possible, sit down to dress. They should be discouraged from standing with one foot resting on a chair. It is wiser to call in a doctor when an old person has had a fall even when there does not appear to be any injury.

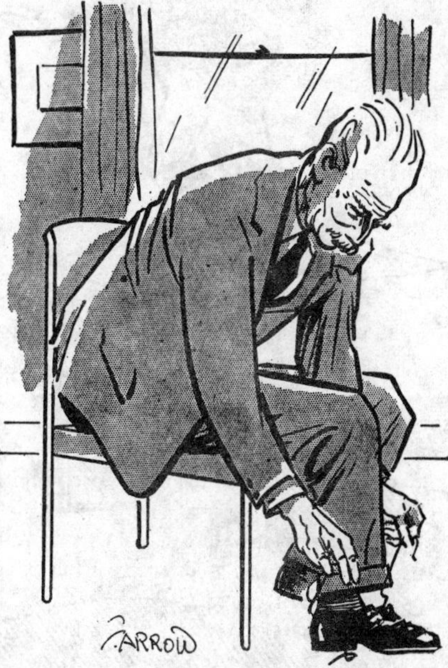

Fig. 10. *TYING UP SHOES. To avoid accidents from overbalancing, old people should sit down to tie up shoe laces.*

Senility

This is by far the most distressing and the most common disturbance in the seventies and eighties and can result in very considerable confusion both to the person concerned and to those caring for him. There can be loss of self-respect and carelessness about appearance, or loss of judgment or of moral standards. Placid people may become apathetic and indifferent. They may laugh or cry for no apparent reason or may talk constantly, repeating the same stories over and over again. They may show a general restlessness and a tendency to wander.

The condition can improve if care is taken. If it has started suddenly following some physical illness such as pneumonia, heart failure, etc., it may improve as the person gets better. It is more usual for this condition to come on slowly but this does not mean that the deterioration will continue. It is important to try to keep senile persons occupied and as active as possible, and it does demand much devoted patience on the part of those who care for these old people.

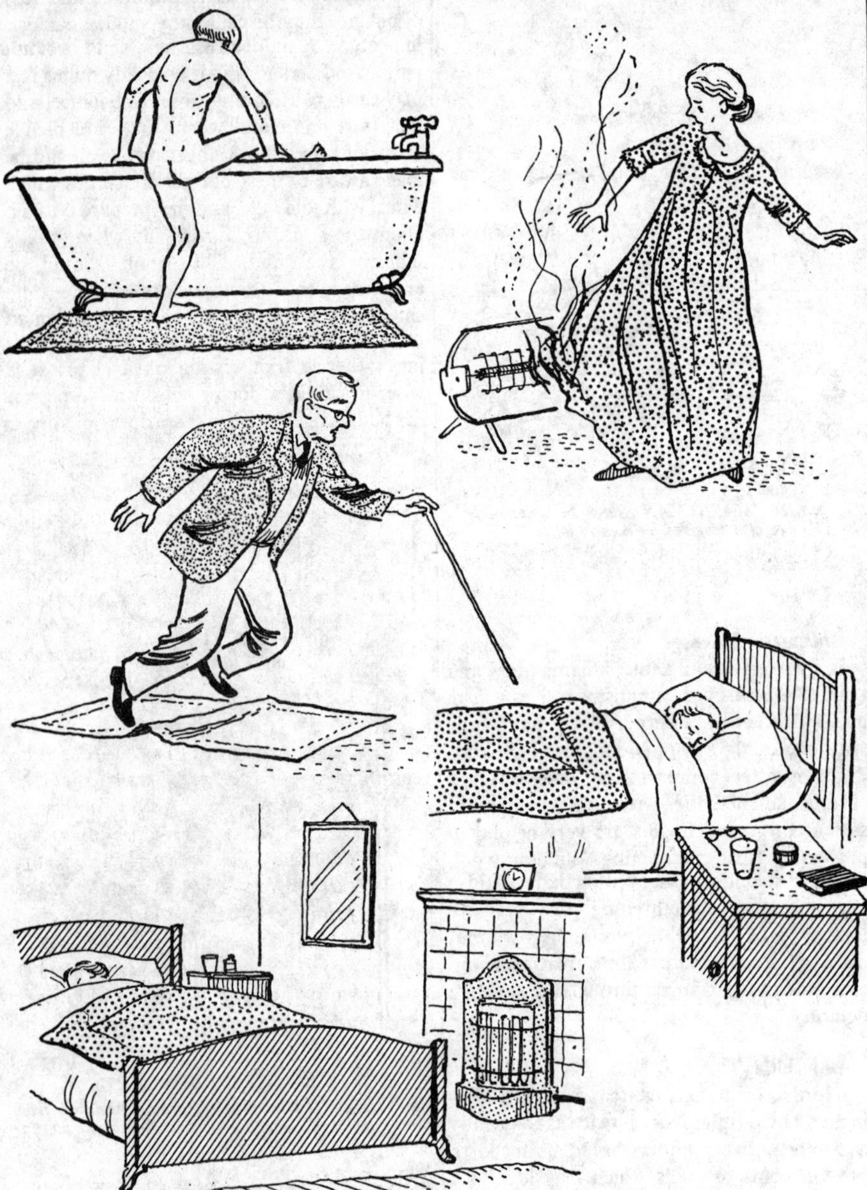

Fig. 11. *DANGERS TO AVOID. High baths; unguarded electric fires; wrinkled rugs; whole box of tablets at the bedside; gas fire left alight in sleeping person's room.*

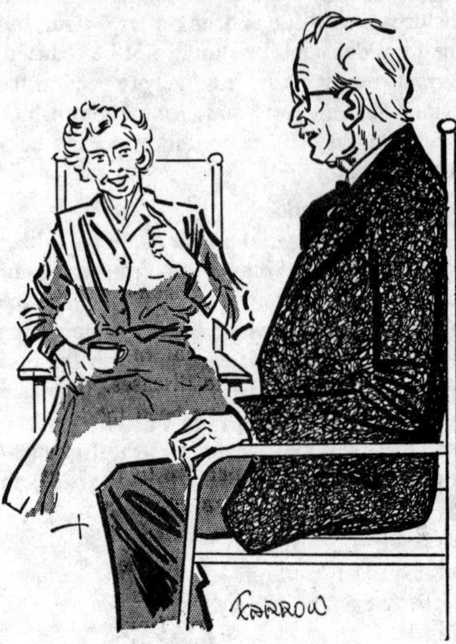

Fig. 12. *AN UPRIGHT CHAIR with arms is usually more comfortable for an older person than the low lounge type.*

Accidents may occur as a result of untacked edges of linoleum, insecure mats, ridges in carpets, a loose stair tread, a dim light on stairs, or no handrail. Small handrails fixed close to the bath and near the toilet give the older person a greater feeling of independence and security.

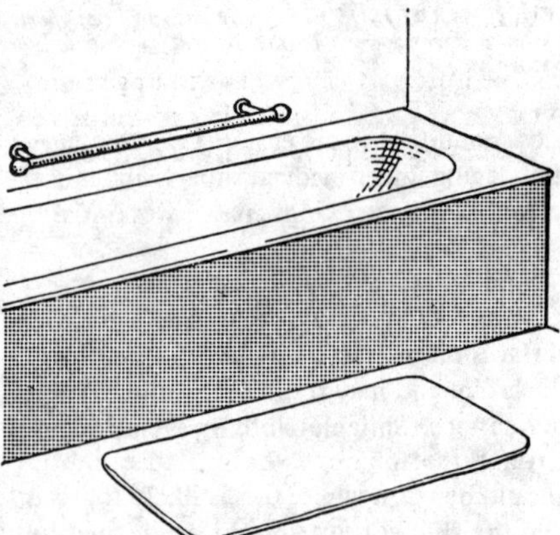

Fig. 13. *A HANDRAIL fixed to the side wall of the bath gives older persons a greater feeling of security.*

DEPRESSION should be taken seriously as there may be danger of suicide. It does not help to tell the sufferer to 'pull yourself together' but tranquilizer drug treatment under the doctor's guidance can often bring great relief. Depression usually passes off if the person is helped medically in this way in the acute stage and is gently encouraged to help in little ways about the house and to go out, or be taken out, for short periods.

DELIRIUM mostly occurs at night and is usually of short duration, and a night-light often helps to avoid its occurrence.

DELUSIONS may result in old persons fearing that others are talking about them, or trying to rob them, but not much can be done to remedy this, and reasoning with them rarely works.

MORAL DETERIORATION may occur in some men. Sexual desire may reawaken and may get the sufferer into trouble. The cause of this is not known, but it is wiser to consult the doctor if disorders of this type are suspected. Great care is needed to deal with this problem. Long-term psychological treatment is not possible and may be undesirable, but it is sometimes of help if the old man has someone to whom he can 'let off steam.'

Aids in the Home

Furniture. Many houses and some furniture are not suited to the needs of the elderly and the old, but a little ingenuity with regard to furniture can make life much more comfortable for them. The whole family will benefit since the old person will thereby gain greater independence. A fairly upright chair with arms is the most suitable, and extra cushions will give height. The fashionable low lounge chairs are not comfortable for the more rigid backs and joints of older people. A low bed can be heightened by an additional mattress.

Hand Aids. A great deal of crippling is caused by the rheumatic diseases. In recent years great advances have been made in the design of gadgets for the use of the disabled. Many of these are expensive to buy but are simple in design and can easily be designed and made at home. For those whose wrists and elbows have become stiff the handles of ordinary articles of use such as spoons and forks can be extended by welding or screwing a strip of metal on (see illustrations in Occupational Therapy, p. 367). When hands have become crippled it becomes extremely difficult to hold utensils but this can often be overcome by fixing bicycle handgrips to the handles of the utensils.

Walking sticks, tripod walking aids (see illustration in Physiotherapy, p. 178), and light metal elbow crutches greatly assist those whose walking has become unsteady.

Nursing the Elderly

At Home

The very old may pick up infections such as colds, influenza, or bronchitis easily and there may be no rise of temperature. Complete rest in bed is seldom needed and should be discouraged wherever possible. Once old people take to their beds it may be difficult to get them up again. It may seem cruel to try to get them up and about but it is for their own good. Continuous lying in bed leads to weakened muscles and joints, to minor ailments and, in some instances, to congestion of the lungs, particularly if the patient is lying flat.

Details for nursing at home are given on p. 49, but it is well to consider the following special points when nursing the elderly.

1. They need a lot of fluids, at least two pints daily. It helps if sugar and a little common salt are given with some of the drinks.

2. Do not leave boxes of tablets in the bedroom. Old people frequently become a little confused and may take too many by mistake.

3. Give them plenty of encouragement to remain as active as possible and keep them in touch with life going on around them.

4. They are frightened of silent consultations with the doctor, and should be drawn into conversation about their own treatment whenever possible.

5. If there is a danger of incontinence a protective pad across the bed may help. Rubber sheets over mattresses are usually advisable.

6. Bedpans should be avoided whenever possible and the patient encouraged to use the toilet or commode.

7. Bedclothes may become heavy on the feet: a pillow, or small stool turned upside down, at the bottom of the bed makes an effective foot cradle (see also Home Nursing, p. 46).

8. It is necessary for people with heart or chest complaints to be propped up in bed. This makes breathing easier. If no back rest is available, cushions will suffice.

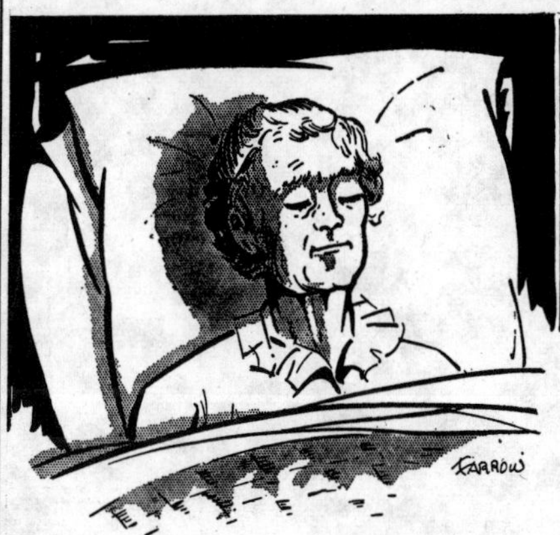

Fig. 14. *WEAK HEART. Persons with heart disorders or chest complaints should sleep propped up with several pillows.*

9. Patients confined to bed should have a good wash daily and a bed bath as often as possible. Where families find this difficult the visiting nurse may be able to help.

Day Hospitals and Geriatric Units

Experience over the last few years has shown that rehabilitation of old people, although slow and laborious, is possible. Where admission to hospital is necessary it should be regarded, as with other age groups, as a temporary measure, and geriatric units are being developed along these lines. Outpatient treatment departments are being extended to give more service to older patients. Day care centers, as the name suggests, provide medical treatment and physiotherapy, and also keep the elderly occupied and active in company with others: the old people return to their homes at night. Social services for the elderly are increasing. Some geriatric units have arrangements to admit people to their convalescence ward for a few weeks to give the family a holiday.

Residential Accommodation. If an old person becomes exceedingly frail and sick, and requires expert care, it may be necessary for him to go to a hospital geriatric unit or into a Home. This has to be arranged by the family doctor. Every effort is made to make the old people as comfortable and cheerful as possible. Although they may be apprehensive about going, most of them quickly settle down particularly if letters and visitors keep them in contact with home.

WOMAN AND BEAUTY

Whatever her age or circumstances, every woman should make the most of whatever beauty Nature has given her, and supplement its deficiencies with Art. She should consider it her duty—to herself, her family and all the people she meets in the course of the day—to put her best face forward, in every sense of the word.

The woman who thinks she has no time for good grooming is only confessing to a feeling of inferiority. She is not only selling herself short, but also her family and her work, be it at home or outside. The world judges much by external appearances, and she who cannot organize her own looks may be thought to be no better at organizing her home, or any other work.

Foundations of Beauty

The foundations of beauty go deeper than cosmetics and are built on simple rules of health and beauty care. Fresh air, exercise, sound sleep and a properly balanced diet help towards a lovely skin, and one of the most important parts of beauty care for every woman is impersonal examination of the good points to be brought out and the poor points which might well be kept in the background. This sincere reflection constitutes an elementary beauty treatment. She who straightens her spine, holds her head up and her chin pressed in instead of forward will eliminate 'sag,' the greatest enemy of beauty.

A well-fitting brassière is no substitute for good deportment, but rather a most valuable support, both physical and moral, to supplement it. 'Well-fitting' is important since no teenager or young woman should flatten her nipples with a tight bra and run the risk of inverting them, thus laying up difficulties for herself when later she may have a baby to nurse.

Foundation garments are of primary importance, as in many women they can literally preserve or ruin the wearer's health. Into this category come elastic stockings, whether of the surgical type, obtainable to measure by prescription, or of the support type now universally on sale. It is false vanity for any woman who needs even the slightest support not to wear suitable stockings, as it would be for her not to wear a brassière.

She must remember that a despondent droop of mind registers itself quickly on the features but at the first hint of renewed interest in life the eyelids lift, the muscles of the cheeks lift and the corners of the mouth cease to droop. The skin too must be given daily attention for it can be the most valuable asset or the most damaging liability to any face.

Beauty Treatment

In recent years, great progress has been achieved in all branches of beauty treatment, so much so, in fact, that it is sometimes difficult to choose the most appropriate.

For the woman of means, it is simple: the great surgeons, and expensive salons are at her disposal. But the less fortunate can also benefit today: in many cases a serious facial defect can be corrected by operation, as also can one of figure. Rejuvenating treatments for the face, once the prerogative of the rich, are now available in budget sizes at local pharmacies but, as the packs contain active biological elements, they should be used with care and certainly by no one under the age of thirty. One should not, however, wait till then before beginning beauty treatment: on the contrary, the proper cleansing and care of the skin should begin in adolescence.

CARE OF THE FACE

Cleanliness is the first essential, for otherwise the skin will become muddy and perhaps infected and no cosmetics can camouflage an impure skin.

A successful beauty treatment must be carried out in a strong light, day or artificial, with the aid of a clear, flawless mirror. Cleansing creams, astringent lotion, powder and make-up should be placed on a table in front of the mirror so that the treatment may be carried out in comfort and relaxation, without the physical effort of jumping up to look for something that has been forgotten.

The head should be tied up in a lightweight cloth so that no stray hair can fall about the face. Wash your hands before touching your face. Carelessness may turn one isolated infected spot into an unpleasant skin eruption.

There are so many makes of cleansing cream available that no rule can specially be advised, except that the cleansing cream must be extremely light and easy to work into the skin, and easy to remove.

For those who prefer something lighter, they are cleansing milks and lotions, and baby lotion or baby oil are also excellent. For those who dislike creams made from animal fats, there are others made with wax and vegetable constituents. Inexpensive cleansing creams and lotions are easily obtainable at the drug and department stores.

Your Skin Type and its Care

Dry Skin

Early in life a dry skin is delightfully trouble free, but later, because the skin produces insufficient oil, it develops fine lines and wrinkles. A dry skin needs gentle care, neglected it ages quickly and become parched and crêpey.

CLEANSING must be thorough but non-drying. Apply cleanser with fingertips, massage gently with upward and outward movement. Allow cleanser to remain on skin for a little while before wiping it off gently with tissues. Soap and water may be used once a day, preferably at night when they can be followed up by skinfood. Do not use very hot water or strongly perfumed soap. Both are drying. A bland soap specially made for dry skins is best. Every scrap of soap must be rinsed away and the skin patted dry, never rubbed. Be especially careful around the eye area, where the skin is most dry and sensitive.

TONING. Use a mild skin tonic once a day. Pat lightly on to the skin with cotton, taking care not to stretch the skin.

NOURISHING is the most vital beauty need for dry skin. Always follow night cleansing with cream. Smooth it on gently upward and outward. Include your neck. Don't put on too much. Skin can absorb only a small amount, the rest is wasted.

Greasy Skin

The constant flow of oil relaxes the pores and, unless the skin is kept scrupulously clean, the pores clog with grease and stale make-up and grime. Blackheads develop, followed by tender fiery spots which can lead to acne.

CLEANSING thoroughly is vital for this type of skin. Liquid cleansers are best, applied with cotton, smoothed over the skin in an upward and outward direction. Soap and water can be massaged in or worked gently in with a soft complexion brush or baby's hair brush, which stimulates the circulation.

TONING. This is extremely important for oily skins as they are often sluggish and need stimulation. After each cleansing apply a good astringent, strong if your skin is very oily, medium otherwise. Soak a pad of cotton in astringent and wipe the face with it. Then hold the pad firmly and slap it against the skin all over the face except around the eye area, which is very sensitive. Astringents remove the last trace of oiliness and pep up the circulation. As a result the skin gets a healthy glow and will keep make-up on for much longer.

NOURISHING. A greasy skin barely needs nourishing as the active oil glands do this adequately themselves. Never use rich cream on this type of skin. It will only clog the pores. The only area that might be dry is around the eyes. If necessary, use a special eye cream or oil at night or before having a bath.

Dual-type Skin

This kind of complexion has a greasy center panel down forehead, nose and chin, while the rest of the face tends to be dry. Dual-type skins are by no means rare, especially among young girls. Later in life the oily panel tends to get drier. With this type of skin, you must treat both parts separately. This may be difficult at first, but you will soon acquire the knack of it.

CLEANSING must be thorough, but the oily area needs conscientious cleansing while the dry area requires gentler cleansing—see dry and greasy skin. This is when a complexion brush comes in handy; it will help to get the lather where it is needed—nowhere else.

TONING. Plenty of vigorous toning for the center panel—less and milder toning for the cheeks. Should you have dilated pores on your nose, soak a piece of cotton in astringent, smooth it over your nose and leave for a few minutes.

NOURISHING. You will probably only need a light skin food for the cheeks and the eye area. Never let the cream reach the oily center panel.

Normal Skin

Normal skin is a rare gift. It looks naturally lovely and poses no problems. Such a treasure is worth guarding. Sensible diet, plentiful rest and wisely-applied make-up will keep it smooth and attractive. But even a normal skin isn't guaranteed for life. Change of climate or health upheavals may cause it to become either greasy or dry. In which case, adjust your beauty routine.

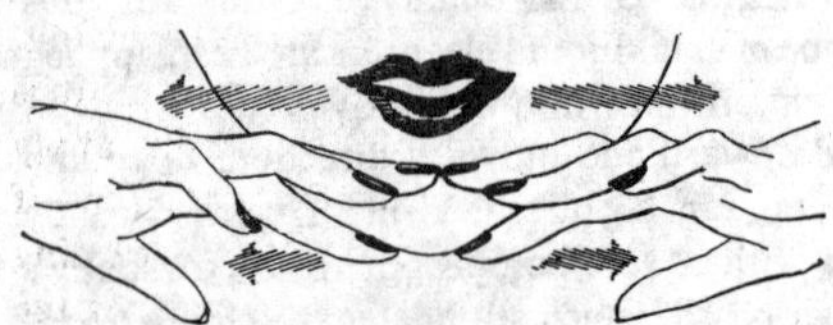

Fig. 1. *TO PREVENT CHIN SAG. Stroke the under-chin upwards and outwards.*

Night Treatment

Bedtime is often suitable for extra beauty care. Try to allow yourself 30 minutes before bedtime—even 10 minutes will be useful—for your basic cleansing, plus one extra beauty task.

Cleanse, tone and nourish your face according to your skin type, working the cream in lightly and firmly with an upward movement starting at the base of the throat, passing to the jaw bones, and then over the cheeks, in towards the nose until the whole face is covered with cream.

The cheeks should then be lifted into a smile until a roundness feels firm to the touch of the finger tips.

At the same time it is a good plan to inhale a deep breath through the nostrils and hold this breath for about five seconds, then exhale it slowly without relaxing any of the muscles of the cheeks. The head should be bent back slowly and then lowered to the original position, and the cheeks relaxed.

Now fresh blood will be flowing through the newly exercised tissues and the pores of the skin slightly opened to release their waste products into the cleansing cream on the surface.

The cream must be removed almost immediately, in the same upward movement always. For this purpose small pieces of old toweling or soft linen are the best cleansers. Tissues or cotton may be used, but there is nothing better than soft toweling to give a firm and thorough pull, without dragging the skin.

The practice of first using a damp piece of cotton is not really a good one. It may feel refreshing, but it is inclined to form a kind of emulsion as it mixes with the cream, and thus clogs the pores. Use a dry remover first and, when the skin is completely free from all traces of shine, then use a damp remover.

It is extremely important always to retain the upward movement in cleaning or drying the face so as to counteract the tendency to sag, which is natural in the delicate tissue of the facial muscles.

A second cleansing, with liquid if cream has been used the first time, is usually needed to remove further impurities.

As soon as the skin is clean, it may be treated with a skin food or moisturizer to prevent it drying up. Inexpensive skin foods and moisturizers usually contain less expensive perfumes but all are equally useful. In the case of the older woman whose delicate tissues have begun to sag, a skin-toning astringent cream should be used. For the upper lids a lubricating eye cream is best and an astringent one for the lower lids.

A rejuvenating preparation will give marvellously youthful results in a very short time but, being biologically active, it may spread an infection from a boil or pimple. So, at the first sign of a spot, it should not be used on the forehead, nose and chin, but confined to the skin at the outer corners of the eyes, taking care not to let any of the cream into the eyes themselves.

Rejuvenating creams, like anti-wrinkle preparations of all kinds, should not be used every day. Three days' treatment, then a rest of a day or two, then three more days' treatment is adequate. These biological creams are usually sold along with a special astringent, which must be used first to prepare the skin to absorb them.

These creams, like moisturizers, will soak into the skin, but the skin foods properly so-called are often so rich in lanolin or some other lubricant that they must be wiped off before retiring for the night, so that the skin may breathe freely.

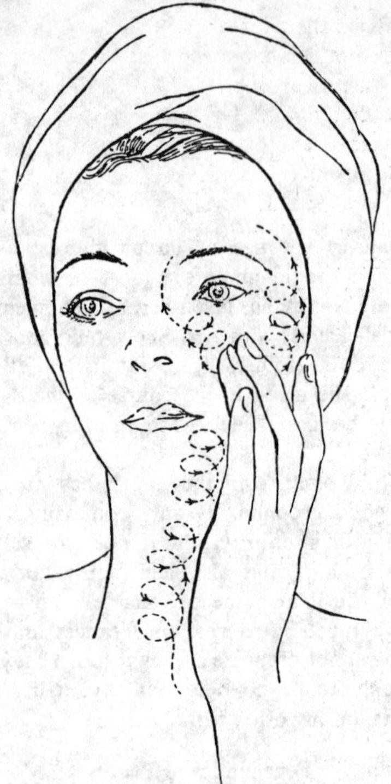

Fig. 2. *THE CORRECT METHOD OF APPLYING CLEANSING CREAM TO THE NECK AND FACE. The upward spiral movement helps to counteract the droop of the small facial muscles particularly those around the eyes.*

Morning Treatment

For morning treatment or at any time immediately preceding the application of make-up, after cleansing, the pores are closed by dabbing the skin gently with a final pad of cotton moistened with astringent lotion, or a small quantity of water to which two or three drops of alcohol have been added.

The eyes should then be wiped with a pad of cotton dipped in cool water containing a pinch of salt or a small quantity of cool (not too cold) weak tea; and then the face is ready for its make-up.

Owing to the atmospheric contamination which is so prevalent today, a sensitive skin, especially in winter, should always be protected, even under make-up, by a moisturizer or germicidal ointment, to prevent chapping. Powder should never be applied directly to the skin: it is drying, and can lead to wrinkles. Some foundation should always intervene, even if it is only a thin layer of cleansing milk.

Masks and Face Packs

Before making-up for a special occasion, it is desirable to stimulate the face and neck with a mask: either a ready-made product of the jelly or cream type which can be quickly applied and easily removed or, if time permits, the more thorough-going home-made pack.

More than an hour should be allowed for the use of the pack or mask, as it must be given enough time to draw the impurities out of the skin, and then be removed.

While the pack dries, it pulls the muscles, therefore it is more satisfactory to lie down, so that the tissues will avoid the dragging sensation that the weight must give. Complete relaxation at the same time is a good plan, so that the nerves and facial muscles will be rested as well as the skin.

When the face pack is perfectly dry, both hands should be pressed over the surface of the face, and the mask will crack and crumble off in small pieces. This cannot be hurried as the tiny particles tend to remain, especially when the face has an inclination to be downy.

Go over the whole face carefully, cracking and dusting off the small pieces and then, if this seems to take too much time and is difficult, a towel may be wrung out of tepid or warm water and held over the face.

Never bathe, nor splash water on a pack. Use as little moisture as possible, and then apply cold cream generously and very lightly in an upward movement.

When the cream has cleared away all traces of the pack the face will feel young and fresh, and it can then be dabbed with a piece of cotton sprinkled with a mild astringent lotion—such as rose water or cooled boiled water containing a few drops of scented essence.

Home-made Packs

A good general rule is to use a drying pack on an oily skin, and an oily pack on a dry skin. Both can be stimulating or bleaching, but they work in different ways.

Fuller's Earth Pack. Perhaps the best known pack is made with fuller's earth. It seems to suit all types of skin and is specially good when there are slight blemishes to be removed. Use not more than once a week.

This healing preparation can also be the foundation for several other packs. For general purposes use:

One tablespoonful of fuller's earth,
One tablespoonful of boiled water, or Rose Water, or witch hazel water.

Mix the powder into a thin paste with the water and rub out all the lumps. It then becomes a 'mud pack,' and is spread over the face with the finger tips, or a bone spatula. The mixture can be made thicker or thinner as preferred, and might have a few drops of castor oil added. As this pack has a rather unpleasant smell a few, but only a few, drops of eau de Cologne may be added. Leave the pack on the face for 10 to 20 minutes, before crumbling it off.

Oatmeal Pack. Oatmeal has been well known throughout the ages as a face cleanser, and may be used successfully as a mask. Take:

One tablespoonful of fine oatmeal,
One tablespoon, or more, of warm water,
One teaspoonful of salad oil.

The ingredients are mixed in a small bowl and smoothed over the face.

Oatmeal with a little honey and water added can also make a delightful mask.

Oil Pack. When oil (almond or olive preferably) is plentiful a small quantity can be warmed in a basin standing in another basin of hot water. To the oil add as much honey as will cover the tip of a teaspoon. The mixture is smoothed over the face, and a thin warm towel is pressed lightly over the face to keep the oil warm.

For 'elderly' complexions this is an extremely beneficial pack, and can be repeated once a week for six weeks. By that time the muscles should be stimulated, and the skin made more supple.

Mashed Potato with two or three drops of light ammonia added can do wonders for a faded neck. It can be used two or three times a week on the neck, and should not be placed much above the jaw line, as it is a drastic pack and should be well tested before trying it on the neck.

Strawberry Pack. This is excellent for toning up the skin. It is made from either a purée of strawberries, or fine slices laid flat on the skin. Cucumber slices may be used similarly.

Yeast Pack. About a teaspoonful of yeast made into a paste with milk and used as a pack is softening and bleaching.

Yolk of Egg. Occasionally the yolk of an egg is advised as a quick pack, but though extremely beneficial, it is a mistaken idea to think it can be used quickly. The benefit is in the drawing together of the pores of the skin, and the pack must be crumbled off when nearly dry. No water should be used for removal.

Homely Skin Aids. When there is no time to prepare a pack a last minute aid from the kitchen may be useful.

All these aids are slightly drying and must be removed by cream or very soft water before retiring for the night.

BEETROOT slices can take the place of rouge before powdering.

RAW POTATO. When a refreshing treatment is needed, a thick slice of raw potato rubbed briskly over the face (always in an upward direction) will have an astringent and bleaching effect.

The moisture should be removed immediately with cotton or soft linen, and the skin will then be ready to take the usual powder and rouge.

MASHED TURNIPS. A generous spread of mashed turnips, as cold as possible, has a bleaching and softening effect on a dry skin. This mash may be rubbed in with the finger tips before removal.

RAW TOMATO JUICE. Raw tomato juice is a good astringent wash.

VINEGAR. Vinegar diluted with a little water is a remedy for rough blotchy skin.

Make-up

Always leave enough time to make up, however simply, having first brushed the teeth and given them any further treatment that is necessary with a toothpick or spool of dental floss.

On occasions when one is not feeling one's best, it may give a sense of freshness to chew chlorophyll breath mints. A liberal application of eau de Cologne or toilet water, perfumed or otherwise, is pleasant for one's escort or friends, and a tonic to oneself.

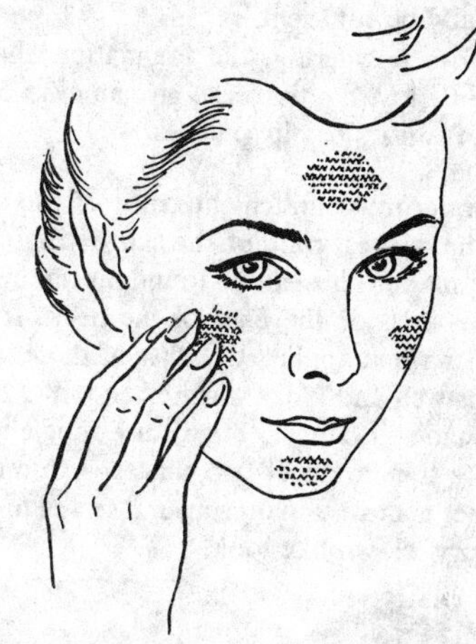

Fig. 3. *HOW TO APPLY FOUNDATION CREAM. The four spots of cream are gently spread over the skin with the fingertips.*

The Base. Some protective base for make-up should be applied first, and there are several creams on the market which incorporate colored foundation, powder and moisturizer combined. Others, again, combine only powder and foundation, and require to be applied over a separate moisturizer or lubricant.

Many of these products are excellent but, on days when the skin is irritated and it is desirable to avoid infection, simply apply loose powder over a separate foundation—if possible a germicidal ointment or cleansing milk. In that way, the dangers of clogging the pores are reduced, and the risk of infection is minimized.

It is worth noting here that sufferers from hay fever or other allergies can obtain a complete range of preparations (hypo-allergic products) free of irritating allergy-producing ingredients; some special lipsticks and lip barrier creams are also free of such ingredients.

There are also day cosmetics, like cleansing creams, free from animal fats. They are made from vegetable mucilages and contain extracts of elderflowers, cucumbers and other plants.

In addition to the protective base, older women may prefer to use a little rejuvenating cream, eye cream or oil under their make-up: this should be patted in with a tissue before applying the foundation, which at that age should never be very dark, to avoid a hot-and-bothered look.

Those who are not using an all-in-one make-up have the choice of liquid or cream base, colored or otherwise. Color, however, demands care in its application. A heavy jawline, for instance, can be shaded out with dark foundation and rouge; a less than perfect nose can be straightened out with a line of pale foundation applied from bridge to tip.

Naturally these extra shades of base mean more expenditure of time and money but, with practice, the application becomes second nature, and a single shade of powder will generally be sufficient.

Before powdering, the foundation should be blotted with a tissue, to give an even base, free of smears or oily patches.

Powder must match the color of the skin and the darkest tone of the skin is the right color shade. This can be found on the inside of the wrist or the base of the neck. If the powder when applied to either of these spots blends well and looks warm, then that will be the shade to choose, but if in doubt always choose the darker of two shades. A too light powder is most unflattering and serves to give a floury, clown-like look.

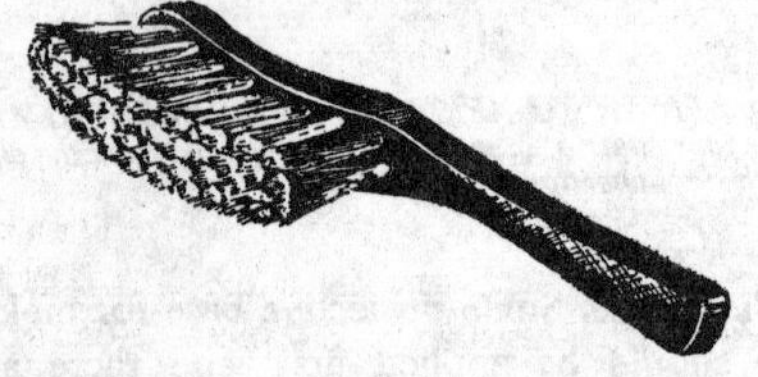

Fig. 4. *THE COMPLEXION BRUSH should have very soft bristles.*

To get the smoothest most velvety finish, powder should be applied plentifully with clean cotton and then brushed into the skin with a very soft-bristled complexion brush. Always brush the powder downwards (this is almost the only downward movement in beauty care).

A large nose should not be over-powdered or the feature will appear to come forward.

Before powdering the nose see that the pores are thoroughly clean and free from grease. The nostrils should be gently pressed if the pores are stopped up. The contents will then come out, and fresh powder must be dusted over, especially where the nostril joins the upper lip.

Rouge. There are two kinds of rouge—dry and cream. Dry is perhaps the simplest to apply, but cream rouge is more natural-looking and lasts longer. Dry rouge goes on after the first powdering and before the second, and cream rouge goes on before a liquid foundation or after a cream one, and always before powder. The right place for rouge can be found by smiling until little 'bunches' come up on the cheeks. Color should be applied deepest here and fanned well outwards for a thin face, and towards the center for a wide one. A hint of rouge on the chin is shortening for a long face, but

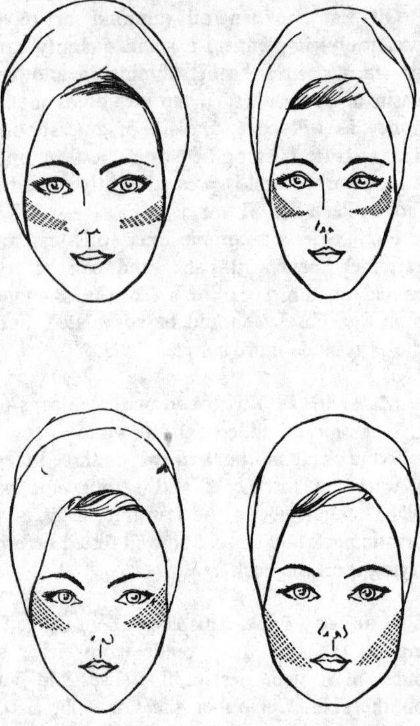

Fig. 5. *THE ROUGE TRIANGLE. For each type of face rouge should be placed in a different position. Top: for the round face and the long face. Below: for the pointed face and the broad face. All hard edges must be shaded away in an upward and outward direction.*

apart from this, color should never be placed below the level of the tip of the nose. One golden rule is to apply rouge in a strong full light, and never in a side light or dark corner.

After application, the rouge should be dusted with powder.

Lip Make-up. There are so many changes in fashion where lipstick is concerned—sometimes it is even dispensed with altogether—that it is difficult to lay down hard and fast rules for its use. Some lip color is necessary to balance the different features of the face: if in doubt choose a shade as near as possible to your own blood coloring; and if that is unobtainable wear a red lipsalve rather than no color at all. Like a lip barrier cream, this is an excellent protective, when the skin is irritated, for wearing under ordinary lipstick.

To avoid stretching and splitting the skin of the lips in cold weather, it is as well to apply the color with a brush, rather than to use the lipstick itself. Should acidity be present on 'off' days, when the chemical balance of the body changes and the skin may look yellowish, any blue in a lipstick will be intensified, with unflattering results.

Bluish lipsticks are often aging, as are the darker reds and, indeed, dark shades of make-up in general. In later life, therefore, one may prefer to abandon the solid reds hitherto used, and choose instead a more coral shade, or a flame-pink with not too much orange, not too much blue, in its composition.

Having chosen your color, trace the outline of the lips with a red liner or brown eyebrow pencil; then go over it and fill in with a brush which has been rubbed on the lipstick, stretching the mouth open slightly to fill in the corners. If desired, blot on a tissue and add a dusting of powder to fix the color.

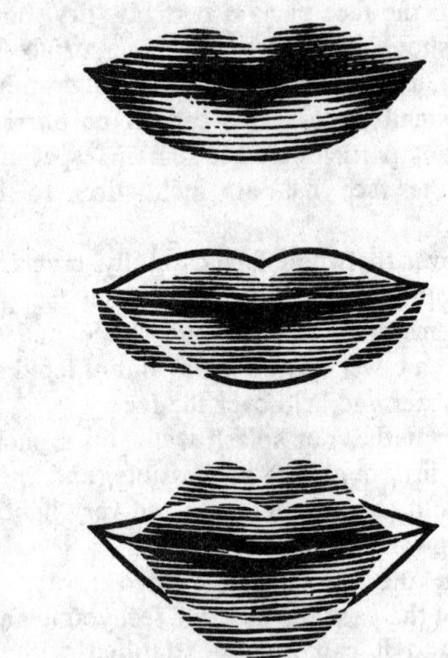

Fig. 6. *THE RIGHT AND WRONG WAY OF APPLYING LIPSTICK. The first illustration shows the correct way following the natural color line of the mouth. The second shows unsuccessful reshaping with the natural line showing through. The third shows an exaggerated shape out of keeping with the natural shape.*

A 'paintbox' of lipsticks is not necessary, but the lower lip can be made to look fuller with a lighter shade, or one with a gold or pearly finish, while a dark outline, filled in with one shade lighter, can look lively and attractive.

Eyebrows and Eyelashes. Eyebrows and eyelashes must be brushed with a special brush kept for them. Often the skin beneath the eyebrow retains dust and dirt. This must be brushed and cleaned away and instantly the eyes appear brighter. Every trace of powder and grease must also be removed with the small eyebrow brush.

Straggling hairs above and below the brows may be plucked out one by one with tweezers and, in spite of being slightly painful to do, the brows should be narrowed and trimmed towards the ends.

Nothing is so aging as superfluous hair straggling down from the outer wings of the eyebrows, which should always be tapered, slightly upwards if possible, into a neat point. As such radical plucking in middle age can be a great strain on the eyesight, it is well worth the expense to get this done professionally. After plucking the eyebrows, eau de Cologne or surgical alcohol should be applied, to close the holes and avoid infection.

The shape can be corrected with soft short strokes of black lead-pencil or eyebrow pencil; a combination of brown and gray pencils, or a brownish-black one, gives a more natural effect than a hard black line.

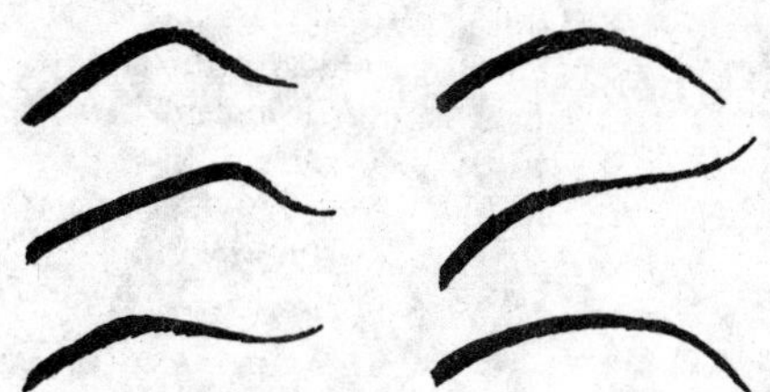

Fig. 7. *EYEBROW SHAPES. Experiment with these shapes to find the one that suits you best.*

MASCARA also can be used to define the brows, but they must make a neat frame for the face, giving an air of youthful serenity.

The eyelashes should be brushed and groomed, either with vaseline or with mascara. This is best applied in cream or liquid form (either is more hygenic than water-black in cake form) with a roller or brush.

Though many colors are on the market the best are still black, brownish-black, dark brown, dark blue or dark gray –the last often very attractive for the older woman.

EYESHADOW, like lipstick, is now an everyday cosmetic. To avoid pressing on the eyeballs and so causing small blood vessels to break in the eyes, it is best to apply eyeshadow with a lipstick brush, not a stick.

It is not necessary that the eyeshadow should match the eyes or the mascara, but women with small, deep-set eyes can make them appear more prominent and sparkling by applying thickly, all over the dome of the lid, gold or silver shadow. Even in daytime this is by no means gaudy; on the contrary, as these are not 'colors' in the strict sense of the word, it is pleasing and neutral.

Here again, a rainbow of shades is not necessary; for most purposes it is enough to paint a thick line along the roots of the eyelashes with dark gray, brownish-black or dark brown. On the right face, black or off-black (a gray-black) is very striking, as also can be dark blue. Dark green can make all the difference to eyelids reddened by the cold.

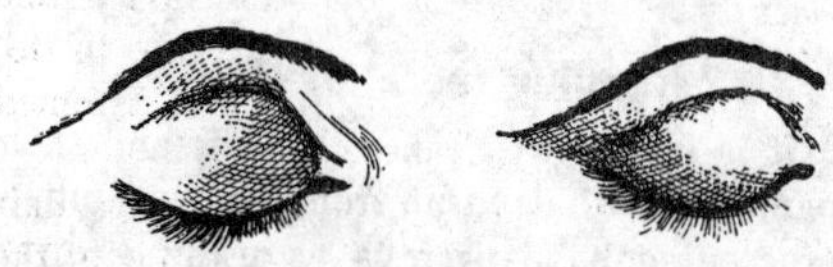

Fig. 8. *EYE SHADOW. For the heavy-lidded eye* (left) *cover entire lid lightly with eye shadow. For the full eye* (right) *place eye shadow low on the eye lid, sweeping it to the outer corner as illustrated.*

Final Touches. The next point of grooming is to see that no powder has been left inside the nostrils. They may be powdered but at the same time thoroughly cleaned, otherwise they appear dark and deep in contrast with the powdered face.

The make-up completed, the head band can then be removed and the hair brushed loosely from the face and rearranged. The general reflection should then be pleasing and gratifying.

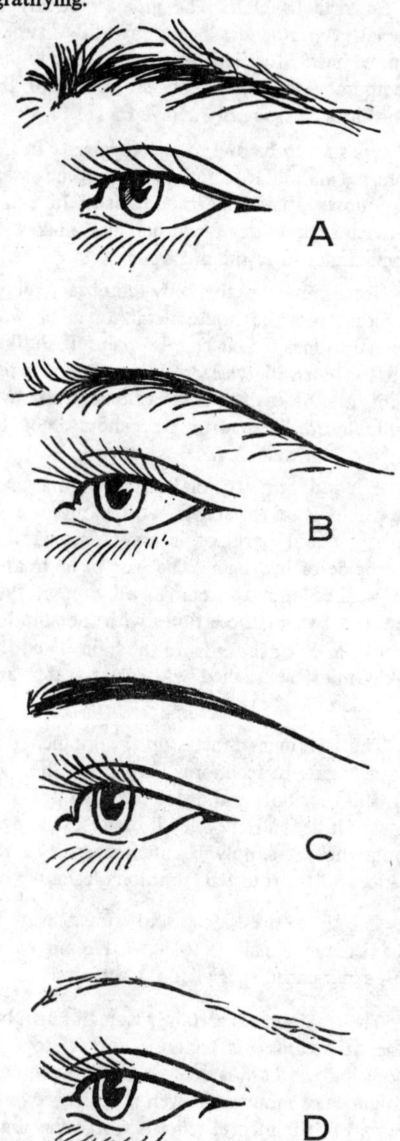

Fig. 9. *EYEBROW TRIMMING.* A. *The natural eyebrow.* B. *After stray hairs have been plucked from the top.* C. *A smoothly trimmed eyebrow with tapering end.* D. *An over-trimmed eyebrow with untidy tuft.*

Facial Blemishes

There are, speaking generally, two kinds of facial blemishes: those which need surgical or mechanical aid, and those which can be regulated and cured at home.

Correction is all that the second kind needs and every care should be taken to deal with them as soon as they appear, for nothing is more damaging to a beautiful exterior than pimples, blackheads, red patches and other temporary eruptions. Pimples may often occur in youth but they are not necessarily part of youth and should be corrected as soon as they begin to appear.

Acne is a common kind of eruption associated with spots and pimples, and is usually more prevalent during puberty. Washing the face with medicated soap often reduces the inflammation. For stubborn cases, see medical treatment in section on Diseases of the Skin.

Pimples or Spots. Pimples generally appear in a specially greasy area, around the chin or the sides of the nose. In all cases they are tiny spots of infection, and the warm greasy bed may be a breeding ground for germs.

Several pimples together denote a patch of infected skin; single spots, which are hard and inflamed, or even throbbing, denote the presence of one germ-infected focus which, if neglected, may lead to a boil, and then one boil leads to another, until a doctor must be consulted. It is unwise to tamper with a boil without medical advice.

In the case of pimples the skin must be kept perfectly clean and dry. No grease at all should be used as grease spreads infection readily. Soap and warm water only is the way to clean a patch of pimples. Sulphur soap should be used, and it is best to use sulphur powder rather than ordinary talcum to dust the back, which may be infected from dandruff in the hair.

If the heads of the spots are to be opened, one small prick with the point of a sterilized needle is enough, and then the pus can be pressed out gently with a piece of cotton.

If the spot is not ready to open, do not try to force it, as the cells are likely to break inwardly and the infection spreads under the skin. Never rub the spots with the fingers, and always dab a spot of antiseptic lotion over the newly cleansed place.

Blackheads. It is helpful to adjust the diet, cutting down firmly on starchy, greasy and fried foods and increasing salads, green vegetables and raw and cooked fruits. Constipation should at all costs be guarded against and as much water as possible should be taken.

Blackheads, small or large, are all tiny centers of infection. Small ones, if neglected, can cause coarse skin or open pores. Large ones if neglected soon turn to throbbing spots, and should never be tampered with.

Many a large spot or pimple was once a small blackhead that was only half removed or driven into the skin. For that reason it will be seen that the removal of blackheads is a serious business and plenty of time must be allowed for it. Never 'dash' at a blackhead just before going out. Wait till the blackhead can be seen in a strong light.

Wash the area in which it is with soap and water; or wring a piece of cotton out of hot water and hold it to the blackhead to loosen the surrounding grease.

Cover one finger of each hand with a cloth and press a certain distance away from the blackhead. Continue to press firmly and the blackhead will gradually appear and drop out. To begin to press close to the blackhead drives it into the skin, and it may never come out again without an operation.

As soon as the pore is empty, dab it with peroxide of hydrogen to prevent infection.

Red Patches. These may be the result of a nervous strain, or an acid condition in the blood. Perhaps one special item of diet is not just suitable at the moment. Shellfish produce red patches on the face in certain individuals who are allergic to them.

All greasy applications must be strictly avoided, and no ointments may be used. Only dry bicarbonate of soda, or damp washes of Epsom salts.

Red Veins. These unsightly veins on the cheeks and bridge of the nose show that the small surface blood vessels are overdilated. A transient flush may be due to dyspepsia but when the dilatation is permanent the blood pressure may be high or there may be some weakness of the heart; a tendency for such veins to appear in middle age seems to occur in some families. Liquids such as strong tea or coffee must be moderated and water drinking reduced until the veins are less noticeable. Extremely hot, damp, but not wet applications help the condition.

These veins are untidy and neglected-looking, and should have special care in make-up. Rouge can be used to harmonize with the color; alternatively, green foundation and powder is now available to tone down the excess red.

Freckles and Moth Patches. Freckles are most commonly seen in young people and often run in families. After the age of twenty they usually die away, but at any age they can be treated with tiny spots of colorless iodine painted on with a brush.

Moth patches come much later in life and are sometimes due to liver irregularities, or to too much sunshine on the unprotected skin.

Moth patches on the hands are especially aging; they can be kept at bay by always wearing gloves out of doors, and by using lemon hand cream.

Moles, either hair-growing or just dark colored, are blemishes that need skilled aid.

Electrolysis is a safe and sure cure for small moles and involves neither cutting nor stitching.

Hair-growing moles take longer to cure, because each hair has to be permanently destroyed before the mole can disappear. It is important to visit an operator who has had extensive experience in this type of work; otherwise a serious burn, leaving a bad scar, may be inflicted.

Where a mole is too large for electrolysis, it can be camouflaged by theatrical make-up in a dark shade.

Superfluous Hair. The greatest enemy of facial grooming is a heavy growth of superfluous hair. Most hair removers are only just temporary removers, and the return of the unwanted hair is only delayed.

It is said to be due to an irregularity in the internal glandular secretions or, in some cases, it follows attacks of rheumatism. In some women superfluous facial hair first makes its appearance after the menopause.

Home remedies give only temporary relief, whether they be liquid depilatories or wax preparations, which can be painful. Pulling out the hair with tweezers does not remove the root of the hair. A safety razor, though suitable for underarm use, should not be used on a woman's face.

A good way to make superfluous hair invisible is to bleach it with a mixture of nearly equal parts of liquid ammonia and peroxide of hydrogen. The part to be treated is washed first to remove all grease, then dabbed two or three times with the solution until the color fades from the hair. Then the skin may be washed with clear water and powdered.

The treatment must stop the moment the skin begins to feel sore. Very often the hair rots at the roots and drops off. This does not mean it is entirely killed because the real nourishment supply is much deeper in the skin, and is protected from the bleach.

Certainly the safest and surest way to banish facial hair is to have it removed by an experienced specialist in electrolysis.

The treatment is certainly a small burn, but the pain caused is bearable and it stops as soon as the hair is removed. A severe case might take months or even a year or two to cure, but the mental relief is worth the slight discomfort, and the happy patient faces the world with poise and confidence.

The greatest care must be observed in treating the skin after the use of electrolysis, as scars may result, not from the burns, but from rubbing the skin before the burns are thoroughly healed.

A face cream containing too much animal fat will encourage the growth of hair, and sleeping with the face covered with cream is also the way to encourage the growth.

Warts can be removed by the application of electrolysis and two or three small treatments are better than one long one. Burning with acid is not recommended, as it can damage the nails. In some cases, your doctor may 'freeze' off the wart with a carbon dioxide 'snow pencil.'

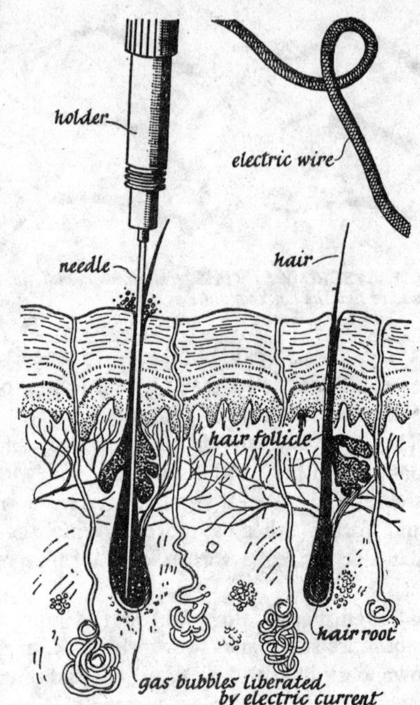

Fig. 10. *REMOVAL OF SUPERFLUOUS HAIR BY ELECTROLYSIS*

CARE OF THE HAIR

To be beautiful, the hair, like the skin, must be healthy and scrupulously clean. Owing to the atmospheric pollution in which we live nowadays, this is almost impossible.

The hair should be protected far more than is customary. Out of doors, the sunshine can fade its color, whether natural or tinted, and indoors, a smoky atmosphere can dull its sheen and sour its smell, destroying in a few minutes the fragrance left by a recent shampoo.

Oils and creams, even when perfumed, are apt to turn rancid after a few days in a smoggy or smoky atmosphere; therefore lacquer is increasingly used for fixing the coiffure. This, however, should be used sparingly, and brushed out each day, if the hair is not to be rendered dull and brittle.

Keeping the Hair Clean

It is useless to cleanse the hair and then reinfect it with dandruff from a dirty comb, a proceeding as dangerous as using a dirty powder-puff. Therefore, if the comb is of the type that cannot be cleaned, it should be thrown away and replaced after every shampoo. A comb, in any event, should always be kept in a case, never exposed to dirt and dust on a dressing table or carried loose in a handbag.

A weekly brushing for at least a quarter of an hour is not too much for long hair, and this should be followed by a tonic shampoo, and more brushing just before the hair is finally dry. It is not good for the hair brush to use it on damp hair but the hair benefits considerably, and a second best brush should be kept clean and dry for this purpose, and washed again immediately after use; then the bristles will settle back into shape.

Several minutes should be spent on brushing the hair where it grows from the temples, as that part needs extra stimulation, and is the first place to show signs of grayness. In this area, dandruff and resulting grayness are all too often encouraged by deposits of soap rubbed into the hairline when washing.

When a shampoo cannot be arranged the hair should be massaged, particularly at the front, with pads of cotton soaked in bay rum, or in vinegar, to clear up dandruff.

Whether the hair is washed once a week or once a fortnight is not important. There is no set rule, but the scalp should be cleaned before the shampoo, and soon—a few days—after the shampoo.

Every moment the small pores of the scalp are throwing off waste products, and as soon as those pores become clogged they cease to convey nourishment to the hair; then they suddenly have a rush of waste matter to discharge and that is too much to deal with, and the hair suddenly becomes greasy and lank. It can become sticky in one night, very often three or four days just after it has been shampooed.

Hair Brushing keeps the scalp clean, and young, because it loosens the dead cells and stimulates the growth of new ones.

The hair should be parted in several places, and the scalp brushed sharply, then the dead skin should be carried away by brushing the long strands of hair.

After brushing, a few strokes of massage, with the finger tips, will give an added stimulation. Polish the hair with a silk scarf or nylon stocking wrapped round the bristles of the brush and lightly pulled through each strand of hair. This will also help to free it of dust and grime, and add soft shine to jaded hair. The hair can then be combed back into its usual dressing.

Shampooing and Setting

Although shampooing and setting are skilled professional jobs there is no reason why hair should not be shampooed and set at home between visits to the hairdresser. The first requisite is a good shampoo which suits your hair. If you can use the one your hairdresser recommends that will be best. Before wetting the hair, brush and comb it well to remove tangles and surface dust. Use half only of the prepared shampoo and rub it hard until there is a thick lather. Rinse away thoroughly the first lathering before applying the second. Then rinse again with several waters, each time with the water a little cooler than the last. Give at least three separate rinses, one with vinegar (or lemon juice for blonde hair). Finish with a cream rinse.

Setting lotion should be used sparingly, choosing a spirit type for greasy hair, and the setting done with rollers for soft curls, or choosing an alcohol type for greasy hair, and the setting done with rollers for soft curls, or bobby pins or clips for flat waves.

Place a net over the head and dry the hair with an electric hand drier if possible, or leave to dry in a warm room. When the hair is quite dry, take off the net and remove the rollers, clips, and pins. Brush the hair carefully into the style required. To give body to the hair a little back combing of the small sections of hair is very professional looking and gives a natural look.

Hair Conditions Needing Special Attention

Falling Hair. Hair may fall out if the bloodstream is in a run-down condition or after a shock. Before shampooing, rub warm oil into the scalp; then wrap the head in a warm towel and hold over a bowl of boiling water to steam the oil into the scalp.

Dandruff and Alopecia. These are both conditions due to infection of the scalp by a minute fungus. A doctor should be consulted in cases of alopecia in which bald patches appear suddenly. A very mild case of dandruff can be helped by using a commercial dandruff shampoo.

Great care must be taken to clean the face directly after the shampooing, as the tiny infected flakes of dandruff can fall on the skin of the face and set up slight inflammation and, if neglected, the condition produces spots which are hard to disperse.

Gray Hair. Gray hair, at whatever age it occurs, indicates that the glands which create the color are decreasing in their activity.

Early grayness may run in families; in some cases it is associated with severe headaches and certain types of rheumatism, which may be inherited. The hair does not lose its quality in grayness, it only lacks the color particles which flow inside the individual hairs.

A sudden attack of grayness may sometimes be checked by skillful hand massage, or electrical massage, of the scalp and back of the neck. This may be accompanied by hot towel application placed at the back of the neck and ears to stimulate the nerves and blood flow.

COLORING GRAYNESS. Graying hair can add distinction to a face but it can also add years to the appearance. Most women want to delay the process of graying as long as possible. For this purpose there are many new color rinses. They are quite harmless and can give a new luster to fading hair. Many of them can be used quite successfully at home, either combined with the shampoo, or applied afterwards. This type of coloring, unfortunately, is liable to rub off in a day or two on collars, towels or pillows, whereas a true dye or tint takes a month to grow out and really stays fast until the next shampoo.

For those who have decided that their hair needs dyeing to bring it back to its natural color it is better to seek professional help if a chemical dye is to be used. To give a natural appearance the tint must be chosen with care and the dye applied professionally to give an even color. There is nothing so sad-looking or so detrimental to good looks as a badly tinted head of hair. The darker the tint, the greater the trouble it is to apply; a very dark tint is really a job for the hairdresser.

A 'test piece' of hair should be treated with the dye first, since in some women an allergic rash may develop. In such cases the dyeing should not be proceeded with.

Bleaching. Continual application of any kind of bleach will gradually weaken the growth unless the hair is treated with tonic and scalp stimulating treatments.

Strong chemical bleach should be used only by the professional but there are 'brightening' rinses which can be successfully used at home.

Peroxide and ammonia in water, bleach and brighten the hair. Lemon juice bleaches, especially if the hair is exposed to strong sunlight while it is drying. The natural color in these cases is lightened, but preserved.

Vinegar or cold tea can be used as emergency rinses for brown hair, if nothing else is available.

Dressing the Hair

Women with regular features can wear severely plain styles, while women with irregular features can wear curls and soft waves.

It is by no means universally true that a long thin face needs width of hair behind the ears, though faces which are inclined to be too old for their real age should have the hair brushed up from the temples. This method is kind to the sides of the face especially if the hair, while being brushed up, is not taken away from the back of the ears.

CARE OF THE HANDS

Brittle Nails. Nails are a clear indication of a condition of health which has been existing for some time—say months or a year or two. The nails we see today are the results of the nails which were growing two or three months ago in a deeper pad under the skin.

A slimming diet, in particular, will slim first the neck, then the face and body, but not till several weeks have passed will the nails show any response to the treatment. They will then begin to split or crack. As a temporary measure to strengthen the nails they should be soaked in hot oil every night. It is better to consult a doctor before repairing the damage caused by excessive dieting.

A deficiency of calcium in the system causes thin threadlike lines on the nails, and, five or six months after a serious operation or a very severe illness, soft ridges appear across every nail on hands and feet.

To aid nails in poor condition, there are special nail foods and creams available.

Hand Care for the Housewife

When small corn-like pieces of skin form on each side of the nail, it can generally be concluded that the hands have been too much in strong detergent or soda water, or the soap used has been too drying.

Flaking nails are usually caused by scouring saucepans with steel wool, instead of using a brush.

If several vegetables have to be peeled together, the potato should be left till last, as its cleaning properties help to remove the other stains, though nowadays by buying vegetables ready-washed and packed it is generally possible to avoid this chore altogether.

For very tired hands, a hand bath in hot Epsom salts and water is often found to be a great relief. After the bath, the hands should be washed in fresh soap and water to remove the traces of the Epsom salt deposit, patted gently dry, and treated with hand lotion. The hands, in short, should be treated with the same tenderness as the face, for they are infinitely more useful, and vulnerable. A work-calloused hand, ingrained with dirt and wrinkled, merely advertises its owner's carelessness.

Hands and wrists should be protected with lotion each time they are washed; for housework, rubber gloves larger than your usual glove size, or gloves with a cotton lining, are desirable, unless a silicone protective or barrier cream is used before tackling each dirty job, and the nails filled with soap.

For weekly repair work, a bleaching lotion may be added after the first wash before the nails are trimmed.

A small toothbrush is better than a hard nail brush for cleaning the nails and finger tips. The hands should not be brushed, but rubbed with a piece of soft cloth and soap if they are dirty or, for more thorough treatment, brown sugar and warm olive oil. It is important, however, not to wrinkle the skin of the hands when washing or drying them. For smooth hands wear gloves summer and winter, every moment that one is out of doors. Wool jersey gloves, extending well over the wrists, give excellent and elegant protection against chapped skin and chilblains.

Much damage is done to the hands by bad habits; taking off one glove, for example, and chewing a knuckle abstractedly can lead not only to chilblains, but to enlarged joints. So can the practice of clutching a purse too tightly.

Strains and Injuries

The hand more than any part of the body needs first aid to keep it in repair; for it is exposed to extremes of heat and cold, and to sudden graspings to catch falling articles of use. By themselves these sudden 'graspings' are strictly non-injurious, but they sometimes cause a slight stab of pain, which may lead to an ache later and, supposing rheumatism is present, there is swelling in the muscle that is strained, and thickening in the bone to which it is attached.

Therefore a strained hand must be attended to as soon as possible. Use a compress made of linen dipped in hot water containing Epsom salts—about a teaspoonful to half a pint of water. The compress must be left on the strained wrist or thumb joint for twelve hours, and then the joint can be exercised and massaged.

Opening a door with a heavy handle, lifting a full saucepan, carrying a suitcase, turning a new cap on a lotion bottle, etc., are all movements which give a slight and sudden wrench to hands. But the most refractory bottle will usually yield either to dipping the neck in hot water, or to pressure from a special rubber ring made for the purpose.

Some occupations lead to thickened ends of fingers—knitting for instance, is inclined to cramp the joints of the fingers, and after the work is put down, the hands should be exercised by straightening them forcibly, and causing the stagnant blood to move.

Manicure

Beautiful hands are a great asset. Allow yourself half an hour each week for a complete home manicure. Assemble everything you need before you begin:

clean hand towel	emery board
bowl of soapy water	nail polish
cuticle remover	polish remover
orange sticks	bottle of peroxide
cotton	cuticle oil

Fig. 11 (1 to 7) illustrates the stages required for a manicure.

1. Working from base to tip of nail, wipe off polish with raw cotton pad soaked in oily remover, taking care not to push the old polish into the cuticle.

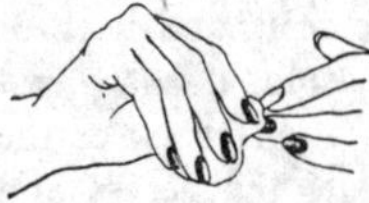

2. While nails are dry and hard, file them into an oval shape with emery board. Good filing should begin at the corner of the nail and sweep—not 'saw'—to the center, first one side and then the other. Do not file the nail too deeply into the corner or the growth will be thickened.

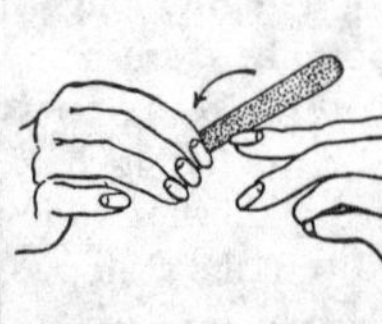

3. Soak the fingertips in warm soapy water to clean the nails and soften cuticles. Clean the nails with an orange stick. Remove stains under the nails with an orange stick dipped in peroxide.

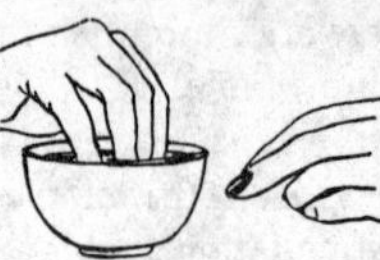

4. Paint the cuticles with cuticle remover or oil. Wrap cotton around the tip of an orange stick and gently work round each nail loosening the cuticle. This should never be hurried because if the cuticle is roughly handled it may cause hangnails, or become infected. Gently reveal the halfmoons.

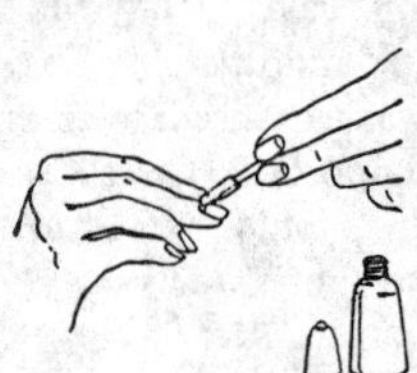

5. When applying nail polish, first apply a base coat. This semi-transparent polish puts a smooth protective layer on the nails and is especially helpful for brittle nails. Use strong brush strokes from base of the nail to the tip.

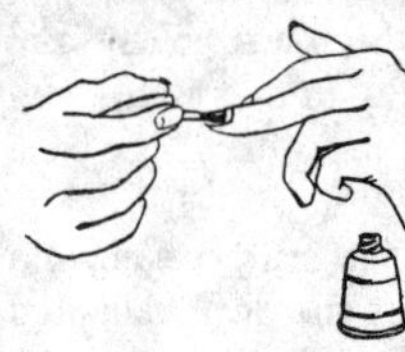

6. When the base is dry apply the polish: several fine coats last longer than a single thick one. Let each coat dry before putting on the next. Brush color right across the base of the nail, keeping clear of the cuticle, then make two strokes along the edges of nail from base to tip. Finally fill in middle with one strong stroke from base to tip. Never go back on wet polish or you will get ridges.

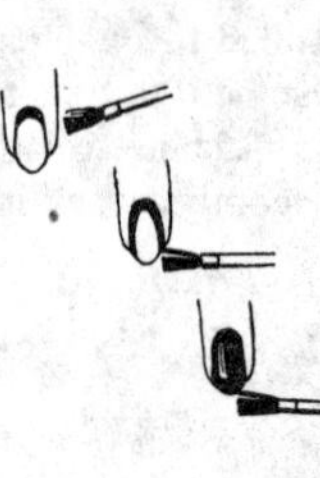

7. After polishing each nail, run the pad of your thumb round the very edge of the nail to leave a hairline free. This delays chipping. If you use a sealer topcoat, leave it for 20 minutes to harden.

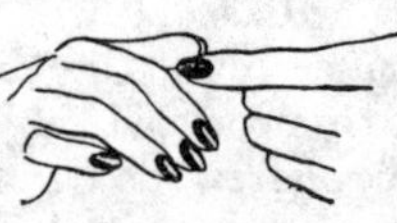

Note: Once the cuticle is trained to grow down from the half moon, cuticle cream or oil will be found satisfactory for everyday use, and the strong cuticle remover reserved for the weekly manicure.

CARE OF THE FEET

Feet and weight are so closely related that it is hardly possible to decide which to care for first. 'Bad' feet make a woman walk badly—she tends to avoid walking, and in consequence will often put on weight!

She grows heavy and middle-aged looking, even when she is under thirty—her feet grow worse—she is no longer attractive.

When a woman has a weight in keeping with her height and figure she will not put much strain on her bony structure, nor undue pressure on the heel, nor on the ball of the foot. Walking is then a pleasure, and old age is not a threatening specter.

Therefore feet, regardless of their size, are vastly important to weight control. Yet they are the most abused part of the human structure and often overloaded, under-dressed, and sadly neglected from the point of view of general grooming.

False balance caused by wearing unsuitable shoes will not only strain the tendons of the feet but will in turn stiffen the muscles of the back, put bones out of alignment and cause severe headaches.

Feet are really so important that any trouble that does not give way to general care should be taken to a doctor. Modern foot surgery has made such wonderful advances that no sufferer need despair.

Wash your feet frequently. Make them feel fresh and tingling by splashing them with cold water, or spray them with Eau de Cologne.

Foot Troubles

Bunions. A bunion is caused by a continued strain on a joint. It is nearly always caused by wearing shoes which are too short and which have pointed toes, or from wearing shoes which throw the weight of the foot in the wrong place, or the result of some earlier injury which has not been attended to. Whatever the cause the unnatural pressure deforms the joint of the big toe, and the sac (or bursa) over the joint where the toe joins the foot may become inflamed and swollen, or pus may form in its cavity.

In the early stages a bunion may be massaged and strapped with adhesive plaster to reduce the pressure. Special shoes may be made to measure, and rest may be taken, but there is very little chance of a complete cure by these means.

Much valuable time and patience can be wasted in enduring an unsightly bunion, when a slight operation could remove the deformity, and the foot, in fact, would be beautiful in a few weeks. A doctor, of course, should advise the operation and it could be done either in a nursing home, or by attending any hospital with an orthopedic department. Then after two, or perhaps three, weeks of absolute rest the bunion is a thing of the past.

'Burning' Feet. Burning sensation on the soles is often due to vitamin lack, especially riboflavine (see p. 69).

Corns. Corns are the result of pressure and irritation in one place. Each corn has a small center of hard skin, which presses down on the soft parts below and causes pain.

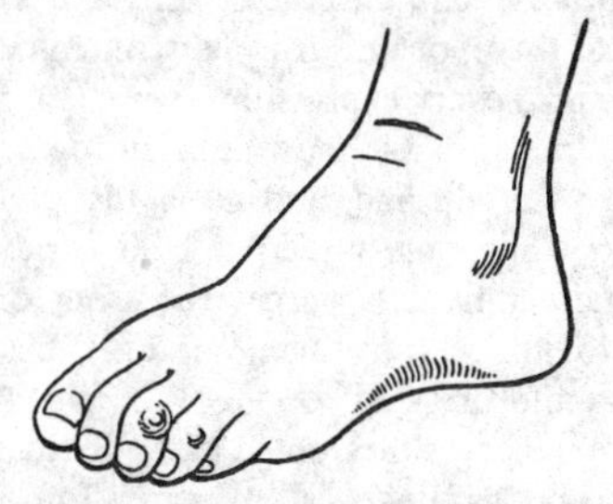

Fig. 12. *CORN. The result of pressure and irritation from a badly fitting shoe, which may be too roomy or too tight.*

Corn solvent can give temporary relief, though the source of pressure can only be removed with the center of the corn itself.

The foot should be soaked in soft soap and water to loosen the skin, then the layers must be scraped off one by one, and never cut. The part from which the corn is removed must be rubbed with glycerin and a mild disinfectant, and powdered with dry sulphur.

Callouses can be treated like corns, layer by layer, and until they are cured. The exposed place should be protected by a layer of adhesive plaster.

Fissures. These are small cuts in the soft skin between the small toes. The feet should be soaked in pale pink potassium permanganate solution and washed; then the fissure should be dressed with an antiseptic lotion and strapped across with adhesive plaster. Often these fissures are due to a fungous infection of the skin, known as 'athlete's foot.'

Footwear for Health

Shoes. With a good shoe you can have both support and style. Heels should fit snugly. Weight should be shared equally along the foot with no cramping of toes. Shoes with hard soles are best avoided by all feet except the very strongest, as such soles put too much strain on the ankle and cause an unnatural pressure of tread.

It is a sensible plan not to wear the same shoes two days running. The change of shape from one pair to another encourages flexibility of the foot and leg muscles. If you are at home all day do not wear sloppy slippers; a low heel will provide the support that is needed—especially when doing sink-side chores.

When shopping for shoes ask to have your feet measured for width as well as length, and ensure the right fit every time. Walk about the shop floor in the shoes before deciding to buy them because it is difficult to judge the fit when sitting down as the feet tend to spread when you stand up. Do not buy shoes when your feet are cold, for the feet are bound to swell a little in warmer weather.

Stockings. In summer, mesh stockings enable the feet to breathe and remain cool; if possible, stockings should be changed during the day. This is particularly important if rubber-soled shoes are worn.

At the first signs of swollen veins in the calves, support stockings should be worn, changing to fancy mesh only for the most formal occasions. The time for made-to-measure surgical stockings is later, when the condition worsens.

Red or purple patches round the ankles are caused by poor circulation. These can be camouflaged by colored make-up.

A coarse-skinned leg looks better in fancy stockings than in sheer nylon. The skin should be given a drastic pack each week, and then soothed with hand or body lotion (baby lotion will do). Hair, too, should be removed from the legs every week; most women require a cream depilatory, though never a razor.

Pedicure. The feet deserve their weekly pedicure, just as the hands their manicure. Thickened toenails can be trimmed only by patient and gentle filing from 'fore and aft' (not from side to side). Ingrowing nails need treatment by a chiropodist, as they may be a possible source of infection.

With good feet, a healthy body retains its elasticity and walking becomes a pleasure at any age.

WEIGHT PROBLEMS

Every woman, whatever her build, has a bone structure which forms the foundation for her figure, and any excess fat must be reduced to the minimum, for the sake of health as well as beauty.

Too Heavy

Where obesity is attributable to a glandular disorder medical treatment is needed, but otherwise overweight is simply the result of overeating—maybe to compensate for dissatisfaction with life in general, or to insufficient exercise.

Diet. The basic treatment is a restriction in diet, especially of starchy foods, and the diet must be rigidly followed every day, no matter how great the temptation to deviate from it. Too drastic a reduction in weight can lead to kidney trouble, or to nervous disease; hence the importance of losing weight gradually.

It is usually advisable for anyone on a strict slimming diet to do so with the advice of her doctor and have regular check-ups.

BREAKFAST should consist of fruit, an egg, a slice of enriched bread with a little butter or margarine.

Black China tea, weak Indian tea, or coffee, with a little milk but without sugar, may be taken as desired.

LUNCH should consist of consommé or fruits, salads or a hot vegetable dish (not potatoes); lean meat or fish (never fried), stewed fruit sweetened with saccharin. No sauces, no mayonnaise—though a little oil and vinegar, or lemon juice, makes an appetizing salad dressing, and SUPPER should be another austere meal on the same lines as lunch.

No liquids should be taken with meals—not even water, and fresh fruit is preferable to canned fruits in syrup, to ice-cream or puddings.

Exercise is important—if possible more exercise than usual—and a glass of water should always be taken before the evening meal. Violent exercise is not necessary as long as the muscles are kept in a comfortably active condition. When one begins to feel 'elegant' the cure has begun, no matter how it has been helped!

Too Thin

Being too thin sometimes carries with it a feeling of bad temper, irritation or nerve strain. Then it may be that a doctor could discover a glandular reason, especially if the frame is large and bony.

To be extremely thin and over-active and still quite happy denotes some special need—possibly more rest and relaxation before meals.

Rest and comfortable relaxation should be taken daily, not occasionally, and it should be an absolute rule to take more than eight hours sleep every night. If you sleep for eight hours normally try to make sure of nine or ten hours in bed—not reading, but thoroughly relaxing, and keeping warm. The rest will help the muscles to take in a little more nourishment during the night, then you will rise without a feeling of too much activity, or panic, and eat a peaceful breakfast.

Relaxation seems impossible in the daily life of busy women, but the mind should be rested for at least an hour every day, by doing entirely different work or, best of all, making the mind blank and erasing all worries.

Foods. The thin, nervous type of woman will find oatmeal in all its forms very soothing to the nerves, while a 'nightcap' of warm milk is truly soporific, and also fattening.

While taking in flesh-formers, overloading with carbohydrates must be avoided. Brown sugar, for instance, is more helpful than white sugar, and there is more bulk in coarse brown bread than in white-flour foods. Use butter generously. Eat more often if you are underweight but do not overload the stomach at one meal.

Get used to putting on weight for a little while, and then stop, as it is easier to stop before fat begins to settle in unwanted places.

OVER FORTY

A middle-aged look often begins to be noticed about the middle thirties. This is not as much a matter of body as of mind.

At Forty, and over, there is the danger of getting into a groove. Either one gets used to comfortable circumstances, and the enjoyment of them, or one grows discontented and shows it in every expression.

Hip line and jaw line will begin to vary, so watch your hip line, and never lose sight of the bone structure underneath. It is possible to retain a flatness across the front of the hips to almost any age, but only by wise dieting and dressing.

If you have not studied diet, do so now, and spend as much as you can afford on a foundation garment or belt that will control that hip flesh.

Study your teeth in a strong light—never be afraid to hold a tiny mirror inside your mouth and reflect the teeth or gums; clean healthy gums mean better health generally, and clean teeth (even or uneven) mean a brighter smile, and a firm smile enlivens and strengthens the muscles of the face. Therefore visit the best dentist you can find. Have dark spaces cleaned and filled, and smile.

Never let the cheeks sag with indifference and discontent. A little rouge applied discreetly can liven dull cheeks and cheat the years. Tone up the skin with face packs, then nourish it with a rich skin food.

At Sixty. The woman of sixty begins to feel she cannot remain young for ever, but she can keep her bones loosely articulated, her muscles firm and therefore her flesh regulated, until there is an interesting air of mystery or wonder about her.

You are as old as your blood circulation. Keep circulation in mind when eating or oversleeping—circulation is life and youth, stagnation is death and decay.

Exercise and Poise

The heart is a powerful muscle, controlling the bloodstream and sending it to every part of the body by means of blood vessels.

The bloodstream must be purified to help the heart to work regularly. Fresh air, breathed in properly, is absolutely necessary to keep the bloodstream free from impurities, and an impoverished bloodstream will show signs of immediate recovery when a course of breathing exercises is begun.

Respiration. A short study of correct breathing will help to straighten the spine and brighten the eye in a very short time, when the study is combined with regular practice.

There are three actions of correct breathing:
Inspiration of breath
Retention of breath
Expiration of breath

An intake of breath raises the collar bones and exercises part of the lungs; but a deeper method of breathing is more beneficial to the lower part of the lungs and the use and control of this fuller, deeper breath, which is called deep breathing, not only lifts the clavicles (collar bones) but also exercises the diaphragm.

The diaphragm muscle, which is a strong dividing sheet between the chest and abdominal organs, is capable of great development when deep breathing is practiced daily. Athletes and people who develop the vocal organs are known to thicken this muscle until it is extremely hard to the touch while it is holding the pressure of the breath.

The lungs are expanded downwards and sideways by taking a deep breath through the nostrils, and at the same time the nervous system is vitalized.

Breathing exercises are best done with the student lying flat on the floor with the head slightly raised at first.

The hands may be placed on the hips or across the ribs, then they will rise and fall with the intake of breath.

One full breath should be taken through both nostrils and the body will gradually seem to fill with air until no more breath can be admitted through the nose. This breath should be held for a few seconds and gradually released, either with or without a 'hiss' through the lips.

The object of the exercise is to learn to retain the breath for several seconds or longer, and then make the exhaling process as long as possible. The exercise should be repeated six times.

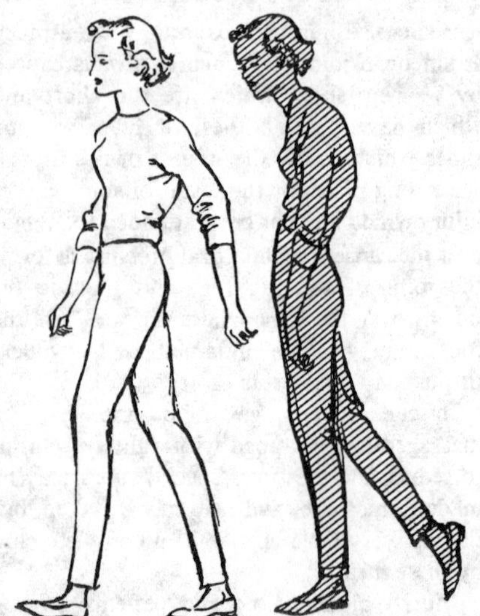

Fig. 15. *WALKING POSTURE. To walk correctly hold head high and the tummy tucked in.*

Walking exercises in the open and before retiring for the night is a good blood tonic, especially if breath-retaining exercises are practiced as well.

For instance, walk ten steps taking a sharp inward breath at every step. Then hold this breath for ten more steps and exhale a puff of breath for the next ten steps and so on for a good sharp walk.

To follow such an exercise with a hot bath and a vigorous friction with a rough towel every day will considerably brighten both eyes and skin.

Poise is more a condition of alert nerves than tense muscles. Poise is hard work at first, for very few people possess it naturally.

A good poise may be practiced by running along a corridor on tiptoe, and then coming to a sudden standstill. How are feet placed? They should be ready to balance the body—but if they are not, straighten them till they do and then lift the head, stretch the spine upward, lifting the ribs out of the hips and run again and stop; continue the exercise until you are used to the feeling of poise, and can adapt it to your daily walk.

Exercise in Middle Age. It is often a serious mistake to begin to do exercises, especially those which call for lying down flat on the back, without a good padding on the floor.

A mat is not always thick enough, and the bones of the shoulders and spine (being less resilient than in youth) grow easily sore and bruised, and the exercises have to be neglected for a week or two, while the inflamed patches of skin recover.

To lie down flat, rise to a sitting position, and lie down again, slowly, is a most valuable brightener to both bloodstream and eyes but it is a severe tax on the abdominal muscles at first and, as the back is lowered, there is an additional strain on the bone structure of the back.

To avoid this pressure, and to make the exercises more attractive, they could be done on a hard bed—or even in bed, as long as the arms are kept close to the body, and are not allowed to act as levers.

When this exercise is thoroughly mastered, the lower abdominal muscles are strengthened by lying quite flat, keeping the legs together and lifting the feet about six inches from the ground, holding them in that position, then lowering them, and repeating the movements several times.

Carriage Faults. Most carriage faults begin in the abdominal region, where sagging of the muscles leads to stooping and round shoulders. It is the easiest thing in the world to lapse into a round, stiff-backed posture for life but most difficult to liberate oneself from it.

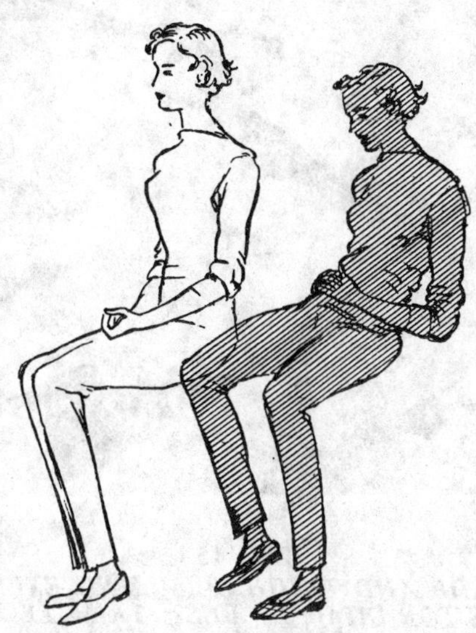

Fig. 17. *SITTING POSTURE. On the left a good sitting posture. On the right the slumped sagging of abdominal muscles.*

When working, therefore, or reading or sewing, it is important to pause now and again, straighten the back, and close the eyes, trying to visualize absolute velvet blackness. This exercise is especially valuable when performed in a noisy, crowded train or bus. It is useful to cultivate the art of making a little retreat, when desired, into a private world of peace and quiet. Then you can come back refreshed, ready to cope with the task in hand as expeditiously as possible.

Fixed attitudes, whether mental or physical, are the worst enemy of youth and beauty; fight them, strive to remain young in heart, and you will find that you remain, for years to come, remarkably young in body!

EXERCISES FOR HIPS AND THIGHS

Fig. 14 (above)

1. Flat on floor, arms above head, roll over and over to the end of room. Roll back.
2. Flat on back with knees bent with arms outstretched swing forward till head touches knees. (Repeat.)
3. Sit on floor, hands on hips, feet straight before you. Pull tummy in and then travel forward on your tail across the room.
4. Clasp knees and rock backward till shoulders touch floor, forward till toes touch floor.
5. Flat on back with hands underneath, knees bent up on chest. Shoot legs skyward; bend to chest again and lower to floor. (6 times)
6. Right knee half bent, revolve fully bent left leg. Repeat in reverse.
7. Sit on table, swing left and right legs alternately.

EXERCISES FOR BUST, LEGS, AND ANKLES

Fig. 14 (below)

8. Raise arms to shoulder level, turning head left and right. Repeat several times.
9. With bust uplifted, shoulders flat, arms shoulder high, clasp hands across chest. Resisting with right arm, use left arm to try to pull it across your body. Now pull other way. Repeat.
10. Stand with arms at sides. Rise slowly on toes, inhaling and raising arms to meet above head. Sink back on heels, exhale and lower arms.
11. On floor with hands on hips, raise legs wide apart, cross left over right leg. Cross right over left leg.
12. Weight on shoulders, lie on back, legs in air. Pedal at imaginary bicycle for 2 or 3 minutes.
13. Stand with heels on ground, toes resting on telephone directory. Raise heels till on tip-toe on directory. Lower heels. Repeat several times.

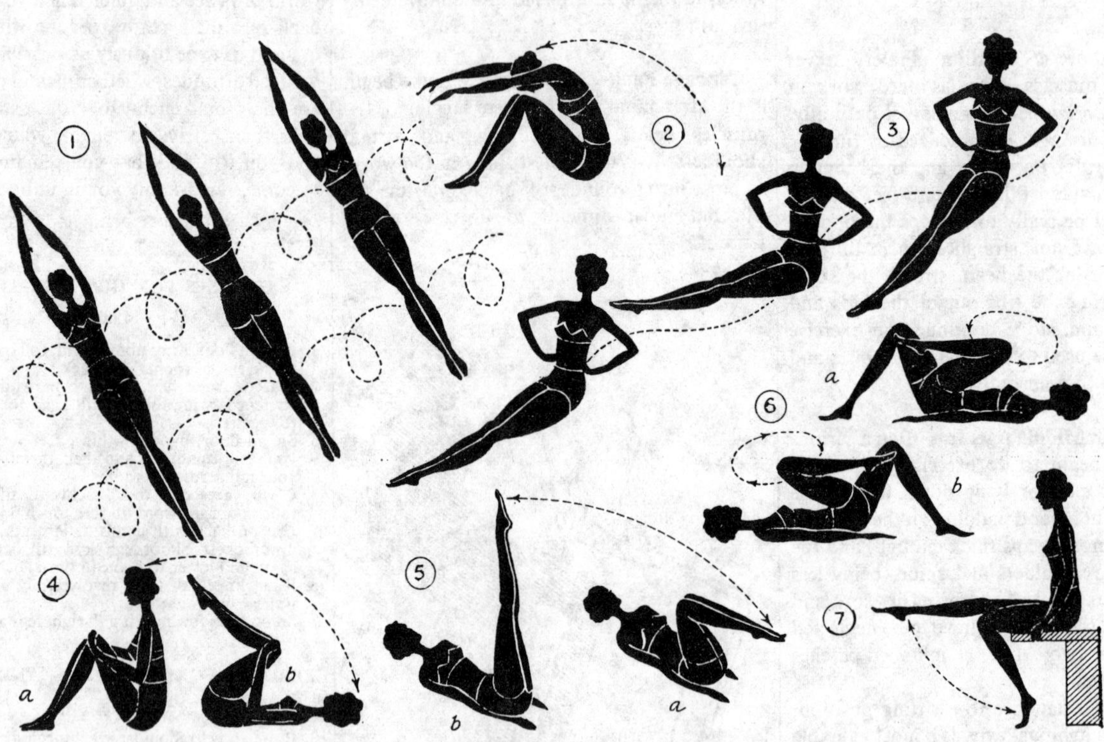

Fig. 15
Above. *HIP AND THIGH SLIMMING EXERCISES*
Below. *EXERCISES FOR SHAPELY BUST, TRIM LEGS AND ANKLES*

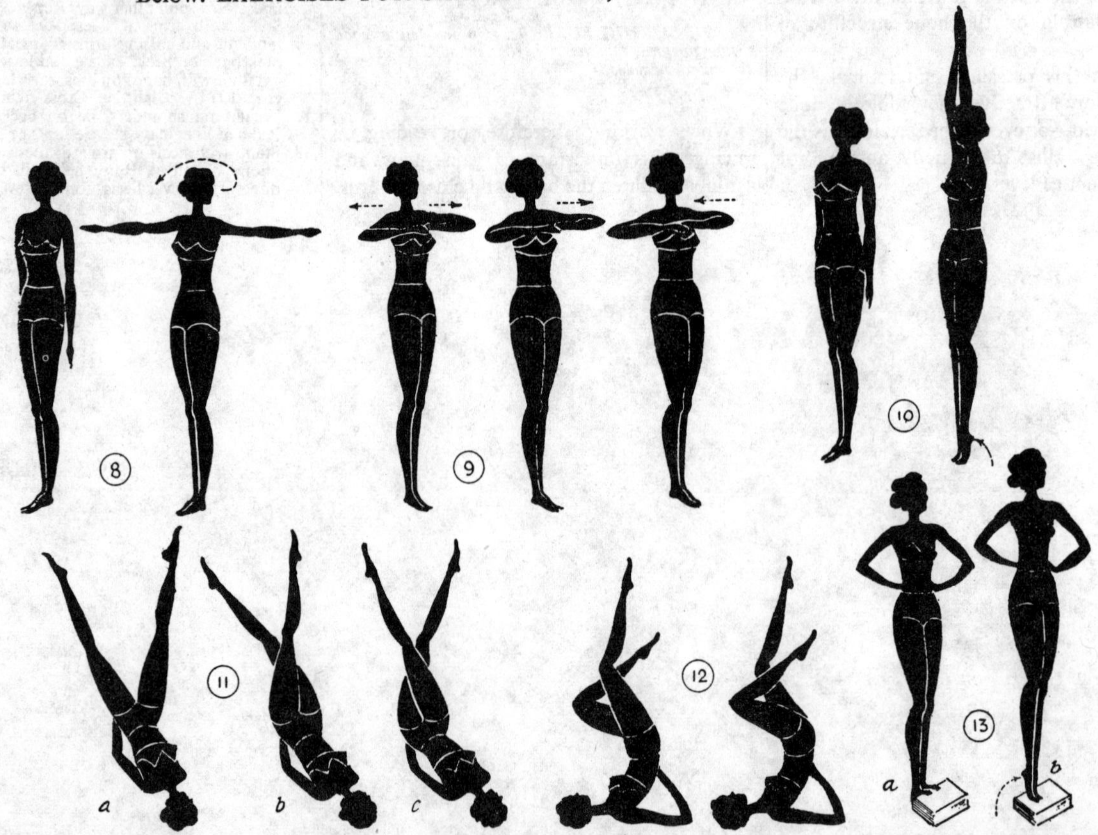

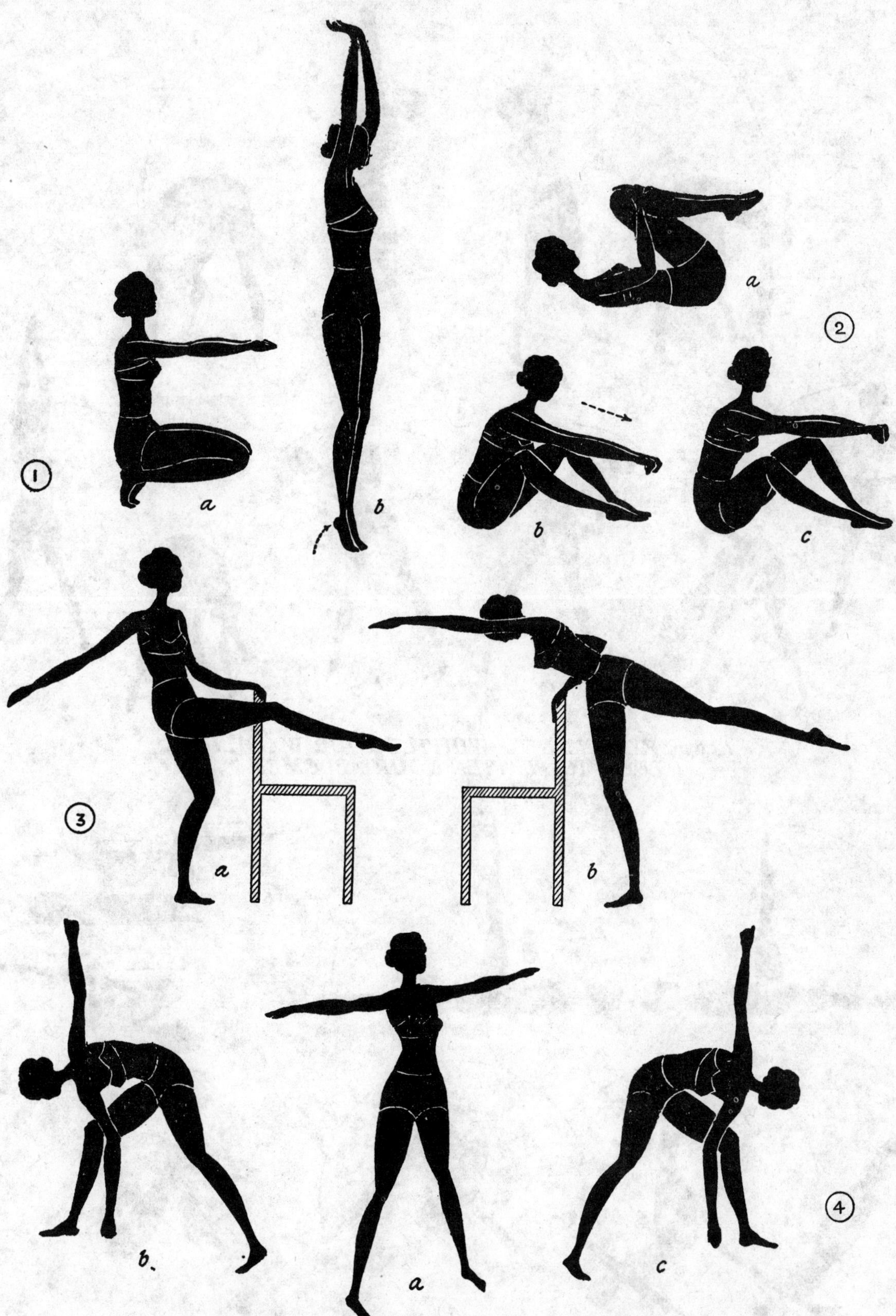

Fig. 16. *EXERCISES FOR CONSTIPATION*

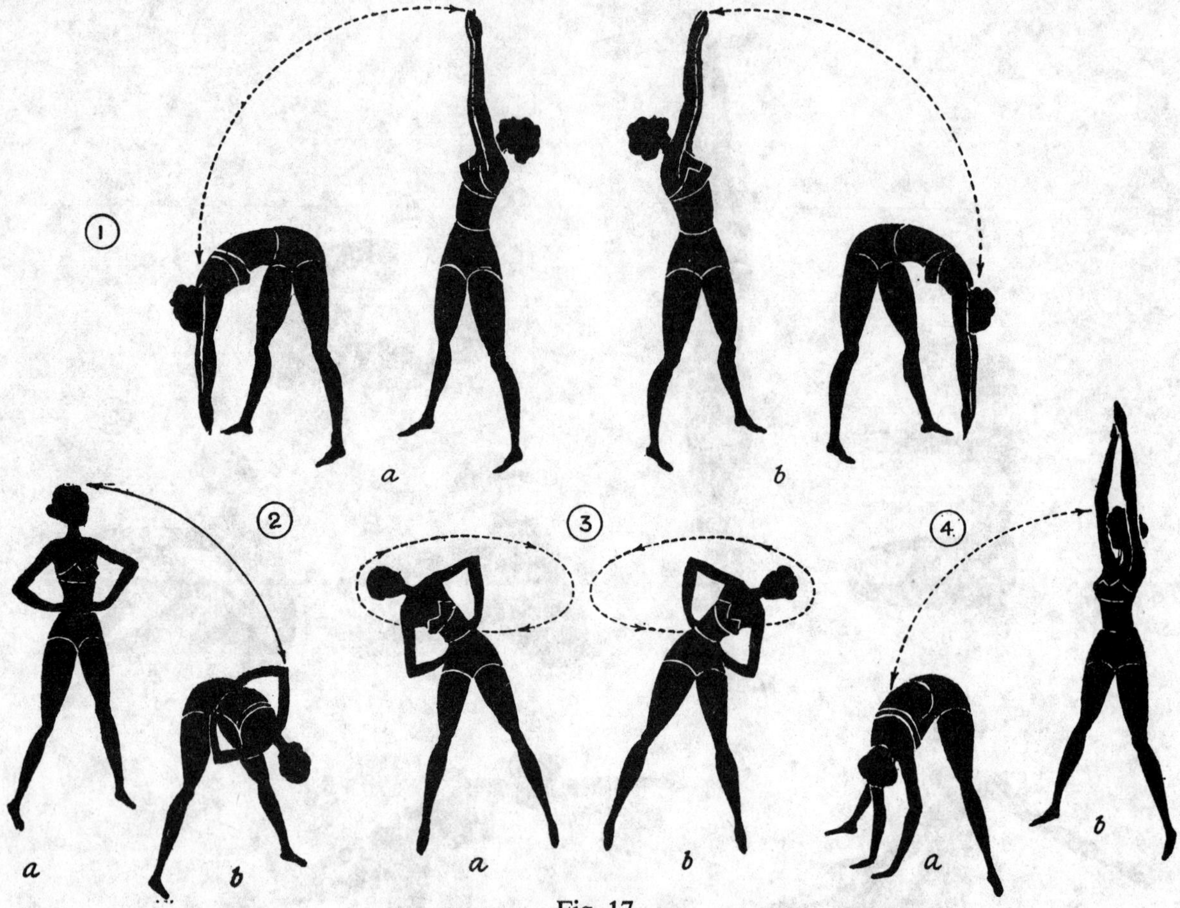

Fig. 17
Above. *EXERCISES TO WHITTLE YOUR WAISTLINE*
Below. *TO FLATTEN YOUR ABDOMEN*

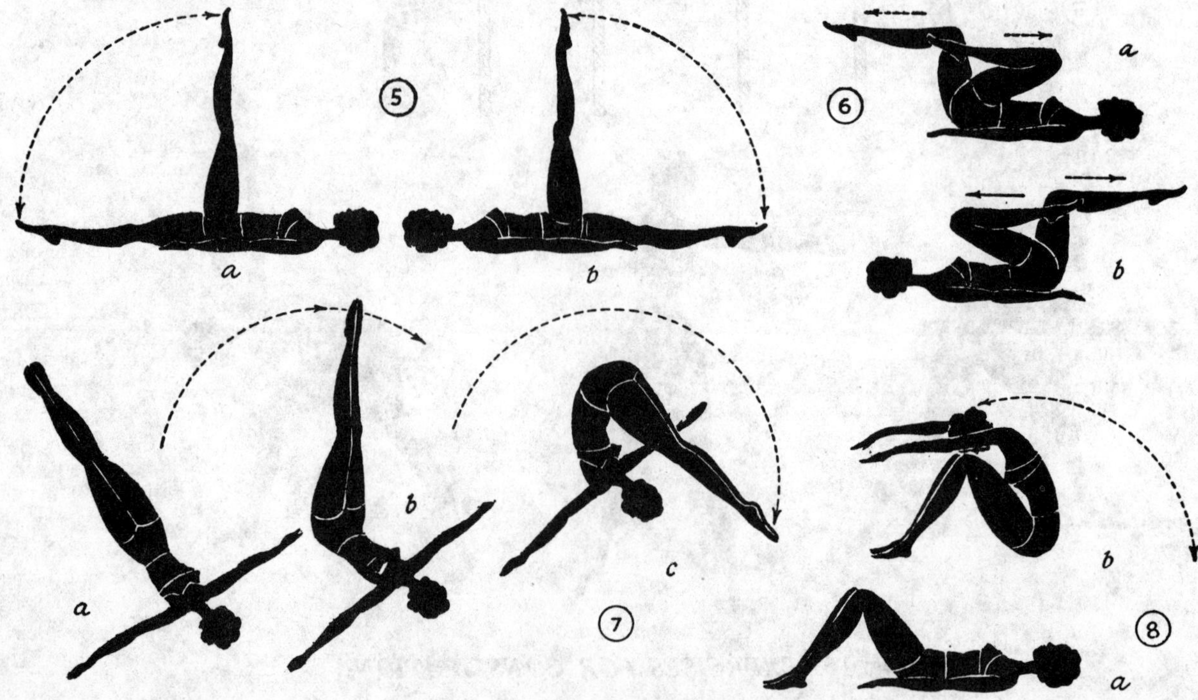

PHYSIOTHERAPY

The art of healing by physical means, that is by a wide range of exercises or by using natural forces such as light, heat, water, and electricity, has made great strides forward during the twentieth century, although the practice of physiotherapy goes back to the very beginning of medical science.

Earlier, it was considered sufficient if the patient was put back on his feet, or his broken arm mended, but nowadays greater regard is given to the patient's functional activities, that is teaching him to re-use the muscles in his legs for walking, how to hold a cup or spoon when part of his hand is missing, how to dress with one arm and so on.

Physical medicine covers a wide field and provides a variety of treatments designed to restore movement and functional activity, to relieve spasm and to promote healing. Massage, electrotherapy, exercises and water-therapy all play their part in the program of treatment and the best results are obtained by a judicious use of all. Treatment, especially in long-term cases, usually begins in the hospital. Some particular method may prove beneficial to people of all age groups and with a variety of complaints. It may help elderly people unable to get about owing to strokes or arthritis, young motor cyclists after accidents, sportsmen after injury, patients recovering from accidents or illness, and even mothers before and after confinement. On the other hand, other methods may have more limited application and will be suitable for certain kinds of disability only.

Physiotherapy today is no longer merely limb-saving but life-saving. It is not an answer to every problem and its results are obtained, not only from the technique, but from the courage and co-operation of the patient. Hope and faith, too, are important allies to both patient and therapist.

Role of the Physiotherapist

The Rehabilitation Team in a hospital or clinic plans a program of treatment for each severely disabled person in its care. Programs include individual and group therapy as well as practice in activities necessary for personal independence. The target must be high to stimulate effort in the patient but within ultimate reach to avoid the disappointments of failure. Young people are encouraged to aim for a full and active life in remunerative employment, but the elderly will probably only desire personal independence in the home and often cannot reasonably hope for more.

The team—doctor, one or more physiotherapist, nurses, occupational therapist, etc. —having worked out a plan or program of therapy for each patient, regard the treatment as a continuous process. Massage, given early in treatment, leads to simple and then to more difficult exercises, and so on. Emphasis is placed upon making the patient increasingly aware of his ability rather than his disability. The physiotherapist therefore selects the exercises and treatments by which stay in hospital can be shortened, return to work hastened, and aid given to many of the incapacitated to enable them to become capable and independent again. This not only saves pressure on doctors and nurses, economizes on national and local expenditure, but restores zest for living to the patients.

Each physiotherapist is not just a figurehead in uniform, but an understanding person who will explain what he or she is doing and hopes to achieve. She will show how apparatus is set up and give any necessary warnings about handling and using equipment, about any discomfort which must be reported, and who will give advice about any special clothing, and so on.

Rehabilitation

Rehabilitation means 'to restore to right or proper condition:' it aims to restore disabled persons to their utmost capacity largely by 'do it yourself' methods. It is a continuous process from onset of injury or sickness to final resettlement in the most suitable work and living conditions. The main stages in rehabilitation are:

1. Individual physiotherapy and underwater exercises.
2. Independent activities.
3. Group work.
4. Recreational activities and sports, social contacts and hobbies.
5. Resettlement.

Sometimes the patient is a child needing special schooling, a disabled housewife, a respiratory polio case, a school dropout, or a wage earner. His problems may sometimes be social ones and the final settlement for adults can often be found through vocational training or a job in a 'sheltered' workshop. The whole team helps to find the way, but the patient gradually becomes the most important member of the team. Treatment is a challenge to him and he gradually realizes, with help, what he cannot do and becomes aware of what he needs to do. The patient who will not accept his disability presents a great

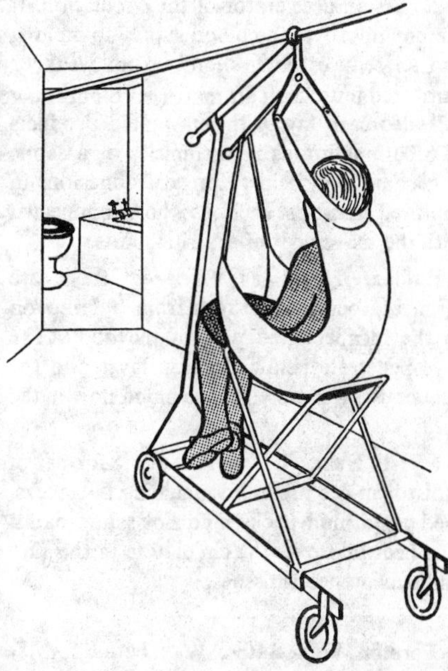

Fig. 1. LEARNING TO GET ABOUT AGAIN. With the aid of hoists, specially adapted chairs, and wide doorways to the bathroom, even a paralyzed patient can achieve some degree of independence.

problem. Even worse is the patient who develops too much faith in his physiotherapist and expects further improvement after his full potentialities have been achieved.

INDIVIDUAL PHYSIOTHERAPY

Massage

Massage, or the manipulation of the soft tissues of the body by the therapist's hands, although a limited part of physiotherapy and not used as widely as formerly, is still of great value if used with discretion. It consists of sustained pressure and relaxation of the tissues; it may be brisk and stimulating if required to produce expectoration; or gentle and soothing when used to induce relaxation of tense muscles. It improves circulation and so helps to disperse swelling, to loosen adhesions, and to check the accumulation of chronic inflammatory products.

The manipulation may be by stroking or kneading, by friction or percussion according to the condition being treated and the result required. Special techniques have also been evolved, e.g. connective tissue massage which utilizes a reflex effect to stimulate wasted tissues. Other special methods can produce active hyperemia (increased flow of blood) by frictions for injuries to ligaments, tendons and muscles; or they can be used to improve local circulation in treatment of ulcers, or to assist plastic repair.

Heat and Electrotherapy

Heat is utilized in two ways:

1. As a sedative to obtain relaxation and relief of muscle spasm and pain, e.g. in acute arthritis.

2. As an accelerator of the circulation. It thereby improves the blood supply to an area and so reduces congestion, e.g. in weak or paralyzed muscles. This increased blood flow will also carry away the unwanted products of inflammation as in carbuncles or a septic finger, and will help to prevent adhesions in ruptured muscles such as those connected with the movement of arthritic joints.

Radiant Heat and Infra-red Rays are given by focusing the rays from a lamp on to the incapacitated part of the body. The rays penetrate below the skin layer and the heat causes a more vigorous blood flow in the area.

Moist Heat. In some cases, forms of moist heat are preferred including hot packs, medicated mud packs, and hot saline baths. The heat improves the circulation in the skin and subcutaneous tissues.

Paraffin Wax Baths. Wax baths for the alleviation of rheumatic stiffness in the hands and feet, and occasionally in other joints, is given for patients both in hospital and in out-patient physiotherapy departments or clinics. The skin must be clean and dry and free from any grease. The patient sits in a comfortable chair near a small table on which stands a small bath of melted wax at about 120° F. For protecting the clothing against drips of wax the patient's lap is covered with a piece of plastic or rubber sheeting. The hands (or limbs) are fully immersed in the softened wax several times until it forms a 'glove.' They are then lifted out gently and the excess wax allowed to drip from the finger tips back into the bath.

In some cases the physiotherapist applies the wax with a brush (like a pastry brush) while the patient spreads his hands on grease-proof paper. The physiotherapist then wraps greaseproof paper or some other protective material around the hands which are then wrapped round with a blanket and rested upon the patient's lap.

After about twenty minutes (first applications will be for shorter periods) the wrappings are removed and the wax is peeled off like a pair of gloves, when the skin will be found to be covered with beads of sweat. The natural heat engendered by the close-fitting wax covering is very soothing to the inner tissues and enables the patient to move the stiffened joints more freely. Other physical treatment is then proceeded with on the warmed limb.

The wax method of giving heat is particularly useful for stiff and scarred hands and feet.

If the doctor has ordered the wax to be applied frequently (sometimes it is used daily), the patient may be given a supply to use at home.

For feet and ankles, warm mud is sometimes applied as an alternative to wax. **But if the patient has any varicose veins the** treatment is dangerous because the heat will induce inflammation.

Short Wave Diathermy. When heating of deeper structures is required short wave diathermy may be given. A special machine is used and a comfortable heat induced in the part of the body by using carefully selected electrodes in the form of rubber-covered pads or special discs which are connected to the machine. If they are correctly placed, the short wave electric current, in passing from one to the other will pass through the part to be treated, causing heat to be generated in the tissues. Short wave diathermy is frequently prescribed for neck and shoulders, as well as for knees and ankles.

The skin must be clean and dry. The therapist fixes the electrode plates (suitably sized according to the part being treated) and after about four minutes a very gentle warmth should be felt.

The therapist will ask the patient if it feels hot. On no account must it feel uncomfortably hot, or the skin will be burned. Sufferers sometimes believe, quite wrongly, that 'hot' treatment will bring speedier relief and so they do not tell the therapist that it feels really hot. Patients should remember that people vary and the therapist can only tell from the patient's description whether or not too much current is being applied.

Short wave diathermy is usually applied for about five to ten minutes the first time, the period being gradually increased until fifteen or twenty minutes is reached. Headaches sometimes indicate that the patient needs shorter treatments or that he has had sufficient treatments, and that is for the doctor to judge, but he can only do so if the patient tells him of any discomforts or disabilities connected with the treatment.

Faradism induces correct function of muscle groups when their action has been temporarily interfered with by injury, disease, or disuse, e.g. in the quadriceps muscle after operation on the knee, or in the small muscles of the feet in cases of flat foot.

The patient puts his foot in a small bath of tepid water. The therapist has two electrodes (small pieces of metal connected to the electrical apparatus) wrapped in wet cloths, one being placed in the water and the other applied to the muscle or joint. Usually the electrode is pressed gently against the flesh, then raised, theopera tion being repeated a little higher, or more to one side, as the toning is required. As the electrode is applied and the current switched on by the therapist, the patient feels a slight prickling sensation which gradually spreads through the limb, and muscular contraction is felt. It helps the therapist to adjust the strength of the current and the position of the electrode if the patient describes just how strong these contractions feel or in which direction they seem to have the strongest effect.

In foot treatment the patient is occasionally allowed to sit for a short time with feet in the water, but should inform the therapist when the current feels stronger or weaker.

In other cases where the extremities are not the focal point, electrodes wrapped in wet cloths are applied simultaneously, again giving a sense of contraction.

At least twenty minutes' rest after each treatment is advisable, since patients attending a clinic, who are well enough to travel home without hospital transport, should not attempt the return journey immediately.

This method is used to teach muscle sense and to restore rhythm, and once the pattern of movement has been re-established the treatment is discontinued.

Other electrical machines provide types of current with different properties. Interrupted galvanism is used to stimulate contraction of paralyzed muscles until recovery begins. Yet other types can assist cases of circulatory disturbances or swelling, or may be used to administer drugs by ionization (see Medical and Technical Procedures).

Artificial Sunlight has stimulating and healing properties and is produced by powerfully bactericidal **Ultraviolet Rays**. The effects are due to chemical changes in the skin and an increase of activity in the tissues, and it is used for cleansing and stimulating the

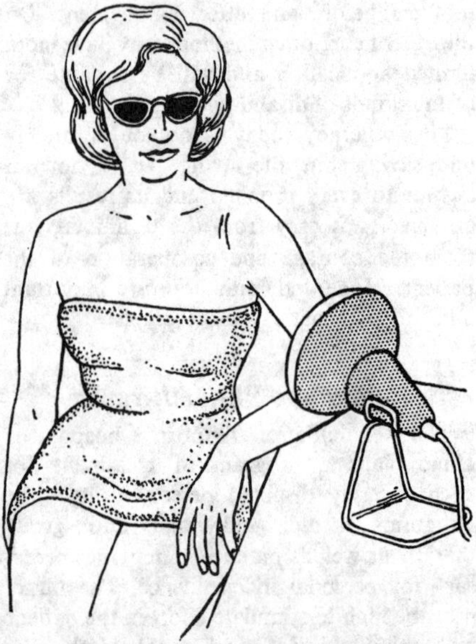

Fig. 2. *QUARTZ LAMP for home use provides a mixture of infra-red and ultraviolet rays. Use only according to the dosage advised by the doctor.*

healing of ulcers, slow healing wounds, pressure sores, some skin lesions, and certain types of baldness. Dosages may be given to produce a mild or a strong reaction. General doses of ultraviolet light may also be used for their tonic effect on the whole body in cases of debility, or to prevent recurrent colds. The patient feels no particular sensation during treatment, but it is necessary to have the eyes protected by goggles from the intensity of these light rays.

Ultrasonic Therapy

Ultrasonics or treatment by ultra-sound therapy is a branch of physical therapy involving new principles. By means of a High Frequency generator, a treatment head (or applicator) and a medium such as oil or water for conduction, it makes use of vibrations which are too rapid to be heard. It is a valuable complement to other physical methods and is superior to them in the treatment of selected patients with fibrositic and certain arthritic conditions, or patients with scar tissue and soft tissue injuries, effusion, sprains, and ligament and tendon injuries.

Passive and Active Movements

Joint movements of all kinds may be performed either by use of passive movements using an external agent such as a piece of apparatus or the hands of the physiotherapist, or by the contraction by the patient of his own muscles, which is called active movement.

Passive Movements have a limited sphere of usefulness but used with discrimination can make a valuable contribution towards recovery, e.g. traction (a form of pulling) to the spine, either manually or with specially designed apparatus, can reduce pain and muscle spasm. They may also be used to maintain a small range of movement in muscles and joints where active movements are impossible and to preserve the patterns of movement while muscles are paralyzed, as in poliomyelitis, or they may be given to correct deformities from birth, such as wry neck and club feet.

Manipulations are a special technique of passive movement particularly designed for alleviating conditions of the spine, including some types of disc lesions.

Active Movements are by far the most important of physical measures used, but they are not always the most enjoyable or the most appreciated! By the active use of the muscles, power, strength and endurance are restored to weak muscles, faulty posture can be corrected, joint range improved, and co-ordination retrained.

When muscles are very weak, the movements can be assisted either by the physiotherapist or by the use of special apparatus with slings on ropes which support the part being treated. A frame known as the Guthrie-Smith Frame has been designed for the purpose of supporting the ropes in any position; this improved form of suspension therapy enables the physiotherapist to give the patient a progressive series of exercises. Assistance is decreased stage by stage and the patient gradually progresses to free unassisted movements. Later, as recovery takes place, the physiotherapist's hand, or springs or weights, are offered as objects of resistance against which the working muscles must make some effort. Later still, practice sessions on various types of equipment may be added.

Proprioception is the power to appreciate one's muscles and joints and this power can easily be lost as a result of pain and stiffness, but function can be re-educated by accurate and careful muscle training. If a wrong movement pattern is built up, e.g. a limp, then great patience is necessary by both patient and therapist to regain the feel of the correct movement and to practice it until it becomes automatic. Muscle can also be re-educated when there is little or no pattern there, as in poor posture or a long-standing stiff joint which has been made movable again by surgery.

Daily activity is made up of habit movements such as walking and touching things. These movements need practically no thought, although they may be very complex, because there is a pattern in the brain for each activity. If even a small part of a movement is lost, the whole unconscious mechanism is put out of action and it is often surprising how great a disability results. In order to restore function, the steps and stages of any activity must be analyzed, and separate exercises need to be worked out for each. When the individual movements are restored then the automatic pattern in the brain can be regained.

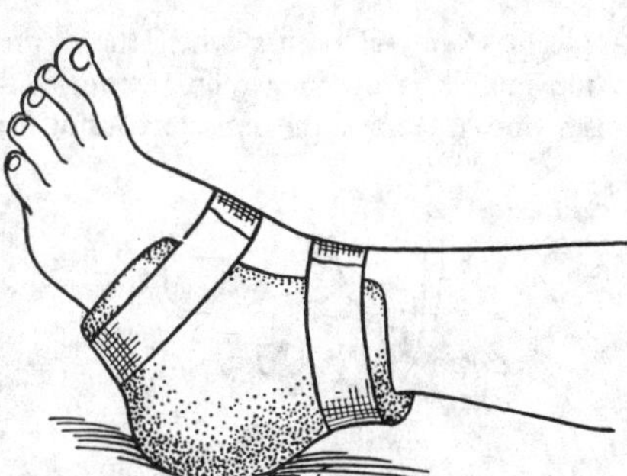

Fig. 3. *HEEL PAD used to prevent bedsores in patients confined to bed for a long time.*

Modern methods of exercise use natural and functional patterns of body movements, although special techniques are still used for retraining the co-ordination of a set of movements, for muscle action, good posture, and relaxation.

Pool Therapy

Pool therapy consists of special exercises with and without the assistance of specially designed equipment and using the buoyancy of water. It is usually given in conjunction with other forms of physical treatment, although it should not be used for patients with certain diseases of the heart, chest and kidneys, or in those with skin disorders, open wounds, or incontinence.

In this form of treatment (which may last from five to thirty minutes each session) the water is not medicated. Its special advantages are the warmth of the water (usually 96° to 98° F) which relieves pain and aids relaxation, the elimination of gravity so that body weight is relieved, and the lessening of friction which makes the patient comfortable and movement easier. Weight-relieving positions and a fine gradation of exercises can be obtained, and the patient finds that changing position is less difficult. The physiotherapist can watch the movements and muscle action more easily, too.

Pool therapy has a recreational value and the patient enjoys it, which gives an increased impetus to recovery. For the severely handicapped the ability to swim may also provide a means of general exercise, recreation and social contacts at a later stage of rehabilitation. The patient is brought into a new environment where all the movements which he has found difficult are made easier, where the temperature and buoyancy of the water ease his pain and give him a feeling of well-being. He senses that he is making progress, his efforts are rewarded, he feels more cheerful and he is stimulated to greater effort.

GROUP THERAPY

Class work is used when a more competitive activity is desirable to make exercises more interesting and stimulating for the patients. Group teaching may range from ward classes to encourage maintenance of muscle tone in the unaffected parts of the body, or ante- and post-natal exercises, to classes in the Physiotherapy Department for those who need remedial exercise for hands, for legs, for shoulders or any other particular body part. Patients whose hands are recovering from injury or disease, or which require re-education after surgery, benefit from the variety and competition obtained by working with others. Patients with weak or damaged feet enjoy working together in groups and in this way games and competitions can aid in retraining muscle function. Those with shoulders, back, and knees affected gain much from watching others and from the realization that they too have a real problem to get their temporarily awkward limbs going again.

Later, as the condition improves, many of the patients progress to eurythmics, dancing, and games and then to full educational gymnastics in order to obtain the best results. At all stages in treatment, the patients are instructed about correct positioning and how and what to practice on their own.

Prophylactic Activity

Physical treatment is usually considered to be for the treatment of conditions already in existence but it is, in fact, often used as a form of preventive or prophylactic activity for both adults and children. Growing children are taught correct posture, and any tendency to flat feet, knock-knees, and spinal curvature is in many instances corrected before it becomes a real deformity. Schoolchildren and students can be taught correct posture, and nurses in training and workers in industry may be instructed in body mechanics and in methods of lifting. In hospital, early exercises and early ambulation often prevent the development of complications in both surgical and medical cases. Chest complications after anesthetics are greatly reduced by pre- and post-operative breathing exercises.

Chest Conditions

Common chest conditions which need remedial treatment are faulty breathing, coughing spasms, defective posture, limited chest movements, or reduced capacity of the lungs with low tolerance to exercise. The therapy may take the form of instruction in correct breathing, postural drainage of the lungs, posture training, or in improved movement of the chest wall. All help to restore the patient's confidence and to facilitate his recovery. Communal games are often used for the children, and frequently the Department looks rather like a playroom with the young patients imitating windmills, playing express trains or blowing ping-pong balls across a tub of water.

Patients with asthma and bronchitis are taught to live with their condition and to control it by learning to relax, to do correct diaphragmatic breathing and to acquire a new breathing rhythm if their earlier pattern was incorrect. Other chest conditions which may benefit are pre- and post-operative chest surgery, pneumonia, or cases of shock. Elderly people are also kept much fitter by breathing exercises and by carefully graduated movements during the period in which their activity is restricted.

Pre-natal and Post-partum Exercises

Exercises and other therapy are given to promote mental and physical well-being during pregnancy and to help the mother to co-operate during labor.

The mothers are given explanations of the need for correct breathing and relaxation during pregnancy and during the birth process itself. This is followed by instruction in relaxation and in breathing control. Afterwards, exercises are taught to correct the mother's posture, to tone up the muscles (especially those of the abdominal wall), or as a preventive against swelling of the legs and feet. Later, if necessary, treatment may be given to relieve breast congestion and to prevent thrombosis in the limbs.

Disabilities in Children

In the treatment of infants and children with muscular and limb disabilities, simpler versions of the routine exercises for adults are widely used. Deformities are now treated quite early in the child's life; special equipment and walking aids are devised to suit different cases, and for general activity much

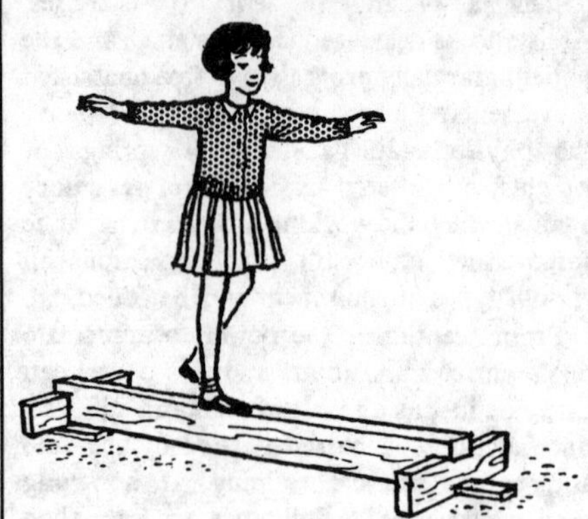

Fig. 4. *BALANCING EXERCISE to improve the child's muscular disability.*

use is made of adapted and carefully graduated toys.

To help children with CEREBRAL PALSY to lead as normal a life as possible, several different methods of treatment are available and the best possible one for each child has to be selected and a full program of treatment carefully carried out. Such children are taken at their own slower pace through all stages of normal development, e.g. rolling, crawling and sitting, however long it takes. They are also educated within their limits and taught to help themselves in feeding, toilet requirements, washing, dressing, and so on.

Nervous Diseases

Among the largest groups of disorders which benefit from physical treatment are those of the nervous system.

Flaccid Paralysis occurs when the nerve to the muscle is no longer conducting impulses and therefore the muscle cannot be made to move; this happens after poliomyelitis or after direct injury to the nerve. Re-education and exercises are then needed to restore power and endurance. A surgical repair of the nerve may be needed before physiotherapy can be given, but in other cases treatment is given to get the part into the best possible state before surgery. Recovery of nerve function is a very uncertain matter. No known treatment influences the rate at which the damaged nerve will recover, but electrical treatment may help the muscle fibers to contract during recovery and so reduce tissue wasting. The muscle fibers themselves contract to the stimulus of a certain strength of current even when the nerve supply is cut off, and so they can be kept somewhat active until the nerve cells and fibers regenerate and become able to function again. For electrical treatment, metal plates with a moist pad between each plate and the patient's skin, or else special padded discs, are placed on the affected muscle for short periods. As soon as there is any sign of nerve recovery, careful re-education of each individual muscle is instituted. Severely affected patients are taught to make the best possible use of muscles remaining active and to walk if at all possible, even if calipers (leg splints), special shoes, crutches, or walking aids have to be used.

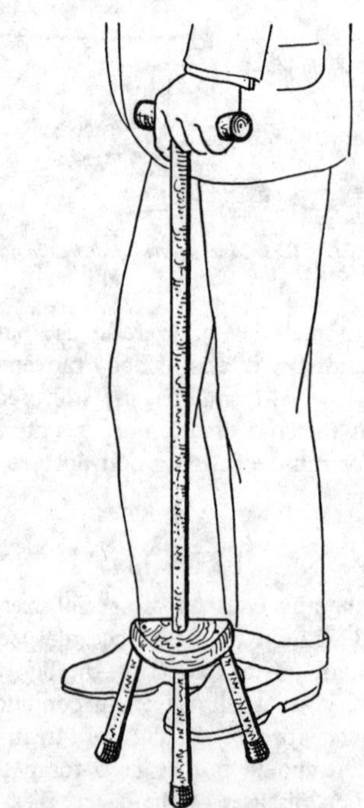

Fig. 5. *WOODEN TRIPOD WALKING AID gives firm balance for the patient who is recovering from paralysis, or a leg injury.*

In the early stages of poliomyelitis complete rest is essential for good recovery, and sometimes constant attendance upon the patient may be necessary if the muscles of breathing are affected and the patient has to be given artificial respiration in a respirator.

Sensory, Cerebellar and Ataxic Conditions occur when certain parts of the nervous system are damaged, making movements of the limbs and trunk clumsy, uncontrolled, and incoordinate. The co-ordinating centers in the patient's brain are no longer receiving stimuli (or messages) from nerves in distant parts of the body and they cannot therefore return instructive impulses to the limbs, or other parts, for the correct movements, as in walking or picking up objects. Such patients need to be taught how to walk by sight instead of by the natural automatic means. Certain of their exercises consist of placing the feet on footprints marked on a strip of matting. New movement is at first very jerky, and music is sometimes used to gain better rhythm in the gait.

In **Hemiplegia,** one arm and one leg of the same side are paralysed, while **Paraplegia** means that both legs are affected. Partial or full paralysis is frequently the result of traffic or industrial accidents which have caused damage to the spinal cord or brain. Treatment is often started as soon as the patient recovers consciousness. Splints of aluminium, plaster of Paris, or plastic, and shaped to suit the injured part of the body may be used to prevent deformities.

Passive movement (see p. 177) is given early to relieve stiffness and to train the feeling of

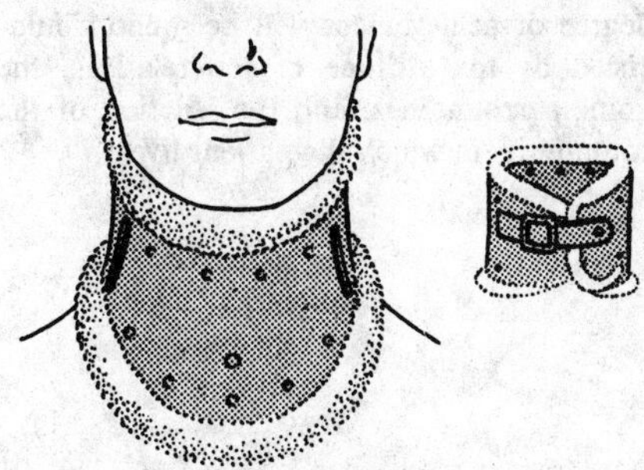

Fig. 6. *NECK SUPPORT shaped to suit the injured part of the body.*

movement, but as soon as possible active movements are started, sometimes using the suspension technique. Treatment is not only given to improve the local condition, but also to encourage self-reliance and the general progress to walking and recreation.

Sciatica associated with a lumbar disc injury causes acute pain which must be relieved as early as possible. Rest in bed is essential for one or two weeks and then hyperextension exercises in bed are often given. The exercises are graduated as improvement occurs. Similarly, the severe pain of brachial neuritis in a busy housewife is first relieved by resting the arm from all activity before exercise is begun.

Amputations and Surgical Cases

For athletic injuries, amputations, reconstruction of damaged hands (including plastic surgery), fractures, and tendon and soft tissue injuries, internal surgical methods of fixation are often used in preference to immobilization for long periods in splints; and movements to re-educate the muscles are also started early in these cases. After a joint repair, constant repetition of each newly obtained movement is essential and the patient has to relearn how to balance, how to remain stable and how to move his muscles in a comfortable way. In the case of the lower limbs he will need instruction in correct weight-bearing and in daily living activities such as getting up steps, and on and off the toilet seat.

Heart Disorders

Techniques used in the treatment of circulatory and heart disorders are very carefully regulated. Precise records are kept in these cases in order to assess gradual progress and to forestall any strain or relapse.

Record and assessment charts are kept of each patient's muscle power and reactions, activities, dosages, and so on in order to modify a plan of treatment, or so that alternative methods may be compared, and new ideas investigated and applied. Progress recorded on the charts is also encouraging for the patient.

Rheumatic and Arthritic Conditions

These include fibrositis, rheumatoid arthritis, osteo-arthritis and ankylosing spondylitis and form a very high percentage of the crippling diseases treated. All these conditions have symptoms of muscle spasm, restricted range of movement in joints, wasting and weakness of muscle and gradual loss of useful activity.

Painful swollen joints need rest, progressing to rest interspersed with exercise. If a patient wears splints, they are usually removed regularly for remedial movements; and the remainder of the body is kept active while the splints are being worn. Even a patient with ankylosing spondylitis may need limited exercise so as to preserve the functioning of his muscles and to restore his independence as much and as soon as possible. Many techniques are devised and used by the physiotherapist to obtain the required results for each of her patients but analgesics (pain-relieving drugs) are not given too often when remedial exercises prove painful because the condition may be worsened by too much activity being done under their protective 'cover.' Arthritic and rheumatic patients benefit particularly from hydrotherapy and spa treatment because the water lightens some of the weight-bearing from the weak muscles and painful joints.

Therapy for the Elderly

Geriatrics is that department of medicine which treats all problems peculiar to aging and old age. It is a great help if a therapist sees and talks to these patients in their home surroundings before admission to hospital. They fear that once they are admitted they will never get out again, and therefore they get emotionally upset and anxious. They are afraid of the strange words used, and fear they will be rejected by their families. For these reasons they are reluctant to call for help until a crisis arises. But once in the care of a physiotherapist and the other members of the team, much can be done to get them going and to relieve their fears. Given enough time and the right approach, however, they will co-operate and so have a chance of improving their powers of activity and mobility which will enable them to return home.

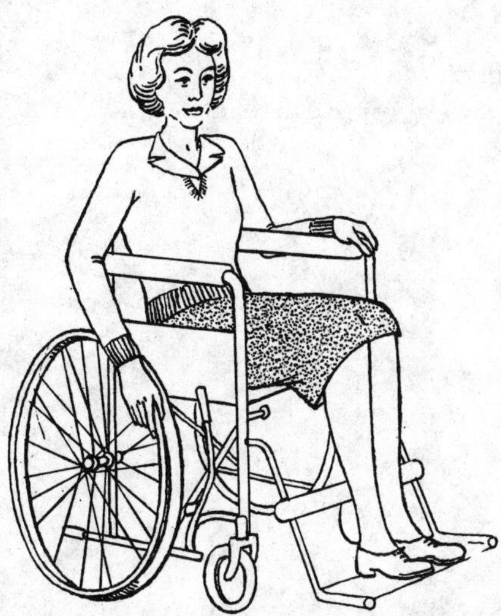

Fig. 7. *MODERN FOLDING WHEELCHAIR. This model is built for comfort and maneuverability.*

HOME TREATMENT

Preparing for the Return Home

The physiotherapist influences the patient's attitude to his future. She endeavors to draw out the maximum capacity of which each patient is capable and she is helped by the co-operation and understanding of the relatives who must be guided by the Rehabilitation Team in handling and managing the disabled person. Over-protectiveness and too much help are just as harmful as lack of help and understanding, but relatives should not attempt to bear too heavy a burden in case they break down.

Before a patient returns home he must learn how to cope with the particular domestic hazards he will face in his home surroundings. A simple daily necessity such as going to the toilet may have become a complicated awkward set of movements to the person with a stiffened hip or with one arm. So the relatives are asked to give accurate and adequate details concerning the layout of the home, kitchen arrangements, width of doors and passages, possible slopes, curbs and ramps. Training under similar conditions in the physiotherapy department is then started, e.g. standing, walking, balancing and management of activities in relation to bed, chair, toilet, bath, steps and stairs.

The bedfast patient needs the greatest possible independence in bed and in sitting; the house-bound need complete independence within the four walls of home, including dressing, bathing and feeding. The ambulant person needs the ability to get about on various surfaces such as grass, gravel, wet pavements, steps and slopes. Some need training in how to use transport—a wheelchair, special vehicle, adapted car, or a public bus or train. The physiotherapist tries to teach the patient maximum independence so that he needs the least possible help once he returns home.

The Rehabilitation Team consider and recommend modifications and adaptations in the home, such as suitable switches, handrails and taps. Relatives are instructed on how to give the necessary physical help in lifting, changing position, using a hoist or assisting with walking. If necessary, they are put in touch with people or local services who will advise and help them with their problems.

Treatment at Home

In some cases, it is considered more suitable for a physiotherapist to give treatment in the patient's own home, or she may continue treatment which had begun in hospital. She works with the general practitioner and consults other members of the team. As in the hospital department, a treatment program is carefully planned for the individual patient. Success or failure depends entirely on the full co-operation of the patient who is the key person and who must know what is involved, and what part he must play in his

own rehabilitation. Therapist, patient and family must have a frank discussion and any suggestions and ideas from the patient and relatives will be considered and tried out if possible. But, of course, what the patient wants is not always the best thing for him. In helping the patient to master his disability and readjust to a different way of life, the degree of achievement will be greatly influenced by the attitude of the relatives, the home surroundings, and the reaction of the community in which the patient lives.

OCCUPATIONAL THERAPY

'Employment is nature's best physician,' wrote Galen in the second century A.D. Since then occupational therapy has been practiced for centuries in one form or another. The Greeks understood and appreciated the therapeutic values of art, drama and eurythmics, while the Egyptians employed simple forms of music and harmony.

At first it was the physician himself who applied the treatment but it is only since the twentieth century, particularly since the Second World War, that occupational therapy has been recognized as a supplementary medical service. It treats the physically and mentally ill by employing varied activities to aid in their recovery from injury or disease. It is the treatment which follows the medical prescription given by a physician for each individual patient and which is administered by an occupational therapist.

Physiotherapists, Remedial Gymnasts, Speech Therapists, Occupational Therapists and medical social workers often work together as a team. For example, a patient who has had a stroke may become partially paralyzed and also lose his speech. As soon as the physician permits, the physiotherapist will begin treatment by retraining the patient to walk. Later, the occupational therapist will teach the patient to feed and dress himself while the speech therapist will concentrate on the re-establishment of communication by speech and writing.

In occupational therapy the range of activities is very wide, and innumerable methods may be employed since no two patients present the same difficulties. All activities, however, must be related to the physical, psychological, social, and economic problems of each patient. Occupation to pass the time and without medical reason is not occupational therapy. Each activity is selected to benefit the patient and improve his condition.

Rehabilitation is the return to the maximum possible function of which the patient is capable.

THERAPEUTIC OCCUPATIONS

In the early acute stage of an illness the patient has little inclination or capacity for even the simplest activity, but once he begins to take an interest again in the people and things around him he may be allowed to have passive therapy which will make little demand on his strength—reading, or being read to, listening to the radio, watching television, dictating letters or joining in guessing games. It is only when the physician decides that the patient has reached the stage when more active occupations will further aid his recovery that a change is made in the routine.

There are five main groups into which active therapy may be divided:

1. The Personal Activities of Daily Living, often referred to by the initials P.A.D.L.
2. Arts and Crafts.
3. Recreational Activities.
4. Industrial and Vocational Activities.
5. Educational Activities.

All of these are used for both physical disabilities and psychological disorders. It is an important part of the occupational therapist's work to assess the individual needs of each person or group under her charge.

Personal Activities of Daily Living

The activities of daily living are feeding, washing and dressing, toilet management and the ability to perform useful tasks. For the disabled patient, aids and adaptations may be necessary and these help towards independence. Built-up cutlery for the weak grip, non-spilling drinking cups for those with tremor, bath hand-rails for the arthritic, or lever handles on taps and doors for the partially paralyzed or hemiplegic patient all aid in giving him the confidence that he can do much to help himself.

In hospitals today there are kitchen units specially designed for disabled patients, and practice in using all the gadgets and adjustments provided in the unit will give confidence to the disabled housewife when she returns home.

Arts and Crafts

Arts and craft activities range from those which are diversional to those which are vocational and which may help the patient to earn a partial living when he has left the hospital. On the whole, hospital handicrafts are undertaken for the enjoyment rather than for the need to learn a new trade, though this may well happen also. Some handicrafts such as weaving and cord knotting are excellent for the re-education of weak muscles and joints.

Some of the arts and crafts activities used in hospitals are:

Basketry	Marquetry	Painting
Book binding	Modelling	Sketching
Embroidery	Pottery	Lino-cut making
Crochet	Mosaic	Drawing
Tatting	Puppetry	Stencilling
Knitting	Rug making	Fabric printing
Lacemaking	Spinning	Carving
Needlework	Caning	Toy making
Leatherwork	Weaving	Netting

Recreational Activities

Music is usually considered as one of the recreational activities so far as the hospital is concerned and it plays an important part in the life of the patient especially during the acute stage of his illness when no effort is permitted. Concerts, sing-songs, radio, television, the phonograph, and a hospital band, create a happy atmosphere from which great benefit may be derived.

Acting, puppet shows, socials, card games or club activities have a social basis and help to keep the patients interested in those around them. Indoor games and outdoor games as well as sports and camping may be included in the recreational activities.

Vocational and Industrial Activities

When time-tables are being planned for the rehabilitation of patients, special consideration must be given to those who have lost a limb, become partially paralyzed, or who have not recovered their former strength or ability. In the larger hospitals the occupational therapy department will provide some light machinery and equipment for training for such work as the following:

Housecraft	Switchboard-operating	Brushmaking
Gardening	Weaving	Draftsmanship
Office routine	Pottery	Photography
Assembly work	Machining (treadle or power)	Printing
Upholstery		Woodwork
		Metalwork

Educational Activities

Most hospitals nowadays possess their own libraries and all patients may become borrowers.

For children there is the hospital teacher who may either attend them in the wards or, if they are up and about, will give group lessons in the hospital schoolroom.

Educational activities also include:

Correspondence courses	Library work
Learning languages	Hospital newspaper
Studying in groups	Hobbies

Planning the Patients' Programs

The range of cases dealt with in general hospitals is so wide that it is only possible to outline programs suitable for the main illness groups. Once the doctor has indicated the particular lines of treatment the therapist's object in planning a program for an individual or a group is to build up work tolerance gradually to the fullest capacity and to avoid fatigue in her patients. Perseverance on the part of the patient is essential to recovery.

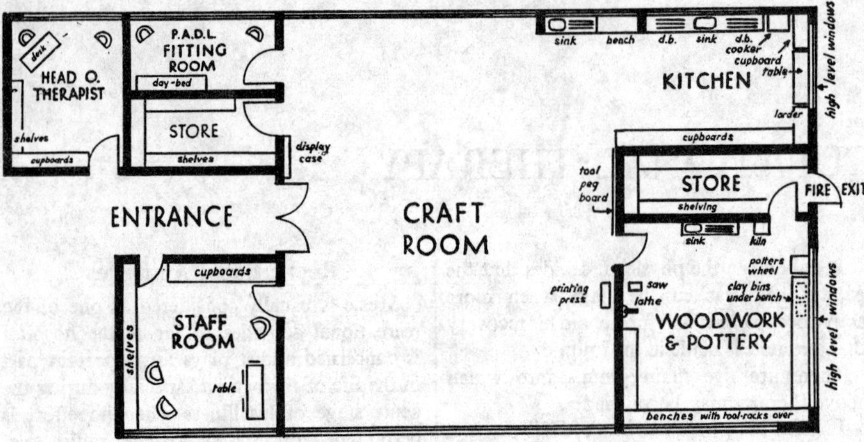

PLAN OF AN OCCUPATIONAL THERAPY DEPARTMENT

Fig. 1. *The design and plan of an Occupational Therapy Department varies greatly from hospital to hospital according to the type of patient, their numbers, ages, and incapacity. The above plan would fulfil the basic needs for a small general hospital.*

In hospitals and institutions, the occupational therapy departments have to deal with patients in varying stages of recovery. There are patients in bed, ambulant ward patients, those who are able to walk to the department and remain there for a working period, and those who can attend in wheelchairs. Some are even brought to the department in their beds!

Bed patients require light activities and as little equipment as possible. Only clean simple materials should be used for handicrafts. A great deal depends on the position and the restriction of movement of the patient. Slings, frames, mirrors and other adaptations may be necessary to help him to do his work. Reading and educational books are useful at this stage; jig-saw puzzles, games and solitaire all have their place. Hobbies, such as stamp collecting, should be encouraged especially for long-term patients.

Patients who can attend the occupational therapy department are able to enjoy a much wider range of activities. Special adjustments for limb injuries and selected work give the patient the first up-grade towards full rehabilitation. All work must be supervised to avoid fatiguing the patient and to prevent strain on healing areas. Well-planned programs help to overcome mental stress, maintain correct physical function, and aid in the restoration of joint and muscle coordination. This in its turn helps to improve the blood circulation and breathing, aids in better posture and improves sleep and appetite.

The old idea that handicrafts would supply sufficient interest and exercise for the disabled convalescent patient has given place to a more realistic attitude. A housewife who develops skills in basketry or fabric printing will not necessarily feel competent to cope with all her duties in the kitchen when she returns home nor may a man who has produced good leatherwork in the occupational therapy department feel assured that he can adequately handle the factory machinery to which he was formerly accustomed. Therefore any activity which leads to a back-to-normal environment should be employed: the housewife needs practice in the kitchen unit, and the man may use treadle or power machines.

A MODERN OCCUPATIONAL THERAPY DEPARTMENT

Occupational therapy departments vary greatly from hospital to hospital. So often in the past, basements, converted outbuildings or even garages were used, but of recent years much thought has been put into the planning of suitable day space departments.

A modern department in a general hospital would ideally be a large airy room on the ground floor with French windows opening on to a veranda where patients could take their work in summertime. Smaller side rooms should lead from the main craft room. These would be used for specific work such as pottery and woodwork, and household jobs in the kitchen unit. A sliding partition fitted across the main room could be used to divide the department into one or two craft rooms as the need arose.

The main craft room needs to be well heated, lighted and ventilated. At least one large sink is required for general use and for wetting cane for basketry. Plenty of cupboard space is essential for materials, tools and finished articles. Peg-boards, within easy reach of the hand, should be fixed to the walls for tools. Chairs should be sturdy yet of light weight and should be stackable. Work tables should be of different heights to suit both walking patients and those in wheelchairs.

In the main craft room one might expect to find large foot looms, hand looms and rug looms, also a bicycle saw, a printing press and book binding equipment, sewing machines, a dressmaker's model, typewriters, and a duplicating machine. A work bench with vises, artists' easels and various types of embroidery frames all make up part of the equipment required to stock an occupational therapy department.

A side room should be kept for pottery as it is extremely messy work: in it will be a sink, modeling bench, large metal bins for the clay, a drying shelf, a potter's wheel and the kiln. The floor should be tiled so that it may be thoroughly scrubbed down occasionally.

Woodwork should also be allotted a separate room as it is noisy and untidy. A large store room is needed to stow away the lengths of wood and the finished goods. In the woodwork room itself carpentry benches fitted with vises, lathes and bench drills, light machinery, and fretsaws will provide for the varied capabilities of the patients.

The kitchen unit is better housed in a side room but it is often only a partitioned-off part of the main craft room. Here the equipment is largely fitted to suit the wheelchair patients. The sink must not be too high, and the stove, whether gas or electric, must be of a suitable height also. The pantry shelves should be at hand level and all kitchen utensils within hand reach. Specially designed ironing boards are made to suit the disabled patient and are usually fixed to the wall.

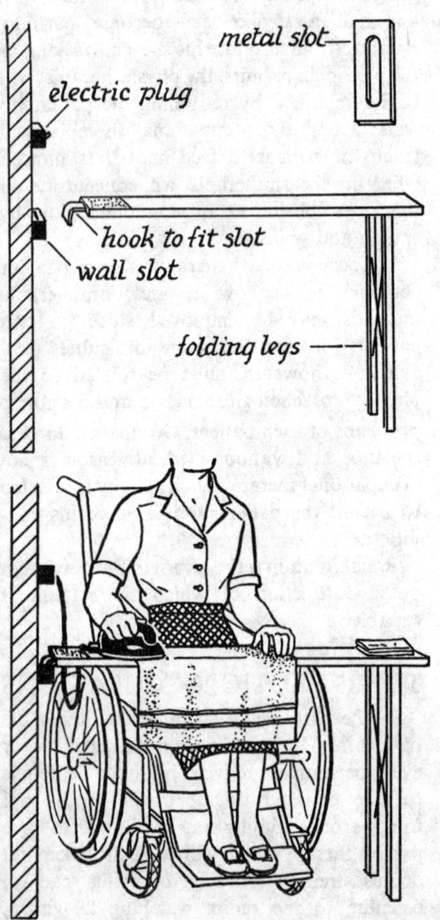

Fig. 2. *IRONING BOARD FOR DISABLED HOUSEWIVES*

Self-aid kitchen gadgets such as can openers for the one-handed person, meat-cutting holders, saw-edged knives, lever tap handles and revolving shelves are all features of the hospital kitchen unit.

Several organizations such as the Red Cross publish illustrated literature describing various aids and the means of obtaining them.

ACTIVITIES FOR SPECIAL CASES

Each disease or disablement has reactions on the patients specific to the disease and these have all to be taken into consideration when planning occupational programs. Those with cardiac diseases quickly suffer from fatigue, and patients with metabolic diseases such as diabetes are inclined to be irritable and must not be over-stimulated. With chest complaints only the lightest therapy is possible and all fluffy materials must be kept away from the patient, or he must wear a mask.

Surgical Cases

The first essential for these patients is to prevent strain in the healing areas; passive occupational therapy is begun as soon as the physician gives his consent.

The psychological aspect in patients who have undergone surgical operations has to be very carefully considered so that they do not suffer from shock, but at the same time they must be helped to become interested in making an effort toward normal function and rehabilitation.

In cases of burns the occupational therapy employed must be directed towards overcoming the stiffness caused by immobility and scar tissue following skin grafting, so that most careful planning and adjustment are necessary.

For patients who have undergone surgery after an accident or industrial injury, for those with limited joint movement, peripheral nerve injuries, spastic hemiplegics, and those suffering from multiple sclerosis, the treatment program should provide:

1. rhythmic and repetitive movements;
2. avoidance of static grips;
3. contraction and relaxation of muscles by graded work; and
4. re-education of poor muscular function.

This will build up work tolerance and avoid fatigue, increase muscle power and range of joint movement, prevent further injury and atrophy from disuse, and develop a healthy psychological outlook.

AMPUTEES. After the shock of surgery, emotional adjustment of the person who has lost a limb is very important. Then, as soon as the physician considers the patient is fit enough, he is given exercises to prepare him to use and control the artificial limb (or prosthesis) with which he will be provided. The amputee must be taught to look at his disability in a healthy way. An artificial limb is not only to be used as a tool but to help with balance and improved personal appearance. Dexterity of the remaining limb should be encouraged and improved so that the artificial limb takes second place.

The Personal Activities of Daily Living may begin when the patient is still in bed. Feeding himself is the first stage, then toilet activities and later dressing movements. Self-help aids may be used for the retraining of the patient.

The occupational therapist must teach the patient how to use his artificial limb correctly and how to apply and fix the harness for the maximum comfort. Persistence is needed by the wearer of an artificial limb and in spite of pain and discomfort he must be persuaded to persevere.

Artificial limbs are now prescribed for amputee children in spite of the fact that they grow out of them but the psychological and physical benefits are well worth the effort.

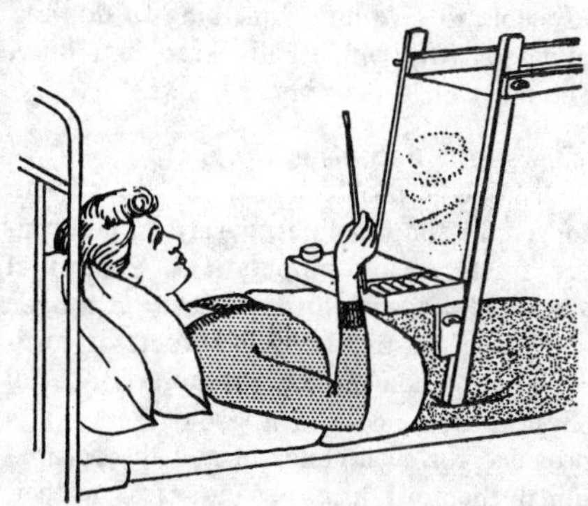

Fig. 3. *EASEL FOR A POLIOMYELITIS CASE. Since there is so much variability in disablement in each case of poliomyelitis, apparatus is usually adapted for each patient's needs.*

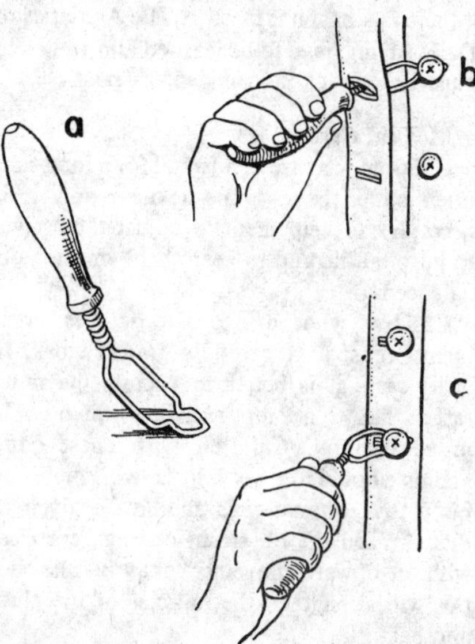

Fig. 4. *BUTTONING A COAT WITH ONE HAND. (a) Shows a specially designed buttonhook; (b) Shows how it is inserted through the buttonhole and around the button; and (c) how the button is pulled into position.*

The bicycle-saw, treadles of looms or sewing machines, potter's wheels and lathes are all mechanical aids to retraining the muscles of foot and leg amputees. Gardening in its many forms may also help in recovery by the use of forks and spades for digging, the sawing of logs or the pushing of a lawn mower.

Arthritic Cases

Heat helps the patient with rheumatoid arthritis considerably and the use of slings, supports and special splinting also gives some ease thus aiding the patient to a better use of his limbs. The Personal Activities of Daily Living are essential for these patients because the functions of feeding, dressing and toilet activities form the basis of restoring them to the routines of everyday life.

For the housewife about to return home, practice in the occupational therapy kitchen unit, with its specially fitted sink, wheeled kitchen trolley, modified cooker and kitchen self-help aids and other gadgets forms the basis for retraining.

Osteoarthritics

Once the patient begins to get up, the utmost care of the joints is essential. Activities such as weaving, which give rhythmic and repetitive movements, are the most valuable in such cases. It is very essential to avoid fatigue. It may be possible for such patients to return to sheltered work, and for them sedentary occupations are best.

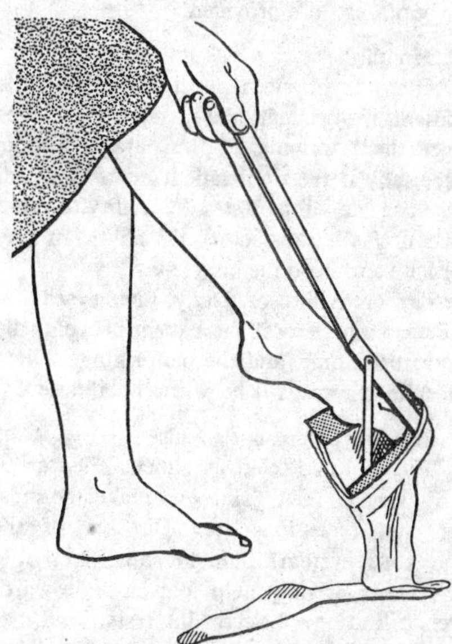

Fig. 5. *STOCKING PULL-UP designed to help the arthritic patient who cannot bend to put on her stocking.*

Poliomyelitis Cases

Since no two cases of poliomyelitis are alike it is necessary to create an individual program for each patient.

Separate appliances may have to be made and a great deal of ingenuity is required in adapting these to the patient's needs. There are special centers for polio cases and these are equipped to suit the disabilities of those attending.

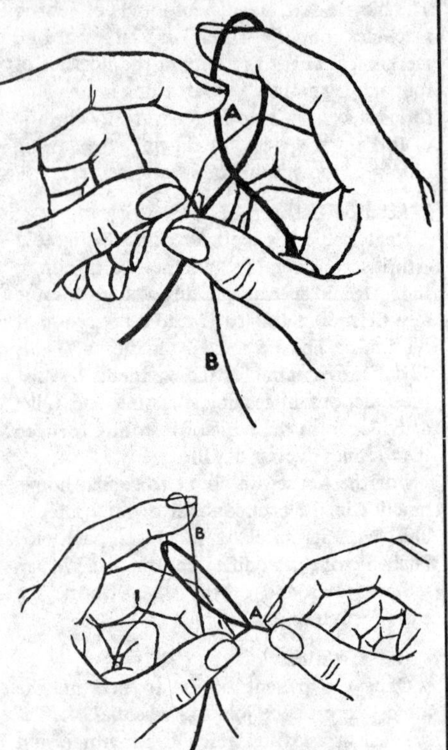

Fig. 6. *FINGER KNITTING is excellent for improving poor muscular function. The top illustration shows how the two threads (A and B) are held, and the lower illustration shows how the knitting stitch is completed. Used to make dressing gown cords, etc.*

For the bed patient with severe paralysis, appliances such as adjustable mirrors, slings, or book-rests are provided.

Hemiplegics

After the physiotherapist has treated the patient, the occupational therapist then takes over the retraining of the paralyzed side, especially if the dominant hand is disabled. The patient will be tested for ability to stand and if this is satisfactory the physician may order exercise on the bicycle-saw.

The Activities of Daily Living are important especially if the patient is eventually to return home, and the performing of light hospital chores will help in rehabilitation.

Multiple Sclerosis Patients

The multiple sclerosis patient must at all cost keep himself going and make the most of any remissions (see Diseases of the Nervous System). The Personal Activities of Daily Living help him also towards rehabilitation. Social interests and recreative activities with their good psychological reactions are of greater value to these patients than craftwork.

Industrial Injuries

Economic worries often beset the industrially injured, especially if the disabled person is the breadwinner. It is therefore necessary that such a patient be restored to his maximum capacity as quickly as possible. When he is on the road to recovery, his work tolerance is tested and, if he is quite unable to return to his former job, new skills by which he earns a living have to be learned.

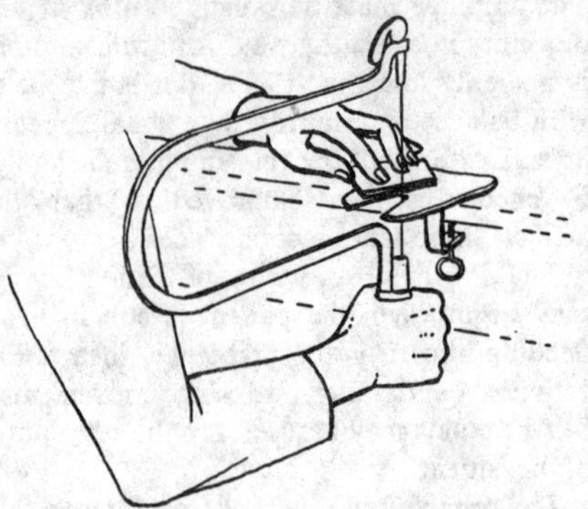

Fig. 7. *SAWING. To strengthen the shoulder after injury, work with a fretsaw is often useful.*

Child Patients

For invalid children (pediatric cases) there are many varied services—children's hospitals (some specializing in one particular branch of medicine), Special Schools for handicapped children, Convalescent Homes, Child Guidance Clinics, and corrective institutions.

The short-stay patient does not necessarily need occupational therapy but it is often advisable to give him something to do, and games or toys will usually keep him busy. The older child may prefer books.

Long-term Patients in Hospital

Orthopedic problems are concerned with congenital abnormalities, paralyses, deformities, fractures, and amputations. Congenital abnormalities, such as the absence of a bone or even of an extremity, clubfoot, or torticollis, are often treated by surgery. Special physical treatment (orthopedic therapy) is provided for such children, and the occupational therapist also has a share in their treatment.

The younger children usually enjoy play therapy, such as singing games, building with bricks, and playing with toys, and older children may be able to join in school lessons if there is a hospital teacher. The Activities of Daily Living have to be learned and the child must become as independent as possible.

Medical Cases

Children who are in hospital for a long time often suffer from home-sickness and it is necessary to help them to adjust themselves to hospital life and to keep them emotionally balanced.

Children who have cardiac or chest complaints must have carefully graded work. In heart cases it is better to occupy the mind rather than to attempt activities which could prove harmful. Children with chest complaints should do very little work and no fluffy toys or materials should be given to them. When the physician permits, exercises with an upward movement may be allowed; this will strengthen the muscles of the chest and back.

Weaving, paper modeling, knotting or jigsaw puzzles, quoits, and pencil and paper games will all hold the interest of young patients.

Nose, Throat, Ear and Eye Cases

Most nose, throat and ear troubles are of short duration and all that is necessary during his hospital stay is to keep the child sufficiently occupied so that he forgets his condition. Drawing, crayoning or painting are always popular pastimes with children. In the case of eye troubles the child may need psychological help and reassurance. Even when the eyes are still bandaged, guessing games by feel may be introduced, and every child enjoys being read to. Later, any form of modeling should be tried, cutting out shapes with scissors, or any activity which concentrates on form.

Psychological Problem Cases

The occupational therapist must gain the trust of the child suffering from any form of mental disorder as quickly as possible. This means an individual approach and behavior faults should be noted. The hostile child who might be destructive will be given activities which provide an outlet, such as modelling with clay, wax or plasticine, hammering nails in wood, finger painting, or educational toys.

As children with psychological problems become more sociable, group work becomes possible and there is more effort to prove their skills to their teacher and to each other.

The Personal Activities of Daily Living are most important for this type of child. Good feeding habits, lessons in dressing, toilet cleanliness and good manners need to be learned and learned again. Training in social behavior is more important than acquired skills.

Music, rhythm, dancing and a percussion band are all within the range of these children and give much enjoyment. 'Dressing-up,' Nativity plays and acting are taken very seriously.

Mentally Handicapped

The mentally-handicapped child has his own aptitudes and these should be drawn out and encouraged. The Activities of Daily Living must take first place in his training, and cleanliness and good behavior insisted upon at all times. Such children sometimes acquire a good standard in repetitive skills and a few may eventually be able to earn their living with the help of an understanding employer. Suitable handicrafts for children with psychological and mental disorders are:

Basketry	Simple rug making	Sewing
Weaving	Knitting and crochet	Knotting
Modeling	Embroidery on canvas	Beadwork

Cerebral Palsy and Spastic Cases

These patients need team-work help from the physiotherapist, occupational therapist, speech therapist and the hospital teacher. Much of the work may have to be done on the floor and the children learn to use educational toys. To strengthen weak muscles the same movement has to be learned over and over again.

The Activities of Daily Living are of

primary importance, and aids and adaptations are often needed. Special drinking cups which do not spill should be used, or drinking straws. Cutlery which is adapted to the needs of the user can be obtained from certain medical

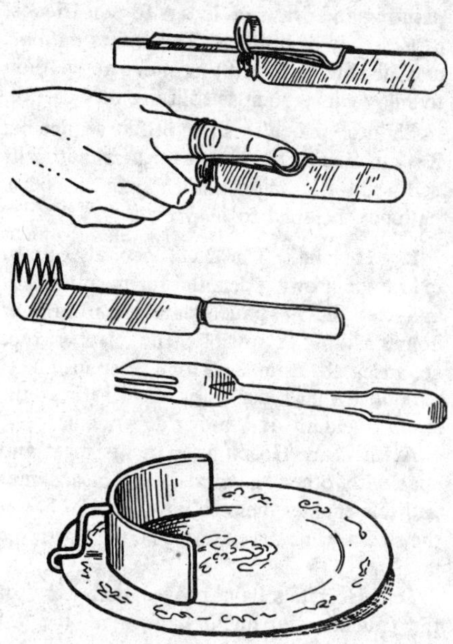

Fig. 8. *MODIFIED CUTLERY. The illustration shows cutlery and tableware adapted to assist patients with disabled fingers and hands.*

appliance suppliers or with a little ingenuity they could easily be made at home using modern plastic molding materials or building up with wood.

Singing, rhyming games, movement to music all help towards rehabilitation of spastic children.

Psychiatric Patients

Today a much more sympathetic outlook on mental diseases is accepted, and this is reflected in the treatment of psychiatric patients. They respond best to a friendly attitude which is combined with firmness. Mental patients are often over-sensitive and those in charge of them need complete self-control.

Psychiatric and neurotic patients soon lose interest in their work and are apt to become inattentive so that concentration must be encouraged. Educational programs are important for psychiatric patients in order to keep their minds from deteriorating. There are many things they are able to do and take a real interest in. In the recreational field alone, music, whether it is in the form of a concert given by an outside group, the patients forming a band, a sing-song, or the Church choir, gives endless interest and pleasure. Most hospitals have regular dances or socials for their patients together with play-acting, indoor and outdoor games, sports day, picnic parties, camping, bus trips and celebrations for special occasions. Much of this is organized by the occupational therapy department.

In the department itself almost any handicraft may be attempted as well as light assembly work, art, gardening or housecrafts. When patients have progressed sufficiently they can be 'promoted' to work in some department of the hospital—the clerical offices, the farm or garden, the hospital laundry, the sewing room, or the stock room.

Most mental patients are able to help on the wards by making their own beds, sweeping or dusting. The occupational therapy department is used as an adjustment center.

Patients who have progressed well may be given vocational training and if improvement continues may be placed in selected jobs outside of the hospital.

THE CHRONIC MENTAL PATIENT is usually a long-term patient and must be carefully watched for behavior changes. Such persons are often highly intelligent and it is important to give them activities which satisfy their needs. As they become more social and concentration improves, music and painting are of great benefit. Work in the library, including book binding, is suitable and, in the occupational therapy department, weaving, basketry, rug making, knitting and embroidery keep hands and mind occupied. Some may be trained for permanent jobs within the hospital.

In senility the most that can be expected of a mental patient is that he will learn the activities of daily living especially with regard to feeding, dressing himself and keeping himself clean and neat.

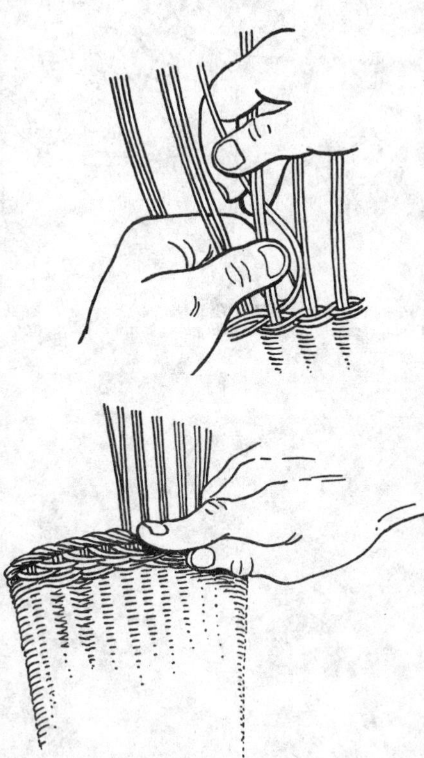

Fig. 9. *BASKETRY is a particularly useful occupation for patients with mental afflictions.*

Encephalitis Lethargica (and Parkinsonism). Such patients should only be given the lightest work and tasks which do not call for too much concentration. Light housework is quite suitable, and pastimes such as painting, embroidery, knitting or basketry. If there is tremor, coarser work will be necessary and embroidery on canvas, frame-loom weaving or polishing will give some occupation.

Epilepsy. Epileptics vary very much. Some are able to live and earn a living outside the hospital, while others must remain permanently in hospital. Their work varies from high grade to the simplest finger activities. It has been proved that handicrafts are helpful, and music and painting restful. Housecraft is also within the scope of these patients.

Mental Subnormality. Within the last few years much greater effort has been made to teach and train the mentally subnormal. Most of them have some latent skills and these are encouraged and developed. It is possible for many of the hospital patients to work in the various departments. The occupational therapy department has an important part to play in the early training so that the young patients may later help in the linen rooms, laundry, kitchens or maintenance work.

It greatly improves the community life if the activities of daily living are well learned, and good habits should be constantly encouraged. Outdoor sports, indoor games, dances and socials should be arranged by the occupational therapy department. Lessons in personal make-up, hair-dressing and social education are very popular with such patients.

Elderly Patients

There is such a demand for beds in geriatric hospitals that more effort is being made to rehabilitate elderly people who are still able to look after themselves or who can return to relatives.

The elderly need a sympathetic understanding; the slowing of mental and physical activities must be accepted by those who live and work with them. The old-age patient often has multiple disabilities and is frequently confused as well.

They enjoy social activities—even a simple get-together for a chat. Group work also assures better standards of behavior, efforts to improve work, and the comfort of companionship.

Personal likes and dislikes have to be considered and patients who are compatible and sympathetic towards each other's disabilities enjoy working together in a group. It is usually better for the older person to keep to familiar work such as knitting, crochet or rug making but there are always the few who will be willing to try new skills.

Comfort, warmth, good lighting and comfortable seating arrangements are necessary for the elderly.

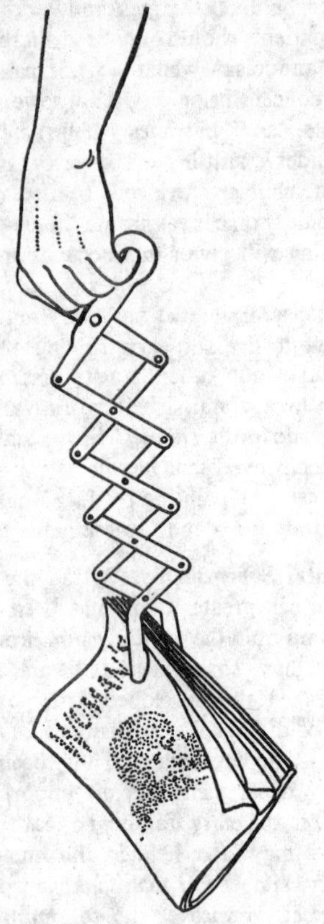

Fig. 10. *EXTENDING PICK-UP. A useful gadget for the elderly arthritic patient.*

Tuberculosis Patients

When the patient with tuberculosis enters the hospital, passive occupational therapy usually commences at once. This may be listening to the radio or television, being read to or reading to oneself. The changeover from passive to active therapy must be gradual, and handicrafts such as embroidery, simple weaving, toy making, knitting, pottery and cord knotting are helpful.

Bed patients find painting a satisfactory medium in which to express themselves and it is not too exhausting.

Once the patient is up, a wider range of activities such as leather work, lino-cutting, modeling, tapestry, sewing, typing and shorthand, netting or basketry may be offered. Sketching, lettering, geometrical design and stick printing are light and suitable pastimes.

Tuberculosis patients often make good students. Those in bed are quite capable of undertaking some form of study which interests them and should be given every form of encouragement. (See also Diseases of the Chest, section on Tuberculosis, p. 350.)

OUT-PATIENT CLINICS

These clinics usually cater for patients who have left hospital to return home yet still need a certain amount of treatment to help them towards full rehabilitation. Amputees, hemiplegics, and poliomyelitis cases all need further training. The out-patient clinic is the stage between the hospital and the sheltered workshop. For housewives the kitchen unit is of the utmost importance and for the disabled workman the work benches and small assembly jobs help towards deciding his future vocation.

SERVICES OUTSIDE THE HOSPITAL

The Sheltered Workshop. These workshops have been usefully employing disabled people for some years. The patient works and is paid according to his capacity.

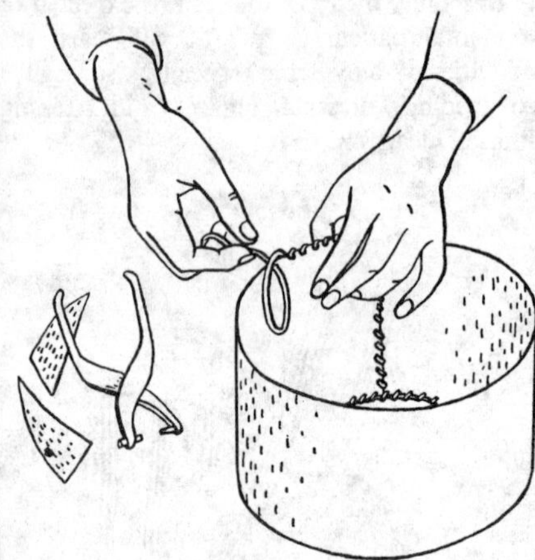

Fig. 11. *LAMPSHADE MAKING is within the competence of patients with many types of disability.*

Homebound Patients. Weaving, basketry, embroidery, typing, knitting and sewing by hand and machine are all activities which may be done at home. Tuberculosis and heart patients who are not able to do anything strenuous may take up music, painting and drawing, letters to pen friends, or a variety of hobbies. The frailer patients may be able to do nothing more active than to enjoy games such as solitaire or patience.

Children may also share in this service but it is much more likely that the local authority will send a teacher rather than an occupational therapist to help them.

Day Hospitals. The Day Hospitals help to relieve the growing demand for hospital beds and keep old-age patients active and in their homes as long as possible. The relatives, too, are released from full-time responsibility making it much easier for them to bear the strain of elderly and failing dependants.

At the Day Hospitals, patients meet and chat with others having similar incapacities and this enables them to have a social life of their own while maintaining contact with the family.

Day Hospitals have proved that many of the patients who might have spent the last years or months of their lives in a hospital bed can now be kept active and interested.

State Prisons. Occupational therapy is now being used in State Prisons and with great success. It has already proved its therapeutic value in the improved behavior of the prisoners and it is obviously a field in which there are great possibilities.

Industrial Therapy. One of the more recent developments is the use of light industry in rehabilitation. Patients who are well enough to put in some 20 to 25 hours of work a week in a small factory producing such items as boxes or ball-point pens, for which only moderate skill is required, go from hospital or home each day.

The patients and the suitability of the machines to their disabilities are studied and the work is supervised by industrial and nursing staff. Patients are paid the proper rate for the job.

SPEECH DEFECTS, SPEECH THERAPY, AND DEAFNESS IN CHILDREN

Nature of Speech Disorders

Speech is an extraordinarily complex form of human activity—a marvelous acquisition which we all take for granted until something goes wrong. It involves a long chain of events beginning with the ability to hear and listen to speech, to interpret its meaning, to remember words and phrases and to organize these intellectually into comprehensible utterance. The processes of decoding and coding messages in communication depend upon normal hearing, emotional stability and intelligence.

Thinking in words what one wants to say is only the first part of the mastery of speech. To produce the voice the vocal cords must be moved in the right manner and the muscles of the tongue and lips must tense and relax in many ways before the words can be pronounced. This executive speech depends upon an intact nervous system, normally functioning muscles, and perfect speech organs with no abnormality in tongue, jaws, or palate. Any irregularity in any section of this complicated mechanism and cycle of events can produce a speech defect, and the different types are as varied and individual as the individuals themselves. It is only possible to refer briefly to some of the more common disturbances which parents may encounter.

Cleft Palate Defect

It must be a great shock to a mother to see this ugly deformity in her baby but she may draw comfort from the fact that it is one of the disasters in development which can be most successfully remedied by plastic surgery. The lip is repaired when the baby is about three months old and the palate at the age of one, before the child begins to speak.

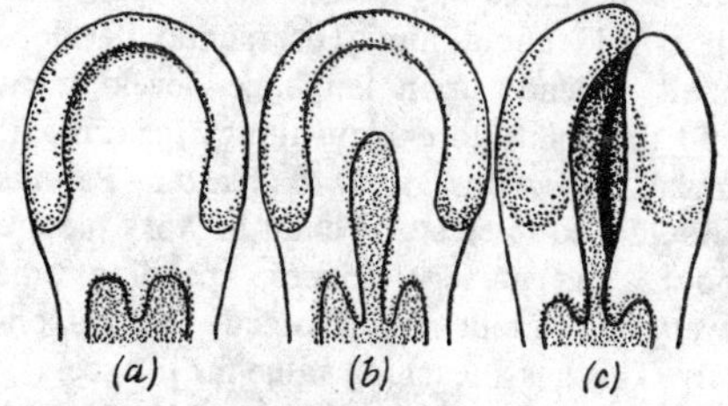

Fig. 1. *CLEFT PALATE. Diagram of the roof of the mouth showing (a) normal soft palate, (b) partially cleft palate, and (c) a fully cleft palate.*

Today the child need not grow up with either a facial disfigurement or a defect of speech. It is found that 80 per cent of cleft-palate children speak normally after surgery, and of the remainder most will acquire normal speech after a further operation and speech therapy. The stigma of 'cleft palate speech,' which is due to the child's being unable to prevent air escaping down the nose while speaking, is now largely a thing of the past.

Adenoidal Speech

The growth of adenoids in the back of the nose above the level of the soft palate causes nasal obstruction and the child snores and snuffles and sounds as if he has a chronic cold in the head. After surgical removal of the adenoids the voice should be quite normal but in some cases a child returns home speaking down his nose because the soft palate does not elevate fully. There is no need for alarm because after a week or so speech begins to improve and should recover in another three or four. A child may be helped to exercise his palate by drinking through straws and blowing bubbles, or a trumpet, or a mouth-organ. If the child continues to speak nasally, the ear, nose and throat specialist should be consulted again. In rare cases the palate functions poorly on account of causes other than removal of the adenoids, the condition having been present all along but concealed by the presence of the adenoids.

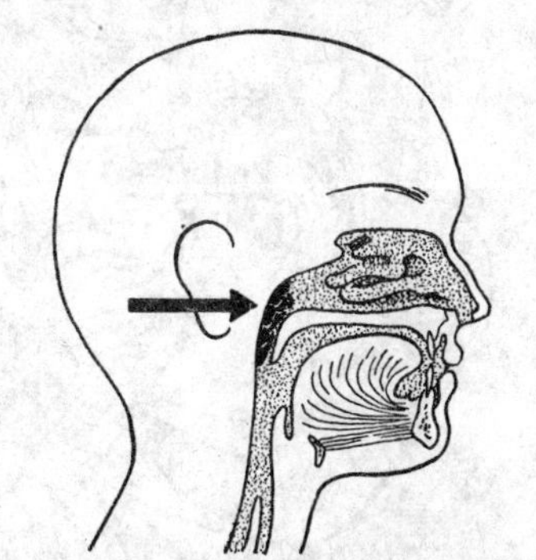

Fig. 2. *ENLARGED ADENOIDS (marked with arrow) blocking the airway between the back of the nose and the soft palate so that speech is impaired.*

Tongue-tie Difficulties

Tongue-tie is commonly believed to cause a child not to speak at all or to speak badly. When the membrane or the frenum which ties or tethers the tongue to the floor of the mouth extends to the tongue tip on the underside it prevents the child elevating or protruding the tongue. This condition is generally discovered at birth when the infant has difficulty with sucking; the frenum is snipped and the tongue freed. Sometimes it is not detected until the child is late in speaking when the tongue-tie is blamed. There is much disagreement among doctors and speech therapists as to whether or not tongue-tie really causes speech disorders. There seems to be a body of evidence to support either contention. Although it is unlikely that the condition can prevent a child speaking altogether, it may well hinder him from speaking distinctly. It would seem advisable therefore that when a child's articulation is much below par for his age, the very small operation of cutting the tongue-tie should be performed, followed by a course of speech therapy. Parents, however, should not press for the operation which necessitates a few days in hospital (always a traumatic experience), until the child is at least four years of age—by which time it is to be hoped that his speech will have improved and no operation will be necessary.

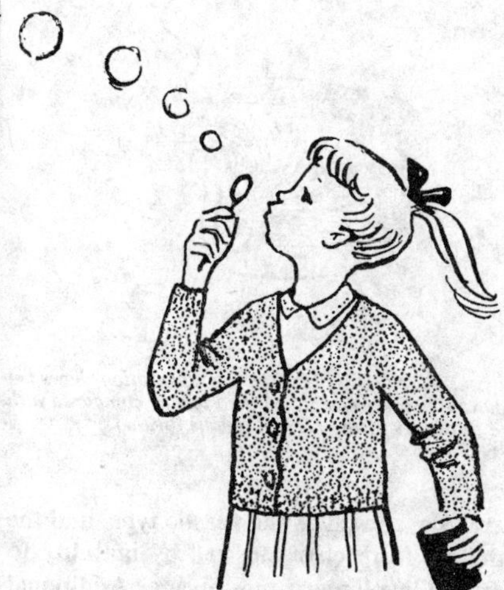

Fig. 3. *BLOWING BUBBLES exercises the soft palate after surgical removal of adenoids.*

Spastic Disorders

Spasticity is the neurological term for rigidity in the muscles encountered in one form of paralysis. In everyday language 'spastic' refers to any child suffering from the kind of brain damage which results in paralysis and in difficulties in muscle movement. Cerebral palsy is actually a better term for describing the lax or flaccid-limbed

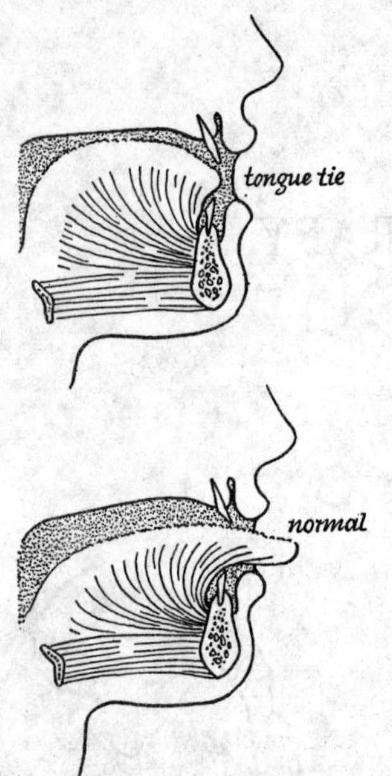

Fig. 4. *TONGUE-TIE. The top illustration shows the limitation of movement of a tied tongue compared with the flexibility of the normal tongue (below).*

paralysis, as well as the spastic type, and the athetoid form characterized by inability to prevent involuntary movements. Additional handicaps of impaired intelligence, hearing and emotional stability may exist also.

Many children with cerebral palsy are so slightly affected that they may hold their own in ordinary schools, while others need years of physiotherapy, speech therapy, and education in special schools where they can benefit from the services of a team of remedial specialists. As regards speech this may be very late in developing and, when it does, it is slurred and labored and the voice monotonous. Co-operation between physiotherapist and speech therapist is essential in developing a child's speech since speech may only be elicited in severe cases after the physiotherapist has taught the child control over posture, swallowing, and breathing. When helping her child, a mother must endeavor to combine the advice and exercises prescribed by both therapists.

STAGES OF NORMAL SPEECH DEVELOPMENT

In order to understand and assess whether a child's speech is retarded for his age it is essential to know something of the normal stages in speech development that the infant passes through. Knowing what to expect of a child and how to help him in learning to speak is the best guarantee that he will speak normally. Only the briefest outline of this very important topic is possible here, but parents are advised to read *Learning to Talk —a Guide for Parents,* by M. C. L. Greene (Heinemann) for a helpful and clear account of infant speech development.

The great majority of children who receive treatment from a speech therapist are those who fail to speak at two and a half to three years, or those who speak at the normal age but retain at school age the infantile articulation and language of the toddler. Some of these speech difficulties are due to causes outside anybody's control, such as mental retardation or poor muscular co-ordination, in which cases speech development depends upon the rate of physical or mental maturation. Many speech difficulties, however, are due to lack of adequate stimulation from the parents especially during the first year when the child is not speaking nor fully understanding. Parents may not realize that babies need to be talked to constantly before they can understand speech and then speak.

At Three Months. As early as three months a child begins to coo and, moreover, to coo when spoken to, and this early vocalizing is undoubtedly the first conversational effort. Later, he begins to babble and utter syllables and it is a fact that babies in hospitals and institutions, who are deprived of being talked to sufficiently, babble far less and talk later and less well than babies receiving the constant attention of their mothers.

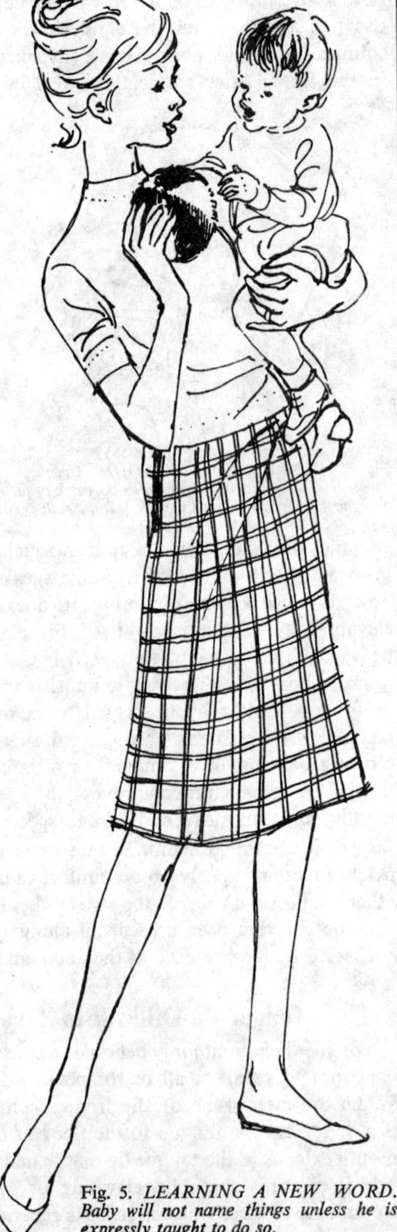

Fig. 5. *LEARNING A NEW WORD. Baby will not name things unless he is expressly taught to do so.*

At Eight Months a baby starts imitating his babble syllables when you say them, and developing concurrently is the understanding of simple instructions and names. Between the twelfth and fourteenth months the first baby words should appear, 'dada,' 'mamma,' 'wowow,' all words emerging from his babble talk and his mother's use of these sounds to name objects. Baby will not name things, however, unless he is taught to do so.

At Two Years. Towards the end of the second year (though children vary enormously regarding the ages at which they do these things) a toddler is imitating almost anything and suddenly becomes very interested in learning new words, constantly demanding, 'What's that?' This is the time of speech readiness when he can be taught many new words a day. His articulation is, of course, far from perfect and for some time his mother is the only person who can understand him. His muscular co-ordination of lips and tongue is still too immature for him to speak 'trippingly on the tongue' and he omits the consonants, especially one of a pair ('poon for spoon) and substitutes one sound for another (t for k, tat for cat; and d for g, pid for pig). It is wrong to pull him up for this and, in fact, dangerous to do so in case he loses his confidence in speech. It is quite enough to speak to him clearly and distinctly yourself and he will correct himself when he is old enough to do so. This will be at the age of three or four maybe, according to his individual rate of development, boys on the whole being later than girls.

About Three Years. Around three years of age the child becomes interested in how things work, what things are for, why this and that happens, and perpetually asks for explanations. Parents, despite the tax upon their patience at this time, should supply simple, clear and sensible explanations because this is the way a child gains insight into the world about him. His mental development depends upon language development and the ability to explain things for himself, make deductions, and to reason. Parents should also interest the child in story picture books and nursery rhymes, spending time every day to talk to him directly and personally. This has a teaching value far in excess of the impersonal relationship established with a television set—on which many children nowadays have to rely. Given adequate help the average three- or four-year-old shows a wonderful mastery of speech.

Between Three and Four years many children pass through a phase of speech hesitation and repetition when it seems their thoughts run ahead of speech. They are often at a loss for words, having difficulty in formulating and expressing what they want to tell you, more especially when excited. This phase is sometimes described as developmental stammering but it should not be thought of as stammering at all and should not be mentioned or corrected, but quietly ignored. In the great majority of children it disappears as greater mastery of vocabulary and language develops, and as speech regains its fluency.

STAMMERING

The phase of hesitation and non-fluency just mentioned is unquestionably an unstable phase in speech development coinciding with great dependence upon the mother as the child becomes less egocentric and more aware of the magnitude of the outside world. It is the stage at which most stammering commences but real stammering is generally precipitated by some emotional trauma, a shock or fright or sudden separation from the mother without due warning. Speech disturbance is accompanied by obvious emotional upset, clinging to the mother, nightmares, bed-wetting, food fads, and so on. A child producing speech repetition rather conspicuously should be carefully handled. Overexcitement should be avoided, a regular routine observed and adequate rest taken, and consistent discipline maintained. An attempt should be made to discover and remove any cause of anxiety and fear and the child should be given extra love and reassurance to build up the security he needs and may have temporarily lost.

If the speech symptoms persist or increase, a speech therapist should most definitely be consulted, especially in the case of a boy. Stammering is rare in girls. An established stammer is very difficult to cure: there is, in fact, no positive cure known. It is therefore better to prevent its establishment rather than to assume that 'the child will grow out of it'. So often he does not, and receives speech therapy too late when repetitive speech has become an ingrained habit and the psychological conviction, based on bitter experience that he will stammer whenever he speaks, has become deeply rooted.

DEAFNESS AND HEARING THERAPY

Before a child can learn to speak he must have normal hearing so that he can first learn to understand what is said, then imitate words and reproduce what he hears. Gradually he memorizes a fund of meaningful words and phrases which he can recall and use in communication. If a child cannot hear, he cannot understand speech, nor imitate it and learn to speak. Fortunately, total deafness is rare. The residual hearing of the partially deaf can be exploited to the full by means of special training with a hearing aid which amplifies sound. Severely deaf children can learn to speak and with modern methods of diagnosis and education will not grow up dumb unless they have some additional handicap.

Early diagnosis of deafness, ideally during the first six months of age, is vital, since the earlier special training commences the greater the chances of the child learning to speak well. Doctors, health visitors and parents should be on the look out for deafness in babies who have been subjected to conditions known to give rise to deafness. Such conditions are certain infections of the mother, especially German measles during early pregnancy; and toxemia of pregnancy. In the infant himself, premature birth, birth jaundice, and severe infections in early infancy such as meningitis, measles and mumps, may impair or even destroy his capacity for hearing.

Diagnosis of Deafness in babies is not at all easy. During the first three months a baby should respond to a loud noise by a 'startle reflex'—blinking and jumping. When this reflex dies down it is difficult to ascertain a hearing loss till about seven months when a normal child begins to respond unmistakably to speech and turns to look when spoken to, even though his mother is out of sight. He also attends to sounds which have meaning for him, like footsteps, the click of a door latch, or the clink of a spoon on a plate, though it is characteristic at this age that the baby may ignore loud sounds, banging on a drum, or a shout from a doctor or nurse which is meaningless for him. His failure to respond to speech, later to understand simple instructions, to imitate words and to speak according to the averages already given under normal infant speech development (p. 188), should immediately raise the question in a parent's mind 'Is my baby deaf?' Should there be any doubt whatsoever about a child's hearing being normal, parents should insist upon seeing an otologist and teacher of the deaf for a careful examination of the child.

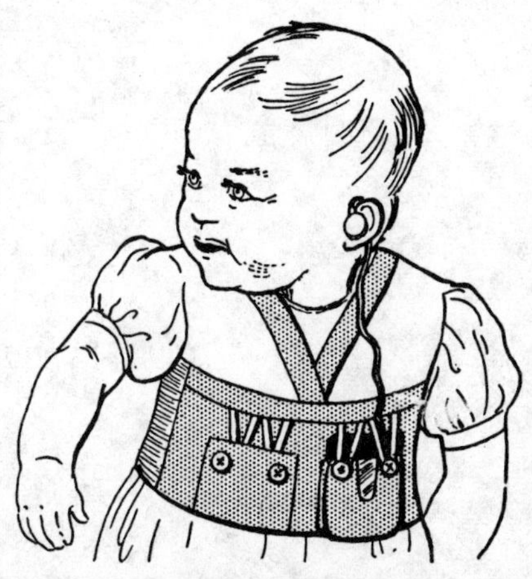

Fig. 6. *DEAF AID FOR THE BABY. The earlier a deaf child begins to pick up sounds through a hearing aid the better chance she has of learning to speak adequately.*

Once deafness is ascertained, even as early as three months, a baby is provided with a hearing aid and the mother is advised how to teach her baby to listen. The teacher of the deaf will see the baby and mother regularly. She watches progress and gives guidance in management of the problem as a whole.

Teaching Deaf Children

It is recognized that the deaf child needs help early if he is to be helped to use every vestige of hearing and to utilize the normal developmental impetus to speak which is inherent in the child even though deaf. Two years old is obviously late to start training a child to listen to speech because the normal child is using hearing and acquiring the foundations of speech probably from the day he is born and at two years of age he is talking.

Teachers of the deaf are now available from hospital audiology units or from the peripatetic staffs of local health authorities to take over hearing therapy for small children and babies with hearing loss, and they will follow the child through to school age. As he approaches the age of five, his educational needs are assessed upon the basis of his language ability and his speech. He may be able to hold his own in the normal school, or may need education in a school for the partially deaf, or he may be better placed in an ordinary school in a special class for partially deaf children with a teacher of the deaf in charge.

The child who is not making sufficient progress with speech will be placed in a school for the deaf. This may be either a day or residential school. Severe deafness is easier to diagnose than partial hearing loss but in emotionally disturbed children and backward children it can still be missed. A child who is severely deaf *will* be difficult, distressed and backward. Some intelligent, well cared-for children, on the other hand, may manage so well with what hearing they have and with lip reading that they appear not to be deaf at all.

Deafness may go undetected for several years and only be suspected when speech remains defective. It is not uncommon for a child to hear sufficiently to understand speech and to speak, while having a high-frequency deafness which renders it impossible for him to distinguish adequately the difference between the high-frequency consonants s, z; sh, ch; j and th. When such consonants are incorrectly articulated poor hearing should always be suspected and be tested carefully.

PARENTAL CO-OPERATION

In cases of cleft palate, cerebral palsy, and obvious deafness the condition is generally diagnosed early and taken care of by the appropriate specialists who bring in the speech therapists and teachers of the deaf, as and when necessary. It is in the less obvious cases of speech defect that parents may be perplexed and anxious. If a child of two is not speaking at all, if a child is stammering, or if his speech is incomprehensible at three years, expert advice must be sought. Parents worried about a child's speech should not hesitate to discuss it with the family doctor so as to obtain a consultation with a speech therapist. She is there to be consulted, and there is no need to fear that she will insist upon giving your child 'lessons' unnecessarily and when he is too young. In any case children under five are not given lessons but are helped through play therapy. Helping a child develop or improve speech is a delicate and skilled procedure needing much psychological insight and technical skill.

It is unwise for parents to try to correct the speech of their child themselves if he is having real difficulty. For this reason it is not the intention here to describe speech exercises or treatment. If speech treatment is necessary, the speech therapist should give it, but she will rely enormously on the co-operation of the mother to carry out her advice and suggestions at home, knowing that the mother is ultimately the real instrument in treating the child through whom she must operate if therapy is to be effective.

SPEECH THERAPISTS AND TEACHERS OF THE DEAF

The work of the speech therapist is frequently confused with that of the elocution teacher or the teacher of the deaf.

The teacher of elocution (speech training and dramatic art) aims at improving speech that is normal but inadequate for certain purposes. Thus she may correct a weak voice, mumbling pronunciation, or teach the arts of public speaking and drama.

The teacher of the deaf, after a course at a teachers' training college or a university, takes a year's special training in the methods of teaching the deaf and hard of hearing. She is skilled in the diagnosis of deafness in children, the provision of auditory training with a hearing aid (hearing therapy), lip reading and teaching the child to speak. She is also qualified to educate the deaf child of school age.

The speech therapist deals only with the real abnormalities of speech, voice, and language due perhaps to structural abnormalities (cleft palate), emotional disturbances (stammering), neurological disorders (spasticity), or the late development of speech in certain children. The speech therapist does not correct the speech of the child who picks up the local dialect from his playmates at school; this is normal speech though it may be annoying to his parents. She does not usually teach the severely deaf child but may have to do so with a pre-school child if no teacher of the deaf is available in the area. She may, however, frequently be called upon to treat a child with a slight hearing loss who has developed adequate language but who has some faults in articulation.

Few speech therapists set up in private practice. The majority work in the school health service and a lesser number in the hospital service. In order to consult a speech therapist it is necessary to ask a doctor to refer your child to her. Some doctors take the precaution of referring a child to a hospital pediatrician first for a thorough check-up, after which the child sees the speech therapist.

RADIO-ACTIVITY: ITS USES AND DANGERS

Sources of Radio-activity

Radiation is the giving off of rays of some kind. For instance, a fire gives off rays of light and heat. The sun gives off these rays as well as some other electrical radiations.

This section is concerned with radio-active radiations which are given off by radium, by X-ray machines, and by various other sources which will be discussed later on. These radiations can be very powerful and may penetrate what we regard as solid objects, including the human body.

One very important source of such radiations is outer space. At present no one can say where in outer space these rays come from. They are called 'cosmic' radiations and are immensely powerful. They can be detected in coal mines at depths of 1,000 feet or more, which means they have penetrated through the earth to that depth.

Strangely enough a very large percentage of these radiations is stopped by the earth's atmosphere. Even so, every living thing on earth has been subjected to them throughout the existence of life here.

Radio-active Rocks

Much of the earth itself is also slightly radio-active. This comes from the fact that uranium and thorium, which are both radio-active, are distributed very widely in the rocks and soil of the earth. Rocks of the granite type have a good deal more of those two elements than other kinds of rock and soil. Everybody is subject to this kind of radiation.

Until fairly recently little was known about these natural forms of radiation and still less about their effects on human beings. With the discovery of the means for making use of the enormous power of atomic energy many other radio-active substances are being produced artificially. Many of these products are immensely useful in various ways, and there is no doubt that vastly greater use will be made of them in the future.

Atomic Piles

Radio-activity is produced in large quantities by atomic piles including those used in nuclear power stations (where they are called, rightly, nuclear reactors). It is also obvious that nuclear power stations will, in time, very largely replace other types of power stations if only because natural fuels, such as coal and oil, will eventually be exhausted.

Obviously, atomic and hydrogen bombs can produce enormous quantities of radio-activity, and there seems little reason to doubt that all-out nuclear war might well destroy the entire human race. For that reason there is not much point in discussing the effects of such bombs. The view taken is that it is more sensible to assume the survival of humanity and to discuss the other forms of radio-activity.

It is very important to make quite clear at this stage that there is a lot of disagreement among scientists about the amount of damage to the human body that can be caused by radiation. Even the processes that cause the damage are not all clear, although a great deal more is known now than was the case in 1950. This is also true of the means for protecting the body from the effects of radiation.

High Radiation Levels in Tibet

One of the great mysteries is how the people of Tibet can keep healthy and show no apparent signs of radiation damage. They live at a height of about 12,000 feet where a lot of cosmic radiation gets through, and the rocks of the Himalayas contain, relatively, a fair amount of radio-active material. The water they drink must also contain some radio-active material, as will the food they eat. Yet not only do they survive, but they flourish, and many of them live to old age.

This suggests the possibility that resistance to some forms of radio-activity may be acquired by heredity. On the other hand, it is believed that the population of Tibet may be static, or declining, but the reasons given for this have nothing to do with radio-activity.

ARTIFICIAL RADIO-ACTIVITY

Atomic piles, or reactors, are charged with uranium metal as fuel. It is likely that other forms of the material will be used for the purpose later on, but at present these forms are experimental. Uranium metal is quite plentiful in nature and is to be found in rocks, particularly some forms of granite. It is radio-active and has a small fraction which is 'fissile,' that is to say, can be split. It is so volatile that its atoms throw off particles which hit other atoms causing them, in turn, to throw off particles. This is the chain reaction. The fissile fraction is the isotope (which will be explained later on) U-235. There is enough of the isotope to set up in the metal a chain reaction which is easily controlled. The fuel in reactors can be 'enriched,' which means it will contain more of the U-235 and less of the inactive elements.

The difference between the chain reaction of an atomic bomb and the chain reaction of an atomic pile, or reactor, can be explained in the following way. If you take a box of matches with the heads all lying at one end and set fire to one match-head the flame will spread almost instantly—like an explosion—to all the other heads. That is an uncontrolled chain reaction. If you take the matches out of the box and lay them side by side so that the head of each just touches the head of the next and set fire to the end one, each match-head in turn will be set off. That is a controlled chain reaction. The first one is like the bomb, and the second is like the reactor.

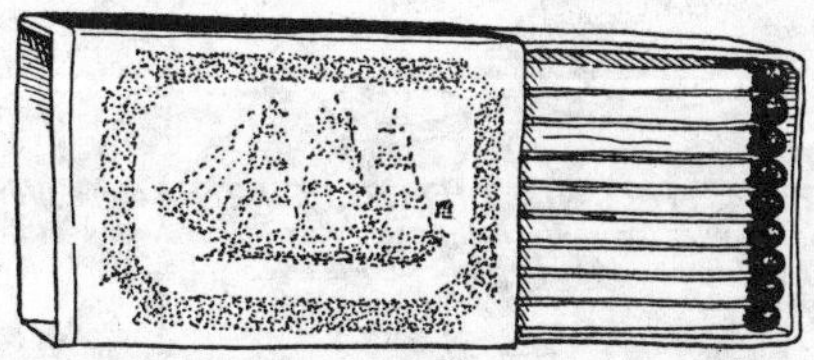

Fig. 1a. *CHAIN REACTION, UNCONTROLLED. Set fire to one match in a box and the flame will spread almost instantly. That is an uncontrolled chain reaction.*

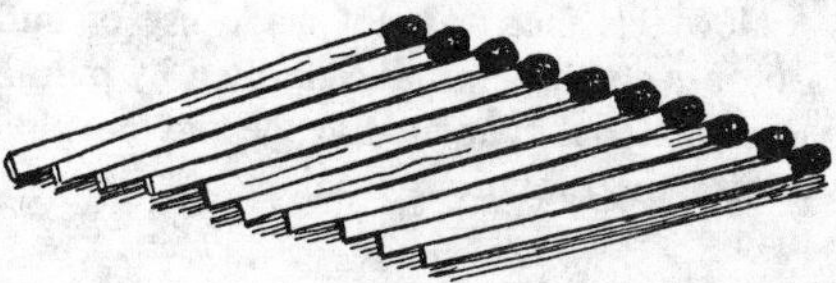

Fig. 1b. *CHAIN REACTION, CONTROLLED. Lay the matches in a line so that each head just touches the next. Set fire to the end one, and each match-head in turn will be set off. That is a controlled chain reaction.*

In a similar sort of way the uranium metal in the reactor goes on generating heat through its chain reaction for a considerable time, and that heat is made to turn water into steam which, in turn, drives the generating plant to produce electricity.

In the course of this atomic reaction a certain amount of radio-active 'ash,' or waste, is produced—just as a coal fire leaves ash behind. The radio-active ash has to be handled with great care because it gives off powerful and dangerous radiations. In all atomic energy plants this careful handling is a first consideration, and the possibility of accidents happening with it is remote in the extreme.

Isotopes

Just as the heat in a furnace can be used to change the chemical properties of some metals—turning iron into steel, for instance—so the radiations in an atomic reactor can change the physical properties of a number of materials and make them immensely useful in many ways. The changes turn atoms of some elements into 'isotopes' of those elements.

Isotopes were first discovered by the Englishman, Professor Soddy, in 1911. He found that atoms of some elements which seemed to be absolutely identical with other atoms of the same elements were, in fact, different in some way. It was like looking for the difference between identical twins. To every chemical test they responded in the same way. Eventually he discovered the truth: the isotope atom was heavier than its identical twin, the ordinary atom. The heavier one is often radio-active.

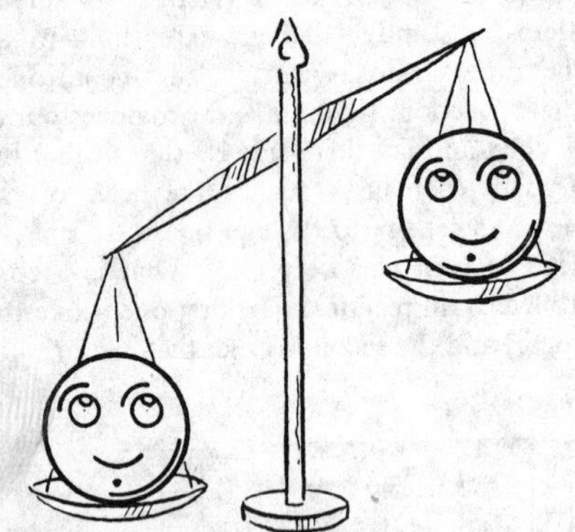

Fig. 2. *THE ONLY DIFFERENCE. The isotope atom is heavier than its identical twin, the ordinary atom. The heavier one is often radio-active.*

Now this fact was not made use of until isotopes could be produced, often by putting some material in an atomic pile and 'cooking' it with the radiations inside.

Isotopes in Medicine

The first and most important uses for isotopes were in medicine. Doctors could give patients, either by mouth, or by injection, substances containing isotopes which could be traced or detected wherever they went inside the body. The tiny bit of radio-activity of the isotopes gives off pulses of energy which enable sensitive detectors to find it.

For Thyroid and Tumors

One substance, iodine, has a particular affinity for the thyroid gland. It is fairly well known that a lack of iodine in the diet—only minute quantities are needed—may cause a malfunctioning of the gland. Cases of goiter are often associated with countries and districts where the water has not enough iodine.

To help doctors study the functioning of the thyroid gland patients are given isotopes of iodine. The body cannot tell the difference between these 'identical twins' of any substance, and so the isotopes travel as ordinary iodine to the thyroid gland. By what happens to them when they get there the doctors can diagnose the trouble, which may not even be in the gland itself.

Other substances have an affinity for tumors, and their isotopes are of enormous value to brain surgeons in locating the positions of tumors inside the brain. Much of the time of these specialists was formerly spent in trying to decide where to operate, so the advantage to them and to their patients is obvious.

Locating a Blood Clot

Quite often in diseases involving the circulation of the blood in, for instance, the leg, it is very difficult for the doctor to discover exactly where there is a stoppage of the circulation. By injecting a small amount of isotopes into the main artery of the leg the blood will carry the isotopes round as part of itself. The flow can be followed through the smaller blood vessels, into the capillaries and then back into the veins. And where the blood stops the isotopes will also stop, and they will go on sending out their minute 'ticks' to the detector.

With his knowledge of anatomy, coupled with the relative strength or weakness of the signals, the doctor can say with certainty which blood vessel is blocked or not working properly. Treatment is then much easier because the problem is clear.

Cancer Treatment

The use of X-rays in the destruction of some sorts of cancer is well known. The beam of X-rays can be directed at the site of the cancer in the hope of burning it out. A difficulty with this treatment is that sometimes the beam also damages surrounding tissues. Now, tiny needles containing isotopes which give off radiations which can destroy cancer can be inserted into the cancer itself, so that the damage is done only to the new growth, and the other parts are hardly touched. This is particularly useful when the cancer is lying near a specially sensitive organ of the body.

Plant Research

It is not only in medicine and surgery that isotopes have proved so valuable, but also in veterinary work and in agricultural research. Enormous strides have been made in recent years in finding out how plants live, take up their nourishment and transform it into the substances of the living plant by feeding them with isotopes mixed in with fertilizers and so on. Through this, and related work, new strains of plants have been grown which give greater yields in all kinds of situations. Plant diseases, too, have been attacked by these methods.

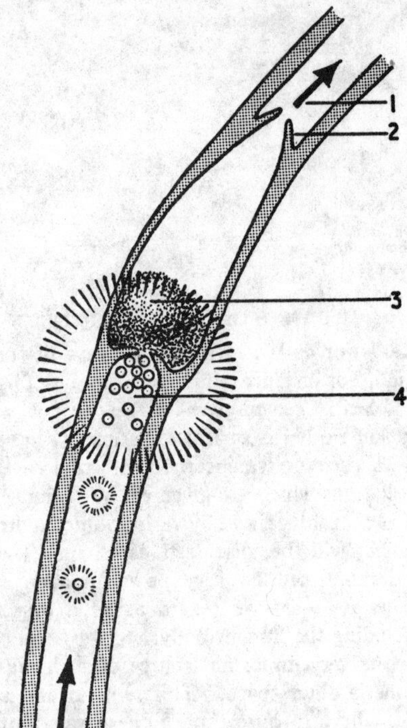

Fig. 3. *ISOTOPES FIND THE BLOOD CLOT. The isotopes, carried along in the bloodstream, are stopped by a clot and congregate there sending out their minute pulses of energy which are heard as 'ticks' from the detector.* 1. *Direction of blood flow.* 2. *Valves of vein which prevent return of blood or clot.* 3. *Blood clot.* 4. *Group of isotopes.*

Isotopes in Industry

The uses of isotopes in industry are immensely varied and growing. They have done much to make some industrial processes safer. For instance, one of the things that isotopes do is to 'ionize' the air. Ionizing gives the air so treated a small positive charge of electricity.

In Paper Mills. A problem in paper mills and other places is the building up of static electricity. This comes about through friction—you can prove it by rubbing the fur of a cat and listening to the crackles—and if there is enough static electricity on a roll of paper there is a risk that the roll will catch fire.

To prevent this happening a small amount of isotopes—carefully shielded so that it will not injure workpeople—is positioned so that its radiations are directed across the paper as it is reeled up. This makes a sort of 'lane' of ionized air along which the static electricity readily travels to a point from which it can be safely grounded.

In Textile Mills 'static' caused another problem. The cloth being woven into reels acquired static electricity through friction, and when the machines were stopped at the end of the day the piece of cloth stretching from the reel to the weaving machine was heavily charged with static. The static collected dirt in the most amazing way, and the dirt was so deeply embedded in the fibers of the cloth that it could never be removed by cleaning. Every day the pieces spoiled by this dirt had to be cut out and thrown away. Now isotopes perfrom their trick of ionizing a path in the air to carry away the static and the cloth stays clean.

In Steel Works. Because the radiations of isotopes can penetrate thin sheets of most substances, they form remarkably useful thickness gauges. Steel is rolled out into sheets of various thicknesses. It is vital that the sheets should be exactly as thick, or as thin, as they are supposed to be. Later on they are used in various manufacturing processes, and the machines used in these processes will work properly only if the sheet steel is right.

In the old days mechanical gauges were employed to test the sheet as it was rolled out, but all sorts of things could spoil their accuracy. When the radiations of isotopes are directed at sheet steel they pass through it, but some are absorbed on the way. If the sheet is the tiniest bit thicker than a set standard, less of the radiations get through. If it is thinner more of the radiations get through. So on the opposite side of the moving band of sheet steel, away from the isotope source, there is a very sensitive detector picking up the radiations that pass through. So long as the detector picks up exactly the right amount of radiations the sheet is all right. The moment it varies the detector records the fact, and sets in train devices which adjust the rollers producing the sheet to correct the fault. This happens so quickly that hardly any of the sheet is lost through being of the wrong size.

These sheets, by the way, must be accurate to hundredths, or thousandths, of an inch.

Detecting Thickness of Paper and Paint. Similar detectors are used now in paper mills to control the thickness of rolls of paper, in plastics factories, and even for measuring the thickness of coats of paint and other coverings. In some of these it is necessary to measure only the paint, or plastic, or other covering, and not what the covering is applied to. Now, a proportion of the radiations directed at sheet metal, for instance, is reflected back. The radiations will pass through the paint and a certain proportion of them will be reflected back from the metal underneath. This is called 'back-scatter,' and the detecting device, which forms part of the isotope gauge itself in this case, measures the amount of 'back-scatter' and, therefore, the thickness of the coat of paint.

Checking Castings. Because of this property of 'seeing through' solid objects isotopes are now used for checking metal castings to see whether there are cracks or other faults in them. Previously this could only be done by using very large and powerful X-ray machines, and that kind of examination was costly. It was also necessary to take careful precautions to ensure that people working near the castings were not endangered. Now it is a common practice to set up a whole ring of castings with an isotope source in the center and a photographic plate behind each casting. The isotopes need not be very powerful because this arrangement can be left standing all night to expose the plates fully. Thus no worker need be exposed to risk since he would have to stand in the way of the radiations a long time to suffer damage; the process is cheap, and little or no time is lost in making a most thorough check.

Safety in Industry. Because the uses of isotopes in industry are now widespread, and likely to become more so in the future, it is important to make several things clear. As has already been said, there are stringent regulations covering the use of isotopes. These regulations ensure every possible protection to people working with, or near, the isotopes.

Space itself is a very great safeguard, and the kind of isotopes used in industry are absorbed by the air at distances of ten feet or so. This means that it is not possible for radiations used in a factory to penetrate to nearby houses.

Most of the isotopes used industrially are very small amounts emitting 'soft' radiations. Some of these sources would have to be carried in a pocket for some time before they caused any damage to the person in whose pocket they were. There is, therefore, no reason whatever for men or women, working in factories where isotopes are used, to suffer in any way from that fact. Even if someone set out deliberately to harm himself with the kind of radiation source in general use he would find it extremely difficult to suffer more than minor damage.

Length of Life of Isotopes

It is one of the most important things about isotopes that the length of time for which they remain active is known quite accurately. They are described as having a 'half-life' of however long it may be. This means that in that time, which may be a matter of hours, days, or weeks, or in some instances, years, they will lose half their activity.

One isotope, carbon 14, which is present in almost every living creature in the world, has a half-life of thousands of years. When animals and human beings die they stop taking in carbon 14, and it is possible for scientists to measure fairly accurately how far the carbon 14 in the body has decayed and so date the historic period at which the body, or skeleton, lived.

Most of the isotopes used in medicine and veterinary work have half-lives of only a few days. Some of the isotopes used in industry have half-lives of some months. Always these sources used in industry must be carefully guarded. It is not so much because they are highly dangerous as because there is nothing to show that there is any danger at all, and without proper precautions people might suffer radiation burns, or minor damage, simply through not realizing that the isotopes were there. The regulations governing their use are extremely strict, and make it almost impossible for people to come into contact with the radiations even if they try to do so.

RADIATION HAZARDS

Although we are all exposed to 'natural' radiation which surrounds us at all times, additional hazards come from the 'fall-out' from atomic tests, which may be brought to an end if international agreement can be reached, and from a very small amount of radiation from all sorts of industrial activity. Then there is what might be called the 'calculated' radiation of hospital treatment by X-rays and radio-active isotopes where the benefits are most likely to outweigh any possible risk by exposure to an increase of radiation. In addition, there is always the possibility of accidents in the use and handling of radio-active material.

The Risks

What, then, are the risks from radio-active radiations?

There is danger of damage to the cells of the body, including blood cells, and the possibility of damage to the testes in men, to the ovaries in women, and to the genes and chromosomes from which infants develop.

Observation on people who have suffered from exposure to heavy radiations, as for instance the survivors of the atomic bomb explosions at Hiroshima and Nagasaki, shows that there can be considerable delayed effects even if they are not quite as bad as at one time seemed likely.

There are four kinds of radiation. These are known as:

ALPHA RADIATION, which has a penetrating power of less than one-tenth of a millimeter in human tissues and therefore irradiates only those cells in the immediate vicinity of the source of radiation;

BETA RADIATION rays which are a little more penetrating than the alpha rays and will penetrate a few millimeters into the body;

GAMMA RAYS AND X-RAYS which have high penetrating power and can irradiate the whole of the body; and

NEUTRONS which can also penetrate deeply into the body.

All types of radiation can be received by exposure to a radio-active source, and the first three types can also be received by being swallowed with food or drink, and by being breathed.

When any of these particles passes through the cells in the body it destroys them, or causes changes in them.

Vulnerable Germ Cells

In the normal and healthy individual millions of cells die every day and are replaced. Obviously, if in addition to these millions a small number of other cells die the consequences would probably not be noticed. It is only when the cells destroyed are of a particular type of which the numbers are small, and which cannot be replaced, that it would be serious. This could happen to the female germ cells in the ovaries, to early developing embryos and to some other tissues. In the ordinary way it might be more serious for cells to be damaged than to be destroyed. These modified cells may divide later on, and this change could be transmitted to later generations of cells in the body of a man, or, if germ cells were affected, in the bodies of his children. But even the damaged cells may be eliminated by the body's normal processes, or the damage may be repaired.

Women are more likely to lose fertility through exposure to radiation than are men. This is because all the egg cells a woman ever has are present in her, in undeveloped form, at birth. If they are destroyed the woman can never be fertile. Men may suffer damage to their reproductive organs, but so long as certain cells remain healthy the damage should be repaired within about two years.

Leukemia

Some isotopes have an affinity for the marrow in bones where they attack the blood-forming cells. From this some experts argue that this particular kind of radiation is one of the causes of leukemia.

Rays from Common Mechanisms

In addition to radiation from X-rays and from the use of isotopes we must add radiation we receive from man-made sources such as shoe fitting (which is very low), luminous clocks and watches (which is thought to be about one or two millirems a year), and television sets, now thought to be almost negligible for viewers but requiring precautions for development and maintenance engineers.

The risks of those who work with radio-active materials of any kind are known and carefully guarded against. They must wear a film badge all the time they are at work, and when the film is developed it shows precisely how much radiation has been received.

'Fall-out'

Then we come to 'fall-out' from atomic and hydrogen explosions. 'Fall-out' is material that is made radio-active by the explosion and thrown high into the air, or into the stratosphere, from which it descends at speeds depending on the size of the particles and the height to which they have been thrown. It will take from minutes to years to reach the ground again. From this source the dose-rates over a long period are said to be about 1·2 millirems per year to the gonads (ovaries and testes), and about 7 millirems per year in bone. For the period of July, 1959, the radiation to the gonads was said to be at the annual rate of 6 millirems a year, and the amount in bone for 1958–9 was about 16 millirems.

It will be seen, therefore, that the amount of radiation from 'fall-out' is very small by comparison with natural radiation. On the other hand, every atomic explosion stores up radiation in the stratosphere from which it descends only gradually. No one knows how far we can safely add to the natural radiation without causing damage to ourselves and danger to future generations. In the opinion of those best qualified to know we should not take the risk of increasing the amount of radiation in the atmosphere at least until we are more certain of its consequences.

PROTECTION

It may seem surprising, in view of what has been said about the penetrating power of radio-active radiations, that any form of protection against them is possible. Yet atomic piles and nuclear reactors function without harming the people who work round them. That is because each pile and reactor is surrounded by a 'biological shield' consisting of several feet of concrete. The workers in atomic laboratories are shielded by lead walls from the dangerous materials they handle. Every care is taken in these establishments to ensure the safety of the workers.

So far as we know the natural radiation to which we are subject has no bad effects on us, and it would seem that only a big increase in radiation from 'fall-out' might be harmful. But if this were to happen, or if, through an accident of some kind a large quantity of radio-activity was released and put the radiation rate up to a dangerous level, could anything be done to protect people from it?

A certain amount of protection can be given by shielding the vital parts of the body such as the gonads, the ovaries, the liver, and so on. But we do not all carry shielding material about with us. Nor would we know exactly where to put it if we did. However, the fact that it has now been found possible to protect the vital parts—even from heavy exposure—is an indication that some kind of protection might be available in an emergency.

Medical scientists are also searching for a drug or drugs that might be used to protect people from radiations. If this sounds a little like the 'pills to cure earthquakes' it is, in fact, a very serious study with a lot more hope of success than that. In the words of one expert. there are good grounds for believing that substances of this kind will be discovered, The reason for the belief is that a lot more has been found out in recent years about the way radiations work to damage, or destroy, the body. When this is fully understood it should be possible to devise means for reducing the risk of those things happening.

One thing is certain. It is that as we all receive a certain amount of radiation every day of our lives none of us is likely to suffer from any kind of 'radiation sickness' in the normal course of things. Since this subject became such a center of attention in recent years a number of people have claimed to be suffering from the effects of radiations. Their symptoms have varied as widely as their imaginations could suggest. None of them has had any condition which could be remotely related to radiation.

So long as the people of Tibet remain proof against these things there is every reason why we, who receive less than a tenth of the radiations to which they are subjected, should likewise remain healthy.

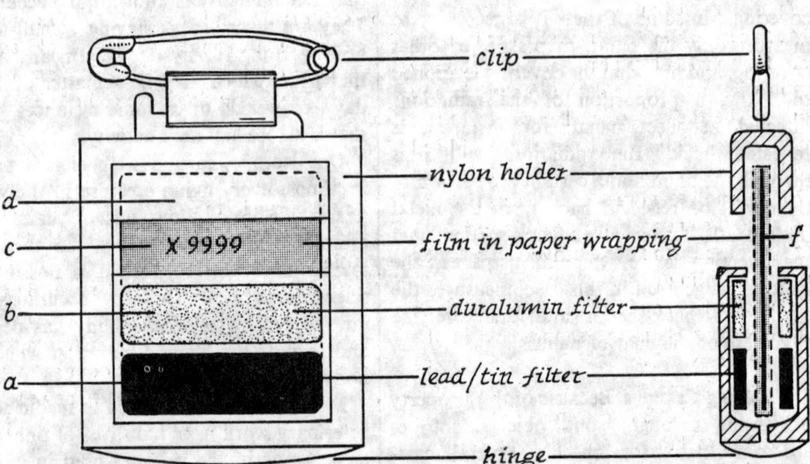

Fig. 5. *A FILM BADGE. A strip of ordinary film (f), wrapped in ordinary paper, is placed in the holder. The film is affected in four ways: at (a) it is covered by a lead-tin covering through which not even radio-active rays can penetrate. At (b) the duralumin covering gives some but not full protection from the rays. At (c) the film is protected from daylight by paper but radioactive rays can penetrate it (this is the most sensitive part of the badge). At (d) only the nylon case gives a modest protection.*

If a worker suspects that he has received a strong dose of radiation, the film is extracted and developed like an ordinary photograph and the four different areas give an indication of the dose received. The blacker the area (c) the stronger has been the dose.

PHYSICAL CULTURE

The following eight tables of simple exercises are so planned as to be suitable for both men and women. They form a normal all-the-year-round routine. No more than fifteen minutes a day need be given to these exercises to ensure the perfect co-ordination of muscle movement, mobility of joints and correct breathing and posture which bring physical fitness and form the basis of good health.

FIFTEEN MINUTES A DAY FOR FITNESS

Physical fitness is a relative term. There are many degrees of such fitness. There is the super-fitness of the super-athlete, the fitness gained by specialized means for a specialist sport. The champion runner, football player, boxer, swimmer, the rower, each attains a high standard of physical fitness in relation to the needs of his own particular sport. But let him step out of his own sport into the competitive field in another and it will be seen that the super-fitness of one sport has no bearing on physical requirements in another.

The ordinary individual who has no pretensions to excellence in sport has no such incentive to seek physical fitness. The athlete is inspired by a love of his sport to adopt every possible method for increasing athletic efficiency. He has a goal.

Much less apparent but just as real is the need for physical fitness in the ordinary person with little or no active interest in any sport. In life there is no such state as that of complete inactivity. Whatever one is obliged to do in one's daily life, expenditure of physical energy always is necessary. In relation to the energy expended it is necessary that the muscles and nerves involved must be trained accordingly.

A practical example of this can be given from one of a thousand simple acts in the lives of everyone. To the child the first steps in the art of learning to use a fork and knife are very difficult. But constant repetition—the training of muscle and nerve to perform a complicated act—produces a skilled performance accomplished with ease. That the technique of eating by means of a fork and knife may be described as a 'skilled performance' may seem ridiculous. The degree of skill is best judged, however, by the clumsy efforts of the fork and knife eater who tries to use chop-sticks for the first time.

Practice Makes Perfect

This is true of most acts performed automatically because of constant repetition early in life, as in the case of writing, which the practiced person does with ease and the individual who writes only one or two letters a year does slowly, laboriously, and with great efforts at concentration.

The novice types slowly, one finger at a time, eyes searching the keyboard for each individual letter. The expert typist's fingers fly across the keyboard without the conscious mind even once having to determine the position of one letter, figure or symbol. The cyclist balances without giving a thought to the actual process of maintaining balance. The beginner alternately falls and wobbles precariously on his way.

In time we learn to use fork and knife, and chop-sticks, too, if we are so inclined, to write and to type, to cycle, to drive a car, and a thousand and one seemingly simple everyday acts. But in the process of learning the methods have always been the same, the synchronizing of muscular action and nerve control, a slow process stretching from the clumsy, tense, energy-wasting efforts of the first attempt to the smooth, relaxed movement of the skilled performer.

It should be so of every natural movement as well as of the movements that civilized life insists that we must learn. There would be fewer round shoulders if the body were educated to maintain correct posture. The possession of a podgy waistline would not be accepted as a dignified decline to old age if we understood its harmful effect on health and the means by which we could prevent its development.

Careless Posture

Immobility is the cause of many human ailments. Because there is little need for much bending, the back, normal in childhood, loses its mobility long before middle-age. Because there is little that is physically strenuous in normal existence the abdominal muscles responsible for holding the abdominal organs in a balanced position lose power and efficiency, sag and stretch under the joint influence of weakening muscle fiber and the weight of the organs. The result is a distended abdomen.

One physical trouble is the forerunner of others. Drooping shoulders influence the development of hollow back. With hollow back comes distended stomach. And with these comes foot trouble due to added body-weight being superimposed on feet the muscles of which are deteriorating along with the rest of the body.

Cure for Those Aches and Pains

To the vast majority physical life is burdened by abnormalities that range between indefinite aches and persistent pain. These are due to neglect of commonsense precautions. They need never arise except as the result of injury. What these precautions are will be outlined in the succeeding pages.

They consist of a series of exercises that can be done in the home. Their effects are several. For instance, constant repetition of these exercises will result in increased mobility of the joints, including the spine. At the same time the movements will improve the quality of the muscles, which is vastly more important than increasing the quantity.

Exercise increases the flow of the blood to the muscles, providing a corresponding increase in the quantity of oxygen normally carried by the bloodstream. It improves, too, respiratory efficiency, including improving the quality of the system by means of which oxygen carried in the blood stream combats the incidence of fatigue in the form of carbon dioxide deposits.

The effect of exercise on the nervous system is not so well known or understood, but it can be said that the reflexes, which play an important part in physical movement, are materially improved, supposedly because of the greater use of these nerve paths and the consequent reduction of resistance to the nervous impulses. An important effect is that of induced relaxation, physical and mental, resulting in, among other things, improved sleep.

No more than fifteen minutes a day need be given to the task of conscientiously going through a table of exercises in the garden or in the seclusion of one's bedroom. In the space of fifteen minutes it is possible to do up to ten exercises thoroughly.

Family P.T. Class

A series of eight tables of exercises has been prepared. Each table should be done for one week. The tables are arranged in such a way that each exercise is more strenu ous than the corresponding one in the previous table. Table VIII is the basis of the normal all-the-year-round activity. But this may be varied by the inclusion of the supplementary exercises which are given at the end as alternatives.

The exercises, with few exceptions, have the advantage of simplicity. They are, again with rare exceptions, not difficult to perform.

They have been so planned that they are suitable for women as well as men, which means that husband and wife may do the exercises together. When this admirable arrangement is followed the children, too, should be encouraged to join in as these mobilizing and strengthening exercises will be of value to them as well.

In addition to exercising muscles and muscle groups, particularly the postural muscles that keep the 'tummy' in shape, stop shoulders stooping, and take excessive hollows out of backs, these movements aim at an increased range of mobility in such joints as the neck, shoulders, spine, hip, knee and ankle, in themselves the seats of many troubles later on in life.

The breathing exercises are given at the end of each table because it is held that these are relatively without value unless preceded by movements accelerating the blood flow and the rate of respiration.

The exercises in each table conform to a sequence throughout, with occasional variation. There are ten exercises in each table. These are given in the order in which they should be done.

Breathing

Breathing exercises may be done standing up or lying down on the back with the knees bent to reduce pull on the abdominal muscles and through them on the floating ribs.

To fill the lungs completely the following method is recommended. In the standing position feet astride, hands on hips, breathe in and push the abdomen out. When it is felt that the lower half of the lungs have been filled continue the inhalation by allowing the upper half to take in the air and push out the chest.

In exhaling, do so in the same order, keeping the chest high while forcing the wind out of the lower part of the lungs. If this is done correctly the abdomen will be drawn inward automatically and the muscles of the abdomen will contract. Having felt the abdominal muscles contract powerfully, allow the chest to fall, expending the last of the air from the lungs.

This in itself is a powerful abdominal exercise and five to ten repetitions at any time will suffice. It can be done either in a standing or a back-lying position. It should be followed at all times by easy, rhythmical breathing in which emphasis is given to relaxation instead of range or depth.

Clothing

These exercises may be done in the morning or the evening. A minimum of clothing should be worn, unless the individual is carrying too much weight and is desirous of inducing perspiration for the purpose of reducing. Ordinarily, however, for the sake of comfort, it is advisable to do the exercises wearing only a pair of shorts. If a carpet is available the feet can be bare.

In warm weather it may be necessary to have a sponge down following the exercises. In winter a vigorous rubbing with towel or the hands is recommended to stimulate the skin after exercise. Another worthwhile addition is that of five minutes' complete relaxation on bed when the morning's table has been run through.

FIRST WEEK (Table I)

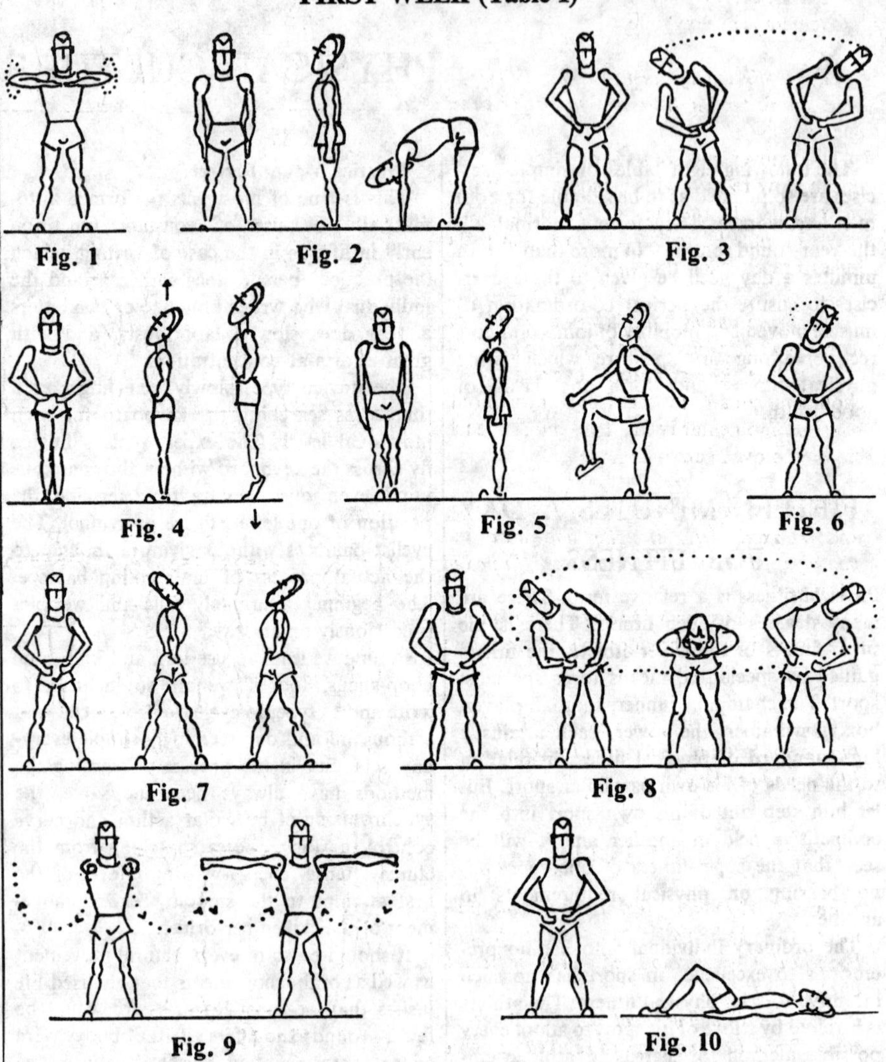

Fig. 1. *Standing, feet astride, arms across bend. Elbows circling forward-up-back-down* (20 *times*).

Fig. 2. *Standing, feet astride, arms at sides. Trunk bending to touch the floor with the fingers, quickly down, slowly up* (10 *times*).

The upward movement in slow time is a relaxed, unrolling of the spine, from the lumbar region (small of the back) to the neck, ending by slowly lifting the chin away from the collar bone with which it should be in contact throughout most of the movement of unrolling.

Fig. 3. *Standing, feet astride, hands on hips* (*not waist*). *Trunk bending from side to side* (5 *times to each side*).

The sideways bend should be sharp, the upward movement slow. Concentrate on contracting the muscles of the side during the sideways bending movement so that the muscles on the side to which one is bending are contracted and the muscles on the other side are relaxed.

Fig. 4. *Standing, feet together, hands on waist. Heels raising and lowering* (10 *to* 15 times).

Note that the starting position is feet together and not merely heels together. This means that the inner sides of the feet should be touching throughout their length. This angle is a natural one. The other is not. With rare exceptions the same foot angle should be maintained throughout these tables of exercises.

Avoid swaying forward and backward in doing this exercise. Let the lower legs do all of the work. Relax elsewhere.

Fig. 5. *Standing, feet together, arms at sides, fingers lightly clenched. Stationary walking with knee raising and opposite arm swinging* (10 *times each leg*).

The knee should be raised to hip level or higher according to individual ability. The arms, straight, should be swung freely, but not necessarily vigorously, to help maintain balance.

Fig. 6. *Standing, feet astride, hands on waist. Head rolling (5 times each way, twice).*

This is not a relaxed movement, but an effort to stretch the head as far as possible in the direction in which it is bent. The movement is in slow time.

Fig. 7. *Standing, feet astride, hands on hips. Trunk turning from side to side (5 times each side).*

This movement consists of a quick turn and a slow re-turn with a momentary pause in returning to the starting position. Allow the back muscles to do the work. Keep the knees braced back throughout.

Fig. 8. *Standing, feet astride, hands on hips. Trunk circling (5 times each way).*

Keep the knees braced back and the shoulders square to the front throughout, pausing momentarily at the end of each circling movement.

Fig. 9. *Standing, feet astride, arms forward relaxed. Arms swinging downward and sideways, downward and forward, relaxed (20 times).*

The arms must be held relaxed throughout. The swing ends at shoulder level in front and at the sides.

Fig. 10. *Standing, feet astride, hands on hips, or back lying, arms at sides, knees bent. Rhythmic breathing.*

SECOND WEEK (Table II)

Fig. 11. *Standing, feet astride, arms sideways stretched, palms up. Arms circling backward (forward-up-back-down) in small circles (15 times).*

Fig. 12. *Standing, feet astride, arms at sides. Trunk bending forward relaxed, to three counts, to touch the floor with the fingers on third count.*

Brace the knees back throughout. Let the weight of the body effect most of the trunk bend, going half way down on the first count, a little farther on the second, and touch the floor on the third. In between each of the three counts the trunk should be allowed to rebound but not to rise to the starting position. At the end of the third count the return to the starting position is a relaxed unrolling of the spine in slow time.

Fig. 13. *Standing, feet astride, arms at sides. Trunk bending from side to side, with one arm reaching down (5 times each side).*

The sideways bend is sharp, the upward movement slow and relaxed, pausing momentarily in the starting position at the end of the upward movement.

Fig. 14. *Standing, feet together, hands on waist. Heel raising, knee bending, stretching and lowering (10 times).*

Keep the body upright. Do not sway forward and backward. Maintain the same speed throughout.

SECOND WEEK (Table II)

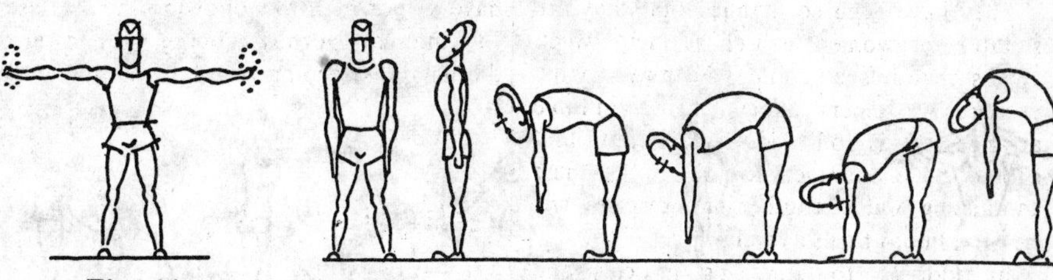

Fig. 11 Fig. 12

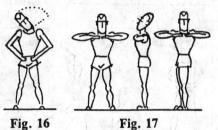

Fig. 13

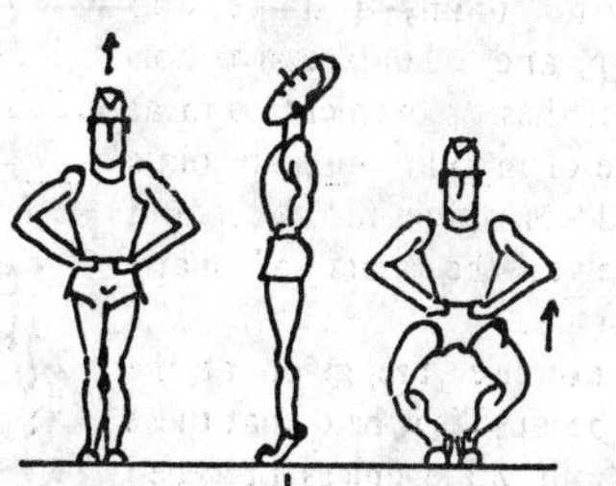

Fig. 14

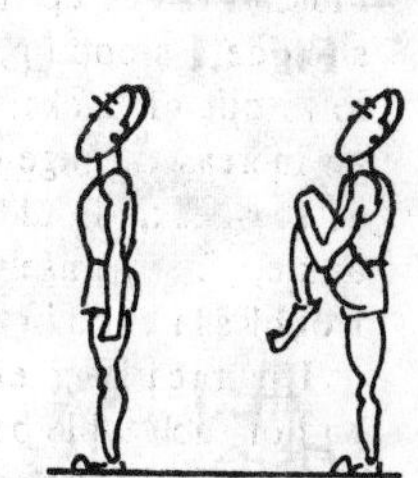

Fig. 15

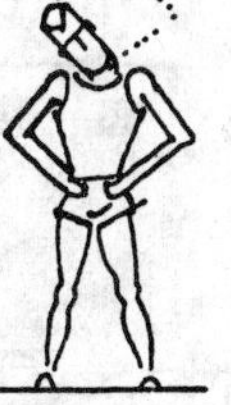

Fig. 16

Fig. 17

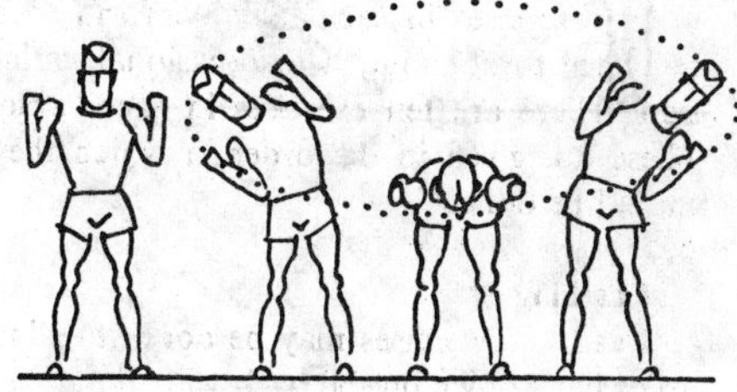

Fig. 18

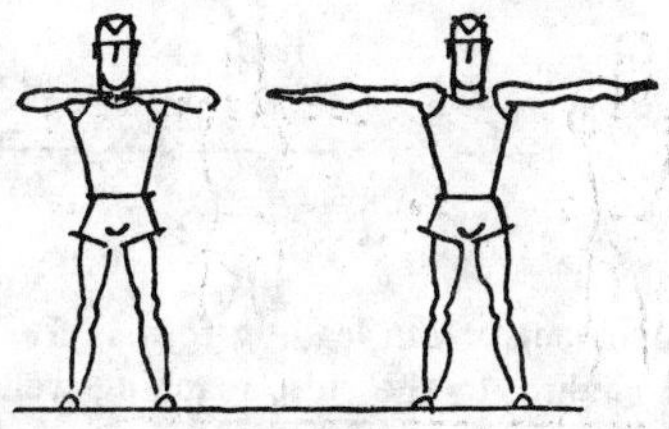

Fig. 19

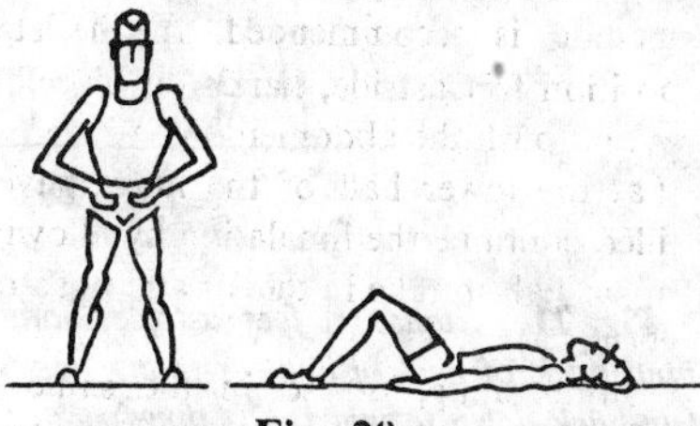

Fig. 20

Fig. 15. *Standing, feet together, arms at sides. Knee raising to chest, with the assistance of the hands (5 times each leg).*

The shoulders should be kept square to the front, the body upright, not bent forward. The leg may be raised by placing the hands across the face of the knee or the fingers under the knee.

Fig. 16. *Standing, feet astride, hands on waist. Head bending from side to side (5 times each side).*

Try to contract the muscles on the side of the neck on the side to which the head is being bent. The movement is a slow one, with a brief pause on returning to the starting position.

This may be followed by the first neck exercise (head rolling) (Fig. 6).

Fig. 17. *Standing, feet astride, arms across bend. Trunk turning from side to side (10 times each side).*

Quick, backward press, slow return, with pause in starting position before turning to the other side. The back muscles should do the work. Brace the knees back throughout.

Fig. 18. *Standing, feet astride, arms upward bend. Trunk circling (5 times each way).*

Shoulders square to the front, knees braced back. Pause on returning to the starting position.

Fig. 19. *Standing, feet astride, arms across bend. Arms flinging backwards and elbows pressing backwards alternately (10 times).*

The arms flinging backwards is a slow movement ending in a quick press in the last foot of travel. The return to starting position also is done in slow time, ending with the elbows pressing backwards movement. Do not allow the body to jerk forward when the press is made at the end of the arms swinging forward movement. Keep the head steady throughout.

Fig. 20. *Breathing.*

THIRD WEEK (Table III)

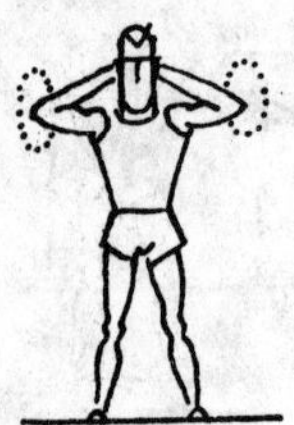

Fig. 21

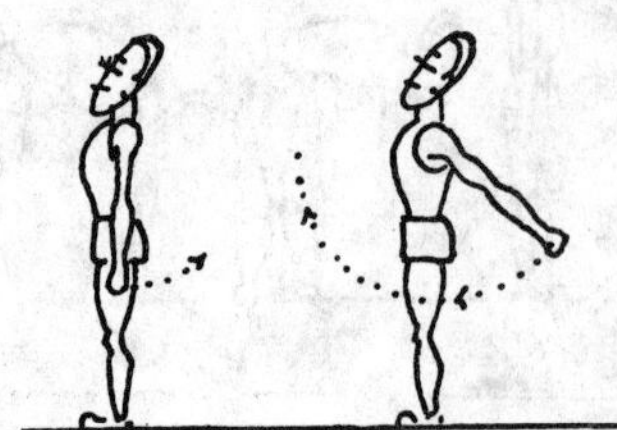

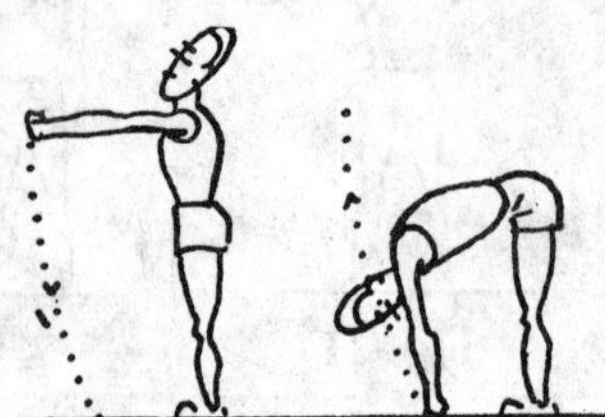

Fig. 22

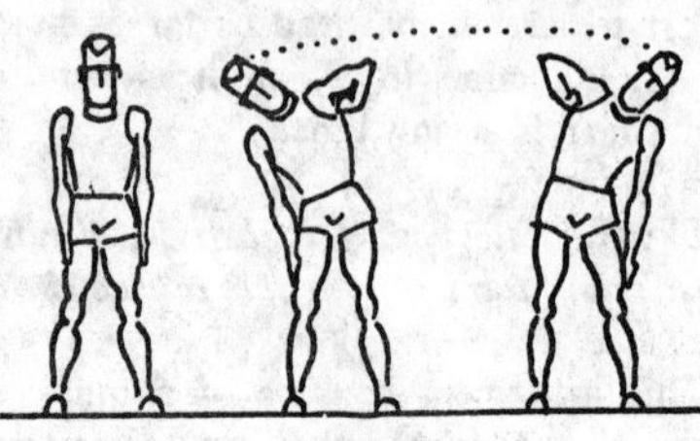

Fig. 23

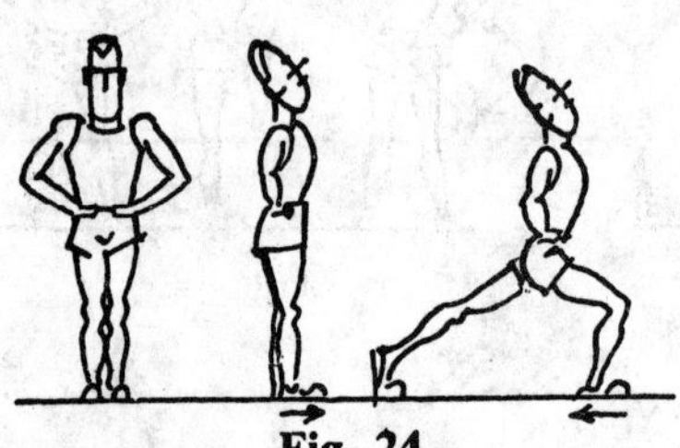

Fig. 24

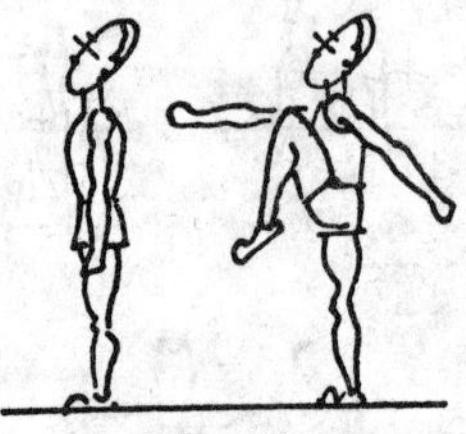

Fig. 25

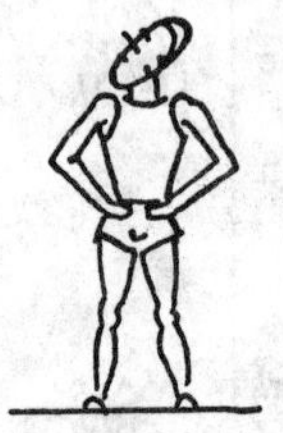

Fig. 26

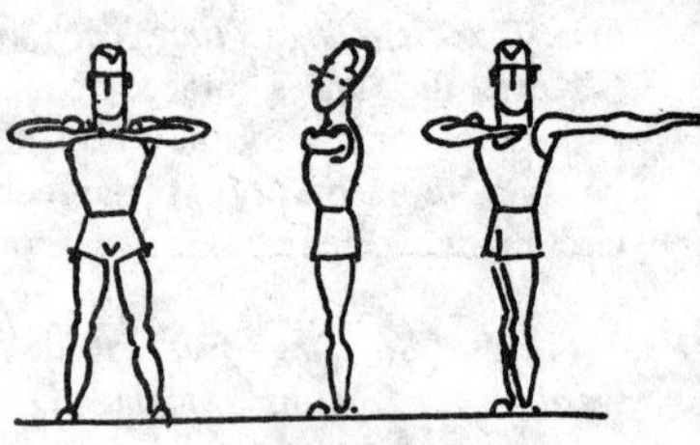

Fig. 27

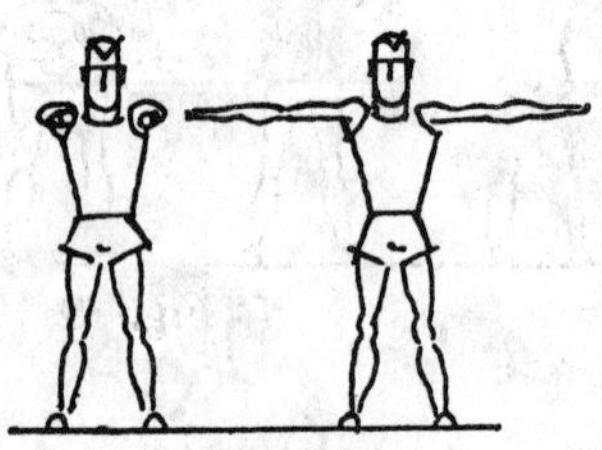

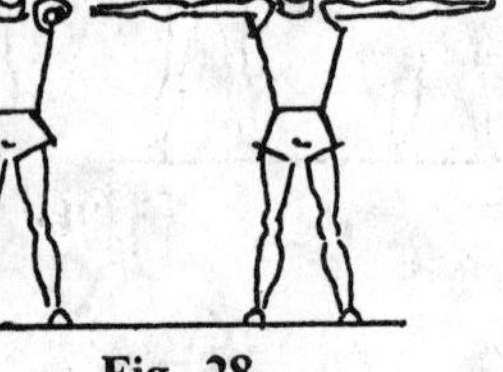

Fig. 28

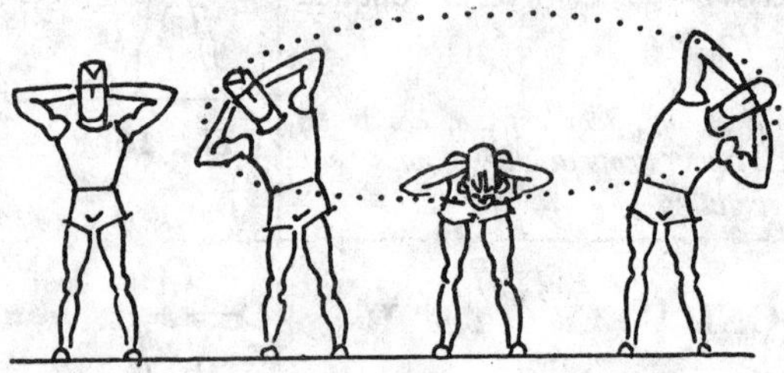

Fig. 29

Fig. 21. *Standing, feet astride, hands behind back of neck. Elbows circling backwards (up-back-down-forward)* (20 *times*).

Fig. 22. *Standing, feet astride, arms at sides. Arms swinging backward-forward to shoulder level, combined with trunk bending to touch the floor with the hands* (15 *times*).

This is a quick movement, done rhythmically. The arms are relaxed, fingers lightly clenched. The trunk bend is done at the end of each forward swing of the arms. The trunk unbending is done at the same speed as the bending movement. The arms are raised forward at the same time as the trunk is raised. The arms are then swung back and forward again. Then the trunk bending is repeated. The knees should be braced back throughout.

Fig. 23. *Standing, feet astride, arms at sides. Trunk bending from side to side, with one arm reaching down, one arm under-bend* (10 *times each side*).

The bend is a quick movement, the stretch a slow, relaxed recovery.

Fig. 24. *Standing, feet together, hands on hips. Alternate foot lunging forward* (10 *times each leg*).

The movement of the leading foot is forward and slightly to the side, reaching well forward. The body is maintained in an

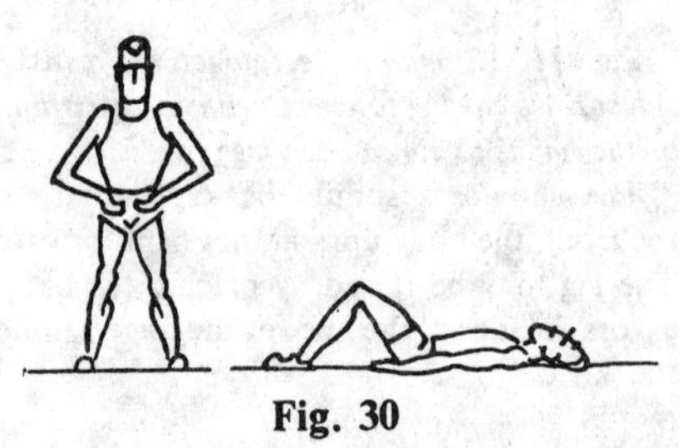

Fig. 30

upright posture. Any tendency to sway forward in stepping back to the starting position must be corrected.

Fig. 25. *Standing, feet together, arms at sides. Knee raising to chest, with arm swinging in time* (10 *times each leg*).

Shoulders must be kept square to the front. Correct any tendency to bend the body forward as the knee is raised to the chest. Swing the arms vigorously, with opposite knee and arm going forward together.

Fig. 26. *Standing, feet astride, hands on waist. Head turning from side to side* (5 *times each side*).

This may be followed by head bending from side to side (Fig. 16).

Fig. 27. *Standing, feet astride, arms across bend. Trunk turning sideways with arm flinging sideways* (10 *times each side*).

Easy trunk turning ending with quick press as the arm is flung into extension. The return to the starting position is relaxed and steady, with a pause in the starting position before turning in the opposite direction. Keep the shoulders back. Brace the knees back.

Fig. 28. *Standing, feet astride, arms forward relaxed, backs of the hands up, fingers relaxed. Rhythmic arm parting* (10 *times*).

This is a slow movement, with a quick press in the last foot of backward travel. The return to the starting position also is slow. Avoid a natural tendency to sway forward as the arms are pressed back.

Fig. 29. *Standing, feet astride, hands behind neck. Trunk circling* (5 *times each way*).

Shoulders must be kept square to the front, knees and elbows braced back. The movement is a moderately slow one.

Fig. 30. *Breathing.*

FOURTH WEEK (Table IV)

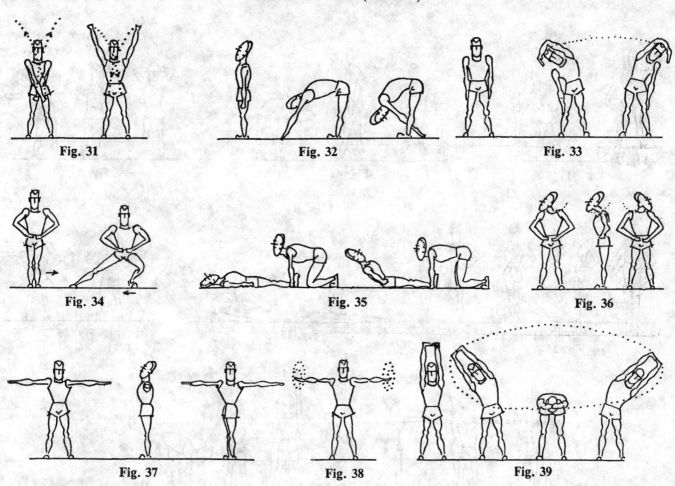

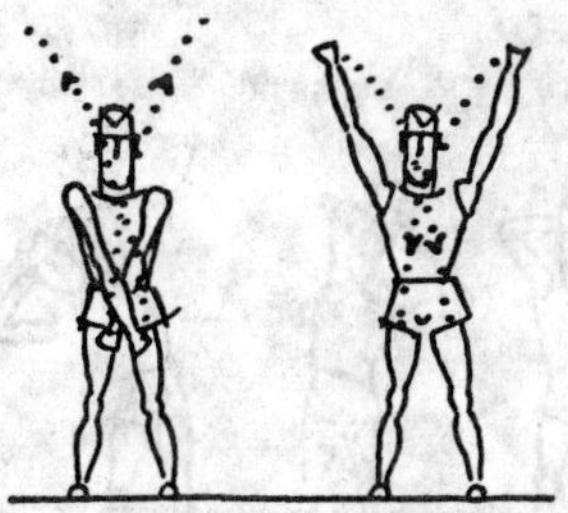

Fig. 31

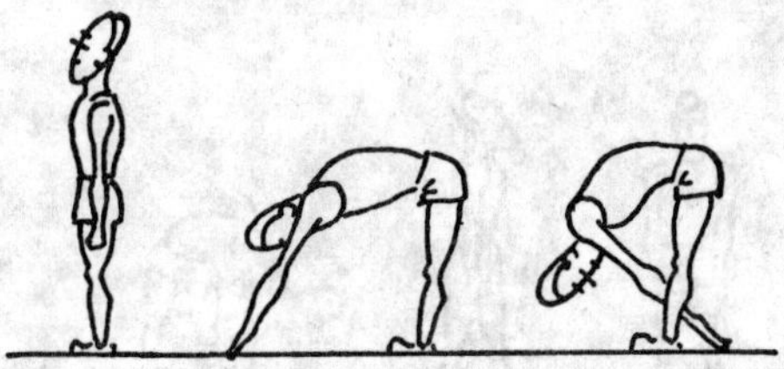

Fig. 32

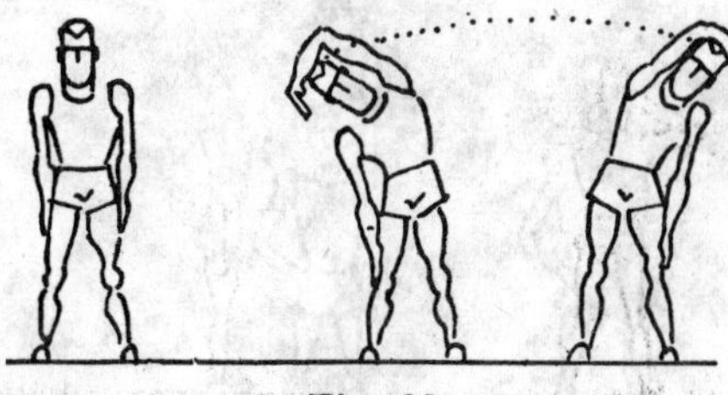

Fig. 33

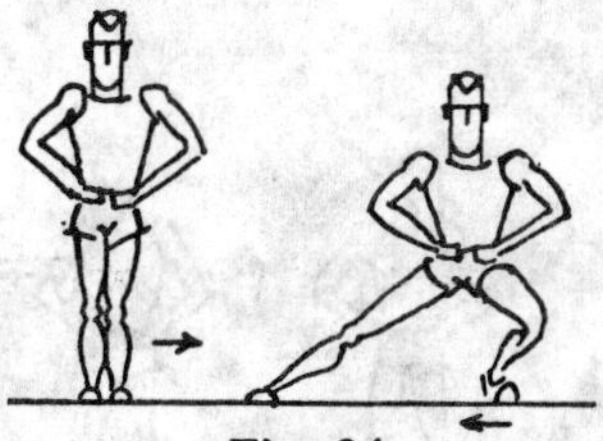

Fig. 34

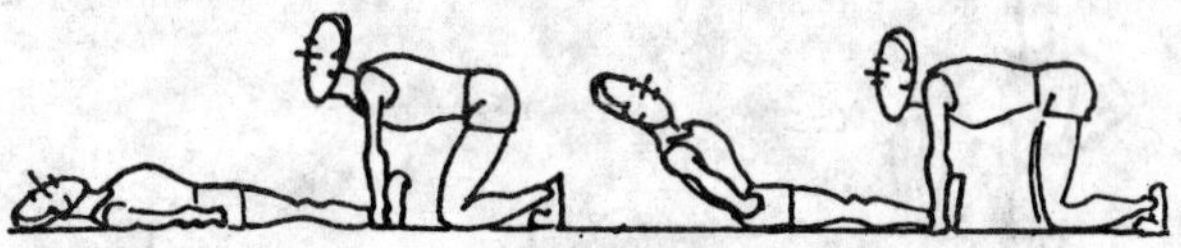

Fig. 35

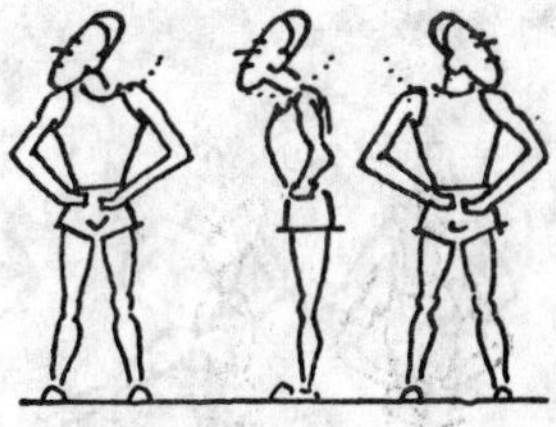

Fig. 36

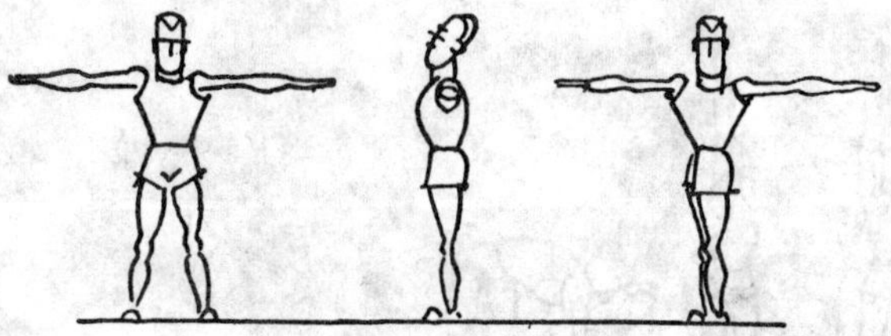

Fig. 37

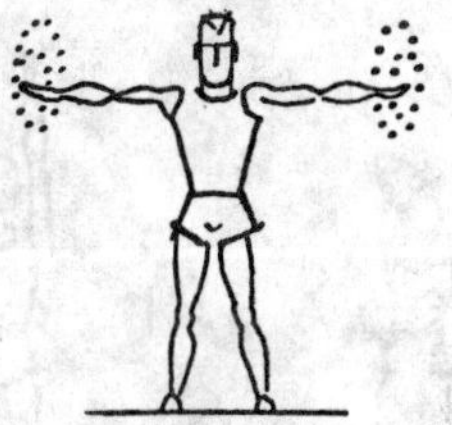

Fig. 38

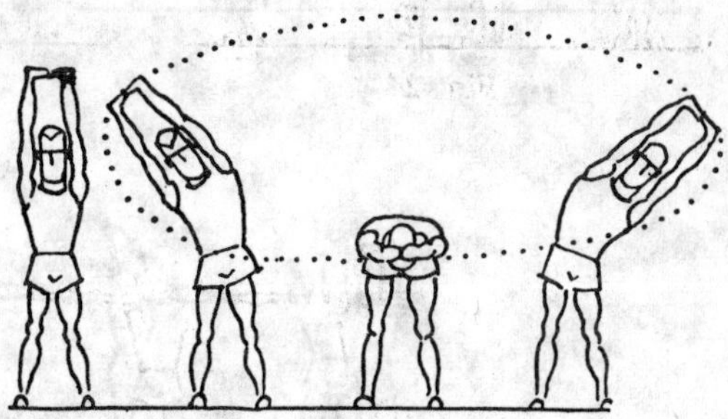

Fig. 39

Fig. 31. *Standing, feet astride, wrists crossed in front. Arms swinging forward to midway-upward* (10 *times*).

The arms are crossed at the wrists. They are swung forward and upward to finish more than shoulder-width apart and as far back as the arms can be pressed. This is a slow starting movement finishing with a quick press. The return to the starting position is made slowly.

Fig. 32. *Standing, feet astride, arms at sides. Relaxed trunk bending to touch the floor (forward and back between the legs) and slowly unrolling* (10 *times*).

Bend down and reaching out as far as possible with the hands (1), back between the legs (2), then slowly unroll in the manner already described for other trunk bending exercises.

Fig. 33. *Standing, feet astride, arms at sides. Trunk bending sideways, one arm reaching down, one arm over-bend* (5 *times each side*).

Fig. 34. *Standing, feet together, hands on hips. Foot lunging sideways* (5 *times each side*).

Concentrate on keeping the body upright and making the legs do all of the work.

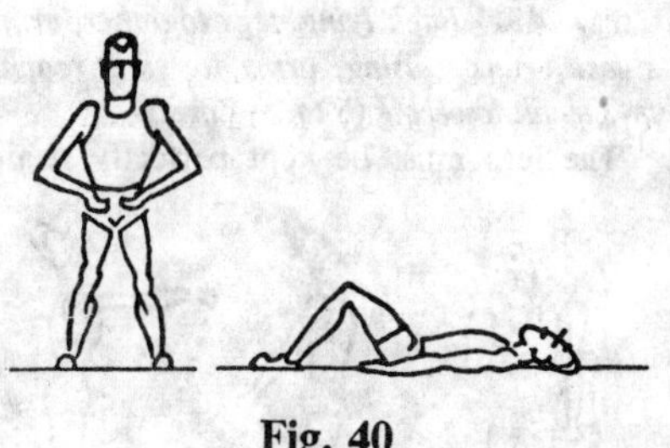

Fig. 40

Fig. 35. *Back lying, legs together, hands on hips, ankles held (if possible). Trunk half-raising and lowering* (5 *times*).

This exercise should be done with the assistance of a partner to hold the ankles. As an alternative it is sometimes possible to put the feet under a heavy article of furniture, such as a dressing table.

Keep the body straight. Half raise slowly, pause, then return slowly to the starting position.

Fig. 36. *Standing, feet astride, hands on waist. Neck stretching sideways-forward-sideways in semi-circle* (5 *times to each side*).

Keep the body perfectly still. Push the chin out as far as possible to one side, then circle the extended chin forward and round as far as possible towards the other side.

Finish by bending the head from side to side (Fig. 16).

Fig. 37. *Standing, feet astride, arms stretched sideways. Trunk turning sideways* (5 *times each side*).

The movement is done moderately slowly each turn ending with an arm press. The return to the starting position is slow and relaxed. There is a brief pause in the starting position each time. Brace the knees back.

Fig. 38. *Standing, feet astride, arms stretched sideways, palms up. Arms circling backward (forward-up-back-down) in small and large circles alternately* (5 *small*, 5 *large*, 5 *small*, 5 *large*).

Fig. 39. *Standing, feet astride, arms raised, fingers interlaced. Trunk circling* (5 *times each way*).

Movement slow, shoulders square to the front, knees braced back.

Fig. 40. *Breathing.*

FIFTH WEEK (Table V)

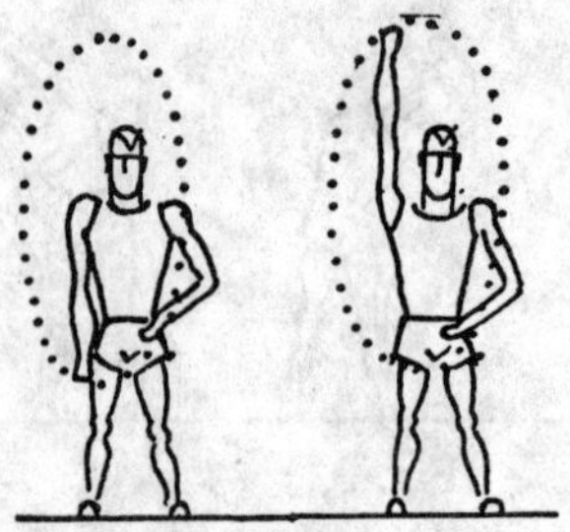

Fig. 41

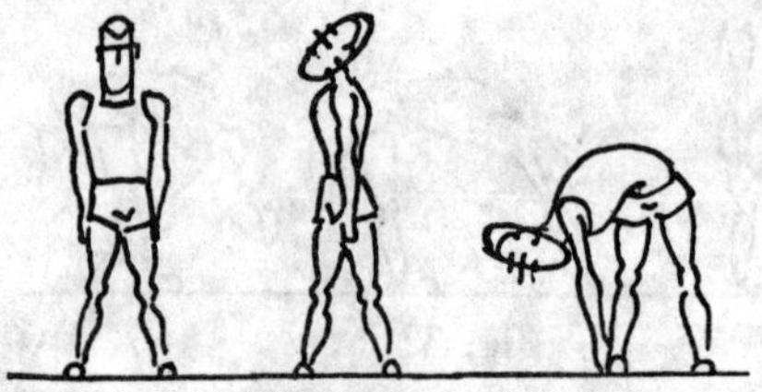

Fig. 42

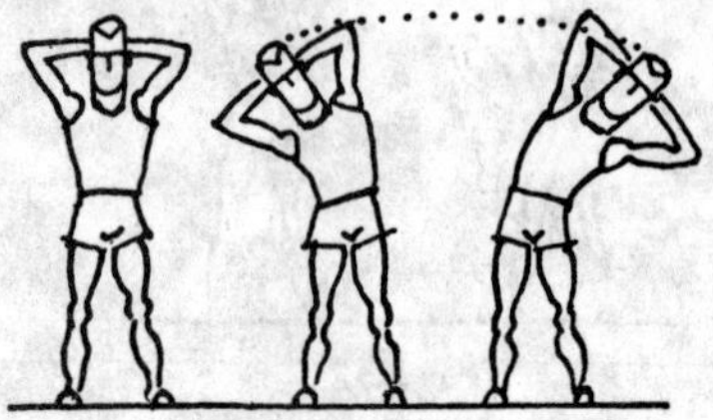

Fig. 43

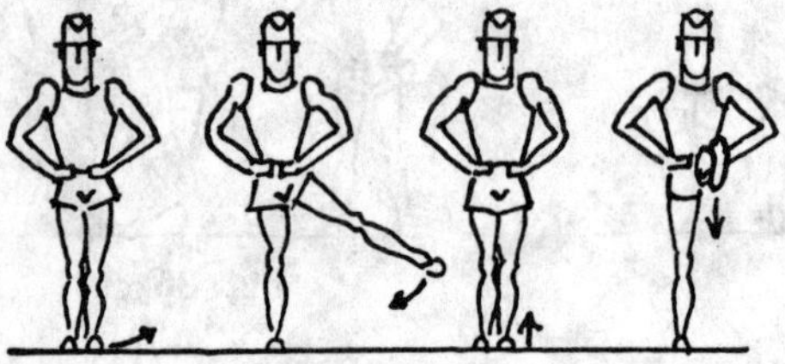

Fig. 44

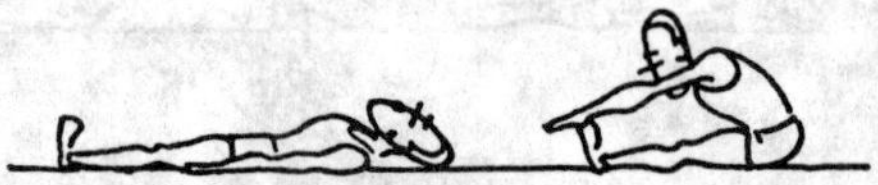

Fig. 45

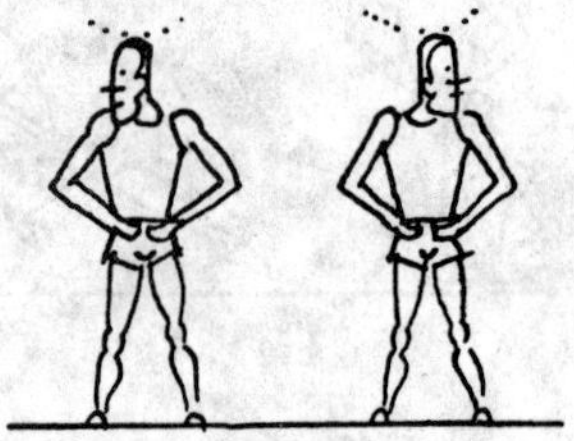

Fig. 46

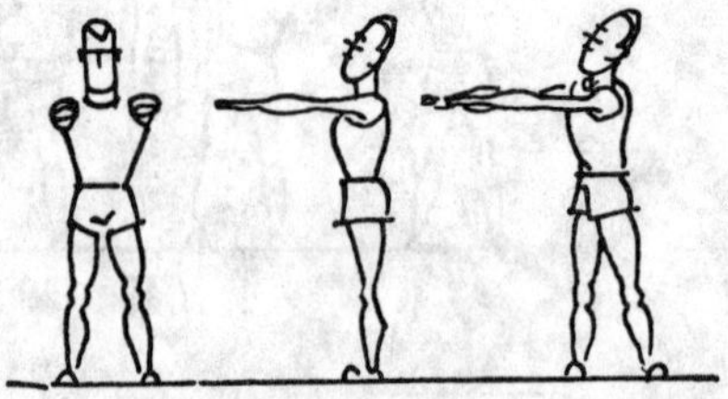

Fig. 47

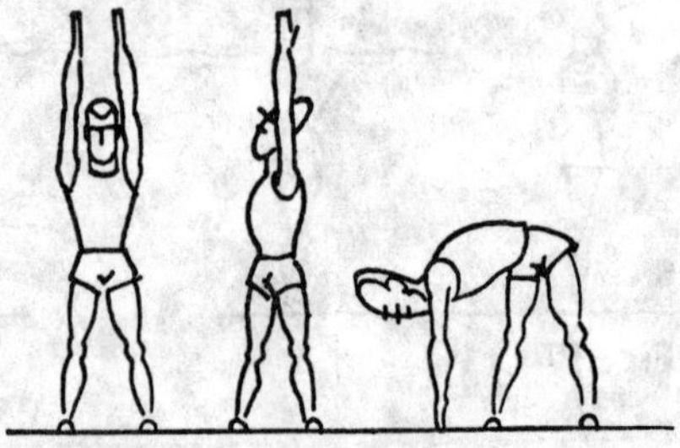

Fig. 48

Fig. 41. *Standing, feet astride, one arm at side, one hand on hip. Arm circling upward-backward* (15 *times each arm:* 5 *times one arm,* 5 *times the other, and so on*).

This is a full arm swing, partly across the body in front. The shoulders should remain square to the front.

Fig. 42. *Standing, feet astride, arms at side. Trunk turning and bending to touch the floor with the hands* (5 *times each side*).

The trunk turn is a smooth one, the trunk bend quick. The return to the starting position is a relaxed one, the return to the upright and the turn to face the front being combined in one movement.

Fig. 43. *Standing, feet astride, hands behind neck. Trunk bending from side to side* (5 *times each side*).

The sideways bend is a quick movement, the return to the starting position slower and relaxed. There is a brief pause in the upright position before bending in the other direction. Keep the shoulders square to the front.

Fig. 44. *Standing, feet together, hands on hips. Leg raising sideways and forward alternately, each leg in turn* (5 *times each leg*).

Keep both legs perfectly straight and body upright.

Fig. 45. *Back lying, legs together, arms at sides. Trunk raising, arms forward reaching, and trunk lowering* (5 *to* 10 *times*).

The legs must be kept perfectly straight.

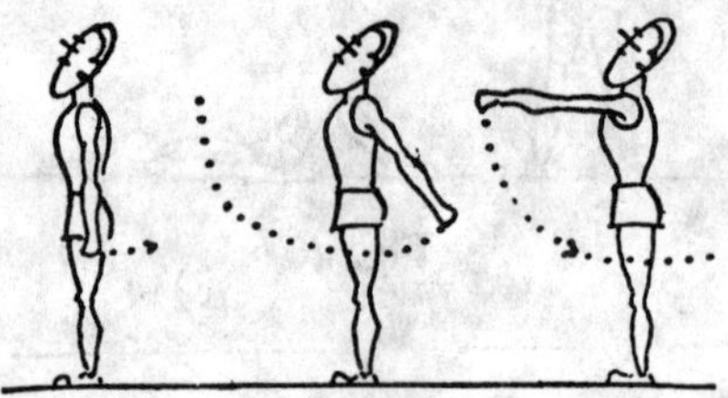

Fig. 49

In reaching forward concentrate on contracting the abdominal muscles. The trunk raising is done steadily, the forward reaching smartly, and the return to the starting position slowly.

Fig. 46. *Standing, feet astride, hands on waist. Head-rolling, with chin scraping collar bone* (5 *times to each side*).

The chin should maintain contact with the collar bone throughout this movement.

Fig. 47. *Standing, feet astride, arms forward shoulder-width apart. Trunk turning from side to side* (5 *times each side*).

The turn in this exercise is effected without the usual pause in the starting position. The finish of the movement is a quick press. The turn is done slowly. The knees should be well braced back.

Fig. 48. *Standing, feet astride, arms stretched upwards. Trunk turning and trunk bending sideways to touch the floor with the hands* (5 *times each side*).

The trunk turning is quick, as is the trunk bending. The return to the starting position is done in two distinct movements by (1) unbending and (2) turning.

Fig. 49. *Standing, feet astride, arms at sides, hands lightly clenched. Arms swinging backward and forward to shoulder level* (20 *to* 30 *times*).

Fig. 50. *Breathing.*

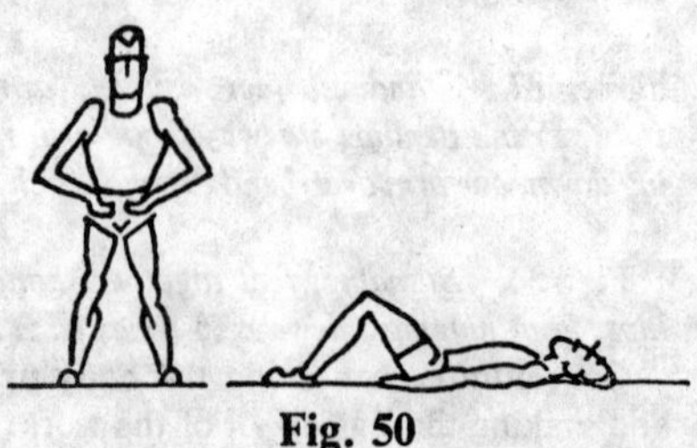

Fig. 50

SIXTH WEEK (Table VI)

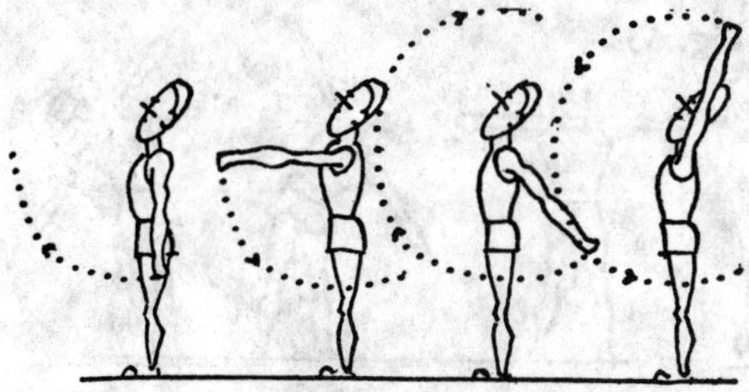

Fig. 51 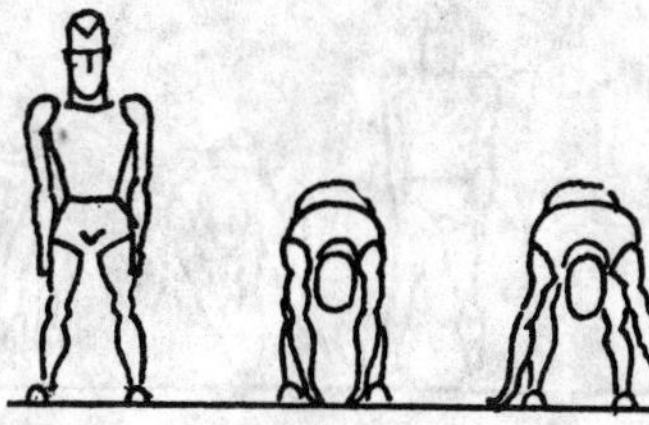 **Fig. 52** 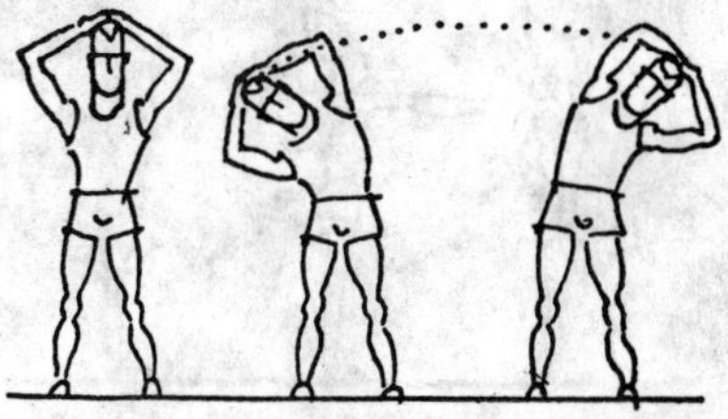 **Fig. 53**

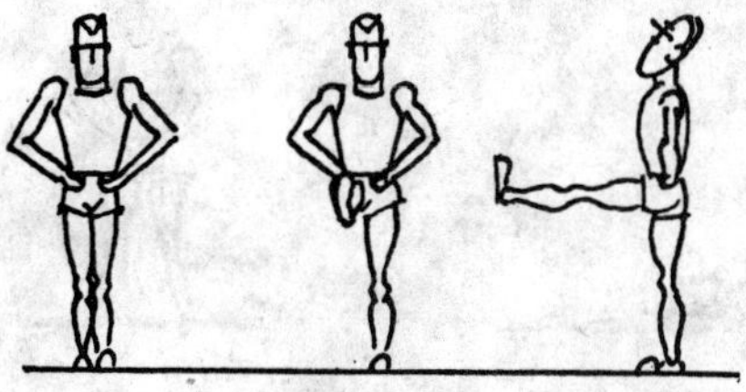

Fig. 54 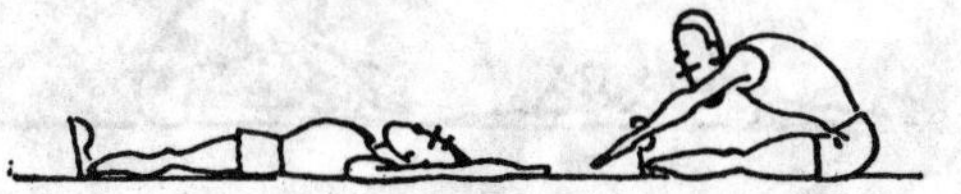 **Fig. 55** 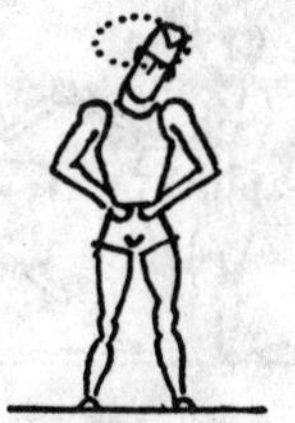 **Fig. 56**

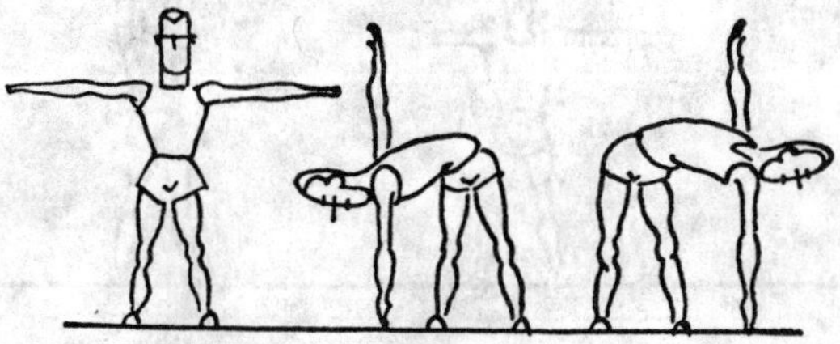

Fig. 57 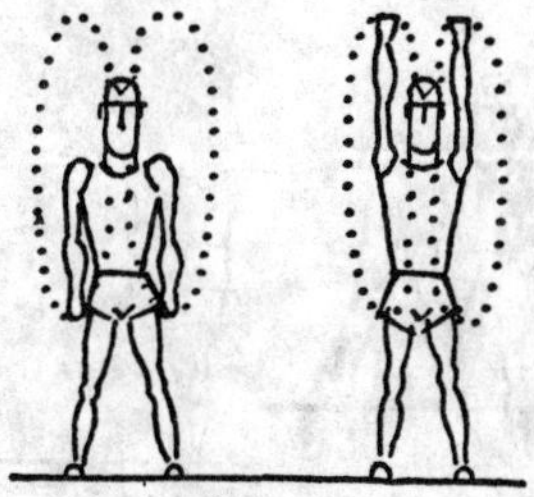 **Fig. 58**

Fig. 51. *Standing, feet astride, arms at sides, hands at sides. Arms swinging backward and forward to shoulder level and overhead alternately* (*10 times*).

The arms are relaxed. Backs of the hands face forward. The swing is a relaxed one. The overhead swing should be carried through to a final pressing movement that will carry the hands back well beyond the line of the shoulders. Avoid hollowing the back.

Fig. 52. *Standing, feet astride, arms at sides. Relaxed trunk bending to touch the floor with the hands between the feet and outside the feet in turn* (*10 times*).

The trunk bend is a quick movement, relaxed in between the touching of the floor in between and outside of the feet so that the body rises and falls slightly from one floor contact to the other. The return to the starting position is a slow unrolling of the spine.

Fig. 53. *Standing, feet astride, hands resting on top of the head. Trunk bending from side to side* (5 *times each side*).

Concentrate on contracting the muscles on the side to which the trunk is bending. Keep the shoulders square to the front and the elbows pressed well back. Do not lean forward. Pause momentarily in the starting position as the trunk returns to the upright.

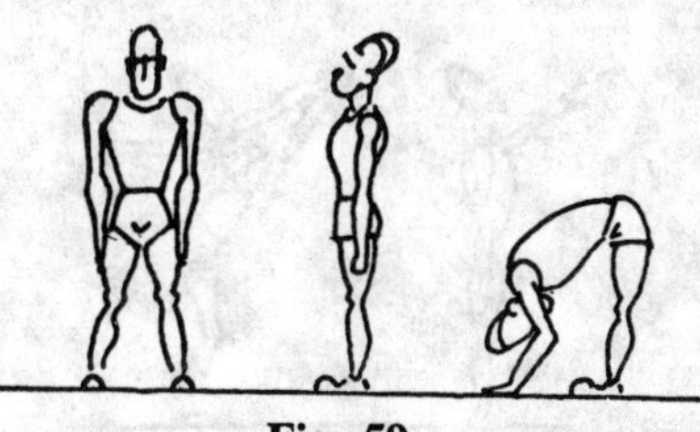

Fig. 59

Fig. 54. *Standing, feet together, hands on hips. Leg raising forward slowly* (5 *times each leg in turn*).

Both knees must be kept straight. Avoid leaning forward.

Fig. 55. *Back lying, legs together, arms stretched upward. Trunk raising with arms swinging forward overhead to forward reach to toes or beyond* (5 *to* 10 *times*).

Fig. 56. *Standing, feet astride, hands on waist. Head rolling* (*as Fig.* 6) (5 *times each way*).

Fig. 57. *Standing, feet astride, arms stretched sideways, fingers extended. Trunk turning and trunk bending to touch the floor beyond the foot with opposite hand* (5 *times to each side*).

The return trunk raise and body turn is done in one movement. There is a pause in the starting position in between each trunk turn.

Fig. 58. *Standing, feet astride, arms at sides, fingers lightly clenched. Both arms circling backwards simultaneously* (*20 times: in groups of five at intervals of five seconds*).

Fig. 59. *Standing, feet astride, arms at sides. Quick trunk bending to touch the floor with the hands* (*15 times*).

Both the bend and upward stretching are done quickly. Brace the knees back.

Fig. 60. *Breathing.*

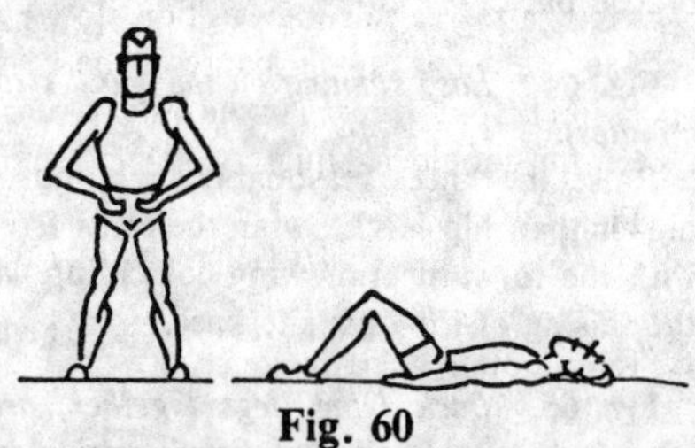

Fig. 60

SEVENTH WEEK (Table VII)

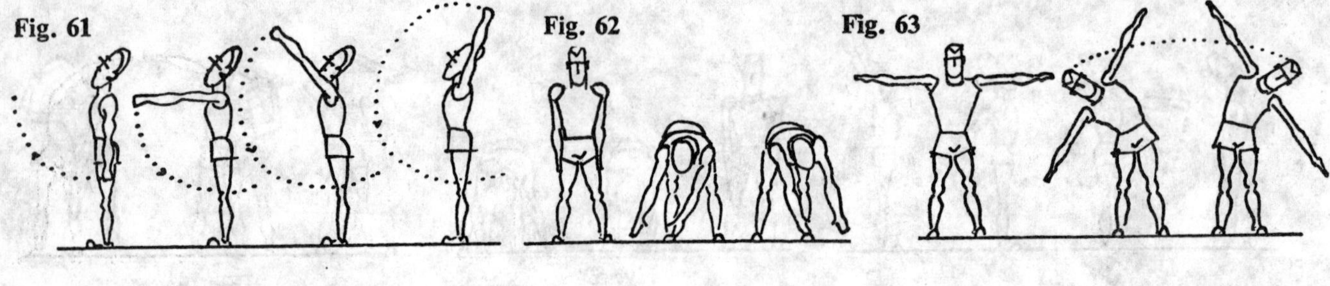

Fig. 61 Fig. 62 Fig. 63

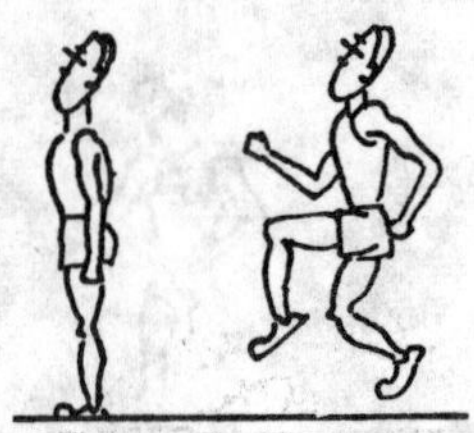

Fig. 64.

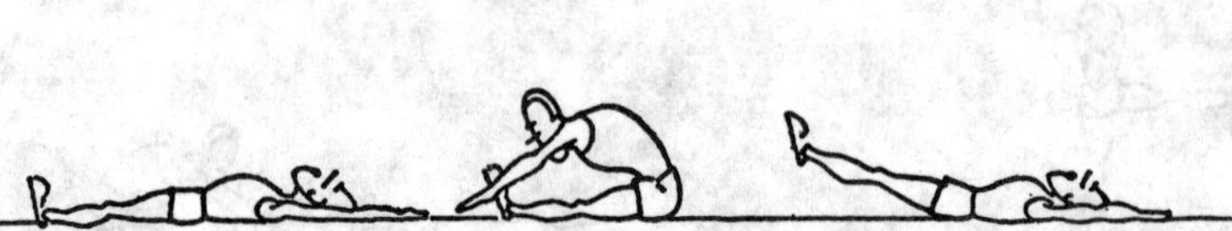

Fig. 65

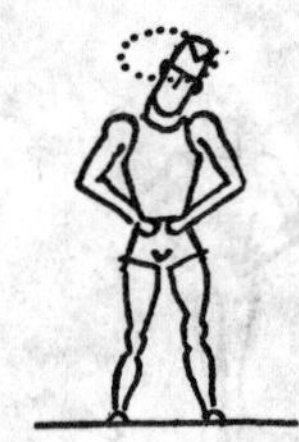

Fig. 66

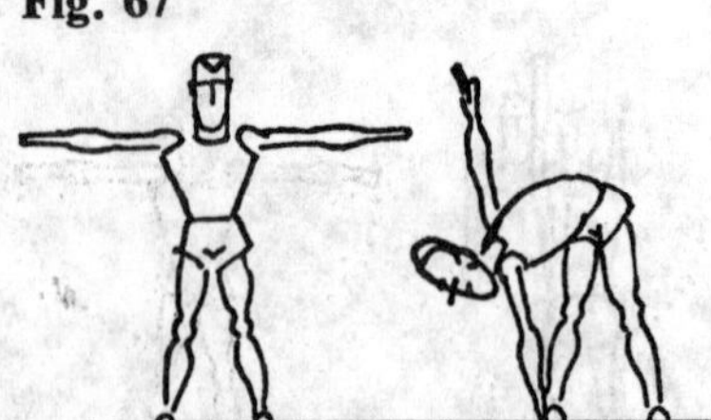

Fig. 67

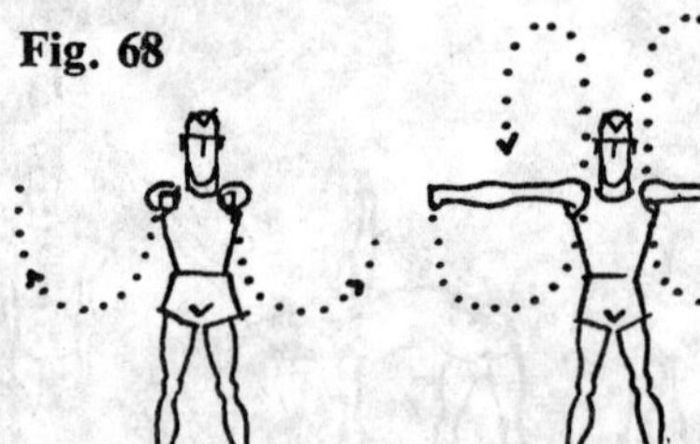

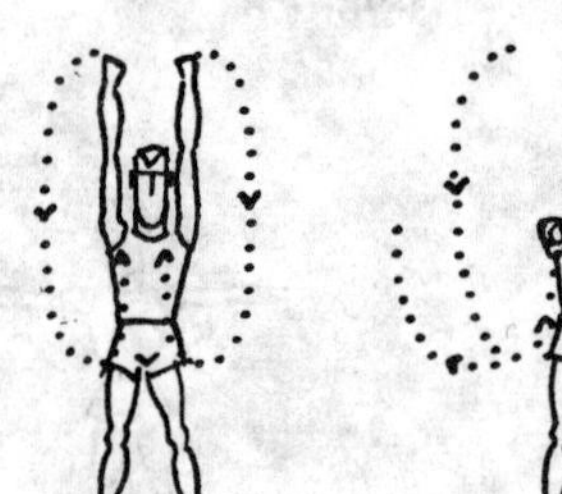

Fig. 68

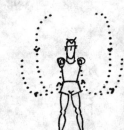

Fig. 61. *Standing, feet astride, arms at sides, fingers lightly clenched, backs of the hands forward. Arms swinging forward, midway-upward, and overhead* (15 *times*).

The arms are swung back and forward to shoulder level, back and forward to midway-upward, back and forward to overhead (this latter being finished with final press to carry the hands back beyond the line of the shoulders).

Fig. 62. *Standing, feet astride, arms at side. Trunk bending to touch each foot in turn with opposite hand and return to standing position* (5 *times*).

Fig. 63. *Standing, feet astride, arms stretched sideways, fingers extended. Trunk bending sideways* (5 *times each side*).

Keep shoulders square to the front and braced back.

Fig. 64. *Easy running on the spot* (1 *to* 2 *minutes*).

Raise the knees reasonably high, but no higher than hip level. Swing the arms freely, with the forward arm swing coinciding with the raising of the opposite knee.

Fig. 65. *Back lying, legs together, arms stretched upward. Alternate trunk-raising-and-arms-forward-reaching with legs half-raising* (5 *to* 10 *times*).

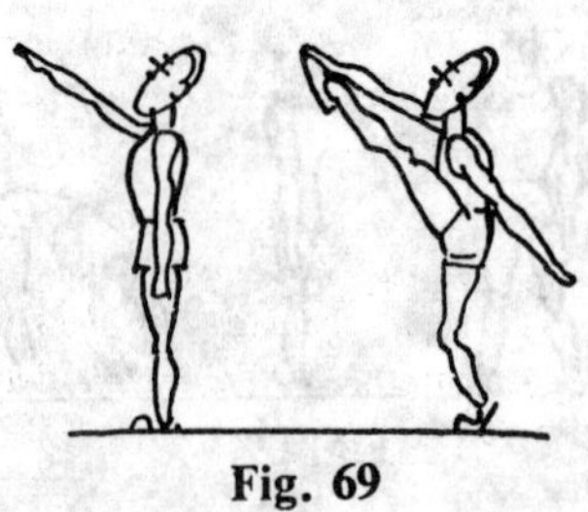

Fig. 69

The trunk raising is smooth. The arms forward reaching is done briskly. The return to the starting position is done smoothly, being followed almost instantly by a slow half-raising of the legs so that the heels are about 12 to 15 inches off the floor. Keep the legs straight.

Fig. 66. *Standing, feet astride, hands on waist. Head rolling with chin scraping collar bone* (*as Fig.* 46).

Fig. 67. *Standing, feet astride, arms stretched sideways, fingers extended. Trunk turning and bending to touch opposite foot with hand* (5 *times each side*).

Keep the knees well braced back.

Fig. 68. *Standing, feet astride, arms forward relaxed, fingers lightly clenched, thumbs uppermost. Arms swinging downward-sideways downward-forward backward-circle to starting position and repeat* (15 *times*).

Fig. 69. *Standing, feet together, one hand at shoulder to head level. High kicking with alternate foot to opposite hand* (5 *times each leg*).

Try to keep both legs straight. Balance by throwing opposite arm backwards.

Fig. 70. *Breathing.*

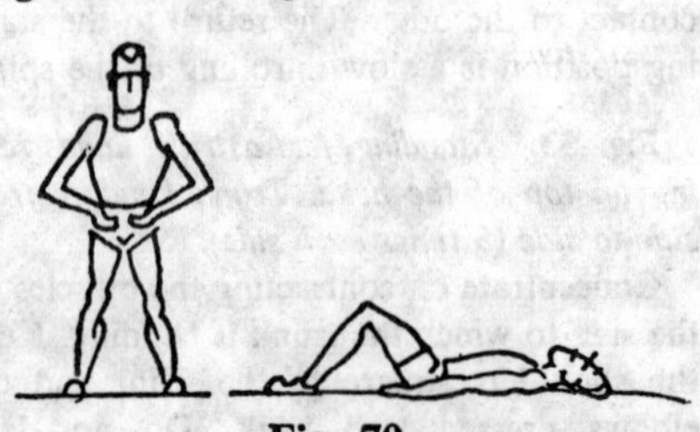

Fig. 70

EIGHTH WEEK (Table VIII)

Fig. 71 **Fig. 72** 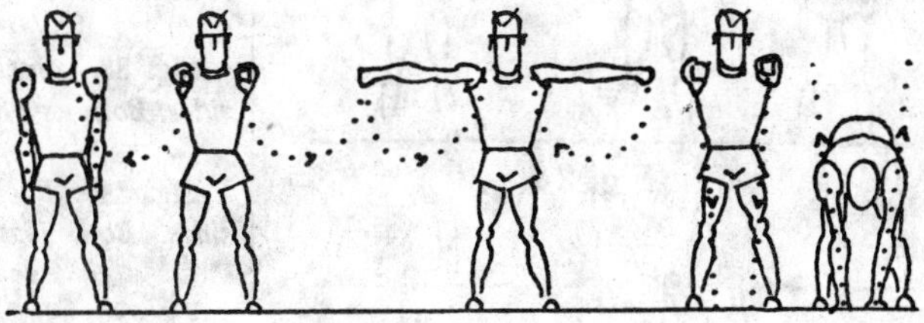 **Fig. 73**

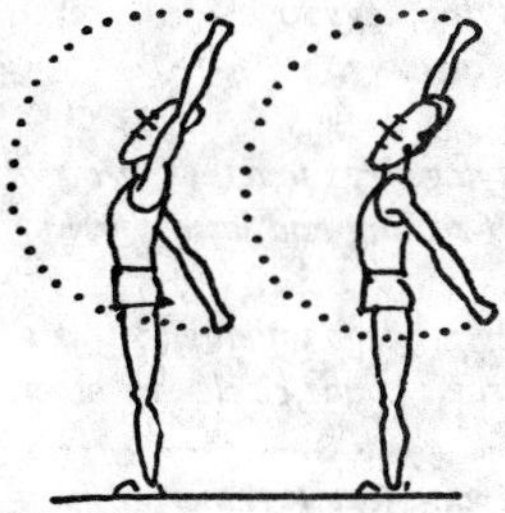

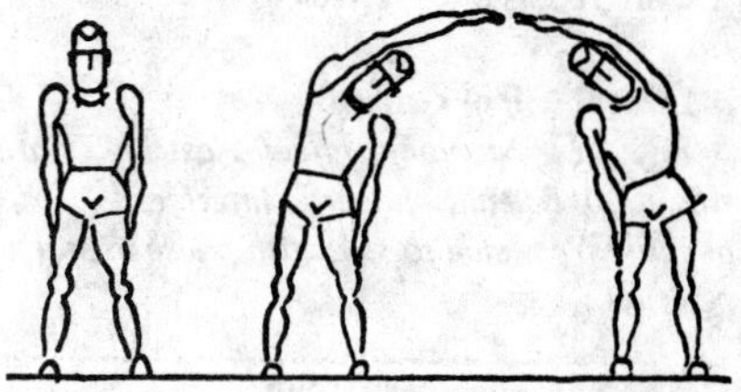

Fig. 74 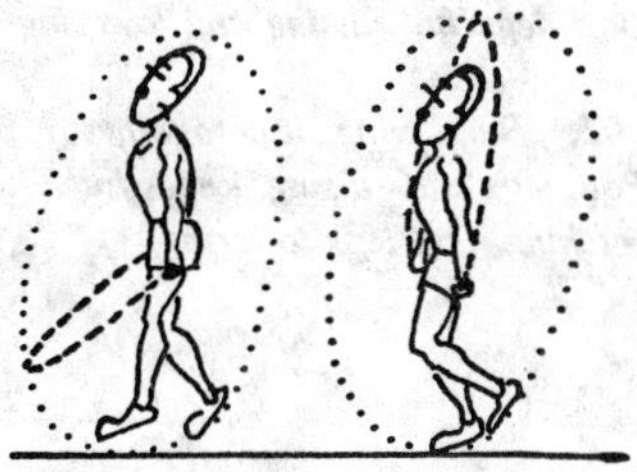 **Fig. 75**

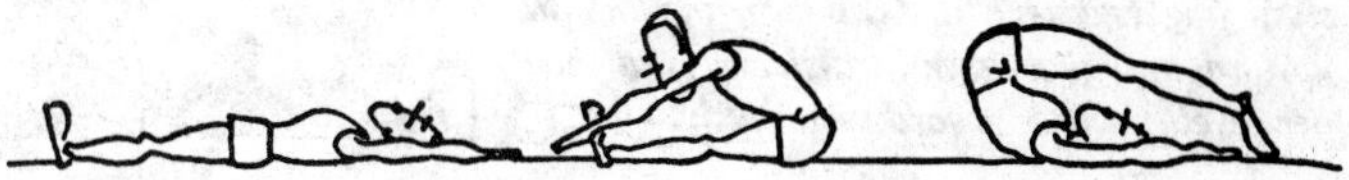

Fig. 76 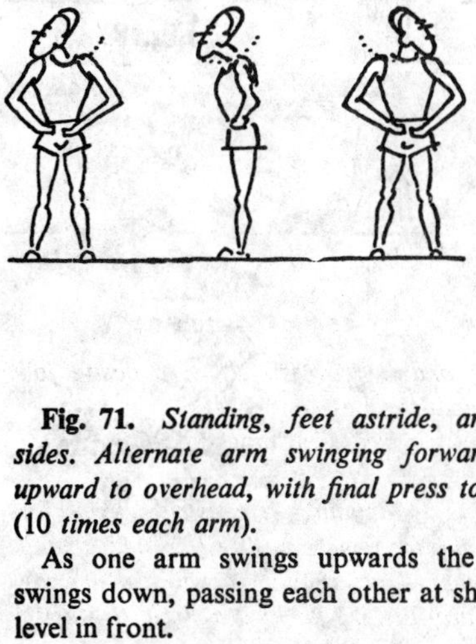 **Fig. 77** 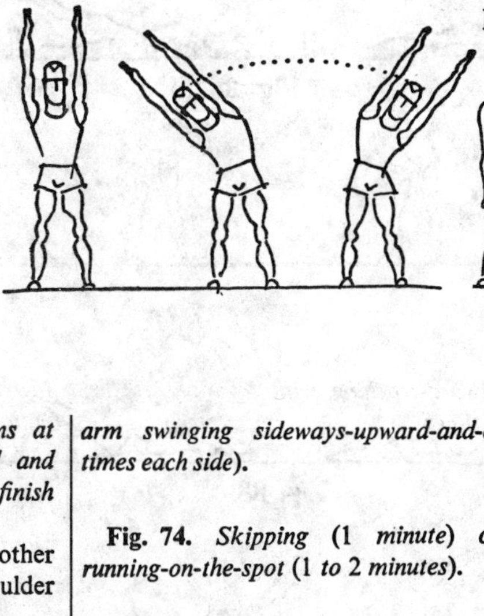 **Fig. 78**

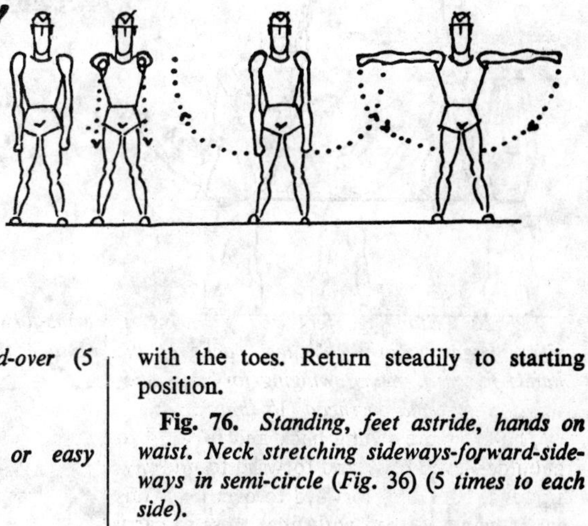

Fig. 71. *Standing, feet astride, arms at sides. Alternate arm swinging forward and upward to overhead, with final press to finish* (*10 times each arm*).

As one arm swings upwards the other swings down, passing each other at shoulder level in front.

Fig. 72. *Standing, feet astride, arms at sides, hands lightly clenched, thumbs uppermost. Arms swinging forward-sideways-forward, trunk bending to touch the floor with the knuckles, rising to arms forward* (15 *times*).

Fig. 73. *Standing, feet astride, arms at sides. Trunk bending sideways, with opposite arm swinging sideways-upward-and-over* (5 *times each side*).

Fig. 74. *Skipping* (1 *minute*) *or easy running-on-the-spot* (*1 to 2 minutes*).

Fig. 75. *Back lying, legs together, arms stretching upward. Alternate trunk-raising-and-arms-forward-reaching with legs raising and swinging overhead to touch the floor with the toes beyond the head* (5 *times*).

Raise trunk steadily, forward reach with the hands smartly, return to starting position steadily, then raise the legs and swing overhead, with knees straight, to touch the floor with the toes. Return steadily to starting position.

Fig. 76. *Standing, feet astride, hands on waist. Neck stretching sideways-forward-sideways in semi-circle* (*Fig.* 36) (5 *times to each side*).

Fig. 77. *Standing, feet astride, arms stretching upwards, fingers extended. Trunk bending from side to side with slight pause in starting position* (5 *times each side*).

Fig. 78. *Standing, feet astride, arms at sides. Arms raising forward and sideways alternately, vigorously* (10 *times*).

The shoulder muscles should be contracted powerfully in raising and relaxed in lowering.

Fig. 79. *Standing, feet astride, arms stretched sideways, trunk bent forward. Trunk turning from side to side to touch opposite foot with fingers* (5 *times each side, twice*).

This exercise should be done vigorously.

Fig. 79

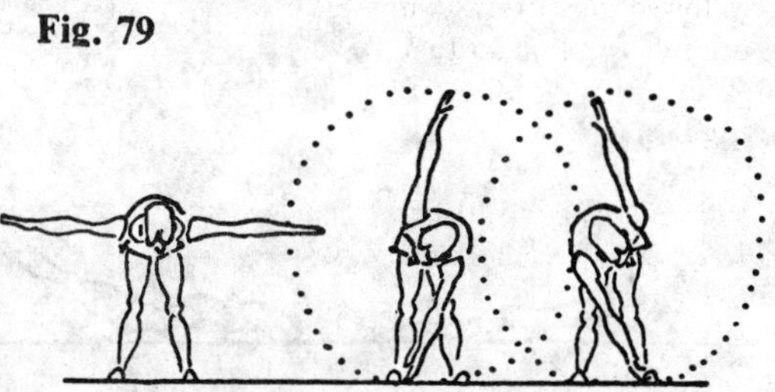

Fig. 80 *Breathing.*

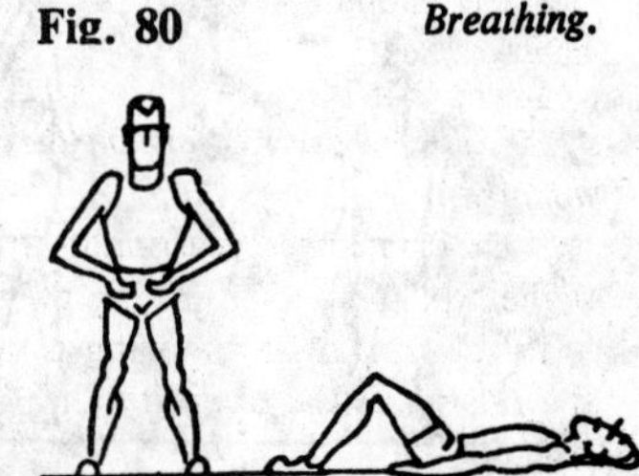

SUPPLEMENTARY EXERCISES

In order that variety may be introduced into tables following the preliminary eight weeks the following supplementary exercises are offered as alternatives.

Lateral (Side) Group

Fig. 81. *Standing, feet astride, arms raised overhead, fingers interlaced. Trunk bending from side to side with pause in starting position.*

Arm and Shoulder Group

Fig. 82. *Standing, feet astride, arms at sides. Arms raising vigorously forward-upwards and sideways-upward alternately.*

Fig. 83. *Standing, feet astride, arms at sides, fingers extended. Arms swinging sideways-upward to clap hands over head.*

Fig. 84. *Standing, feet astride, arms at sides, fingers extended. Arms swinging forward-upward, swinging downward-sideways at shoulder level, inward-upward, vigorously.*

Fig. 85. *Standing, feet astride, arms overhead, fingers lightly clenched. Arms swinging forward-downward sideways-upward.*

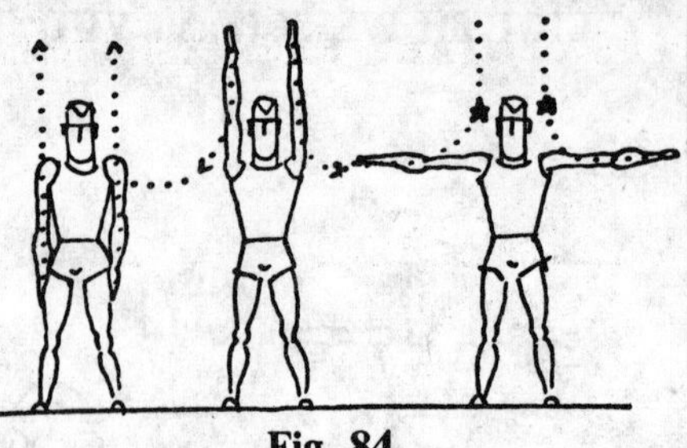

Fig. 84

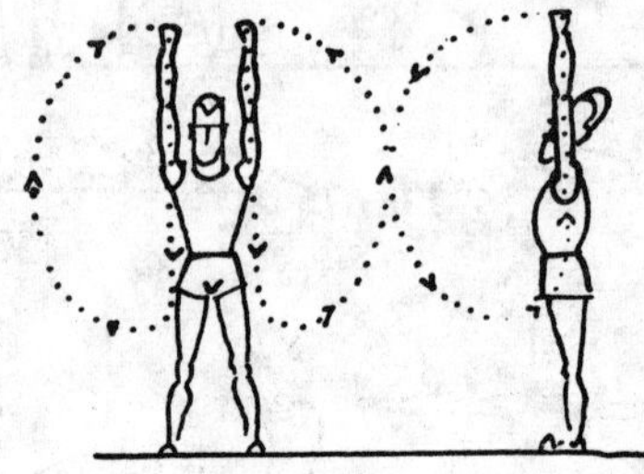

Fig. 85

Abdominal Group

Fig. 86. *Back lying, legs together, arms at sides. Alternate leg half-raising and lowering.*

Fig. 87. *Back lying, legs together, arms at sides. Alternate leg circling.*

Fig. 88. *Back lying, legs together, arms at sides. Both legs half-raising and lowering.*

Fig. 89. *Back lying, legs together, arms at sides. Both legs raise and circle together.*

Fig. 90. *Back lying, legs together, arms at sides. Alternate leg full-raising and lowering.*

Fig. 91. *Back lying, legs together, arms at sides. Both legs full-raising and lowering.*

Fig. 92. *Back lying, legs together, arms at sides. Both legs half-raising, knees full-bending and stretching, and legs lowering.*

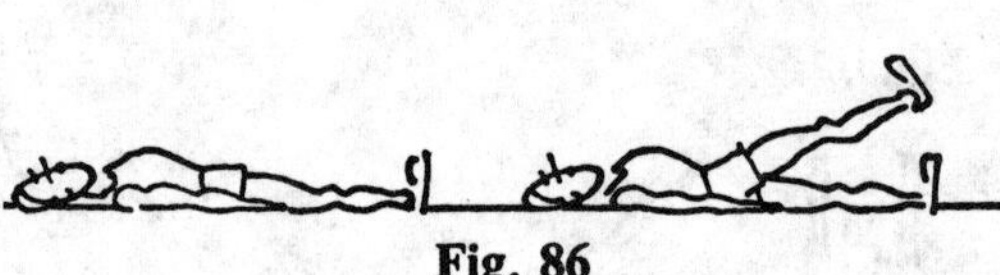

Fig. 86

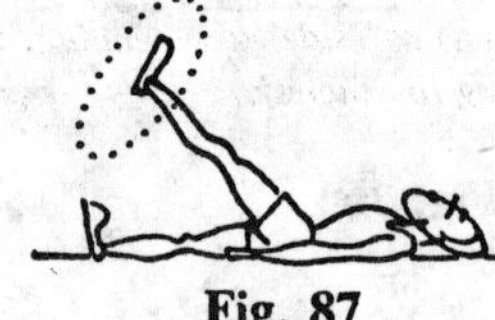

Fig. 87

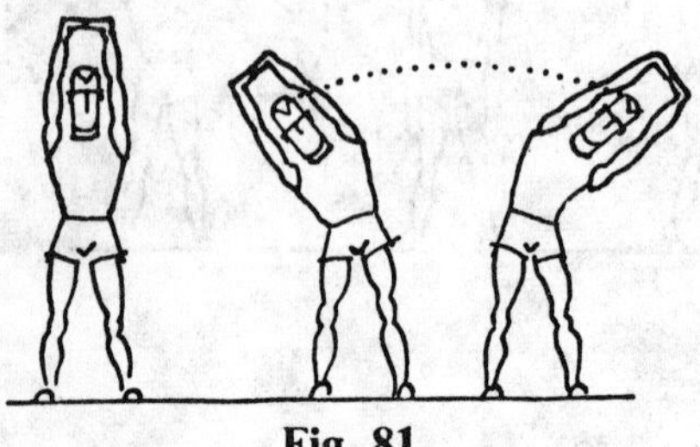

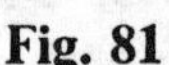

Fig. 81

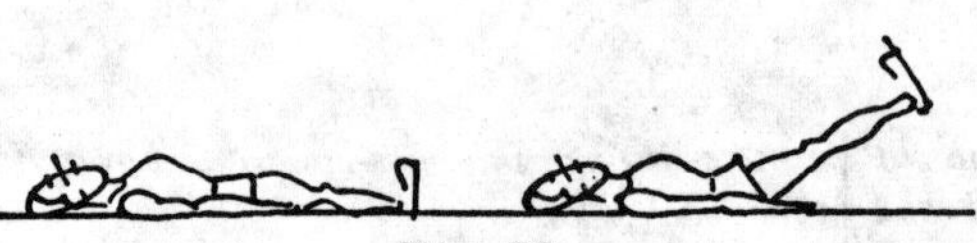

Fig. 88

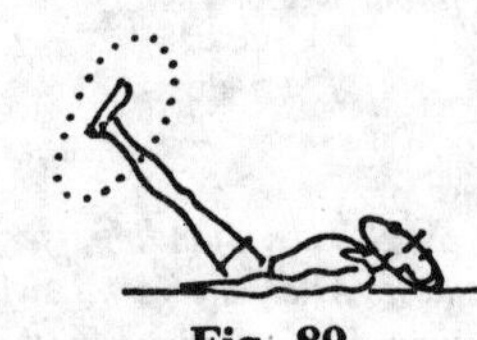

Fig. 89

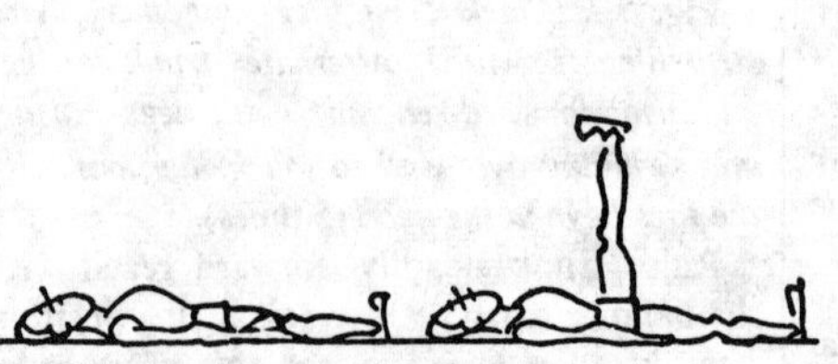

Fig. 90

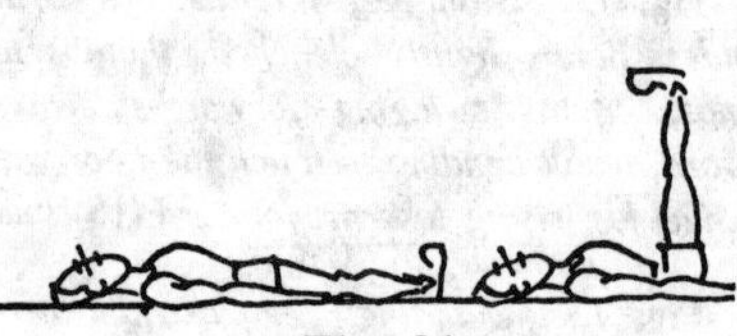

Fig. 91

Fig. 82

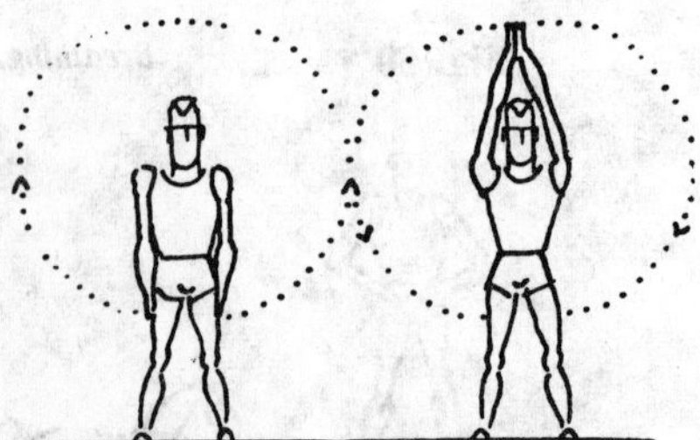

Fig. 83

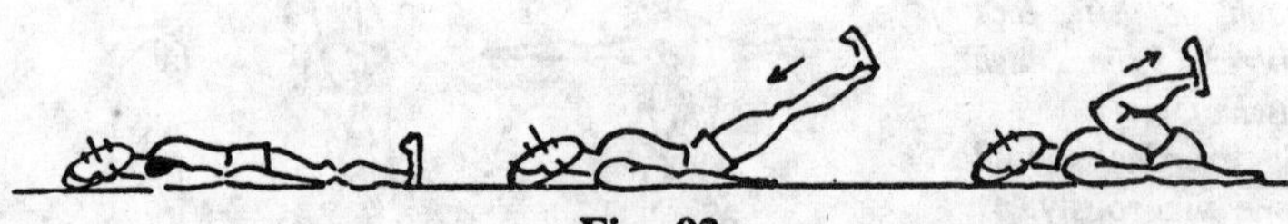

Fig. 92

SUPPLEMENTARY EXERCISES contd.

Fig. 93. *Back lying, arms at sides. Cycling.*

Fig. 94. *Back lying, legs together, arms at sides. Leg raising, leg criss-crossing in wide sweeps.*

Fig. 95. *Back lying, legs together, arms at sides. Legs full raise. Legs swinging from side to side.*

Fig. 96. *Back lying, arms at sides, knees bent to right-angle, feet off floor. Leg swinging from side to side.*

Fig. 97. *Standing, feet together, arms at sides. Running on the spot, with bursts of high knee-raising.*

Fig. 98. *Standing, feet astride, arms stretching sideways, fingers extended. Trunk turning, sideways bending, rolling over, bending to other side, rolling over and continuing.*

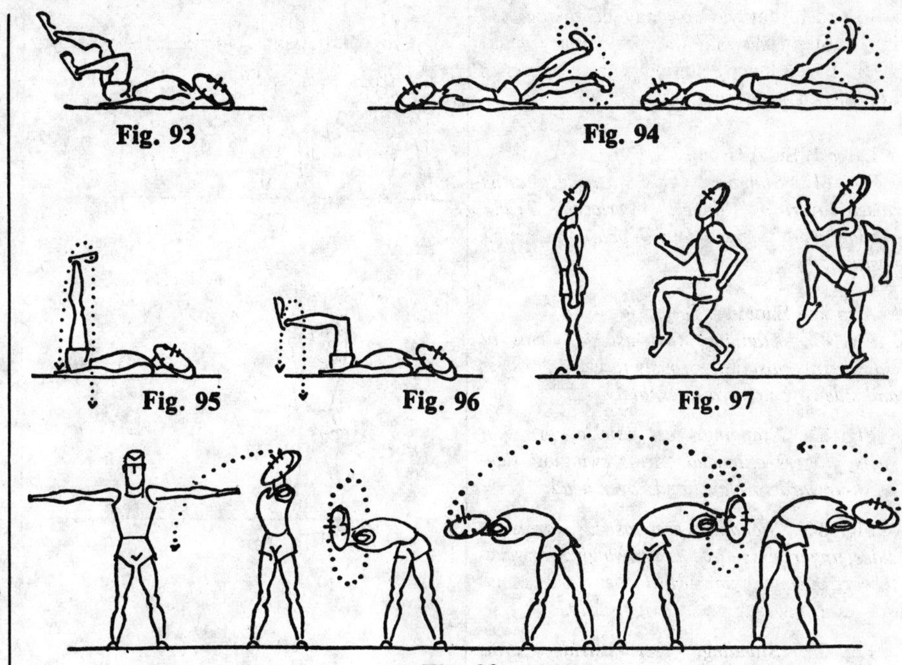

Fig. 93 Fig. 94 Fig. 95 Fig. 96 Fig. 97 Fig. 98

UNARMED COMBAT

SELF-DEFENSE SIMPLIFIED

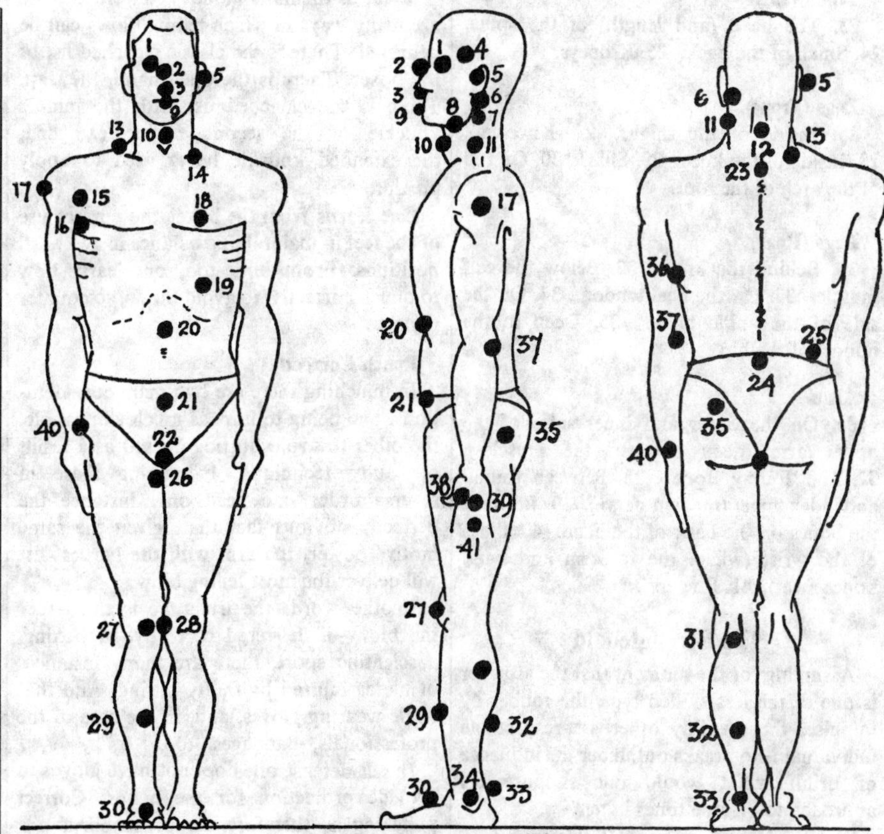

VULNERABLE POINTS

The ability to defend oneself against unprovoked attack is a simple science which should be acquired by all. It has long since ceased to be a mystery. Ju-jitsu, forerunner of self-defense methods, never was very popular with ordinary people who did not have the time to give to mastering its intricacies. The few who have become masters in the Judo art are undoubted experts in self-defense. But theirs has been a long road.

These are the exceptions. The average individual is not interested in self-defense as a science and is not prepared to give the time necessary to master it as such. Few, however, will be so uninterested that they will not be prepared to consider at least the simplest of the defense methods explained in this section.

Even 'A Little Knowledge . . .'

Mastery of half a dozen tricks of defense will give confidence to anyone. A complete study of the methods outlined here will leave the student with little more to learn in the way of self-defense.

Success of the application of the various methods depends to a great extent on quick-thinking and cool-headed speedy action. In selecting the various methods for inclusion in this series first consideration was given to simplicity so that little time need be spent in practicing the moves.

The numerous illustrations which accompany the descriptions show the demonstrators in athletic costume so that the action may be made as clear as possible. Practice should be done in soft-soled shoes and on wrestling or gym mats indoors or on soft turf out of doors.

Defense Weapons

The boot, knee, elbow, fist and head are the stock-in-trade weapons in defense. The use of these may seem ruthless, but as they are often used in unprovoked attack they should be considered and used in such situations.

The knock-out areas if the blow is delivered correctly and with sufficient force, are the side of the chin, the solar plexus and the heart. There are, in actual fact, many similar, equally vulnerable although less well-known points where the application of blows of varying strength can be effective.

Where it Hurts

The boxers' 'point' is the narrow groove in the edge of the jaw bone about an inch and a half from the angle of the jaw bone and through which passes one of the principal nerves of the face.

There is, too, the 'mark' or solar plexus, just above the navel, the most congested area in the whole of the body's intricate nervous system. And there is the heart, guarded by the ribs against any normal outside force, but vulnerable to blows correctly applied.

There are, in addition to these, many more accessible nerves and arteries, as, for instance, the carotid artery under the ear and behind the angle of the jaw bone, where pressure may range in result from extreme discomfort to complete unconsciousness.

Few of us need to be told just how uncomfortable it can be to receive a blow on the protruding part of the throat we know as the 'Adam's Apple.' Given sufficient force behind the blow it is quite possible for a person to choke without other force or pressure following.

Any punch to the kidneys is forbidden in boxing because of its possible disastrous effects, for even in the strongest of men no one can forecast the possible outcome of such a blow, breath-taking at its lightest and fatal in certain circumstances.

Vulnerable Points

Head and Neck

1. Eyes. 2. Bridge of the nose. 3. The cartilage dividing the nose and forming the partition between the nostrils. 4. The temples. 5. Ears. 6. Behind the lobes of the ears. 7. Behind and above the angle of the jaw. 8. The 'point' of the jaw (actually about $1\frac{1}{2}$ inches from the angle of the jaw bone) where one of the main facial nerves passes through a narrow groove in the lower edge of the bone. 9. Lips. 10. Protruding part of the throat known as the 'Adam's Apple.' 11. Sides of the neck. 12. Back of the neck.

Trunk (Front)

13. In the big muscle that stretches along the shoulder from the neck down to the apex of the shoulder. 14. Behind the collar bone. 15. On the point of the shoulder at the top of the arm. 16. Armpits. 17. On the side of the shoulder. 18. On the big chest muscle above the heart. 19. The heart. 20. The 'mark' or solar plexus, just above the navel. 21. Below the navel (known better as 'below the belt'). 22. Between the legs or crotch.

Trunk (Rear)

23. The head (and length) of the spine. 24. Small of the back. 25. Kidneys.

Legs (Front)

26. Inside of the thigh. 27. Knee-cap. 28. Inside of the knee. 29. Shins. 30. On top of the arch of the foot.

Legs (Rear)

31. Behind the knee. 32. Below the calf muscle. 33. On the heel tendon. 34. On the side of the ankle bone. 35. Deep in the hollow of the hip.

Arms

36. On the outer and inner sides of the upper arm (deep between the muscles). 37. The 'Funny Bone.' 38. Between thumb and index finger (median nerve). 39. Between the bones on the back of the hand. 40. Sides of the wrist (where the forearm and hand bones meet). 41. Fingers.

The Stranglehold

Assuming for the moment that the attacker is one of the less skilled type, the robber by impulse, the possibly otherwise respectable individual who breaks out under the influence of drink, what would one suppose his approach to be nine times in ten?

Watch a couple of men of this type in a brawl. Some instinct directs them to each other's throat.

Against an unskilled and frightened opponent the would-be strangler can succeed. But calm consideration of both positions, that of the attacker and the defender, will show that, in actual fact, the advantage is not with the strangler but in the hands of the other.

While both of the strangler's hands are fully occupied the defender is relatively free to use both arms and both legs.

The human hand can be very powerful. It has made fortunes for boxers. But it has a lot of weaknesses because it is not one bone but many, and the majority of them small, easily damaged, and weak in themselves, both as regards structure and the delicacy of the muscles that control them.

Collectively the bones of the hand form a hard-hitting mass. Individually they are very weak and vulnerable.

Confidence

Have someone of ordinary normal weight and strength apply a neck hold from the front, applying full pressure. Put the palms of the hands on his chest. Give a powerful, sharp push. The release will have been effected.

There is your first practical lesson. It does not relate, except incidentally, to the subject of releases from strangleholds. It shows that, before all, it is necessary to have self-confidence. The novice would grapple, probably in vain, to wrest the fingers away from his throat. The expert would apply one of dozens of counters, coolly, but at terrific speed.

So far as the hand alone is concerned there are many ways in which telling blows can be delivered. There is the classic clenched fist of the boxer. There is the open hand, the slap. There is the clenched fist with the middle knuckle of the second finger extended, the extended knuckle being used to apply pressure.

One learns from the boxer the correct use of the feet in maintaining balance in awkward positions. From him, too, one learns how to punch correctly, to avoid blows, to counter punches.

Punch Correctly

In punching there are two main considerations, one being to hurt as much as possible, the other to avoid hurting oneself as a result of faulty technique. Examining these in reverse order one need only instance the perfectly obvious fact that, given the same motive power, the arm with the hardest fist will deliver the most telling blow.

In other words, the firmer the fist the harder the blow—if delivered correctly. In boxing, a scientific sport, there are many instances of hands injured by faulty hitting. And that while wearing gloves, and, in the case of the professionals, bandages, too.

In self-defense one does not have gloves to provide protection for the hands. Correct punching is, therefore, doubly important.

In both boxing and self-defense the blows must be delivered in exactly the same way—with the knuckles formed by the bones of the hand and those of the fingers. To clench the fist correctly for punching, first clench the fingers, then fold the thumb across the middle of the three bones forming the index finger and its immediate neighbor. This will keep the thumb well away from the punching part of the fist.

On Guard

Now for the correct poise of the body from which an effective blow may be struck, the correct 'on guard' position (Fig. 1) of the trained boxer. This is not necessarily the correct attitude for tackling a rough-house adversary, but it is one the mastery of which, and the ability to move from which, will give the poise from which spring rapidity of movement, quick recovery of initiative, and crisp delivery of blows.

In moving forward always do so by moving the leading foot first in short, quick steps. In moving back bring the leading foot back first. In moving sideways avoid crossing the legs. In going to the left, step sideways with the left foot first; if to the right, lead with the right foot.

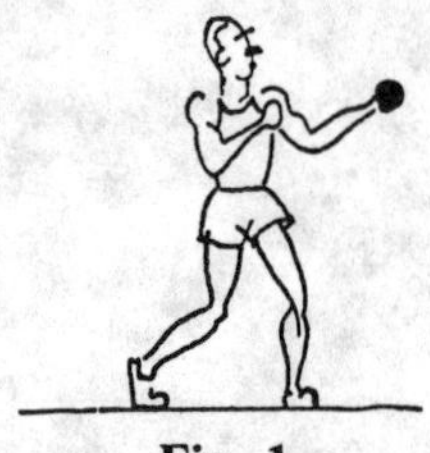

Fig. 1

Orthodox types of blows, guards, parries and counters are given as a matter of interest. For clarity the fist delivering the effective blow, and the hand or arm blocking or deflecting, are pin-pointed in black. Thus in Fig. 2 the straight left to the chin has the left hand in black.

Against the straight left as a defensive measure there is the block guard (Fig. 3), which is much more effective with a boxing glove than with bare hand receiving bare fist. There is, too, the right hand deflection (Fig. 4), in which the left lead is pushed (not slapped) aside. In other circumstances it is possible to slip aside from a left lead to the head without using a right hand deflection. And in both it is possible to counter with a left hand punch to the body (Fig. 5).

Straight Left

Another orthodox blow is the straight left to the body (Fig. 6), beaten by a right forearm deflection (Fig. 7), followed by a left to the chin (Fig. 8). Again it is possible to slip a left lead, swaying to the left and countering with a right hook (Figs. 9 and 10).

The uppercut may be delivered with either hand at close quarters, legitimately (Fig. 11) or illegally, as when pinning one of one's opponents arms to one's side (Fig. 12), or by pulling on the back of the neck with one hand and hitting with the other (Fig. 13).

The 'rabbit punch' to the back of the neck is a boxing illegality quite likely to crop up in rough-house fighting either in the form of an unassisted blow to the back of the neck from any angle or in the more blatant form where the head is pushed or held down while the blow is delivered (Fig. 14). The 'below the belt' blow (Fig. 15) is an obvious one and perhaps the commonest of all in fights outside of a boxing ring.

Close-quarter work or in-fighting is suggested (Fig. 16) as a point of passing interest, passing scrutiny in the ring so long as there is no holding.

Off Balance

Caught off balance even the expert is open to counter-attack. Causing an opponent to lose balance is, therefore, part of self-defense. And it is really astonishing how often this can be effected even in practice. The attacker, initiating action, makes himself

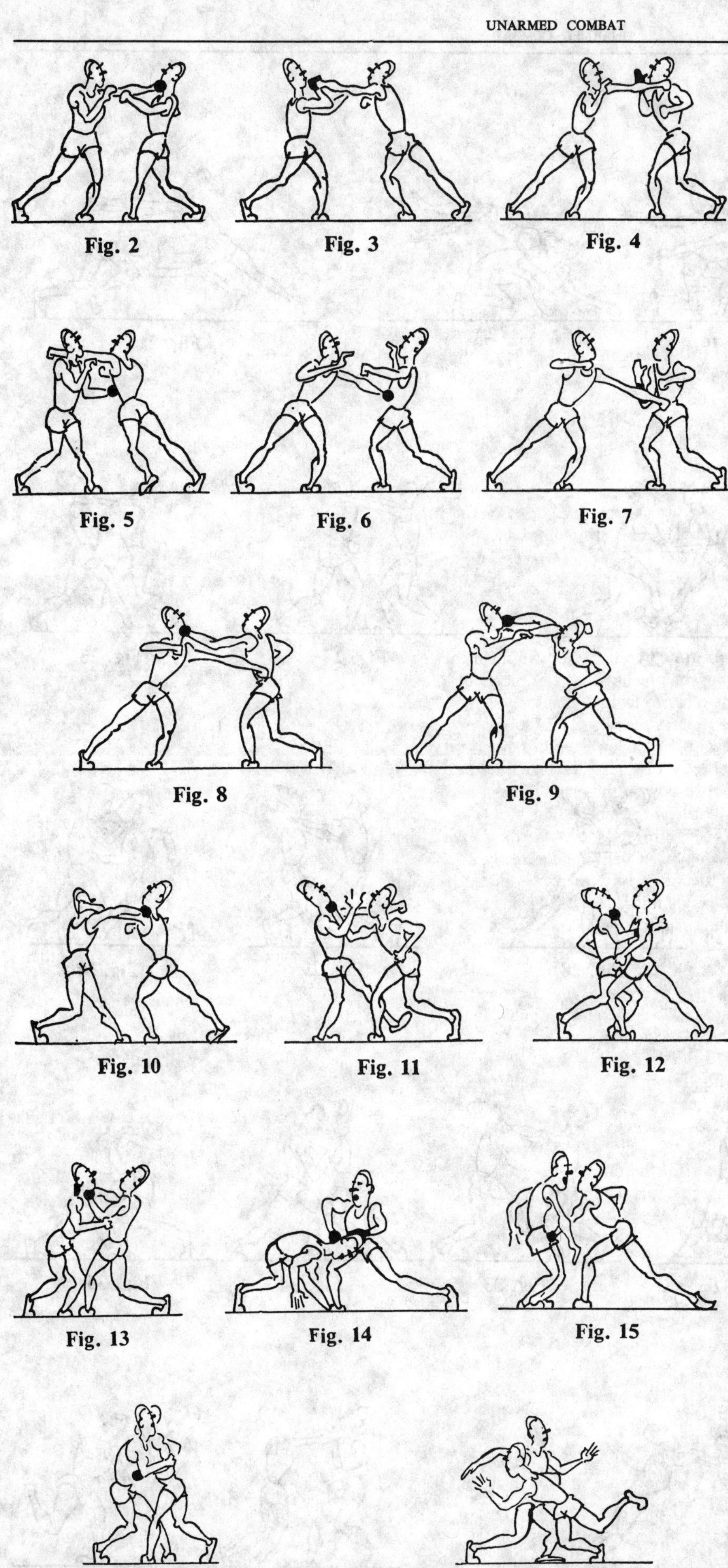

Fig. 2 Fig. 3 Fig. 4 Fig. 5 Fig. 6 Fig. 7 Fig. 8 Fig. 9 Fig. 10 Fig. 11 Fig. 12 Fig. 13 Fig. 14 Fig. 15 Fig. 16 Fig. 17

open to this initial phase of defense. A practical example can be given:

The defender stands perfectly still as the attacker rushes in, then, when he is almost on top of him the defender neatly steps aside (Fig. 17), and the attacker stumbles forward trying to recover balance, balance having been lost because the subconscious mind had already accepted the assumption that something solid—in this case the body of the defender—would end the attacker's forward drive.

Boxing has already provided several fine examples of the effect of disturbing an opponent's balance by means of body sway, hand and forearm deflections of blows, ducking and stepping out of reach. If these succeed in a sport where body control and balance are of first-rate importance it is obvious that they will be even more successful when used against an unskilled opponent in unorthodox fighting.

The use of hand and arm for deflection can be used just as easily and effectively in self-defense (Fig. 18); and ducking, as used in boxing simply to avoid a blow and sometimes to initiate a counter punch, can be made the opening for a robust counter in the form of a shoulder charge (Fig. 19).

Duck!

Alternative to the shoulder charge or obstruction to somewhere around the middle of the body is an even lower ducking of the body to take the full force of the charge on the attacker's thighs (Fig. 20), ending in the attacker being sent sprawling on his face many feet to the rear. Another alternative, one which probably calls for a little more courage than the others, is to butt the attacker in the stomach (Fig. 21), but here one must take the risk of a chance smack in the face from the attacker's knees.

At this point, however, it is inadvisable to consider these as other than lessons in the technique of disturbing an opponent's balance. Later, with practice, they will become instinctive defense moves or opening moves for more advanced forms of defense.

The elbow is a very vulnerable point. A slap or push on the elbow will rarely fail. The attacker may be swinging a blow at his opponent or reaching out for neck or shoulder when a smart elbow push (Fig. 22) will send him off in another and quite unexpected direction. To this may be added a sharp tap on the ankle.

Now we come to consideration of countering attempts at strangling. All things being equal the would-be strangler simply does not have an earthly chance against a cool-headed defender with some notion of defense.

Instinct Wrong

As the majority of counters are directed against the head these will be dealt with first. An outline drawing of the head, with vulnerable points dotted and numbered in accordance with the text of the 'Head and Neck' sub-section of the section headed 'Vulnerable Points', is given on p. 207.

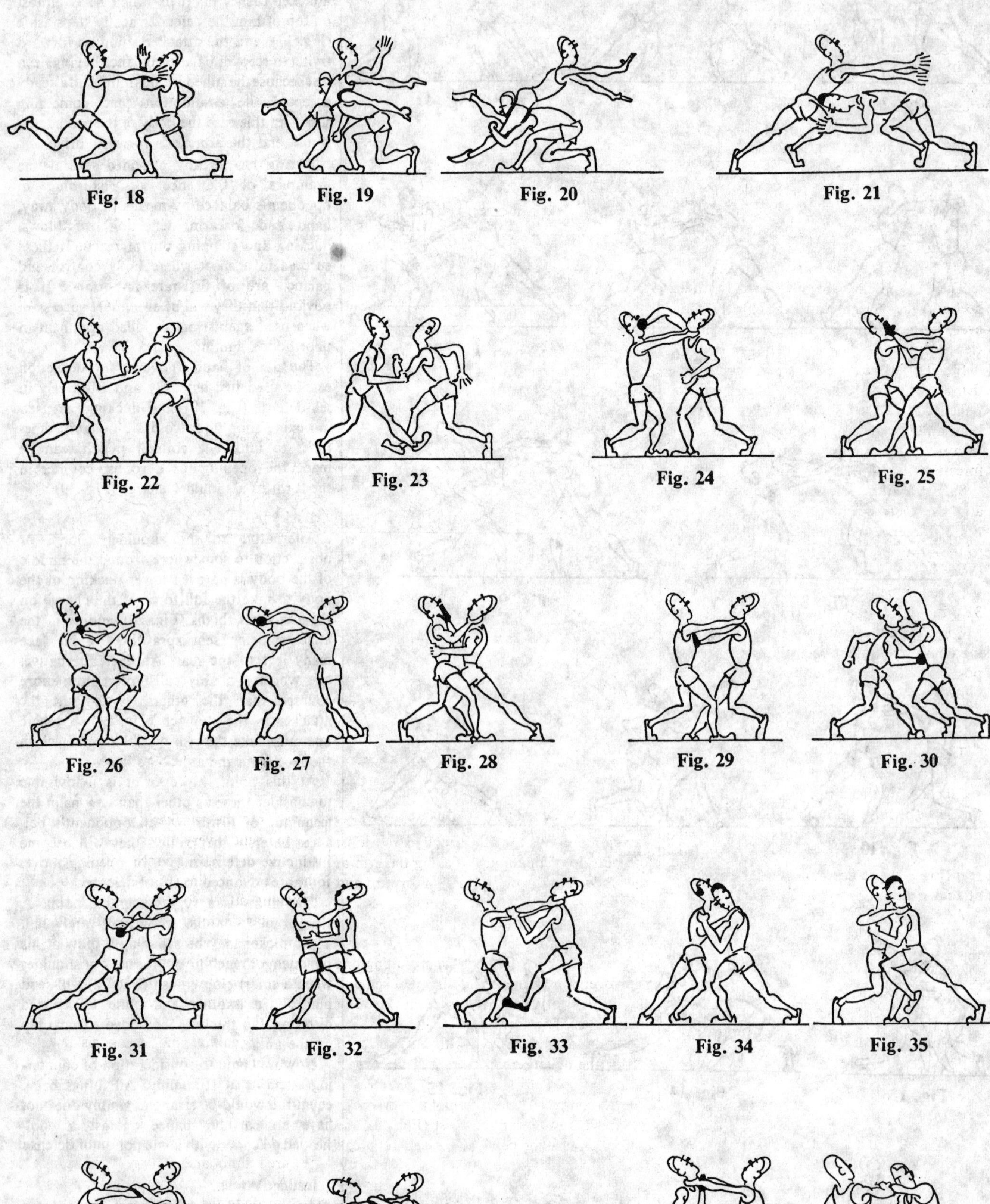

Fig. 18 Fig. 19 Fig. 20 Fig. 21

Fig. 22 Fig. 23 Fig. 24 Fig. 25

Fig. 26 Fig. 27 Fig. 28 Fig. 29 Fig. 30

Fig. 31 Fig. 32 Fig. 33 Fig. 34 Fig. 35

Fig. 36 Fig. 37 Fig. 38

Instinct in the face of imminent strangulation dictates that the attacking hands should be dragged away from the throat. That is instinct. But instinct is often far from being efficient. The attacker must be hurt before he can be forced to release his grip. Instead of tugging at his hands, hit him in the face with the clenched fist (Fig. 24). Such a direct and vigorous counter attack is far more effective in making him release his hold than the comparatively weak hold afforded by dragging to release his hands around your throat.

That is the opening lesson in defense against attempted strangulation. Attack by direct means. Direct sharp counters can be made to the nose (Fig. 25), to the Adam's apple (Fig. 26), or the ears (Fig. 27).

There is, too, the vigorous chin-jab with the heel of the hand right under the chin (Fig. 28), every bit as effective as an uppercut with the clenched fist.

Finally, so far as the head is concerned, there is the very vulnerable mouth, to be punched with the fist, cut with the edge of the hand, or the lips which can be seized between thumb and forefinger and twisted forcefully.

Still tackling releases from the front attempted stranglehold there is the very simple but effective push (Fig. 29), the punch to the stomach (Fig. 30) or to the kidneys or lower ribs (Fig. 31), a well-chosen drive with the knee in between the attacker's legs (Fig. 32) or a kick to the shins (Fig. 33).

These do not exhaust the releases. By pulling one's antagonist sharply forward it is possible in certain conditions to deliver a blow with the forehead to his face (Fig. 34). This, too, can be combined with a knee-drive in between the legs (Fig. 35).

Two other counter moves to evade the strangler may be made by applying the body-weight in another direction. Jump clear of the ground, raise the feet, and drop forcibly down with the arms across those of the attacker (Fig. 36), or throw the legs to the rear (Fig. 37) and drop down on the extended attacking arms.

A very simple and effective release-counter is that (Fig. 38) in which, from in between the attacking arms, the defender drives hard against the inner side of one wrist. This breaks the throat-hold, partially or fully, but the attacker resists automatically by pressing the dislodged hand back in the direction of the throat. The defender follows up the first move by seizing a firm hold on the wrist,

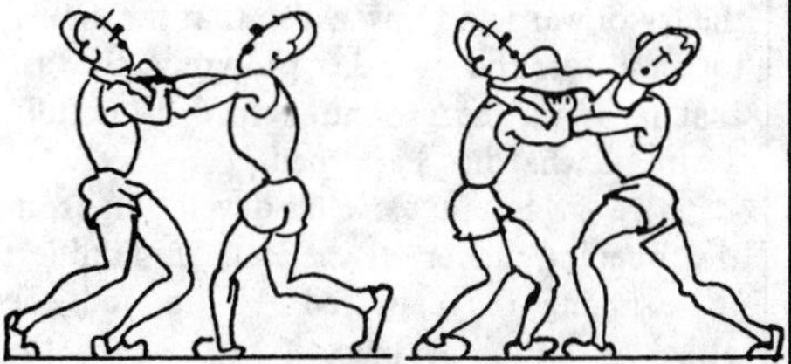

Fig. 39

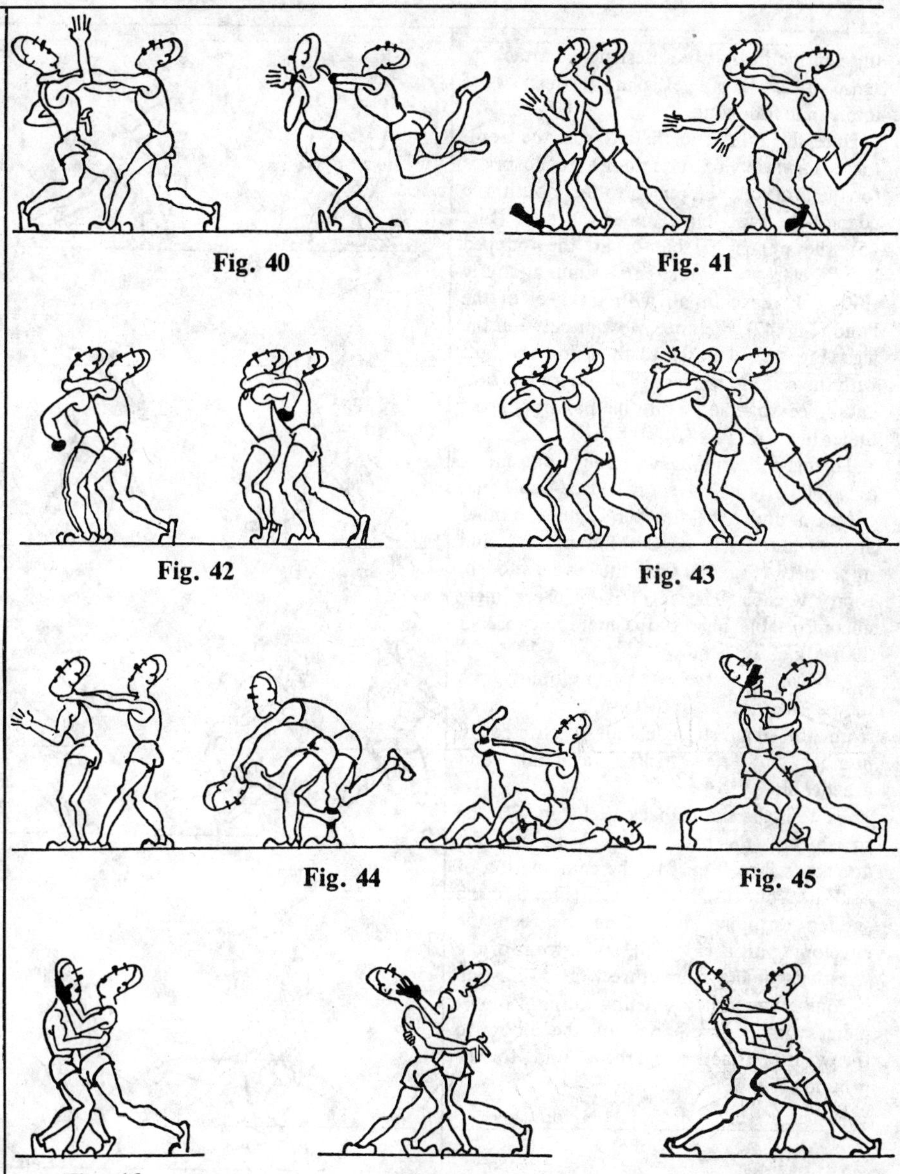

Fig. 40 Fig. 41

Fig. 42 Fig. 43

Fig. 44 Fig. 45

Fig. 46 Fig. 47 Fig. 48

pulling back in towards the neck, and, at the same time, drives the other hand hard against the outside of the elbow, locking the arm at the elbow and throwing his man forward and down.

Having got him down the obvious follow up is to jump on him.

Yet another release consists of putting one arm over the near arm of the attacker and the other arm under his other arm (Fig. 39), interlacing the fingers, and pressing up with the under arm and down with the over arm.

For the agile person there is a very spectacular release-counter in which one arm is thrown completely over both of the attacker's arms low down near the wrist (Fig. 40), the action of turning being continued to break the hold and continue into a fast fall.

Rear Stranglehold

Getting away from a rear stranglehold is not quite so simple. If the attacker is close up it is possible to use the elbow by a quick half-turn, driving the elbow hard into the ribs. Sometimes the back of the head can be driven into the attacker's face. But not often as the result is very uncertain.

One can take a chance with a kick with the heel to the shins (Fig. 41) or a two-handed punching attack to the lower ribs (Fig. 42). But by far the most effective move is to seize the attacker by each of his little fingers and, having got a secure grip, to bend them back away from both neck and hand (Fig. 43).

Having secured the release in this way lift one of the attacker's arms over your head, turn to face him, and, using his fingers as levers, force him to the ground.

Sometimes it is possible to make a quick body bend, reach through between the legs and seize the attacker by the lower leg (Fig. 44), at the same time pulling on the captured limb and falling back heavily on the attacker's stomach as he topples over backwards to the ground.

Arms pinned to Sides

Akin to the stranglehold, both front and rear, is the equally unscientific attempt to pin the arms to the sides from front or rear, unscientific in that in a destructive attacking sense it is devoid of plan in respect of immediate follow-up.

Here, as in the stranglehold from the front, there is a variety of quite unpleasant surprises for the attacker: the punch to the mouth, the edge-of-the-hand blow under the nose (Fig. 45), the punch to the throat, the 'cupped hand' clap to both ears simultaneously (Fig. 46), the chin-jab with the heel of the hand (Fig. 47), the knee blow in between the legs (Fig. 48), the kick to the shins, the butt with the head to the face (Fig. 49), or the butt and knee together, and the poking fingers under the ears (Fig. 50).

To this collection can be added one more, a particularly effective one. Place one hand, palm up, under the attacker's chin, the other around the back of the lower head and upper neck (Fig. 51). Give the head a sudden, rotary wrench. The effect is an exceedingly uncomfortable one, and is more unexpected than a kick or a blow.

Attacked from the rear by enveloping arms the releases are, as in the case of the releases from the rear strangleholds, restricted in number but, nevertheless, available and practicable.

There is the simple back-heel (Fig. 52), the smash with the back of the head into the attacker's face (Fig. 53), the combination of back-heel and use of the head (Fig. 54), the sudden dropping away from between the enveloping arms (Fig. 55), and a form of the wrestler's 'flying mare' throw, a strong grip on one elbow and a twisting, turning movement, with a strong pull on the elbow to throw the attacker overhead and to the ground (Fig. 56).

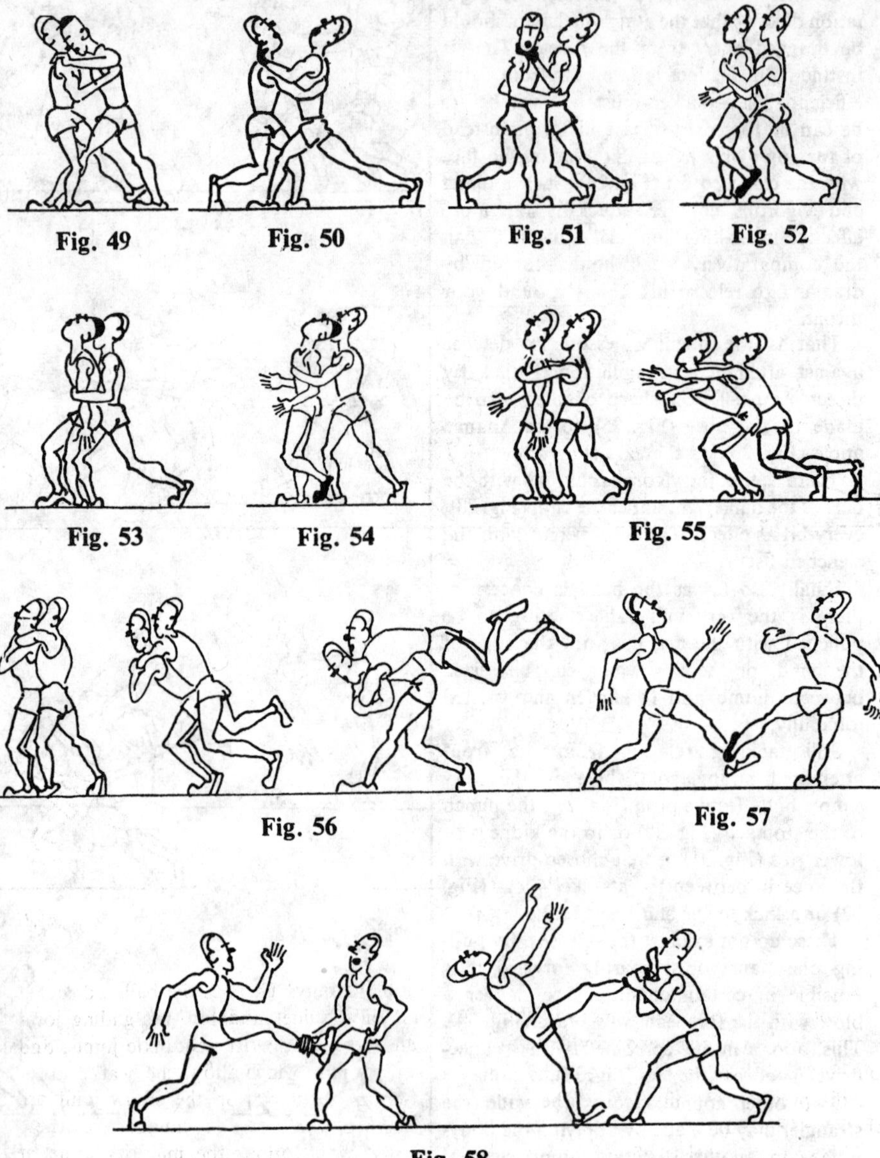

Fig. 49 Fig. 50 Fig. 51 Fig. 52

Fig. 53 Fig. 54 Fig. 55

Fig. 56 Fig. 57

Fig. 58

The Boot in Defense

One of the most powerful weapons of defense and attack is the boot or the shoe. Many rough-house battles start and finish with boot duels. Here we are concerned with defense against kicks on the one hand and the use of the boot as a measure of defense on the other.

It is almost impossible to ward off a kick at close quarters. One can often see the beginning of even a short-range blow with the fist. Not so the kick. Vision is completely obscured by the fact that the antagonists are close together. The range is short. The kick is made at speed with only a short distance to travel.

But outside of fighting range it is easy to see the start of a kick and, given the knowledge, equally easy to counter it. The long-range kick is unscientific. And the obvious way to beat it is to get out of the way. Which, in fact, is the first principle of defense against the long-range kick.

Evasion is only half of the defense, however. Just as the boxer is not content merely to duck or sidestep a blow, so must the self-defense student learn to go beyond the mere act of stepping out of the way of a kick. He must block the kicks and turn them to his advantage by counters.

Shin Jab

Just as the boxer blocks a left lead with his glove, so can the defender against a kick block a leg lead. But he can go farther than that. Block a punch in boxing does not hurt the attacker's fist. Block a leg lead in close combat should definitely hurt the attacker's leg, and hurt hard.

Here is how it is done. As the attacker swings in his powerful kick the defender turns inwards, the sole of his shoe being jabbed hard against the shin of the oncoming leg (Fig. 57). Here the attacker is quite likely to kick himself into hospital with a broken leg.

A neat side step from a kick can be turned to advantage (Fig. 58) by grasping the ankle by one or both hands and, taking full advantage of the impetus of the swing, continue the leg onward and upward so that the kicker topples over backwards, probably so fast that he is on the ground before he is fully aware of what has happened.

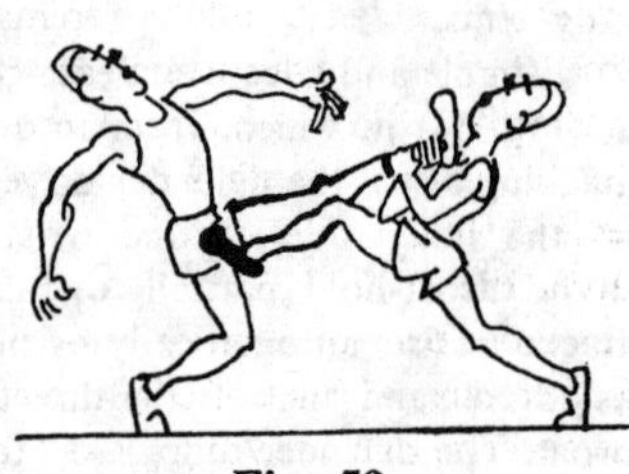

Fig. 59

There are several varieties developing from the opening under discussion. In addition to swinging the captured leg up and the attacker on to his back it is open to the defender at the same time to give vent to his feelings with a well-directed kick (Fig. 59).

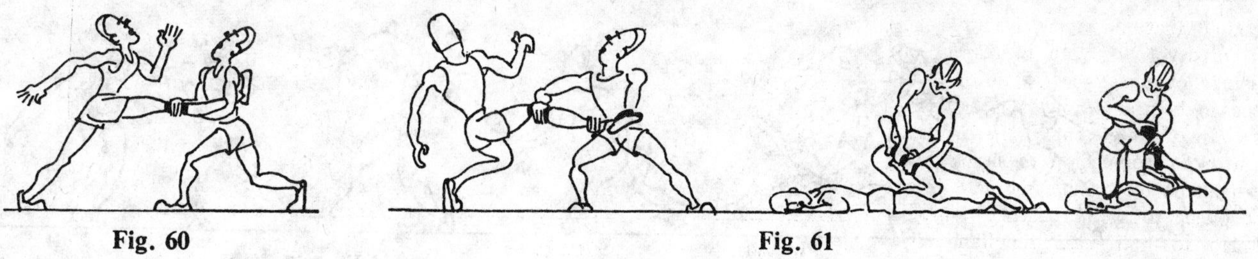
Fig. 60
Fig. 61

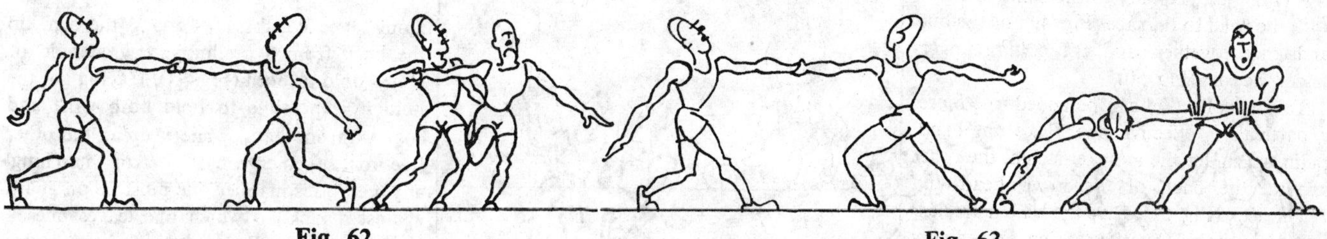
Fig. 62
Fig. 63

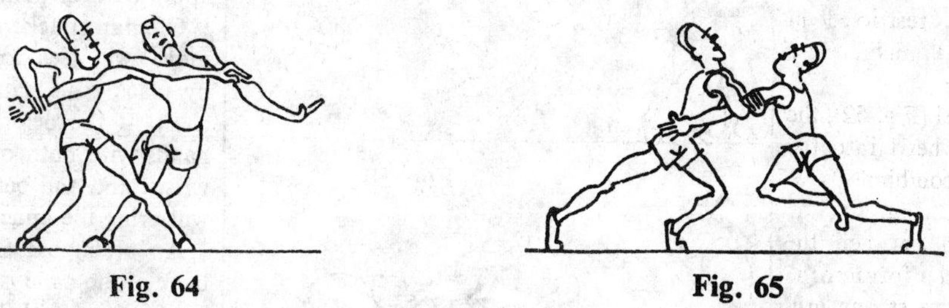
Fig. 64
Fig. 65

Leg Lock

Another way, but this is more difficult, is to jump ahead of the oncoming leg, seize it, pin the ankle under one arm, and apply terrific pressure speedily against the joint of the knee (Fig. 60).

Yet another consists of seizing ankle and knee almost simultaneously, rotating the leg inwards so as to cause the attacker to turn and fall face downwards. Retaining possession of the captive leg as the attacker falls, the defender goes down with him, forcing the heel of the captive leg against the hip. From there an effective hold can be made, crossing one lower leg under the other and applying pain pressure with the upper leg by pressing downwards (Fig. 61).

Close combat being a form of self-defence in which there are no rules of conduct which one must observe, one naturally looks for the most effective means of success without so much regard to the niceties.

Study the Joints

Take the skin and muscle wrappings off the skeleton and we can get down to study of yet another branch of the self-defense business, the exploitation of joints.

There are several types of joints. There is the hinge joint common to elbow, knee, finger and toe and permitting movement in one plane only. There is the ball-and-socket joint of shoulder and hip, the gliding joint found below the wrist and ankle joints, and the pivot joint which allows the head to turn.

So far as attacks on the elbow joint are concerned there are a number of these worthy of attention, the majority done at speed and with some force. There is the straightforward 'arm break' in which the arm is seized by the wrist, often when an attacker is running in, the attacker being pulled forward sharply and the defender turning towards him, pulling back with the hand and driving forward with the chest against the back of the locked elbow (Fig. 62).

Arm Breaks

Another form consists of applying pressure with the free hand (Fig. 63) instead of with the extended chest. One can also use a more advanced arm break in which the free arm is thrown across the attacker's chest and the near leg across the front of his legs (Fig. 64).

An attacker diving for a waist hold may be pinned and even have his elbows injured by a quick-witted adversary applying inward pressure to both elbow joints simultaneously (Fig. 65). A fast and dangerous 'arm break' and throw consists of seizing one wrist with both hands, turning about and bringing the captive arm over one shoulder, elbow down (Fig. 66).

Remembering that an attacker will rarely be dressed only in gym costume there is another attack on the elbow joint worthy of recalling. This consists of seizing the right wrist with the right hand, or left wrist with left hand, quickly sweeping the other hand underneath the arm to get a tight hold on shirt or jacket, the elbow meanwhile being pressed firmly back against the defender's chest (Fig. 67).

Yet another consists of seizing an arm by the wrist and swinging the arm upwards and over the head, the defender at the same time bobbing down under the up-coming arm, finishing with the arm across his shoulders with the outside of the elbow resting on his shoulders (Fig. 68).

The 'come along' hold, for some unknown reason probably the best known of all self-defense holds, is best followed by sketch (Fig. 69). One point that might be mentioned here is that many elbow breaks, throws and locks are more easily effected if preceded by a quick downward jerk of the captive arm as is suggested in the first sketch in Fig. 67.

A spectacular but difficult elbow lock throw is shown in Fig. 70. This requires much practice and self-confidence.

'Frog March'

One of the old favorites of the 'come

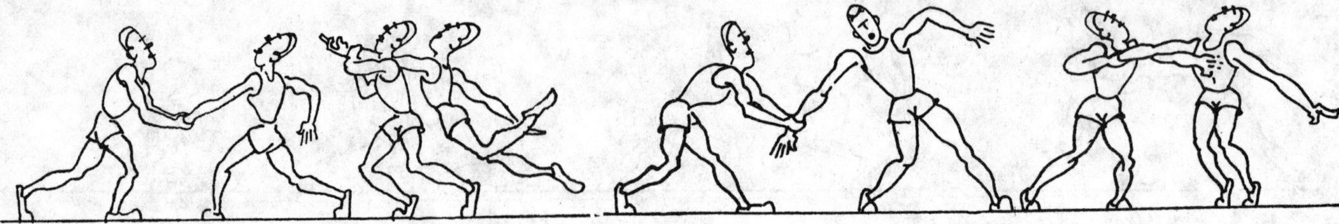

Fig. 66 Fig. 67

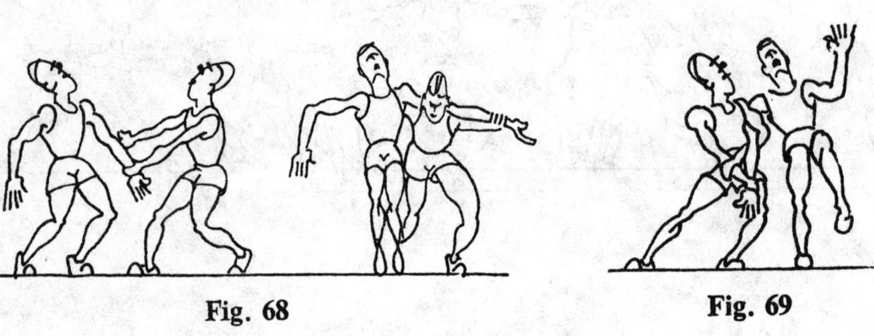

Fig. 68 Fig. 69

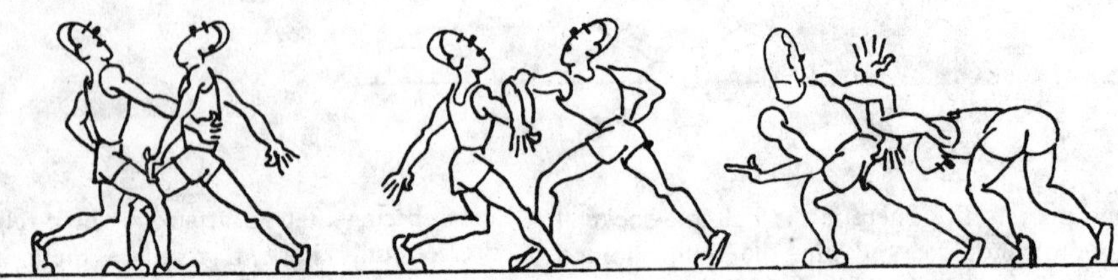

Fig. 70

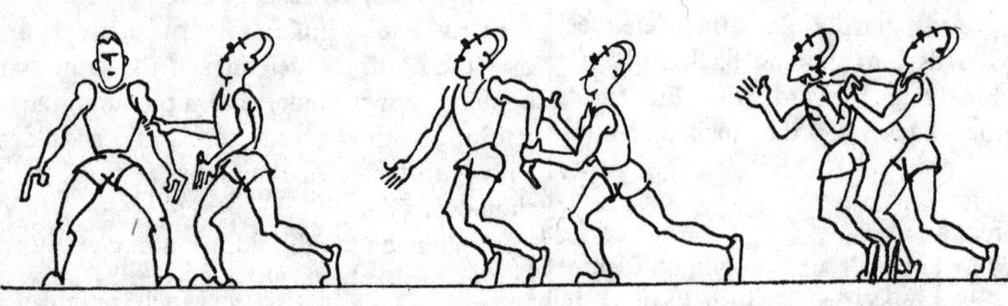

Fig. 71

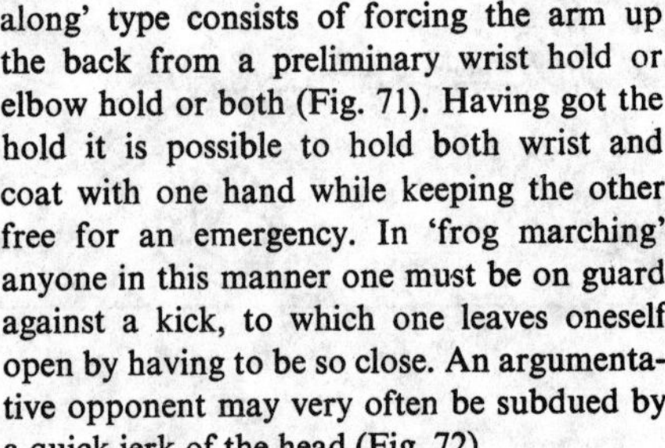

along' type consists of forcing the arm up the back from a preliminary wrist hold or elbow hold or both (Fig. 71). Having got the hold it is possible to hold both wrist and coat with one hand while keeping the other free for an emergency. In 'frog marching' anyone in this manner one must be on guard against a kick, to which one leaves oneself open by having to be so close. An argumentative opponent may very often be subdued by a quick jerk of the head (Fig. 72).

The wrist presents many openings for the application of painful counters and holds.

Often an attacker, following an unsuccessful move, will seek to push the defender away by placing his hands flat on the defender's chest. If the defender covers the attacker's hands with both of his own, just above the wrist joint, and bends forward and down he will bring the attacker to his knees (Fig. 73).

An attempted slap to the face with the back of the hand is easily countered (Fig. 74) with a two-handed grip, forcibly flexing the wrist beyond its normal range. In fact, if done speedily, there is no need to use two hands. One does just as well (Fig. 75), leaving the other free for a punch or for the quick application of a hold.

Here is an example of what can be done as a follow-up to the one-hand hyper-flexion of the wrist joint. Assuming that the attacker's left hand has been seized by the defender's right hand and the wrist flexion grip applied, he then proceeds to swing the left arm up behind the attacker's left, gripping the wrist and pressing the forearm back and down (Fig. 76).

The gliding joints of the feet are particularly vulnerable to heavy blows behind which there is the full bodyweight, blows such as those involving stamping on the feet or jumping on them.

Neck

An example of what can be done in attacking the pivot joint of the neck has already been given (Fig. 72). Another con-

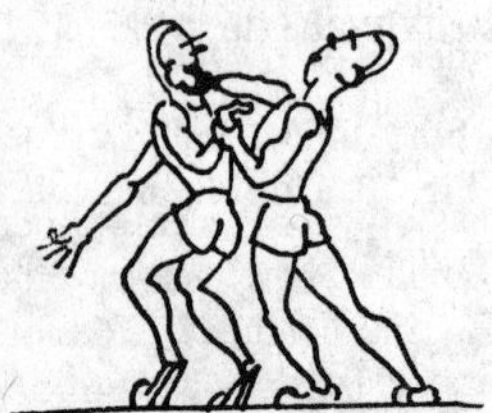

Fig. 72

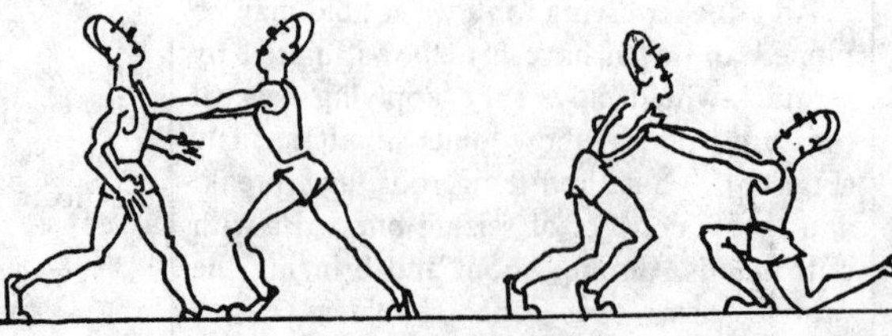

Fig. 73

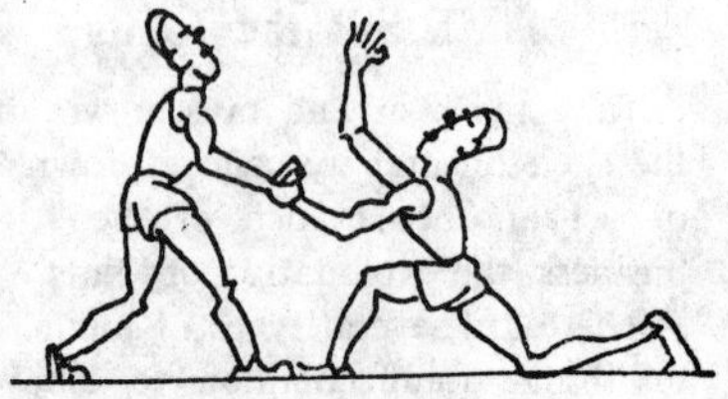

Fig. 74

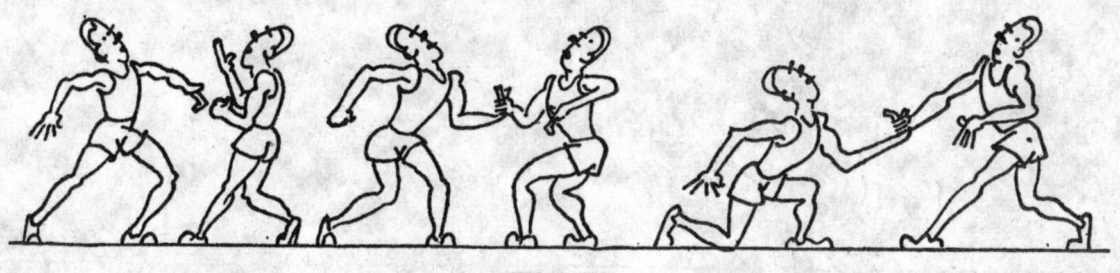

Fig. 75

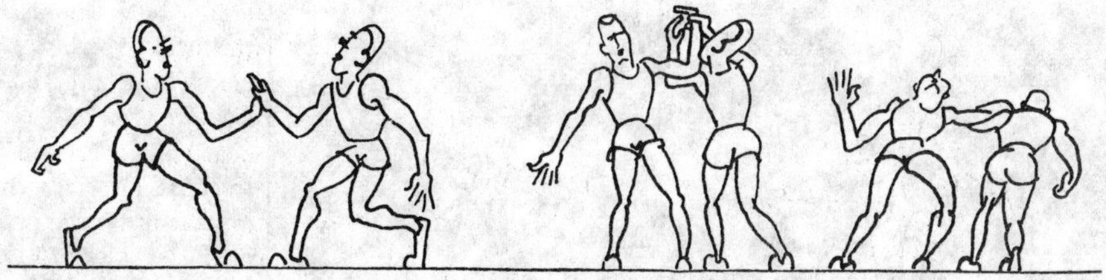

Fig. 76

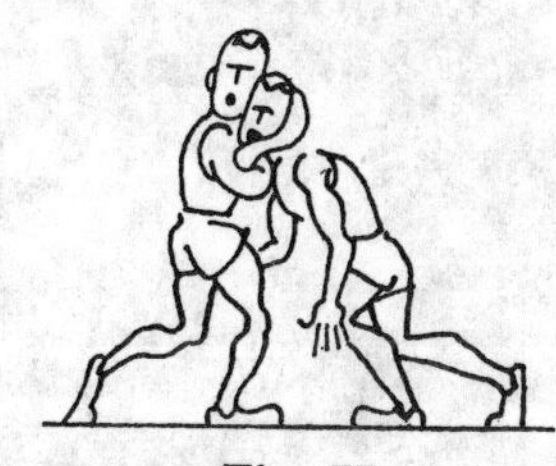

Fig. 77

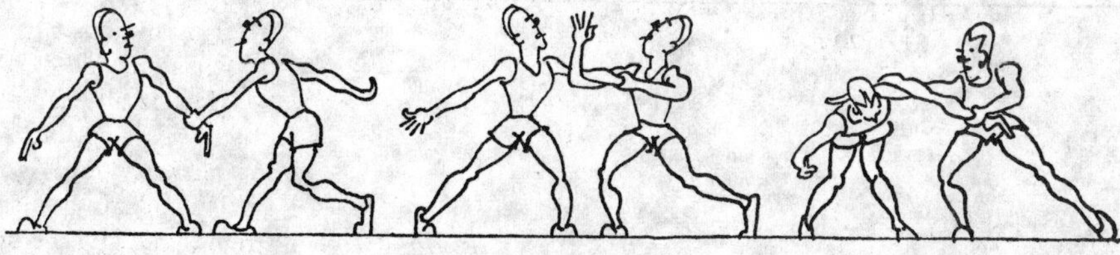

Fig. 78

sists of encircling the neck with one arm (Fig. 77) and pulling on the chin with the hand while pushing against the other shoulder with the other hand.

The neck, although not in any pivotal sense, is involved in this movement (Fig. 78). Grasp the left wrist with the left hand. Swing the right arm up and forward from behind the opponent's left arm, finishing with the right hand on the back of his neck. The extended elbow joint is forced back against the defender's chest at the same time as pressure is brought to bear on the back of the neck. As the attacker is forced to the ground the knee can then be brought into his face.

Worthy of memorizing: Grasp an opponent by the lapels of his jacket, turning the coat outside in as far as the elbows with a quick movement (Fig. 79). If an opponent dives for your legs, pick him up with a rear waist-hold (Fig. 80) and throw him face down on the ground, preferably dropping on top of him.

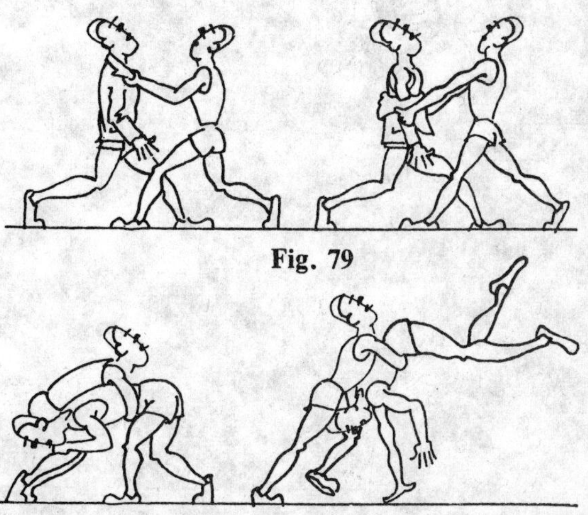

Fig. 79

Fig. 80

So to the end of the lessons and the beginning of experience. Much practice is needed for it is only by constant repetition that the application of these so-called tricks of self-defence can be applied confidently and quickly. A measure of physical fitness will come from this practice, but it is better that this physical fitness should come from a table of well-balanced exercises and be used as a background to the practice of close combat.

ANATOMY

Anatomy describes the structure and organization of living creatures.

Physiology describes the uses or functions of each part and organ and how they are integrated to work as a whole.

Pathological Anatomy describes the alterations occurring in different organs as a result of disease. It is more especially the concern of the doctor and pathologist.

To know one's self physically is to gain a new insight into the wonderfully skillful adaptation of structure and function throughout all Nature. Without this knowledge one cannot know how to take care of health, and without health life loses most of its value.

Early Stages of Development

Bodies begin their growth as a single cell which is formed by the union of the male sperm and the female egg. The product is a delicate little bladder or mass of soft living substance called protoplasm, which contains a denser central portion called the nucleus; this again contains a small body called the nucleolus. The nucleus governs the growth and life-processes of the cell, and carries the genes which are responsible for the transmission of inherited characteristics.

In the human, the male sperm fuses with the nucleus of the female egg or ovum, which is thus fertilized and made capable of further growth. This proceeds by repeated division of the single nucleus and protoplasmic mass into two, four, eight, sixteen, etc., cells, so that finally a multicellular mass results. This is at first spherical in shape, but gradually becomes differentiated into the embryo and its supporting tissues. Finally the embryonic cells produce the skin, muscles, bones and all the organs of the fetus which, by the end of the normal term of pregnancy, develops into the viable infant.

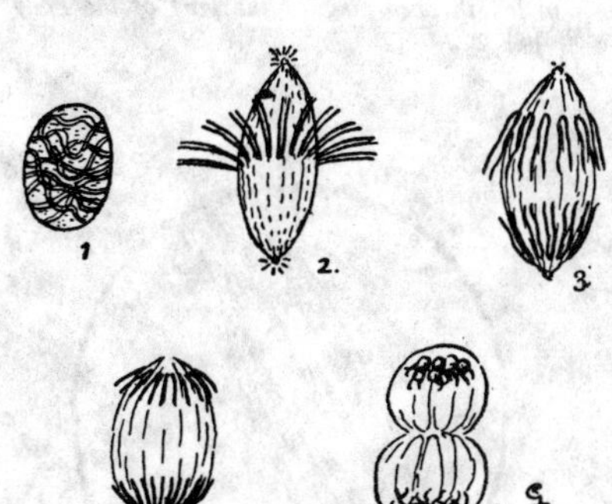

Fig. 1. *CELL DIVISION.* 1. *Nucleus of single parent cell, with chromatin filaments.* 2. *Chromosomes, with centrosomes connected by the achromatic spindle.* 3. *Daughter chromosomes.* 4. *Diaster, or double star formed by daughter chromosomes.* 5. *Two new daughter cells, formed by division of parent cells.*

Structure of the Body

The human body is composed of millions of cells and various fluids, each designed for special functions. The cells are joined together in masses to form different types of tissues and organs with different structures. Most of the cells in the body consist of protoplasm, a jelly-like substance, with a central nucleus which controls the life and functions of the cell. The fluids of the body are concerned in the nourishment and lubrication of tissues and the removal of waste products, and their composition varies according to their role.

Chemical Properties of the Body

The exact chemical structure of living protoplasm has not yet been determined although more and more detail is being discovered every year. All cells contain the complex substance protein which is composed of carbon, hydrogen, oxygen, nitrogen, sulphur, with a large admixture of water. These elements, together with traces of phosphorus and other minerals such as iron and iodine, compose most of the soft tissues of the body. The bones of the skeleton consist mainly of calcium salts such as calcium carbonate (chalk), calcium phosphate and calcium chloride. The body also contains traces of the salts of potassium, calcium and magnesium.

The body of a man weighing 150 pounds contains about 91 pounds of water, 18 pounds of dried albumen, 9 pounds of gelatin, 21 pounds of fat, 3 ounces of sugar and glycogen, 8¼ pounds of calcium phosphate, 1 pound of calcium carbonate, 6 ounces of magnesium phosphate, 4 ounces of calcium fluoride, and a few ounces of sodium chloride (common salt) and a fraction of an ounce of iron.

Living protoplasm in the human body requires water, oxygen and warmth to enable it to manifest its vital properties; these include the utilization of oxygen for the continuous combustion of food products, with the liberation of energy in the form of heat, movement and nervous impulses. The protoplasm also has to repair its own substance, that is to maintain its own nutrition, and to carry on the vital processes of growth.

THE TISSUES

There are many types of cells in the body and they vary in size and structure according to the work they are required to do. All cells which serve the same function are grouped together to form tissues.

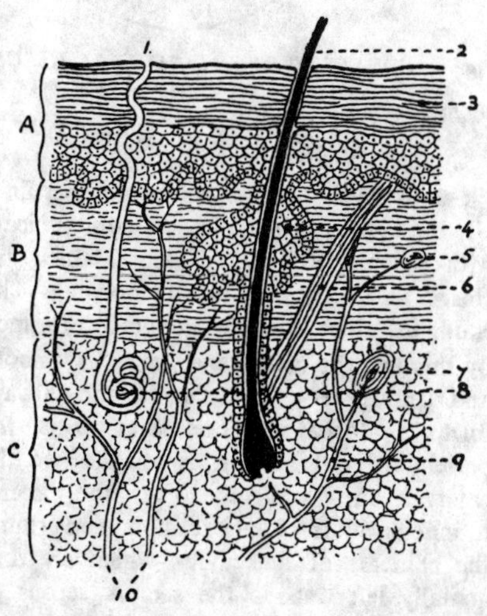

Fig. 2. *SECTION OF SKIN.* A. *Epidermis.* B. *Corium.* C. *Subcutaneous fatty layer.* 1. *Duct of a sweat gland.* 2. *Hair.* 3. *Horny layer.* 4. *Sebaceous gland.* 5. *Nerve ending.* 6. *Muscle for erecting hair.* 7. *Nerve ending.* 8. *Sweat gland.* 9. *Nerve.* 10. *Blood vessels.*

Epithelial Tissue covers the whole of the outside of the body and lines the various cavities within. The outer covering forms the **Skin** or dermoid tissue which is composed of two main layers (1) the cuticle or epidermis, and (2) the corium or dermis. The epidermis is the outer horny layer and is protective in function; it varies in thickness in different parts of the body and the outer cells are being continually rubbed off and replaced by cells from the deeper layers. The dermis has a rich nerve supply which enables one to appreciate many different sensations. It also contains many blood vessels and sweat glands which assist in regulating the temperature of the body. Hairs arise from the dermis, each hair having a root and a shaft. The shaft is lubricated by fatty material secreted by sebaceous glands which are found in the dermis in close association with the hairs.

Mucous Tissue, or mucous membrane, is epithelial tissue adapted for lining all the cavities which communicate with the air, as in the nose, mouth, stomach, bowels, lungs, esophagus, and so forth. It contains numerous small glands, which secrete a sticky kind of fluid called mucus to protect the surface from any injury which might be inflicted by irritating substances in contact with it, or by friction.

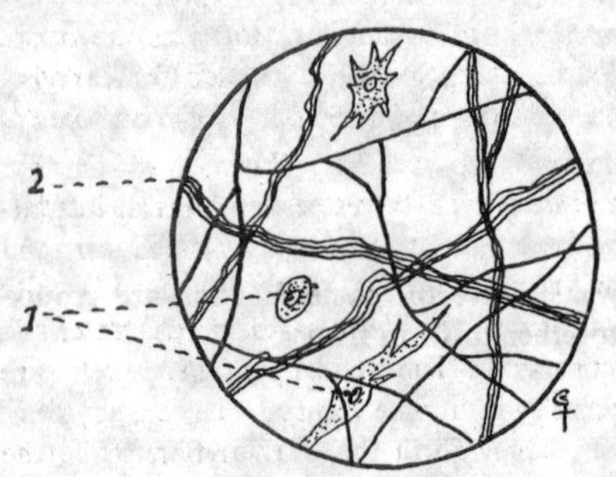

Fig. 3. *CONNECTIVE, OR AREOLAR, TISSUE.* 1. *Cells.* 2. *Fibers. The spaces in this loose network are filled with tissue fluid.*

Serous Tissue, or serous membrane, lines all the cavities which do not communicate with the air, that is, all those which are closed and have no outside opening. The skull, the chest, and the abdomen are lined by this kind of membrane, which is smooth and transparent. The membrane always forms a closed sac; one layer of it, the parietal or outer layer, is attached to the cavity it lines, while the other, the visceral or inner layer, is folded back upon and around the contents of the cavity, which are thus actually left outside the sac. A serous or watery fluid oozes from the inner surface of the sac to make its two layers glide easily upon each other. When any disease causes this fluid to be exuded in excess so that it fills or partly fills the cavity, it causes a meningeal effusion, pleural effusion, or peritoneal effusion, as the case may be.

Connective Tissue, commonly called areolar tissue, is loose but strong, and is made up of small fibers and cells woven together into a sort of network while the spaces between the cells and fibers are filled with tissue fluid. The use of connective tissue is to give support to parts and organs so that they may not be bruised and injured by shocks and pressure; connective tissue also carries the blood vessels from one part of the body to another.

Fibrous Tissue is abundant throughout the body, and is of two kinds. White fibrous tissue consists of fibrous cells grouped into bundles, and is a dense unyielding structure; it forms the tendons and ligaments which join the muscles and bones together in the body. Yellow fibrous tissue is elastic and is present in the walls of the arteries and in some ligaments.

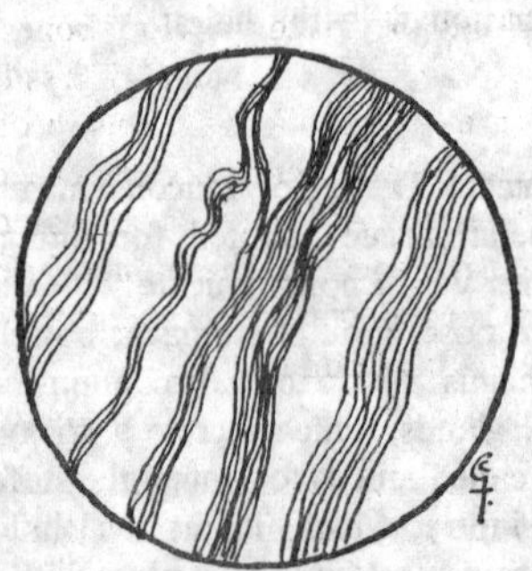

Fig. 4. *FIBROUS TISSUE*

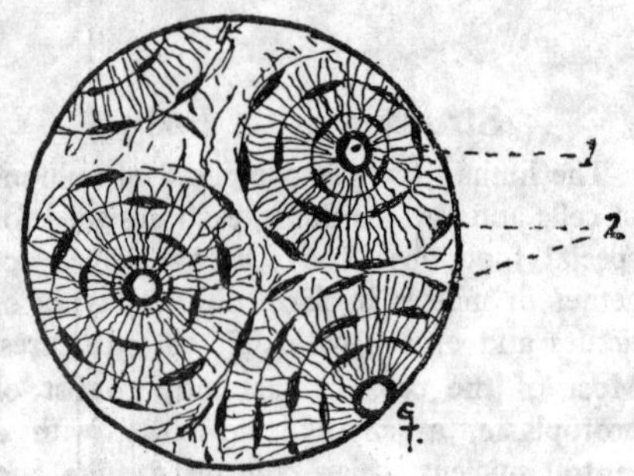

Fig. 5. *BONE, OR OSSEOUS, TISSUE.* 1. *Haversian canal.* 2. *Bone cells.*

Bone, or Osseous Tissue, forms the framework or skeleton of the body. It consists partly of fibrous tissue, and partly of calcium phosphate and calcium carbonate. Its density and strength vary according to its composition, and according to the age of the person.

In the central portion of most bones there is a space known as the medullary or marrow cavity. This cavity contains blood vessels, fat and fibrous connective tissue necessary for the nutrition and repair of bone. In addition it contains special cells which develop into red and white blood corpuscles, and these are carried by small vessels into the bloodstream.

At birth all the bones of the body contain red marrow tissue which is actively producing blood cells, but as the demand for new blood becomes less the red marrow of the long bones is replaced by fatty tissue and becomes yellow marrow. In the adult, only the bones of the thoracic cage, vertebrae, pelvis, and skull contain red marrow.

Muscle Tissue consists of many small fibers which, when stimulated, contract and shorten and so can perform mechanical work such as turning the head, or walking.

Two types of muscle are known:

1. STRIPED or VOLUNTARY muscle which consists of numerous fibers with cross striations grouped into bundles or fasciculi, many fasciculi making up a whole muscle. It forms the bulk of muscular tissue in the body and is found in the limbs, back, abdominal wall, face, etc. The activity of this type of muscle is under the control of the will.

2. UNSTRIPED, INVOLUNTARY, or visceral muscle. The fibers of this smooth muscle lack the cross striations of voluntary muscle and are arranged in sheets lining the walls of hollow organs, e.g. alimentary canal, blood vessels, the bladder, etc. A special variety—cardiac muscle—is found in the heart. The function of smooth muscle in general is to squeeze hollow organs and expel their contents. Its activity is not under the control of the will.

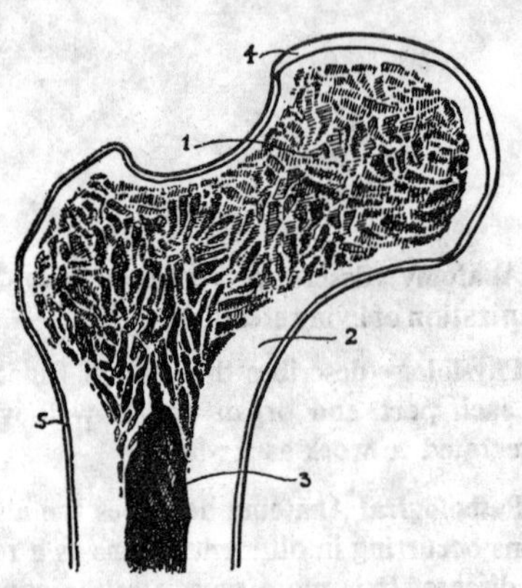

Fig. 6. *STRUCTURE OF BONE (head of long bone).* 1. *Cancellous or spongy tissue.* 2. *Compact or hard tissue.* 3. *Marrow cavity.* 4. *Joint surface covered with cartilage.* 5. *Periosteum, the fibrous sheath surrounding bone.*

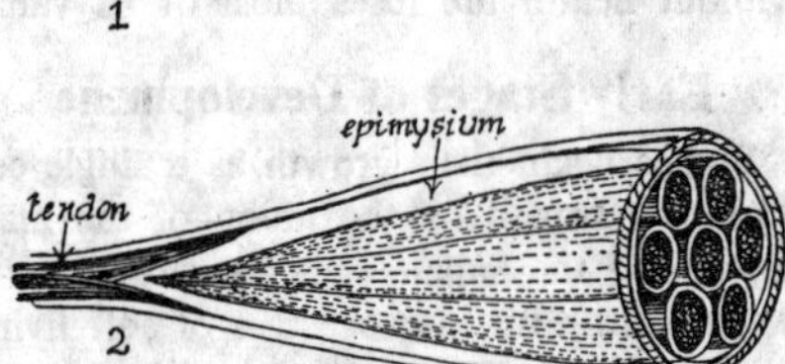

Fig. 7. *MUSCLE BUNDLES, OR FASCICULI.* 1 *Individual fibers of a fasciculus, running parallel to one another, are grouped within a connective tissue sheath (perimysium).* 2. *A number of fasciculi, held together with further connective tissue (epimysium), form a muscle. This narrows to a tendon attached to bone.*

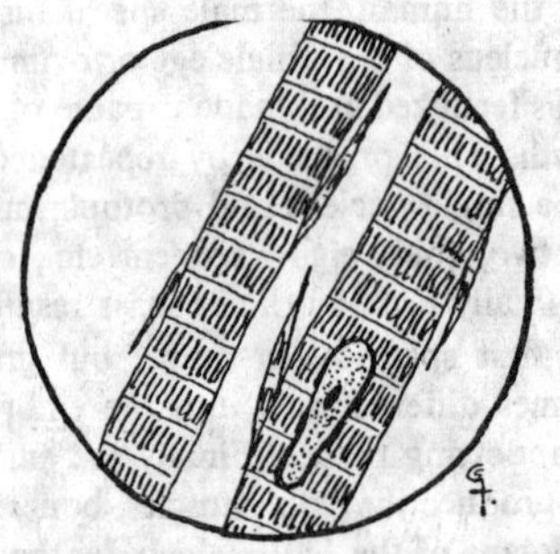

Fig. 8. *STRIPED (OR VOLUNTARY) MUSCLE FIBERS. Because of their strengthening cross striations they are also known as striated fibers. They vary in length according to the part of the body in which they occur.*

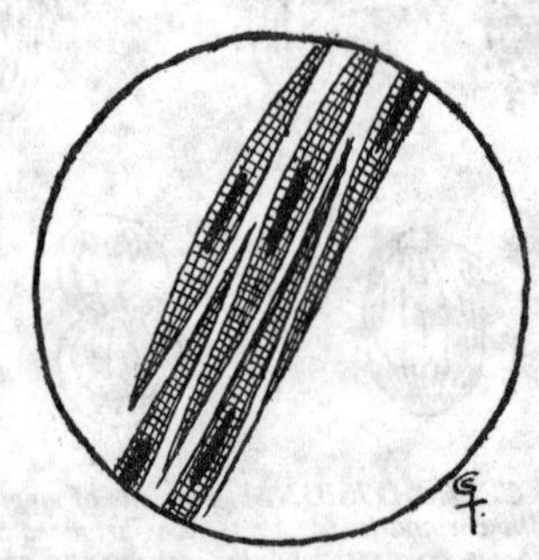

Fig. 9. *UNSTRIPED (INVOLUNTARY) MUSCLE FIBERS. These fibers lack cross striations.*

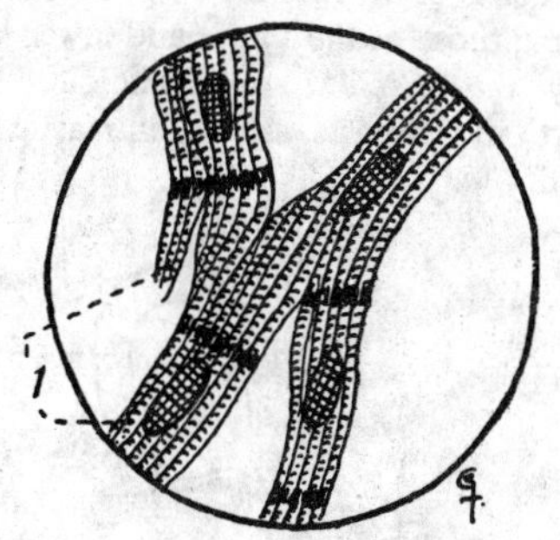

Fig. 10. *HEART MUSCLE TISSUE.* 1. *Striated muscle fibers.*

Cartilaginous Tissue or cartilage covers the ends of the bones where they come together to make a joint. It enables the joint to move easily, being smooth, hard and pliant.

Adipose Tissue or fat occurs in the connective tissue under the skin and round the various organs. It forms a soft protecting layer, and gives roundness and beauty to the body. It prevents sudden loss of heat, and is an important reserve of food. At the normal body temperature fat is semi-fluid. By the increase of this tissue, persons may become extremely obese without having their muscles at all increased in size. Such a condition is to be deplored, the body having become merely the storehouse of huge deposits of fat.

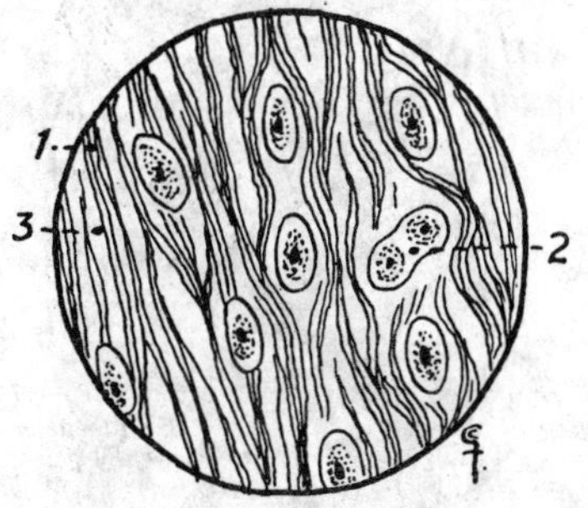

Fig. 11. *CARTILAGE TISSUE.* 1 *and* 3. *Connective tissue fibers.* 2. *Cartilage cells in hyaline matrix.*

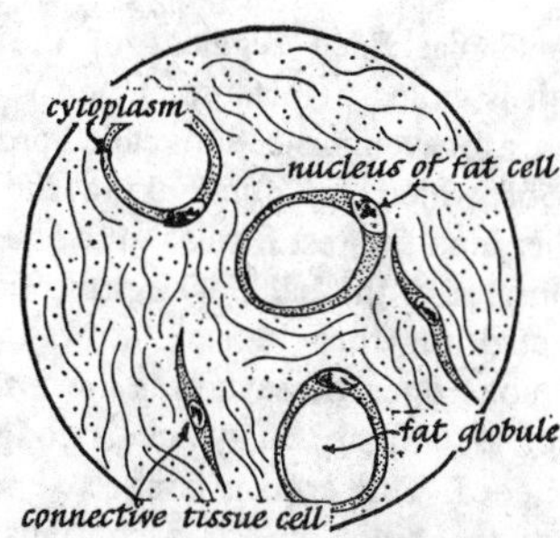

Fig. 12. *FAT (OR ADIPOSE) TISSUE*

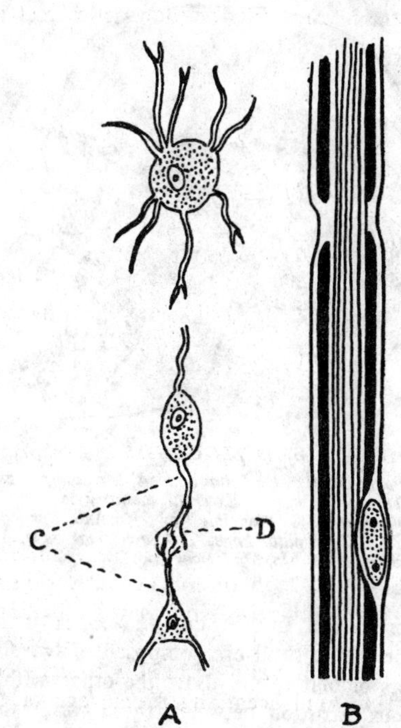

Fig. 13. *STRUCTURE OF NERVE TISSUE.* A *Typical forms of nerve cells.* B. *Medullated nerve fiber.* C. *Nerve axon.* D. *Synapse: where the nerve endings intercommunicate with those of the next nerve.*

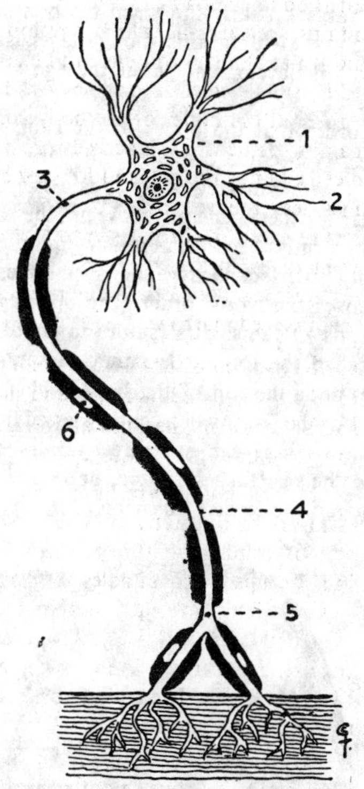

Fig. 14. *A NERVE CELL WITH AXON AND NERVE ENDINGS.* 1. *Nerve cell with nucleus.* 2. *Dendrons (dendrites).* 3. *Axon of nerve fiber.* 4. *Node of Ranvier.* 5. *Axis cylinder.* 6 *Nucleus in myelin sheath.*

Nervous Tissue is composed of irregularly shaped cells which have one or more processes arising from the body of the cell. The processes are known as dendrons (see Fig. 14) and in some nerve cells one process is very much elongated and is known as the axon. The cells are specially adapted for carrying messages (or nerve impulses) from one part of the body to another; those in which the impulse travels fastest have a special insulating layer of fatty material or myelin around the axon (Fig. 14). The myelin is white and gives to nerves their characteristic appearance. The majority of nerve cells are found within the central nervous system, where they form the gray matter, while the myelinated axons form the white matter. Nerve cell processes both enter and leave the central nervous system grouped together into paired nerves—twelve pairs arising from the skull and thirty-one pairs from the spinal cord. They carry messages from sense organs all over the body to the central nervous system and from the latter to muscles and glands. The spinal nerves also carry unmyelinated or gray fibers of the automatic nervous system; the cell bodies from which these fibers arise lie in groups or ganglia which form a chain on either side of the vertebral column or are scattered in the walls of viscera. The nerve fibers from the ganglia form extensive plexuses which innervate glands and involuntary muscle all over the body. The autonomic nervous system regulates the activities of organs such as blood vessels and digestive glands, which are not controlled by the will.

ANATOMY OF THE SKELETON

The human skeleton is composed of over two hundred bones, the teeth not included.

The bones are to the body what the frame is to the house; they support, protect and retain the other parts in their proper places. They furnish protuberances or points of attachment for the muscles and ligaments, to hold the different parts of the body together, and to give them motion. They also furnish strong bony cavities to protect delicate organs such as the eye, the brain and the heart.

The bones are supplied with nutrient blood vessels. In infants they are comparatively soft and cartilaginous; after a time, in the young child, they begin to develop bone cells at certain places called centers of ossification. Bones are covered with a strong fibrous membrane called the periosteum which contains blood vessels. A somewhat similar covering on the cartilages has the name of perichondrium, and that which covers the skull is called the pericranium.

The bones are mainly composed of calcium carbonate and calcium phosphate, and as such they also act as storehouses of these materials for the functioning of other organs.

The outer layer of both the long bones, such as are found in the limbs, and of the flat bones such as the shoulder blades, is formed of compact or cancellous bone and resembles ivory. Inside the ends of the long bones and between the hard outer layers of the flat bones is formed the spongy bone of looser texture. In the hollow parts of the long bones is the bone marrow, which also occurs in the small spaces of the spongy bone. The cylindrical form of the long bones increases their strength and lightness, while the spongy bone inside acts as a supporting structure. The blood vessels which nourish the bones and bone marrow run through the outer periosteum and pass into small canals in the bone substance.

The bones of the skeleton are divided into those of the head, comprising twenty-two; of the spine, twenty-six; of the ribs and breastbone, twenty-five; of the upper limbs, sixty-four; and of the lower limbs, sixty-two.

The Bones of the Head

The bones of the head are divided into those of the cranium, the ear, and the face, including the jaws. The skull or cranium encloses and protects the brain and has

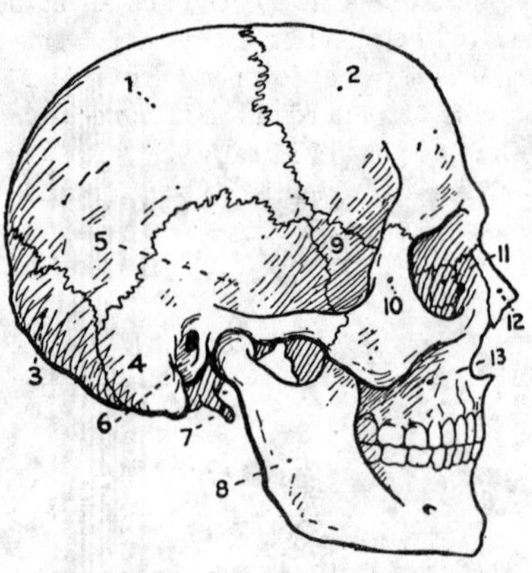

Fig. 16. *SIDE VIEW OF SKULL.* 1. *Parietal bone.* 2. *Frontal bone.* 3. *Occipital bone.* 4. *Mastoid process.* 5. *Temporal bone.* 6. *External auditory meatus.* 7. *Styloid process.* 8. *Mandible (lower jaw).* 9. *Sphenoid bone.* 10. *Zygomatic bone.* 11. *Lachrymal bone.* 12. *Nasal bone.* 13. *Maxilla (upper jaw).*

fifteen bones. In the adult the bones of the dome of the skull are composed of two flat layers or plates, one above the other, with a porous partition between; these two plates protect the brain against injury, the outer one being fibrous and tough, the inner one hard and resistant. The middle layer has the name of diploe; it is spongy in texture and thus reduces the effects of blows upon the outer table. In early life when the bones are tender and yielding, this spongy layer is not present; it develops at about the age of ten years.

In order that the bones of the skull may not easily become displaced they are dovetailed together in irregular lines called sutures. In later life these generally close up, the bones uniting firmly together; in infancy the sutures are not interlocked and the firm bones do not cover the whole brain. The openings at the ends of the sagittal suture in childhood are called the fontanelles; they present soft places upon the top of the head, which may be felt by the finger when gently pressed down.

The internal ear has three small bones, called the malleus, the stapes and the incus. These aid the sense of hearing.

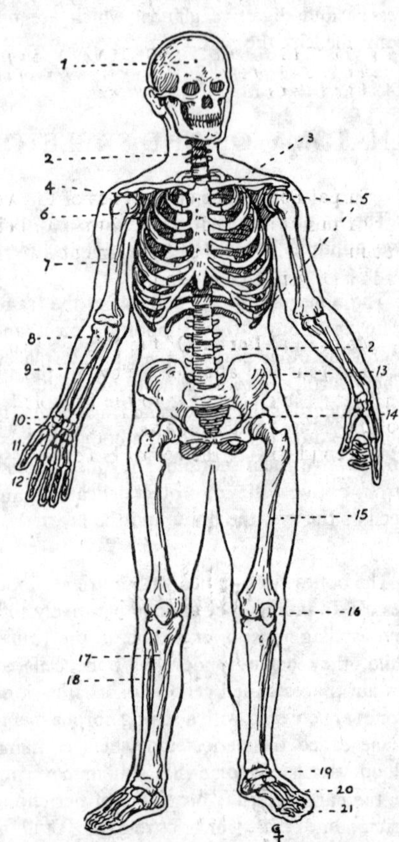

Fig. 15. *THE SKELETON.* 1. *Skull.* 2. *Spinal Column.* 3. *Clavicle, or collar-bone.* 4. *Scapula, or shoulder blade.* 5. *Ribs.* 6. *Sternum, or breast-bone.* 7. *Humerus.* 8. *Radius.* 9. *Ulna.* 10. *Carpals.* 11. *Metacarpals, or bones of hand.* 12. *Phalanges, or bones of fingers.* 13. *Pelvis.* 14. *Sacrum.* 15. *Femur, or thigh-bone.* 16. *Patella, or knee-cap.* 17. *Tibia.* 18. *Fibula.* 19. *Tarsals, or ankle bones.* 20. *Metatarsals, or bones of foot.* 21. *Phalanges, or bones of the toes.*

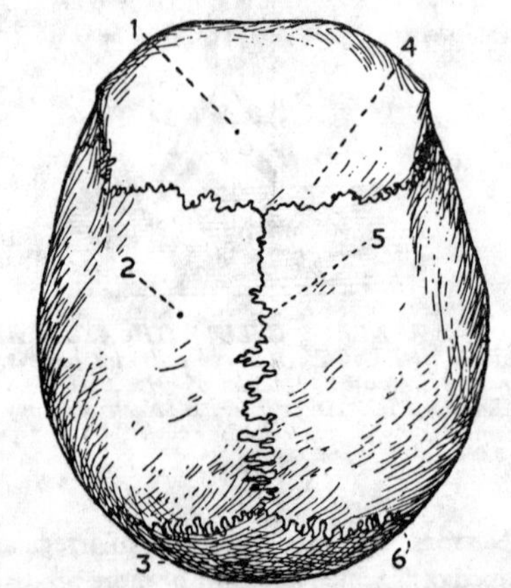

Fig. 17. *DOME OF SKULL.* 1. *Frontal bone.* 2 *Parietal bone.* 3. *Occipital bone.* 4. *Coronal suture.* 5. *Sagittal suture.* 6. *Lambdoidal suture.*

The bones of the face are seven in number, including those of the upper and lower jaws, namely the maxilla and mandible. They support the soft parts, and aid in mastication of food.

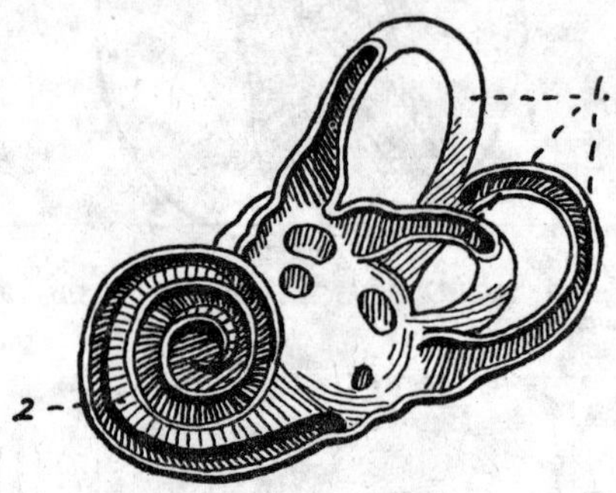

Fig. 18. *INNER EAR (labyrinth).* 1. *Semicircular canals.* 2. *Cochlea.*

The Bones of the Trunk

Connected with the trunk there are twenty-four ribs; there are twenty-four segments or vertebrae in the backbone or spinal column, and four bones in the pelvis and hips; the breast-bone is called the sternum. These bones support two great cavities, namely the thorax or chest, and the abdomen or belly.

The Ribs. The ribs, all connecting with the backbone behind and some with the breast-bone in front, form the thorax which contains the lungs and heart. Fig. 19 shows the natural form of the healthy chest.

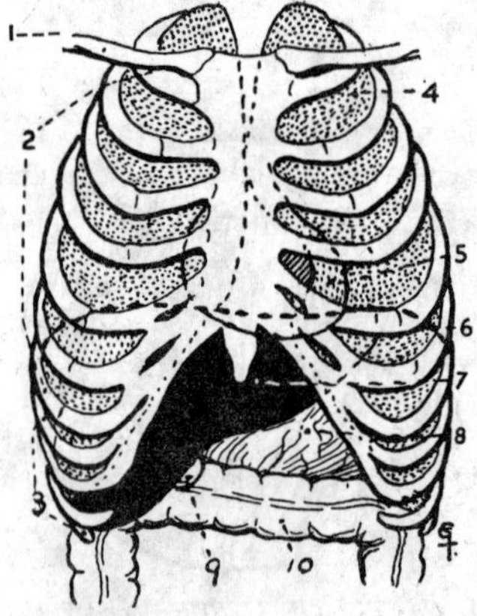

Fig. 19. *THE THORAX.* 1. *Clavicle.* 2. *Ribs.* 3. *False or floating ribs.* 4. *Lungs.* 5. *Heart.* 6. *Diaphragm.* 7. *Liver.* 8. *Stomach.* 9. *Gall-bladder.* 10. *Transverse colon.*

The Spine. Each segment of the spinal column is called a vertebra. Upon each one of these are seven projections called processes, some of which are for linking the bones together, and the rest furnish attachments for the muscles of the back. The projections are connected together in such a way that a continuous open passage runs down through the spinal column, in which is lodged the spinal cord. This cord is connected with the base of the brain, and is a continuation of the nerves originating in the brain.

Between all the vertebrae are cartilaginous pads or discs which are resilient and protect the brain from being injuriously jarred by running, leaping or other movements.

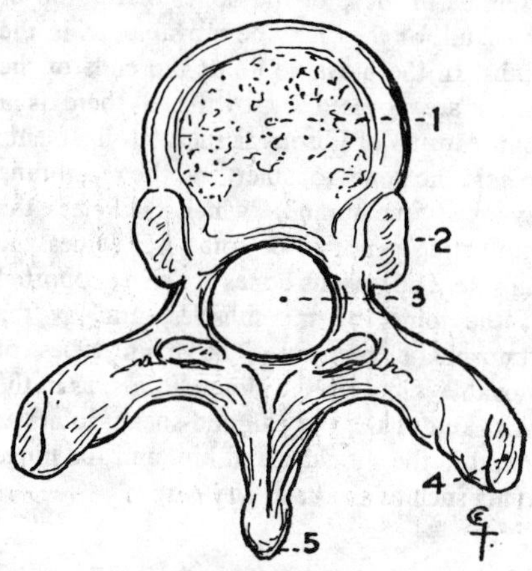

Fig. 20. *A TYPICAL VERTEBRA.* 1. *Body.* 2. *Articular surface.* 3. *Spinal canal.* 4. *Transverse process.* 5. *Spinous process.*

The pelvis, or pelvic girdle, is made up of two hip bones, the sacrum and the coccyx. Each hip bone is large and irregular in shape, and is formed by the fusion of three bones—the ilium, the ischium, and the pubis. In its outer wall is a deep smooth cavity called the acetabulum which holds the round head of the thigh-bone, or femur. The sacrum and coccyx are triangular in shape and are formed by thè fusion together of the bones of the lower part of the vertebral column.

The Bones of the Upper Limbs

The shoulder blade (scapula), the collar-bone (clavicle), the bone of the upper arm (humerus), the two bones of the forearm

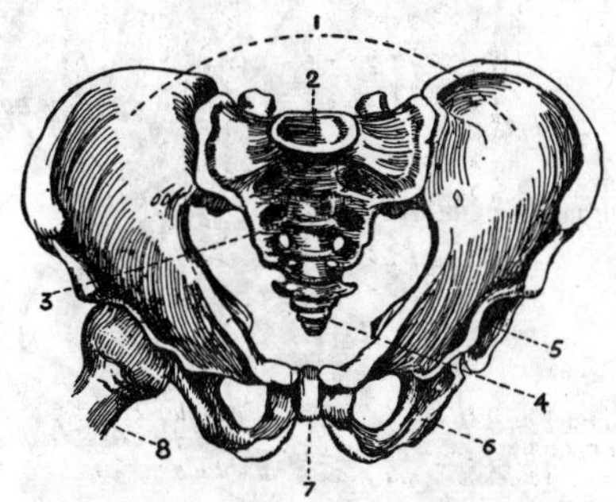

Fig. 21. *THE PELVIS (front view).* 1. *Ilium, or hip-bone.* 2. *Union of sacrum and lower end of spine.* 3. *Sacrum.* 4. *Coccyx.* 5. *Acetabulum or socket for head of femur.* 6. *Ischium.* 7. *Symphysis pubis, or pubic bone.* 8. *Femur, or thigh bone.*

(ulna and radius), the bones of the wrist (carpal bones), the bones of the palm of the hand (metacarpal bones), the bones of the thumb and fingers (phalanges), comprise the bones of each upper limb. The scapula and clavicle comprise the shoulder girdle, while the remainder form the arm, forearm and hand.

The Collar-bone is joined by ligaments to the breast-bone at one end and at the other end to the shoulder blade; it prevents the shoulders from dropping forward. Many persons become round-shouldered by faulty habits of posture in early life; this happens if children are allowed to sit habitually in a stooping posture.

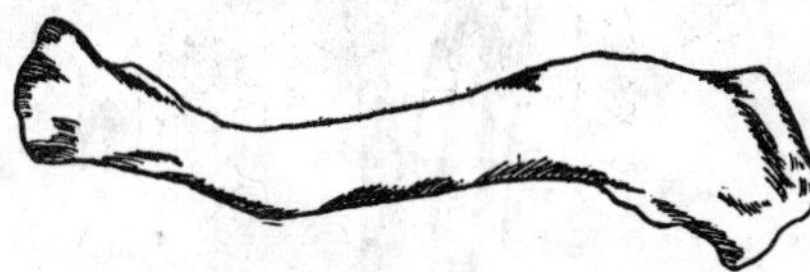

Fig. 22. *COLLAR-BONE, OR CLAVICLE*

The Shoulder Blade (scapula) lies upon the upper part of the back, forming the shoulder. It has a shallow cavity (glenoid cavity), into which is inserted the head of the upper arm-bone. Several strong ligaments and muscles are attached to the elevations of this bone, which keep it in its place and move it about as required.

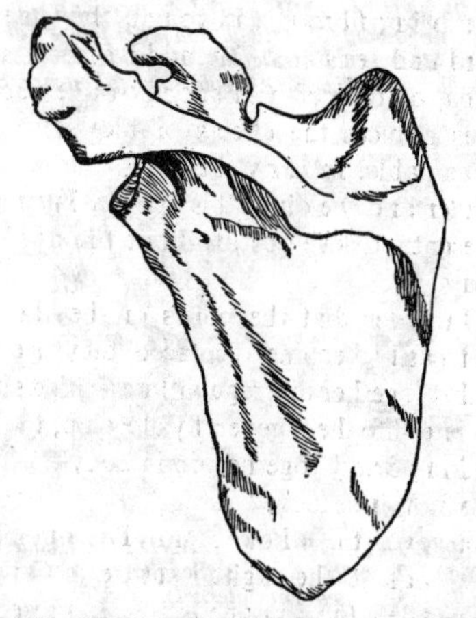

Fig. 23. *SHOULDER BLADE, OR SCAPULA*

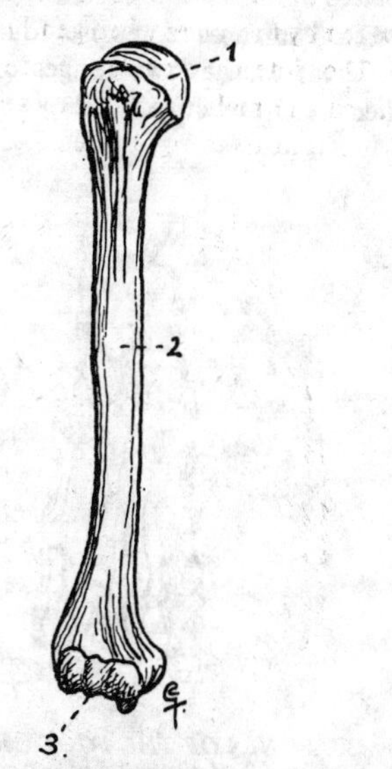

Fig. 24. *THE HUMERUS.* 1. *Head.* 2. *Shaft.* 3. *Surface which articulates with the ulna, at the elbow joint.*

The bone of the upper arm, or **Humerus** (Fig. 24), has a rounded head which fits into the shallow glenoid cavity of the scapula, to the edges of which it is attached by the capsular ligament. The shoulder joint has a great range of movement but it is not very stable and is easily dislocated, since the socket into which the head of the humerus fits is very shallow. At its lower end the humerus articulates with the **Ulna** and **Radius** to form the elbow joint. The radius and ulna articulate at their lower ends with the carpal or wrist bones (Fig. 25).

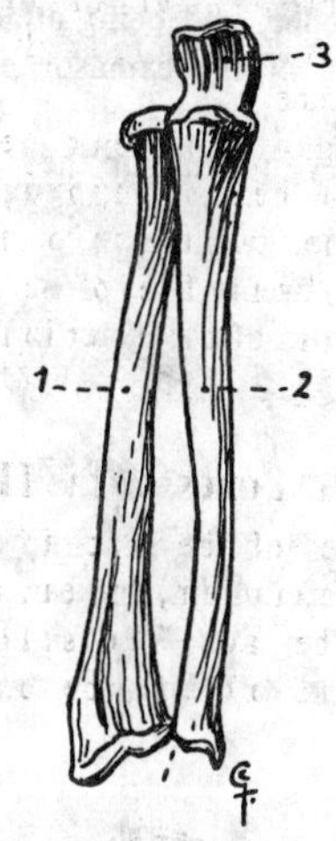

Fig. 25. *THE RADIUS AND ULNA.* 1. *Shaft of radius.* 2. *Shaft of ulna.* 3. *Olecranon process of ulna.* 4. *Articulation surface with wrist bones.*

Carpal Bones. The eight bones of the wrist or carpus are ranged in two rows and, being bound closely together by ligaments, do not admit of very free motion.

Metacarpal Bones. Of the five metacarpal bones, four are attached below to the first phalanges and the other to the first phalanx of the thumb, while all articulate above with the second row of the carpal bones.

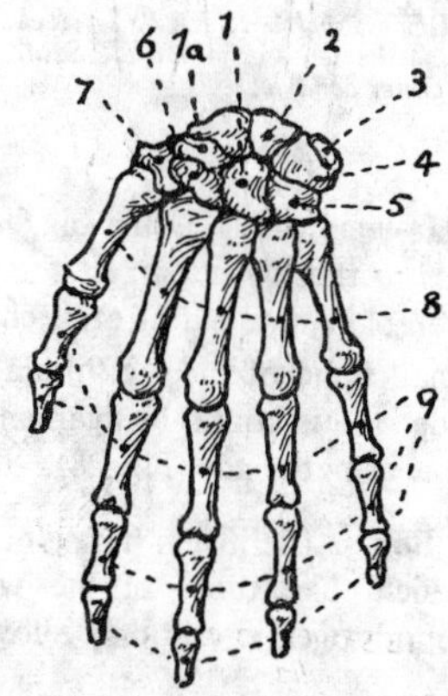

Fig. 26. *BONES OF THE HAND.* 1. *Os magnum.* 1a. *Scaphoid.* 2. *Semilunar.* 3. *Pisiform.* 4. *Cuneiform.* 5. *Unciform.* 6. *Trapezoid.* 7. *Trapezium.* 8. *Metacarpals of the hand.* 9. *Phalanges of fingers and thumb.*

The Bones of the Lower Limbs

These are the thigh-bone (femur), the knee-cap (patella), the shin-bone (tibia), the small bone of the leg (fibula), the bones of the instep (tarsal bones), the bones of the middle of the foot (metatarsal bones), and the bones of the toes (phalanges).

The Thigh-bone, or femur, is the longest bone in the body. Its head, which is large and round, fits into the cavity called the acetabulum in the hip-bone and forms a ball-and-socket joint (Fig. 33).

The Knee-cap (patella) is placed on the front of the knee, and being attached above to the tendon of the extensor muscles and below to the tibia by a strong ligament, it acts as a pulley in lifting up the leg.

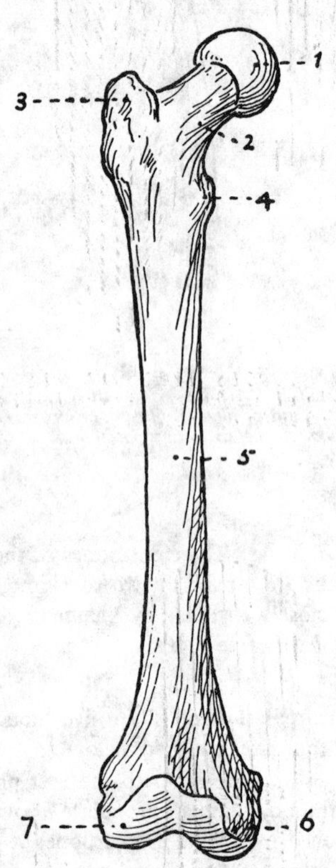

Fig. 27. *THE FEMUR.* 1. *Head.* 2. *Neck.* 3. *Great trochanter.* 4. *Lesser trochanter.* 5. *Shaft.* 6. *Inner condyle.* 7. *Outer condyle.*

The Shin-bone (tibia) is the bigger of the two bones in the lower part of the leg, and is considerably expanded at each end.

The small bone of the leg (fibula) lies on the outside and is bound by ligaments to the larger bone at both ends (Fig. 28).

Tarsal Bones. The instep (tarsus) has seven bones which, like those of the wrist, are firmly bound together and only allow limited motion.

The Metatarsal Bones, corresponding to the metacarpals of the hand, are five in number and unite at one end with the tarsal bones, and at the other with the first range of the toe bones (phalanges). The tarsal and metatarsal bones form an arch, the spring of which, when the weight of the body descends upon it in walking, prevents injury to the organs above (Fig. 29).

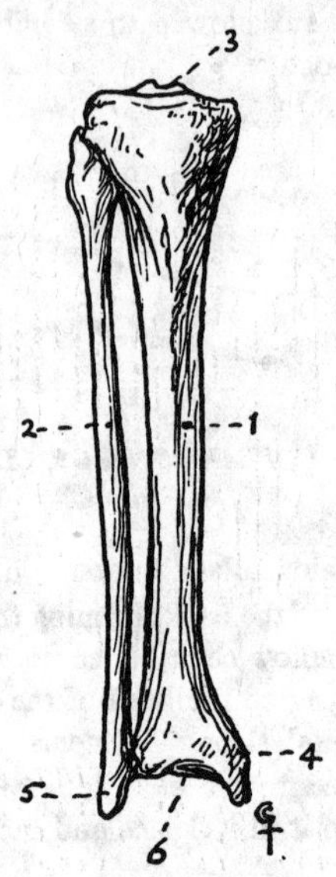

Fig. 28. *TIBIA AND FIBULA.* 1. *Shaft of tibia.* 2. *Shaft of fibula.* 3. *Articulation with femur (at knee joint).* 4. *Internal malleolus of ankle.* 5. *External malleolus of ankle.* 6. *Articulation with tarsal bones.*

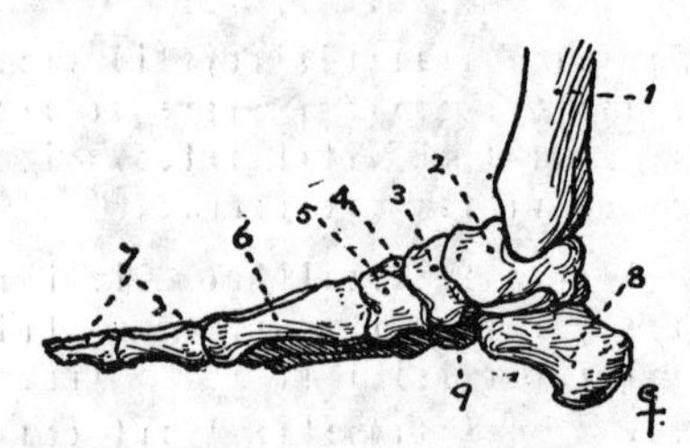

Fig. 29. *BONES OF ANKLE AND FOOT (side view).* 1. *Tibia.* 2. *Astragalus.* 3. *Scaphoid.* 4. *Cuneiform (middle).* 5. *Cuneiform (internal).* 6. *Metatarsal bone of foot.* 7. *Phalanges of toes.* 8. *Os calcis.* 9. *Cuboid.*

The Phalanges comprise fourteen bones. The great toe has two ranges of bones; the other toes have three.

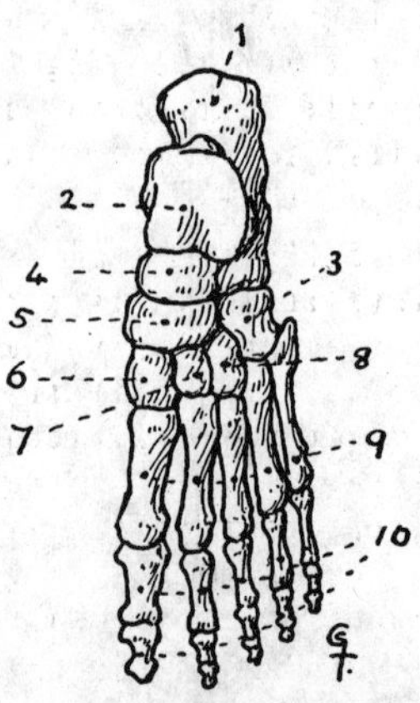

Fig. 30. *BONES OF THE FOOT (seen from above).* 1. *Os calcis.* 2. *Articulation of astragalus with tibia.* 3. *Cuboid.* 4. *Body of astragalus.* 5. *Scaphoid.* 6. *Internal cuneiform.* 7. *Middle cuneiform.* 8. *External cuneiform.* 9. *Metatarsal bones of foot.* 10. *Phalanges of toes.*

The Joints

A joint or articulation is the connection between two or more parts of the skeleton, either of bones or cartilage. Joints may be fixed, as in those of the bones of the top of the skull, or they may be movable, as in the limbs. In the movable joints the ends of the bones are covered by cartilage, there is a joint capsule of fibrous tissue with ligaments to hold the bones together, and the membrane (synovial membrane) which secretes the lubricating synovial or joint fluid lines the capsule. The various bones are also supported at the joints by the muscles, and by the atmospheric pressure. The main types of movable joints are the gliding joints, as in the wrist and ankle, the ball-and-socket joints as found in the shoulder and hip, and the hinge joints such as the knee and elbow.

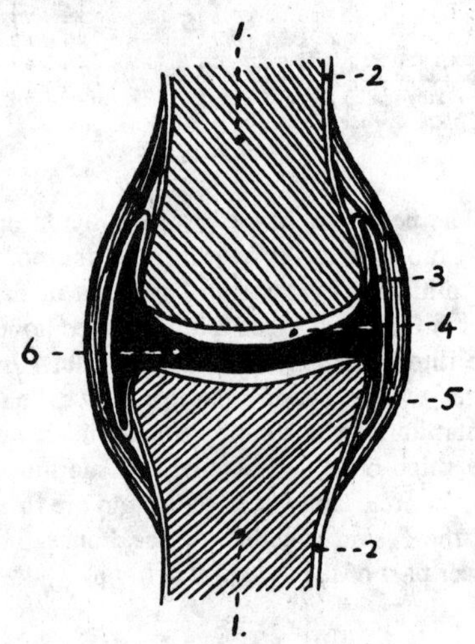

Fig. 31. *SECTION THROUGH A TYPICAL GLIDING JOINT.* 1. *Bone.* 2. *Periosteum.* 3. *Synovial membrane.* 4. *Cartilage.* 5. *Ligament.* 6. *Joint cavity.*

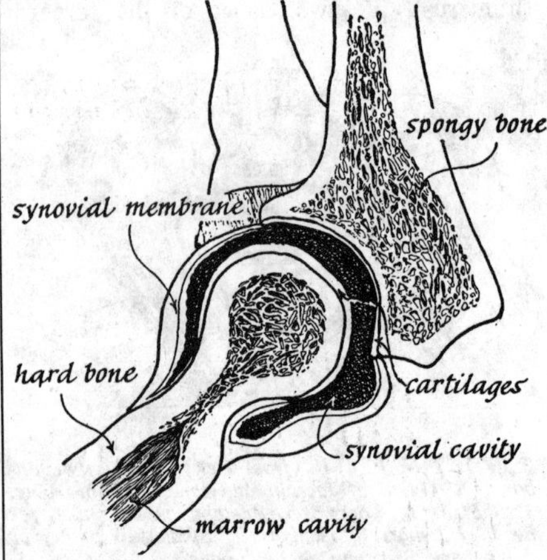

Fig. 32. *A BALL-AND-SOCKET JOINT, in section, to show how the arrangement of the cartilage coverings and the synovial fluid cavity protect the bony ends of he joint from jarring upon one another.*

Fig. 31 shows a joint with the intervening cartilages.

Cartilage becomes thinner, harder and less elastic in old age; hence old people are not quite as tall as in middle life and are a little stiffer in their joints.

Around the bony prominences of the joints are small sacs called bursae which are lined with synovial membrane and filled with synovial fluid.

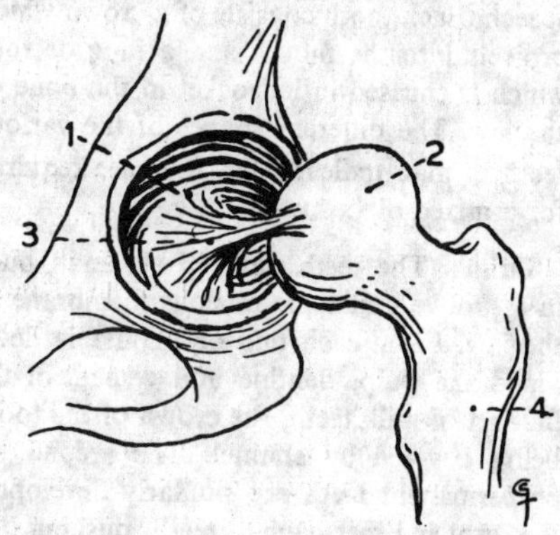

Fig. 33. *INTERIOR OF HIP JOINT (a ball-and-socket joint). 1. in Socket hip-bone, or acetabulum. 2. Head of femur (thigh-bone) shown dislocated to demonstrate its relationship to the socket. 3. Ligament of femur attached to head. 4. Upper end of femur.*

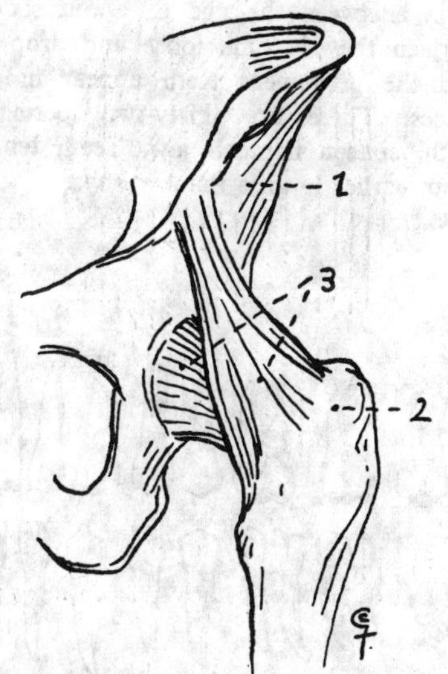

Fig. 34. *LIGAMENTS OF THE LEFT HIP JOINT. 1. Hip-bone (Ilium). 2. Femur. 3. Ligaments extending between the two bones.*

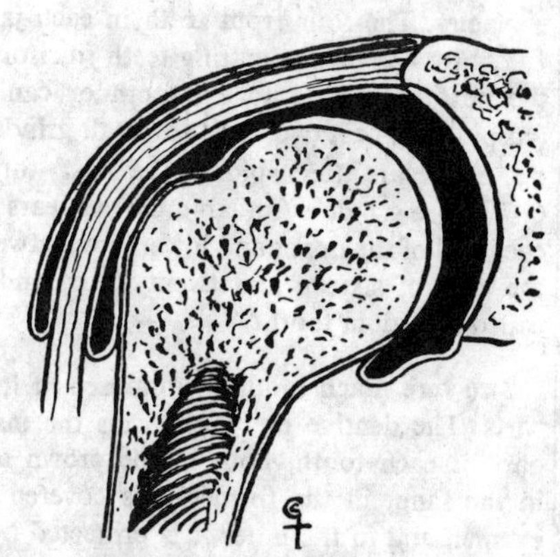

Fig. 35. *SECTION THROUGH A JOINT SHOWING A BURSA*

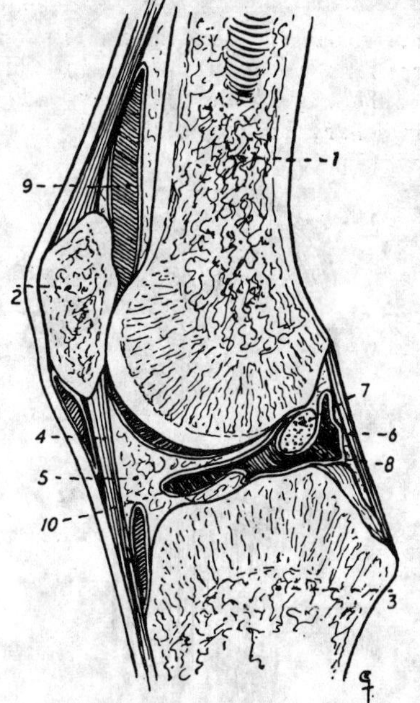

Fig. 36. *LIGAMENTS OF THE KNEE JOINT (a hinge joint). 1. Femur. 2. Patella. 3. Tibia. 4. Ligament of patella. 5. Infra-patellar pad of fat. 6. Capsular ligament. 7. Anterior cruciate ligament. 8. Posterior cruciate ligament. 9. Supra-patellar bursa. 10. Synovial membrane.*

THE MUSCLES

That part of an animal's body which we call lean meat is composed of muscle and comprises about 40 per cent of the body weight. There are two main types of muscle.

1. **Voluntary** or **Skeletal Muscle.** The fibers of this type of muscle are striped and their action is controlled by the will. Voluntary muscle is found attached to all parts of the skeleton and is responsible for the movements of the limbs, movements of facial expression, and so on. The shape of the muscle varies with its situation: some typical arrangements of voluntary muscle are illustrated in Fig. 37. At each end the muscle merges with a different type of tissue—the tendon whose strong inelastic fibers attach the muscle to bones.

See also Figs. 8 and 9, p. 218. Fig. 7 illustrates a muscle bundle tapering to form a tendon.

Every muscle is supplied with many nerve fibers; each nerve fiber branches and supplies up to 100 individual muscle cells. Stimulation of the nerve causes the muscle to contract and shorten, thus causing movement of the joint which is spanned by the muscle. Contraction of one muscle is accompanied by relaxation of the antagonist or muscle which causes the opposite movement. For example, flexion of the elbow joint is accomplished by contraction of muscles which are attached to the front of the humerus and the radius and ulna: the biceps is the most powerful of this group. As these muscles contract there is at the same time relaxation of other muscles which would, if stimulated, cause extension of the elbow joint (mainly the triceps muscle). Thus movement of a limb is accomplished by both contraction and relaxation of opposing groups of muscles.

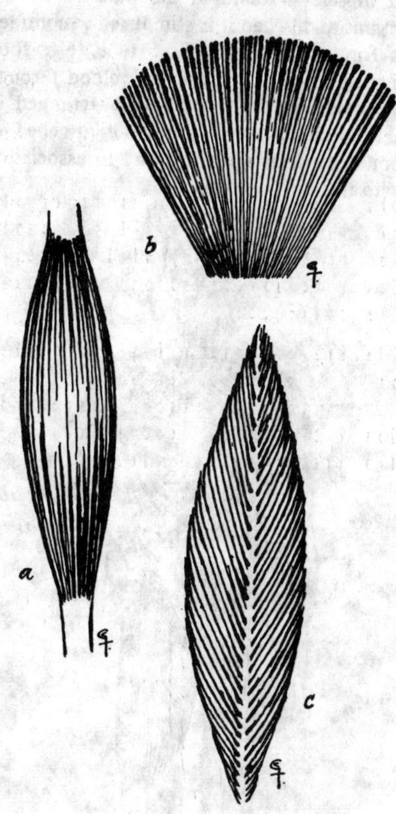

Fig. 37. *VARIOUS TYPES OF MUSCLES. a. Spindle-shaped or fusiform muscle. b. Fan-shaped muscle c. Penniform muscle.*

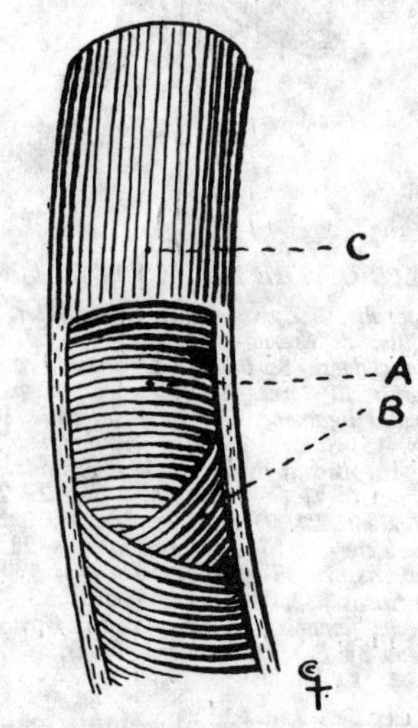

Fig. 38. *SECTION OF THE ESOPHAGUS OR GULLET.* A and B. *Circular muscle fibers.* C. *Longitudinal muscle fibers.*

2. Involuntary or **Smooth Muscle.** This type of muscle is found in the walls of hollow organs and, when it is stimulated to contract, it forces fluid through a tube, e.g. food through the alimentary canal, blood through the heart, etc. The fibers are arranged in sheets, and since they are not attached to bones, tendons are not found in association with this type of muscle.

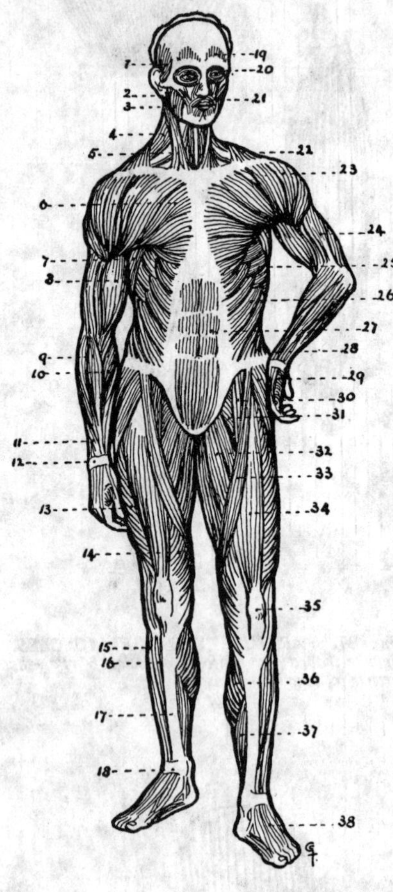

Fig. 39.
MUSCLES OF THE HUMAN BODY (front view).

1. *Temporalis.* 2. *Zygomaticus.* 3. *Masseter.* 4. *Splenius capitis.* 5. *Sterno-mastoideus.* 6. *Pectoralis.* 7. *Latissimus dorsi.* 8. *Biceps.* 9. *Brachio-radialis.* 10. *Pronator radii teres.* 11. *Extensor carpi radialis.* 12. *Annular ligament.* 13. *Vastus lateralis.* 14. *Vastus medialis.* 15. *Sulcus.* 16. *Peroneus longus.* 17. *Crest of tibia.* 18. *Annular ligament.* 19. *Frontalis.* 20. *Orbicularis oculi.* 21. *Orbicularis oris.* 22. *Trapezius.* 23. *Deltoideus.* 24. *Triceps.* 25. *Serratus anterior.* 26. *Obliquus externus.* 27. *Rectus abdominis.* 28. *Extensor carpi ulnaris.* 29. *Tensor fasciae latae.* 30. *Iliacus.* 31. *Pectineus.* 32. *Adductor longus.* 33. *Sartorius.* 34. *Rectus femoris.* 35. *Patella.* 36. *Gastrocnemius.* 37. *Soleus.* 38. *Extensor tendons of toes.*

In the wall of the alimentary canal there are two distinct layers of muscle: an inner layer where the fibers are arranged in a circular manner, and an outer layer where the fibers are arranged longitudinally (Figs. 38 and 41). At intervals the circular coat is thickened to form a sphincter which, when it contracts, completely blocks the tube.

The activity of involuntary muscle is not under the control of the will. It is innervated by nerve fibers from the autonomic nervous system.

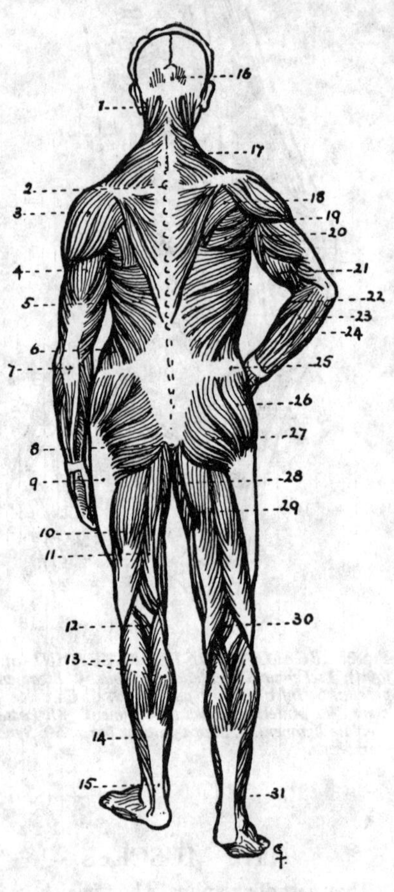

Fig. 40.
MUSCLES OF THE HUMAN BODY (back view).

1. *Sterno-mastoideus.* 2. *Vertebra of spine.* 3. *Deltoideus.* 4. *Triceps.* 5. *Latissimus dorsi.* 6. *Obliquus externus.* 7. *Olecranon process.* 8. *Coccyx.* 9. *Fascia lata.* 10. *Biceps femoris.* 11. *Semi-tendinosus.* 12. *Plantaris.* 13. *Gastrocnemius.* 14. *Soleus.* 15. *Tendo achillis.* 16. *Occipitalis.* 17. *Trapezius.* 18. *Infraspinatus.* 19. *Teres major.* 21. *Biceps.* 22. *Extensor carpi radialis longus.* 23. *Flexor carpi ulnaris.* 24. *Extensor carpi ulnaris.* 25. *Crest of ilium.* 26. *Gluteus medius.* 27. *Gluteus maximus.* 28. *Adductor magnus.* 29. *Semi-membranosus.* 30. *Semi-tendinosus.* 31. *Peroneus longus.*

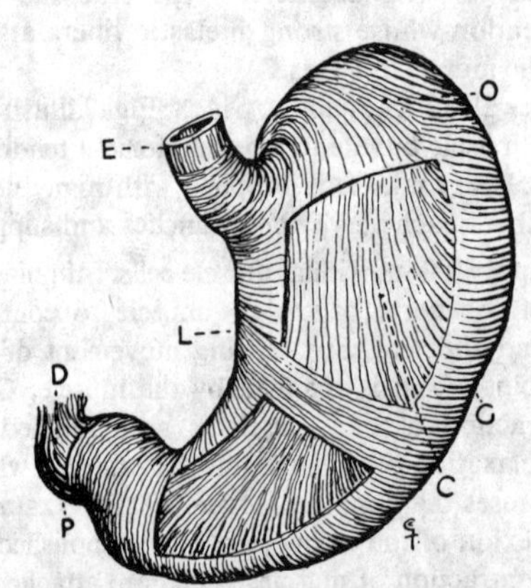

Fig. 41. *MUSCLES OF THE STOMACH WALL.* E. *Esophagus, or gullet, lower end.* O. *Muscle fibers of fundus.* C. *Muscle fibers (oblique).* D. *Beginning of the duodenum.* P. *Pylorus.* G. *Greater curvature of the stomach.* L. *Lesser curvature of the stomach.*

THE TEETH

The teeth are hard bodies embedded in sockets in the jaw bones, which serve for biting and chewing food and to assist in speech. Each tooth consists of a crown which projects into the mouth and a fang or root which is encased in its socket in the bone of the jaw. The different shapes of the various teeth in man indicate that they are required for a mixed diet.

Origin. The teeth develop as small buds in a groove under the mucous membrane of the jaw. From each bud or papilla is developed the pulp, dentine and cement of the first set of milk teeth, the crown of the tooth being covered by enamel. The second set or permanent teeth are similarly developed, the growing permanent teeth pushing the crown of the milk teeth out, while the fangs are absorbed.

Number. The first temporary set of teeth are called the milk teeth; there are twenty of them. Between the age of about six and thirteen they become loose and drop out, and the permanent teeth appear in their places. There are thirty-two permanent teeth, sixteen in each jaw. Teeth tend to erupt earlier in girls than in boys.

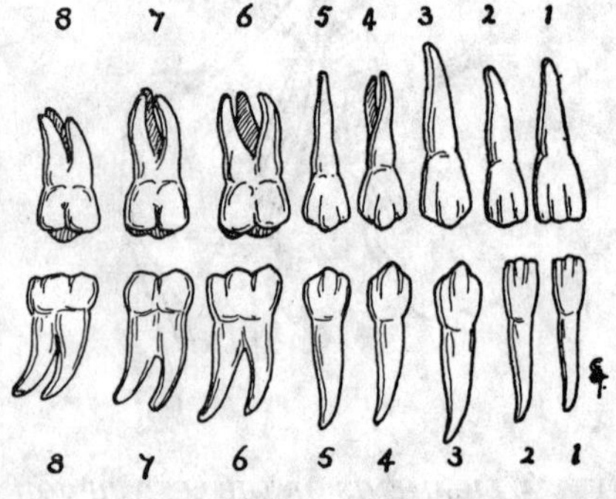

Fig. 42. *THE HUMAN TEETH (half set in upper and lower jaws).* 1. *Central incisor.* 2. *Lateral incisor.* 3. *Eye-tooth (canine).* 4. *Bicuspid.* 5. *Bicuspid.* 6. *Molar.* 7. *Molar.* 8. *Molar.*

Names. The four front teeth in each jaw, 1, 2, Fig. 42, are the cutting teeth (incisors); the next one, 3, is an eye-tooth or canine (cuspid); the next two, 4, 5, are small grinders or premolars (bicuspids); the last three, 6, 7, 8, are grinders (molars). One appears on each end of the upper and lower jaws between the ages of sixteen and twenty-four, and is called a wisdom tooth.

Structure. Each tooth is composed of four parts. The dentine or ivory forms the main part of each tooth, both in the crown and in the fang; in the former it is covered by enamel, and in the latter it is protected by a layer of cement. Enamel is the hardest tissue in the body and is a translucent white, but in old persons the biting surfaces of the teeth become worn and flattened in use. The cement is a thin layer of bone covering the root. The pulp in the central cavity of the tooth is soft and contains blood vessels and nerve fibers which pass into the dentine and render it sensitive.

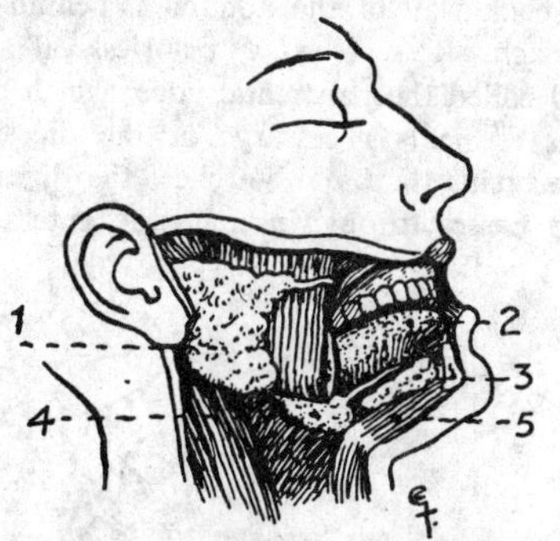

Fig. 43. *SALIVARY GLANDS OF THE MOUTH.* 1. *The parotid gland, and duct.* 2. *The tongue.* 3. *The sublingual gland.* 4. *The submaxillary gland and duct.* 5. *Hyoid muscle of floor of mouth.*

Use of the Teeth. The incisors bite the food apart; the molars break it down into smaller fragments and grind it to a fine smooth consistency for the stomach. In masticating the food the lower jaw has two movements, an up-and-down motion like a pair of shears, and a lateral or grinding motion; these two movements are performed by different sets of muscles. Flesh-eating animals have only the up-and-down motion; vegetable-eating animals have only the lateral or grinding motion; while man has both the up-and-down and the lateral movements. This seems a clear intimation that he requires both flesh and vegetables in his diet.

The teeth aid in articulating words, and they give roundness and symmetry to the lower part of the face. When well formed and kept in good condition they add much to the beauty of the face, and their decay is an irreparable loss.

THE DIGESTIVE ORGANS

The alimentary or digestive organs comprise the mouth, the teeth, the salivary glands, the pharynx, the gullet (esophagus), stomach, bowels (intestines), sweetbread (pancreas), chyle vessels (lacteals), liver and gall-bladder.

Salivary Glands

The preparatory process of digestion, the mastication of food, takes place in the mouth where the food is mixed with saliva, a secretion of the salivary glands. There are six of these glands, three on each side of the mouth.

The Parotid Gland lies near the angle of the jaw, in front of the ear; it has a duct opening into the mouth opposite the second molar tooth of the upper jaw. This is the gland that swells in the disease called mumps, hence the disease is also called parotitis.

The Submaxillary Gland lies on the floor of the mouth near the sides of the jaw. Its duct opens into the mouth by the side of the bridle of the tongue (frenum lingua). On each side of this string or bridle and under the mucous membrane of the floor of the mouth lies the **sublingual gland,** which pours its saliva into the mouth through several small ducts.

The Tongue

The tongue is a muscular organ covered with mucous membrane. The muscles pass in three directions so that it is very mobile. It serves to mix the food with the saliva and to force the food into the back of the pharynx in the process of swallowing. Taste buds are distributed over the mucous surface, each taste bud being the end organ of nerve fibers which carry the sensation of taste to the brain.

Pharynx and Gullet

The Pharynx is the cavity into which the mouth and nose open, and lies just below and behind the soft palate. The two passages to the nose (posterior nares), the gullet (esophagus) passing down to the stomach and the passage to the lungs (larynx and trachea) all meet in this cavity. Embedded in the walls of the upper pharynx are the tonsils which are part of the lymphatic system.

The Gullet or esophagus is a long tube descending behind the windpipe, the lungs, and the heart, and passing through the diaphragm into the stomach. It conveys food and fluids from the mouth to the stomach and is composed of three coats, the inner one being mucous, and the outer muscular with a central layer of connective tissue. The two sets of fibers composing the muscular coat are arranged circularly and longitudinally (see Fig. 38). The esophagus conveys food from the pharynx to the stomach by a wave-like rhythmic contraction of the muscular coat called *peristalsis.*

The Stomach

The stomach lies in the upper part of the abdomen on the left side. It is a sac-shaped organ, the upper end being the larger and being called the fundus. The esophagus passes into the stomach at an opening known as the cardiac orifice. The lower smaller end of the stomach connects with the first part of the small intestine, called the duodenum; the junction of the stomach and duodenum is called the pylorus. The two curved sides of the stomach walls are referred to as the greater and lesser curvatures (see Fig. 41). The walls consist of muscle, lined with mucous membrane and the outer surface is covered by serous membrane, the peritoneum. The glands of the mucous membrane secrete the gastric juices.

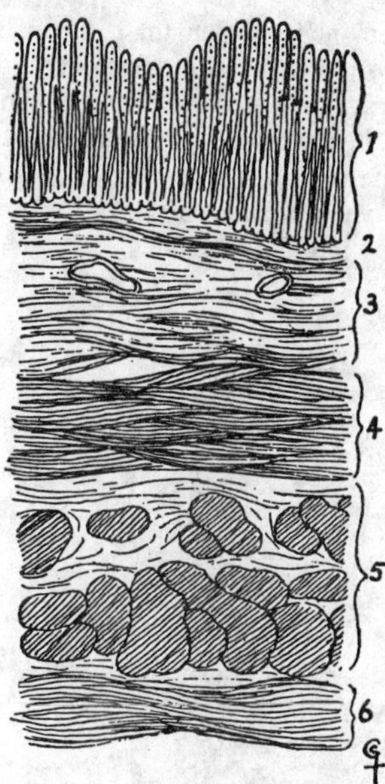

Fig. 44. *SECTION THROUGH THE STOMACH WALL.* 1. *Mucous membrane lining.* 2. *Lamina muscularis.* 3. *Submucous layer.* 4. *Circular muscular layer.* 5. *Longitudinal muscular layer.* 6. *Serous coat.*

The fundus, which is separated from the heart by the thin central tendon-sheet of the diaphragm, usually contains a little gas. Digestion takes place mainly in the lower part of the stomach, just before the pyloric junction.

The Intestines

The intestines, or bowels, consist of the small and large intestines. The small intestine has a length of about twenty feet and is divided into three parts, the duodenum, the jejunum, and the ileum. Of these three divisions, the duodenum is the widest and is

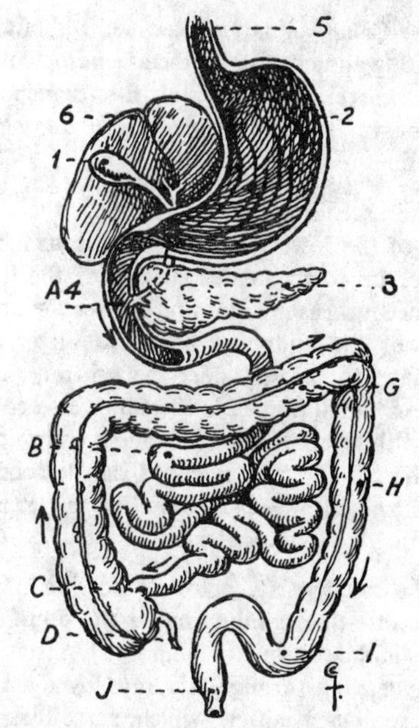

Fig. 45. *THE ALIMENTARY CANAL.* 1. *Gall-bladder.* 2. *Stomach.* 3. *Pancreas.* 4. *Duodenum.* 5. *Esophagus.* 6. *Liver (turned upwards).* A. *Duodenum.* B. *Small intestine.* C. *The junction of the small intestine with the ascending colon.* D. *The appendix.* G. *Transverse colon.* H. *Descending colon.* I. *Sigmoid flexure.* J. *Rectum.*

about ten inches in length. It begins at the pyloric orifice of the stomach, and passes backward to the under surface of the liver, whence it drops down perpendicularly in front of the right kidney and passes across the abdomen behind the colon, where it is continued into the jejunum.

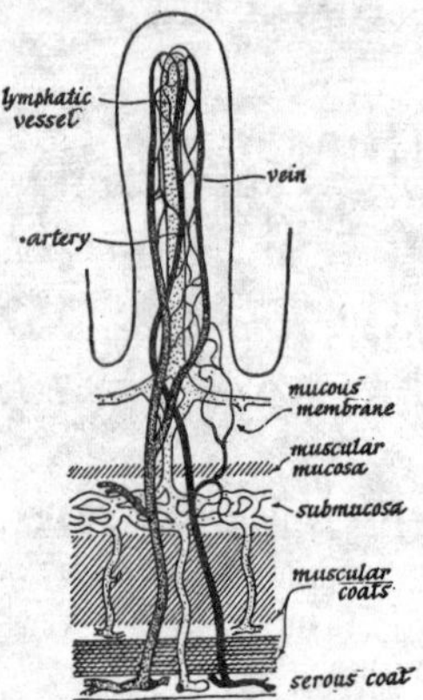

Fig. 46. *A VILLUS OF THE INTESTINAL WALL. The blood vessels in these innumerable minute finger-like projections on the intestinal wall absorb digested food, while the lymphatic vessels take in digested fat.*

The Jejunum is about eight or nine feet long and terminates in the ileum.

The Ileum is a continuation of the jejunum and opens in the lower part of the abdomen on the right side, into the colon. A valve located here prevents the backward passage of the bowel contents from the colon into the ileum. At this point the large intestine begins and connected with it is the cecum, a blind pouch or cul-de-sac attached to which is the appendix vermiformis, a worm-shaped tube about one-third of an inch in diameter, and from one to eight inches long.

The Colon, or large intestine, is about six feet long and consists of the ascending colon, the transverse colon and the descending colon. It is much wider than the small intestine.

The ascending colon rises from the right side of the lower part of the abdomen and passes up to the under surface of the liver, whence it turns inwards and crosses the upper part of the abdomen below the liver and stomach to the left side; the portion which crosses the abdomen is the transverse colon. From this point on the left side it turns down to the left hip and is called the descending colon; here it makes a curve like the letter S, forming the sigmoid flexure.

The Rectum is the lowest portion of the large intestine, terminating at the anus. The feces in the rectum are temporarily restrained from leaving through the anus by the ring-like sphincter muscle which surrounds the opening.

The Lacteals are small lymphatic vessels which arise in the villi (Fig. 46) of the mucous membrane lining the small bowel. From here they pass in the layers of the mesentery to small glands, from which larger lymphatic vessels run to other groups of glands and finally pour their contents, chyle, into the thoracic duct.

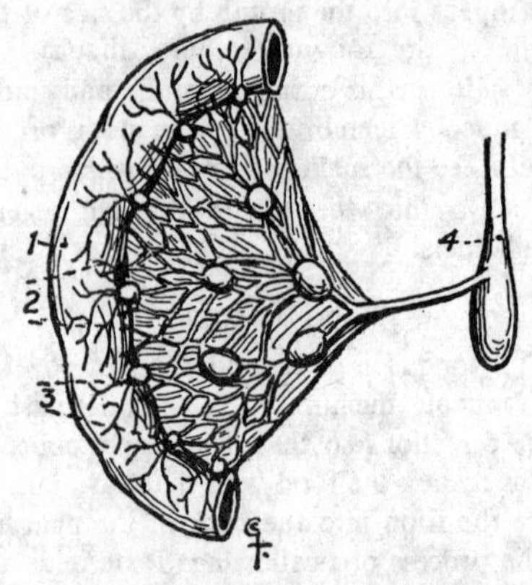

Fig. 47. *LACTEAL VESSELS AND MESENTERIC GLANDS. (1) The intestine where the lacteal vessels of the villi absorb nutriment. It is then conveyed by the small lacteals (2) to the mesenteric lymphatic glands (3), and thence via larger lymphatic vessels to the thoracic duct (4) near the neck.*

Other Organs Associated with the Digestive System

The Mesentery of the abdomen is a double sheet of membrane formed by several folds of the peritoneum, and spreads out from the back wall of the abdomen like a fan. The small intestine is attached to its edge and is supported by it, at the same time having free motion. Between its layers are the mesenteric artery and vein with their branches, and a great number of lymphatic glands.

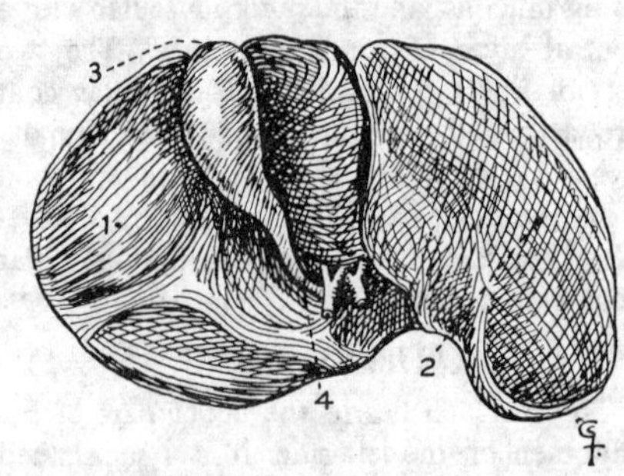

Fig. 48. *THE LIVER (under surface).* 1. *Right lobe* 2. *Left lobe.* 3. *Gall-bladder.* 4. *Cystic, or bile, duct.*

The Liver is a large solid gland lying under the short ribs on the right side of the upper part of the abdomen below the diaphragm; it is convex on the upper surface and concave below, and is composed of four lobes. The liver has many functions, including secretion of bile, storage of glycogen or animal starch, and conversion of waste products into urea and uric acid for excretion.

The Gall-bladder is a small sac which lies on the under side of the liver; bile passes into it from the liver and becomes concentrated before it is transported along the bile duct to the duodenum to assist in the digestion of fats.

The Pancreas, Fig. 49, is an elongated secreting gland which lies transversely across the back wall of the abdomen, behind the stomach. It secretes a colorless alkaline fluid called the pancreatic juice, which contains ferments necessary for the digestion of proteins, fats and starches; the digestive fluid passes through a duct and enters the duodenum near the opening of the bile duct. The hormone insulin, which prevents diabetes mellitus, is also secreted by special cells in the pancreas.

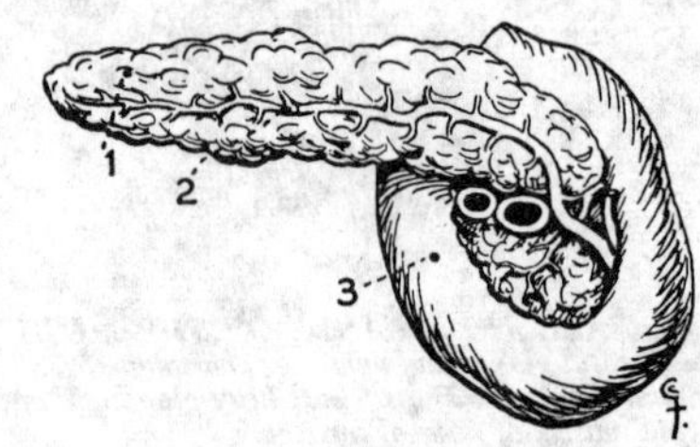

Fig. 49. *THE PANCREAS (back view).* 1. *Body of pancreas.* 2. *Pancreatic duct.* 3. *Duodenum.*

The Omentum is a long fold of the peritoneum. It is loaded with fat and lies in front of the bowels in the abdominal cavity and is attached to the stomach. It protects and keeps the bowels warm; hence it is often called the apron.

THE URINARY SYSTEM

The organs of the urinary system form urine from blood and convey it out of the body. These organs comprise the two kidneys, the ureters, the bladder and the urethra.

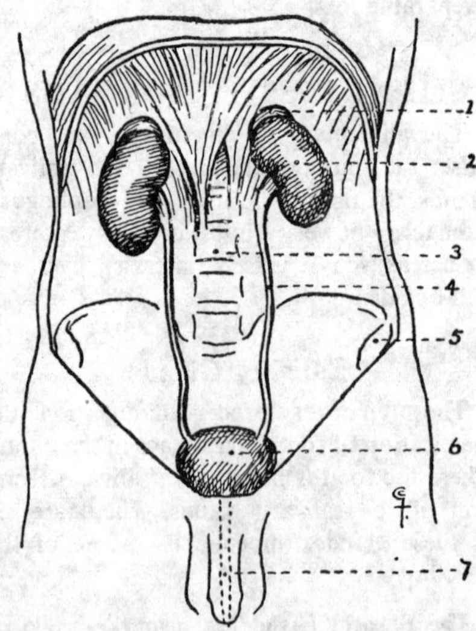

Fig. 50. *MALE URINARY SYSTEM.* 1. *Left adrenal gland.* 2. *Left kidney.* 3. *Vertebra of spinal column.* 4. *Left ureter.* 5. *Crest of ilium.* 6. *Bladder.* 7. *Urethra in penis.*

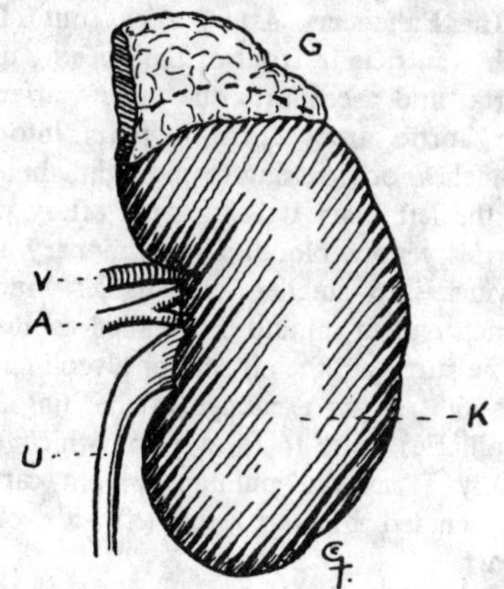

Fig. 51. *THE KIDNEY.* A. *Renal artery.* U. *Ureter to bladder.* G. *Adrenal (or suprarenal) gland.* K. *Kidney* V. *Renal vein.*

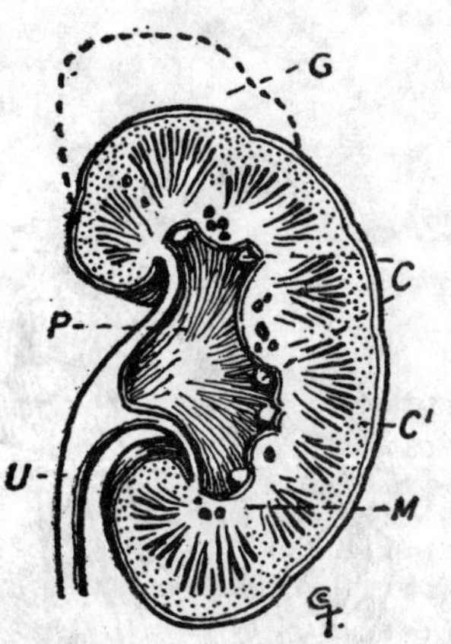

Fig. 52. *INTERNAL STRUCTURE OF THE KIDNEY.* G. *Capsule of adrenal gland.* C. *Papillae of calices of kidney.* P. *Pelvis of kidney.* U. *Ureter.* C[1]. *Cortex, or outer zone of kidney.* M. *Medulla, or inner zone of kidney.*

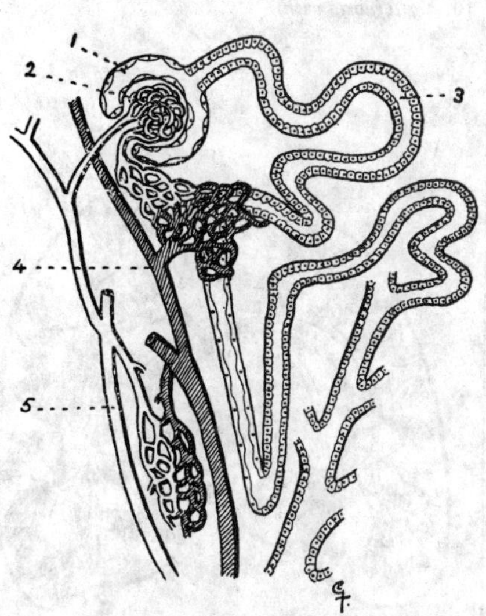

Fig. 53. *CIRCULATION WITHIN THE KIDNEY.* 1. *Capsule containing blood vessels.* 2. *Coil of blood vessels (glomerulus).* 3. *Tubule secreting urine.* 4. *Vein.* 5. *Artery.*

The Kidneys lie one on each side of the backbone in the lumbar region, behind the peritoneum. They are about four inches long, and two and a half inches broad. They are shaped like the kidney-bean and weigh about four to five ounces each. On the inner concave side is the pelvis of the kidney, which tapers like a funnel and unites with the ureter which conveys the urine to the bladder. Each kidney is covered by a tough fibrous capsule; the tissue of the kidney is divided into two zones, the outer layer or *cortex* being about one-half of an inch thick, and the internal zone or *medulla.* The cortex contains the expanded ends of the renal tubules (or nephrons) each containing a small knot of capillaries, which give the cortex its dark red color. The medulla contains parallel rows of renal tubules which carry the fluid, which has been filtered from the blood into the nephrons, to the ureters; as the fluid passes through the tubules in the medulla it becomes altered by the tubules and so urine is formed.

The Ureters are membranous tubes about the diameter of a goose quill and twelve to eighteen inches long, which run down the back wall of the abdomen behind the peritoneum to the bladder, into each side of which they open obliquely; they carry the urine from the kidneys to the bladder.

The Bladder lies in the pelvis, in front of the rectum. The wall consists of three coats; the external covering is serous, the middle layer muscular, and the internal is composed of mucous membrane. The external coat is strong and fibrous; the internal mucous layer is drawn into wrinkled folds; it secretes mucus which prevents it from being injured in cystitis. The urine is retained in the bladder by means of a circular muscle called a sphincter, which closes the mouth of the organ. When the quantity of urine (about twelve ounces) is so increased as to cause some uneasiness or pain, this muscle by reflex stimulation relaxes and the urine is passed. The bladder is attached by several ligaments to the rectum, to the hip bones, to the peritoneum and to the navel. In the female the womb lies between the bladder and the rectum.

The Urethra is a membranous canal which leads from the neck of the bladder; it is composed of three layers, mucous membrane, a submucous layer and a thick muscular layer. Through this passage the urine passes out of the body.

The structure of the urethra is different in the male and female. The male urethra is longer and passes from the neck of the bladder right through to the tip of the penis. It forms a common pathway for urine and the secretions from the reproductive organs. The female urethra is about 1½ inches long and empties between the labia minora in front of the vaginal opening.

THE RESPIRATORY SYSTEM

These organs consist of the nose, pharynx, larynx, windpipe (trachea), the branches of the windpipe (bronchi), and the lungs with their alveoli or small air sacs.

When air is breathed in through the nostrils it passes into the nasal cavity on the sides of which are three scroll-like processes of bone covered with mucous membrane. These are the turbinates or conchae which act as radiators, warming the air and moistening it. The hairs in the nostrils function as sieves to remove dust particles. The inhaled air (via either the nose or mouth) then passes into the middle or oro-pharynx which is a hollow tube shared by both the respiratory and alimentary tracts. The air is drawn into the larynx which is protected by a flap of elastic cartilage, the *epiglottis,* against invasion of food particles going via the back part of the pharynx into the esophagus. From the larynx (voice box) the air continues through the trachea into the bronchi and the bronchioles where it comes into intimate contact with the large absorbing surface of the small air sacs or alveoli of the lungs (see Figs. 54, 56 and 57).

The Trachea (windpipe) extends from the larynx, the organ of the voice, to the third dorsal vertebra, where it divides into two tubes called bronchi. It runs down the front of the throat, and the esophagus behind runs between it and the spinal column; it is composed mainly of rings of cartilage, one above another, so that it resists closure by pressure.

The Bronchial Tubes are formed by the division of the trachea, and are two in number, but they divide and subdivide until they become very numerous, and branch into small bronchioles.

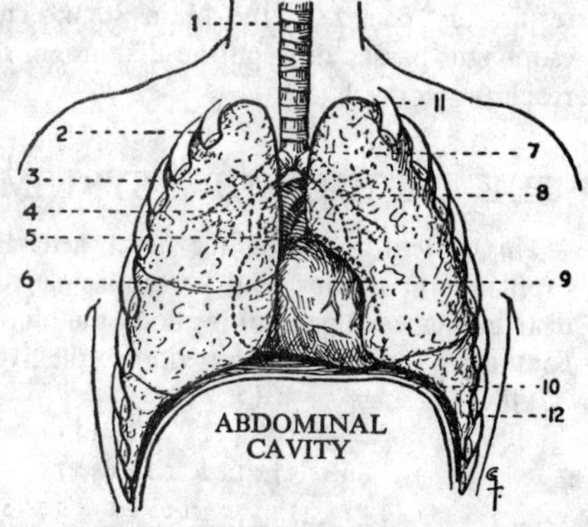

Fig. 54. *LUNGS, TRACHEA AND HEART IN RELATION TO ABDOMINAL CAVITY.* 1. *The trachea.* 2. *Ribs cut away.* 3. *Right lung, exposed.* 4. *Right bronchus, branching in lung.* 5. *Arch of the aorta.* 6. *Right border of heart.* 7. *Left lung, exposed.* 8. *Left bronchus, branching in lung.* 9. *Heart.* 10. *Diaphragm (cut through).* 11. *Apex of lung.* 12. *Base of left lung.*

The Air Sacs or **Alveoli** of the lungs are small bladder-like expansions at the ends of the bronchial tubes. They are expansile and dilate when the air passes into the lungs at each inhalation.

The Lungs

The lungs fill the greater part of the chest, the heart being the only other organ which normally occupies much space in the thorax. The size of these two organs varies according to the capacity of the chest. Each lung is cone-shaped, with its base resting upon the diaphragm and its apex lying behind the collar-bone. The lungs are concave below where they are in contact with the diaphragm, which is convex on its upper side. The right and left lungs are separated from each other by the mediastinum which is a space formed by two portions of the pleura, a smooth serous membrane attached behind to the spine and closely enveloping each lung; the heart is covered by the pericardium and lies in the center between them.

The right lung is divided into three lobes; the left is composed of two lobes. Each lobe of the lungs is divided into a great many lobules which are connected by cellular tissue; these lobules are also divided into very fine air sacs or alveoli. The lungs also contain innumerable fine blood vessels and capillaries, nerves and lymphatics.

Before the lungs of a newborn baby have been filled with air they are solid and heavy, but, after their cells have once been filled with air and breathing has been established, they are light and spongy and float upon water. Complete opening of the air sacs of the lungs is not attained until the infant is between two and three weeks old.

The Diaphragm

The chief muscles used in breathing are the diaphragm and the small muscles between the ribs. The diaphragm (see Fig. 54) is a large, thin, dome-shaped muscle dividing the chest and abdominal cavities. Rhythmic breathing throughout life is under the control of the respiratory center in the brain stem. The esophagus passes through the diaphragm to reach the stomach.

THE CIRCULATORY SYSTEM

This system comprises the heart, arteries, capillaries and veins, and is responsible for distributing to all parts of the body the blood containing food and oxygen vital to the lives of all the tissues.

The Heart

The heart lies obliquely in the chest, with one lung on each side, and it is enclosed between the two walls of the mediastinum. Its form is like a cone or pear, with its base turned upward and backward in the direction of the right shoulder, and the apex lying forward and to the left, occupying the space between the fifth and sixth ribs, about three inches from the breastbone and above the diaphragm. It is surrounded by a membranous sac called the pericardium and is lined by the endocardium.

The human heart is a four-chambered hollow muscular organ and has its fibers interwoven so that it is endowed with great strength. It has two sides, a right and a left, which are divided from each other by a muscular partition called a septum. The right side receives the venous blood from all over the body and sends it for aeration to the lungs; the left side receives oxygenated blood back from the lungs and distributes it to the entire system. Each side is divided into two chambers, an auricle and a ventricle, and these communicate with each other by a valvular opening, through which the blood passes from the auricle above to the ventricle below, the valve preventing regurgitation. (See also Fig. 8, p. 242.)

The Auricles have thinner walls than the ventricles, being reservoirs to hold the blood until the ventricles force it along into the arteries for transmission through the body.

The Ventricles have fleshy columns on their inner surfaces, called columnae carneae. The walls of the left ventricle are much thicker than those of the right, being required to contract with more force. Each of the four cavities will contain from one and a half to two ounces of blood.

The Tricuspid Valve is situated between the auricle and ventricle on the right side, and consists of three folds of a thin triangular membrane. The mitral valve occupies the corresponding position on the left side. Small white cords called chordae tendinae pass from the floating edge of these valves to the columnae carneae, to prevent the backward pressure of the blood from carrying the valves into the auricles.

The pulmonary artery is the outlet of the right ventricle; the large artery called the aorta passes out from the left ventricle. At the opening of these arteries are membranous folds called semilunar valves.

The Arteries

The arteries are the blood vessels which carry the red oxygenated blood from the left side of the heart to every part of the body. The walls of arteries are elastic, dilating each time the heart beats and pumps the blood through them. They have three coats: an external fibrous coat, a middle coat of elastic tissue; and an internal coat of smooth endothelium like that lining the heart. After the arteries have divided and become much smaller they are termed arterioles; these vessels have smooth muscle instead of elastic tissue in the middle coat of the vessel wall. The muscle is innervated by the autonomic nervous system and when it contracts the arteriole becomes much smaller thus restricting the flow of blood through the vessel. In this way the flow of blood to any particular organ can be regulated by alteration in size of the arterioles.

The Pulmonary Artery opens out of the right ventricle in front of the opening of the aorta, and ascends to the under surface of the aortic arch where it parts into two branches, one passing to the right, the other to the left lung. It is the only artery which carries venous blood. The pulmonary artery divides into smaller and smaller branches which end in minute thin-walled capillaries; these surround the air sacs or alveoli and are the site of gas exchange in the lungs. The capillaries unite to form veins which eventually form the pulmonary vein carrying oxygenated blood to the left side of the heart.

Fig. 55 shows the heart and great vessels: 1, is the right auricle; 2, the left auricle; 3, the right ventricle; 4, the left ventricle; 5, 6, 7, 8, 9, 10, are the vessels which bring the blood to and carry it away from the heart.

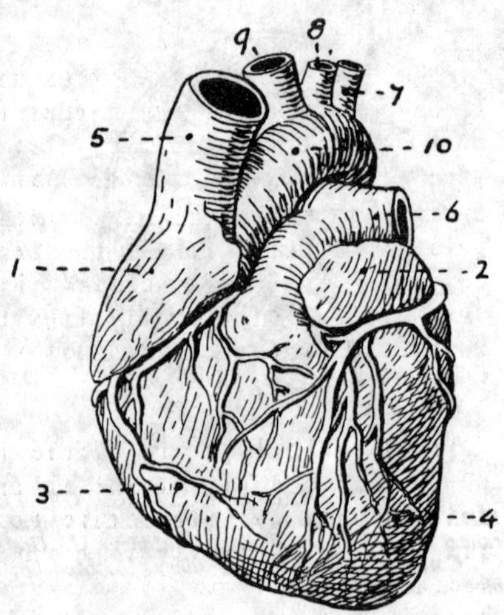

Fig. 55. *THE HEART.* 1. *Right auricle.* 2. *Left auricle.* 3. *Right ventricle.* 4. *Left ventricle.* 5. *Superior vena cava.* 6. *Pulmonary artery.* 7. *Left subclavian artery.* 8. *Common carotid artery.* 9. *Innominate artery.* 10. *Aorta (aorta arch).*

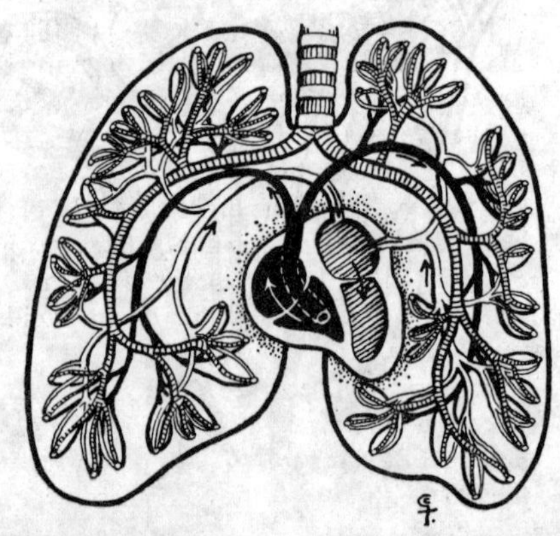

Fig. 56. *CIRCULATION OF HEART AND LUNGS. The dark venous blood returns to the heart and is pumped into the lungs, whence it returns re-oxygenated for circulation through the whole body.*

The Aorta is the largest artery in the body. After leaving the heart it curves down in the chest, this curve being called the arch of the aorta; from it are given off the arteries which carry the blood to the head and arms. It then descends into the thorax and abdomen along the side of the backbone, and at the bottom of the abdomen it divides into two arteries called the iliac arteries, one passing to each of the lower limbs.

The Veins

The veins carry the dark purple or venous blood which contains carbon dioxide. Having been oxygenated by the atmospheric air in the lungs, and then being conveyed in the arteries to every part of the body, the blood gives up its oxygen in the capillaries, and returns in the veins to the heart for re-oxygenation in the lungs. The veins are more numerous and are generally nearer the surface than are the arteries; they have thinner walls and when empty these collapse or fall together. The veins are formed by the union of the capillaries and, joining together, they grow larger and larger, and finally form the great trunks which pour the dark blood into the right auricle. The veins are composed of three coats similar to those of the arteries, except they are thinner and more delicate. These vessels have valves all along their inner surface to prevent the back-flow of the blood.

Vena Cava. The large vein which receives all the dark blood from the head and arms and pours it into the right auricle is called the superior vena cava; the vein which brings it back from the lower part of the body and transmits it to the same chamber is the inferior vena cava.

The pulmonary veins bring the red oxygenated blood from the lungs to the left auricle, and are thus exceptional, being the only veins which carry red blood.

The Capillaries are minute blood vessels whose walls are only one cell thick; it is through these vessels that exchange of fluid between the blood and tissues takes place. The capillaries form an extensive network in the tissues connecting the arterioles with the smaller veins.

Fig. 57 is a good diagram of the whole circulation. From the right ventricle of the heart, 2, the dark venous blood passes into the pulmonary artery, 3; and its branches, 4, 5, carry it to both lungs. In the capillary vessels, 6, 6, the blood comes into contact with the air and becomes red and oxygenated. Thence it is returned to the left auricle of the heart, 9, by the veins, 7, 8, and passes into the left ventricle, 10. A forcible contraction of the left ventricle sends it forward into the aorta, 11, whose branches, 12, 13, 13, distribute it to all parts of the body. The arteries terminate in the capillaries, 14, 14. From these the blood gives up its oxygen and goes back to the right auricle, 1; by the superior vena cava, 15; and the inferior vena cava, 16. The tricuspid valves, 17, prevent the return of the blood from the right ventricle back into the right auricle. The pulmonary valves, 18, prevent the blood from passing back from the pulmonary artery to the right ventricle. The mitral valves, 19, prevent it flowing back from the left ventricle to the left auricle. The semilunar valves, 20, prevent the return flow from the aorta into the left ventricle.

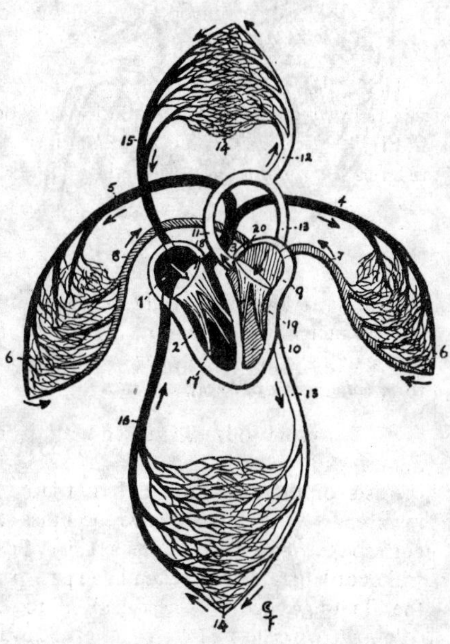

Fig. 57. *CIRCULATORY SYSTEM OF THE BODY showing oxygenation of the blood within the lungs.* 1. *The right auricle of the heart.* 2. *The right ventricle of the heart.* 3. *The pulmonary artery.* 4. *Left branch of the pulmonary artery.* 5. *Right branch of the pulmonary artery.* 6. *Capillary blood vessels of the lungs.* 7. *The left pulmonary vein.* 8. *The right pulmonary vein.* 9. *The left auricle of the heart.* 10. *The left ventricle of the heart.* 11 and 13. *The aorta.* 12. *Branches of the aorta.* 14. *Capillary blood vessels of the body.* 15. *The superior vena cava.* 16. *The inferior vena cava.* 17. *The tricuspid valves.* 18. *The pulmonary valves.* 19. *The mitral valves.* 20. *The semilunar valves.*

The passage of the blood from the right heart through the lungs and back to the left heart is called the lesser, or pulmonary circulation; its passage from the left heart through all parts of the body and back to the right heart is the greater or systemic circulation.

The Blood

The blood is the fluid circulating in the arteries and veins through the different organs and tissues. It consists of fluid or plasma, together with cells or corpuscles which are of three varieties, namely the red blood corpuscles or erythrocytes, the white blood corpuscles or leucocytes, and blood platelets.

The fluid plasma contains salts and soluble food substances, waste products which are carried round to the kidneys for filtration, and endocrine secretions or hormones.

The Red Cells contain hemoglobin, an iron compound which is the oxygen-carrrying substance of the blood. Each is shaped like a biconcave disc, and consists of a cell without a nucleus about 1/3000th of an inch in diameter; when blood is allowed to stand these cells adhere together and form chains or rouleaux. There are about 5,000,000 red cells in every cubic millimeter (a *very* small drop) of blood in a healthy person.

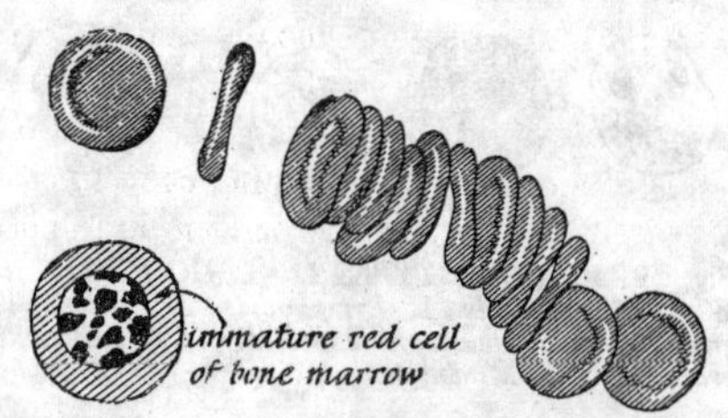

Fig. 58. *ERYTHROCYTES, or Red Blood Cells. Front and side views, and cells in clumped rouleaux formation.*

The White Cells or leucocytes are nucleated cells of several different types, some containing characteristic granules in the cytoplasm. Leucocytes have the ability to pass through vessel walls into the tissues where they assist in the repair of injury, destroy bacteria and absorb dead tissue. There are normally only about 7,000 leucocytes in every cubic millimeter of blood but the numbers may increase considerably in certain diseases. When large numbers of white blood cells die in conflict with bacteria or germs, their dead bodies form pus such as is found in boils, abscesses and discharging wounds.

Blood Platelets or thrombocytes are somewhat oval in shape and about one-third the size of red corpuscles. They are derived from giant cells in the bone marrow and have no nuclei. They provide thromboplastin, a substance which initiates blood clotting after hemorrhage.

THE LYMPHATIC SYSTEM

The lymphatic system consists of a network of delicate vessels draining most tissues and communicating with each other through collections of lymph glands which are to be found in axillae, groins, and in special sites in the neck, thorax and abdomen. In the lymph glands a special type of white cell, known as a lymphocyte, is formed. The glands also act as filters, preventing bacteria from passing into the blood from an infected area. When local infection such as a boil occurs, the lymph glands draining the area become enlarged and tender.

The lymphatic vessels draining the small intestine are called lacteals and are concerned with the absorption of fat; following a fatty meal the lacteals become filled with a milky fluid called chyle, which consists of an emulsion of fat particles. The lymphatics all over the body finally unite to form one large vessel, the thoracic duct, which passes up through the diaphragm and then empties into the jugular vein in the neck.

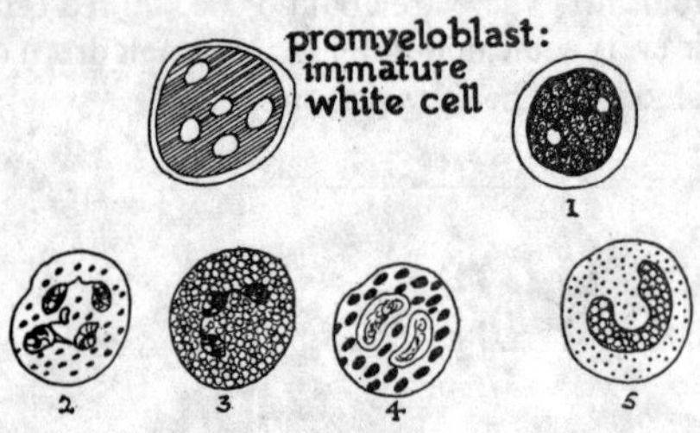

Fig. 59. *VARIOUS TYPES OF LEUCOCYTES, or White Blood Cells. 1. Lymphocyte. 2. Eosinophilic granulocyte. 3. Neutrophilic granulocyte. 4. Basophilic granulocyte. 5. Monocyte.*

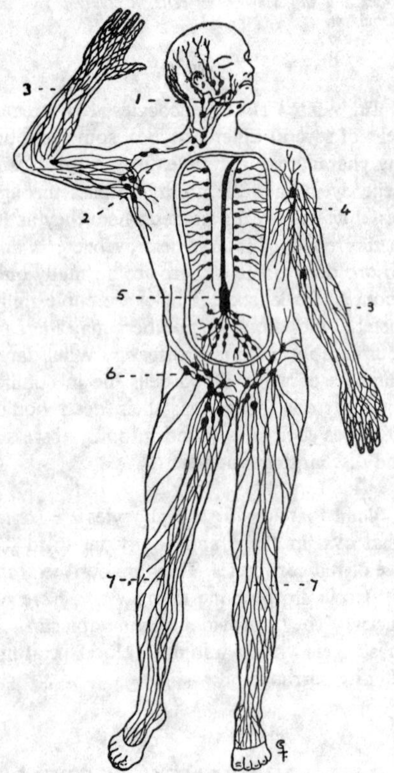

Fig. 60. *THE LYMPHATIC SYSTEM. 1. Glands of the face and neck. 2. Axillary glands. 3. Lymphatic vessels of the arm. 4. Thoracic duct. 5. Chyle reservoir. 6. Inguinal glands. 7. Lymphatic vessels of the leg.*

The Tonsils are aggregations of lymphatic tissue lying on either side of the upper or oral pharynx. They form part of a ring of lymphatic tissue protecting the oral and nasal openings. The adenoid tissue lying in the upper back wall of the pharynx is part of this ring of tissue.

The Spleen, a dark purplish, soft, crescent-shaped organ of lymphatic tissue about six inches long, lies on the left side of the abdomen in its upper part, just under the diaphragm and close to the stomach and pancreas. It contains a great number of blood vessels and assists in the production of white blood cells, while useless worn-out red blood cells are broken up in the spleen. In infections caused by bacteria or tropical parasites, the spleen becomes greatly enlarged.

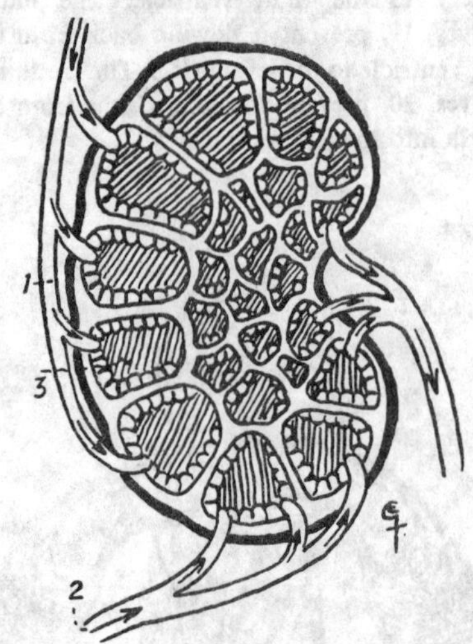

Fig. 61. *A LYMPHATIC GLAND.* 1 and 2. *Lymphatic vessels. 3. Lymphoid tissue.*

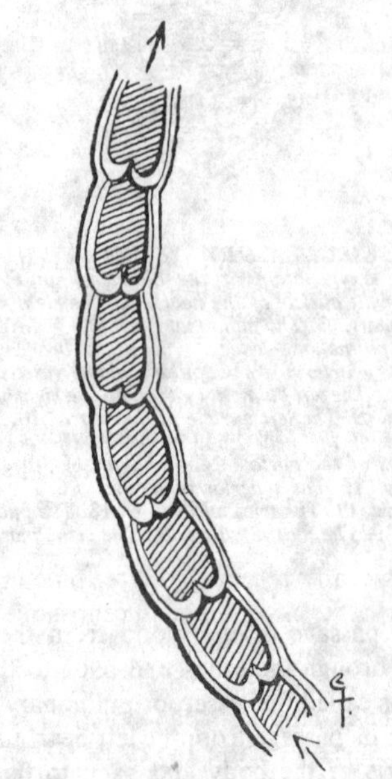

Fig. 62. *A LYMPHATIC VESSEL. Arrows show the direction of flow of lymph.*

THE NERVOUS SYSTEM

The brain and spinal cord are, in structure and function, so integrated as to form a continuous organ. This **Central Nervous System** is a hollow tube filled with cerebrospinal fluid and enclosed throughout by protective layers of tissue known as meninges. The cerebrospinal fluid between two of these layers gives added protection, cushioning the very delicate and vital nerve tissue against shocks or violent movements. Connected with the brain are twelve pairs of cranial nerves which, with thirty-one pairs of spinal nerves, form the **Peripheral Nervous System.** These nerves are distributed thoughout the body.

Parts of the body which work automatically, e.g. the liver, the heart, and the skin, are controlled from the central nervous system via outlying nerve cells grouped into ganglia which, together with the nerve fibers arising from the ganglia, form the **Autonomic Nervous System.** The latter is also known as the involuntary, visceral, or vegetative system. Here the functioning is divided into the work of the *sympathetic system*—preparing the body for activity—and that of the *parasympathetic system*—controlling the body at rest and rebuilding tissue.

The nerve fibers of the autonomic system travel with the peripheral nerves and are connected with ganglionic plexuses (networks) found in the head, neck and trunk.

The Brain

The brain consists of five main divisions, the cerebrum or fore brain, the basal ganglia, the mid brain, the cerebellum or hind brain, and the medulla oblongata. It is covered and protected by three membranes, the meninges, which are separated by fluid. These three membranes are known as the dura mater, the arachnoid, and the pia mater.

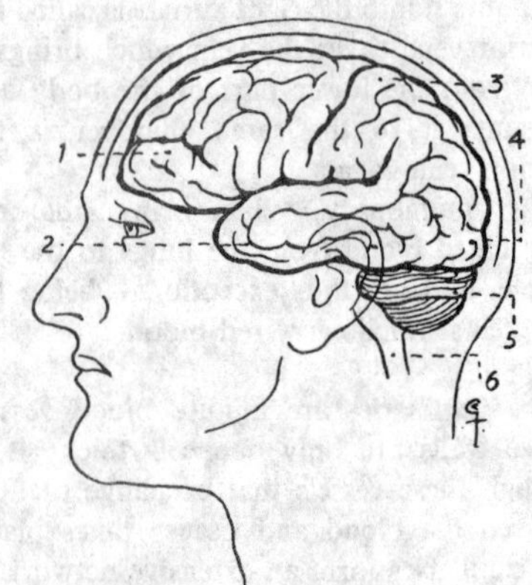

Fig. 63. *THE BRAIN. 1. Frontal lobe. 2. Temporo-sphenoidal lobe. 3. Parietal lobe. 4. Occipital lobe. 5. Cerebellum. 6. Medulla.*

The Cerebrum is the upper and larger portion of the brain, and occupies the whole of the vault or dome of the cranium. It is divided into two cerebral hemispheres by a deep cleft or fissure; a portion of the dura mater dips into this cleft and from its resemblance to a sickle is called the falx cerebri. It thus supports each half of the brain and prevents it from pressing upon the other half when the head inclines to one side. The undulating surface of the cerebrum is formed by what are called convolutions or gyri, with their intervening sulci or grooves. The cerebrum is divided into four main lobes, the anterior or frontal, the middle or parietal, the posterior or occipital, and the lateral or temporal lobes.

The surface layer of the cerebrum is called the cortex and is of a gray color, being cellular; the central portion called the medulla is white and consists of nerve fibers. Deeply embedded in the white matter are masses of gray matter know as basal ganglia, the largest being the *thalamus* which is the main subconscious center.

The cerebrum is associated with the intellectual faculties and controls the other parts of the central nervous system and the muscular system.

The Cerebellum is about one-sixth the size of the cerebrum. It lies just under the posterior lobe of the cerebrum, and is separated from it by an extension of the dura mater called the tentorium cerebelli. It is composed of white and gray matter; when the former is cut it resembles the trunk and branches of a tree, and is called the *arbor vitae.* The cerebellum regulates the muscular movements and postural equilibrium.

The Medulla Oblongata is the lowest pyramidal part of the brain, and in structure resembles the spinal cord with which it is continuous. It is about one and a quarter inches long and contains centers which control various important functions such as respiration, digestion, and the action of the heart.

The Meninges

The Dura Mater is a strong fibrous membrane which lines the skull and spinal column, and sends folds or processes inward to support the different lobes of the brain and the nerves which go out from the brain and spinal cord.

The Arachnoid Mater is a serous membrane and, like all other serous membranes, is a closed sac. It is reflected upon the inner surface of the dura mater.

The Pia Mater is a vascular membrane and lies next to and invests the whole surface of the brain, enfolding its convolutions. It transmits blood vessels to the brain.

The Cranial Nerves

The cranial nerves pass out from the brain in twelve pairs. In reading a description of them, let the reader keep his eye on Fig. 64.

The First Pair, the olfactory nerves (6), pass through several small openings in the ethmoid bone, and are distributed to the mucous membrane which lines the nose. If they are cut or destroyed the sense of smell is lost.

The Second Pair, the optic nerves (7), pass through the base of the skull, and enter the orbit where they spread out over the inner surface of the wall of the eye, namely the retina. Disease of these nerves may impair sight, or cause total blindness.

The Third Pair, the oculomotor nerves (9), pass through the sphenoid bone to the muscles of the eye and control their movements.

The Fourth Pair, or trochlear nerves (10), pass to the superior oblique muscle of the eye.

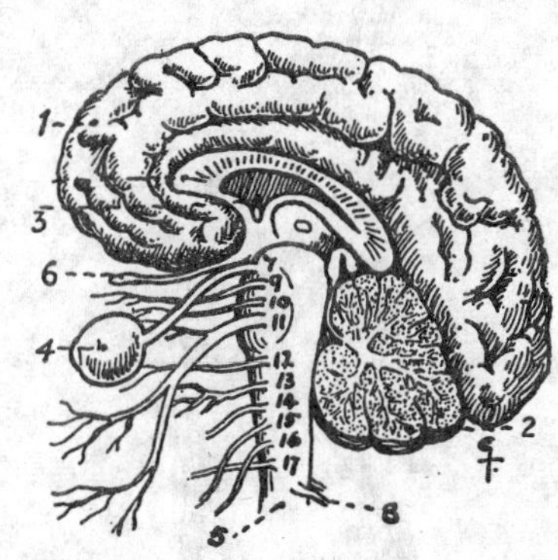

Fig. 64. *SECTION OF THE BRAIN SHOWING SPINAL CORD AND CRANIAL NERVES.* 1. *Frontal lobe.* 2. *Cerebellum.* 3. *Corpus callosum (cavity).* 4. *Globe of eye.* 5. *Spinal cord.* 6. *Olfactory nerves (1st Pair).* 7. *Optic nerves (2nd Pair).* 9. *Oculomotor nerves (3rd Pair).* 10. *Trochlear nerves (4th Pair).* 11. *Trigeminal nerves (5th Pair).* 12. *Abducent nerves (6th Pair).* 13. *Facial nerves (7th Pair).* 14. *Auditory nerves (8th Pair).* 15. *Glosso-pharyngeal nerves (9th Pair).* 16. *Pneumogastric or vagus nerves (10th Pair).* 8. *Spinal accessory nerves (11th Pair).* 17. *Hypoglossal nerves (12th Pair).*

The Fifth Pair, the trigeminal nerves (11), like the spinal nerves have two roots, and each nerve divides into three branches, one going to the eye, forehead, and nose, called the ophthalmic branch; another supplies the eye, the teeth of the upper jaw, etc., and is called the superior maxillary nerve; and the third goes to the ear, the tongue, and the teeth of the lower jaw, and is called the inferior maxillary nerve. Disease of the branches of the fifth pair gives rise to the neuralgic affection called tic douloureux.

The Sixth Pair, the abducent nerves (12), pass through the opening by which the carotid artery enters the cavity of the skull, and go to the external rectus muscles of the eye.

The Seventh Pair, the facial nerves (13), are distributed over the face and send filaments to the muscles.

The Eighth Pair, the auditory nerves (14), supply the structures in the internal ear.

The Ninth Pair, or glosso-pharyngeal nerves (15), pass through the same opening as the jugular vein and are distributed upon the mucous membrane of the tongue and throat.

The Tenth Pair, the vagi (16), supply the pharynx, larynx, gullet, lungs, spleen, pancreas, liver, stomach and bowels.

The Eleventh Pair, or spinal accessory nerves (8), connect with the ninth and tenth pairs, and are distributed to the muscles of the neck.

The Twelfth Pair, the hypoglossal nerves (17), go to the tongue and are the motor nerves of this organ.

The Spinal Cord

The spinal cord is about sixteen or eighteen inches long and extends from the medulla oblongata, which is continuous with the brain, down to the second lumbar vertebra, lying within the spinal column. The upper end of the cord presents a bulbous swelling or enlargement; another swelling is found where the nerves are given off which go to the upper extremities, and a third occurs near the end of the cord where the nerves which go to the lower extremities begin.

The cord is cylindrical in shape and is about as thick as the little finger, being slightly flattened from front to back. It is covered by extensions of the three membranes that surround the brain, namely the dura mater, the arachnoid mater and the pia mater. The cord consists mainly of white nerve fibers, but there is some gray matter in the center.

The cord is fissured or grooved in front and behind, and is thus divided into two lateral parts, which are united by a thin layer of white substance. These lateral parts are divided by furrows into anterior, lateral, and posterior columns; the anterior column is the motor column, the posterior contains sensory fiber and the lateral column is mixed. The cord ends in a sheath of nerves called the cauda equina.

The Spinal Nerves

The spinal nerves are given off from the cord in pairs, of which there are thirty-one. Each pair (Fig. 65) has two roots: a motor root, 4, arising from the anterior columns of the cord, and a sensory root, 3, springing from the posterior columns. 1, is a section of the cord, surrounded by its sheath, with two spinal nerves, formed by the union of the motor and sensory roots.

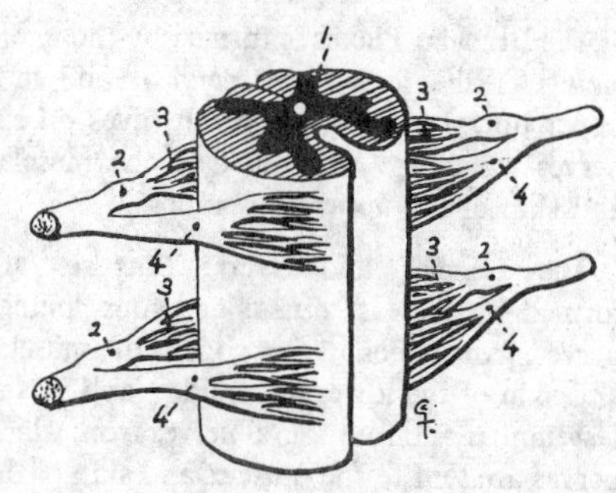

Fig. 65. *THE SPINAL CORD.* 1. *Cross section of the spinal cord, showing gray and white matter.* 2. *Dorsal root ganglia.* 3. *Sensory nerve roots (posterior).* 4. *Motor nerve roots (anterior).*

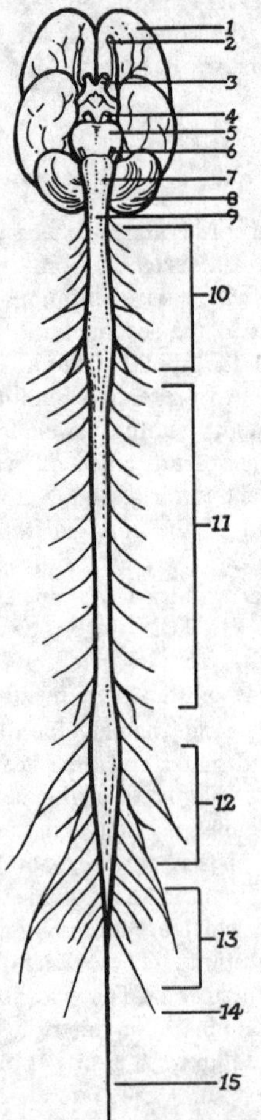

Fig. 66. *THE BRAIN AND SPINAL CORD, WITH CRANIAL AND SPINAL NERVES.* 1. *Left hemisphere of brain.* 2. *Olfactory nerve.* 3. *Optic nerve.* 4. *Oculomotor nerve.* 5. *Pons variolii.* 6. *Abducens nerve.* 7. *Medulla oblongata.* 8. *Cerebellum.* 9. *Spinal cord.* 10. *Eight cervical nerves.* 11. *Twelve thoracic nerves.* 12. *Five lumbar nerves.* 13. *Five sacral nerves.* 14. *Coccygeal nerve.* 15. *Filum terminale.*

After the union the nerve, with its motor and its sensory branches divides and subdivides as it passes on, and is distributed to the tissues of the part which it supplies. The thirty-one pairs of spinal nerves are divided into eight pairs of cervical, twelve pairs of dorsal (or thoracic), five pairs of lumbar, five pairs of sacral, and one pair of coccygeal nerves.

The Brachial Plexus is formed by the interlacing of the four lower cervical and first upper dorsal pairs of nerves. It gives off six nerves which are distributed to the muscles and skin of the upper extremities.

The Lumbar and **Sacral Plexuses** are formed by the last dorsal and four lumbar nerves, from which nerves go into the muscles and skin of the lower extremities, and by the last lumbar and four sacral nerves from which nerves are sent to the muscles and skin of the hips and lower extremities.

Fig. 67 represents a plexus, showing how the filaments of one nerve pass to be enclosed in the sheath of another.

The Autonomic Nervous System

This division of the nervous system controls the activities which function independently of the will, e.g. secretion of glands, activity of intestinal muscle, etc. It is divided on an anatomical and a functional basis into the **sympathetic and the parasympathetic nervous systems.**

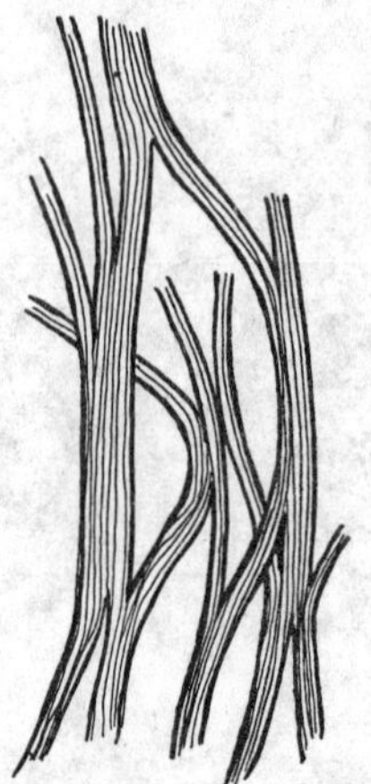

Fig. 67. *A NERVE PLEXUS*

The Sympathetic Nervous System consists of nerve fibers which run from the spinal cord in the thoracic and upper lumbar region to groups of nerve cells or ganglia which form a chain on either side of the vertebral column; this is known as the thoraco-lumbar outflow. The nerve cells in the ganglia give rise to fibers which pass to other ganglia in the neck and pelvis and to nerve plexuses which eventually supply individual organs of the body.

The Parasympathetic Nervous System consists of ganglia whose nerve fibers originate in the brain or the sacral part of the spinal cord. At the plexuses the fibers often intermingle with those of the sympathetic fibers. Parasympathetic ganglia do not form a chain but are close to each organ they supply.

These two systems have contrasting functions on the same organs, e.g. the sympathetic nerves reduce the activity of the intestines whereas the parasympathetic nerves stimulate them.

SPECIAL ORGANS

The Vocal Organs

Vocal sounds are produced in the larynx, but these sounds are grouped or formed into articulate speech by the pharynx, the nasal cavities, the tongue, the hard and soft palates, the teeth and the lips.

The Larynx is a box-like cavity at the top of the trachea, formed by the union of five main cartilages—the thyroid, the cricoid, the two arytenoid cartilages and the epiglottis. Connecting ligaments form two pairs of vocal cords, the upper or false cords and the lower or true vocal cords.

The Thyroid Cartilage is the largest cartilage in the larynx and is composed of two parts; it is connected with the bone at the base of the tongue above, and with the cricoid cartilage below.

The Cricoid Cartilage is shaped like a ring and hence its Greek name. It is narrowest in front and broadest behind, and connects with the thyroid cartilage above and with the first ring of the trachea below.

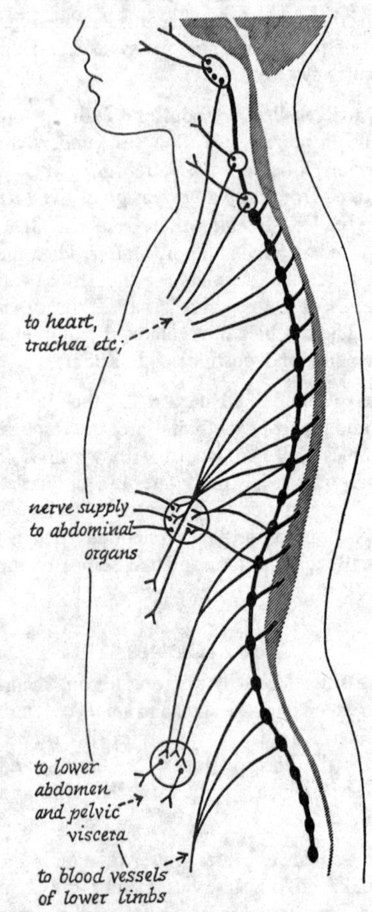

Fig. 68. *THE SYMPATHETIC NERVOUS SYSTEM. Spinal cord and brain shown in gray. Sympathetic nerve fibers in black.*

Fig. 71 is a back view of the cartilages and ligaments of the larynx.

The Arytenoid Cartilages are joined to the hind part of the cricoid cartilage and are connected with the thyroid cartilage by the vocal cords.

The Epiglottis is a fibro-cartilaginous lid shaped like a leaf, which covers the upper opening of the larynx. It is connected by a cartilage to the hyoid bone and to the thyroid cartilage. During respiration it opens and shuts, and during swallowing it closes down over the top of the larynx to prevent food and drink from passing down the windpipe.

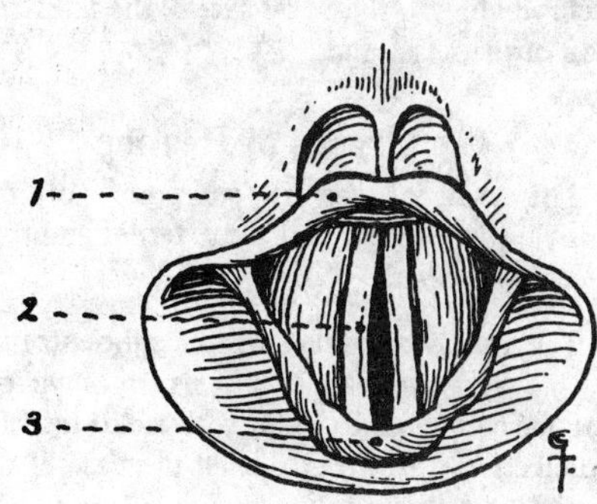

Fig. 69. *THE LARYNX (seen from above)*. 1. *Epiglottis* 2. *Vocal chords*. 3. *Arytenoid cartilage*.

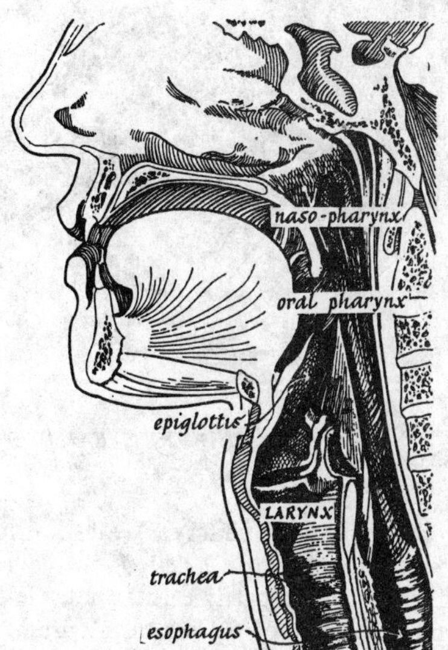

Fig. 70. *THROAT SHOWING ANATOMICAL POSITION OF THE LARYNX*

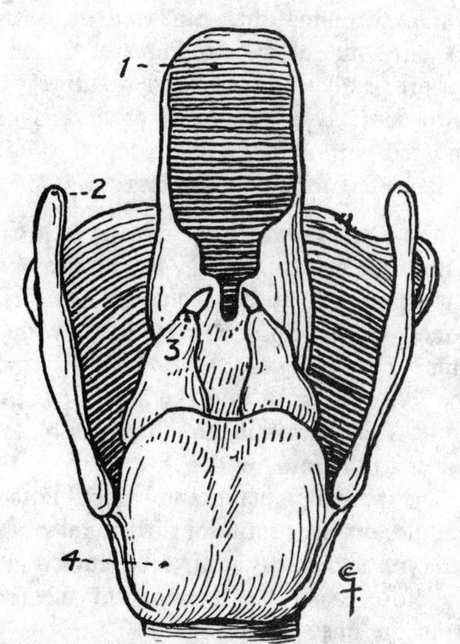

Fig. 71. *THE LARYNX* (*back view*). 1. *Epiglottis*. 2. *Thyroid cartilage*. 3. *Arytenoid cartilage*. 4. *Cricoid cartilage*.

The Vocal Cords, two ligaments formed of elastic fibrous tissue enclosed in a fold of mucous membrane, are inserted behind into the anterior projection of the arytenoid cartilages and, passing forward, are attached to the anterior angle of the thyroid cartilage. There are four ligaments crossing the larynx, two superior and two inferior, the latter being called the true vocal cords; the space between them is the glottis. The depression between the superior and inferior ligaments is the ventricle of the larynx. The muscles which are attached to the cartilages control their tension and can thereby change the shape of the laryngeal cavity in various ways; thus they enlarge or diminish the size of the glottis and relax or tighten the vocal cords. The vocal cords vibrate in different notes and produce the various fundamental sounds of speech. Tightening and approximating the cords, for example, raises the pitch of the voice.

The Organs of Sight

The organs of vision are:

the optic nerve, with its connections in the brain;
the eyeball, with its various structures;
the muscles of the eye;
the lachrymal or tear apparatus; and
the organs of protection, or lids.

Many of the tissues concerned with the production of vision are of a highly specialized nature, and they are extremely fine and delicate, so that they need the protection afforded by the bony prominences of the forehead, nose and cheek bones around the optical orbit.

The Optic Nerve originates in two roots at the base of the brain, the fibers from which meet as they pass forward, and some of them cross each other. The two nerves then separate and enter the back part of the eyeball and spread out over the retina. Fig. 72 shows the globes of the eyes and the crossing of the optic nerves.

The Eyeball is a better constructed optical instrument than man has ever made. Its interior is filled with what are called refracting humors or media, which are surrounded and held in their place by membranes of the wall of the eyeball. The wall has three coats: the sclera or sclerotic including the cornea, the choroid including the iris and the ciliary body, and the retina.

The Sclerotic Coat or Sclera is a fibrous membrane covering all the globe, except where the optic nerve enters behind. To this membrane the muscles are attached, and it is the part which is called the white of the eye. It is modified in front where it becomes the cornea.

The Cornea is the circular transparent part of the sclera which projects in front, and forms about one-fifth of the globe. It lies in front of the iris and pupil and permits the light rays to pass through to the retina.

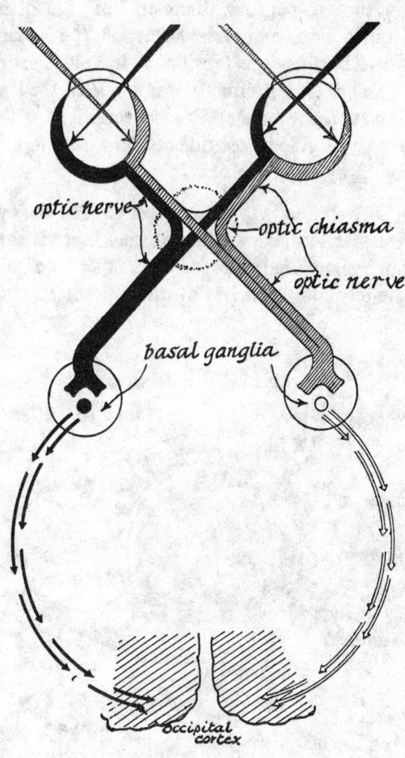

Fig. 72. *THE OPTIC NERVES in relation to the eyeballs and the sight-center in the occiput (see text).*

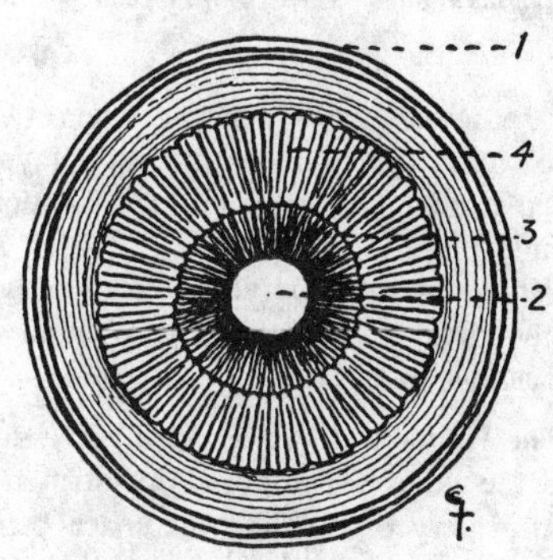

Fig. 73. *SECTION OF FRONT OF THE EYE*. 1. *The cut edges of the sclera and the choroid*. 2. *The pupil*. 3. *The iris*. 4. *The ciliary body*.

The Choroid Coat, or uvea, is a vascular membrane; its color is brown externally, and black within. It is connected with the sclerotic coat externally and with the retina internally, and is composed of three layers.

The Iris is the colored portion of the eye (blue, brown, green, etc.) and is part of the choroid coat. It is the partition between the anterior and posterior chambers of the eye and has a circular opening in the center called the pupil. It is made up of two sheets of smooth muscle fibers. The anterior radiating fibers dilate the pupil while those of the circular sphincter reduce the size of the pupil in bright light.

The Ciliary Body is a thickening of the anterior portion of the choroid coat and consists largely of the ciliary muscle attached to the suspensory ligament of the lens. Contraction and relaxation of the ciliary muscle adjust the tension in the suspensory ligament and, indirectly, the shape of the lens and its focal power. This is necessary for the eye to be able to see objects both near to and far away from the observer.

The Retina is the innermost coat of the eye and has ten layers. The external layer is thin and pigmented; the central layers contain the terminal branches of the optic nerve, and

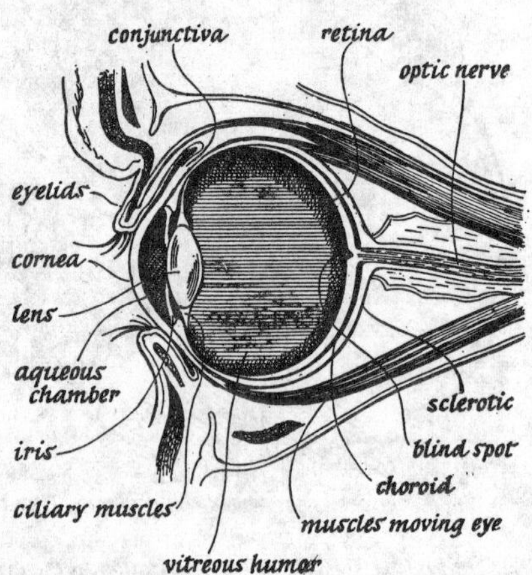

Fig. 74. *A SECTION THROUGH THE EYEBALL and the adjacent tissues. The optic nerve runs from the back of the brain to the back of the eyeball, opposite the lens.*

the rods and cones which are sensitive to light and colors. The internal layer is vascular and consists of a ramification of minute blood vessels.

Where the optic nerve fibers all converge at the back of the eyeball is a 'blind spot' insensitive to light.

The Humors of the Eye are the aqueous and the vitreous humors; the former is a clear watery fluid filling the space between the cornea and iris, while the vitreous humor is a jelly-like substance which fills the posterior four-fifths of the eyeball.

The Lens is immediately behind the pupil. It is convex both on the posterior and anterior surface and is supported and controlled by the ciliary muscle and suspensory ligament.

The Muscles of the Eye are six in number and are attached by their tendons to the bones of the orbit behind, and to the sclerotic coat in front. In Fig. 75, six of the muscles are indicated to show the attachment to the related structures (see 2, 3, 4, 5, 6, 7). The optic nerve (number 8) lies at the back of the eyeball.

The Orbits are the bony sockets which contain the eyes. The optic nerve to each eye passes through a hole at the back of the cavity.

The Eyebrows are the projecting arches over the upper orbital margins and are covered with short hairs. They prevent the sweat from running down into the eyes, and also shade them from strong light.

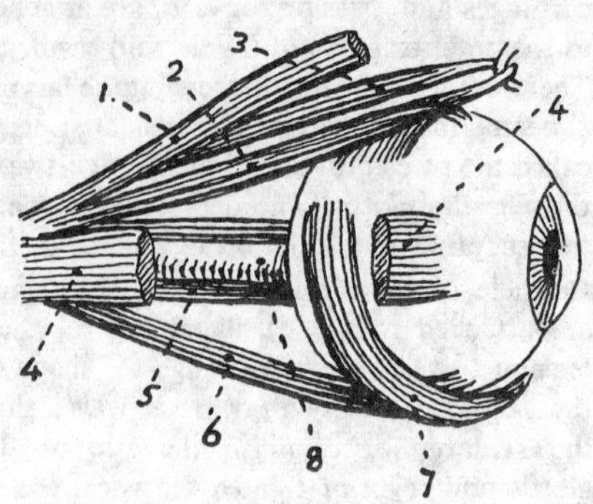

Fig. 75. *MUSCLES OF THE EYEBALL (right). 1. Muscle which raises the upper eyelid. 2. Muscle which turns the eye upward (superior rectus). 3. Muscle which rotates the eye clockwise. 4. Muscle which rotates the eye outward (external rectus). 5. Muscle which rotates the eye inward (internal rectus). 6. Muscle which rotates the eye downward (inferior rectus). 7. Muscle which rotates the eye anti-clockwise. 8. Optic nerve.*

The Eyelids cover the eyes in front when the eyes are closed. The smooth membrane which lines them is called the **conjunctiva;** it secretes a fluid which makes the eyelids open and shut easily. The eyelashes project from the free margins and protect the eye from foreign particles. In the eyelids are the meibomian glands.

The Lachrymal Gland, in size and shape like an almond, lies at the upper and outer angle of the orbit; several small ducts from it open upon the upper eyelid, through which the tears run down upon the conjunctiva, over the eye, escaping by two small openings near the internal angle of the eye, which communicate with the nasal duct.

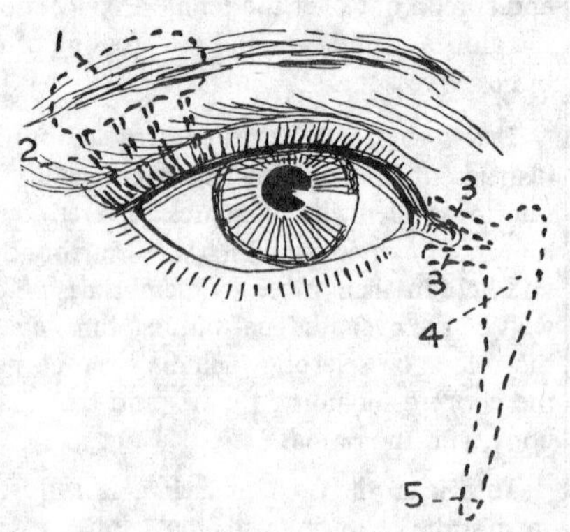

Fig. 76. *THE LACHRYMAL ORGANS. 1. Lachrymal gland. 2. Ducts leading to eyelid. 3. Tear points. 4. Nasal sac. 5. Termination of nasal duct in nose.*

The Naso-lachrymal Duct is a canal about three-quarters of an inch long, which runs down from the inner angle of the eye to the interior of the nose.

Fig. 76 shows these organs: 1, being the lachrymal gland; 2, the ducts leading to the upper eyelid; 3, 3, the tear-points (puncta lachrymalis); 4, the nasal sac; 5, the termination of the nasal duct.

The Organs of Hearing

The external ear is composed of the auricle (the pinna), and the external auditory meatus or canal.

The Auricle or pinna surrounds the entrance to the auditory canal. It consists of yellow cartilage covered by skin, with small muscles connecting it to the scalp. At the base of the auricle is a fleshy lobe (see Fig. 77).

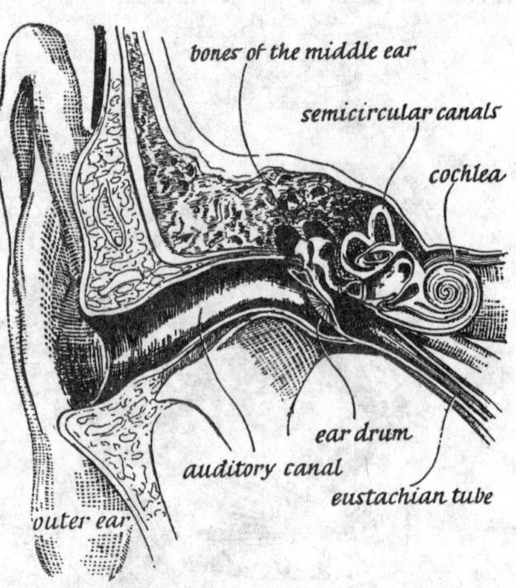

Fig. 77. *THE RIGHT EAR*

The External Auditory Meatus is a cana about an inch and a half long in the adult, partly bony and partly cartilaginous, leading from the pinna of the ear to the drum. The lining cells secrete the waxy substance found in the canal. In young children the canal is much shorter.

The Drum of the Ear (tympanic membrane) is a thin oval-shaped membrane at the inner end of the auditory canal. Normally it is white, glistening and somewhat transparent, so that some of the structures of the middle ear are partly visible when viewed through an auroscope. It is composed of fibrous tissue covered with skin on the external side and mucous membrane on the inner.

The Tympanum or middle ear is a cavity within the temporal bone. It contains several important structures, including three small bones which connect the drum with the internal ear; they are the *malleus* or hammer, the *incus* or anvil, and the *stapes* or stirrup bone. They transmit the vibrations of sound waves to the inner ear.

The mucous membrane which lines the middle ear is continuous with that of the pharynx and mastoid air cells. Infection can therefore easily travel along the membrane from the nose or throat.

The Eustachian Tube (auditory tube) is a channel of communication between the tympanum and the upper part of the pharynx. It admits air from the throat to the tympanum and so maintains an equal pressure on both sides of the drum.

The Labyrinth or internal ear is a series of chambers through the petrous bone, comprising the vestibule, separated from the middle ear by a membranous oval window; the cochlea, which makes two and a half turns spirally around an axis called the modiolus, and which contains the organ of Corti where the sound vibrations are transmitted to the hearing nerve fibers; and the semicircular canals. These three canals are set at right angles to each other and delicate hair cells within them are affected by sudden movements, change of direction, or balance of the body.

THE SKIN

The skin is a supple membrane composed of two principal layers which covers the outer surface of the body. It joins with the mucous membrane lining the various orifices. The outer layer is the epidermis; the inner layer is the true skin, dermis or corium. These layers differ in their structure and uses (see also p. 217).

The Cuticle or **Epidermis** varies in thickness in different parts of the body, being thickest where friction occurs. It consists of four layers, namely the horny or keratinized layer, the clear layer, the granular layer (often absent) and the layer of germinal cells (Malpighian layer) which contains soft living cells. There are no blood vessels in the cuticle but small sensory nerves enter the germinal layer. A blister is formed by a collection of fluid forming between the germinal layer and the outer layers.

The lower germinal layer is the pigmented zone. Some cells here contain a pigment (melanin) incorporated with the elementary granules, which give to the various races their several shades of color; the depth of hue is dependent entirely on the amount of coloring matter present.

The True Skin or **Dermis** is a fibrous layer which contains many sensory nerves and blood vessels which nourish the skin and regulate the temperature of the body; it also contains the hair follicles and the oil and sweat glands. Below the true skin is loose connective tissue and fat. Upon its upper surface is the sensitive or papillary layer composed of blood vessels and nerves which form little prominences called papillae.

The arteries, veins and nerves are spread so profusely over the true skin that it is impossible to push the point of a needle into it without piercing a blood vessel and a nerve. The lymphatic vessels are also very numerous in the skin.

The Sebaceous or **Oil Glands** are embedded in the true skin and communicate with the surface by small ducts. They are most abundant on the face, nose and ears.

The Sweat Apparatus. The sweat glands or sudoriferous glands are very numerous, being present in the skin all over the body, and they are rather more deeply placed than the sebaceous or oil glands. Each consists of a long coiled tube from which a duct passes up to the skin surface. The openings of the sweat ducts can be easily seen through a magnifying glass; there are from 400 to nearly 2,800 of these pores in every square inch of the skin.

The sweat glands play an important part in the heat regulating mechanism of the body. Water vapor is lost continuously through the cells of the epidermis (insensible perspiration) and is independent of the activity of the sweat glands. When the environmental temperature rises the sweat glands become active and secrete a watery solution of sodium chloride and small quantities of other minerals. The evaporation of this fluid from the skin causes it to become cool and so prevents a rise in body temperature in a hot environment.

The wax-secreting glands of the ear are modified sweat glands.

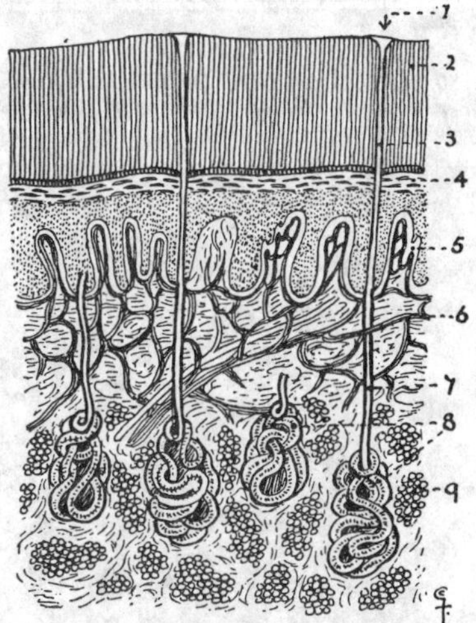

Fig. 78. *STRUCTURE OF THE SKIN.* 1. *Pore of skin.* 2. *Outer skin or cuticle.* 3. *Sweat duct.* 4. *Dermis or true skin.* 5. *Nerve endings.* 6. *Blood vessels.* 7. *Sweat ducts.* 8. *Sweat glands.* 9. *Fatty tissue.*

Hair and Nails

The hair and the nails are special modifications of the skin. Hairs are found on most parts of the skin surface, but may vary in consistency in different areas. Each hair grows from a root arising in a hair follicle. Variation in the coloring of hairs is due to different pigments in the shafts; when hair turns white the pigment is replaced by tiny air bubbles.

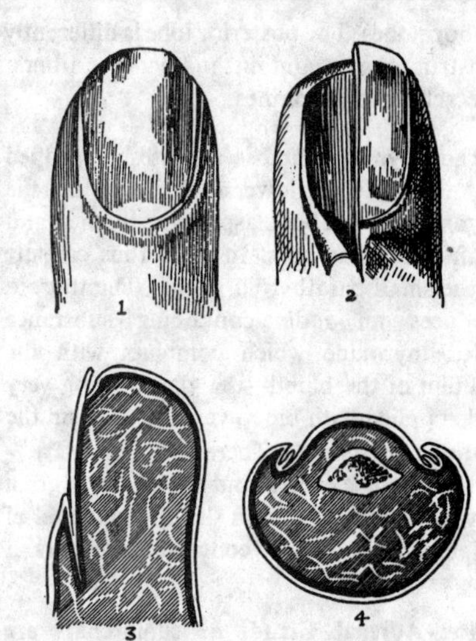

Fig. 79. *FINGER NAILS.* 1. *Normal finger nail.* 2. *How nail is embedded (front view).* 3. *Side view.* 4. *Section across finger tip showing proximity of the bone to nail bed.*

Nails are horny plates which grow continuously throughout life on the dorsal side of the toe and finger tips. Their function is protective.

In healthy young adults the nails should be smooth, quite free from ridges, and neither too soft nor too brittle. In old age they become more brittle, somewhat opaque and thickened.

THE ENDOCRINE SYSTEM

The glands of the body are of many different kinds. The term 'gland' includes the liver, pancreas, and kidneys, as well as the small lymphatic glands, the mucous and skin glands, and the endocrine glands. The skin is furnished with oil and sweat glands, while the salivary glands, the small mucous glands in the mucous membrane of the stomach and intestines secrete digestive juices, and the breasts or mammary glands secrete milk during lactation.

In various parts of the body there are a number of important glands which form the endocrine system. They secrete hormones which are chemical substances required for the chemical regulation of the body, some hormones being essential for life itself. The endocrine glands have no duct or outlet such as the pancreas or salivary glands are furnished with. Instead, their secretions are absorbed directly into the bloodstream or lymph stream.

Pituitary Gland. Of first importance is the pituitary gland or hypophysis cerebri whose hormones control the activities of the other endocrine glands. The pituitary is a small oval mass about the size of a large pea, and is suspended by a slender stalk to the underside of the brain. It has an anterior lobe well supplied with blood vessels and it secretes six hormones. The posterior lobe is differently constructed and contains many nerve fibers; it secretes two hormones.

The Thyroid Gland is a horseshoe-shaped organ lying in the lower neck just below the larynx, its two lobes clasping the trachea and uniting their surfaces. In its fibrous capsule lie the small parathyroid glands. The thyroid produces an iodine-containing substance called thyroxine which combines with the globulin of the blood—the glands being very well supplied with blood vessels—to form the thyroid hormones. There are four **Parathyroid Glands** each about the size of a grain of wheat. They maintain the calcium level of the blood. Death in convulsions occurs if they are removed.

The Adrenal Glands or suprarenals are yellow, cap-like bodies which lie on the top of each kidney. Within the fibrous capsule a thick cortex of glandular epithelial cells surrounds a medulla intimately connected with nerve fibres of the sympathetic system. The cortex is essential to life and produces the corticosteroid hormones; the medulla produces adrenaline and noradrenaline under conditions of stress, but it is not vital to life.

The Pancreas (see also p.226) is a compound gland; its duct pours pancreatic juice for digestion into the duodenum, but lying among its pale cells are nests of red cells called the Islets of Langerhans. These islets behave independently as an endocrine gland secreting the hormone insulin which is necessary for the proper utilization of carbohydrates in the body. Lack of insulin is the cause of diabetes mellitus.

The Thymus Gland in a newborn child is about half an inch long, and it develops until about the eighth year, but at puberty it regresses and remains so throughout adult life. The gland, which lies between the trachea and the great aorta of the heart, is thought to influence growth and maintain muscle function; it also makes lymphocytes.

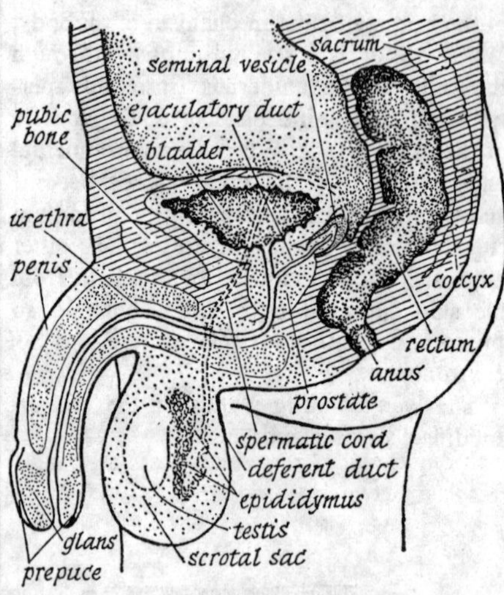

Fig. 80. *SEXUAL ORGANS OF THE MALE showing their position in relation to the urinary and rectal excretory organs.*

The Gonads, or sex glands, are the testes in the man and the ovaries in the woman.

The two oval, walnut-sized, white **testes** lie within the scrotal sac in the perineum. Each testis contains seminiferous tubules lined with special cells from which the male elements, the spermatozoa, develop. The tubules unite to form a long, very narrow, convoluted tube known as the epididymus which joins the testicular artery, veins and lymphatics to form the spermatic cord in the lower pelvic cavity. In addition to producing spermatozoa, other cells of the testes produce the hormone testosterone which, jointly with the hormones of the anterior lobe of the pituitary gland and of the adrenal, is responsible for the secondary sexual characteristics of the male, e.g. deepening of the voice, growth of hair on the face and pubes, and strong bone and muscle.

The two **ovaries** each lying to left and right in the pelvic cavity, correspond to the testes in the male. Each ovary is about the size of an almond, grayish-pink in color, and is attached to the broad ligament of the uterus. The germinal epithelium of the ovary produces the immature ova or eggs which mature in Graafian follicles in the core of the ovary. The ripened ovum (one at each cycle) bursts through the follicle into the peritoneal cavity on its way to the uterus. Hormones secreted by the ovary under the control of the pituitary gland produce secondary female characteristics such as the menstrual cycle, the growth of breasts and pubic hair.

PHYSIOLOGY: HOW THE BODY FUNCTIONS

The human body is like a piece of delicate machinery. The machine is a very remarkable one for it works for seventy years or more without replacements. Each part of the machine has a special job to do, and all the separate parts work together to make a complete animal. The scientific study of the way in which the organs work is called Physiology.

Body Function is Chemical Change

When the function of any part of the body is looked at closely, we find that most of the changes are really concerned with chemical reactions. In order to be able to understand this section more easily, a few simple chemical terms are first explained.

Atoms and Elements. All matter is made of atoms. An atom is the basic unit of an element. There are about 100 different elements which, when combined in various ways, form all the matter of which our earth is composed. Each element has a special symbol: oxygen=O; carbon=C; hydrogen=H; nitrogen=N; etc. Each element consists of atoms which are alike, but which are different from those of all other elements.

Molecules. Atoms can join together to form a partnership; this partnership is called a molecule. The atoms in a molecule may be alike, e.g. O_2 represents a molecule of oxygen; or the atoms in the molecule may be from different elements, e.g. CO_2 represents a molecule of carbon dioxide which has one carbon atom + two oxygen atoms. A molecule of water is written H_2O; this is made from two hydrogen atoms and one oxygen atom (Fig. 1).

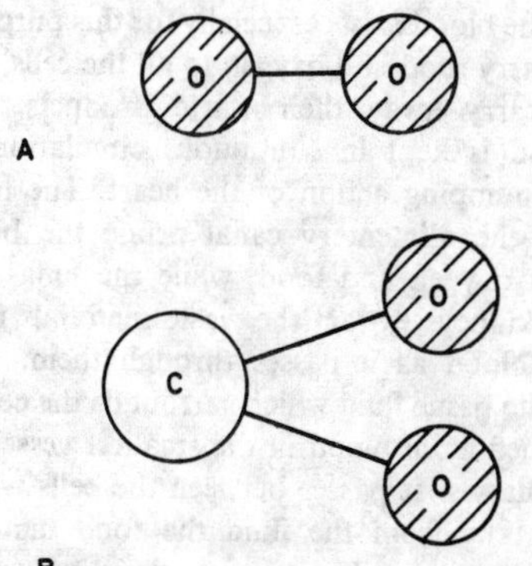

Fig. 1. A. *An oxygen molecule of two oxygen atoms.* B. *A carbon dioxide molecule of one carbon and two oxygen atoms.*

Compounds. Molecules made from a variety of different atoms are called compounds. There are two main groups of these compounds, organic and inorganic.

Organic compounds contain mainly carbon, oxygen, hydrogen and nitrogen in their molecules. Small numbers of atoms of other elements may take part as well. Under natural conditions, organic compounds are made by living organisms—both animal and plant.

Inorganic compounds may contain atoms of any of the elements. Usually their molecules are smaller and less complicated than those of organic compounds.

The body contains very many different compounds, both organic and inorganic. Most of these are in solution, or dissolved in water. Water actually accounts for 60 to 70 per cent of the total weight of the body. Water forms the medium or background in which our chemical reactions take place, and so plays a very important part in the life and health of the body.

Millions of Cells

Cell Structure. The body is made of millions of tiny units called cells. All cells are basically alike. Fig 2 shows a typical cell. It

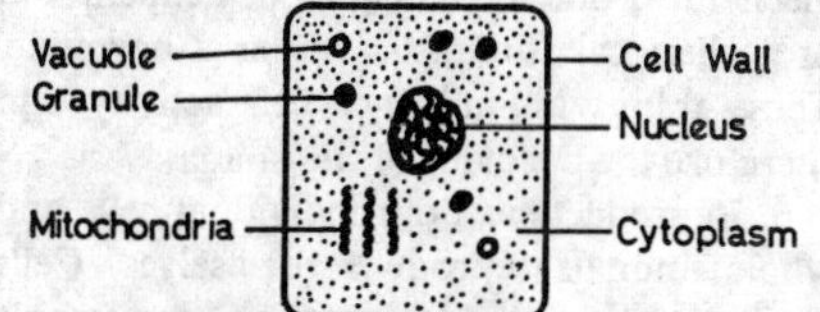

Fig. 2. *THE STRUCTURE OF A TYPICAL CELL*

consists of a jelly-like material, the cytoplasm, which is surrounded by the cell membrane. Cytoplasm is a very complicated mixture of organic and inorganic compounds.

Nucleus and Genes. There are several special structures embedded in the cytoplasm. The most noticeable one is the nucleus. The nucleus seems to direct the rest of the cell, controlling its activities. It also contains the genes. These are particles which are handed on from parent to child and are important in heredity. The cell nucleus actually decides the physical characteristics of the whole body.

Food Granules. The cytoplasm may also have granules in it. These are often food stores. Some cells store glycogen (animal starch); others hoard iron until needed by the body. The granules in some cells are special materials manufactured by the cell as part of its job.

Other Cell Contents. There are vacuoles filled with fluid in the cytoplasm of many cells. Usually there are also mitochondria, which look like little rods and seem to be concerned with the chemical reactions which release energy inside the cell.

All the cells in the body have the same basic structure. But of course, if a cell is needed to do a particular job it naturally develops special characters of its own. Some of the different cell types are described in the Anatomy section, pp. 217-219.

The Water of Life

Cells live surrounded by water. Dissolved in the water are food materials and oxygen needed for life. Waste materials from the cells are unloaded into the outside fluid which carries them away. Water is vital to life. The inside of the cell is separated from the outside world by the cell membrane. This protects the cell and helps in deciding which materials can travel into the cytoplasm from the outside.

Diffusion. How do materials pass back and forth between the cell and its watery home? Particles in solution move through the fluid by diffusion (Fig. 3). They spread out and move away from a place where they are closely packed together until they are evenly spaced through the liquid.

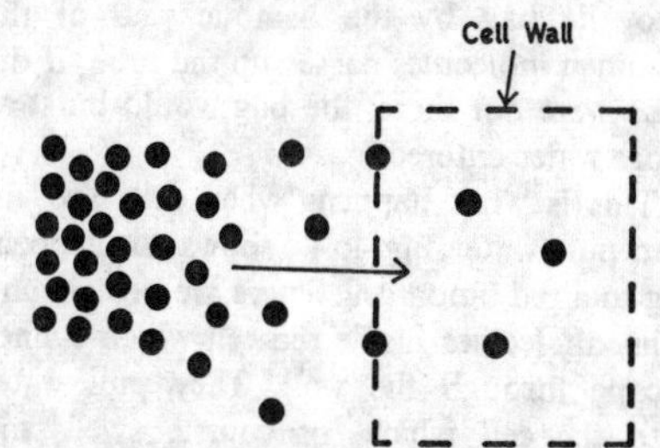

Fig. 3. *DIFFUSION OF MOLECULES INTO A CELL. When particles are concentrated at one point in a liquid, they invariably separate until they are evenly spaced out. The molecules in the diagram are moving into the cell because there is a bigger concentration outside the cell than inside.*

Particles will diffuse into a cell from the outside if there is a bigger concentration outside the cell than inside. The cell wall behaves like a sieve with holes in it. If the molecules are bigger than the holes in the wall, they cannot get into the cell.

At other times the cell seems to be able to concentrate particles inside itself, drawing them in from the outside fluid. This is the very opposite of diffusion, and requires much hard work from the cell.

Osmosis. The ease with which a cell wall lets particles pass through it is called its

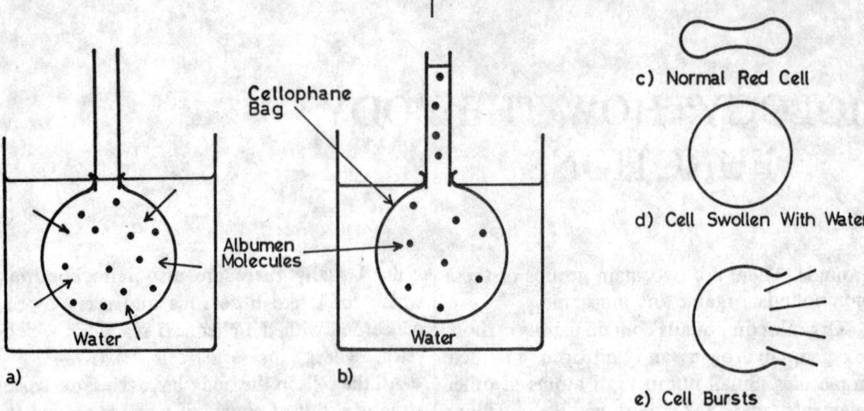

Fig. 4. *OSMOSIS.* (*a*) *Water is pulled into the cellophane bag by the osmotic attraction of albumen molecules, and* (*b*) *it rises in the tube.* (*c & d*) *Water is pulled into a red blood cell (placed in water) by the osmotic attraction of protein molecules, and* (*e*) *the cell bursts because there is no escape tube.*

permeability. Cell walls are semipermeable: they let some things through but not others. Water molecules pass in and out of cells very easily.

Cellophane is a material which, like the wall of a cell, is semipermeable. It can be made into a bag and the bag filled with a protein solution, for example egg albumen (egg white). The albumen molecules are very large, much bigger than the holes in the cellophane. They are retained inside the bag. If the bag is put into water, it swells up. The albumen molecules cannot escape, and they attract water into the bag. This process is called osmosis. The attracting force which the albumen molecules have for the water is called their osmotic pressure. If there are many albumen molecules in the bag, there will be a big osmotic pressure.

Fig. 4 illustrates the process of osmosis. In this diagram a glass tube projects from the top of the bag. The water which is sucked into the bag by the osmotic pull of the albumen molecules passes up the tube. If the tube were not there, the bag would burst as more water entered.

This is what happens when cells are put into pure water. Fig. 4c—e shows this happening to a red blood cell. There are protein and other molecules inside the cell which cannot escape through the wall. They pull water into the cell which, of course, swells up. Eventually the pressure inside the cell is so great that the wall cannot stretch any more and the cell bursts.

Osmosis plays a very important part in our lives. It controls the movement of water into and out of cells. Osmosis also helps to regulate the flow of fluid between the blood and tissues.

THE PROPERTIES OF LIFE

If we look closely at the way in which different animals live, we find that they have many things in common. In fact there are certain activities which seem to be essential for living.

1. **Food Intake and Digestion.** Food is a source of energy. It also provides the raw material for building new body tissue. After food has been eaten by the animal, it must be broken down or digested. Digestion changes the food into a simpler form and makes it easier to use.

2. **Metabolism.** This term covers all the complicated chemical reactions occurring in the body when the food gives up its energy and is converted into new cell material. In this way growth occurs.

3. **Respiration.** Chemical reactions which release energy from food also involve the use of oxygen and the production of carbon dioxide. This is termed respiration.

4. **Excretion.** If waste products were allowed to accumulate they would harm the animal. They must be regularly removed from the body, or excreted.

5. **Irritability.** This is the ability to react or respond to a stimulus. The stimulus may be a mechanical one, or a change in temperature, or a chemical stimulus, such as a hormone. These things all influence cell activity and therefore the behavior of the animal.

6. **Reproduction.** Both individual cells and whole animals reproduce themselves. Cells usually simply divide into two, but whole animals reproduce by a sexual process. In this two special cells, the gametes, combine to form a completely new individual.

Amoeba: A Simple Form of Life

The activities described above make up what we call 'life.' They are all carried out by large complicated creatures, such as man, and also by very simple forms of animal life, such as the amoeba.

This tiny animal (Fig. 5) is made of only one cell. It lives in fresh water ponds. The cell is an irregularly shaped blob of cytoplasm surrounded by a membrane. The cytoplasm contains a nucleus, granules, and one or more vacuoles.

Food Intake and Digestion. It can change its shape by forming 'arms,' or pseudopodia. In this way it catches food particles which are taken into the cytoplasm. Here the food is digested, the nutrient material used by the cell, and the unwanted portions returned to the water.

Respiration. The amoeba respires by taking dissolved oxygen from the pond water, and passing carbon dioxide into the water as it is formed.

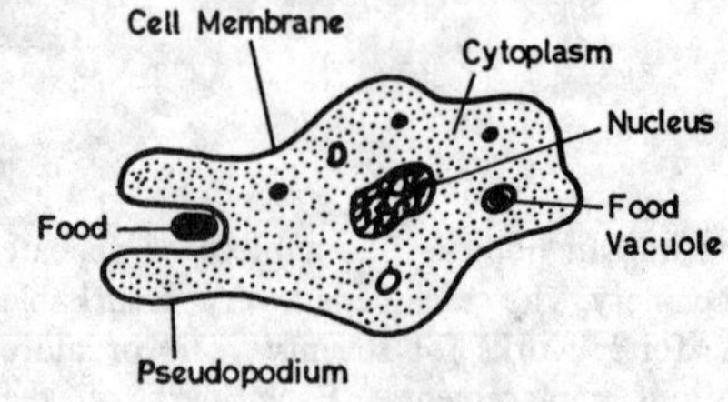

Fig. 5. *AN AMOEBA. A simple single-celled form of animal life.*

Irritability. The animal is sensitive to changes in its surroundings and will respond to these. If it is touched it will 'creep' away from the stimulus by changing its shape. If the pond water dries up, the amoeba responds by forming a protective coat around itself.

Reproduction. It reproduces by dividing its nucleus and cytoplasm into two and forming a cell wall around each half. The life of this animal is very restricted; it is extremely susceptible to changing conditions in the pond and has very little defense against adversity.

Man Compared with Amoeba

Man is obviously very different from amoeba. His body is composed of many millions of cells. He lives surrounded by air and not by water.

Tissue Fluid. However, each individual cell in his body is surrounded by a special fluid, the tissue fluid. This replaces the pond water in which the amoeba lives.

Tissue fluid is a solution of salts containing oxygen and food waste products. It is formed from the blood. The food and oxygen come primarily from the outside world but special organs have been developed to take these materials into the body. Here they are dissolved in the blood and so carried to the cells.

The blood exists especially for this purpose; to carry food and oxygen to all the cells, and to carry away their waste products. The blood is kept in continuous circulation by the pumping action of the heart. The lungs and the alimentary canal prime the blood with oxygen and food, while the lungs and the kidneys extract the waste materials from the blood as it passes through them.

The tissue fluid which surrounds the cells is formed from blood in the smallest vessels or capillaries. It passes between the cells which can take from the fluid the food material they need, and discharge their unwanted waste products into it.

Although tissue fluid resembles the pond water of the amoeba in its function, it is very different in some ways. The pond water is continually changing in temperature, acidity and in chemical composition. The amoeba is at the mercy of such changes which it cannot control. Chemical reactions are very much affected by all these disturbances, and so the amoeba lives a 'stop—go' kind of life.

Man's Internal Environment. To avoid such erratic variations in activity, the tissue fluid in man is kept as constant as possible in every way. This means that the cells are not continually disturbed by changes in the composition of the fluid surrounding them.

Many of the body's activities are concerned with keeping this fluid, or internal environment, constant. It is this stability which enables man to be so independent of his external conditions. This was first recognized by the great French physiologist Claude Bernard when he said 'The constancy of the internal environment is the condition of a free life.

BLOOD AND CIRCULATION

In order to live, cells need food, oxygen, and a means of disposing of the waste products of their metabolism. In the human body, most of the cells live far from the source of the essential materials but food and oxygen are carried to the tissues in the blood. This circulates around the body in a system of closed blood vessels, driven by the pumping action of the heart.

See Anatomy, Fig. 57, p. 229, which shows diagrammatically the main centers of the circulatory system; and Fig. 7, p. 241, which shows how the blood is pumped around the body.

Blood consists of cells of several different kinds suspended in a liquid called plasma. Some of the plasma forms tissue fluid which leaves the circulation by passing through the walls of the tiniest blood vessels, or capillaries. Tissue fluid passes between the cells, carrying food and oxygen to them, and taking away their waste products. Blood is the transport system of the body. An average-sized adult has about 10 pints in his body.

PLASMA

Plasma is the fluid part of the blood and there are about 6 pints of it in the body of an adult. It consists of water in which are dissolved many minerals (chiefly sodium chloride), proteins, food materials such as glucose and fat, and many waste products. Oxygen, needed for cell respiration, is also dissolved in the plasma.

The Plasma Proteins

There are many proteins in the plasma. They all have very large molecules compared with those of the salts and substances like glucose. They have several very important functions.

1. They act as regulators, allowing only a necessary amount of tissue fluid to be formed from the plasma. Because protein molecules are very large, they cannot pass freely through the capillary wall into the tissue spaces, but water, glucose, salt, and many other substances with small molecules can easily pass through. Because they are confined inside the capillary by their large size, protein molecules prevent the escape of all the water from the vessels into the tissue spaces. This is osmosis (p. 238) in action. The capillary wall is the semipermeable membrane, and the protein molecules lie on one side of this, inside the blood vessel. Their osmotic action tends to keep fluid inside the circulation. If the plasma has too little protein, too much fluid leaks out of the capillaries and the tissues become waterlogged.

In this way, the plasma proteins are important regulators of the volume of plasma in the circulation.

2. They act as carriers. The proteins can join on to other chemicals in the blood and carry them around the body.

3. One group of proteins, the gamma globulins, help the body to resist disease. They form the antibodies which help to put out of action the bacteria which cause disease.

4. Some proteins help the blood to clot after injury.

5. The proteins can act as food for the cells in extreme starvation.

6. Many of the proteins are hormones or enzymes which help to regulate the functioning of many organs.

These are some of the main functions of the plasma proteins. They are extremely important to the body.

THREE TYPES OF BLOOD CELLS

There are three main types of blood cell: red cells or erythrocytes; white cells or leucocytes; and platelets (Fig. 6). They are all made in the bone marrow. The spleen and lymph glands also produce some white cells.

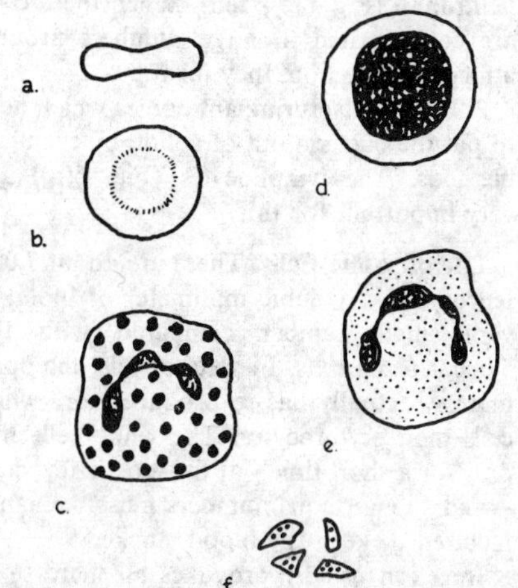

Fig. 6. *BLOOD CELLS.* a. *Red cell (side view).* b. *Red cell (from above).* c. *Eosinophil white cell.* d. *Lymphocyte white cell.* e. *Neutrophil white cell.* f. *Platelets.*

During childhood the marrow of all the bones is busy making blood cells. In the adult the marrow in the long bones of the limbs is no longer a 'factory' for blood cells. The blood-forming tissue is replaced by fat and the bones are filled with yellow marrow. The yellow marrow can change back to red marrow, and make blood cells again if the body suddenly needs them.

RED BLOOD CELLS

The erythrocyte, or red cell, is biconcave (Fig. 6) (a and b) but, unlike most other cells in the body, it has no nucleus.

Hemoglobin. The cell is red because it contains hemoglobin. This is a pigment containing the metal iron combined with a protein. Hemoglobin has a special liking for oxygen. It picks up oxygen in the lungs and carries it to the tissue cells. It also helps to carry carbon dioxide (the main waste product) away from the tissues to the lungs. The peculiar shape of the cell helps it in its job as an oxygen carrier.

Life of Red Cells. There are about 5 million red cells in 1 cubic millimeter of blood (a *very* small drop). Although each cell lives for about 120 days, about 10 million new red cells pass into the bloodstream every second. These replace the worn-out cells which die.

Transforming Old Cells. At the end of its life, the erythrocyte is engulfed, or 'eaten' by special scavenger cells in the spleen, liver and bone marrow. These phagocytes break up the hemoglobin molecules, and carefully preserve the iron and protein to make new cells. The pigmented part of the hemoglobin molecule travels in the blood to the liver which excretes it as bilirubin into the bile. Bilirubin gives the bile its greenish-brown color.

Anemia: a Red Cell Disorder. When a person's blood contains too little hemoglobin, he is anemic. There may be too few red cells in the blood, or there may be a normal number of cells, with each one having less than its proper amount of hemoglobin.

Blood Groups

It sometimes happens that a person needs to be given a blood transfusion. Before doing this, the doctor needs to know something about the quality of the blood of the person who is providing the blood (the donor) and of the person who is receiving the transfusion (the recipient). This vital information concerns the blood group.

Antigens and Antibodies. The red cell carries certain factors known as antigens (or agglutinogens). The plasma contains other factors which are known as antibodies (or agglutinins).

The cell antigens are called A and B; the plasma antibodies are α and β. If the A cells meet the α antibodies a chemical change takes place. The cells stick together in clumps: they agglutinate. The cells then break up, spilling their contents into the blood. If this happens inside the body, serious or even fatal consequences are certain to ensue.

The blood of each person contains two of the total of four factors: A, B, α and β. There is either one cell antigen and one plasma antibody; or two cell antigens and no plasma antibodies; or two antibodies and no antigen.

Agglutination of A cells is caused by α antibody, and B cells by β antibody. Therefore A and α cannot occur in the same person, nor can B and β. If they did the cells would be agglutinated inside the body by the person's own antibodies and impede the circulation.

The blood group to which a person belongs is named from the cell factors. Table 1 shows the different blood groups and the corresponding antigens and antibodies.

TABLE 1

Factors in ABO Blood Groups

Blood Group	*Cell Antigen*	*Plasma Antibody*
A	A	β
B	B	α
AB	AB	None
O	None	αβ

Blood Transfusion

Before a blood transfusion is given to a patient, it is necessary to know the blood group of both the donor and the recipient. The blood group of both must be the same, or the donors may be of blood group O.

Blood group O is known as the universal donor, because this blood can, in theory, be given without harm to anyone. There are no cell antigens, and so the cells cannot be agglutinated.

In practice, whenever possible, some cells from the donor's blood are mixed with plasma from the recipient. If no agglutination occurs, then it is safe to transfuse the patient. This test is called the direct cross match. It takes some time to complete. If the emergency is very great, there may not be enough time to do the test, so blood of group O is used.

The Rhesus Factor. The A and B antigens are not the only cell factors. Others exist, but none is so important as the Rhesus antigen. This was discovered during some experiments involving Rhesus monkeys, and so was given this name. The rhesus antigen has no natural antibody. If a person has the rhesus antigen in his cells, he is Rhesus positive (Rh+). A Rhesus negative person (Rh−), however, has neither the cell factor nor a plasma factor. About 85 per cent of the population is Rh+ and about 15 per cent Rh−.

The rhesus antibody (plasma factor) can be made by the tissues of a Rh− person, if he is given a transfusion of Rh+ cells. His body treats the Rh+ cells as invaders, and makes an antibody which will agglutinate and destroy the red cells. Actually, several transfusions of Rh+ cells must be given to a Rh− person before he forms enough antibody to cause dangerous agglutination. Because of the extreme care taken in cross matching blood, this situation is unlikely to occur nowadays.

Pregnancy and the Rhesus Factor. It is quite common for a woman who is Rh− to bear a child who is Rh+, if the father is Rh+. The mother has no antigen in her blood cells, nor any antibody in her plasma. But the child (fetus) growing inside her womb, has the Rh antigen in his body. The blood cells of the fetus seem to be able to cross the placenta into the mother's blood. Here, the Rh antigen in the baby's cells provokes the mother's tissues into producing the Rh antibody. This of course, is deadly to the cells of the fetus. If enough antibody is made by the mother, this can actually travel back to the baby and destroy its red cells.

Fortunately only small amounts of antibody appear during each pregnancy. With each successive pregnancy the risk is greater. Actually the danger today to the child is small. The blood of the Rh− mother is tested very carefully during pregnancy. If the amount of antibody in the mother's blood rises above a safe level, preparation is made to transfuse the blood of the fetus in the womb (by puncturing the mother's peritoneum with a hollow needle) or to exchange the blood as soon as the baby is born.

WHITE BLOOD CELLS

The different types of white cell are illustrated in Fig. 6. These cells help to defend the body against bacterial invasion. They do this in at least two ways.

1. By migrating through the capillary walls and into the tissue spaces where they engulf the noxious bacteria. This is the job of the neutrophil (Fig. 6(e)) cells. When these cells are concentrated in large numbers around a focus of infection, they form pus.

2. By manufacturing antibodies which help to put the bacteria out of action by chemical methods. The lymphocytes (Fig. 6(d)) are very important for this.

Life of White Cells. There are about 7,000 leucocytes in 1 cubic millimeter of blood, a very small number compared with the 5,000,000 red cells. In spite of this, the bone marrow actually has to produce more white cells than erythrocytes. The white cells live only for a short time—at the most a few days —and so enormous numbers must be manufactured to keep the blood stocked.

Infection usually provokes an increase in the number of white cells in the blood. The particular type of cell selected for increase depends on the kind of infection.

Leukemia: A White Cell Disorder. Rarely, the leucocytes may be produced in enormous numbers for no apparent cause. This condition is know as leukemia. The bone marrow is so busy manufacturing white cells, it has no room for the red cells. The patient then becomes severely anemic and ill. At present we know very little about the reasons why the bone marrow should become so overactive. The disease is usually fatal.

BLOOD CLOTTING

When tissues are damaged, they usually bleed. The bleeding soon stops (unless an artery is cut) and a blood clot forms over the wound. The clot is a fine network of interlacing threads of a protein called fibrin. Entangled in the threads are all kinds of blood cells.

Formation of the Fibrin Clot. The fibrin threads are formed from a protein dissolved in the plasma. This is fibrinogen. Many chemical factors are needed to bring about this change from a soluble protein to the network of threads. The actual conversion is made by an enzyme, thrombin, which forms in plasma when tissues are damaged. Damaged cells release many chemicals which together are called 'thromboplastin.' Already in plasma is a protein, prothrombin, just waiting to be changed into thrombin when there is sufficient thromboplastin around to help it. The blood platelets (Fig. 6(f)) seem to provide some of the essential factors in this process. The steps in blood clotting are as follows:

Prothrombin (a protein dissolved in the plasma)
+Calcium (dissolved in plasma)
+Thromboplastin (formed from damaged tissues and platelets)
= Thrombin

Thrombin (an enzyme)
+Fibrinogen (a protein dissolved in plasma)
= Fibrin clot

Work of the Platelets. Blood clotting is only one factor which helps to stop bleeding. Immediately following injury, the platelets (Fig. 6(f)) stick to the walls of the damaged vessels and help to plug the holes in them. The platelets also liberate a substance called serotonin which makes the vessels close down, thereby reducing the bleeding. This is followed by blood clotting, and so the wound is sealed, and further bleeding prevented.

Drugs to Prevent Clotting. Blood clotting can be prevented by giving drugs which interfere with prothrombin action. These are called anticoagulant drugs. Such drugs are often used by a doctor to prevent a clot from spreading. Their use may prevent the spread of a coronary thrombosis, or clotting in the big veins which sometimes follows a surgical operation.

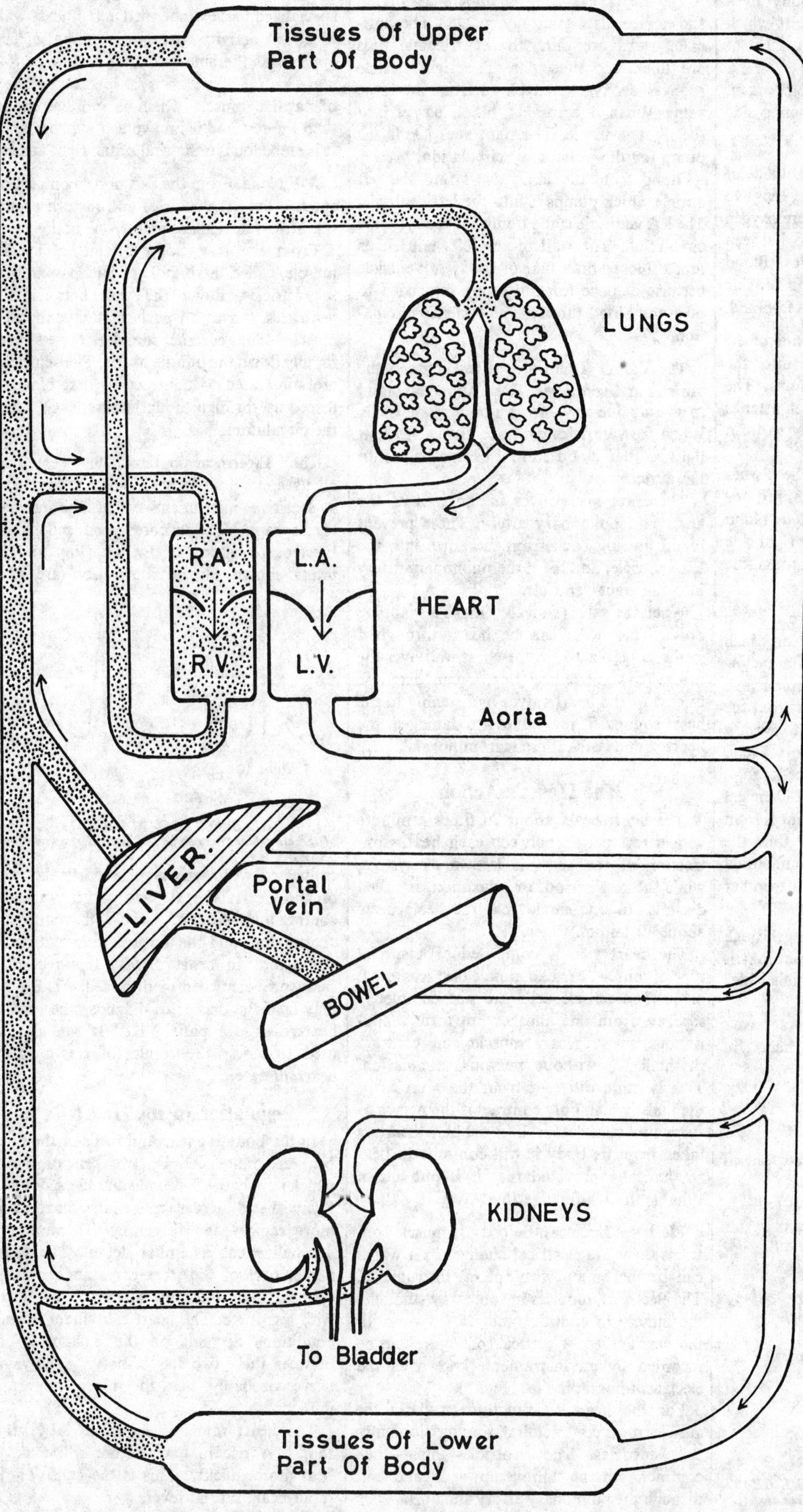

Fig. 7. *HOW BLOOD IS PUMPED AROUND THE BODY*

To enable blood to circulate and serve every tissue in the body, six important processes are ceaselessly at work.

(1) *The left ventricle (L.V.) pumps blood into the aorta which distributes it through the arteries to all parts of the body.*

(2) *In the tissues blood gives up its oxygen and takes up carbon dioxide.*

(3) *Blood which has given up its oxygen returns to the right auricle (R.A.) of the heart in the veins.*

(4) *The right ventricle (R.V.) pumps blood through the lungs, where it loses carbon dioxide and replenishes its oxygen supply and returns to the left auricle (L.A.).*

(5) *Food enters the blood from the bowel, then travels in the portal vein to the liver.*

(6) *Waste matter is excreted as the blood flows through the kidneys.*

THE CIRCULATION

Blood is driven around the body in a system of closed vessels by the heart which acts as a pump. The general arrangement of the circulation is shown in Fig. 7.

The heart is a hollow muscular organ, which actually behaves as two pumps side by side.

1. **Pulmonary Circulation.** The right side of the heart pumps blood through the lungs to form the pulmonary circulation. Here oxygen and carbon dioxide are exchanged between the blood and the air in the lungs. Blood leaving the lungs and traveling to the left side of the heart is thus red, or oxygenated blood.

2. **Systemic Circulation.** The left side of the heart pumps oxygenated blood into the largest artery in the body, the aorta. The aorta distributes blood to the lesser arteries and thence to all parts of the body to form the systemic circulation.

The arteries deliver blood to the tissues where food and oxygen are exchanged for waste products. The deoxygenated blood then travels in the veins back to the right side of the heart, to be pumped again through the lungs.

SPLANCHNIC CIRCULATION. There are two special parts of the systemic circulation which are very important. The blood traveling through intestinal vessels (the splanchnic circulation) absorbs food materials from the intestine. The intestinal veins join to form a large vein going to the liver—the portal vein. Inside the liver, blood gives some of its food to the liver cells, which act like a chemical factory and manufacture new substances from these raw materials. At the same time the liver cells give some of the manufactured products to the blood to be carried to other tissues.

RENAL CIRCULATION. Blood flowing through the kidney vessels (the renal circulation) is cleansed of some of its waste materials which pass out in the urine.

Blood from the liver and kidneys travels with other venous blood to the heart for recirculation.

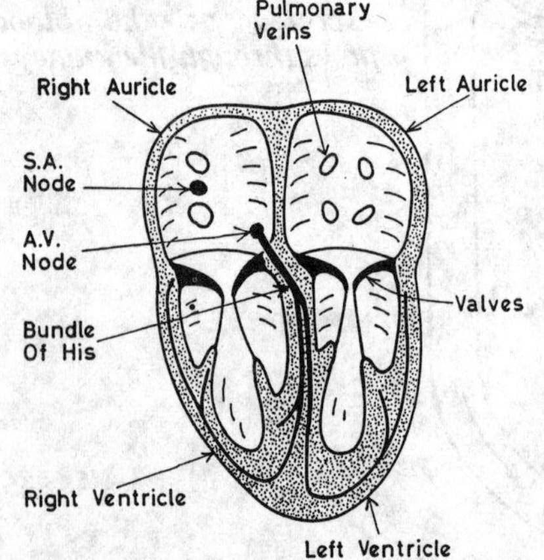

Fig. 8. *THE FOUR CHAMBERS OF THE HEART, AND THE CONDUCTING TISSUE. See text.*

THE HEART

The heart has four chambers as Fig. 8 shows (see also Anatomy, p.228). The auricular walls are thin; the ventricular walls are thick and muscular. The right auricle receives deoxygenated blood from the large veins. When it contracts, blood passes into the right ventricle. The right ventricle is the pump for the pulmonary circulation.

Blood from the lungs flows into the left auricle which pumps it into the left ventricle. The left ventricle is the pump for the systemic circulation. The wall of the left ventricle is much thicker than that of the right ventricle because a more forceful pump is needed to push the blood through the systemic circulation.

The Valves. There are valves between the auricles and ventricles. These allow the blood to go only one way—from auricle to ventricle. When the ventricles contract, the valves shut tight so that blood cannot escape back into the auricles.

There are also valves in the wall of the aorta and pulmonary artery. These prevent blood flowing back from the aorta into the left ventricle, and from the pulmonary artery into the right ventricle.

When the valves shut they make a snapping noise. This noise can be heard through a stethoscope placed on the chest wall over the heart. An experienced doctor can diagnose disease of the heart valves by listening to the heart sounds. If the valves are damaged, the heart sounds are different from normal.

The Heart's Action

The heart beats about 70 times a minute with a rest period between each beat. Contraction of the heart is known as systole, while the rest period, or relaxation, is called diastole. In one single year the heart beats about 40 million times.

The heart wall is composed of a special type of muscle, cardiac muscle (see Anatomy, p.219). The muscle cells are not completely separate from one another but form a continuous sheet. Heart muscle can contract rhythmically without nervous stimulation. This is quite different from the muscles of the limbs which only contract if the nerves to them are stimulated. If a rabbit's heart is taken from its body it will continue to beat rhythmically provided that it is put into a suitable fluid with sugar and oxygen.

Electrical Impulses. Before any muscle contracts there are electrical changes in it which can be picked up with special instruments. The electrical impulses in some way stimulate the muscle to contract and do its work. In the heart these electrical changes can be recorded by an instrument, known as the electrocardiograph (see Fig. 9).

For the heart to function properly the auricles must contract first, forcing blood into the ventricles. The ventricles must then contract, forcing blood upwards and out through the pulmonary artery and aorta.

The 'Pacemaker' or S-A Node. The action of the heart is co-ordinated by the activity of specialized tissue embedded in the heart wall. Electrical activity (the cardiac impulse) first appears at the sino-auricular node (the S-A node in Fig. 8). This is a specialized piece of cardiac muscle which is more excitable than the rest and is known as the pacemaker. It is embedded in the wall of the right auricle.

A-V Node. From the S-A node, contraction spreads over the auricles and in turn excites the atrio-ventricular node (A-V node).

From the A-V node a band of special muscle, called the bundle of His, passes from the auricles, down the wall between the ventricles and to all parts of the ventricular muscle. The cardiac impulse travels very rapidly down the bundle of His. The ventricles are stimulated to contract so that blood is forced up through the large arteries and into the circulation.

The Electrocardiogram. The electrical changes mentioned above can be recorded on a sensitive instrument called the electrocardiograph. The record produced is an Electrocardiogram, or E.C.G. (Fig. 9). The peaks shown in the illustration are each

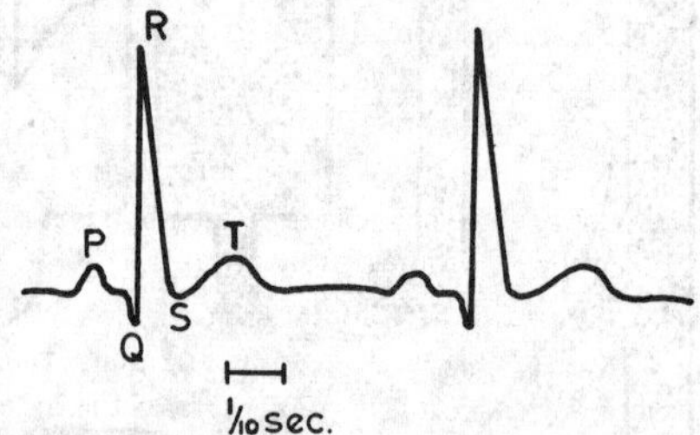

Fig. 9. *THE ELECTROCARDIOGRAM. A record of the electrical changes in the heart during two heart beats. See text.*

connected with activity in a particular part of the heart: the P wave with auricular contraction, the QRS wave with ventricular contraction, and the T wave with ventricular relaxation. In heart disease this record is frequently disturbed or distorted. An E.C.G. may help the doctor to diagnose the type of heart disease a patient has. It can also be used to assess the results of treatment of heart disease.

Regulation of the Heart Rate

In the body the rate and force of the heart beat are influenced by two sets of nerves which supply the S-A node and the A-V node. Sympathetic nerves make the heart beat more rapidly and forcefully. The hormone adrenaline has a similar action. The vagus nerve, part of the parasympathetic nervous system, makes the heart beat more slowly and with less force. The heart rate under normal conditions depends on the balance struck between these two sets of nerves. The vagus nerve probably has the more important influence.

The heart rate is also affected by other things. A rise in temperature will make it beat more quickly. This is the cause of the rapid heart rate in fever.

BLOOD PRESSURE

The Cardiac Output. In one minute, the left ventricle pumps about 10 pints of blood into the aorta for distribution around the body. This quantity of blood is called the cardiac output, and it depends first upon an adequate blood volume. After a hemorrhage, when blood has been lost from the body, the cardiac output falls.

The blood must also flow freely back into the heart from the veins. The return of blood to the heart is helped by two factors.

(a) Expansion of the chest when breathing in: this helps to suck blood into the thorax.

(b) Contraction of the muscles of the limbs: this squeezes the veins and helps to force blood through them.

During exercise a person breathes more deeply and rapidly, and his limb muscles contract very vigorously. Both these actions help to hasten the flow of blood back to the heart. In severe exercise the heart beats much more rapidly, and the cardiac output may rise from 10 pints per minute, at rest, to as much as 50 pints per minute.

Systolic Pressure. Each beat of the heart forces blood into the aorta, causing the pressure inside the artery to rise. A similar rise of pressure occurs in all the arteries of the body. The highest pressure recorded inside the artery is called the systolic blood pressure. The systolic blood pressure is about 120 millimeters of mercury (mm. Hg), as recorded on a manometer, Fig. 10.

The arterial wall contains much elastic tissue. When blood is pumped into the artery from the heart, the blood cannot flow away at once so the artery wall stretches to accommodate the extra fluid. When the ventricle relaxes, the stretched artery walls spring back to their proper size. In doing so, they help to push the blood further along the vessels.

Diastolic Pressure. During relaxation (or diastole) of the heart, the pressure of blood inside the arteries gradually falls. It is increased again when more blood is pumped in. The lowest level of pressure recorded in the artery is the diastolic blood pressure. It is usually about 70 mm. Hg.

The Peripheral Resistance. The heart decides the level of the systolic blood pressure. If the cardiac output is high, the systolic pressure will be high. The value of the diastolic pressure depends on how freely the blood can flow out of the arteries. If it could escape at once from the arteries the pressure would fall to nothing between heart beats.

Blood does not escape very quickly from the arteries because it is prevented from doing so by the small vessels, the arterioles, which branch off at the end of the arteries. The arterioles act like stopcocks. When they are tightly shut blood escapes slowly and so the diastolic pressure is high. If they are wide open the blood runs away quickly and the diastolic pressure is low. The arterioles act as a resistance to blood flow. They provide what is often called the peripheral resistance.

The cardiac output and peripheral resistance together determine the blood pressure.

Regulating the Stopcocks. The arterioles are very important vessels. They can change the arterial blood pressure if a large number constrict or dilate (relax) together. They also regulate the amount of blood flowing to each individual organ.

NERVE CONTROL. The muscle in the walls of the arterioles is supplied by nerves from the sympathetic division of the autonomic nervous system (see Anatomy, pp. 230, 232). These nerves take their orders from a special collection of nerve cells—the vasomotor center—found in the medulla of the brain.

When these nerves are stimulated, the erterioles constrict, or narrow. The vessels expand when stimulation from the brain is reduced. There is, normally, always some activity in the nerves, so the arterioles are usually semi-constricted.

EFFECT OF TEMPERATURE. There are other act ors which alter the amount of constriction, or tone of the arterioles. A rise in temperature of the blood will dilate the vessels, and cold causes constriction. This is easily seen in the skin. On a hot day the skin is warm and pink, the vessels are expanded and much blood flows through them. On a cold day the skin is pale and cold because the arterioles are constricted and a smaller amount of blood is flowing through the skin.

HORMONES, such as adrenaline, will also alter the size of these vessels, and so influence the blood flow and even the general arterial pressure.

Measurement of Blood Pressure

The blood pressure is usually measured in the main artery of the arm, the brachial artery. Fig. 10 shows how this is done with a sphygmomanometer. An inflatable rubber bag confined within a cotton sleeve is wound around the arm just above the elbow. The bag can be blown up with a hand pump. When this is done, the bag presses on the arm and squashes the artery against the humerus (the bone of the upper arm). The pressure inside the bag is measured on a mercury manometer connected to the bag. A stethoscope is placed over the brachial artery and the pressure inside the cuff lowered. As the pressure falls a number of sounds can be heard coming from the artery. By listening to the sequence of sounds one can judge the level of the systolic and diastolic blood pressure.

The systolic blood pressure in a healthy young adult is about 120 mm. Hg and the diastolic pressure about 70 mm. Hg. But there is a lot of variation from person to person.

The elasticity of the arterial walls will also affect the height of the blood pressure. As old age approaches, the artery walls 'harden' and lose much of their elasticity. This is the reason why elderly people have a higher blood pressure than young people.

High Blood Pressure

The blood pressure in a healthy person stays fairly steady. It tends to rise gradually with advancing years but sometimes a young

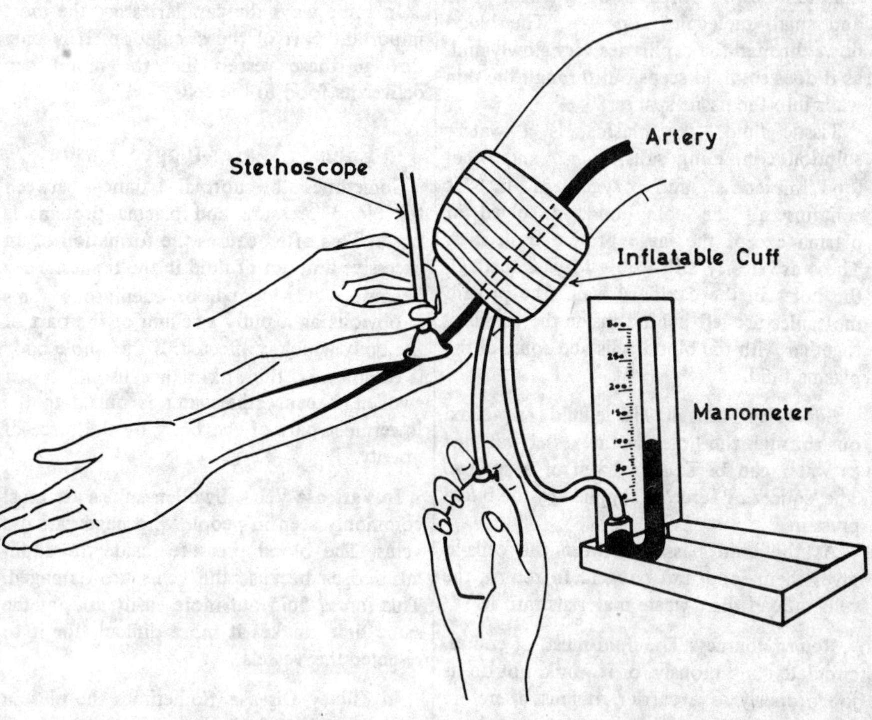

Fig. 10. *MEASUREMENT OF BLOOD PRESSURE. The artery is compressed against the bone of the arm when the cuff is inflated by the hand pump. The pressure inside the cuff is registered on the mercury manometer. The doctor listens through the stethoscope for sounds which tell him the level of the systolic and diastolic blood pressure.*

person develops a high blood pressure, or hypertension. This is abnormal, and will certainly shorten the life of the person concerned. Its cause is quite unknown. It seems fairly certain that the arterioles are more tightly closed than in normal people. This makes the blood pressure rise. But we do not know why the arterioles behave like this.

Because the blood pressure is so high, the heart must work harder to pump blood out into the circulation against such a big resistance. Eventually the heart fails from overwork.

Lowering the Pressure. The blood pressure can often be lowered by giving the patient drugs which depress the nerves controlling the arterioles. The vessels, released from their commanding nerves, open up and the blood pressure falls. This will prolong the life of the patient.

THE CAPILLARIES AND TISSUE FLUID

Although the circulation is used to deliver food and oxygen to the cells, and to carry away their waste materials, the blood stays inside the vessels, while the tissue cells lie outside them.

Delivery of Food. How does the food travel from the blood into the tissue? It does this by means of the tissue fluid which is formed from blood in the capillaries, the smallest blood vessels in the body. Some capillaries are so small that the red cells have to travel in single file through them. The wall of a capillary is very thin and delicate, and only one cell thick. Between the cells there are minute holes, or pores, through which water and small molecules can pass. The blood flows through the capillaries very slowly and, as it does so, fluid seeps out through the thin walls into the tissue spaces.

Tissue fluid, like plasma, is a watery solution containing salts, sugar, and other food materials, and oxygen—in fact it contains all the compounds dissolved in plasma except the large protein molecules. These are nearly all too big to pass through the holes in the capillary wall. The protein molecules are left behind inside the capillary together with the blood cells and some of the plasma fluid.

Squeezing Through. Tissue fluid is squeezed out through the holes in the vessel wall just as water can be squeezed out of a sponge. The 'squeezing force' is supplied by the blood pressure.

As the fluid passes between the cells it gives them food and oxygen. In return, the cells unload their waste materials into it.

Return Journey. The fluid must, of course, circulate continuously, or it would not do its job properly as a carrier. It must therefore return to the circulation in order to pick up more food and oxygen, and to deliver the waste materials to the kidneys and lungs.

The plasma proteins which have been left behind inside the capillaries play an important part in attracting tissue fluid back into the capillaries by their osmotic action (see p 238). Just as egg albumen pulls water through a cellophane bag, so do the plasma proteins pull tissue fluid back into the blood vessels.

Tissue fluid returns to the circulation at the ends of the capillaries just as they join up to

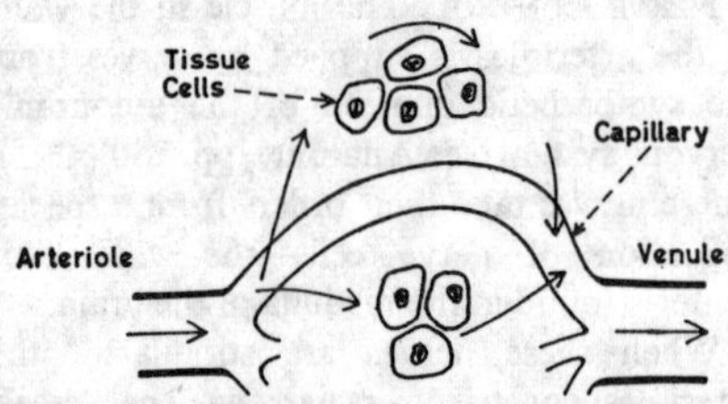

Fig. 11. *THE CIRCULATION OF TISSUE FLUID. Fluid filters through the wall of the capillary as it leaves the arteriole where the blood pressure is high. Fluid from the tissue cells returns through the capillary walls and into the venule where pressure is low.*

form the thicker walled venules. At the end of the capillary the blood pressure inside the vessel is much lower than at the beginning.

A Tug-of-War. There are two forces at work on the tissue fluid (Fig. 11). The blood pressure trying to drive fluid out of the vessel, and the osmotic attraction of the proteins trying to pull it back again.

At the beginning of the capillary, the blood pressure wins this tug-of-war and fluid is pushed out into the tissue spaces and percolates around the cells. At the end of the capillaries where they join to form the veins, the plasma proteins win and the fluid re-enters the circulation.

In some ways the capillaries are the most important part of the circulation. It is only through these vessels that the blood can deliver its food to the cells.

Edema: Water-logged Tissue

Sometimes the normal balance between the blood pressure and plasma proteins is upset. This often causes the formation of an excessive amount of fluid in the tissues. They become water-logged, or edematous. This is obvious as a puffy swelling of the part of the body which is affected. If the whole body is edematous, the ankles are usually most swollen, because the water is pulled to the lowermost part of the body by the force of gravity.

In Varicose Veins. Swollen ankles are most commonly seen in people who have varicose veins. The blood pressure inside the capillaries rises because the veins are damaged. This forces fluid out more easily and, at the same time, makes it more difficult for it to re-enter the vessels.

In Kidney Disease. Sometimes the plasma proteins are at fault. In patients who have chronic kidney disease, the amount of protein in the blood may be very low since the blood loses its protein into the urine through the damaged kidneys. The osmotic force pulling tissue fluid back into the vessels is then too small to recover the normal amount, and the tissues become water-logged.

In Local Inflammation. If the capillaries become more than usually porous, the holes may be big enough to allow large amounts of the big protein molecules to leak out into the tissue spaces. The proteins then help to pull fluid out of the capillary. This helps to cause the swelling found around a local inflammation such as a boil. The capillaries become more 'leaky' because of powerful chemicals which are released during the infection.

Dehydration

Too little tissue fluid is formed only when the whole body is short of water. In severe dehydration, such as may occur in constant vomiting or chronic diarrhea, or in hot dry climates, the skin loses its elasticity, the cheeks become sunken and the person looks as if he has lost weight—as indeed he has. The whole body shares in this dehydration, and less fluid than usual is found in the tissues.

THE VEINS

From the capillaries blood passes into the veins. These vessels distend very easily, and carry blood under low pressure back to the right auricle of the heart.

The veins are very capacious and hold a large amount of blood. In fact, about 65 per cent of the total quantity of blood in the body is in the veins. They act as a blood reservoir. After a hemorrhage the veins can become very much smaller, squeezing blood out into the rest of the circulation where it is sorely needed.

The blood in the veins is deoxygenated and bluish in color. It has parted with much of its food and oxygen to the tissues, and carries a big load of waste materials. The veins eventually empty into the right side of the heart, to be pumped by the right ventricle through the lungs. In the lungs, carbon dioxide 'waste' is exchanged for oxygen and the blood flows into the left ventricle for recirculation around the body.

Varicose Veins

There are valves at intervals along the veins. These lie so that blood can only flow toward the heart, and not backward away from it. Often the valves become damaged and no longer do their job properly. The veins then become swollen and distended with blood, and appear as varicose veins. In many women, varicose veins first appear during a pregnancy. The baby, lying inside the womb, presses on the veins at the top of the mother's leg, and distends them. The prolonged pressure damages the valves and so permanent varicose veins may develop.

RESPIRATION

The Combustion Process. The tissues of the body need energy to do work. This energy comes from food, and is set free when the tissues burn their food. Oxygen is used up during this combustion or burning process. Another gas, carbon dioxide, is formed during the process and it must be excreted.

Glucose + oxygen = water + carbon dioxide + energy

$$C_6H_{12}O_6 + 6\,O_2 = 6\,H_2O + 6\,CO_2 + \text{energy}$$

The burning process is summarized in this chemical equation. 6 molecules of oxygen are needed to burn 1 molecule of glucose: 6 molecules of water and 6 of carbon dioxide form. The energy locked up in the glucose molecule is set free and can be used by the cells.

Carbon dioxide is an acidic substance; it combines with water to make carbonic acid. The tissues are very sensitive to acid, and can tolerate only very little of it. The carbon dioxide must therefore be excreted quickly, before it poisons the tissues.

Respiration is the study of the ways and means of supplying oxygen to the tissues, and ridding the body of carbon dioxide.

How Oxygen Enters the Lungs. The oxygen used by the body comes from the air, which is a mixture of gases, 20 per cent of it being oxygen. Table 2 shows the exact composition of atmospheric air. Notice that there is very little carbon dioxide.

How does oxygen get into the blood from the air? This happens in the lungs. The respiratory system is described in Anatomy, p.227. With each breath, air is drawn into the lungs, passing first through the nose, where it warms up to the temperature of the body and is moistened.

Deep in the chest, the tiny bronchioles lead to little air sacs, alveoli, whose walls are very thin. Each alveolus is enveloped by a network of capillary blood vessels. The capillary wall is also very thin, so that gas passing from the alveoli into the blood has only to cross two layers of cells.

Exchange of Gases. The gas inside the alveoli is called alveolar air. It is different from atmospheric air since it contains less oxygen and more carbon dioxide (Table 2). Blood takes oxygen from alveolar air and gives up carbon dioxide in exchange.

With each breath, a person sucks about 500 milliliters (over a pint) of air into his lungs. This mixes with the gas in the deeper parts of the lung, supplying it with oxygen. As he breathes out, carbon dioxide from the alveoli escapes into the atmosphere.

The normal respiratory rate is about 16 breaths a minute. During that time, about 250 milliliters of oxygen enter the blood, to be used by the tissues. Over the same time the body manufactures about 230 milliliters of carbon dioxide which is excreted through the lungs.

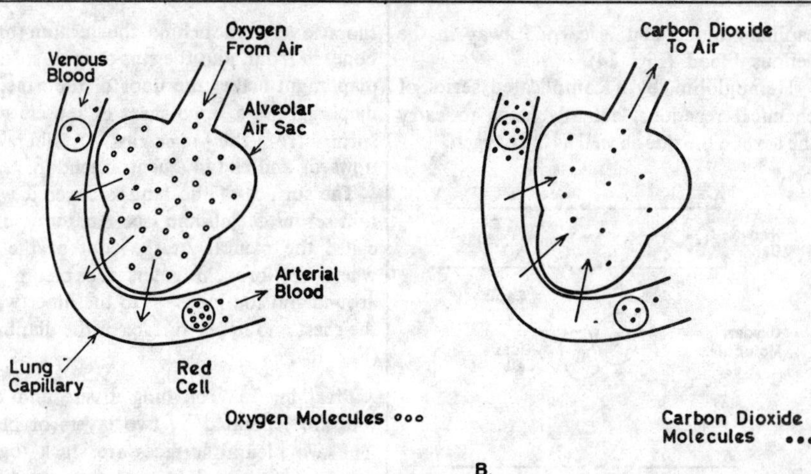

Fig. 12. *GAS EXCHANGE IN THE LUNGS.* A. *Alveolar air contains a higher concentration of oxygen molecules than venous blood. Oxygen diffuses from alveolar air into the blood.* B. *Alveolar air has a lower concentration of carbon dioxide than venous blood. Carbon dioxide diffuses from the blood into the alveoli of the lungs.*

TABLE 2
Percentage Composition of Dry Atmospheric Air and Alveolar Air

Gas	*Atmospheric Air*	*Alveolar Air*
Oxygen	20·95	14·2
Nitrogen	79·00	80·3
Carbon dioxide	0·05	5·5

Increasing the Exchange Rate. Of course, the amount of oxygen taken into the body depends upon how hard the tissues are working. When a man is running he uses more energy, and his need for oxygen increases too. This is supplied by an increase in the depth and rate of respiration. When a person is at rest, he breathes about 8 liters of air in and out of his lungs in one minute. In vigorous exercise this may increase to 70 liters per minute.

Respiration, then, is geared to the body's demand for oxygen and its need to excrete the waste product, carbon dioxide.

Oxygen Revitalizes the Blood. The right side of the heart pumps blood into the lungs (see Fig. 7). This is venous blood collected from all parts of the body. Venous blood has a low concentration of oxygen, and a high concentration of carbon dioxide.

As the blood flows through the lung capillaries it gives up carbon dioxide and takes in oxygen. These changes occur because the concentration of oxygen molecules in alveolar air is greater than their concentration in the venous blood. Oxygen molecules diffuse (see p. 237) from alveolar air into the blood (Fig. 12A).

The concentration of carbon dioxide molecules in blood is greater than that of alveolar air, and so carbon dioxide moves out of the blood into the alveoli (Fig. 12B).

Table 3 shows the amounts of carbon dioxide and oxygen in 100 milliliters of blood in an artery and in a vein. As each 100 milliliters of blood flows through the lungs it gives up 6 milliliters of carbon dioxide and takes in 56.5 milliliters of oxygen.

TABLE 3

Gas	*Arterial Blood*	*Venous Blood*
Oxygen	19	12·5
Carbon dioxide	50	56

(milliliters of gas per 100 milliliters of blood)

Hemoglobin: the Oxygen Carrier

Role of Iron. Hemoglobin is a protein with the element iron in its molecule. The iron can pick up oxygen when the oxygen pressure is high, and hold on to it very loosely. When blood passes through the tissues where the oxygen pressure is low, the hemoglobin gives up its oxygen. Oxygen molecules then diffuse from the blood into the tissue fluid, to be used by the cells.

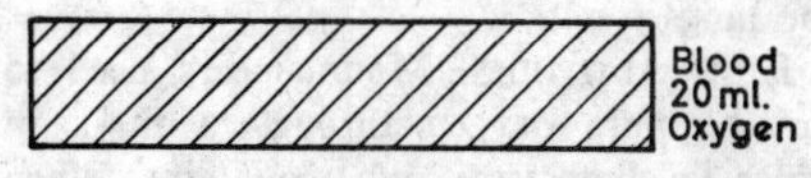

Fig. 13. *OXYGEN TRANSPORT A comparison of the amount of oxygen taken up by 100 milliliters of plasma and 100 milliliters of whole blood. This shows the importance of red blood cells in oxygen transport.*

As in the lungs, oxygen molecules travel by diffusion from a region of high oxygen pressure (in the blood) towards the tissues where the oxygen pressure is low (Fig. 14).

Removal of Carbon Dioxide. Carbon dioxide travels in the opposite direction. The cells make carbon dioxide which dissolves in the tissue fluid around them. The arterial blood flowing into the capillaries has a low pressure of carbon dioxide. The tissue fluid has a high pressure of carbon dioxide. So carbon dioxide diffuses from tissue fluid to capillary blood and is carried away in the venous blood (Fig. 14).

Hemoglobin, by a complicated series of chemical reactions, actually helps to carry the carbon dioxide as well as the oxygen.

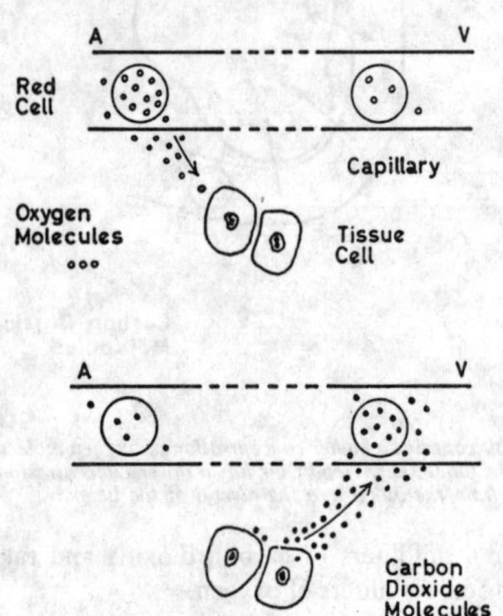

Fig. 14. *GAS EXCHANGE IN THE TISSUES. Arterial blood (A) has a high concentration of oxygen and a low concentration of carbon dioxide. As the blood flows through the capillaries the cells take up oxygen (top) and exchange it for carbon dioxide (bottom). Venous blood (V) has a low concentration of oxygen and a high concentration of carbon dioxide.*

How Oxygen Shortage Causes Fast Breathing

A shortage of oxygen in the body, anoxia, may have several causes.

In a stuffy room the air entering the lungs may have too little oxygen in it. On the other hand, the oxygen pressure is low at high altitudes so that the alveoli cannot get enough oxygen into the blood for the body's needs. To overcome this, the respiration rate increases in an attempt to take more air into the lungs.

High Altitudes. Mountaineers need to breathe pure oxygen through a mask in order to climb very high mountains. When flying in an aircraft at very high altitudes, the inside of the aircraft is pressurized to keep the oxygen pressure up to a normal value and so allow comfortable breathing.

In Pneumonia. Patients with pneumonia become very breathless, because they too are short of oxygen. There is enough oxygen inside the lungs, but the gas cannot easily get into the blood. The alveoli are filled with pus and fluid which prevent the easy diffusion of gas into the blood.

Anemia. In a patient who is anemic, there is too little hemoglobin in the blood to carry enough oxygen for the cells' needs. His heart beats more rapidly and so pumps the available hemoglobin more quickly around the circulation. This usually supplies the tissues with enough oxygen when the patient is resting. If the patient takes even mild exercise, he usually becomes breathless.

How Breathing Takes Place

The Breathing Apparatus. The lungs lie inside the thorax, a bony cage formed by the thoracic vertebrae behind, the sternum (breastbone) in front, and the ribs at each side. The diaphragm makes the floor of the cage. The diaphragm is a large sheet of muscle which springs from the lower ribs. Its fibers arch upwards and end in a central tendon.

The surface of the lung is covered with a thin serous membrane (see Anatomy, p.228) called the pleura. At the root of the lung where the bronchi enter, the pleura curls around and continues on to the inner wall of the chest and upper surface of the diaphragm (Fig. 15).

Breathing In. The lung tissue and chest wall are separated by two layers of pleura. The two pleural surfaces are stuck together by a thin film of fluid, and are very difficult to separate. This is very important. When the chest wall moves outward during inspiration, the pleura lining the chest wall pulls on the membrane covering the lungs. This, in turn, drags on the lung tissue and so the lungs expand.

How does the thorax get bigger during inspiration? The lower ribs lie rather like the handle of a bucket. They swing upwards and outwards during inspiration. This makes the thorax bigger from side to side. The movement of the upper ribs pushes the breastbone forwards, deepening the chest from back to front. Contraction of the intercostal muscles, connecting the ribs one with the other, causes these movements.

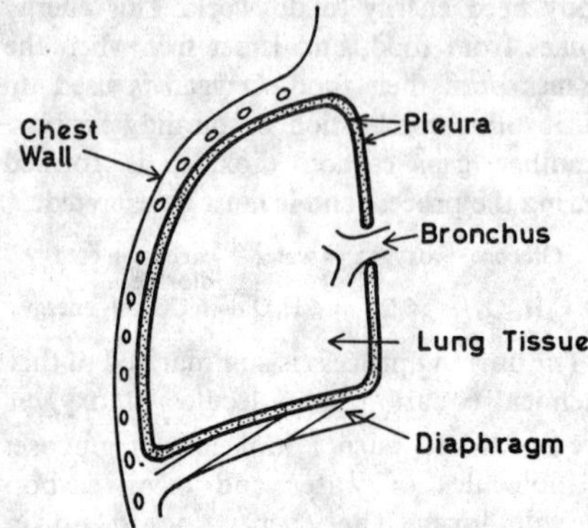

Fig. 15. *THE PLEURA. A thin membrane lining the chest wall and covering the lung surface.*

The diaphragm, when it contracts, pulls the thoracic floor downwards towards the abdomen. Thus, during inspiration, the thorax becomes much bigger (Fig. 16). The elastic lung tissue is pulled outward by the movement of the chest wall, and so air rushes into the lungs.

Breathing Out. Expiration (breathing out) is passive. The intercostal muscles and diaphragm relax. The elastic tissue in the lungs springs back to its normal size and air

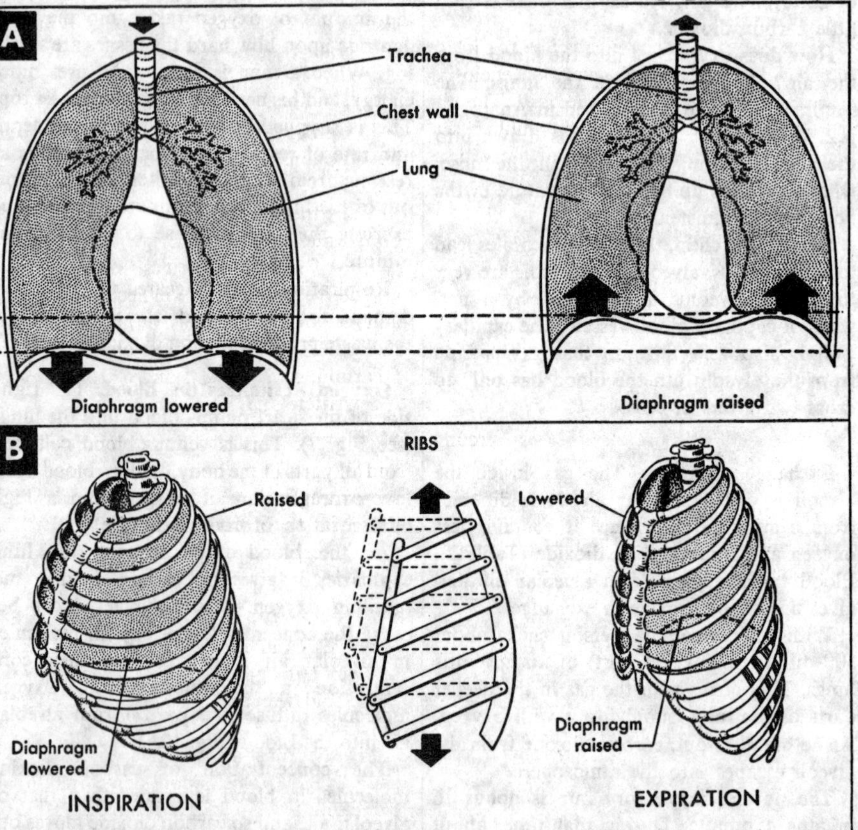

By courtesy of Routledge & Kegan Paul, from *Life: An Introduction to Biology* by G. G. Simpson, C. S. Pittendrigh, and L. H. Tiffany.

Fig. 16. *MECHANICS OF BREATHING. Movement of air in and out of the lungs is due to the bellows-like action of the thoracic cavity in which the lungs lie. Air is forced into the lungs when the cavity is enlarged by inspiration. Air is forced out of the lungs when the cavity is reduced in volume by expiration. The central diagram indicates the way in which the ribs are loosely joined to the spinal column and breast-bone.*

is forced out through the trachea into the atmosphere.

About 500 milliliters (about a pint) of air passes into the respiratory 'tree' with each inspiration. This is called the *tidal volume.*

Respiratory movements not only ventilate the lungs. Inspiration also helps to suck blood into the chest from the veins, and so assists the circulation.

ARTIFICIAL RESPIRATION

At any time one may be faced with an emergency in which a person has been electrocuted or drowned. The victim's respiration has stopped, but his heart is still beating.

First Aid. Prompt artificial respiration (see First Aid, p. 19) may then save a life. It is essential to keep the blood oxygenated until the victim begins to breathe again on his own. Speed is all important for success.

There are many different methods of artificial respiration. They can be learned by any lay person in a very short time. The best and simplest is probably the mouth-to-mouth breathing method.

Every responsible person should know how to apply artificial respiration in an emergency.

Artificial Respiration by Machine. Sometimes artificial respiration must be given by machine to a patient for a very long time. This may happen during an attack of poliomyelitis, or following an overdose of barbiturates.

IRON LUNG. The patient may be put inside an iron lung. This is a metal box enclosing the whole body except for the head. The box is made airtight with a light rubber seal around the neck. At regular intervals air is sucked out of the box. This pulls the patient's chest wall outward and draws air into his lungs. Some patients have lived for years in an iron lung, but the general nursing care of the patient is rather difficult.

PORTABLE MACHINES. Today it is more common to use a machine which inflates the lungs through a tube in the windpipe. The machine is small and portable, and there are no special nursing problems to be overcome.

Brain's Control of Breathing

The normal respiratory rate of an adult at rest is about 16 breaths a minute. This supplies the body with the oxygen it needs and allows it to excrete all the carbon dioxide formed. During inspiration the intercostal muscles and diaphragm contract. During expiration the muscles relax. The muscles are 'commanded' to contract by their nerves. These, in turn, are controlled by the respiratory center which is a special collection of nerve cells in the brain and is vital to life.

The respiratory rhythm is affected by many things. Respiration stops when the person swallows. His rhythm alters when he speaks. The respiratory center is particularly sensitive to the pressure of carbon dioxide in the blood. If this rises, respiration immediately increases. The extra carbon dioxide quickly passes out into the atmosphere.

A low pressure of oxygen in the blood also stimulates respiration. More fresh air enters the lungs and so the blood takes up more oxygen to satisfy the extra demand.

In this way, the respiratory rate alters to meet the changing needs of the body.

NUTRITION AND METABOLISM

The energy needed to finance the vital activities of the body comes from the food we eat. A normal diet contains the three main classes of foodstuffs: fat, carbohydrate and protein. These are complicated organic materials which are built up by other organisms, both animals and plants. As they are made, energy is locked up in their molecules.

To obtain this stored energy for our own purpose, we must break down, or 'unlock,' the molecules. The unlocking process begins during digestion. The large complicated molecules eaten in the food are chopped up chemically in the intestine. The smaller molecules set free pass into the bloodstream. They are then carried in the blood to the tissues. In the tissues the small molecules are finally disrupted, giving up all their stored energy.

As well as supplying fuel to the body, food also provides the raw materials for building new body tissues.

THE COMPOSITION OF FOOD

1. **Carbohydrate.** This type of compound has carbon, hydrogen and oxygen in its molecules. Sugar and starch are both carbohydrates. The more complicated carbohydrates, e.g. starch, are made of long chains of simple molecules, or units, joined together. The glucose molecule forms the unit, or 'brick,' in many large carbohydrate molecules. Each glucose molecule contains 6 carbon, 12 hydrogen and 6 oxygen atoms. It is written $C_6H_{12}O_6$.

2. **Fat.** Fats also have carbon, hydrogen and oxygen in their molecules. These atoms are arranged in quite a different way from those in the carbohydrate molecules. The main energy stores of the body are formed from fat.

3. **Protein.** Protein molecules have carbon, hydrogen, and oxygen atoms plus NITROGEN in them. Nitrogen is essential for building new tissue and we cannot do without protein in our diet.

The diet must also contain water, minerals and vitamins. This is considered fully in the section on Food and Nutrition, p. 65).

ENERGY VALUE OF FOOD

When food burns, or is oxidized, in the body a definite and measurable amount of energy is liberated. This all ultimately appears as heat. Waste products also appear. Fat and carbohydrate form carbon dioxide and water. Protein forms, in addition, nitrogen-containing waste products such as urea.

The chemical reaction describing the burning or oxidation of glucose is written:

$$C_6H_{12}O_6 + 6\,O_2 = 6\,CO_2 + 6\,H_2O + \text{Heat}$$

Glucose + oxygen = carbon dioxide + water + ENERGY

Each molecule of glucose needs 6 molecules of oxygen to burn it. Six molecules of carbon dioxide and six of water form, and a certain amount of heat is set free.

Calories. Heat is measured in units called calories, just as weight is measured in grams or ounces. 1 calorie is the amount of heat needed to raise the temperature of 1 kilogram of water by 1°C.

When 1 gram of glucose burns, 4.1 calories are set free.

When fat burns, carbon dioxide + water + heat are also formed. However, 1 gram of fat produces 9.3 calories of heat, weight for weight, so fat has an energy value more than twice that of sugar.

When 1 gram of protein is burned in the body, 4.1 calories of heat appear. Protein and sugar have about the same energy value, weight for weight (Fig. 17). The end products of protein combustion contain nitrogen.

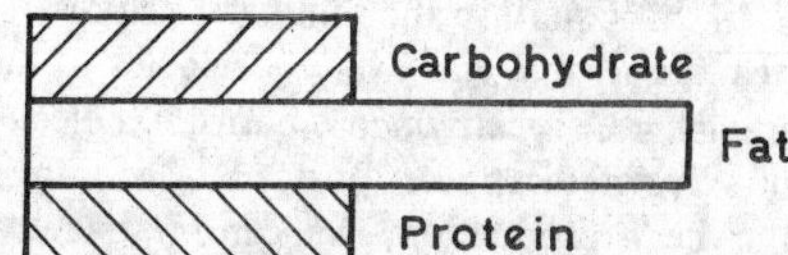

Fig. 17. *ENERGY VALUES. Fat contains more than twice as much energy as the same weight of carbohydrate or protein.*

Three things stand out from what has already been said.

1. **Energy Released.** Each type of foodstuff has an energy value which can be measured.

2. **Oxygen is used up** when food burns. Oxygen is supplied by respiration.

3. **Waste Produced.** When food burns, waste products appear. These must be excreted. If they remained in the body, they would poison the tissues.

The main waste product is carbon dioxide. This is an acidic substance which leaves the body as a gas through the lungs. Other acids are formed in much smaller quantities. These are not gaseous and so cannot be excreted through the lungs. They leave the body in the urine. Nitrogen-containing substances, chiefly urea, formed from protein breakdown also pass out in the urine.

The metabolic activities of the cells are supported and indeed made possible by the processes of digestion, absorption, respiration and excretion.

How Much Food? How much food does a normal person need to eat? This question is simply answered: enough to cover his energy and growth requirements. To answer the question properly we must be able to measure our energy and growth needs. The energy value of each kind of foodstuff is known, and so it is easy to calculate the weight of food needed to supply any number of calories.

ENERGY NEEDS OF THE BODY

Even when asleep, a person uses energy. This is needed to keep the heart beating, the respiratory muscles working, and most of all to keep the temperature of the body at the high level of about 37° C (98° to 99° F).

Basal Metabolic Rate. The energy used by the body when completely at rest, not digesting food or doing work of any kind is called the Basal Metabolic Rate, or the B.M.R. All the energy used by the body in this basal, resting condition eventually appears as heat.

Therefore, to measure the minimum resting energy usage by the body, we need only measure the amount of heat formed under resting conditions. This sounds simple, but is actually very difficult, and so the problem must be tackled in another way.

Let us look again at the chemical equation which describes the combustion of glucose.

$$C_6H_{12}O_6 + 6\,O_2 = 6\,CO_2 + 6H_2O + X\text{Calories}$$
$$\text{glucose} + \text{oxygen} = \text{carbon dioxide} + \text{water} + \text{heat}$$

In this equation the number of calories of heat is called X. Each time X calories of heat are given up when glucose burns, 6 molecules of oxygen disappear. Instead of measuring the heat production, we can measure the amount of oxygen which is used. This enables us to calculate the amount of heat set free, because we know how much oxygen is exchanged for the heat.

Measuring the Fire of the Body. The B.M.R. is the fire of the body when it is burning most slowly. The amount of heat given off by this fire can be calculated by measuring the amount of oxygen used by the body. This measurement is often made in hospitals when the doctor suspects that his patient's basal energy production is abnormal. The patient lies quietly at rest in warm comfortable surroundings. No food is eaten for 12 hours before the test, as digestion uses up energy and so upsets the result. The patient then breathes normally from a tank filled with oxygen. After half an hour the amount of oxygen which has disappeared from the tank into the body is measured. The heat production of the patient during the period of the test can then be calculated.

Thyroid Control of B.M.R. The diet of an adult must supply 1,800 calories to provide energy for basal activities. In other words, the B.M.R. of an adult is about 1,800 calories per day. Men need more calories than women. In proportion to their size, children need more than adults, because they are growing rapidly and building new body tissue. For the same reason, pregnant women need more than those who are not pregnant.

The resting energy consumption of the body seems to be controlled by the thyroid gland. This is an endocrine gland which makes a special chemical, or hormone, called thyroxine. Thyroxine is delivered to all the cells of the body by the blood. In some way it stimulates the cells, making them work hard to produce heat and use up oxygen.

THYROTOXICOSIS. Sometimes the thyroid gland produces an excessive amount of thyroxine. The cells of the body work harder and produce more heat. The patient's B.M.R. goes up above normal levels. This condition is called thyrotoxicosis. The patient's skin is warm and flushed in an attempt to get rid of the extra heat. The person usually loses weight because the body's food stores are being used up as the cells work harder.

MYXEDEMA. The thyroid gland may be underactive, and produce too little thyroxine. The B.M.R. is then lower than normal and, as the cells are not working so hard, they produce less heat and use less oxygen. In an adult, this condition is called myxedema. In a child, underactivity of the thyroid may produce a cretin (see Diseases of the Endocrine Glands, p. 401).

The doctor uses the B.M.R. measurement to check that his patient's energy consumption is normal. If it is abnormal, thyroid disease may be suspected.

FOOD FOR WORK

The average adult needs 1,800 calories each day for basal requirements. It would be difficult to do much physical work on a diet of this size without losing weight. One must eat extra food to provide energy for work.

Scientists have made many measurements of the amount of energy used up in doing different kinds of job. We know therefore how many extra calories are needed for typing, scrubbing floors, walking upstairs and many other activities. For example, 30 calories per hour are needed for dressing and undressing; 25 calories per hour for sewing; 175 calories per hour for polishing floors; while swimming, one uses up about 400 calories per hour. See also p. 72.

The energy needs of a person in almost any job can be calculated from measurements of this kind. It is usually estimated that a housewife needs about 2,200 calories to cover all her activities, while a coal miner needs about 5,000 calories per day.

Importance of Proteins. We now know how many calories each type of food can supply. Fat, carbohydrate and protein all provide calories. However, there are very good reasons for taking a mixture of all three kinds of food in the diet.

Only protein can supply the nitrogen needed to build new tissues and the special secretions of many cells.

AMINO ACIDS. Proteins are made from chains of 'bricks' called amino acids. There are about 20 different amino acids occurring naturally. About half of these can be manufactured inside the body. The rest must be supplied in the diet and are called essential amino acids because they are essential for health and growth. Animal proteins have a greater number of essential amino acids in their molecules than plant proteins do.

The average person takes about 70 grams of protein each day in the diet. This provides about 300 calories.

TABLE 4
Calories from Food

	Weight in grams	*Calories*
Protein	70	300
Fat	70	630
Carbohydrate	360	1440
	Total	2370

Fat, too, is necessary for health. It contains some essential growth factors, and carries the fat-soluble vitamins A and D. Because each gram of fat yields many calories a small portion will provide a great deal of energy. Fat is important too because it makes the diet palatable and more interesting. In most diets fat provides about a quarter of the total calorie intake.

The remaining calories are supplied by carbohydrate, the cheapest of the foodstuffs. **Table 4 shows the number of Calories** provided by each type of food in the average balanced diet. The balanced diet of course includes minerals, such as iron and calcium, and plenty of fluid. This is considered in Food and Nutrition, p. 65.

KEEPING THE BODY WARM

Most of the heat produced by the cells is used to keep the temperature of the body at about 37° C or about 99° F.

Variations in Temperature. The actual temperature depends upon where the thermometer is placed. The deeper parts of the body, where most of the heat is produced, are warmer than the surface of the body. The temperature is usually about 98·4° F in the mouth, a degree lower in the armpit, and a degree higher in the rectum. It is a mistake, however, to think that the temperature must be 98·4° F in the mouth. Normal people do not all have exactly the same temperature. Each day the body temperature varies a little. It is lowest at about 6 a.m. and a degree or so higher at 6 p.m.

The temperature of the body remains fairly steady even though the temperature of its surroundings may change very considerably in the course of a single day. How does the body temperature stay so constant? It does so because the body is able to strike a fine balance between the amount of heat produced in the body and the amount of heat lost to the outside world.

The Source of Heat. The body is like a slow-burning fire. All the time the tissues are consuming food and producing heat. This slow-burning fire we have called the Basal Metabolic Rate. During exercise, or physical work of any kind, the tissues make more heat; that is to say, the fire burns more fiercely. When it is very cold, we actually use exercise as a way of making more heat to keep us warm.

Shivering—one of the body's responses to cold—is a mild form of exercise. The muscles contract involuntarily and, in doing so, provide the body with more heat.

COOLING DOWN

Heat produced in the body is lost through the skin to the outside world. Because the temperature of the surrounding air is lower than the temperature of the body in most parts of the world, we lose heat all the time. The body temperature stays steady because we lose just about as much heat as we produce in our tissues.

The body loses heat in four ways: by conduction of heat when a colder surface is touched; by radiation, like an electric fire; by convection; and by sweating (see below).

Conduction, Radiation, and Convection. In the first process, the hot skin warms the air next to it. The warm air rises and moves away, to be replaced by a layer of cold air.

When the skin is much warmer than the surrounding air, it loses a lot of heat by radiation to the air. This cools the body down. On the other hand, when the skin is at almost the same temperature as the air, very little heat can be lost. This means that the temperature of the skin is very important in regulating the heat loss.

The temperature of the skin depends upon the amount of blood flowing through it. When a lot of blood flows through the skin it looks red and feels warm. A pale cold skin has a much smaller blood flow. The blood vessels in the skin can be opened or shut by the nerves of the sympathetic system. On a cold day the nerves are active and 'instruct' the skin blood vessels to shut down.

Sweating. On a hot day, although the skin blood flows very rapidly through the skin bringing all the heat it can to the surface of the body, this probably will not cool the skin sufficiently. The body then falls back on a fourth method for losing heat. This is the evaporation of water from the skin. When water evaporates, it absorbs heat from the skin, and so cools it down. The sweat glands secrete a fluid through the pores of the skin where it evaporates. If the air is very damp, the sweat will not evaporate nor cool the body. This is why people cannot easily tolerate a hot humid climate. In a hot dry climate, on the other hand, the sweat can evaporate and cool the body.

THE THERMOSTAT IN THE BRAIN

The body regulates its temperature with the help of the brain. In the brain there is a special collection of nerve cells which acts as a thermostat. If the blood temperature rises, as it may do after exercise, the nervous system 'commands' the skin blood vessels to open so that they can lose more heat. Alternatively, if the body temperature drops slightly on a cold day, the nervous system stimulates the blood vessels to close and causes shivering.

It is a remarkable fact that the body temperature stays nearly constant (excluding illness) throughout the year, whatever the weather. This illustrates the power of the body to adapt itself to changing conditions in its surroundings without disturbing its own, internal, environment.

DIGESTION

Between being eaten and surrendering its energy in the tissue cells, food must travel a long journey and undergo many chemical changes. These changes—the breaking down of the large and complicated molecules of the foodstuffs into small molecules which the tissue cells can use—form the process known as digestion.

Digestion of starch releases glucose molecules which are small enough to pass through the wall of the intestine and enter the bloodstream. Big protein molecules are broken into small units called amino acids, and fats into fatty acids.

Enzymes as Aids to Digestion

The chemical reactions which liberate molecules during digestion can all be performed in the laboratory. If starch is boiled in acid for many hours, glucose eventually appears. Food cannot be boiled inside the body, which has a temperature well below that of boiling water. Such a reaction would take far too long to be useful to the body.

But in the intestine there are special chemical helpers, or enzymes, which speed up the digestion of food. Enzyme action enables food to be digested quickly. Each type of foodstuff has a special enzyme to help digest it.

The enzymes are manufactured by the digestive glands which pour their secretions into the intestine. As the food passes through the alimentary canal it meets the secretions of each of these glands in turn and so is gradually broken down.

Digestion in the Mouth

When food is eaten, it is thoroughly chewed and mixed with saliva. This sticky fluid is secreted by the salivary glands (Fig. 18).

Function of Saliva. Saliva has many functions. It moistens the food and so helps in swallowing. It moistens the lips and tongue, and aids speech. The chemicals which give food its flavor dissolve in the saliva, which in this way helps us in tasting the food. Saliva also has in it an enzyme which speeds up the digestion of starch.

Food usually stays in the mouth for only a short time. When it has been chewed and thoroughly mixed with saliva it is swallowed, and slips down the gullet (esophagus) into the stomach.

Digestion in the Stomach

In the stomach, food mixes with gastric juice. This is a very acid juice which contains an enzyme, pepsin, for digesting protein.

The juice is made in numerous tiny glands embedded in the stomach wall. As soon as food enters the mouth these glands begin to secrete gastric juice. Taste buds in the mouth send messages to the central nervous system and this in turn causes stimulation of the nerves supplying the salivary glands, the gastric glands, and even the pancreas. The whole digestive mechanism is put into gear by the act of eating.

The gastric glands continue to secrete gastric juice for a very long time after food has been eaten. The glands are stimulated by a hormone, a chemical, which passes in the bloodstream to the gastric glands. The juice is released from the wall of the stomach and the intestine while food is being digested. This means that as long as there is food in the stomach, there will be gastric juice present to deal with it.

Digestion in the Intestine

The ceaseless movements of the stomach wall mix up the food and gastric juice.

In the Small Intestine. Gradually all the stomach contents pass into the duodenum, which is the first part of the small intestine. If the meal contains a lot of fat, the stomach empties much more slowly than when a non-fatty meal is eaten.

In the small intestine food mixes with pancreatic juice, bile and succus entericus (the juice from glands in the intestinal wall) (Fig. 18).

The intestinal and pancreatic glands between them contain a mixture of enzymes which hasten the breakdown of fat, carbohydrate and protein. The large molecules are split up into smaller ones. The small molecules pass into the blood and travel in the portal vein to the liver.

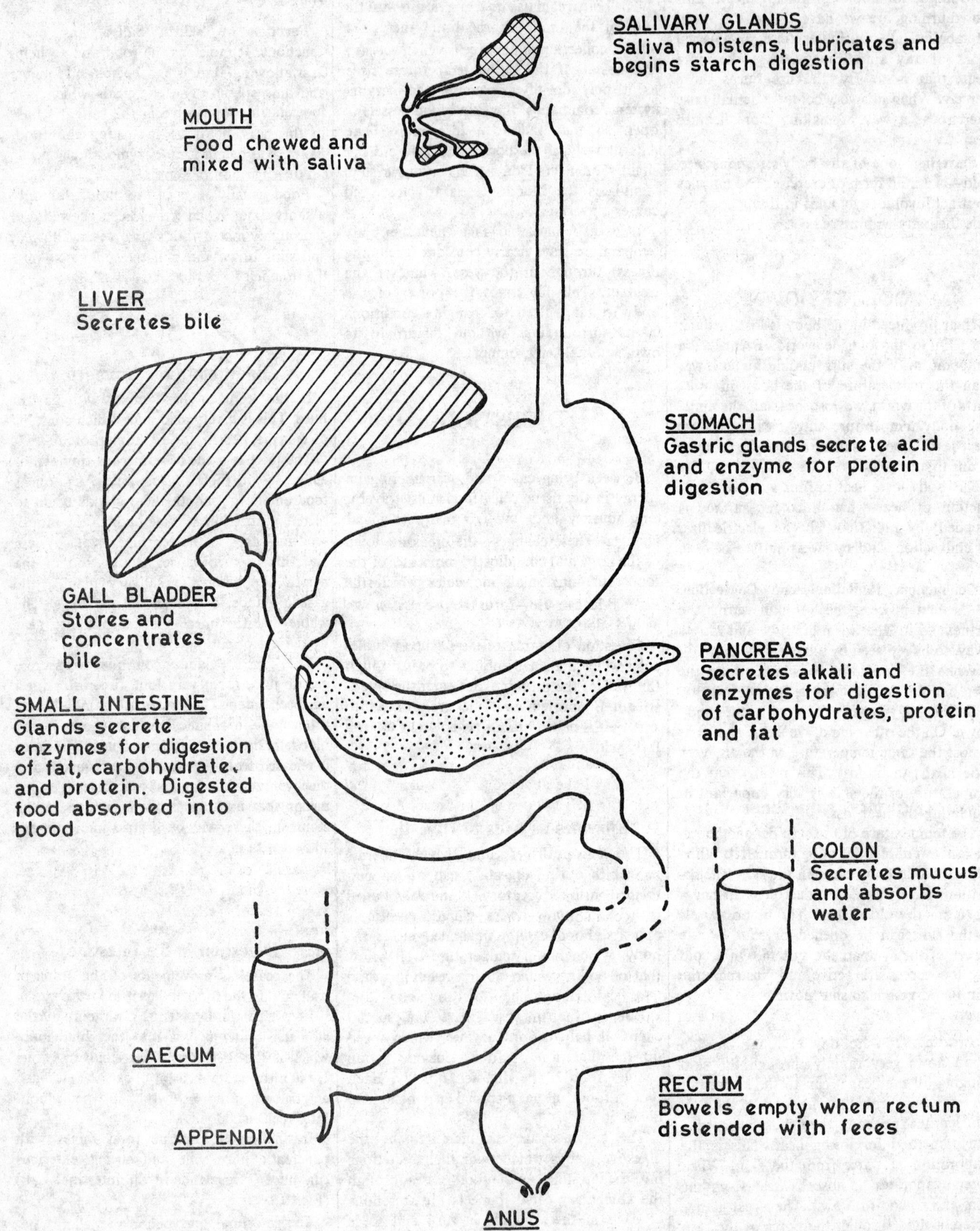
SALIVARY GLANDS
Saliva moistens, lubricates and begins starch digestion
MOUTH
Food chewed and mixed with saliva
LIVER
Secretes bile
STOMACH
Gastric glands secrete acid and enzyme for protein digestion
GALL BLADDER
Stores and concentrates bile
PANCREAS
Secretes alkali and enzymes for digestion of carbohydrates, protein and fat
SMALL INTESTINE
Glands secrete enzymes for digestion of fat, carbohydrate, and protein. Digested food absorbed into blood
COLON
Secretes mucus and absorbs water
CAECUM
RECTUM
Bowels empty when rectum distended with feces
APPENDIX
ANUS

Fig. 18. *HOW THE ALIMENTARY CANAL FUNCTIONS. A diagram to illustrate the physiology of the gastro-intestinal tract.*

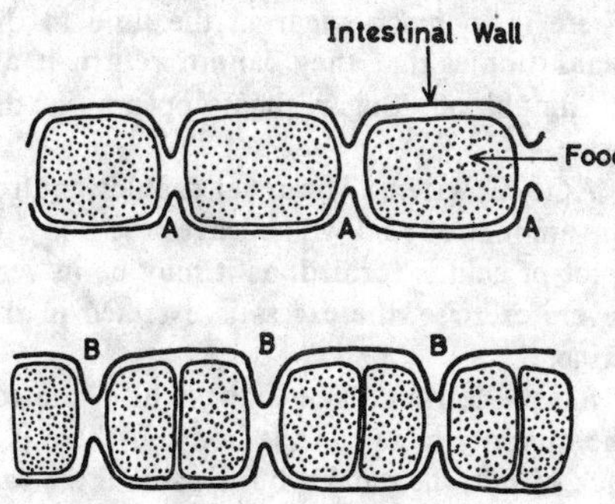

Fig. 19. *SEGMENTATION MOVEMENTS IN THE INTESTINE. The circular muscle in the intestinal wall first contracts at* A. *It then relaxes, and the muscle contracts at point* B. *Segmentation helps to mix up the food in the intestine.*

Gall-bladder and Bile. Bile is secreted by the liver. It contains no enzymes, but the very important bile salts. These help the fat-splitting enzyme, lipase, of the pancreatic juice to do its job. They also help in absorbing fat from the intestine. The dark color of bile is due to the pigments biliverdin and bilirubin. These are waste materials made from the hemoglobin of broken-down red blood cells.

There is a slow continuous secretion of bile from the liver. In between meals this is stored in the gall-bladder, a little sac lying beneath the liver. When food is eaten, the gall-bladder contracts and squeezes bile down the bile duct into the duodenum.

Sometimes a gall-stone forms in the bile duct and blocks the flow of bile into the duodenum. When this happens, the patient becomes jaundiced; fat digestion is also very much upset.

Movement of the Intestinal Wall

Movements and contractions of the intestinal wall aid in mixing the food and digestive secretions thoroughly. The wall has two layers of muscle: an inner layer arranged in rings around the intestine, and an outer coat whose fibers run lengthwise along the intestine.

The food mass is broken up into segments when contraction rings appear in the circular muscle (Fig. 19). At intervals this set of contraction rings (A) disappears, and fresh ones appear in different places (B). This movement is called *segmentation*. It breaks up the food and helps it to mix with digestive secretions, but does not push it along.

Peristalsis. Food travels along the intestine by the action of peristalsis. This is illustrated in Fig. 20. The circular muscle contracts at one point and the contraction ring passes along, pushing the food mass in front of it. This type of contraction always travels in a direction away from the mouth and towards the anus.

Formation of Feces. By the time the food

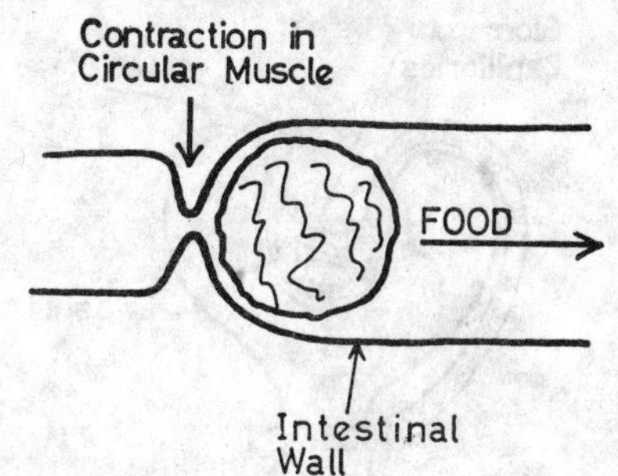

Fig. 20. *PERISTALSIS IN THE INTESTINE. A contraction ring in the circular muscle sweeps along the intestinal wall pushing the food before it.*

reaches the end of the small intestine, all the useful material has passed into the blood. The unwanted residue is in a semi-liquid state and passes into the colon. In the large intestine, most of the water passes back into the blood, leaving behind the soft solid feces.

The feces are made up of indigestible material (such as cellulose), some fat, minerals, dead bacteria, and epithelial cells shed from the lining of the intestine.

Evacuation of the Bowel

Several times a day a peristaltic wave travels the whole length of the large intestine, sweeping the contents before it. At the end of the large intestine is the rectum which is normally empty. When it becomes filled with feces, following peristalsis, the rectal wall is stretched, and the person feels the need to pass a bowel movement.

Stretching the wall of the rectum sets off a nervous reflex: the sphincter muscle guarding the anus relaxes, the diaphragm and muscles of the abdominal wall contract and help the peristaltic wave in the wall of the intestine to push out the feces.

Constipation. The defecation reflex can be suppressed by an effort of will. If it is inconvenient to have a bowel movement when the rectum becomes distended, the person can wait a while. Unfortunately, if this happens too often, the rectum becomes used to distension and then may not empty properly. This is a common cause of constipation, and shows how important it is to respond to the urge to defecate whenever possible.

Need for Bulk. Constipation may follow if the diet has too little bulk in it. Plant foods contain much cellulose—a substance which cannot be digested by man. Cellulose gives bulk to the feces. The rectum needs to be well filled to stimulate evacuation. Bulky plant foods, such as cabbage, provide 'roughage' and so help to promote good bowel habits.

Food Enters the Blood

The Villi. The small molecules of sugars, amino acids, fatty acids, vitamins and mineral salts which are absorbed into the blood in the upper or small intestine do so by the aid of tiny finger-like projections, the villi, which line the intestinal wall (Fig. 21). Near the surface of each villus lies a rich network of capillary blood vessels busily taking in the absorbable food particles which then trave via the portal vein to the liver.

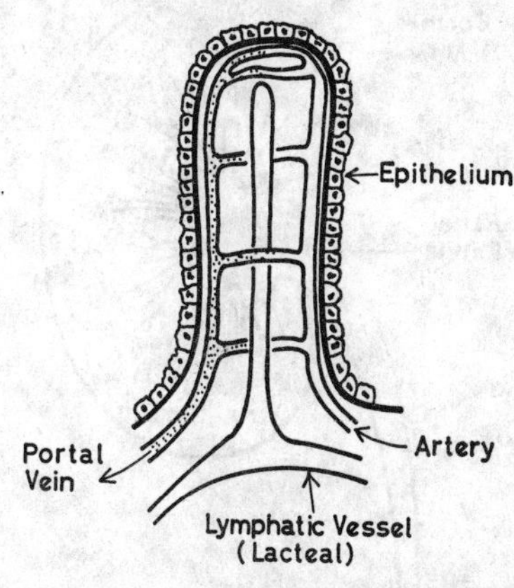

Fig. 21. *A VILLUS OF THE INTESTINAL WALL The rich network of capillary blood vessels takes in absorbable food particles, the amino acids and sugars passing into the portal vein and fats into the lacteals.*

The Lacteals. Much of the fat is separated out in the villi and is carried away in lacteals or lymphatic vessels. This fatty fluid, or *chyle*, is emptied into a large vein in the neck and then passed to fat depots in the body for storage. These depots are found mainly under the skin.

Function of the Liver

The Chemical Factory. The food-laden blood from the gut goes to be processed in the liver which is like a huge chemical factory, making new materials, breaking up unwanted compounds, and converting one substance into another. Glucose is changed into glycogen, or animal starch. Vitamins are stored. Amino acids are built into new proteins suitable for human tissues. Excess proteins are broken up and converted into urea, then sent to the kidneys for excretion.

Food Depot. The body can draw on these food stores in the liver when it needs them. If the diet contains more calories than are needed for daily activities, much of the extra food is converted into fat and stored.

EXCRETION AND THE KIDNEYS

The waste materials formed in the body must be excreted or they would poison the tissues. Carbon dioxide, one of the main waste products, leaves the body through the lungs. The feces, formed from undigested food mixed with bile and dead cells, are voided from the intestine. All other waste materials are excreted by the kidneys and leave the body in the urine.

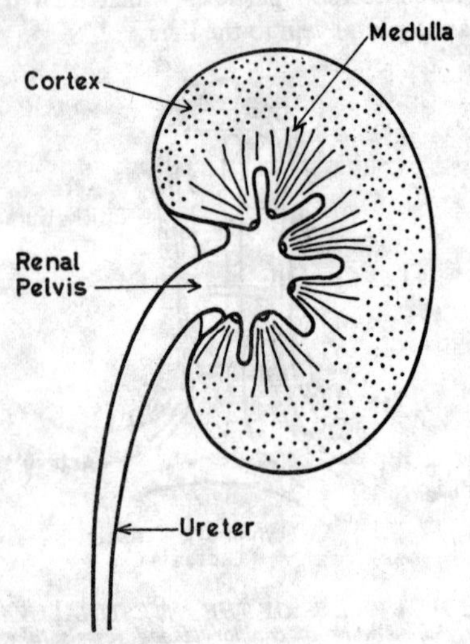

Fig. 22. *THE STRUCTURE OF ONE KIDNEY CUT IN HALF.*

The kidneys not only excrete waste material but they also regulate the amount of salt and water in the body, and many other things. They are organs which have a very great influence over the quality of the tissue fluid which forms our 'internal environment.'

The Structure of the Kidney

Fig. 22 shows the structure of a kidney which has been sliced down the middle (see also Anatomy, p. 227).The outer part is the cortex and is dark red because it holds much blood. The inner lighter part is the medulla. Passing through the medulla from the cortex are lines which end in projections—the renal papillae. There are about nine papillae in each kidney. They project into a hollow bag, the renal pelvis.

Urine is made in the kidney and runs from holes in the renal papillae to collect in the pelvis. Each pelvis is connected by a hollow tube, or ureter, to the bladder. The urine runs down the ureters and into the bladder where it is temporarily stored.

The two kidneys excrete 2 to 3 pints of urine each day. The bladder usually empties when it contains about one-third of a pint.

HOW THE URINE IS MADE

Each kidney is really a collection of tiny tubules, or nephrons. One end of each tubule lies in the cortex. It is hollowed out into a cup, or capsule (Fig. 23). Inside the cup sits a little knot of capillaries carrying blood from the renal artery. The other end of the tubule opens into a large collecting duct. This carries the urine from the tubules to the renal pelvis. One collecting duct drains many tubules. Between the capsule and the collecting duct the tubule coils and winds in a complicated manner. There are about one million tiny nephrons in each kidney.

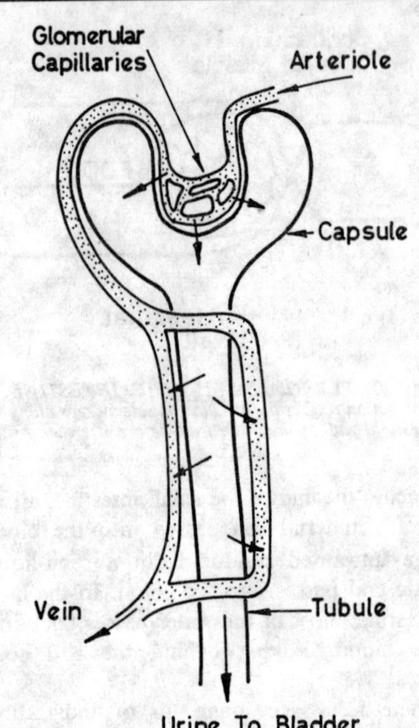

Fig. 23. *A SINGLE NEPHRON (much simplified). Fluid filters from the blood flowing through the glomerular capillaries and passes along the tubule.*

Glomerular Filtrate. The cup at the end of each tubule acts as a filter. Fluid filters from the blood as it flows through the capillaries lying in the capsule. It is driven out by the pressure of the blood inside the capillaries. This fluid, the glomerular filtrate, is very like tissue fluid formed from capillaries elsewhere in the body. It is plasma without the protein molecules which are too large to pass through the holes in the filter.

Each day 320 pints (182 liters) of fluid pass through the kidney filters yet only about 3 pints of urine enter the bladder. Most of the fluid which flows through the renal tubules passes back again into the blood.

The renal tubules seem to select some materials and return them completely to the blood. Others are partly returned, or are rejected completely.

Composition of Urine. Urine is a watery solution of salts formed from the blood, the main waste product being urea, a nitrogenous compound formed from protein breakdown. Urine also contains much acid which would seriously upset the working of the body if it were not excreted.

SUGAR IN URINE. Usually all the sugar passes back into the blood as it flows through the vessels surrounding the tubules. There is normally no sugar in the urine. Sometimes the amount of sugar in the blood is unusually high. This is the case in a patient suffering from diabetes mellitus, or sugar diabetes. There is so much sugar in the fluid in the renal tubules that they cannot return it all to the blood. Sugar then appears in the urine.

ACID CONTROL. The renal tubules control the amount of acid which leaves the body. If a lot of acid is formed, as it may be in very severe exercise, the excess is excreted in the urine.

SALT CONTROL. The kidneys also control the quantity of salt in the body. If there is a lack of salt, the renal tubules pass all the salt in the tubular fluid back into the blood. If a large amount of salt is eaten, the excess leaves the body in the urine.

The kidney also regulates the amount of calcium, potassium, phosphate, and other minerals leaving the body.

BALANCING THE WATER ACCOUNT

One of the kidney's biggest tasks is to control the amount of water leaving the body. Each person normally takes in about 6 pints of water each day in food and drink. Water leaves the body in the urine, in the sweat, in the feces, and is breathed out as vapor with other gases from the lungs.

TABLE 5
The Daily Water Balance

Volume in (milliliters)		*Volume out (milliliters)*	
Drink	1,300	In expired air	400
Food	850	In feces	100
Formed in body	350	Sweat	over 500
		Urine	1,500
Total	2,500	Total	2,500

This water loss is unavoidable and inevitable, and we can do little to control it. Unwanted water passes out in the urine.

On a very hot day, when the body perspires excessively, the kidneys form only a small volume of urine. If a person drinks more than usual the extra water is quickly passed in the urine.

Osmotic Pressure. The kidneys work to strike a balance between the amount of salt and the amount of water in the body. In fact, they regulate the two together. The purpose seems to be to keep the osmotic pressure of the body fluids constant. This is very important, since changes in osmotic pressure would disturb the movement of water between the cells and the tissue fluid bathing them (see p 238). If the osmotic pressure of the tissue fluid fell, water would pass into the cells. This would make them swell and perhaps burst. If the osmotic pressure rose above the normal level water would pass out of the cells, and they would shrink.

Kidney Regulators

The kidneys, of course, do not work alone. They are controlled in turn by other organs. Kidney function does not seem to be much affected by nervous control. It is much more regulated by the endocrine organs. These are glands which secrete chemicals, or hormones, into the blood. The hormones, traveling in the bloodstream, control the activity of other organs.

Posterior Pituitary Gland. This gland regulates water excretion. If it is destroyed by disease the patient has the condition of diabetes insipidus (not to be confused with diabetes mellitus in which sugar metabolism is upset). He cannot control his water excretion and may pass 40 pints of urine a day. Of course he must drink an equivalent amount of fluid to make up for this severe loss. The condition is controlled by giving the patient an extract of the posterior pituitary gland.

Adrenal Gland. Hormones from the adrenal gland regulate the excretion of salt. If the adrenal gland is destroyed (Addison's disease) large amounts of salt leave the body in the urine. Again, by giving the patient the appropriate hormones, this loss can be controlled.

The endocrine glands co-operate with the kidney in helping to regulate the blood's composition.

THE BLADDER

Ureters and Urethra. As urine forms in the kidneys, it passes down two tubes, or ureters, into the bladder (see Anatomy, p. 227, Fig. 50) which is like an elastic bag with muscular walls. It in turn empties the urine through another tube, the urethra. The urethra is usually kept closed by two rings of circular muscle, or sphincters.

Nerve Control. The nerves to the bladder come from the autonomic nervous system, and the most important are the parasympathetic nerves. When these nerves are excited the sphincter opens and the muscle in the bladder wall contracts. This pushes the urine out of the bladder through the urethra to the outside.

Micturition

The act of emptying the bladder is called micturition. In health the bladder empties by the operation of a nervous reflex. As urine runs into the bladder its wall at first relaxes to accommodate the fluid. When the bladder holds about one-third of a pint of urine the muscle in its wall begins to contract feebly. This is a reflex response to stretching the bladder wall (Fig. 24). If it is inconvenient to pass urine the reflex can be inhibited by an effort of will. The pressure inside the bladder falls and more urine flows into it. Eventually the bladder can hold no more fluid. Further attempts to prevent micturition voluntarily cause a feeling of intense discomfort or even pain. It then becomes impossible to delay micturition any longer. The sphincters open, the bladder muscle contracts and the bladder empties.

Learning Bladder Control. In babies and young children the reflex operates unchecked by voluntary control. As soon as the bladder becomes distended it empties. As the child grows it learns to control the reflex. The age at which this occurs is extremely variable. Many children are 'dry' both by day and night at four years of age. Others do not achieve full bladder control until a much later age.

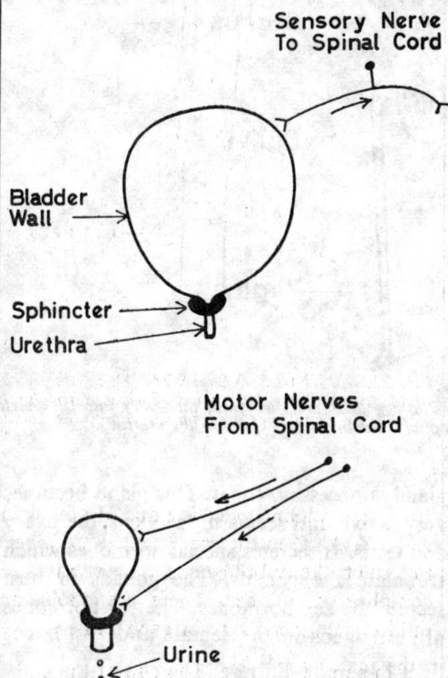

Fig. 24. *MICTURITION. A full bladder with its exit closed by a sphincter. When the bladder needs emptying, a message travels in the sensory nerves running from the bladder wall to the spinal cord. Below: in response to this message, motor nerves from the spinal cord stimulate contraction of the bladder wall and opening of the sphincter. The bladder empties. This is a reflex.*

REPRODUCTION

The life of a human being begins inside the womb of its mother. Here the mother's germ cell joins with the germ cell of the father. The two cells fused together form the zygote. This cell divides very rapidly, and eventually grows to form a new human being.

The Vital Gonads. Every person carries inside him- or her-self the germ of a new life. The germ cells come from the gonads. These are the ovaries in the female, and the testes in the male. The ovary forms the female germ cell, or ovum (Fig. 25). The testis forms the male germ cell, or spermatozoon (Fig. 26).

Chromosomes Carry Hereditary Factors. Each germ cell has only half the amount of nuclear material of ordinary cells. When the ovum and spermatozoon fuse, their nuclei join together to make a whole cell nucleus again. The nucleus carries the chromosomes. These particles transmit special characters from one generation to the next. They determine the sex of the child, the color of its eyes, its blood group, and many other characteristics. The nucleus of the *zygote* (fertilized egg) decides the make-up of the next generation. Mother and father give equally to this new nucleus.

Female Reproductive System

OVARIES. The ovaries lie inside the abdomen. Each ovary contains thousands of egg cells. These are in the ovary when the child is born, but they do not mature until adult life. The ovary also secretes hormones (see p. 236) which play a big part in reproduction.

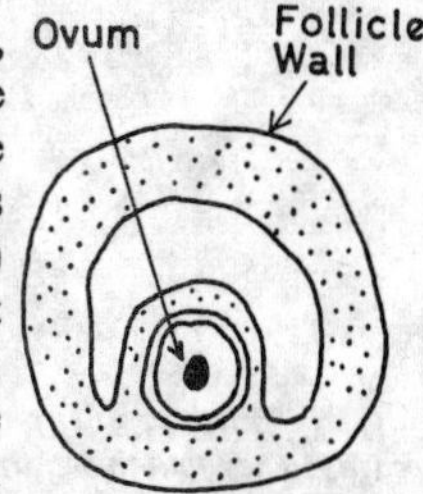

Fig. 25. *THE OVUM: FEMALE GERM CELL. This lies within a double layer of cells to form the Graafian follicle.*

WOMB. The female has other organs which help in the essential function of child-bearing. The womb, or uterus, is a hollow muscular organ which houses the developing child (the fetus or embryo) during pregnancy (Fig. 27).

FALLOPIAN TUBES. From the top corners of the uterus, two tubes arise. These are the Fallopian tubes, and they stretch sideways, like arms, towards the ovaries. The Fallopian tubes have open ends, ready to catch the ova as they leave the ovary. The neck of the womb, or cervix, projects downward into the top of the vagina.

BREASTS. The breasts of the female are important in reproduction. They secrete milk for the nourishment of the infant.

Male Reproductive System

TESTES. The male germ cells, or spermatozoa, develop in the testes. Each testis is a mass of tubules in which the spermatozoa mature and are stored (see Anatomy, p. 236).

URETHRA AND PENIS. To reach the outside, the spermatozoa must travel through a long tube to the urethra. The urethra runs through the penis; it also carries urine away from the bladder. When intercourse occurs, the penis becomes large and hard, for introduction into the female vagina.

THE SPERMATOZOA, as they travel from the testes, are mixed with secretions from the seminal vesicles and the prostate gland which help to nourish the spermatozoa. This fluid with the spermatozoa is called *semen.*

Once inside the vagina, the sperm make the difficult journey into the womb and up into

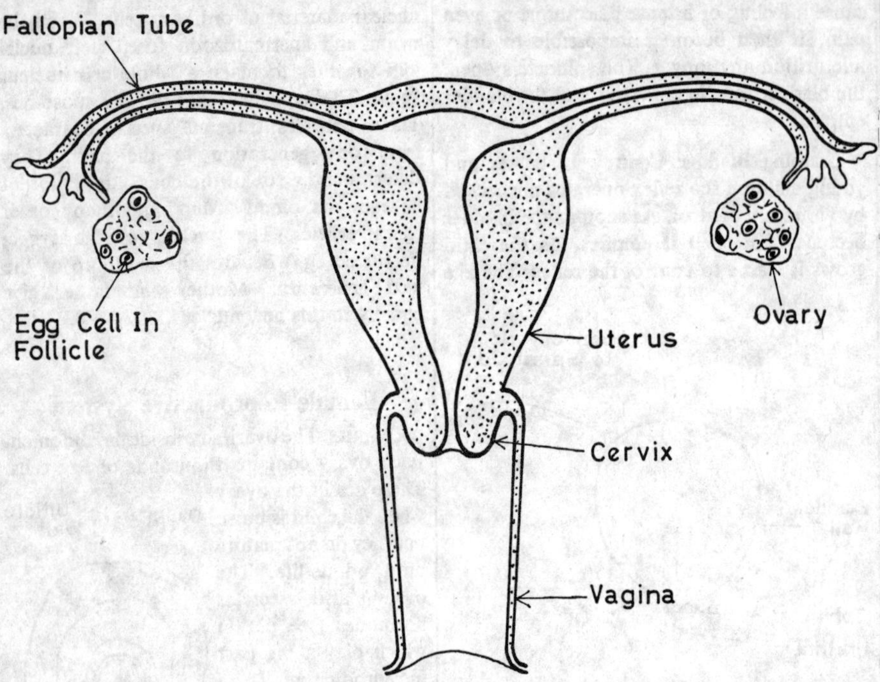

Fig. 27. *THE FEMALE REPRODUCTIVE ORGANS. The egg cells are shed from the ovary into the pelvic cavity. They find their way into the open ends of the Fallopian tubes and travel down to the uterus.*

the Fallopian tube. This is where fertilization usually takes place. The spermatozoon travels by making lashing movements with its tail.

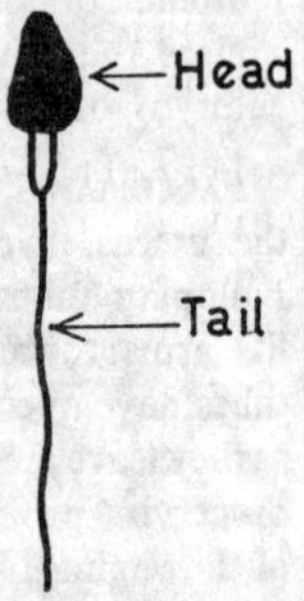

Each ejaculation discharges several million spermatozoa. The wastage is tremendous, but the large numbers make sure that fertilization will take place if there is a ripe ovum in the genital tract.

The spermatozoa survive for about four days. The egg has a much shorter life —probably no more than a day or so.

Fig. 26. *A SPERMATOZOON: MALE GERM CELL. The head alone fertilizes the egg.*

MALE SEX HORMONES. The testis, as well as producing spermatozoa, has a second function as an endocrine gland (see p. 262). It secretes the male sex hormones, or androgens. The androgens stimulate the typical changes which occur at puberty in the boy—the change in the voice and the growth of the skeleton and hair are due to the influence of the sex hormones.

PREPARING FOR PARENTHOOD

In children and other young animals the reproductive organs are underdeveloped, but at a certain age, however, changes occur in the growth and behavior of the animal, preparing it for parenthood. This period of change from child to adult is puberty. In humans it happens in the early teens.

Awakening the Ovaries and Testes. No one knows what causes puberty to occur when it does. We do know that the anterior pituitary gland is necessary for it. This gland becomes very active and seems to 'awaken' the ovary and testis. It secretes special hormones which stimulate the gonads. The gonads in turn secrete the sex hormones. The sex hormones are estrogens in the female and androgens in the male.

Secondary Sex Characters. The growth changes occurring at puberty are actually due to the sex hormones. Estrogens stimulate breast growth and cause the menstrual cycle to begin. Androgens stimulate the growth of hair on the young man's chest and face, and cause his voice to break. These features which distinguish the male and female after puberty are called the secondary sex characters. If the sex glands *or* the anterior pituitary gland are damaged, the typical changes do not appear.

The Adult Patterns. Once the testis becomes active it continues to make spermatozoa for many years. There does not seem to be any special cycle of activity. In the female, there is a definite cycle of change called the menstrual cycle. The eggs are shed at about monthly intervals and changes occur in the womb, culminating each month in the monthly period.

The pituitary gland and the gonads work together to produce these changes. They are dependent on each other. If the pituitary gland fails, the gonads do not function properly.

THE MENSTRUAL CYCLE

The reproductive period in the female lasts about thirty years. During this time, her reproductive organs go through a cycle which is interrupted only by bearing a child.

When a baby girl is born, her ovaries contain about 70,000 egg cells. These lie dormant until puberty. Then, driven by the anterior pituitary gland, the egg cells begin to ripen.

Egg Cell and Follicle. At about monthly intervals, an egg cell pushes its way to the surface of each ovary. As it does this, it is encased in a covering of special cells (Fig. 25). The developing egg in its cover is the Graafian follicle.

The Endometrium Prepares. As the follicle with its egg cell ripens, the ovary secretes estrogen. This hormone, traveling in the blood to the womb, causes the lining, or endometrium, to thicken and grow more blood vessels.

After about ten days, the follicle splits open, sending the egg cell down into the Fallopian tube. The follicle cell, empty of the egg, then makes another hormone, progesterone. This stimulates the endometrium even more. It becomes very thick and spongy. Special food stores appear in the lining of the womb, together with many glands. The endometrium is thick, and full of blood and food ready to shelter and feed a tiny embryo.

The egg meanwhile journeys down the Fallopian tube to the uterus.

The Fertilized Egg Settles. If it has been fertilized by a spermatozoon en route, the zygote quickly burrows into the endometrium. From the blood flowing so freely through the endometrium, the tiny embryo can take the oxygen and food it needs for survival. Eventually a special organ (the placenta) grows from the tissues of mother and embryo. The placenta allows the developing child, or fetus, to feed on the mother.

The Unfertilized Egg Dies. What is the fate of the unfertilized egg? It dies inside the womb. This happens to most egg cells. Only a few eggs are fertilized during the lifetime of one woman. After the egg has died, the ovary temporarily loses interest in the uterus.

The Womb Sheds its Lining. The hormones which were secreted in order to prepare the womb for an embryo are no longer formed. The growth of the endometrium is dependent on these hormones. As they wane in the blood, the lining of the womb changes very dramatically. Almost the whole thickness peels off and is discarded. At this point, the monthly period begins. The discharge consists of blood and tissue shed from the wall of the uterus, tissue which was prepared for an embryo and which is no longer required.

The Cycle Repeats. The ovary produces ripe ova at approximately monthly intervals throughout the thirty years or so of a woman's reproductive life. Each time an egg cell leaves the ovary, the womb prepares to receive an embryo. If the egg remains unfertilized, no embryo can develop, and so the lining of the womb is discarded. It is rebuilt as the next egg cell develops inside its follicle.

The menstrual cycle is interrupted only when an embryo implants itself in the endometrium so carefully prepared for it. Then the ovary produces no more egg cells until the embryo (or fetus) has completely developed and a child is born. After the birth of the child the cycle begins again.

Changes in the Breasts. The ovarian hormones, progesterone and estrogen, also affect the breasts, stimulating the glandular tissue. During each menstrual cycle, the breasts vary a little in size. They are usually largest just before the beginning of a period when there is most hormone in the blood.

Premenstrual Tension. The hormones have other actions, and probably cause the feeling of tiredness and anxiety—called premenstrual tension—which many women experience just before a period begins.

Pituitary Control

The ovary is awakened by the anterior pituitary gland at puberty. Throughout reproductive life the pituitary drives the ovary by means of the trophic hormones which it secretes. These make the ovary produce estrogen and progesterone. The pituitary gland is, indirectly, responsible for the menstrual cycle. If the anterior pituitary is damaged, the menstrual cycle stops altogether. This of course makes child-bearing impossible.

THE MENOPAUSE

Reproductive life ends at the menopause. For most women, this occurs in the forties.

Irregular Periods. The periods become irregular, and may be very scanty or extremely heavy. The amount of bleeding at each period seems to depend on the balance of estrogen and progesterone in the blood. If the normal balance is upset, bleeding may be very heavy.

As the ovary fails, it secretes its hormones in a rather erratic manner. This interferes with the menstrual cycle, making it irregular, and causing the heavy periods.

Uterine Operation. Since it is the uterus which bleeds, heavy periods at the menopause can be stopped by removing the womb. This is a major operation, and is not desirable unless the bleeding is making the patient anemic. It is not usually necessary, since the periods stop naturally when the ovary ceases to function altogether.

Hot Flushes. Menopausal women often feel emotionally upset. They have 'hot flushes' and other inconveniences which may be very disturbing. Some doctors think that these symptoms are caused by a change in the estrogen secretion. They may often be relieved by small doses of estrogen given for a short time.

After the menopause the reproductive organs atrophy, and the woman usually grows fatter.

Male Climacteric. There is no such abrupt ending to the reproductive life of the male. His gonads may continue to produce healthy spermatozoa when he is in his sixties.

PREGNANCY

In the last section we saw how the fertilized egg buried itself in the prepared lining of the womb. The hormones of the ovary, estrogen and progesterone, cause the uterus to make this preparation for the embryo. They continue to act on the uterus in the early months of pregnancy, making it grow with the fetus. These hormones are essential throughout pregnancy but they are formed in the ovary only during the first sixteen weeks. After this the placenta supplies all the hormones needed.

The Placenta

As soon as the embryo burrows into the lining of the womb, a new organ begins to grow. This is the placenta which mother and fetus make together for the nourishment of the developing child. The placenta is a red spongy structure which at the end of pregnancy is about the size of a dinner plate. It is really a vast collection of blood vessels.

Umbilical Cord. The fetus is attached to the placenta by the umbilical cord. This contains large blood vessels which carry blood between the fetus and the placenta. It is the fetal life-line.

The Sinuses. In the placenta blood from the mother flows through large thin-walled channels, or sinuses. The fetal blood vessels dip into the sinuses. The two bloods do not actually mix, but are separated by the thin sinus walls.

Food for the Fetus. As the blood flows through the channels, oxygen and food in the maternal blood diffuses into the fetal blood (Fig. 28). In exchange, the fetus passes on to the mother the waste products formed inside its own body.

Since the baby is shut up inside the womb of the mother, it must rely on her for all its needs. The developing child has first call on everything. This is why some dietary deficiencies often show in pregnancy. The child takes from the mother what it needs. If her diet is short of some particular foodstuff, the mother will suffer from the deficiency, not the child. Naturally she must eat extra amounts of food in pregnancy to build body tissues for her child.

Bag of Waters

As the fetus grows, the womb enlarges too. The fetus lies in a bag filled with a liquid called amniotic fluid. The wall of the bag is made from membranes formed by the fetus (Fig. 29). The amniotic fluid acts as a shock absorber. The fetus kicks and moves around inside the bag of waters. When the child is born, the membranes break and the amniotic fluid drains away.

BIRTH OF THE BABY

A human pregnancy usually lasts about 280 days, or approximately nine calendar months.

The Womb Contracts. At the end of her pregnancy, the mother feels uncomfortable contractions in the uterus, she goes into labor and her womb expels the baby.

We do not know what makes labor begin.

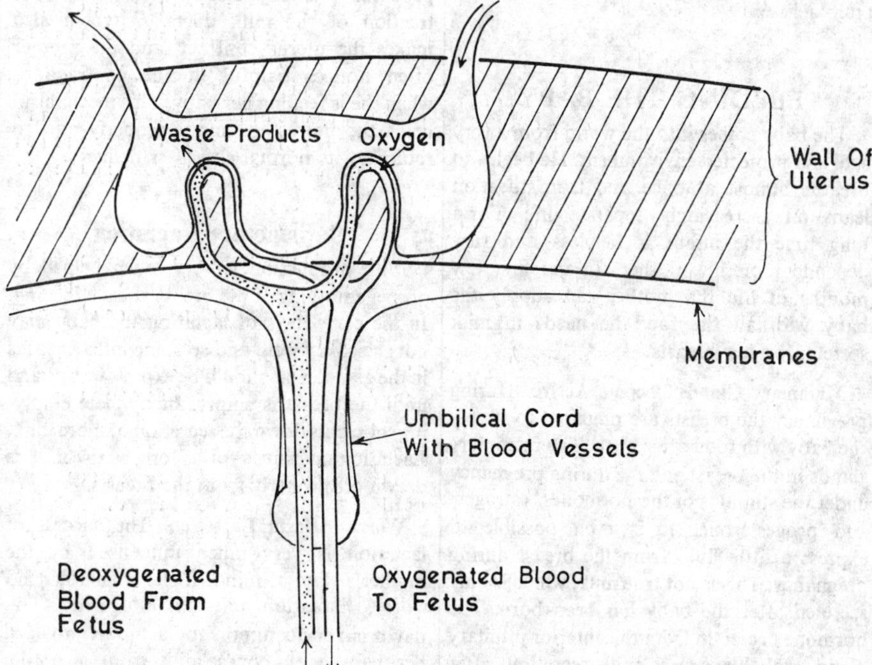

Fig. 28. *THE PLACENTA. A simplified diagram to show how the mother nourishes the developing baby inside the uterus. The fetal blood vessels dip into blood 'lakes' in the uterine wall. Food and oxygen pass from the mother's blood into the fetal blood. Waste material from the baby is carried away in the venous blood of the mother.*

Perhaps the posterior pituitary gland (see p. 260) plays a part since this gland secretes a hormone, oxytocin, which will make the uterus contract towards the end of pregnancy. Oxytocin is often used to start labor when it seems to be delayed.

The Cervix Opens. At the same time as the contractions begin, the neck of the womb (cervix) opens up. When the cervix has fully opened, the mother feels the need to 'bear down.' The resultant straining movements raise pressure inside the abdomen and help the contracting uterus to expel the baby.

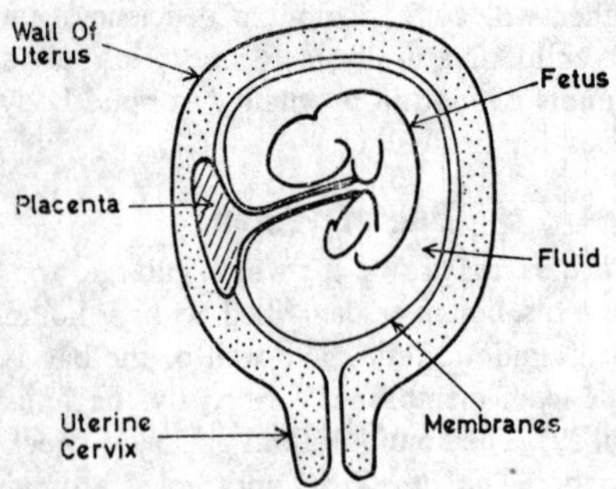

Fig. 29. *FETUS IN UTERUS. The fetus lies inside a membranous bag filled with fluid. The umbilical cord connects the fetus to the placenta.*

Delivery of the placenta closely follows the baby. The placenta is of no further use once the baby has been born and its umbilical cord tied. A powerful uterine contraction usually pushes out the placenta within half an hour of the baby's delivery. There is some bleeding at the same time. This stops as the uterine wall contracts and closes the open blood vessels left at the placental site.

There is a little bleeding for a week or more after delivery.

FEEDING THE BABY

The baby comes into the world from a very safe and protected environment. He begins to breathe almost at once and from then on leads an increasingly separate life. For a long time the infant is helpless and very dependent on his mother. In the first few months of life the mother can supply the baby with all the food he needs in milk secreted by her breasts.

Mammary Glands Become Active. During pregnancy the breasts are prepared to supply the baby with food after birth. The mammary glands in the breast enlarge during pregnancy under the stimulus of the hormones, estrogen and progesterone. It is even possible to express a little fluid from the breast during pregnancy. This is not true milk, which is only secreted after the baby has been born. The hormone prolactin from the anterior pituitary gland probably causes milk secretion, after the breast has been 'prepared' by estrogen and progesterone.

In the first days of the puerperium (the period after delivery) the breasts secrete a yellow fluid called *colostrum*. There is only a small amount of it but it contains a lot of protein. By the third day after delivery the breasts are usually secreting enough milk to satisfy the child.

Early Weight Loss. The baby loses a little weight in the first few days of its life before lactation (milk production) is properly established. This weight loss is normal and the baby regains it as soon as the mother is producing a good supply of milk.

The mother needs plenty of fluid and extra food, especially protein, because she is manufacturing food to give to the baby in the milk.

Human v. Cow's Milk. The composition of human milk and cow's milk is shown in Table 6. Cow's milk contains more protein and less sugar than human milk. The calf grows much more rapidly than the baby, and so it needs more protein.

TABLE 6

Comparison of Human and Cow's Milk (in grams per 100 milliliters)

	Human milk	*Cow's milk*
Protein	1·2	3·3
Fat	3·5	3·6
Carbohydrate	6·5	4·7

Lactation Affects Uterine Contractions. When the baby is put to the breast the ducts of the gland contract and help to squeeze out the milk. The hormone oxytocin (from the posterior pituitary gland) causes this contraction of the milk ducts. Oxtyocin also makes the uterus contract, and the mother often notices painful uterine contractions when she is feeding her baby. This mechanism helps the uterus to empty properly and so return to its normal size after delivery.

Satisfactory Lactation

Milk production is very much helped by proper emptying of the breast at each feeding. In the early days of lactation the baby may not suck very well, and so some milk remains in the gland. This should be expressed by hand until the breast is empty. Incomplete emptying soon cuts down the secretion of more milk. Lactation continues for as long as the milk is drawn off properly from the breasts.

Worry Affects Lactation. The success of lactation is very much influenced by the mother's state of mind. If she is anxious and worried lactation may fail altogether. Today it is very common for a mother to feed her baby with cow's milk from a bottle. While many people feel that both mother and child are happiest when the baby is breast fed, the baby can get all the substances it needs from cow's milk modified to the proportions of human milk. Extra vitamins may be needed too. A woman who is worn out and anxious should not be persuaded into breast feeding if this is a source of fatigue and worry to her.

As the baby becomes more mature, his digestive system can cope with other foods. He is gradually weaned on to a mixed diet. There follows a long period of childhood and adolescence before complete maturity is reached.

CONTROLLING THE MACHINE

The individual organs do not function alone. They co-operate and work together for the good of the whole individual. This means that the body must have some way of controlling the function of each part so that all the activities harmonize. This is done in two ways: control by a system of nerves and also by hormones of the endocrine system.

Nervous Control of Function

The neurones, or special cells of the nervous system, are designed to carry messages very rapidly from one part of the body to another. The message, or nerve impulse, travels through the cell and is handed on to another neurone. A message may be sent through the whole length of the body in this way. Eventually it arrives at a muscle or gland which promptly alters its activity according to the sort of command it receives.

The nervous system provides a rapid means of communication between one part of the body and another.

Hormone Control

The bloodstream is also used for sending messages. The endocrine (or ductless) glands in various parts of the body make chemical substances, or hormones, which are 'posted' into the bloodstream. The hormones travel in the blood to the organ whose activity they control.

Messages carried by hormones travel more slowly than those carried by nerves. The nervous system comes into action when a rapid response is needed. The endocrine system is used for slower and more long-lasting reactions.

THE NERVOUS SYSTEM

Nerve Cells. The basic cell of the nervous system is the neuron. Each neuron has a cell body with a nucleus and cytoplasm. From the cell body arise many processes or dendrites (see also Anatomy, p. 219). One very long process, the axon, carries messages away from the cell body to the next nerve cell.

Some axons have a covering sheath of white fatty material called myelin. This acts as an insulator. Myelinated nerves carry impulses much more quickly than those without a sheath.

Large numbers of axons grouped together in a bundle form the nerves. They are white because of the myelin in the nerve sheaths.

There are three basic types of nerve cell: (1) Sensory neurons, which carry messages from sense organs (in eye, ear, etc.) to the central nervous system; (2) Motor neurons carrying messages from the central nervous system to the motor organs (the glands and muscles of the body) (Fig. 30); and (3) Interconnecting neurons which carry messages between sensory and motor nerve cells.

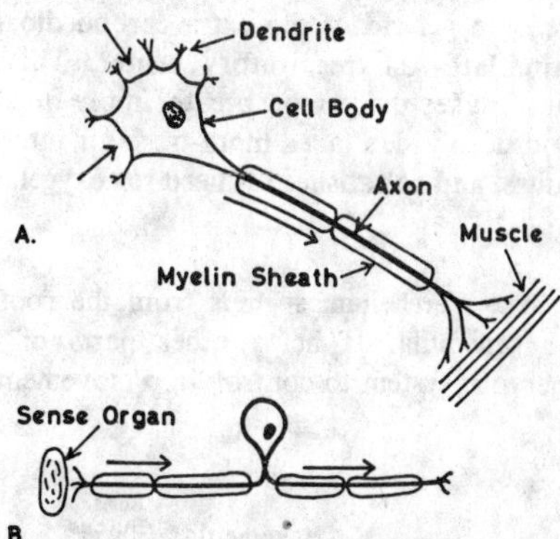

Fig. 30. *NERVE CELLS. The motor neuron* (A) *is stimulated by other nerve cells: its axon travels in a spinal nerve to a muscle. The cell body lies in the spinal cord. The sensory neuron* (B) *is stimulated by a sense organ. The message is handed on to other nerve cells. The cell body lies in the ganglion of the spinal nerve root.*

Passing The Message. The message, or nerve impulse, carried by the neuron is a little electrical disturbance which travels the whole length of the cell from one end to the other. There is no actual contact between nerve cells. They are separated from one another by a gap, called the synapse. The nerve impulse, carried by the neuron is a another across the gap. This is done by chemical means: one nerve cell forms a powerful chemical which travels across the gap to the next cell. This chemical stimulates the second nerve cell to produce a nerve impulse. When the impulse reaches the end of the second cell, it, in turn, forms the chemical. This stimulates other nerve cells sitting near the end of the axon.

Effect of Drugs. Nerve action can be stopped by giving drugs which interfere with the chemicals formed by nerve cells. This is often done in the treatment of people with high blood pressure. In these patients the small blood vessels, or arterioles, seem to be more tightly closed than in normal people. The closure of the arterioles is controlled by nerves. When the nerves are blocked by drugs, the arterioles open and the blood pressure falls.

The Central Nervous System

The cell bodies of neurons are mainly grouped together in the central nervous system. There is no myelin around the cell bodies, and so they look gray in contrast to the white nerves.

The central nervous system is housed in the skull and vertebral column. The skull protects the brain. The vertebral canal houses the spinal cord.

The bony skull has many holes in it. Through the holes run nerves from the brain to structures in the head. Between the vertebrae there are openings through which nerves travel to and from the spinal cord.

A 'Telephone Exchange.' The central nervous system is like a telephone exchange. It receives information from many parts of the body. The information is sorted out, added together and passed on to other parts of the exchange. If necessary, the muscles and glands take action in response to the information received.

The Sense Organs

The body has a special system of 'receivers.' These are the sense organs. Each sense organ responds to a different type of stimulus. The eye responds to light, the ear to sound, and receptors in the skin respond to pain, to changes in temperature, or to touch.

Inside the body, buried in joints and muscles and in the walls of internal organs, there are many tiny sense organs which supply the central nervous system with information about the state of the internal organs. We are usually quite unaware of this internal information. The knowledge of it does not enter our consciousness. In spite of this, our body adjusts itself to the messages which come from the sense organs. This is done by reflex action described opposite.

The Spinal Cord

Fig. 31 shows the spinal cord cut across. From each side of it two nerve roots arise. (There are altogether thirty-one pairs of nerve roots coming from the spinal cord: only one pair is shown here.)

Sensory Nerves. Nerves carrying messages to the spinal cord from the sense organs are called sensory nerves. They enter the back of the cord by the posterior root. On the posterior root there is a little bump, or ganglion, in which lie the cell bodies of the sensory nerve fibers.

Motor Nerves. Nerves carrying messages to muscles and glands are the motor nerves. They leave from the front of the spinal cord, by the anterior nerve root. The cell bodies of the motor nerves lie inside the spinal cord while the long axons, protected in their myelin-covered sheaths, reach far afield to their appropriate receptors in the muscles or glands.

Gray Matter. The spinal cord is roughly divided into two parts. In the center is the gray matter where the cell bodies of many neurons lie close together. Running through the gray matter is the spinal canal. It contains cerebrospinal fluid which helps to nourish the central nervous system, and also acts as a shock absorber.

White Matter. Around the outside of the cord lies the white matter which consists of nerve fibers only. They are arranged in bundles, or tracts. Some carry messages up to the brain, others carry messages down from the brain to the nerve cells lying in the spinal cord.

Reflex Action. What happens to the messages which travel along the sensory nerves to the spinal cord? Some of them pass

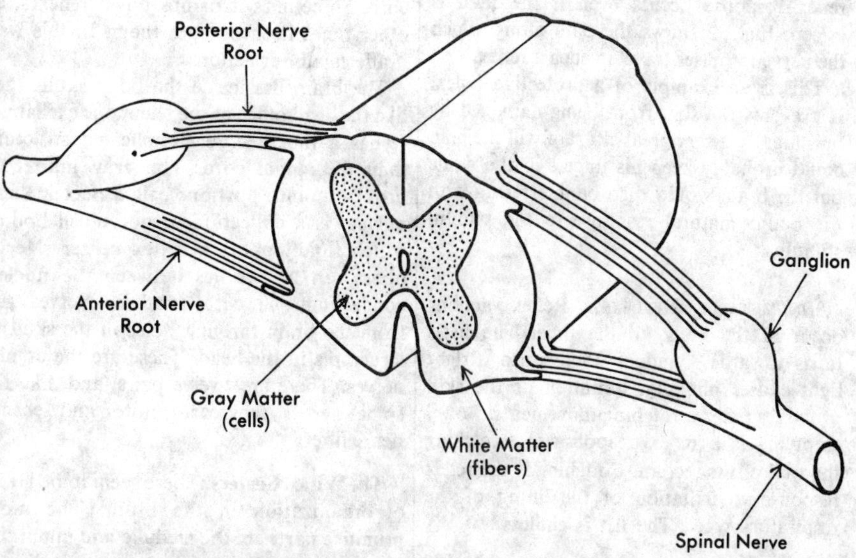

Fig. 31. *SEGMENT OF SPINAL CORD AND ONE PAIR OF SPINAL NERVES.*

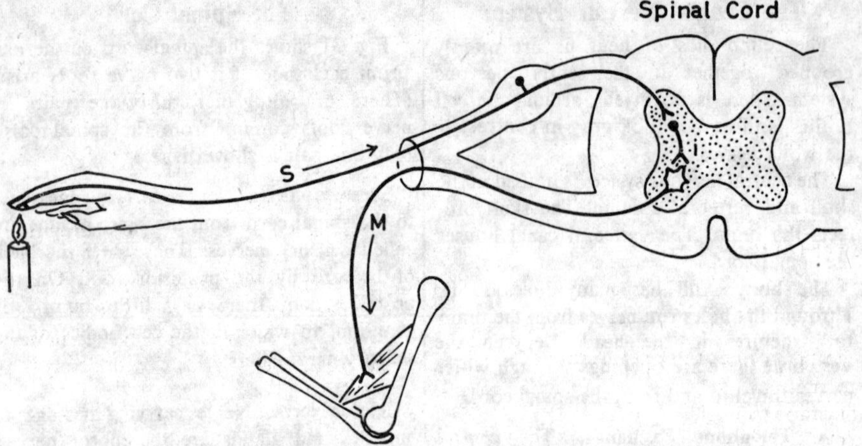

Fig. 32. *A PROTECTIVE REFLEX. The hot flame stimulates pain fibers* (S) *traveling from the finger to the spinal cord. The motor neuron* (M), *stimulated by the sensory neuron via an interconnecting fiber* (I) *causes contraction of the flexor muscles of the arm. The hand moves quickly away from the hot flame.*

through the nerves running to the brain and eventually they reach consciousness. We then become aware of them. Sensations of touch and pain and temperature from the skin are examples. We may take some action in response to these stimuli, such as removing the hand from the hot water to stop the pain. Other messages travel to the brain, but do not enter our consciousness. Some messages travel to the spinal cord and do not go to the higher centers.

Nearly all the messages which travel to the central nervous system produce a change in the activity of our muscles and glands. A muscle may contract, or a gland secrete, or the activity may be slowed down. These changes are called reflexes. A reflex is a movement or some other action made automatically in response to a message from a sense organ.

Touching a Hot Flame. If someone accidentally touches a hot flame with his finger, he at once withdraws his hand. This is an automatic response and he does not have to think about it. It is a reflex action. If the painful stimulus is sufficiently strong, the reflex response occurs even if the man is asleep. Fig. 32 shows the path along which the nerve impulses travel in such a reflex.

This is an example of a protective reflex. It prevents the skin from being damaged by burning. By a very great effort of will the man could probably keep his fingers in the flame but the brain would then be interfering with the body's natural response to the painful stimulus.

Innumerable Reflexes. Reflex actions occur in the body all the time. The head turns towards a sudden loud noise. Bright light causes blinking. Irritation of the skin provokes reflex scratching movements. Bowel emptying is a reflex response to stretching the wall of the rectum. Coughing is the reflex response to irritation of the lining of the respiratory tract. The list is endless.

Brain not Essential For Reflexes. We are quite unaware of many of the reflexes operating in the body. When we eat food, not only do the salivary glands secrete, but also those of the stomach and pancreas. This happens entirely without our knowledge. We are even kept in the upright position because of reflex action.

Experiments with animals and studies of patients with spinal injuries show that the brain is not essential for many reflexes. A man whose spinal cord has been damaged in the chest region can still empty his bladder and bowels. This happens even though the nerve cells in the spinal cord controlling these organs are cut off from the brain's influence. Of course, they function imperfectly, and the patient has no voluntary control over their activity. But bowel and bladder still empty from time to time when they are sufficiently full.

The Brain

The brain acts as a regulator. All the time it is sending messages down to the spinal cord. Sometimes it damps down reflexes, at other times it encourages them. In this way it affects all our actions.

The brain lies inside the bony skull. It is like the head office of the telephone exchange. It has a much more complicated structure than the spinal cord. The gray matter is broken up into portions called nuclei. Each nucleus is a collection of nerve cell bodies which functions as a reflex center. Nerve fibers run in bundles between the nuclei, connecting one with another. Nerves run from the brain through holes in the skull to structures in the head. These are the cranial nerves. There are twelve pairs, and, like the spinal nerves, they carry motor and sensory nerve fibers.

The 'Vital' Centers. There seem to be levels of organization in the brain. The most primitive parts are the medulla and midbrain. Here there are collections of nerve cells, or 'centers,' controlling respiration, heart rate and blood pressure. These centers are vital, or essential to life.

The medullary vital centers, in addition, respond to messages from other parts of the body. Sensory stimuli can alter the heart rate, blood pressure and respiration. For example, when a person gets out of bed in the morning, both the heart rate and blood pressure alter. The change in posture, from lying down to standing up, sets off reflexes which make the heart beat faster and the blood pressure rise. The medullary centers are involved in both these reflexes.

When a person exercises, his respiration increases. The demand for oxygen and the need to get rid of the extra carbon dioxide stimulates the respiratory center. This in turn makes the person breathe more quickly and deeply. He takes more fresh air into his lungs, and so satisfies his need for oxygen.

The Cerebellum springs from the roof of the medulla. It helps other parts of the nervous system to control limb movements.

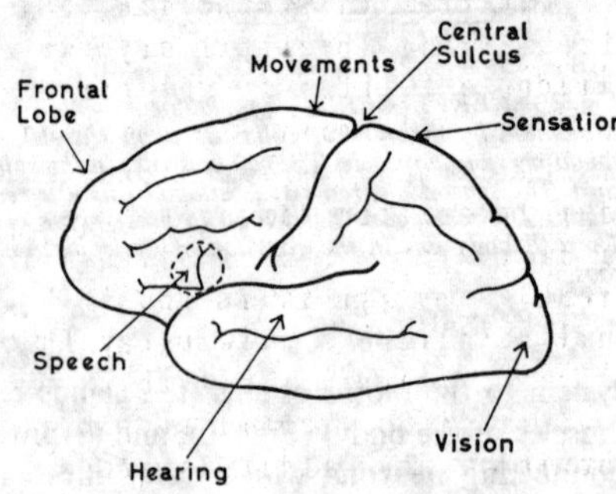

Fig. 33. *THE LEFT CEREBRAL HEMISPHERE (from the side). Certain functions are connected with particular parts of the brain cortex. The frontal lobe may have some connection with the intellect and personality.*

The Hypothalamus. This forms the floor of the most forward part of the brain. There are several nuclei in the hypothalamus, which regulates many functions. The hypothalamus seems to control the intake and loss of water from the body as well as the appetite and food intake; it also regulates body temperature. It probably also controls some of the functions of the anterior pituitary gland.

The Cerebrum. The two cerebral hemispheres form the largest part of the brain. The cerebrum is best developed in man and apes—the most intelligent members of the animal kingdom.

The Cortex. The surface of the cerebrum, or the cerebral cortex, is divided by folds, or sulci (Fig. 33). One very large sulcus runs transversely across each hemisphere dividing it roughly into front and back portions.

The part behind the central sulcus is concerned with sensation. There are definite areas associated with special sense organs.

The occipital cortex has something to do with vision, and the temporal cortex with hearing.

In front of the central sulcus lie the great motor areas. The nerve cells which command voluntary movement lie in the ridge just in front of the central sulcus. There is a special center for speech, another for eye movements, and so on.

It is very difficult to discover what the cerebral cortex actually does. We know that damage to certain parts of it interferes with normal function. If the occipital cortex is damaged, the person may not be able to see, even though his eyes are quite healthy. This, of course, tells us nothing of how the cortex is concerned in vision.

Sometimes injury to a part of the cerebral cortex produces no obvious change in the animal. This may be because one cerebral hemisphere can completely take over the function of the other.

The Forebrain. The most forward part of the cerebral cortex is the frontal area. It is probably concerned with social behavior. Occasionally a patient is in a state of severe nervous tension which cannot be relieved by medical treatment. The surgeon may decide to cut some of the fibers running from the frontal cortex to the deeper parts of the brain. This is the operation of *frontal leucotomy*.

After the operation, the nervous tension goes, but the patient is often indifferent to the needs of the people around him. He may be unable to plan and organize his day. This disability may of course be preferable to the nervous tension. But since such an operation is irreversible, the advantages and disadvantages must be carefully weighed before it is done.

The cerebral cortex is probably concerned with adding together and correlating information from all levels of the nervous system. It may act as the final regulator of all that we do.

HOW MOVEMENT IS PERFORMED

Role of Muscle

The movements which we make are due to contraction of the skeletal muscles. Skeletal muscles are formed from bundles of striped muscle fibers (see Anatomy, pp. 218, 223) held together by connective tissue. Most muscles are attached at each end to a bone. The belly of the muscle spans a joint. When the muscle contracts it shortens and the joint moves.

Bending the Elbow. Fig. 34 shows how the elbow joint flexes when the brachialis muscle contracts. Every joint is covered by at least two muscles which have opposite actions. In this diagram the triceps muscle opposes the action of the biceps muscle. When the biceps contracts to bend the elbow, the triceps muscle must relax and lengthen to allow this movement. Movement of a joint therefore involves contraction of one muscle and relaxation of the opposing muscle.

The elbow joint can only bend and straighten. Other joints have a bigger range of movement. For example, in the hip joint, the head of the femur can also rotate inwards and outwards inside the socket formed by the pelvic bones.

Role of Nerves

The nerve fibers to skeletal muscles come from motor nerve cells in the spinal cord. Stimulation of these nerves makes the muscles contract. The motor nerve cells in turn are influenced by a great many other nerves.

Stretch Reflex. Even when we are 'at rest' our skeletal muscles are contracting a little. This slight contraction is called muscle tone. It is due to a special reflex called the stretch reflex. Fig. 35 shows the pathway for this reflex. Buried in the muscle are sense organs called stretch receptors which send nerve impulses to the spinal cord when the muscle is stretched. This causes a reflex contraction of the muscle. Its effect is to prevent the muscle from being stretched any further.

When the doctor taps the muscle tendon below the knee cap with a rubber hammer, the leg swings out. This is a stretch reflex in action. As the tendon is tapped, the muscle stretches. This pulls on the stretch receptors and provokes a reflex contraction of the muscle (Fig. 35).

The stretch reflex is very important to us. The slight continuous contraction in the muscles of the back and neck, and the extensor muscles of the legs, keeps us upright. Otherwise the joints would flex under the weight of the body and we should then fall to the ground.

Muscle Tone. Damage to either the sensory or motor nerves of a muscle destroys its 'tone.' The muscle becomes flabby and soft and quite unlike a normal muscle. If the stretch reflex becomes more active than usual, it makes the muscles contract more and the limbs then move with difficulty—they are 'stiff.'

Some of the nerve fibers which pass from the brain to the spinal nerve cells restrain the activity of the spinal motor neurons while others 'pep up' the neurons, making the stretch reflex more active. Damage to either of these systems affects the stretch reflex which in turn affects the muscle tone.

Voluntary Movement

Commands from Cortex Cells. How does a person make a voluntary movement? The nerve cells responsible for this lie in the cerebral cortex. They send very long axons from the brain down to the nerve cells in the spinal cord. When the person wishes to bend his elbow, a command travels from the cerebral cortex down to the spinal nerve cells supplying the biceps muscle. This stimulates the motor nerve cells, and the biceps muscle contracts. At the same time, the opposing muscle (the triceps) receives a command to relax. So the elbow bends.

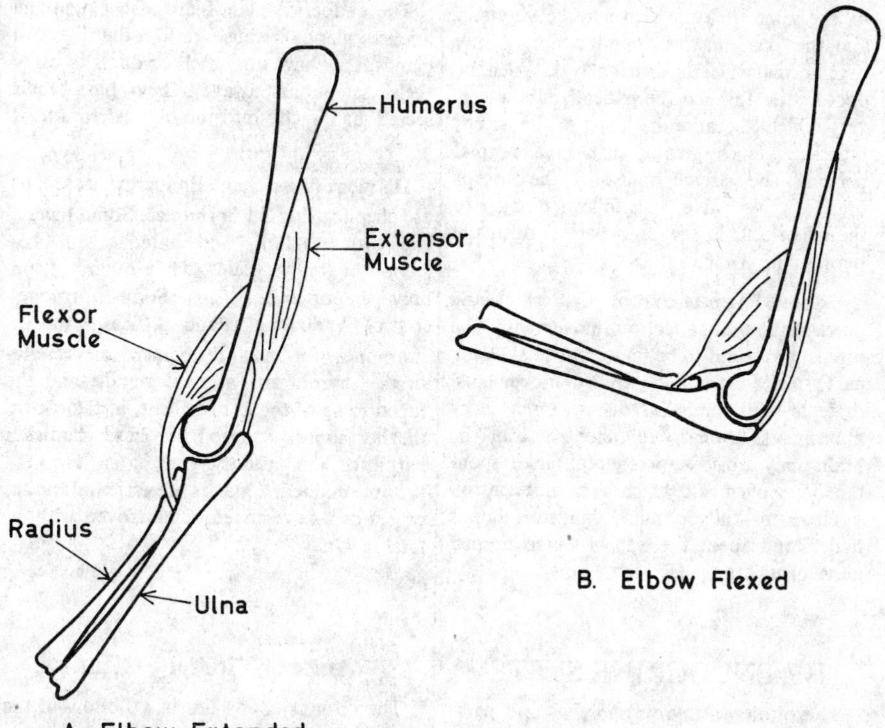

Fig. 34. *MUSCLE MOVEMENT. When the elbow bends, the flexor muscles contract and shorten. The extensor muscles at the same time relax and lengthen.*

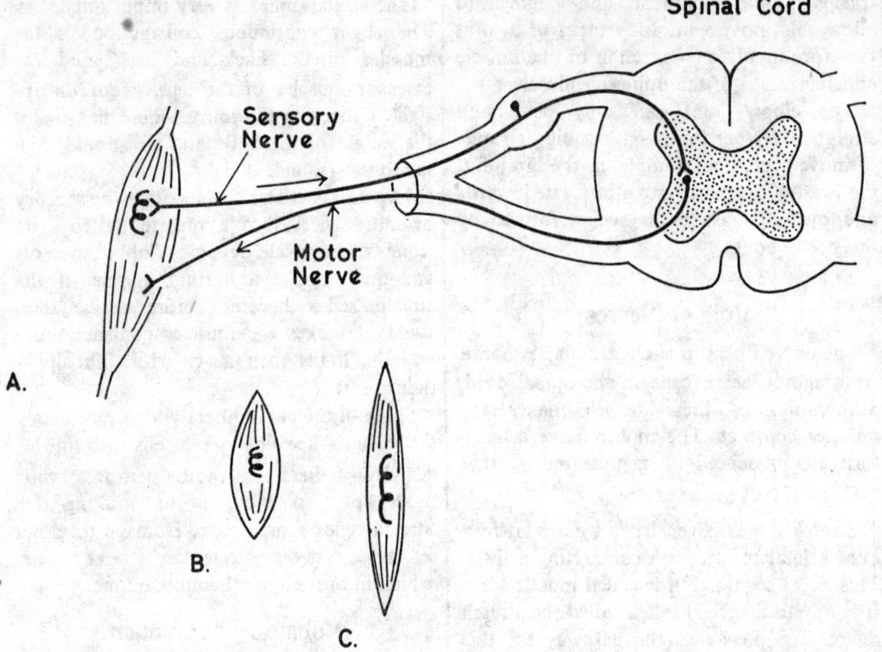

Fig. 35. *PATHWAY OF STRETCH REFLEX.* (A) *Skeletal muscles contain sense organs which are stimulated when the muscle is stretched. The sensory nerves carry messages to the spinal cord. Here the motor neuron is stimulated and makes the muscle contract and so resist further stretching.* (B) *Muscle at rest.* (C) *Muscle stretched. This shows how the sense organ is stretched when a muscle is pulled.*

Effect of Brain Damage. It sometimes happens that an elderly person has a little hemorrhage in the brain. This is a 'stroke.' If the hemorrhage is not severe, he recovers. However, his movements may be imperfect after this. Perhaps his arm is affected. He may not be able to move his arm voluntarily—at will. This indicates that the nerve fibers from the cerebral cortex have been damaged. At the same time the arm may be very stiff and the arm muscles contract more firmly than normal when the arm is at rest. When the doctor tries to bend the patient's elbow it is very difficult because the 'tone' of the triceps muscle is much greater than in a normal person. The stretch reflex in the triceps muscle is overactive. This follows damage to the nerve cells in the brain which normally depress the stretch reflex.

Other Movement-control Centers. Many parts of the brain affect our movements. The cerebellum seems to be important in allowing us to make smooth controlled movements. Patients with cerebellar disease make jerky movements. Damage to other parts of the brain may cause a person to make spontaneous movements which he cannot control.

There are still very many things we do not understand about the way in which normal movements are made.

THE ENDOCRINE SYSTEM

The pituitary, thyroid, adrenal and parathyroid glands, special islets cells in the pancreas, and also the sex glands (ovaries and testes), although widely separated in the body, form the endocrine system. This, together with the nervous system, controls the functions of all other organs and tissues, knitting together all the activities of the body. The nervous system comes into action when adjustments need to be made very rapidly, while the slower endocrine system is used for responses which must be kept going for a long time.

The endocrine glands are also called the ductless glands because, unlike the digestive glands, they have no vessels or ducts to carry their secretions away. They pass their secretions directly into the bloodstream as it flows through them.

Hormone Messengers. Endocrine secretions are chemicals called hormones. Some have a widespread action, and influence the behavior of many tissues, while others act on only one or two organs. Some hormones control endocrine glands. The pituitary hormones, for instance, control the activity of the thyroid and adrenal glands, and the functioning of the gonads. But, in their turn, the hormones produced by these glands in part affect the pituitary.

Some endocrine glands are essential to life; others can be removed or destroyed without fatal results.

Anterior Pituitary Gland

The pituitary body lies in a hollow in the skull beneath the brain. It has two parts—the anterior and posterior pituitary, and each functions quite separately (Fig. 36). The

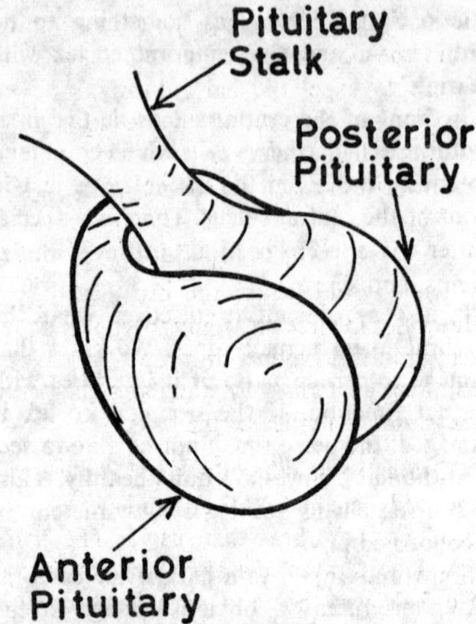

Fig. 36. *THE PITUITARY GLAND. The posterior pituitary is connected to the brain by nerves running down the pituitary stalk. The anterior pituitary gland is quite separate from the posterior pituitary.*

anterior pituitary has been called 'the leader of the hormonic orchestra,' because it controls so many other endocrine glands. It secretes several hormones.

THE GROWTH HORMONE. This is necessary for normal growth and development. If the growth hormone is deficient in early life the child becomes a dwarf. When too much hormone appears in a child he may grow to an enormous size and become a giant. If the pituitary begins to produce too much growth hormone in an adult, only the hands, feet and jawbones grow excessively. This produces the condition known as *acromegaly*. The growth hormone also controls the amount of sugar in the blood. Patients with an overactive pituitary have a high blood sugar level.

TROPHIC OR STIMULATING HORMONES. This group of hormones controls the activities of the thyroid gland, the adrenal cortex, the ovary and testis. If any one of these hormones is produced in excessive quantity, the person will suffer from overactivity of the gland concerned.

PROLACTIN. This hormone helps the breasts to secrete milk when a woman has a baby.

The anterior pituitary gland is partly controlled by the brain. There are no nerves to the gland from the brain; it is regulated only by chemical means.

Posterior Pituitary Gland

This gland is connected to the brain by nerves (Fig. 36). The nerves control the activity of the gland. The posterior pituitary secretes two hormones.

The ANTIDIURETIC HORMONE regulates the amount of water put out by the kidney. When the body needs to save water the posterior pituitary secretes a lot of the hormone. The kidney then forms only a little urine. When the body needs to lose water—as after a large drink—less antidiuretic hormone enters the blood. The kidney then excretes the extra water.

OXYTOCIN is another hormone secreted from the posterior pituitary. This helps the womb to expel the baby during labor. It also causes contraction of the ducts in the breasts when these are producing milk for the nourishment of the infant.

Thyroid Gland

The thyroid lies in the neck, in front of the windpipe (see Anatomy,p 236).The gland secretes the hormone, thyroxine, which seems to affect all tissues. It stimulates the general metabolic activities of the cells.

Overactivity. When the gland is overactive, the cells use more food and oxygen and produce more heat than usual. The patient then has Graves' disease, or thyrotoxicosis. He feels very hot and sweats profusely, his pulse is rapid, and he is restless and anxious. Very often the eyeballs protrude.

The gland can be depressed by drugs, but if they do not work satisfactorily, a part of the gland can be removed surgically.

Underactivity. Sometimes the thyroid gland fails and produces too little thyroxine. If this goes untreated in early life the child is underdeveloped both physically and mentally and becomes a cretin. In adult life a similar glandular failure causes myxedema. The patient puts on weight and becomes very slow mentally. There are many other changes which point to a general slowing down of cell activity all over the body. Myxedema can be cured by giving extracts of the gland.

Two-way Control. The thyroid gland is controlled by a hormone secreted by the anterior pituitary. Thyroxine in turn influences the anterior pituitary, and so, indirectly, the thyroid regulates its own activity.

The Adrenal Glands

There are two adrenal glands. One lies above the right and the other above the left kidney. Because of their position, they are also known as the suprarenal glands. Each gland is made of two separate tissues, a cortex and

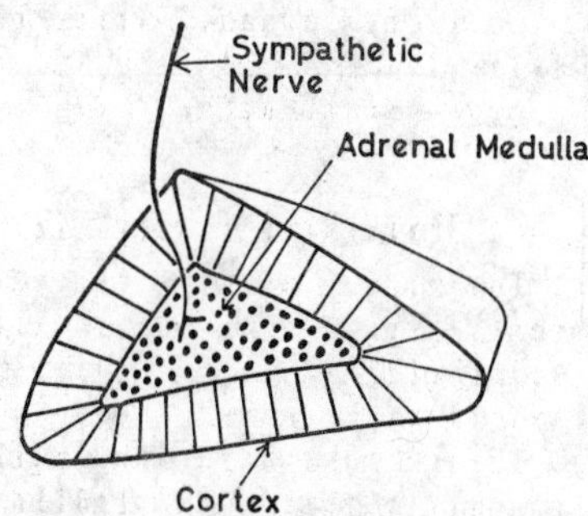

Fig. 37. *SECTION THROUGH ADRENAL GLAND The medulla lies inside the cortex. The two parts of the gland secrete different hormones and function quite independently.*

a medulla (Fig. 37). The adrenal cortex and adrenal medulla are quite separate during early life but come to lie one inside the other. The two tissues are quite different anatomically and have totally different functions. The cortex is essential to life, the medulla is not.

The Adrenal Cortex

Several hormones are produced in the adrenal cortex. There appear to be three main types of hormone.

(a) Those which affect sugar and protein metabolism raise the level of sugar in the blood and thus counteract the effect of insulin (see below).They also increase protein breakdown. The *cortisone* hormone has these actions.

(b) Those which affect the amount of salt excreted by the kidney. *Aldosterone* is one such hormone. If this is lacking, large quantities of salt pass out in the urine. With the salt goes water, and serious consequences follow if they are not replaced.

(c) Small amounts of the *sex hormones* are formed in the adrenal cortex.

Overactivity. Since these hormones regulate many aspects of body function, serious disturbances will occur if anything goes wrong with the gland. Tumors of the adrenal cortex cause it to produce far too much of some or all of the hormones. This occurs in Cushing's disease. The muscles waste, but the patient puts on weight because he retains too much salt and water. There may also be changes in sexual function.

Underactivity. On the other hand, when the adrenal cortex is destroyed by disease and produces too little hormone the reverse happens. This is seen in Addison's disease in which the body is very short of salt and the blood sugar is low. The blood pressure also tends to be low and the patient may have fainting attacks. There is also a curious pigmentation of the skin. The disease can be cured by giving hormones of the cortex.

The cortex seems to be partly controlled by the anterior pituitary, but we do not know what influences the secretion of the remaining hormones.

Cortisone Against Inflammation. Apart from its effects on sugar and salt metabolism, the important cortisone hormone has a very dramatic effect on inflammation. When the tissues are injured in any way they respond by becoming swollen and red—in other words, they are inflamed. This may be useful at times and is part of the body's defensive reaction. In some diseases, however, many parts of the body become inflamed, and we do not know why. This happens in rheumatoid arthritis. Joints become inflamed, swollen and stiff, causing the patient great pain and disability. Cortisone reduces this inflammation and very dramatically relieves the swelling and pain.

Unfortunately, cortisone will also lower the patient's resistance to infection, and has other side-effects which may be very undesirable. Also, when an arthritic patient has been given cortisone treatment and the medication is stopped, the disease may reappear, unless it has died down naturally in the meanwhile. Cortisone will not suit every patient and is therefore only given in certain selected cases.

The Adrenal Medulla

This gland lies enclosed by the adrenal cortex (Fig. 37). It is supplied and controlled by nerves from the sympathetic nervous system. The gland produces two hormones, adrenaline and noradrenaline. But the sympathetic nerves can also make these hormones so that stimulation of the sympathetic nervous system and the adrenal medulla will produce very similar results.

'Fight or Flight.' Adrenaline and noradrenaline together cause an increase in the heart rate, and a rise in blood pressure; the blood sugar level rises, the pupils dilate and the blood flow through the muscles increases. All these are responses which prepare the body to meet and cope with an emergency such as a sudden attack or danger. The adrenal medulla and the sympathetic nervous system then work together in preparation for 'fight or flight.'

Parathyroid Glands

Embedded in the back of the thyroid gland lie four parathyroid glands, each the size of a pea. They control calcium and phosphorus metabolism. These two elements form a very important part of bone structure. Calcium has other important functions: it helps in blood clotting and in nervous activity.

If the parathyroids are diseased, the bones may become soft and fracture easily.

The Pancreas

The pancreas is primarily a digestive gland. It secretes pancreatic juice which travels through a duct into the intestine.

Insulin. Embedded in the gland are scattered islands of cells which have quite a different function. They secrete a hormone, insulin, into the blood.

Insulin plays a very important part in sugar metabolism. Together with hormones from the pituitary and adrenal glands, insulin helps to control the amount of sugar in the blood. If insulin is injected into the bloodstream, the sugar level falls. The person begins to feel hungry and very faint. If the blood sugar falls very low, he may even lose consciousness. This can be prevented by eating sugar quickly.

Diabetes Mellitus. In the disease called diabetes mellitus there is not enough insulin. The sugar level in the blood is very high. A lot of sugar appears in the urine, taking water with it. This means that the patient must empty his bladder frequently.

The cells, however, do not seem to be able to use the sugar when it is present in such large amounts in the blood. Instead, they burn fat to obtain their energy. The body is not equipped to deal with fat combustion on such a large scale. The waste or residue from fat metabolism accumulates in the body and 'poisons' the tissues. If the disease is unchecked, the patient may go into a diabetic coma.

Diabetes is treated with injections of insulin and a well-controlled diet.

The Gonads

Ovaries. The ovaries in the female and the testes in the male are known as the gonads. The ovary forms the egg cells, or ova. It also secretes hormones which regulate the function of the uterus and cause the menstrual cycle.

The Testes produce the male cells, or spermatozoa. They also secrete the male hormone, testosterone.

The hormones secreted by the gonads cause the development of the secondary sex characters at puberty when the child becomes an adult.

The function of the gonads has been considered more fully in the section on Reproduction on p. 254.

FEVERS AND INFECTIOUS DISEASES

CLASSIFICATION OF THE COMMONER INFECTIONS

I. Diseases Due to Bacterial Infection

Anthrax. *Woolsorter's disease: Malignant pustule*
Cerebrospinal fever. *Meningitis: Spotted fever*
Cholera
Diphtheria
Dysentery, Bacillary
Erysipelas
Glanders
Gonorrhea (See Venereal Diseases)
Leprosy
Plague
Pneumonias
Puerperal fever (See Index)
Scarlet fever
Septicemia and Toxemia
Tetanus. *Lockjaw*
Tuberculosis (See also Chest Diseases)
Typhoid and Paratyphoid fever. *Enteric fevers*
Undulant fever. *Brucellosis: Malta fever*
Whooping-cough: *Pertussis*

II. Diseases Due to Fungus Infection

Actinomycosis

III. Diseases Due to Protozoan Parasites

Dysentery, Amoebic (See Intestinal and other Parasites)
Leishmaniasis. *Kala-azar*
Malaria and Blackwater fever
Toxoplasmosis
Trypanosomiasis. *Sleeping Sickness*

IV. Diseases Due to Rickettsias

Typhus fevers
Q fever
Scrub Typhus

V. Diseases Due to Spirochetes

Leptospirosis. *Weil's disease*
Relapsing fever. *African tick fever*
Syphilis (See Venereal Diseases)
Yaws

VI. Diseases Due to Viruses or to Unknown Agents

Acute colds. *Coryza: Acute rhinitis*
Chickenpox. *Varicella*
Dengue
Encephalitis lethargica. *Sleeping sickness*
German measles. *Rubella*
Glandular fever
Herpes simplex (See Disorders of the Skin)
Infective hepatitis. Viral hepatitis (See Diseases of the Digestive System)
Influenza
Measles. *Morbilli*
Mumps. *Epidemic parotitis*
Pneumonias: Virus and Rickettsial
Poliomyelitis (See Diseases of Nervous System)
Psittacosis
Rabies. *Hydrophobia*
Rheumatic fever
Sandfly fever. *Phlebotomus fever*
Sarcoidosis
Shingles. *Herpes Zoster* (See Diseases of Nervous System)
Smallpox. *Variola.* Varioloid
Yellow fever
Other Virus Diseases

FEVER

Fever, or pyrexia, is a rise in the temperature of the body with increased waste of the body tissues; it is generally caused by some infection by micro-organisms or by their toxins. In other cases, such as during convalescence, in neurotic persons or drug addicts, in severe cases of anemia, cancer, and other disorders of bodily function, irregular fever may occur without serious significance. Fever is thus a response or reaction of the body to infection, and is characterized by increased circulatory activity, increased heat, a dry hot skin, diminished strength and often exaggerated thirst.

Pulse Rate. The degree of circulatory excitement is measured by the state of the pulse. Of this state, there are two characteristic indications, namely *frequency* and *strength.* A pulse is frequent when its rapidity exceeds that of health; it is strong when its stroke resists with unusual force the pressure of a finger or thumb held on it.

In health, the pulse of an adult beats from sixty to eighty times in a minute; the pulse rate of children is more rapid. The pulsations of the heart of the unborn infant, as heard through the body of the mother, are one hundred and fifty in a minute. After birth the pulse gradually decreases from one hundred and forty down to the standard of adult age. To appreciate the tension of a pulse, experience is absolutely necessary.

The great activity of the circulation in fever is intimately connected with the patient's heat and thirst, and tends directly to waste the energies and consume the tissues of the body. The toxemia of fever reduces and changes the secretions or different fluids of the body such as the urine and sweat, and is the cause of the dry skin, scanty and high-colored urine, etc., to be noted in feverish cases.

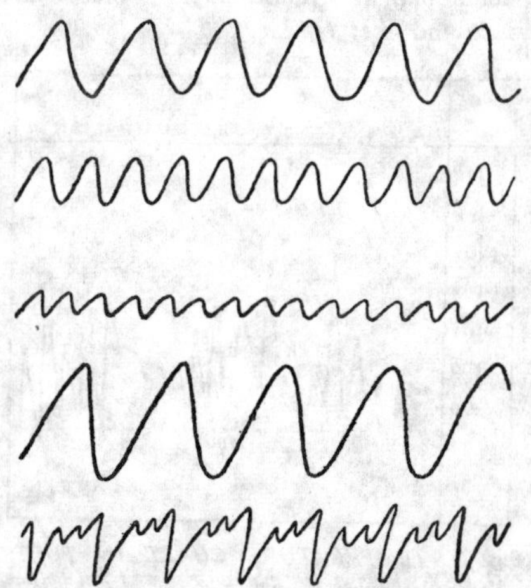

Fig. 1. *VARIATIONS IN PULSE TRACINGS.* 1. *Normal regular pulse; Normal rate—about* 72 *beats per minute.* 2. *Rapid pulse,* 130 *beats per minute.* 3. *Rapid feeble pulse.* 4. *Full bounding pulse.* 5. *Irregular pulse. Each tracing is for a 5-second period.*

A Crisis of fever is that period in its course when unfavorable symptoms may change to those of returning health. Perspiration breaks out on the forehead and sometimes over the whole body, and within about 24 hours the temperature of the patient falls to normal.

Symptoms. Fever or pyrexia is characterized by a great variety of symptoms and signs, the most common being the following.

1. A Rigor, or attack of shivering which occurs in the early stages of many fevers. Repeated rigors suggest malaria or some deep-seated infection of the body organs. The patient feels cold, the expression is anxious, and the teeth may chatter. The temperature is subnormal, but generally rises rapidly.

2. Increased Pulse Rate, or tachycardia, occurs particularly in scarlet fever and tuberculosis. In meningitis, however, the pulse is slow. As a general rule the pulse rate is increased by 8 beats per minute for each degree rise in temperature in adult patients, and 15 beats per minute in children.

3. Breathing is Rapid, especially in pneumonia and inflammatory conditions of the air passages.

4. Anorexia. The appetite is decreased, but thirst persists. The bowels are constipated and the urine is scanty and dark in color.

5. Delirium is common in high fever, and the patient may be partly comatose, or very restless.

Types of Fever

The course and nature of the fever is often a help in diagnosis.

1. **Rise of Temperature** is sudden in pneumonia and erysipelas, whereas in typhoid fever and tuberculosis it is less abrupt but increases daily for several days.

2. **The Course** of a fever may be continuous, remittent, or intermittent.

CONTINUOUS FEVER is noted in lobar pneumonia, in typhoid fever in the second week, and in erysipelas.

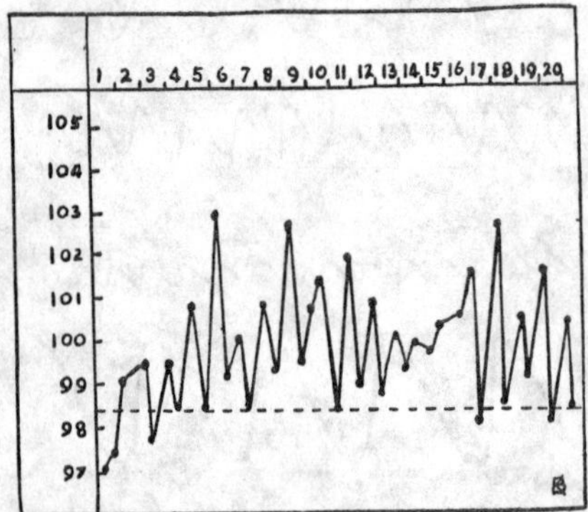

Fig. 2. *TEMPERATURE CHART IN TUBERCULOSIS showing the marked rise and fall between morning and evening temperatures of a remittent fever.*

In REMITTENT FEVER there is a daily rise and fall, with marked difference between morning and evening temperatures; this type of fever occurs in various forms of septicemia and pyemia, in deep abscesses (as in the appendix), and in tuberculosis.

INTERMITTENT FEVER is seen in malaria. Mixed types of fever are also common.

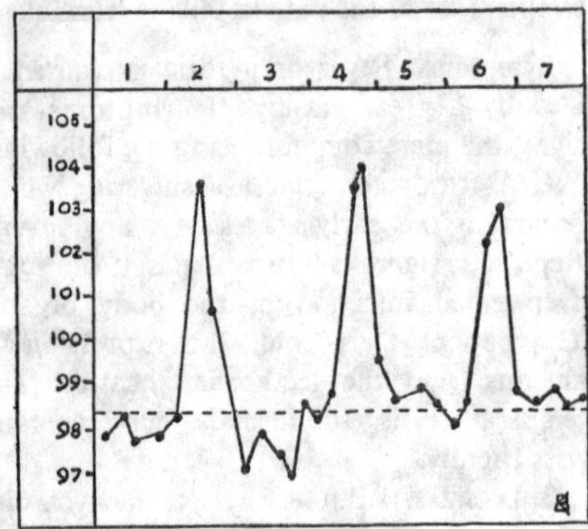

Fig. 3. *TEMPERATURE CHART IN MALARIA showing the high fever alternating every other day with near-normal temperatures. An intermittent fever.*

3. **Fall in Temperature.** BY CRISIS. Fever may end suddenly, the temperature falling to normal within 6 to 24 hours, this being called a crisis; a pseudo-crisis may occur before the actual crisis. In lobar pneumonia the temperature often falls by crisis at about the 7th or 8th day. With the use of antibiotics, a crisis is now much less common.

BY LYSIS. When the temperature takes several days to subside the reaction is known as lysis, and this terminal condition is commoner than a crisis, and is seen in most acute fevers.

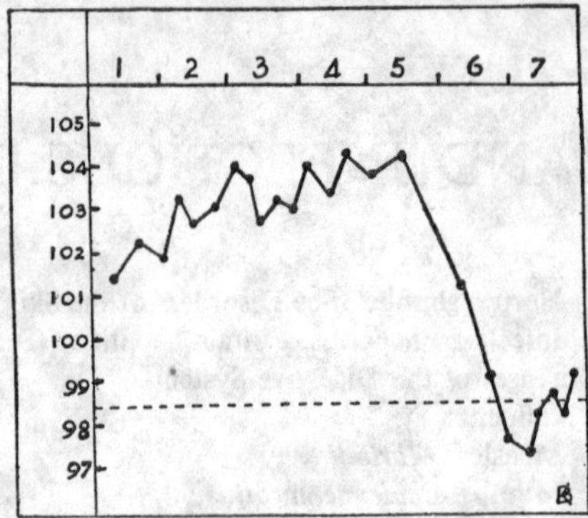

Fig. 4. *TEMPERATURE CHART IN LOBAR PNEUMONIA showing how the temperature falls suddenly and steadily by crisis.*

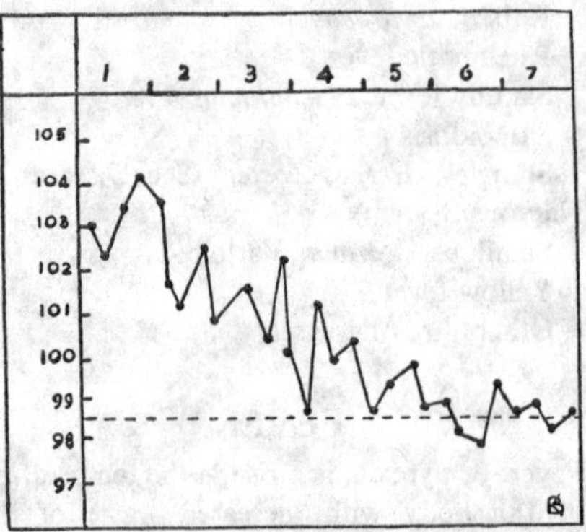

Fig. 5. *TEMPERATURE CHART IN BRONCHO-PNEUMONIA showing how the temperature falls by irregular risings and fallings over several days. This is a fall by lysis.*

General Care of Fever Cases

The chief requirements of patients during fever are: rest, skilled nursing, a suitable diet (see Invalid Cookery, p. 59), plenty of water, fresh air, the relief of symptoms or pain as they develop, and the prevention of complications and serious side-effects.

REST. Rest in bed is necessary as long as fever persists, that is while the temperature is raised, and must be continued until the patient is convalescent and can make a gradual return to normal activity. In diphtheria and typhoid fever the patient should be kept lying flat in bed to ease the strain on the heart caused by the general toxemia.

A firm mattress and light bed-clothes are required for comfort. A quiet room is essential, and the patient should be kept free from worry and disturbance.

NURSING. The temperature of the room should be about 15° C (59° F), although in the case of infants or old persons it may be about 16° to 18° C (60° to 65° F).

Soft furnishings should as far as possible be removed from the room. Those which are kept in the room may need to be disinfected later in certain fevers.

A white coverall should be worn in the patient's room by the attendant, and a bowl of disinfectant should be kept for scrubbing the hands.

The patient should be kept clean by daily tepid sponging, and powdering.

Food should be given at regular intervals, and cold water, or fruit juice with glucose, supplied plentifully. Food not eaten by the patient should be removed, and burned.

If dry the lips should be greased with vaseline or cold cream.

Swabs used for removing nasal, aural, or other discharges must be promptly burned.

VENTILATION. Fresh air in the bedroom is essential for the patient's comfort and well-being. In a close atmosphere the patient will tend to be restless.

DIET. In acute fevers a very light or fluid diet is generally required, but in prolonged cases the strength must be supported by a liberal supply of light nourishing food, which must be appetizing and varied. Glucose is valuable in acute fevers, and lemonade is palatable and cooling. At least 4 pints of water during every 24 hours should be given to adults in most cases.

Treatment of Symptoms

FEVER. Sponging with warm or tepid water may be carried out when the patient's temperature is high. Blanket baths (windows closed) are very refreshing (see p. 47).

HEADACHE. Headache is a common symptom in fever, and may be relieved by aspirin.

RESTLESSNESS AND INSOMNIA should be reported to the doctor or nurse, who may give sedatives such as chloral hydrate, or phenobarbital, but these should only be administered on medical orders.

Sometimes straightening of the sheets, a fresh pillowcase, and a hot lemon or milk drink will bring ease.

VOMITING is also common in fevers, especially in the early stages. An enema should be given in most cases (but not in suspected appendicitis or certain other bowel diseases until a medical diagnosis has been made), and glucose drinks containing a little sodium bicarbonate may be given. Ice may be sucked. Severe vomiting may necessitate removal of the patient to hospital.

CONSTIPATION is common during fevers, and a gentle laxative may be given in mild cases. Senna, or milk of magnesia are suitable for children. In severe illness the bowel may require an enema.

Leucocytosis

Leucocytosis is the name given to a condition of the blood in which the leucocytes or white corpuscles in the blood plasma are increased in number. These leucocytes are minute protoplasmic cells, which have the power of movement and can pass out of the smallest capillary blood vessels into the surrounding tissues. They act as scavengers, and play an important part in the destruction and removal of bacteria in the body, a process known as *phagocytosis*. The leucocytes are of different types (see Physiology, Fig. 6, p. 239), and normal blood contains a fairly constant proportion of each type. In infection or inflammation the leucocytes become greatly increased in number; the leucocytes which are killed in the attack on the bacteria form pus.

White Cell Count. One cubic millimeter of normal blood contains between 5,000 and 7,000 leucocytes. A small increase in numbers is found in so many of the more common diseases that an examination of the blood and a count of the white cells are often made as routine diagnostic measures. In many cases, for instance, of appendicitis, the white corpuscles increase to between 15,000 and 20,000 per cubic millimeter; in pneumonia they increase sometimes to 40,000 per cubic millimeter. In other more common diseases such as tonsillitis or sore throat, in erysipelas, smallpox, and inflammatory diseases such as septicemia, boils, bone diseases and pyemia, a greater or less increase is always found.

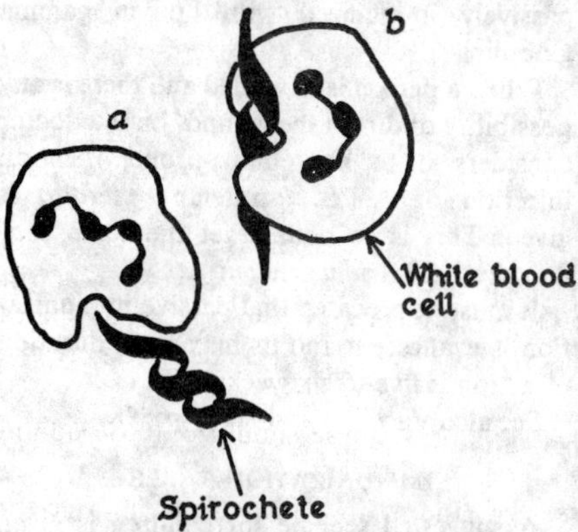

Fig. 6. *PHAGOCYTOSIS.* a. *The scavenging white blood cell approaches the invading micro-organism—a spirochete—and changes shape to engulf it.* b. *The white cell proceeds to destroy the invader by digesting it.*

In whooping-cough a marked leucocytosis occurs, which may confirm a doubtful diagnosis.

In other diseases absence of an increase often enables the right diagnosis to be made, since in typhoid fever (which might in the early stages be mistaken for appendicitis) there would be no increase in the early stage of the disease, but it would probably be marked in the later stages.

Bacteriology

Cause of Infection. Every infective disease is due to the introduction into the body of the specific cause of that disease. The specific cause is some form of organism or micro-organism such as bacteria, parasites, viruses and fungi. Pneumonia is often due to invasion of the lung by the *Pneumococcus.* Measles is caused by a minute virus. Actinomycosis is due to a fungus.

Toxins. During the life processes of these micro-organisms in the body a poison is commonly formed, called a toxin, which has a marked influence on the course which the disease runs, and in many instances it is the toxin rather than the primary invading organism which causes the symptoms of the disease. The membrane of diphtheria in many instances is not great enough to cause the severe effects seen in this disease, and persons sometimes die when relatively little membrane is present in the throat. This is the result of the toxin or poison generated by the bacteria which, during their circulation through the body, cause toxemia and paralysis of various nerves so that swallowing is difficult and the action of the heart or diaphragm is impaired.

The toxin of tuberculosis is called tuberculin.

Transmission of Infection

CONTAMINATED DUST. A disease such as tuberculosis is often spread through contaminated atmospheric dust, which is also true of many other infective diseases, namely diphtheria, pneumonia, influenza, scarlet fever, measles, whooping-cough and smallpox. By breathing in such dust the patient contracts the infection which is most often spread from the nose and throat.

CARRIERS. It must be explained that the disease organisms which are prevalent in the air are often to be found upon the mucous membranes of the nose and throat of persons not ill with the disease; such persons are called 'carriers.' The more numerous the germs and the greater their virulence, the greater is the danger that they will infect another person if he is susceptible—this is the term used when a person is especially liable to contract a particular disease.

DROPLET INFECTION. In coughing, expectorating, sneezing, and sometimes in speaking, little droplets of infected saliva or a fine moist spray which contains micro-organisms are thrown out into the general atmosphere where they may be inhaled and thus spread the disease to many people.

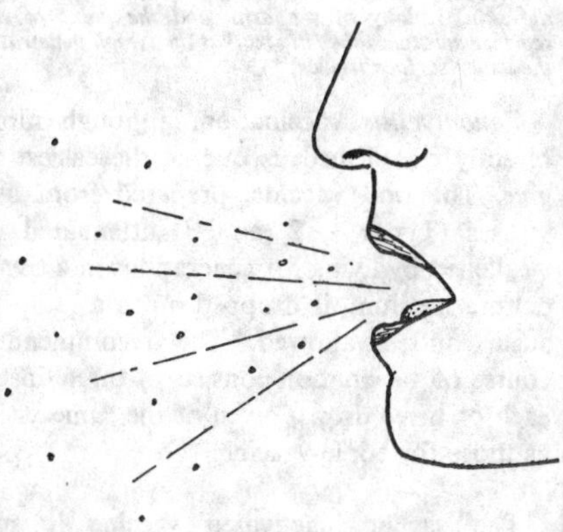

Fig. 7. *DROPLET INFECTION. How some infectious diseases are spread by coughing or sneezing.*

FLIES, CONTAMINATED FOOD, ETC. Other methods of transference of diseases are by rats, by fleas which infest rats, and by flies conveying by their feet bacteria or viruses from contaminated sputum, excreta, sores, etc. Contaminated water, milk and foods are also sources of infection for various diseases.

Prevention of Infective Diseases. It is necessary to understand methods of prevention of different diseases as well as the causes and treatment.

The life history of some bacteria is quite complicated. In malaria, for instance, the *Plasmodium* lives certain stages of its life in a mosquito and others in man, so that prevention of the disease must include getting rid of the mosquitoes, draining swamps where they breed, using mosquito nets over beds at night, as well as researching for drugs which will combat the particular phase of the *Plasmodium* in the infected patient's bloodstream.

HEALTH AND HYGIENE. The prevention of infection also includes keeping people fit and healthy because all micro-organisms are more prone to attack the poor 'soil' offered by a weak, unhealthy, ill-fed, and neglected body. The various ways of keeping fit and healthy are dealt with in some detail in the section on Health and Hygiene. Cleanliness in all its aspects, from the disposal of sewage to the washing of hands before eating meals, is of primary importance. Fresh air, regular exercise, well-balanced diets and adequate sleep are all aspects of the prevention which is better than cure.

IMMUNIZATION as a method of prevention has been known since 1798, when Jenner published reports about smallpox. He noticed that dairymaids whose fingers had the sores of cowpox did not contract smallpox because the milder cowpox had caused their bodies to produce a protective antitoxin which also enabled them to resist the related disease of smallpox. They had been immunized.

Immunity and Immunization

By immunity is meant the ability of a person to resist a disease. When a disease organism gains admittance to the tissues of the body it will multiply and either destroy local tissue or produce poisons which will affect the whole body, or both. The ease with which it can do this depends upon the person's immunity.

Immunity may be natural or acquired.

Natural Immunity is the resistance a person possesses to ward off an infectious disease with which he has never before been in contact. This is partly hereditary and partly due to the state of his health. Nature attempts to counteract antigens, that is invading micro-organisms or other foreign protein substances, by producing its own special protective protein known as antibodies. To counteract the poisons (toxins) produced by invading micro-organisms, the body also makes antitoxins which are a special kind of antibody. For each toxin a separate specific antitoxin has to be made.

Our resistance today to tuberculosis is great. It no longer is the scourge of Europe. Those of our ancestors who had no natural immunity died early from the disease, often before having children, and we are mainly descended from those who had the ability to survive. When Europeans first contacted the Pacific Islanders they brought tuberculosis and measles (as well as other diseases) to these people for the first time. The effect was devastating.

Our natural immunity may be enhanced by getting sufficient sleep and by eating a well-balanced diet including eggs, fish, meat, fruit and milk.

Acquired Immunity. In some diseases we can reinforce a person's natural immunity by vaccinating him so that his body is stimulated to produce plenty of antitoxins which will protect him against that particular disease. This gives ACTIVE IMMUNITY because the patient's tissues actively co-operate in the process.

A short-lived form is known as PASSIVE IMMUNITY. The patient is given an injection of serum containing antibodies or antitoxins when there is little or insufficient time for his body to produce the antibodies by the vaccination process.

Active Immunization. The patient's blood and tissue cells are encouraged to produce antibodies against a particular disease by the administration of killed or attenuated (weakened) micro-organisms, usually in the form of vaccines.

As we all know, some diseases give lasting immunity. One attack of smallpox, tetanus, or whooping-cough will prevent the person from ever catching the disease again. Other infections like the pneumonias, boils, influenza, and colds do not give lasting immunity. Therefore we can only provide lasting active immunity against the former diseases and not against the latter. In the case of whooping-cough, the patient may become infected later by a related organism, *Parapertussis*, and appear to have a mild 'second attack' of whooping-cough.

Today we may actively immunize against certain bacteria, viruses, and rickettsias.

1. BACTERIAL DISEASES. Whooping-cough, tetanus, diphtheria, cholera, typhoid, plague, and to some extent tuberculosis (using B.C.G.).

Immunization against whooping-cough, (pertussis), tetanus, and diphtheria is usually (but not necessarily) performed with a triple vaccine containing all three disease antigens, and may be commenced at 3 months of age; a second and third injection are given after two months then after six months; a booster dose of diphtheria and tetanus vaccine being given at school entry age.

2. VIRUS DISEASES. Smallpox, yellow fever, rabies, poliomyelitis, and measles vaccines are available.

Smallpox vaccination is commonly performed with calf lymph. The cowpox virus in the lymph has been weakened by giving it in repeated doses to the animal until its tissues have produced plenty of protective antibodies. The weakened virus antigens are located in the serum which is then used for human vaccination. Primary vaccination should be performed early in the second year of life. The lymph inoculated on a small scratch on the skin produces a large pustule indicating that the infant's body has produced antibodies against the weak virus antigens. This confers immunity of a high degree for two to three years and of a lesser degree for many years.

Revaccination should be undertaken when one is going into an endemic area. This is performed in a manner similar to that for infants and only a slight papule with some itching results.

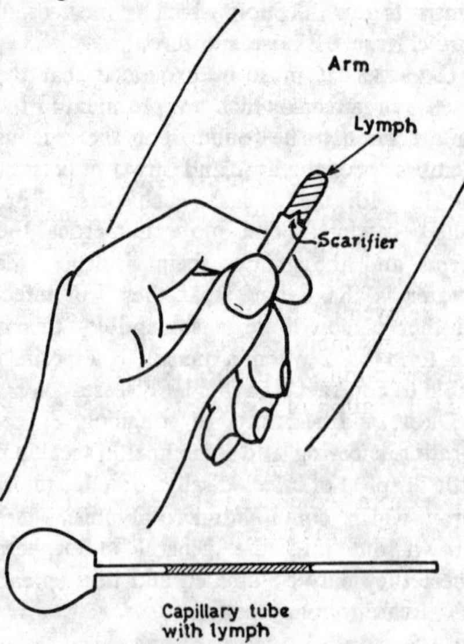

Fig. 8. *IMPLEMENTS FOR SMALLPOX VACCINATION. The lymph is squeezed from the tube on to the skin, usually of the arm, and the point of the scarifier scratches the skin so that the lymph penetrates the under-surface tissues.*

Poliomyelitis vaccination, although more recently established, is one of the easiest to give. The oral vaccine, prepared from live viruses (Types 1, 2, and 3) attenuated or weakened by living for generations in a tissue culture medium, is dropped on to a lump of sugar and swallowed. The recommended course of vaccination consists of three doses, each of three drops, given at the same visits as those for triple vaccine.

The earlier inactivated vaccine is still sometimes given by injection.

Measles vaccination need not be given until a baby is about a year old since it is immune to measles for six months or more due to the presence of maternal antibodies in its serum.

3. RICKETTSIAL DISEASES. One may be immunized against typhus if one is traveling through or living in an endemic area.

Passive Immunization. This is performed by injecting serum which has been prepared, usually in horses, by actively immunizing an animal against a specific disease. Sometimes one may use a serum from a convalescent patient. The serum contains antibodies or antitoxins against a particular organism or toxin. This form of immunization is sometimes of great use in an epidemic.

If a pregnant woman (6 to 12 weeks pregnant) who has not had German measles has contracted, or is in contact with cases of German measles, then it is a wise precaution to passively immunize her. This will prevent her getting the disease and so affecting the fetus.

Another instance of its use is against poliomyelitis. Queen Elizabeth II, when touring Australia, was forced to travel during an epidemic of poliomyelitis and so she was passively immunized with human gamma globulin.

When a person is wounded and there is any possibility of dirt in the wound, or the doctor considers it to be tetanus-prone, then an injection of A.T.S. (antitetanus serum) is given. This is to counteract the toxin produced by *Clostridium tetani*.

It must be repeated that passive immunization is evanescent and its maximum duration of action is five to six weeks.

See also Vaccines and Sera, p. 598.

IMMUNIZATION TABLE

A suggested scheme for children is given below:

Age	*Vaccine*	*Visit No.*	*Interval*
3 months (pref. 6 months)	Triple vaccine (Dip/Tet/Pert) and oral Polio vacc.	1	—
		2	6 to 8 weeks
		3	6 months
early in 2nd year	Smallpox	4	
"	Measles	5	1 month
5 years or school entry	Dip/Tet oral Polio	6	
	Smallpox revaccination	7	1 month
12 to 13 years	B.C.G. (for tuberculin-neg. cases only)	8	
15 to 19 years	Polio booster Tet booster	9	
	Smallpox revaccination	10	

Chemotherapy

This is the name given to treatment of infective diseases by means of chemical substances which, when introduced into the body tissues, act specifically against the invading bacteria without damaging the body cells. The sulphonamide drugs, and the antibiotics such as the penicillins, streptomycin, and the tetracyclines, are the main chemotherapeutic agents available at present. It is important to note that the majority of these drugs either inhibit or stop the growth of bacteria and that only a few destroy the very minute viruses which are the cause of such diseases as the common cold, German measles, influenza, poliomyelitis and smallpox.

For fuller details about the uses, actions, dosages, side-effects and contraindications of sulphonamides and antibiotics, see section on Pharmacy, pp. 595–6; 597–8.

I. Diseases Due to Bacterial Infection

Anthrax

(*Malignant Pustule: Woolsorter's Disease*)

Anthrax is a disease of animals occurring in humans as an acute infection of the skin, causing the so-called malignant pustule. There is also a pulmonary form known as 'woolsorter's disease,' and occasionally intestinal anthrax infection is seen. Anthrax generally attacks persons who work with hides, hair or wool, but may be spread by infected bristles in shaving brushes. The skin lesion is a black ulcerating vesicle, the patient being ill, and developing septicemia within a few days unless treatment is given.

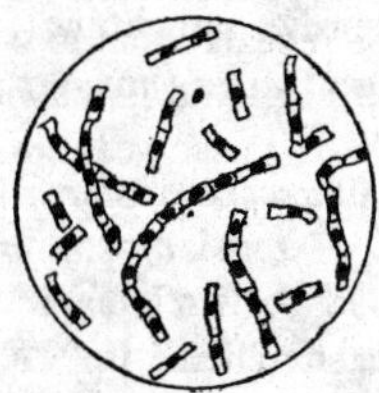

Fig. 9. *ANTHRAX BACILLI from a malignant pustule of the skin.*

Treatment. The patient should be kept in bed.

Better results are now obtained in anthrax of the skin by intramuscular injections of penicillin. Improvement begins to show within twenty-four hours. Tetracyclines are often given in addition. The ulcer may take two to three weeks to heal. In woolsorter's disease the prognosis is very grave.

Cerebrospinal Fever

(*Meningococcal Meningitis: Spotted Fever*)

This is an acute infectious disease often occurring in epidemics, especially in camps, or where persons are living in crowded conditions, and carriers are sometimes responsible for spreading the disease. It is most common in young children, especially in children under 5 years of age.

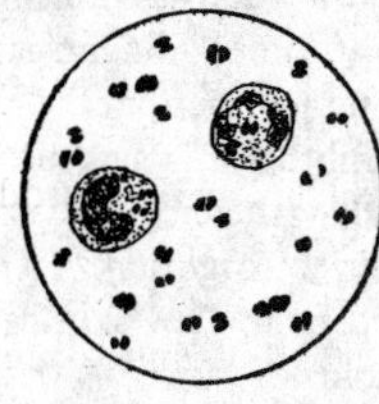

Fig. 10. *MENINGOCOCCI, with two large white blood cells. The white cells remove the cocci by digesting them.*

The fever is caused by the *Meningococcus*, which probably gains entry through the nose or pharynx. The incubation period is from three to seven days.

Symptoms. The onset is usually sudden, with headache, vomiting, high temperature, stiffness of the neck with retraction of the head, pain in the limbs, restlessness and irritability. The pupils are large and squinting may be noted. In children convulsions are common. The patient may become confused or delirious, with twitchings or spasm of different parts of the body, and a rash often develops early in the course of the disease, but this varies in different outbreaks of the disease.

Course. Some attacks of the disease are mild but if treatment is not started early the patient is likely to become comatose; death may follow in a few hours or days. In other cases the disease is more chronic and may leave defects such as blindness, deafness, hydrocephalus and mental deficiency. This disease is the most common cause of meningitis in young children under 3 years of age.

Diagnosis. The disease must be distinguished from typhoid, pneumonia, influenza, abscess of the middle ear, other types of meningitis, poliomyelitis or acute rheumatic fever. Some forms resemble septicemia and may give rise to pericarditis or endocarditis, nephritis, and inflammation of the testes. Pneumonia occasionally develops and is a serious secondary disease in infants and old persons. Arthritis is seen in some cases as a complication but recovery is the rule.

Treatment. Isolation and a search for 'carriers' are essential immediately the disease is suspected. A doctor must be called because the outlook is serious and treatment must be started as soon as possible. Lumbar puncture should be performed by a doctor for diagnosis and prompt treatment. Sulphadiazine, sulphadimidine and penicillin are given early in the attack, and are extremely efficacious; they have greatly reduced the mortality rate and prevent serious consequences. For those who are resistant to penicillin, the tetracyclines are used.

The patient is kept warm and very quiet and sedatives may be required. Nasal tubal feeding may be necessary to maintain nutrition. The fever is treated on general principles. The death rate is high in cases not given penicillin and a sulphonamide, but with these drugs most cases are cured within 6 to 10 days. A few cases relapse and skilled nursing is essential. A long period of convalescence (up to 8 weeks) is required. Blindness, when it develops, is often permanent.

Cholera

This disease is generally water-borne and is most common in tropical countries, being especially prevalent in India, but at the present day the strict vigilance of sanitary boards has done much to prevent its spread and mitigate its terrors in Europe. It is propagated by a micro-organism called Koch's comma bacillus or *Vibrio cholerae*, which is present in contaminated water. It is also transmitted by unhygienically handled food and by flies. Poor sanitation and heavy rainfall aid the spread of epidemics. Cholera is spread by 'carriers' and by persons who are only mildly affected and who mingle with the general population. The efforts of investigators are now being directed to the discovery of an agent that will destroy this organism and thus control the disease. The incubation period varies from a few hours to a few days, generally being from 2 to 7 days.

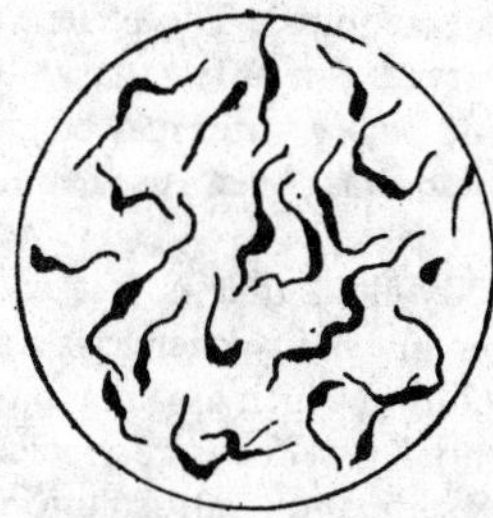

Fig. 11. *CHOLERA VIBRIOS from contaminated water. From their shape they are also known as the 'comma' bacilli.*

Symptoms. The preliminary stage is marked by colic, headache and vomiting, pain in the loins or knees, twitching of the calves of the legs, impaired appetite, thirst, and frequent bowel movements; these symptoms continue from a few hours to several days. For several days before the attack the pulse is often reduced to forty or fifty beats in a minute.

THE FIRST STAGE or stage of evacuation is marked by watery vomiting, by the evacuation of a thin colorless fluid looking like rice-water, and by severe cramps in the hands and calves of the legs, which also attack the bowels and stomach. Restlessness and collapse follow, with blueness and coldness of the skin, and the blood pressure is low (55 to 70 millimeters of mercury). The tongue is and the pulse is feeble; the breathing is hurried, with distress about the heart; there is great thirst, a feeling of internal warmth, and the secretion of urine is diminished or absent. The patient becomes increasingly exhausted.

The thin colorless discharges by vomiting and purging are derived from the serum or watery portion of the blood which oozes through the blood vessels. When so much serum is lost that the blood cannot circulate freely, the second stage is reached.

THE SECOND STAGE or stage of collapse (algid stage) is characterized by great prostration; the pulse is rapid and hardly perceptible; the skin is cold and wrinkled; the face blue or purple, and the eyes are much sunken; the hands are dark-colored and sodden, and the muscular cramps are agonizing. There is a sense of great heat in the stomach and intense thirst. The temperature may be subnormal and the patient is semi-conscious. In unfavorable cases circulatory failure leads to uremia and death, but in less severe cases reaction follows, the blood pressure rises, and the diarrhea abates.

THE THIRD STAGE, or stage of reaction, occurs in favorable cases after or before the second stage. There is rapid improvement with returning consciousness, and the stools become less frequent. Convalescence is usually rapid but there may be relapses or subsequent complications, such as hyperpyrexia (high fever), pneumonia, or uremia.

During epidemics cholera vaccine should be used to prevent infection, and gives immunity for six months.

Treatment. Rest in bed and additional warmth are required. The patient should be nearly starved for a few days, but water, glucose and barley water may be given freely. Tetracycline has been used but without marked effect.

The body fluid that is lost contains not only water but many chemicals and electrolytes in solution which are vital to the patient. It is essential that they are replaced quickly and many liters of salt solution, sodium bicarbonate solution, and dextrose solution are given intravenously until the kidneys begin to function freely. Then the potassium loss can be made good by the intravenous or the oral route.

When the urinary output is satisfactorily established, fluids are still required in plenty but they can be taken by mouth. Milk, milk foods (cereal puddings, egg custard, milk jellies: see Invalid Cookery, p. 59) and other bland foods may be taken as the patient feels able to take them. Protein foods are only given when the kidneys are able to cope with protein excretion products.

Convalescence is usually rapid provided that kidney damage has not occurred.

Personal Cleanliness. It is important that persons handling cholera patients or their beds and belongings be scrupulous about washing and disinfecting their hands after tending the patients and before eating. All drinking water and milk must be freshly boiled and food protected from flies. Raw fruit and vegetables should be temporarily avoided. Cholera vaccination gives protection for six months.

Diphtheria

Diphtheria is an acute contagious and infectious disease in which the characteristic feature is the formation of a membrane of fibrinous exudate upon a mucous surface, usually in the pharynx or larynx. The disease is especially dangerous to children under 5 years, particularly young infants. Diphtheria must be notified to the local health authority. The incubation period is two to five days. Although quarantine is not now considered necessary, a period of 12 to 14 days may be advisable as a precautionary measure for the isolation of contacts.

Cause. Diphtheria is caused by a germ known as the Klebs-Loeffler bacillus or *Corynebacterium diphtheriae.* It begins as a local disease, often as a sore throat, but later affects the whole system as the toxins or poisons are absorbed into the body.

Three forms of diphtheritic infection are recognized: *mitis* is mild with little toxic effect on the body but usually produces more membranous involvement of the throat, *gravis* produces severe toxemia often with intense swelling and edema of the throat resembling quinsy, and *intermedius* is less severe than gravis.

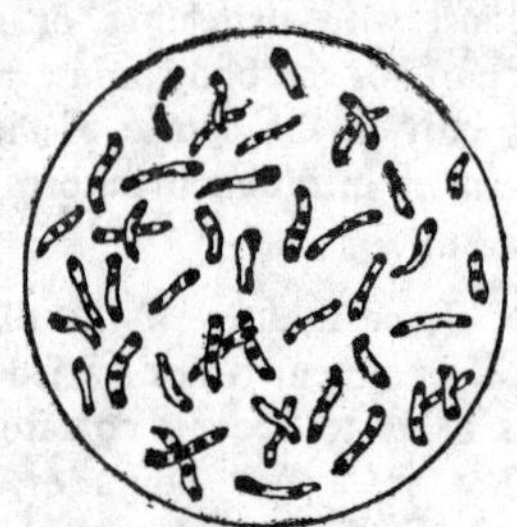

Fig. 12. *DIPHTHERIA BACTERIA. They vary greatly in virulence and are usually located in the nose and throat.*

'False' membrane inflammation of the pharynx such as occurs in Vincent's angina, scarlet fever, tonsillitis and syphilis, cannot always easily be distinguished clinically from diphtheria except by taking swabs from the throat and testing in the laboratory; in diphtheria the *Corynebacterium* is always present. On the other hand, there are cases of true diphtheria so mild in character and showing so little membrane as to pass unnoticed, but which on bacteriological examination prove to be diphtheria.

Propagation. The germs are transmitted for the most part by droplet infection, that is by the minute moist particles given out in breathing or sneezing.

The disease may be also conveyed by 'carriers,' that is, healthy persons who carry micro-organisms in the throat or nose without showing signs of the disease. Epidemics have been caused by infected milk supplies. From 1937 onwards, as a result of the immunization scheme for all children from 3 months to 15 years, the notified cases of diphtheria have fallen phenomenally and deaths are now few and far between.

Symptoms and Diagnosis. The characteristic feature is the pharyngeal or faucial membrane, which is of a glistening pearl-gray color, and is raised and adherent, often being present on the tonsil or throat, spreading gradually and becoming thicker and darker with a well-defined edge.

To distinguish diphtheria from simple follicular tonsillitis, which is so common, is often difficult and frequently impossible without a bacteriological examination. The membrane of simple tonsillitis is white, beginning as little white specks like the curd of milk, and is usually easily removed without bleeding. In the early stages of tonsillitis the temperature is usually higher than in diphtheria (101° to 104° F) and the patient is more flushed.

LOCATION. The tonsils, uvula, pharynx, nasal passages and the larynx are the sites where the grayish diphtheritic membrane is generally formed, but it may be found less commonly on the conjunctivae, border of the anus, vagina, prepuce, respiratory tract, skin or ears. The lymphatic glands of the neck may become much enlarged when the throat is involved.

NOSE AND TONSILS. When the membrane extends to the nostrils the breathing is more labored, and bloody mucus may be seen in the nostrils, which hardens, forming crusts, or it may run down on to the upper lip and cause excoriation. This discharge is highly infectious. As the tonsils grow larger and the nose becomes plugged, sleep is more and more restless and disturbed by snoring and difficulty in breathing, and there may be pain on swallowing.

In nasal diphtheria the disease may cause comparatively mild symptoms even when there is extensive membrane formation. In nasopharyngeal cases, however, the outlook is more grave.

LARYNX. When there is involvement of the vocal cords of the larynx one sees a truly terrible malady, distressing in the extreme, especially in children. Involvement of the larynx may be suspected when the voice becomes husky and hoarse; finally it may be reduced to a whisper. The glands of the neck become swollen and tender. In some cases the membrane may be limited to the larynx alone, as in so-called membranous croup, which with hoarseness and croupy cough generally occurs in children under 4 years of age. The symptoms of this affection are at first local and, if treatment is delayed, difficulty in breathing with laryngeal spasm become more and more marked and distressing till death may ensue from suffocation unless tracheostomy (see under Treatment) is performed. The face becomes blue or leaden, the chest heaves with deep labored respirations, the nostrils dilate, and the hollows below the collar-bones are depressed and the lower ribs drawn in, in the effort to breathe, until death occurs from asphyxia.

The severity of any case depends much on the amount of absorption from the throat, nose, or pharynx of the toxin produced by the growth of the micro-organisms on the one hand, and prompt diagnosis and specific treatment on the other hand. The odor of the breath in diphtheria is sickening and characteristic and, when once experienced, is generally never forgotten. The face is often puffy and ashen. The skin is dry and the limbs are cold.

TEMPERATURE. In simple cases this seldom rises above 38·3° C (101° F), but in severe cases it may be abnormally low, or only slightly raised, with great prostration and languor. The degree of fever, however, is no indication of the severity of the case. Delirium and restlessness accompany severe cases with great absorption of toxin. There are malaise, headache, loss of appetite, and soreness of the throat. The face is pallid and there may be hoarseness.

HEART. The heart is usually rapid, with a feeble soft pulse, but in many severe cases there is a very slow irregular or imperceptible pulse which is an unfavorable sign. The heart muscle in diphtheria is always the uncertain element, many patients dying suddenly and unexpectedly from heart paralysis, either within one or two weeks after the onset, or even during recovery. Albumin often appears in the urine, and is usually evidence of involvement of the kidneys, but subsequent chronic nephritis after convalescence is rare.

Complications. Bronchitis and broncho-pneumonia may occur in severe cases, especially when the larynx is affected. Heart failure is a fatal complication in neglected cases. Relapse may occur at a late stage, but is rare.

The most common and the most characteristic sequels of diphtheria are: (1) paralysis which develops in about 15 to 20 per cent of cases in the third or fourth week, especially in children, and (2) cardiac failure.

PARALYSIS in different forms lasts from a few days to some weeks, though it may last for months. It is not always related to the severity of the disease, but is often proportional to the extent of membrane present, and is usually local rather than general, involving various parts of the body, particularly the palate, eyes, pharynx, larynx, causing a nasal twang to the voice and the regurgitation of food through the nose and affecting the muscles of deglutition and speech. Paralysis may also involve the legs, arms, diaphragm, trunk and rib muscles and the sphincter muscles of the bladder and rectum. Diphtheritic paralysis is never permanent. In the very rare cases in which the diaphragm and respiratory muscles have been involved a mechanical respirator may be required.

CARDIAC FAILURE may occur early, or in the first two weeks of the disease owing to the severe poisoning of the blood by the toxins from the infecting micro-organisms. Blood pressure falls, the pulse is feeble and irregular, the complexion is pallid and urinary output scanty, and the heart becomes enfeebled. Sudden heart failure may follow from heart block.

Prognosis. The prognosis varies according to the age and health of the patient, the severity of the symptoms, the site of attack, the efficacy of treatment, which should be started *early*, and the degree of virulence of the particular infecting bacterium. Nasal and laryngeal complications, because of the large area of mucous membrane involved, increase the risks to the patient. The mildest cases may terminate fatally from relapse. The heart may fail at any stage, and death may occur suddenly when apparently all is going well. Unfavorable symptoms are great pallor, prostration, vomiting, and inability to take much nourishment, weakness of pulse with great rapidity or slowness, hemorrhages into the skin, restlessness and delirium. A profuse nasal discharge, marked enlargement of the glands, and severe albuminuria are also ominous signs.

Treatment. The essentials in general treatment are (1) intramuscular injection of diphtheria antitoxin as soon as the diagnosis is made; (2) absolute rest and recumbency for some weeks, which varies according to the severity of the disease; (3) good nursing; (4) plenty of glucose, sometimes by injection; and (5) early tracheotomy (tracheostomy) when the larynx is involved.

NURSING. If the patient cannot be treated in hospital, complete isolation in a room supplied with as little furniture as possible, is necessary. Isolation is generally necessary for at least 4 to 6 weeks, or until three bacteriological examinations at intervals of one week have proved negative. All utensils and dishes must be thoroughly disinfected before being taken out of the room, and all discharges must be received into a vessel containing lysol. All clothing should be boiled when possible, or should be otherwise sterilized or destroyed.

Attendants should wear gauze face masks (which must be changed often and washed in disinfectant) over the nose and mouth, and their hands must be frequently washed with antiseptics. They should gargle with antiseptic solutions frequently after attendance. Children of the family should not play with others in the neighborhood, although they should be kept out of doors liberally.

The temperature of the room should be about 18° C (65° F), and plenty of fresh air and sunlight admitted. The clothing and bedding should be changed frequently, and a completely recumbent position without exertion be insisted on in order to reduce the risk of heart failure.

DIET. The diet should be at first liquid and given every two to three hours, but with a minimum of disturbance and in definite quantity, not exceeding the amount the patient can easily digest. Bouillon, ice-cream, jellies, egg and milk, are suitable foods to be administered. Glucose lemonade should be given freely; glucose is an important dietary aid in diphtheria. During convalescence light solid foods may be given.

LOCAL TREATMENT. The throat may be gently syringed with warm normal saline, or painted with either potassium chlorate or boracic acid solution. Light warm wet cloths may be applied to the neck.

TRACHEOSTOMY (incision of the trachea for the insertion of a special tube to aid breathing) may be required suddenly in laryngeal diphtheria, although antitoxin and large doses of penicillin generally afford considerable relief.

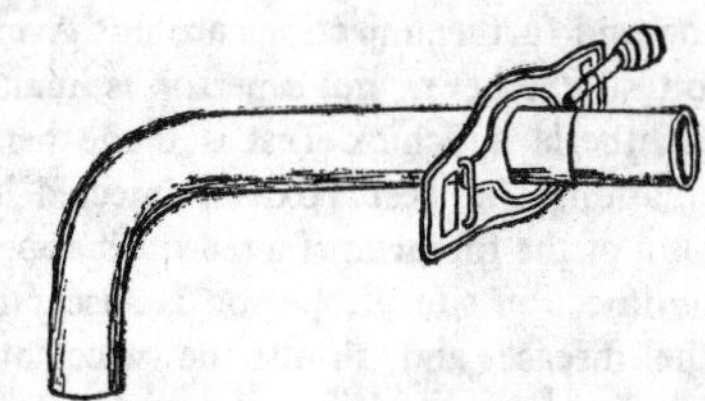

Fig. 13. *TRACHEOTOMY TUBE to assist breathing: for insertion into a hole made in the front of the throat of a patient with diphtheritic obstruction of the larynx.*

CONVALESCENCE. Complete rest, with the patient lying absolutely flat, without a pillow, must be continued for at least three weeks after the membrane has disappeared, or after the disappearance of all symptoms. Convalescence must be very gradual, and the pulse carefully observed when the patient first sits up, because of the risk of heart failure. If this threatens, the foot of the bed should be somewhat raised and the patient laid flat.

Specific Treatment

ANTITOXIN. Once a case of diphtheria is suspected and a throat swab sent for bacteriological examination, diphtheria antitoxin serum should be injected intravenously immediately without even awaiting the bacteriologist's report because delay increases the spread of the toxin. Only the tissues unaffected by the toxin are able to utilize the serum to counteract the poison. Modern antitoxic serum is much purer than the earlier forms and it is now very rare to find patients showing allergic reactions to the serum.

The essential features of serum treatment consist in the injection of doses of antitoxin proportionate to the age of the patient, the severity of the disease, and the time elapsed since the onset of the symptoms. The dosage varies with all these conditions. The repetition of the dose depends on the amount of improvement in the membrane.

IMMUNIZATION. For preventive treatment or immunization, diphtheria antitoxin and diphtheria vaccine are both used. When a case of diphtheria has been confirmed in a community such as a school or hospital ward it is advisable to give all contacts passive immunization which has short-term effectiveness and also active immunization which is long-lasting. Antitoxin gives immediate aid to tissues threatened by the diphtheritic toxin but it gradually passes out of the body. Diphtheria vaccine on the other hand stimulates the tissues to produce their own antitoxin and it remains effective for about five years, repelling any invasions of the *Corynebacterium diphtheriae*. Three injections are necessary to secure an adequate production of antitoxin.

In children, booster doses are given five years later, and often repeated after another five years. A small number of children and adults may show an allergic reaction to the horse serum in the vaccine at the first injection and further injections are not given.

To test whether or not a person is immune to diphtheria a Schick Test is made before vaccination. The Test Toxin is injected into the skin of the forearm: if a red flush appears at the injection site the person is susceptible to the disease and should be vaccinated. Schick Tests are made on children over the age of eight; younger children should all be immunized.

To prevent an unnecessary number of injections in young children, mixed vaccines are sometimes preferred for immunizing. Diphtheria and Pertussis Vaccine; Diphtheria and Tetanus Vaccine.

ANTIBIOTICS. Benzylpenicillin assists antitoxin treatment because it helps to kill the diphtheria micro-organisms and will also eliminate other organisms lurking in the nose and throat which might give rise to secondary diseases such as tonsillitis. Erythromycin has been used when the patient cannot be given penicillin.

CARRIERS of diphtheria infection must be isolated and any septic focus of the mouth or throat treated. Sulphonamides and penicillin are used for this purpose.

Dysentery, Bacillary

Dysentery is associated with diarrhea and the passage of mucus and blood. It can be caused in varied ways, but the term is generally used for two bowel infections: bacillary dysentery and amebic dysentery, which are caused by two entirely different organisms. Amebic dysentery is dealt with in Intestinal Parasites, p. 385.

Bacillary dysentery is a very infectious disease caused by *Shigella* organisms (*Sonne*, *Shiga* and *Flexner*) which occur in impure water, contaminated food and excreta, and are often conveyed by flies or by 'carriers.' It can also be spread by personal contact. The incubation period may be only a few hours, and is seldom more than seven days. The disease is prevalent where unsanitary conditions occur, and epidemics are common especially in the tropics.

Symptoms. The disease develops suddenly with loss of appetite, lassitude, fever, shivering, colicky pain, and a quick pulse. These are followed by contraction pains in the bowels, and a constant desire to evacuate, and prostration. In general the stools are small and slimy, composed of mucus mixed with blood. Defecation is attended and followed by severe contractions and inclination to strain, which is know as tenesmus; in the early stages they are sometimes attended by nausea and vomiting. The natural feces are passed in the first few evacuations. Tenesmus continues and perhaps increases for several days, the discharges being mostly blood in some cases, and chiefly mucus in others. Having generally but little odor at first, these discharges become, as the disease advances, exceedingly offensive. Vomiting is common, and there may be a high or low temperature, with headache. The disease may be severe or moderate in its course. In severe cases there are thirst, muscular pains, blueness of the face, extreme tenderness of the abdomen, hiccup, prostration, incontinence and a high mortality rate. In mild cases the symptoms abate after four or five days.

Treatment. The patient must be isolated in bed, and a bedpan used to prevent contamination of lavatory seats. Warmth is essential. Bland fluids should be given at frequent intervals for the first two days. Light non-stimulating and low-residue diet may then be given. Milk foods, buttermilk, egg custard, weak tea, toast, biscuits or jellies are suitable. Foods should have a high content of proteins and vitamins. In severe cases give chicken broth and milk. Alcohol should not be given. Small quantities of boiled water may be given every ¼ to ½ hour. Intravenous saline injections are given to prevent salt depletion. Two pints of urine should be passed daily.

In more severe cases the patient should not be allowed to sit up; a bedpan must be used. The patient must be kept warm and allowed a very light diet, such as cornstarch (well boiled), rice water, etc., or grated raw apple and weak tea, with plenty of water or other bland fluids.

DRUGS. In mild cases sodium sulphate, one teaspoonful daily for 5 days, often reduces the tenesmus and purging. In other cases morphine may be given for relief.

Sulphonamides of the less soluble type, such as phthalylsulphathiazole, give satisfactory results since they produce little crystalluria and other reactions in the dehydrated patients. Even better results are now obtained with the tetracycline antibiotics. In patients infected with *Shigella* organisms which have become resistant to sulphonamides, it is usually better to give combined treatment using two or more antibiotics. The choice of antibiotic will depend upon the results of sensitivity tests of the infecting *Shigella*.

Dysentery Antiserum (Shiga) is useful against the *Shiga* form of infection but is valueless for the others. It is now only used as an adjunct to antibiotic or sulphonamide treatment.

Convalescence. After severe attacks convalescence is slow. The diet must be very light, easy of digestion, and nutritious. Various complications such as arthritis, iritis, boils, piles, and neuritis may develop, and must be treated appropriately.

Oxytetracycline should also be given to all 'carriers' of bacillary dysentery until stool cultures give negative results in tests for bacteria.

Erysipelas

This acute infection of the skin and its underlying tissues is highly contagious; it follows scratches, abrasions or wounds, by the penetration of streptococci into the deeper layers of the skin. Infection is favored by debilitated states. The disease is often recurrent; a chronic 'erysipeloid' form also occurs.

The eruption most often occurs on the face, and is preceded by malaise, headache, fever, dry tongue, and vomiting; the affected area is of a bright red color, with a shiny surface, and usually starts with a single patch with definite raised edges and irregular outline, which spreads rapidly. There is much swelling, and vesicles may appear; if the outbreak is on the face the disease may spread into the mouth, and the glands of the neck become enlarged. The rash lasts from about three or four days to a fortnight or longer, and then abates, unless the infection extends into underlying structures, causing cellulitis. There is no suppuration in the skin eruption, and the disease is seldom fatal except in infants, debilitated persons, diabetics, or old people.

Treatment. The patient should be isolated and kept in bed. A light and fluid diet is required for the first couple of days.

Penicillin generally produces a rapid cure so that local treatment of the skin is not now necessary. The temperature is usually down to normal within 48 hours of taking the first dose of the penicillin, but it is advisable to continue treatment for a week since recurrences may develop in some stubborn cases. Sulphadimidine is often used for those who are sensitive to penicillin.

Glanders

Glanders is an uncommon disease caused by *Pfeifferella mallei* which occasionally affects persons working with horses. The incubation period is from one to five days. The disease may be acute or chronic. In acute glanders there is an eruption of papules on the face as well as in the nose, which soon become pustular, with fever and malaise; later, ulcerating nodules develop in the nose and cause a foul discharge. The disease is sometimes mistaken for smallpox. Abscesses are formed in the lymph glands and skin and the patient collapses with high fever and often bronchopneumonia. Death follows within ten days in a high proportion of cases.

ACUTE FARCY is a form of glanders which begins on the skin. An inflamed patch develops, followed by nodules beneath the skin (farcy buds) which quickly ulcerate. The patient becomes very ill and the sequence follows that of acute glanders.

Treatment. In acute cases sulphadiazine has been tried, with erratic success. In the chronic cases, which may persist for years, the abscesses are incised and eased with antiseptic dressings.

Leprosy

This is an infective disease due to *Mycobacterium leprae.* It runs a very chronic course and occurs in two main forms. In lepromatous nodular leprosy there are bouts of fever, with nodules in the skin and mucous membranes. In tuberculoid leprosy there are at first areas of redness over the body, with a macular rash, malaise, chills and vague pains, and later areas of numbness develop, with insensibility to touch, heat and cold, and pain. In later cases of both types ulceration is common, and in tuberculoid leprosy there may be loss of fingers and toes or other parts from gangrene. In lepromatous leprosy the mucous membrane of the nose and mouth is involved, with loss of speech, and ulceration and scarring of the lips and tongue. The skin becomes dry like parchment, and the general expression is grave and heavy. The disease is very chronic.

Leprosy is transmitted from man to man through prolonged personal contact. It is not hereditary.

Without treatment there may be remissions or arrest of symptoms, but more commonly death occurs from tuberculosis, exhaustion, or renal failure after twenty years or more.

With treatment by the sulphone drugs, the outlook for leprous patients has changed from one of hopeless misery to one of steady but sure struggle against the bacteria.

Treatment consists in sanitary conditions, scrupulous cleanliness, nourishing diet, and medicinal treatment by the sulphone drugs, dapsone (DDS) and solapsone, by mouth and sometimes by injection. Iron and vitamin B should be given when patients are being given sulphone drugs. Treatment must be continuous over long periods, and permanent cures have been effected after five years in patients with tuberculoid leprosy.

Ditophal ointment has been used with some success. When it is rubbed on the skin it releases in the body a volatile substance which is lethal to the *Mycobacterium.* It is best used in conjunction with dapsone therapy and in courses of three months.

Physiotherapy and graduated exercises are of great help in keeping patients in better general health. Surgical treatment of various kinds may be necessary for amputation, eye operations, etc.

Plague
(*Bubonic Plague*)

Plague is also known as pest, and malignant adenitis, the characteristic features of the disease being fever with general swelling of the glands throughout the body. The infecting micro-organism is the *Pasteurella pestis.*

History. The disease has been known since time immemorial and has ravaged Europe during earlier and less hygienic centuries. The Great Plague of London in 1664–5 killed some 70,000 of the city's population of 480,000. Today it is more prevalent in India, China, Africa, and South America. It occurs in epidemics which are rendered more likely by the insanitary conditions still prevailing in tropical countries.

Plague is primarily a disease of rats and other rodents and it is carried by rat fleas to man. The fleas on rats dying of plague transfer to other warm-blooded animals such as cats and dogs, and so the infection reaches the human host. Small outbreaks originating in camels have occurred as recently as 1953 and 1957 in Central Asia. Camel fleas were the carriers of the infection.

When a case of the disease appears in any locality its extension sometimes takes place very slowly. If not completely eradicated at once, later on a few isolated cases will be discovered, and after a period of one or more years the disease then spreads with alarming rapidity, usually among the poorer classes and later becoming epidemic with all classes.

Symptoms. There are several varieties of the plague; the most common one is known as bubonic plague; the septicemic plague (which is a type of blood poisoning) is, if possible, more severe than when the glands alone are affected. The third type recognized is the so-called pneumonic type in which the lungs seem to be affected more seriously than the rest of the body and death usually results. A fourth type known as pestis minor occurs, where either the resistance by the patient is very great, or in the conveyance of the organism its virulence has been attenuated so that the disease is simply strongly suspected.

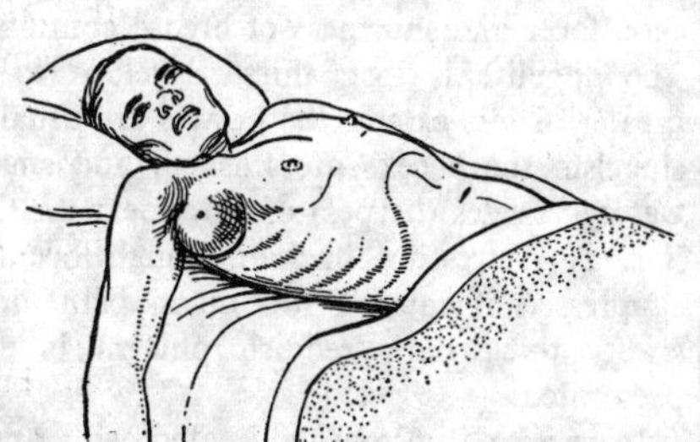

Fig. 14. *A CASE OF PLAGUE. A characteristic feature of the disease is the swelling of the glands of the armpits and groins.*

The onset is sudden, the disease usually developing within 2 to 8 days after exposure to contagion. Dizziness, profound muscular weakness, fever, malaise and pallor are accompanied by headache and backache, nausea, vomiting and diarrhea. Nose-bleeding often occurs. The fever rapidly becomes very high, even reaching 107° F. At this stage the disease resembles severe typhus fever. Within two or three days swellings, or buboes, appear throughout the body, affecting the glands of the groin in the majority of cases, those in the axilla or armpit in about half the cases, and those in the neck in relatively few; the swellings or inflamed glands reach a size from a pigeon's egg to that of a lemon. They are extremely tender and often suppurate. If recovery is to take place, the height of the disease is reached within about a week or so. The pneumonic and septicemic types are always fatal within a few days unless treated with sulphonamides, streptomycin, or tetracyclines.

Treatment. The advent of the sulphonamide drugs and then the antibiotics has greatly changed the prognosis for plague sufferers. Formerly, treatment consisted in careful nursing of the fever, compresses for the buboes, ice applications to the head, and the early administration of anti-plague serum for the bubonic form of the disease. Sulphadiazine has been used with great success if given intensively. Even greater success is obtained with the antibiotic streptomycin since it has a strong bacteriostatic action on *Pasteurella pestis.* Usually both streptomycin and a sulphonamide are employed. For patients with the pneumonic form of the disease who are slow in responding to the combined treatment, either chlortetracycline or chloramphenicol may be given in addition.

IMMUNIZATION against the disease is not required by any country for persons entering it but it is advisable to be vaccinated if one is planning to stay in the interior of one of the countries where plague is endemic. Two inoculations are usually given and, because the protection only lasts about six months, it is best to have booster doses every four to six months.

General Prevention. Since rats are such a widespread pest, prevention of plague begins with rat extermination and the protection of food and grain stores against the invasion of these rodents. To prevent rats from climbing into or out of ships special precautions are required to be taken by the ship owners and master. For control of the fleas there are now many efficient insecticides available.

The Pneumonias

The name pneumonia is given to various types of lung inflammation. Until recently these were classified according to the part of the lung affected, i.e. lobar pneumonia in which the micro-organisms invade deep into the lobes of the lung, and bronchopneumonia in which the upper lungs are patchily infected. With recent increased knowledge of how bacteria, cocci and viruses behave, the grouping of pneumonias is made according to the type of micro-organism which causes the inflammation.

Specific pneumonias are caused by specifically known organisms, each giving rise to a typical form of infection. They may be due to bacteria or viruses. The most common infecting organism is the *Pneumococcus* which is the chief cause of lobar pneumonia. Others are the staphylococci, tuberculosis bacteria, and certain streptococci. The virus infections include those of influenza, psittacosis, typhus fever and others as yet unidentified.

Pneumonias: virus and rickettsial; see p. 285.

Aspiration pneumonias are caused by the extension into the lungs of a mouth or throat infection, giving rise to bronchopneumonia, or by inhaling blood, vomit or septic material from infected teeth, tonsils or sinuses, particularly after operations in those areas. The micro-organisms involved are those commonly found in the upper respiratory tract or mouth, and they are usually of lower virulence. In bedridden or elderly patients the inability to cough up mucus and fluid often leads to hypostatic pneumonia.

Pneumococcal Pneumonia

(*Lobar Pneumonia*)

This acute lung inflammation is commonly due to infection by *Streptococcus pneumoniae,* commonly known as the *Pneumococcus,* of which there are several strains with differing virulence. It is therefore now known as pneumococcal pneumonia.

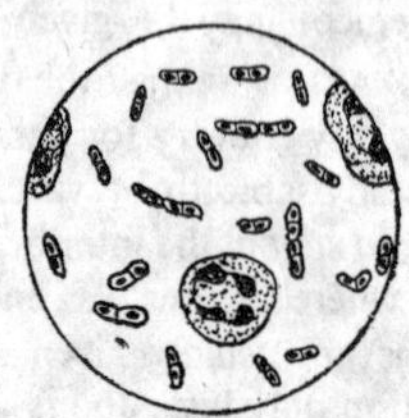

Fig. 15. *STREPTOCOCCUS PNEUMONIAE, or PNEUMOCOCCUS, with white corpuscles from the sputum of a patient with lobar pneumonia.*

If the disease runs it full course it goes through three stages which form the classical picture of all types of pneumonia.

First Stage. This stage of congestion often lasts about 36 hours. The lung tissue is engorged with blood and some of the blood escapes into the air cells. Tapping upon the chest (percussion) gives out a duller or less hollow sound than usual. On applying a stethoscope to the congested area a minute crackling sound is heard, as the air passes in and out during breathing. It is caused by small bubbles of air being forced along the small tubes and it is heard only while the breath is being drawn in.

Second Stage. If the inflammation progresses to the second stage of consolidation no air entry occurs in the affected part, and it becomes solid and useless for the purpose of breathing. In general appearance it resembles a piece of liver; hence it is called the stage of red hepatization. This stage continues for a few days.

With increased solidity there is increased dullness on percussion. The general symptoms increase in severity. When consolidation is extensive there is great difficulty of breathing and the phlegm is more gluey; delirium may occur, and the patient grows weaker.

Third Stage. During this period the lung changes from red hepatization or red softening to gray hepatization or gray softening, and the exudate contains more leucocytes and fewer red corpuscles. The percussion sounds are much the same as in the second stage. The sputum raised is thinner and more liquid, generally streaked with red, or 'rusty;' when it looks like prune-juice, the outlook is unfavorable. The third stage is the stage of resolution during which, in favorable cases, the lungs are gradually cleared of the consolidated blood by absorption. In less favorable cases there is collapse from heart failure or other complications.

Degree of Involvement. Most commonly only one lung is affected, that is in about 80 per cent of cases, and generally the right lung is the region involved. The unaffected lung is usually also somewhat congested. The pleura or membrane covering the lungs is also inflamed (pleurisy is present) if the congestion extends to the lung surface.

Symptoms. Some cases of pneumonia follow a so-called cold or influenza, which may have been present for two or three weeks. In others the onset is sudden, the first symptom being a chill or rigor, mild or severe, which has no influence upon the severity of the disease that is to follow. The temperature rises, and there is so-called pleuritic pain over some portion of either lung, often over the nipple of the side affected, or it may develop in the lower chest or even in the back or abdomen. Shortness of breath then develops, caused by the pain when a deep inhalation is attempted, and although the pain in the chest may diminish, which is frequently the case, fever and shortness of breath continue. The appetite is lost, thirst develops to a greater or less extent, the bowels are usually sluggish, the cheeks are flushed, and small watery vesicles (herpes) often appear on the lips. A distressing hacking cough occurs, suppressed if causing too much pain, and scanty thick dark reddish phlegm is expectorated.

In cases not promptly treated with antibiotics or sulphonamides these symptoms continue, varying in severity according to the gravity of the case. About the fourth day a *false crisis* may occur, the temperature falling somewhat, but rising again until the sixth or seventh day, when it may fall suddenly within six to twelve hours, this being the true *crisis.* If the fall in temperature is extended over thirty-six hours the fall is said to be by *lysis* (see p. 264). Profuse sweating often precedes the crisis, and the patient falls asleep. On waking the breathing is easier and the general condition improved.

During the course of the disease the pulse progressively increases, and varies from about 100 to 130 per minute. A pulse rate of over 140 is a poor omen. The patient is often delirious, and may pass into a sinking state.

Complications may set in when treatment is delayed and often cause a fatal ending. They include heart failure (indicated by very rapid pulse and blueness of the face or lips), pleurisy, empyema, pericarditis, endocarditis, meningitis, and septicemic conditions such as pulmonary abscess or gangrene, abscess of the middle ear, arthritis, jaundice, peritonitis, and rarely phlebitis. Pneumonia is especially serious in children, or in old or feeble persons.

Treatment. Since the pneumococcus is susceptible to the penicillins, the tetracyclines, chloramphenicol and the sulphonamides, the doctor's choice of treatment will depend upon his patient's individual needs. For those over fifty years of age and for those with severe illness, penicillin should be given intramuscularly. This should reduce the temperature and improve the clinical condition within twenty-four hours, although the treatment should be continued until all symptoms have disappeared and then for a further four days. In patients not responsive to penicillin, ampicillin or tetracycline may be prescribed.

General Treatment. The room must be well ventilated, but moderately warmed at about 18° C (65° F). Hot-water bottles may be placed in the bed to warm the feet. The diet should consist of bland fluids (water, lemonade, glucose, bouillon, custard, chicken broth, beaten-up eggs, etc.), and milk (3 pints a day), given every 2 to 3 hours, with eggs, or light cereal foods. The bowels should be attended to. Tepid sponging is advised daily. The patient should rest in an inclined position; elderly patients should have the position changed frequently to prevent accumulation of secretions in the lower lungs. Coughing up sputum regularly should be encouraged; hot drinks may assist the coughing.

For insomnia, the barbiturates or chloral hydrate may be given and for older patients two tablespoonfuls of brandy or whiskey diluted with water is often helpful.

Good nursing is most important and for chronic bronchitics or the elderly it is often better for them to be treated in hospital.

In delirium (temperature above 39° C) the patient must be carefully watched; icebags should be applied to the forehead, and tepid sponging of the body started. It may be necessary to administer paraldehyde. Oxygen administered by means of an oro-nasal mask or an oxygen tent often gives considerable relief if the patient has much difficulty in breathing, and reduces the strain on the heart.

Convalescence is generally fairly rapid, although some heart weakness may persist for some time. Deep-breathing exercises should be started as soon as the temperature has fallen to normal to promote full expansion of the lung. This is most important in children. The patient should be allowed to get up for increasing periods when the fever has gone. He is usually fit to return to work in three weeks although in old and weak persons a convalescence of two months may be needed.

Bronchopneumonia

This is the more usual form of the group of aspiration pneumonias. The inflammation results from an extension of infection from the upper respiratory tract into the small air sacs (alveoli) of the lesser bronchi.

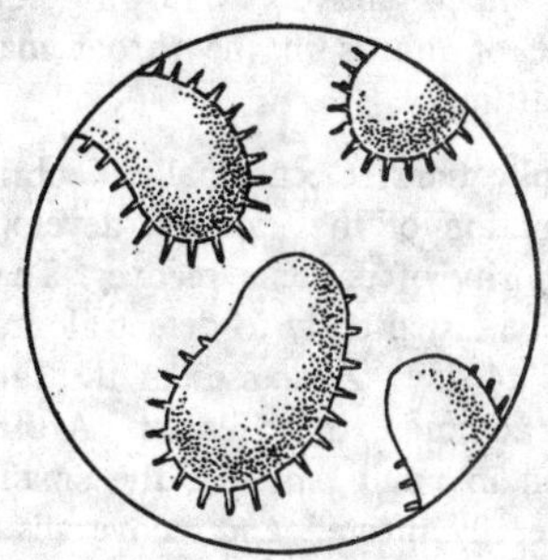

Fig. 16. *KLEBSIELLA PNEUMONIAE. One of the many micro-organisms which cause pneumonia in man.*

Diffuse aspiration bronchopneumonia is sometimes known as lobular pneumonia and is a distinct disease from pneumococcal (lobar) pneumonia. It is the ordinary type of pneumonia of children, and is commonly seen in young children especially under the age of three years. It may be primary, but is often secondary to measles, diphtheria, whooping-cough and so forth. It is especially liable to occur in debilitated or rickety infants.

In adults this type of pneumonia is often an extension of a severe bout of influenza and it is commonly found in chronic bronchitics and in elderly persons. Sometimes it is a sequel to operations which have necessitated the patient's lying in bed; the infection spreads because the lungs are inadequately ventilated. It is a more serious illness than pneumococcal pneumonia.

Symptoms. In the very young the only symptoms are fever, prostration and rapid breathing and may resemble those of acute bronchitis. There may be no cough and no physical signs, but if the disease is neglected it is often fatal within a few hours or days. The patient is often blue and restless, and in unfavorable cases passes into coma.

There is a great difference in the early stages of the disease in different cases, the severer cases being ushered in by one or more convulsions, by rapid rise of temperature, vomiting, difficulty in breathing, and delirium; milder cases begin with lower temperature, less malaise, moderate prostration and shortness of breath.

The height of the temperature is, as a rule, in proportion to the severity of the disease. Cases with temperatures of over 40·5° C (105° F) are usually fatal. The pulse reaches 150 per minute in adults, and even higher in children—so high, in fact, that it cannot be taken; the respiration rate varies from 40 to 80. Sleeplessness, restlessness and even delirium are often present. The face is flushed, the tongue coated, and diarrhea and vomiting commonly occur. Pallor is a grave sign. Cough is usually present but may be feeble, and in young patients the sputum is swallowed. The urine is often albuminous and contains casts. Between the second and fifth days signs of consolidation and pleurisy appear, namely dullness on percussion, bronchial breathing and bronchophony with crepitant rattles. The lips may be cyanosed in serious cases.

The duration of the disease at all ages varies. In the great majority of cases which recover the course varies from one to three weeks, although many persist for six weeks. The softening and absorption which occurs in all pneumonia cases that recover occupy a much longer period in bronchopneumonia than in pneumococcal pneumonia.

Many cases of bronchopneumonia are complicated by cerebral symptoms of convulsions, delirium, stupor, vomiting, etc., even before any marked lesions develop in the lungs; as these subside the signs of lung involvement appear. Many cases are protracted for a long time, and although they may terminate favorably at last, they are apt to develop chronic hardening (fibrosis) of the lung which lasts for years; or there is recovery with permanent consolidation of the lung.

Treatment by penicillin and other antibiotics has greatly reduced the mortality and complications. But antibiotics alone will not work a miracle. It is most important that vigorous measures be taken to get the lungs cleared of foul sputum. Patients must cough it up and do so regularly. Postural drainage (p. 346), if the patient is not too debilitated, is most important.

In emergencies which may occur at any time during the course of the disease and must be watched for especially at the crisis of the disease, oxygen should be given by mask or tent for periods long enough to relieve the cyanosis and the labored breathing. If emphysema has developed the oxygen must be administered at a low flow-rate since in such cases there is a danger of carbon dioxide narcosis. In severe cases where the patient has become too exhausted to expectorate it may be necessary to perform a tracheostomy and remove the sputum by suction through the inserted tube.

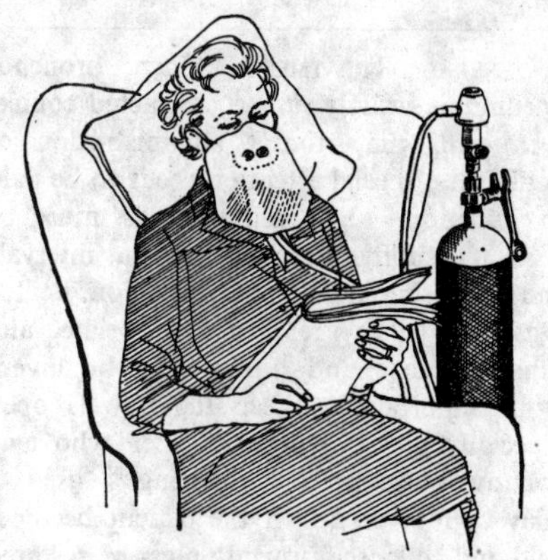

Fig. 17. *A LIGHTWEIGHT OXYGEN BREATHING SET FOR HOME USE. For sufferers from bronchitis, tuberculosis, or pneumoconiosis.*

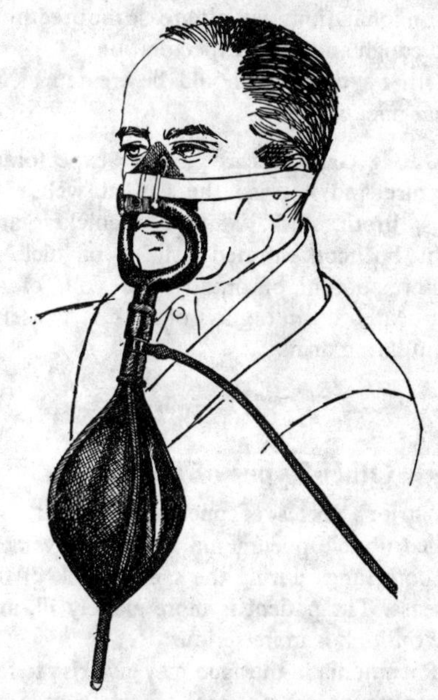

Fig. 18. *NASAL INHALER FOR OXYGEN ADMINISTRATION TO FULLY CONSCIOUS PATIENTS.*

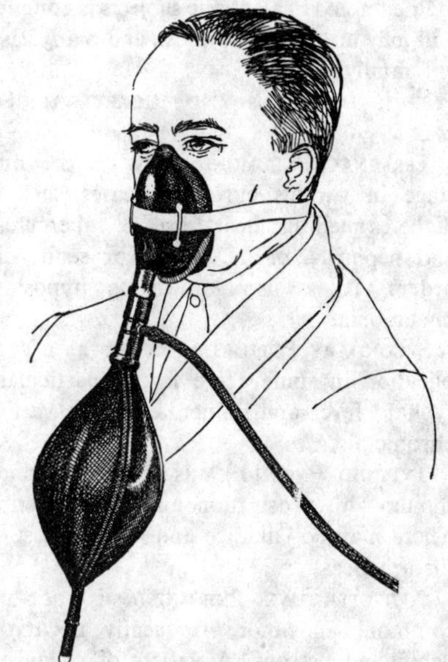

Fig. 19. *MOUTH-NOSE INHALER FOR OXYGEN ADMINISTRATION WHERE NASAL PASSAGES ARE IMPAIRED.*

Courtesy Oxygenaire London Limited

General Treatment. Since broncho-pneumonia usually runs a protracted course, even with the prompt administration of antibiotics, special attention needs to be paid to nutrition. Light milky foods must be given plentifully at regular frequent intervals and water should be given in addition. Beaten eggs and jellies are also appropriate, and sugar, glucose and honey may be given. It is important to keep the bowels open especially in very young children who may swallow sputum. Cool sponging is used to allay high fever but, if the patient becomes cold and collapsed, warmth must be restored by hot water bottles between blankets, not directly on the patient. A vaporizer in the room or the old-fashioned bed-tent with steam inhalations will often ease the breathing and cough and assist expectoration.

Other symptoms should be treated as in lobar pneumonia.

During convalescence give an expectorant mixture and nourish the patient well with eggs, broth, milk, white fish, chicken, and light but concentrated articles of diet. A dessertspoonful of brandy and yolk of an egg beaten up in a glass of milk is a useful stimulating drink.

Other Types of Pneumonia

Various forms of pneumonia occur. So-called double pneumonia is the involvement of both lungs during the same attack of the disease. The patient is more gravely ill, and the outlook is more serious.

Pneumonia in the aged may give rise to few acute symptoms or signs, apart from prostration, but in such cases the mortality is high.

Pneumonia in alcoholic subjects is common and may also be non-typical, and many cases end fatally.

Pneumonia: Virus and Rickettsial. See p. 285.

Terminal Pneumonia may be the final stage in various chronic diseases such as diabetes mellitus, heart disease, tuberculosis and nephritis, or in wasting or senile disorders. It is also known as hypostatic pneumonia.

Secondary Pneumonia occurs as a complication in some acute fevers, particularly typhoid fever and influenza, and in various chronic diseases.

Typhoid Pneumonia is a form of pneumonia with prostration and little reaction. There may be jaundice and gastro-intestinal disturbances.

Post-operative Pneumonia is not uncommon, and more frequently occurs in debilitated persons. A variety of organisms may cause the infection but the most common in these cases is the staphylococcus. The illness runs a course similar to broncho-pneumonia, and antibiotic treatment should be given at the onset.

Scarlet Fever

(*Scarlatina*)

This is an acute illness due to infection by streptococcal bacteria, with sore throat, a generalized rash that causes peeling of the skin, and fever. Inflammation of the middle ear and kidneys are common complications. Epidemics vary considerably in their virulence. In many parts of the world today, scarlet fever is a mild disease although at the beginning of the century it was one of the most serious infectious diseases known. Infection is conveyed by direct contact through 'droplet infection' from patients, by infected articles, by 'carriers' and more rarely by milk or ice-cream.

Symptoms. The incubation period is from one to six days. The fever usually develops between the third and fourth day after exposure. On the second day of the disease the eruption appears in the form of very small points and pimples of a bright scarlet color, either in patches or causing a general redness, and developing at first behind the ears, then on the chest, neck and shoulders, and later spreading to the trunk and limbs. It is most intense in the flexures of the arms and legs.

The disease begins suddenly with sore inflamed throat, vomiting, languor, pains in the head, back and limbs, and with drowsiness, nausea and chills or rigors; these are followed by heat and thirst. In children convulsions and abdominal pain may occur. When the redness of the skin appears the pulse is very quick and the patient is anxious, restless and sometimes delirious. The eyes are red, the face is flushed though the mouth is pale, the tongue is covered in the middle with white mucus, and is studded with elevated points of extreme redness resembling an unripe strawberry. The tonsils are swollen and the throat is red, with swelling and tenderness of the glands of the neck.

The greatest intensity of the rash is often reached on the evening of the third or fourth day from its beginning; it is of a vivid scarlet color with small red scattered spots. Then the disease begins to decline, the temperature falls gradually by lysis, with itching of the skin which is shed in branny scales (desquamation). Peeling usually takes about four weeks, although it may take longer. In some cases there is a total absence of rash; the child feels well and runs about, and only subsequent peeling of the skin suggests that he has had an attack of scarlet fever. Such cases are dangerous carriers of infection, and may cause school epidemics.

Tongue and Throat. In the first stage of the complaint the tongue, as stated above, is covered with fur, but as it advances the fur peels off leaving a glossy fiery-red surface, *strawberry tongue* which, with the entire mucous membrane of the mouth, is sore and tender.

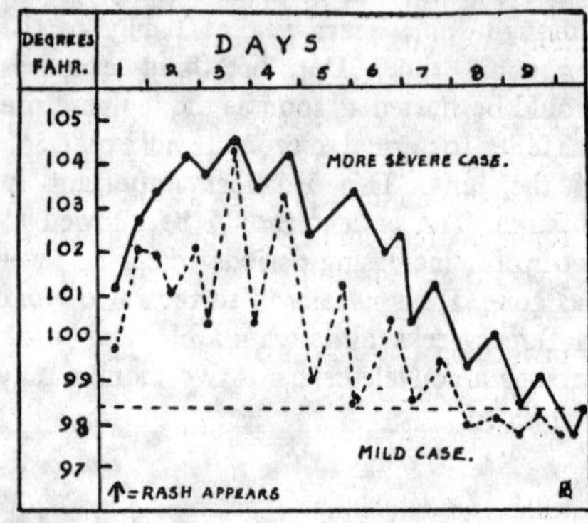

Fig. 20. *TEMPERATURE CHART IN SCARLET FEVER. The temperature has fallen by lysis in both the mild and the more severe case.*

On pressing down the tongue the pharynx is seen to be swollen and of deep red color. On the tonsils may be seen white or gray ulcers, which make swallowing difficult. Increase of mucus in the throat may also cause rattling.

Complications. Occasionally nephritis, or inflammation of the kidneys, develops, but the majority of patients recover. The urine should be tested daily to detect albumen for at least 24 days. Abscesses of the ears used to be common in children. Arthritis is common in adult patients; the small joints are generally affected, and recovery is usually satisfactory. Glandular swelling in the neck is common and occasionally proceeds to suppuration or sloughing. Heart failure occasionally occurs during convalescence; it is very sudden and death may occur without any warning signs. Bronchitis is common among children, and bronchopneumonia is generally present in cases that end fatally.

Scarlet fever somewhat resembles measles in the early stage, but may be distinguished from it by the absence of cough; by the eruption being finer and of a more scarlet color (see p. 284); by the rash developing on the second day instead of the fourth; and by the ulceration in the throat, and the characteristic appearance of strawberry tongue.

In adult persons the appearance of a scarlet rash due to sensitization to an antibiotic or sulphonamide may at first be mistaken for scarlet fever, especially as fever sometimes occurs too. A careful investigation of the patient's medical history should reveal the sensitization. A throat swab may also be helpful in identifying the offending streptococci.

In very severe or septic cases the patient sinks rapidly; typhoid symptoms show themselves, with great prostration, diarrhea and delirium. The skin changes to a purple or mahogany color, or the eruption may be absent altogether. The tongue is deep red or has dark brown fur, and the ulcers in the throat become putrid. This is called the malignant form of scarlet fever, and is a severer form of the same disease, with a high mortality rate.

Treatment. For mild cases, penicillin 200,000 units by mouth every 4 hours for six to seven days usually clears the infection. In more severe cases injections of benzathine penicillin are required for about two weeks.

Passive immunization by scarlet fever antitoxin confers immunity for about fourteen days, but penicillin is more effective. Such prophylaxis is only used for schools or institutions.

Child contacts should be kept from school for one week and a quarantine period of one week is essential for adult contacts handling milk, foodstuffs, or working with children. Such adults should be given full therapeutic doses of penicillin.

GENERAL TREATMENT. In ordinary cases when the disease develops, the patient must be isolated and kept in bed; the room should be kept cool and well ventilated, and the bed-covering should be light. The whole body should be sponged with tepid solution of soda bicarbonate (1 teaspoonful to 2 pints) daily, and the patient be given cooling drinks. The hair should be cut short. The throat should be sprayed or painted with weak antiseptics, or the tonsils may be swabbed with dilute hydrogen peroxide, and ice may be given to suck. Should the bowels be constipated they may be opened by some mild laxative.

No solid food should be allowed during the acute stages of fever; milk, fluids and other milk foods should be given. Lemonade in a tumbler filled with water, and sweetened, may be given to a child in teaspoonful doses and is a good remedy. When the temperature is normal, boiled fish, cereals and semi-solids are allowed. Meat should not be given in cases of nephritis.

Aspirin will relieve headache.

In uncomplicated cases the patient may be allowed up in 7 days but isolated from general contact for four weeks from onset.

TREATMENT OF COMPLICATIONS. Nephritis, a kidney disease, is one of the most serious complications of scarlet fever. If nephritis develops, give a warm bath twice a week, and encourage perspiration by covering the patient with hot blankets, and giving drinks of hot tea or lemonade. A milk and cereal diet only is permitted until the urine is normal when tested for albumen.

The severe effects of nephritis (see p. 409) are greatly mitigated by the treatment of the main fever with penicillin.

Malignant scarlet fever must be nursed in hospital.

Septicemia, Pyemia and Toxemia

These conditions are due to infection, giving rise to constitutional symptoms. There may be localized inflammation in some part of the body, with or without suppuration.

SEPTICEMIA. In septicemia living bacteria gain entry into the circulating blood and often cause the grave symptoms associated with blood poisoning. The site of entry of the infecting germs is often not obvious, but severe symptoms commonly develop within a short time, often about twelve hours. Small hemorrhagic patches may be seen in the skin. The patient has rigors and sweats profusely. The temperature rises but may be swinging; the appetite is lost, the bowels are inactive, and the patient soon wastes and becomes prostrated, and may be delirious in severe cases. The face becomes ashy, the skin cold, breathing is labored, and coma supervenes. Vomiting and diarrhea are grave signs. The disease may occur as a terminal event in other acute infections.

PYEMIA. In pyemia numerous abscesses are formed throughout the body, the bacteria being deposited in the various tissues after some primary infection. In pyemia there is generally some obvious center of suppuration, or pus, with secondary abscesses forming in other parts of the body. The general symptoms are similar to those of septicemia but, if abscesses develop in vital organs, such as the liver, brain, lungs and so forth, these also cause further evidence of disease.

TOXEMIA. In toxemia bacteria are localized in some area but their toxins or poisons are carried around in the blood and give rise to various disturbances and symptoms, such as occur in specific fevers, e.g. diphtheria.

Treatment. Supportive measures are essential. The patient should be given plenty of fluids by mouth. Any obvious source of infection must be treated by prompt surgical methods as may be required, to provide drainage of pus or infected fluid. Blood cultures or cultures of pus should be examined to identify the infecting germ, and the corresponding antitoxin or antiserum may then be used.

The antibiotics have come to the fore in the treatment of septicemia and have proved of immense value in arresting or relieving grave symptoms of these conditions. If the infection has become penicillin-resistant, tetracycline or erythromycin should be prescribed by the doctor.

Tetanus

(Lock-jaw)

This is an infective disease with spasmodic contractions, and rigidity or stiffness of the voluntary muscles caused by *Clostridium tetani*. Sometimes this rigidity is confined to the jaw and neck, in later stages it involves the whole body. It is due to the toxin of the tetanus micro-organisms, which attacks the nervous system.

The tetanus organisms are present in soil, animal excrement, road dirt, etc., and occasionally in commercial gelatine. They enter the body through an external wound or injury to the skin. The incubation period is very variable, but is commonly from one to two weeks. The condition somewhat resembles strychnine poisoning, but the spasms do not entirely disappear in tetanus, as they do in strychnine convulsions.

Symptoms. General malaise is followed by irritability and then by painful muscular contractions and twitchings. At first there is difficulty and uneasiness in turning the head, with inability to open the mouth easily; then the jaws close gradually, but with great firmness. Swallowing becomes difficult and a pain, starting from the breast-bone, pierces through to the back—probably caused by cramp of the diaphragm. The cramps extend to the muscles of the abdomen, trunk, the limbs, face, tongue, etc., which pass into a state of rigid spasm. At times the abdominal muscles are so tense as to make the abdomen as hard as a board. Sometimes the patient is bent backward so that his head is extended towards the heels (*opisthotonus*); at other times he is drawn forward (*emprosthotonus*). All the contractions are attended with intense pain, which may be so violent that the teeth are sometimes broken, and the tongue is often bitten. The appearance of the sufferer is frightful; the forehead is wrinkled, the eyes half closed, the nostrils dilated, the corners of the mouth drawn back, the set teeth exposed, and all the features fixed in a ghastly grin (*risus sardonicus*). Death may occur from asphyxia and suffocation, due to spasm of the diaphragm and heart failure.

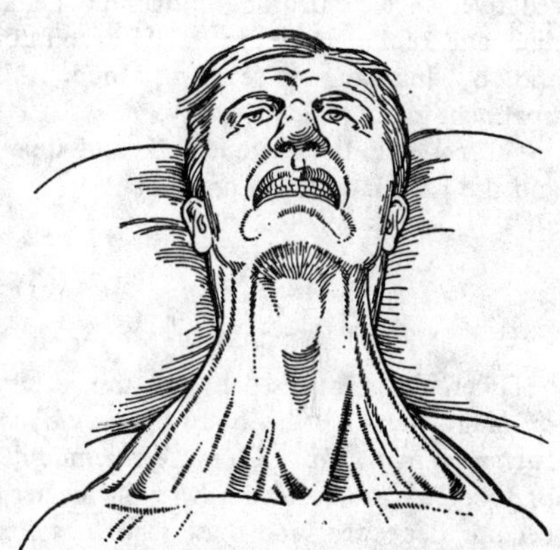

Fig. 21. *RISUS SARDONICUS IN LOCKJAW. The painful spasm and rigid contractions of the jaw and neck in a case of tetanus.*

The prevention of tetanus can be accomplished: (1) by thorough disinfection of all wounds, especially those due to gunpowder accidents and to implements around stables and manure heaps, or to road accidents; (2) by tetanus antitoxin, which should be given as soon as possible after the injury; and (3) by active immunization with tetanus vaccines. The good protection given by immunization is of particular importance to gardeners, demolition workers, soldiers and others who are exposed to constant contact with soil. Three doses are usual, with a booster dose every four to five years.

Prevention is very important because treatment is complex. All children should be given triple vaccine in infancy (see p. 266).

Treatment. Today treatment is concentrated in special centers which have intensive-care units since recovery demands close hospital collaboration of doctors, anethetist, surgeons, nurses, and laboratory tests. This has reduced fatalities from some 75% to nearly 1%.

When a person has incurred a wound which is likely to be infected through soil or dirt, tetanus antitoxin and penicillin should be injected at once after testing for horse serum sensitivity in order to prevent the poison involving the nervous system. The wound should not be closed or allowed to heal before it has been thoroughly cleaned and drained. If disinfectants are not available it is much better to leave the wound exposed to the air, since the growth of the organisms causing the disease is favored by exclusion of air.

If the jaw muscles contract so that food cannot be taken, it may be necessary to feed the patient by means of a small rubber tube passed through the nostril into the stomach, or even by the rectum, but a physician will of course have charge of the case. Ether and chloroform in desperate cases may be administered to ease the struggles of the patient.

In very severe cases the patient is paralyzed with a curare drug to stop the spasms, given sedatives such as pentobarbitone and pethidine, and kept alive by the use of a respirator and by intravenous feeding. Under this treatment many patients survive.

The room must be kept dark and quiet, and the patient watched continually.

Tuberculosis

Tuberculosis is caused by infection of one or many parts of the body by the *Mycobacterium tuberculosis.* Characteristic nodules or tubercles are formed where the bacteria become deposited, and these tend to soften in the center (*caseation*) and become cheesy,' with possibly ulceration in the later stages. If the disease is arrested the original tubercle may become chalky, or calcified, and the spread of the bacteria to other parts is thus hindered. The tubercle bacterium is very resistant to disinfection and destruction, and can survive outside the body in dried particles of infected sputum and in dust for some months. (See. p. 350.)

Causes. There are various types of tuberculosis, namely the *human* variety, *bovine* (in cattle), *avian* (in birds) and *piscine* (in fish). The usual causes of tuberculous infection in man are the inhalation of infected particles of sputum and drinking tuberculous milk, the latter being especially dangerous for young children who have little or no natural immunity to the disease.

Unhygienic environment, overcrowding, poor diet, and bad ventilation are important factors in promoting the risk of infection; inherited susceptibility also occurs in some persons with poor chest development and low vitality. Sometimes tuberculosis develops after some other acute disease, for example, influenza, measles, or typhoid fever, and it may occur in the late stages of chronic diseases such as diabetes mellitus, nephritis, and cirrhosis of the liver. Occupations involving the inhalation of dust or irritating particles increase the liability to tuberculosis of the lungs. Pregnancy may accelerate untreated tuberculosis, relapse occurring after parturition.

The disease may occur at any age, but in children under twelve years of age there is a particular tendency to tuberculous infection of glands, brain, bones and joints. In older persons tuberculosis of the lungs is more commonly seen, and is most common in young adults between 18 and 30 years of age. Improvement in social conditions and diagnosis methods in this country have greatly reduced the mortality rate.

Diagnosis. The diagnosis of tuberculosis must be made by X-ray examination, by identification of the tubercle bacteria in the sputum or other fluids or tissues of the body, by inoculation tests with tuberculin, and other specialized examinations. (For fuller details, see Diseases of the Chest, p. 341.)

Treatment. The treatment of tuberculosis of different parts of the body is dealt with under the various systems or organs which may be involved

The main lines of attack are *preventive*, protective measures being of the highest importance to prevent spread of infection, and *curative* treatment in cases in which the disease is already established. Healthy surroundings, fresh air and sunshine, adequate meals with fresh dairy foods and vegetables, are valuable aids in prevention. Prevention of infection is also promoted by avoidance of contaminated sputum from other tuberculosis sufferers and by the use of tuberculin tested milk. Cure of the established disease consists in improvement in general hygienic conditions with a full and nourishing diet, combined with such specific treatment as is indicated in particular cases. Fuller details are given in Diseases of the Chest, p. 352.

Typhoid Fever

(*Enteric Fever*)

Of the different kinds of fever, this is one of the most widely prevalent. The name typhoid is from two Greek words which mean 'like typhus.' The word typhus, from a Greek word signifying stupor, means stupid, dull or low, and when applied to a fever implies that it is characterized by great debility and depression. Infection is by the *Salmonella typhi* which may occur in water, infected feces or foodstuffs, or may be conveyed by flies. Milk, ice-cream, salads and oysters are foods likely to become infected.

Some persons are typhoid 'carriers,' the micro-organisms being discharged in the feces, and such carriers are sometimes the source of epidemics.

Symptoms. The incubation period is generally about ten to fourteen days. The disease often has precursory symptoms. For several days before its actual acute onset, the patient may attend to his various duties but does not seem well. He is low-spirited and languid, indisposed to any exertion, with pains in the head, back, and extremities. He loses his appetite and his sleep is interrupted and unrefreshing at night. There may be nose-bleeding or bronchitis. In the first five days the temperature rises in steps of two degrees each evening, and falls one degree each morning; at the end of this period it reaches 39·4° to 40° C (103° to 104° F), and remains so until the tenth or the fourteenth day. The disease chiefly attacks the lower part of the small intestine, but may spread into the gall-bladder, lungs, or kidneys and into the bloodstream.

FIRST WEEK. The patient during the first week shows increased heat of the skin surface, and a slower pulse rate than one would expect from the height of the temperature, furred tongue, restlessness and sleeplessness; he has headache and pain in the back, and sometimes diarrhea and swelling of the abdomen with nausea and vomiting. A test known as Widal's test is used to confirm the diagnosis. A low white-cell count is characteristic.

SECOND WEEK. In the second week an eruption of small rose-colored spots often develops upon the chest and abdomen; they fade and disappear on pressure. A crop of little watery pimples appear upon the neck and chest, having the appearance of minute drops of sweat on the skin. The tongue is dry and black, or red and sore, and the gums are foul; there may be delirium and dullness of hearing. The abdomen is distended (meteorism) and the symptoms generally are more serious than during the first week. Diarrhea is common, but is very variable in duration and severity. The stools are like pea-soup, may contain blood, and have a peculiar offensive odor. Occasionally at this stage the bowels are perforated by ulceration, or hemorrhage occurs, and the patient suddenly collapses.

THIRD WEEK. If the disease proceeds unfavorably into the third week, there is low muttering and delirium, great exhaustion, sliding down of the patient towards the foot of the bed, twitching of the muscles, bleeding from the bowels, and red or purple spots upon the skin.

If, on the other hand, recovery takes place, the temperature falls by lysis, the pulse moderates, the delirium is less severe, the tongue is less furred, and the discharges become less foul. The patient is much

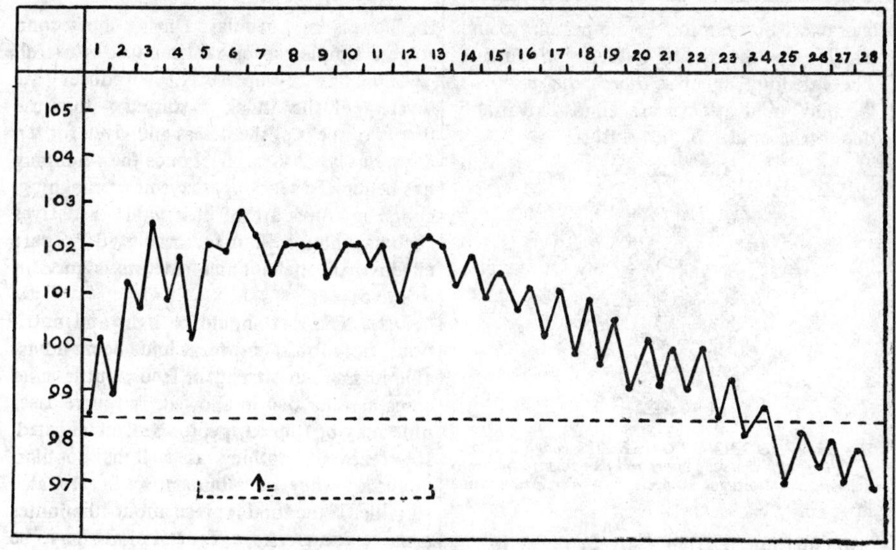

Fig. 22. *TEMPERATURE CHART IN TYPHOID FEVER, showing fall by lysis.*

wasted, the tongue cracked, and he lies in apathy. There may be muttering in a form of coma known as *coma vigil*, in which the eyes remain open.

In patients given antibiotics, particularly chloramphenicol, or in cases which improve spontaneously, convalescence begins about the fourth week; the condition improves rapidly and the appetite returns, although the patient is still very weak, and many weeks may pass before there is complete recovery. No patient should be considered to be non-infective until the stools and urine give negative tests for bacteria.

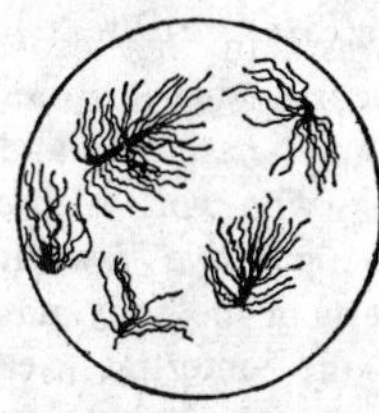

Fig. 23. *SALONELLA TYPHI which cause typhoid fever. Note the flagellae which enable them to 'swim' in water or fluids.*

Treatment. The patient should be isolated and must lie completely recumbent. The sick-room should be large, airy, well-ventilated and without unnecessary furniture. The bed should be where the light may come to it from the side, rather than having the direct rays of light coming over the foot of the bed and shining in the patient's eyes. The temperature of the room should be kept at 18° C (65° F).

DIET. The diet should consist chiefly of milk and enriched milk foods for the first week, two or three pints a day being served at two-hourly intervals. Lemon and glucose drinks may be given freely between feeds. Cornstarch, beaten-up or lightly boiled eggs, jellies, ice-cream, junket and minced chicken may be added as soon as the fever has gone; soon after, the patient should be put on a nutritious diet with at least 70 grams (1½ ounces) of protein daily. No vegetables or other roughage should be given. Severe diarrhea requires modification of the diet.

DRUGS. Special symptoms such as insomnia, bronchitis, persistent headaches, require treatment accordingly. Stimulants are sometimes necessary. For severe diarrhea daily starch and opium enemata, give relief. If constipation occurs the bowels should be opened by a soap enema. Under no circumstances should purgatives be employed.

Chloramphenicol (Chloromycetin) has altered the prognosis of typhoid fever. Treatment is 1 gram by mouth followed by 0.5 grams every 4 hours until fever has settled, and then 6-hourly for one week. Ampicillin is also active against typhoid organisms and is especially effective in the treatment of carriers.

CONVALESCENCE. Relapses are fairly common and the patient should stay in bed for at least fourteen days after the temperature has become normal.

Complications include hemorrhage from the bowels in the second to fourth weeks, perforation of the bowel wall in the third to fifth weeks, heart failure, thrombosis of the veins, abscesses in the bones or other organs, and pneumonia. If hemorrhage occurs food must be withheld (temporarily), and only ice given to suck. Blood transfusion may be necessary. In cases of perforation surgical treatment must be given immediately. Inflammation of the gall-bladder (cholecystitis) is a common sequel, chronic infection causing the patient to become a 'carrier.'

Prevention. Vaccination to prevent typhoid fever infection is carried out successfully and a high degree of immunity follows—about two weeks after the final injection. Immunity lasts for some eighteen months; persons who live or are going into an area where typhoid is common require a booster dose every one or two years. The vaccine should not be given during late pregnancy.

GENERAL MEASURES. Since typhoid is often a water-borne infection, a clean water supply and efficient sewage disposal are of importance in preventing its spread. Control of houseflies and protection of foodstuffs from rats and mice are also necessary. Infection may also easily be spread from the linen of typhoid patients and from the hands of those who care for them, if proper precautions are not taken. During epidemics, milk and water for drinking should be boiled and then cooled.

DISINFECTION. Lime is an efficient disinfectant; it is easily obtained, safe and cheap. By strict sterilization of the hands and wrists of nurses and attendants, danger will be prevented.

Any linen that is soiled by stools or urine should be removed at once, not only for the sake of keeping the patient clean and free from the risk of bedsores, but also to prevent the possibility of the attendants being infected. Linen articles should be soaked for 2 hours in 1 : 20 carbolic lotion and then boiled.

CARRIERS. People who carry the germs of the disease in the intestines or urinary system, and pass infected feces or urine are the so-called typhoid carriers. Such persons, when known, should be strictly isolated until rendered innocuous. Treatment with ampicillin plus probenecid given for three months will often cure the condition. In other cases, a combination of penicillin and sulphathiazole has proved successful. Typhoid carriers must be scrupulously careful in their personal hygiene and habits, and should never work in an occupation requiring handling of food.

Paratyphoid Fever

There are three types of paratyphoid fever with somewhat different geographical distribution. The first one, caused by *Salmonella paratyphi A*, is found in many parts of the world, including Germany and India, but rarely in England. The second variety, due to *S. paratyphi B*, is more common in England, Germany, and America. The symptoms are similar to those of ordinary typhoid fever, although generally less severe, since complications and fatalities are uncommon. Treatment is also on the same lines.

The third type is *S. paratyphi C*. It is rare, and occurs in British Guiana.

The disease can be prevented or modified by previous immunization.

Undulant Fever

(Brucellosis)

The undulating temperature is characteristic of animals or patients infected with the *Brucella* micro-organisms. In Great Britain the form usually encountered is due to drinking raw milk or handling cattle infected with *Br. abortus*. It is more likely to be acquired by veterinary surgeons or cowmen.

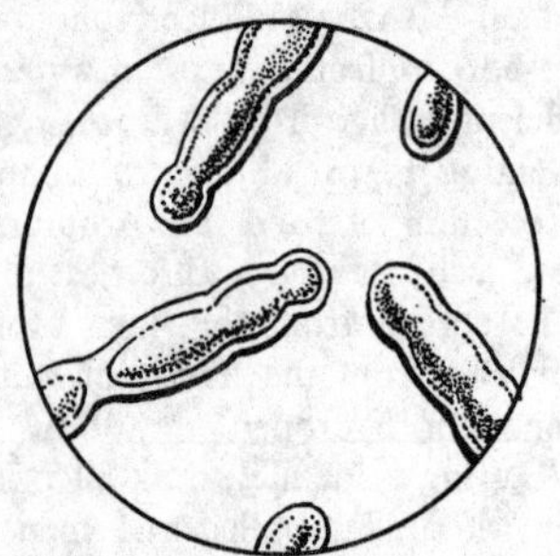

Fig. 24. *BRUCELLA MELITENSIS, the micro-organism which causes the form of undulant fever known as Malta fever.*

Because of the widespread pasteurization of milk, the infection rarely reaches the consumer. In Malta the disease is caused by *Br. melitensis* which infects the milk of goats: hence the name Malta Fever or Mediterranean Fever. In the U.S.A. and other countries, inadequately cooked pork infected with *Br. suis*, or the handling of infected pigs, may spread the infection in man.

The incubation period is about fifteen days and when once the disease is established it may persist for six months or even for years with periods of quietude and renewed fever. The patient becomes weakened and depressed but the mortality is low.

Symptoms. The symptoms are those of general fever with sweating, weakness, headaches, lack of appetite, aching limbs, rigors, and sore throat. The specific feature is that the patient often feels well in the morning but by the afternoon he is sweating profusely and has a temperature of 39·4° C (103° F). Sometimes the spleen is palpable and a rash occurs in about 10 per cent of cases. Malta fever is usually more severe than the other forms of brucellosis. The diagnosis can usually be confirmed by blood culture and agglutination tests.

Treatment. Several antibiotics have been used successfully in controlling the symptoms but once treatment is stopped there is often relapse. For early cases of the disease, 250 milligrams of tetracycline every six hours is usually effective, but for chronic cases a combination of tetracycline, streptomycin and chloramphenicol is indicated for fourteen days.

By boiling or pasteurizing milk for human consumption, undulant fever can largely be prevented since the micro-organism is destroyed by heat.

Whooping-cough

(*Pertussis*)

This is an infectious disease which often occurs in epidemics; it is commoner in childhood, being particularly dangerous to infants under one year of age. It generally occurs only once in the same individual. The characteristic symptom is the peculiar cough which gives the disease its descriptive name. The infecting agent is *Bordetella pertussis*. 'Second' mild attacks are almost invariably due to the milder *B. parapertussis*.

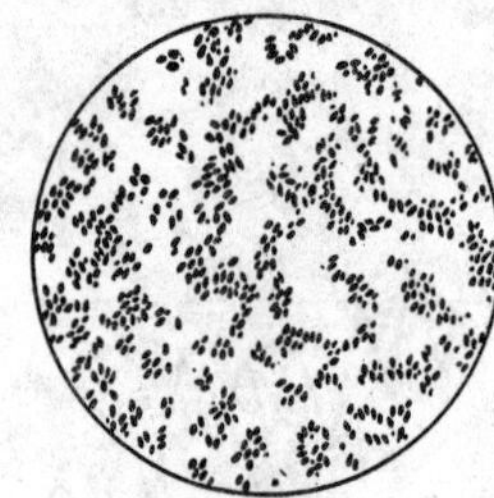

Fig. 25. *WHOOPING-COUGH. The cough is due to infection with the very short rod-like micro-organisms known as* Bordetella pertussis, *or* Hemophilus pertussis.

Incubation is from 7 to 14 days. In the catarrhal stage the child may be feverish and has a persistent cough. The third stage is characterized by a convulsive paroxysmal cough, occurring especially at night and attended by long-continued hissing convulsive breathing with rattling in the air passages. This is succeeded by several short efforts to expel the breath, following each other in quick succession. The long convulsive breathing, attended by the whooping sound or crowing, is immediately repeated; these paroxysms continue until a small quantity of thick slimy ropy mucus is thrown up by expectoration or vomiting, then the breathing again becomes free. During these paroxysms the patient appears to be about to suffocate, with congestion of the face, shedding of tears, sweating about the head and forehead, and such distress that he often lays hold of something for support. Blood sometimes starts from the nostrils and a child may involuntarily pass water or evacuate the bowels. The disease is most commonly seen in spring and autumn. It is not generally dangerous except in young children under five years of age, but is especially to be dreaded in young infants.

Child contacts should be in quarantine for three weeks.

Complications. In infants, the development of bronchopneumonia, lung collapse, convulsions, and gastro-enteritis are serious and may cause death. Ear and heart complications are not common. Chloral elixir should be given to a child with convulsions. For bronchopneumonia, antibiotics will be necessary.

Treatment. Patients should be kept isolated for at least six weeks, or four weeks after the whoop develops. For the first few days the child should be kept indoors or quietly in bed. Later, in warm weather, the child may be allowed in the garden, if the temperature is normal and the child is over four years of age. When the paroxysms are frequent, or there have been previous attacks of bronchitis, the child is better in a warm peaceful bedroom. Excitement must be avoided, and the bowels kept regular. During the second stage a simple expectorant mixture is useful.

Ampicillin syrup, B.N.F., reduces the severity of the attack if started within the first two weeks of the illness and given for ten days, but it has little effect once the whooping has begun. To relieve paroxysms of coughing, cough mixtures are of little value. Sedatives such as chloral elixir for infants, B.P.C. are effective and belladonna tincture is good in severe cases.

DIET. The diet should be light and nutritious, milk foods and meat juice being advisable in small and frequent feeds, but in mild cases a fuller diet is allowed. In severe cases milk may be diluted, peptonised, or citrated. Ice-cream is soothing as well as popular. Glucose, whey or albumen water are also suitable. If the food is given about 10 minutes after a paroxysm, regurgitation may be prevented. Dry crumbly foods should be avoided, since they cause irritation.

During convalescence great care should be taken to prevent chills; cod-liver oil and iron tonics are beneficial. A change to seaside air is often beneficial.

Prevention. The modern treatment of preventive immunization confers a fairly high degree of immunity in children, and modifies the severity of the disease if an attack follows. Babies of three months old may be immunized, the injections being given during the first year of life (see p. 266).

II. Diseases Due to Fungous Infection

Actinomycosis

(*Madura Disease*)

Actinomycosis, due to the ray fungus, occurs in domestic animals, and occasionally human beings who work with cattle become infected. Suppurative swellings develop in certain parts of the body, namely the neck and jaw, the intestines—especially the appendix and large bowel—and the lungs. Secondary abscesses are often formed in other adjacent organs. The pulmonary type of disease resembles chronic bronchitis or tuberculosis and is generally fatal, although the disease runs a long course. In the other types the outlook is more hopeful.

Treatment consists in incision to drain abscesses or remove the swellings where possible. X-ray irradiation may be used for surface swellings, and potassium iodide is sometimes given by mouth in large daily doses for a prolonged period. Sulphonamides and thymol have been given with only moderate success, but penicillin is the mainstay of treatment.

Farmer's Lung

This is a dust disease caused by the breathing in of dust from moldy hay, chaff, or grain. It is not believed to be a specific fungous infection but is more likely to be caused by hypersensitivity to the inhaled spores of the molds, including *Candida albicans*. Cowmen and men working on threshing machines are the more likely farm-workers to be affected.

Symptoms. The respiratory symptoms resemble those of bronchitis with asthma, with cough, thick sputum, breathlessness on exertion, and fever in some cases. In chronic cases a low-grade bronchopneumonia often develops which leads to lung fibrosis.

Treatment. Sufferers from farmer's lung should be removed from dusty work.

For the cough, methadone linctus will give relief. An antibiotic may be given to control secondary infection from bacteria.

III. Diseases Due to Protozoan Parasites

Leishmaniasis

This is a disease caused by certain protozoa (one-celled organisms) transmitted by the sandfly. The Leishmaniae are in appearance somewhat similar to the trypanosomes. There are two forms of this disease, genralized (kala-azar) and localized (cutaneous tropical or oriental sore)

Kala-azar

This disease has an incubation period of about a month and is ushered in insidiously or as a high fever. The fever is often intermittent. In white people the skin becomes noticeably browner. The spleen becomes enormously enlarged and the liver mildly so. There are usually symptoms of profound anemia.

Diagnosis is confirmed in the laboratory with blood tests or specimens from the bone marrow or spleen.

Treatment. Antimony is the most effective drug, and pentavalent antimony compounds are the best. General health needs building up with a well-balanced diet.

Oriental Sore

This disease commences as a small itching spot on the face or arms where the sandfly has bitten. Later, it becomes larger and ulcerates. The sore heals after 6 to 12 months and leaves a permanent deep scar.

A slightly different form occurs in South America where the mucous membranes of the nose, pharynx and mouth are affected.

Treatment. These conditions are successfully treated with antimony compounds.

Prevention is by attacking the sandfly and its breeding places, and by spraying the inside of rooms with DDT powder or aerosols.

Malaria

(*Ague: Intermittent Fever*)

The three main forms of malaria are due to infection by different types of *Plasmodium*. (1) Benign tertian malaria is caused by the *Plasmodium vivax* and *P. ovale*. (2) Quartan malaria is due to infection by *P. malariae*. (3) Malignant tertian malaria is caused by infection from *P. falciparum*.

The different varieties of malaria take their name from the length of the interval of the ague attacks in each case.

The interval in quotidian (daily) ague is twenty-four hours.

The interval in benign tertian (third-day) ague is forty-eight hours.

The interval in quartan (fourth-day) ague is seventy-two hours.

The interval in malignant tertian is irregular, generally about forty-eight hours.

Malignant tertian fever has various forms: (a) regular intermittent; (b) irregular and remittent; (c) pernicious: the comatose and cerebral type, the algid type, bilious remittent fever, malarial cachexia, and latent infections and relapses.

Cause. About 1880 Laveral discovered a parasite in the blood by persistently investigating the blood of persons suffering from malaria. He found that the plasmodium parasite multiplies enormously in the blood of infected persons. But how does the parasite get into the blood?

About 1897 Professor Ross discovered that water-breeding mosquitoes—the *Anopheles*—do not ingest the parasites from decayed vegetable or animal matter, but by sucking the blood of persons already suffering from malaria. These parasites multiply rapidly in the stomach of the female mosquito and, when such a mosquito bites another human being, that person also becomes infected with malaria. Therefore malaria is not caused, as previously supposed, by decayed vegetable matter and low marshy districts containing stagnant water, except in so far as these are the breeding places of the infected mosquito that spreads the disease. On entering the bloodstream the malarial organisms penetrate the red blood cells and breed in them.

Symptoms. In benign tertian and quartan fevers, the period of incubation is from 2 to 15 days, but symptoms may develop immediately. The disease begins with headache and malaise, followed by ague. This has three stages, the cold, the hot, and the sweating stages. In the cold stage, which lasts up to two hours, the patient has a headache and feeling of debility with nausea and sometimes vomiting; he has no appetite, and does not wish to move. The face and extremities become pale and blue, with generalized 'goose-flesh' and rigors, the patient shivers and his teeth chatter. During this phase the temperature rises to 104° or 105° F. After a short time these symptoms decline and the hot stage follows, characterized by various symptoms of headache and thirst. There is often an eruption of herpes around the mouth and bronchitis is common. This stage lasts from half to six hours.

When the fever passes off it is followed by the sweating stage, during which perspiration breaks out, often with profuse sweat. The temperature returns to its normal level, the pains and aches disappear, and a feeling of health returns until the next paroxysm. Each paroxysm lasts for less than twelve hours. (See Temperature Chart, p. 264.)

During the cold stage the blood is driven inward from the surface and particularly congests the spleen which, in longstanding cases, becomes swollen and permanently enlarged. This swelling may be plainly felt and is often quite perceptible to the eye; it is called 'ague-cake.'

Ague fits begin at different hours of the day, generally between midday and midnight. A quotidian attack usually begins in the morning; a tertian at noon; and a quartan in the afternoon. The severity of the paroxysm varies considerably.

The cold stage is shortest in quotidian, and longest in quartan fever. Thus the longest fit has the shortest interval and the shortest cold stage; while the shortest fit has the longest interval and the longest cold stage.

There are also double tertian and double quartan fever wherein the attacks repeat themselves, sometimes on the same day, at other times on alternate days.

Tertians are more common than either quotidians or quartans.

In malignant tertian fever the disease may by similar to the above types, but more often causes irregular fever, the patient becomes more ill, and may pass into a typhoidal condition. Mental or intestinal disorders may develop, with severe diarrhea in the latter type of case.

Agues are more prevalent in spring and autumn. Autumn agues are the most severe types of case.

Diagnosis. The disease must be distinguished from other tropical fevers, such as typhoid fever, heat stroke, yellow fever, and tuberculosis. The diagnosis is made by the microscopic confirmation of malarial organisms in the blood.

Treatment. The patient must be kept in bed, with hot water bottles in the cold stage. He should be wrapped in warm blankets for warmth and comfort.

In the hot stage give cooling drinks and tepid sponging.

Chloroquine, amodiaquine and primaquine are the best drugs for a malaria attack. Dosage of chloroquine for adults is 4 tablets (160 milligrams each of base) followed by 2 tablets in 6 hours, then 2 tablets daily for two days. These drugs do not prevent relapses in vivax malaria because the drugs seem unable to get at the parasites in the liver.

Injections of quinine are given in acute complicated falciparum cases. When there is intolerance to the drug, noises in the ears, nausea or vomiting (*cinchonism*) may occur. Give quinine by slow intravenous injection

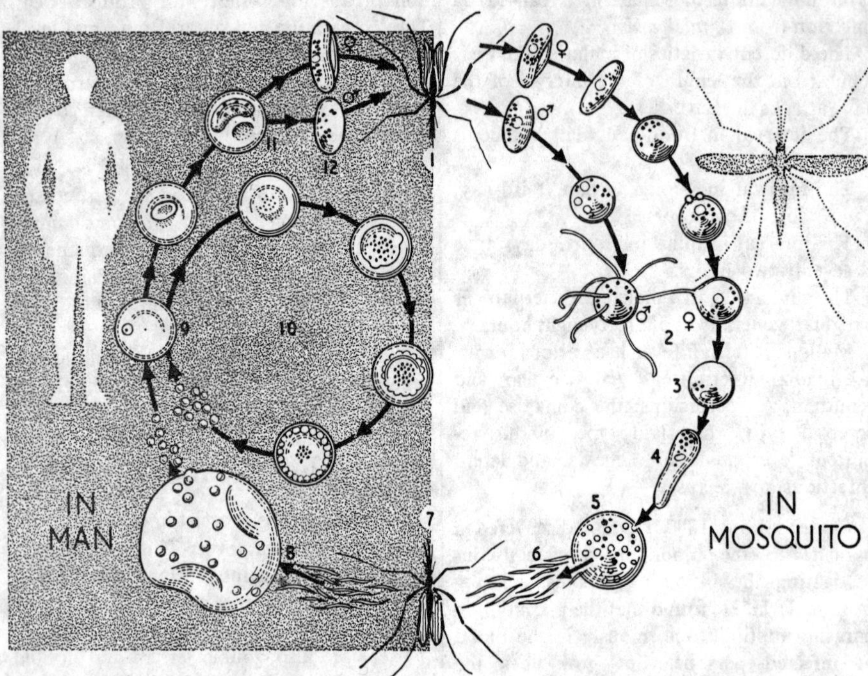

Fig. 26. *LIFE CYCLE OF MALARIAL PARASITES. The mosquito* (1) *having bitten a malarious man and sucked in male and female Plasmodiums with the blood, acts as their host as they mature and mate* (2). *The resultant fertilized parasites, known as zygotes* (3), *develop* (4), *and form cysts on the stomach wall of the mosquito. The cysts burst* (5), *releasing sporozoites* (6), *which enter the mosquito's salivary glands and escape into man's bloodstream when he is bitten by the mosquito* (7). *The sporozoites travel to the liver* (8) *where for about seven days they grow enormously. Some of them migrate into the red blood cells* (9), *where many parasites (now called merozoites) multiply* (10) *and destroy the cells. The freed parasites enter other red blood cells and set up a 'vicious circle'* (10). *As they mature* (11) *they develop into sexual forms* (12) *and the cycle begins again.*

in doses of 500 milligrams for adults every 4 to 6 hours till 2 grams have been taken, then give quinine tablets by mouth for the remainder of the illness.

Malarial cachexia requires removal of the patient from the infected district, and iron and arsenic are given internally.

RELAPSES. For relapses, which are fairly common, primaquine tablets (7·5 milligrams each of base) three times a day, may be taken for about two weeks. Proguanil is too slow-acting to be of great value in an acute attack in non-immune subjects.

Prevention. Malaria can be largely prevented by drainage of breeding sites of mosquitoes, by the use of insect sprays for destroying mosquitoes and larvae in dwellings and pools, isolation of malarial cases, and screening of windows, beds and doors.

For suppression of malarial attacks, protective doses for adults are 1 tablet of proguanil (100 milligrams) each day, or 1 tablet of pyrimethamine (25 milligrams) once a week, to be taken while the subject is in a a malarious area. The first tablet should be taken the day before entering the area. Chloroquine and amodiaquine may also be used for this purpose.

Recently, inoculations have been given to prevent malarial attacks.

In fever and ague districts it is important to avoid the hot sun, and the damp evening and morning air.

Blackwater Fever

This disease is secondary to tertian malignant malaria, and develops after irregular malarial treatment. The attack is frequently provoked by the taking of quinine. The patient has fever, rigors, jaundice, vomiting, pain in the loins, and thirst, and for one or two days passes dark urine. Recovery may follow, or death may occur from exhaustion, high fever or suppression of urine. Large doses of potassium citrate (2·5 grams) given 4-hourly may prevent suppression.

Treatment consists in absolute rest in bed, copious administration of fluids, and heart stimulants. Ice is given to suck, fomentations or hot bottles are applied to the loins, and quinine should be withheld. Blood transfusion is given in the early stages. Chloroquine is given if the malarial parasites are still present in the blood.

Toxoplasmosis

This is a protozoal infestation which has been recognized only in recent years.

The adult type is mild with some enlargement of the lymph glands and a slight fever lasting from days to months. Diagnosis is made only by special tests of the patient's serum. Cases of glandular fever may sometimes resemble the glandular involvement in toxoplasmosis.

The congenital type occurs hen the child is in the uterus and the pregnant mother acquires the infection. Abortion or stillbirth often occurs, but if the child is born alive, the most common damage done to the child is eye disease, often associated with lesions in the brain, muscles, and liver. In children who survive, a mental defect is common.

Treatment. A combination of sulphonamides and pyrimethamine is used. The course is continued for one month.

Prevention, of course, is to keep pregnant women away from people suffering from toxoplasmosis, and from other possible sources of infection.

Trypanosomiasis

(*Sleeping Sickness*)

The parasites which cause this disease are called trypanosomes. *Trypanosoma gambiense* was discovered in 1902 and *T. rhodesiense* in 1910.

The disease is spread by various flies called *Tsetse* flies, and the parasites live in the intestines and salivary glands of infected flies; when they bite a human being the parasite is transferred to the wound and thence to the patient's blood.

The disease is confined principally to Africa and South America, where whole native districts are said to have been depopulated.

Symptoms. An inflamed patch develops round the bite, and is followed within seven to fourteen days by fever. There is a long latent period after infection, and the onset is slow and insidious, with intermittent fever. The patient suffers from headache and weakness, and sometimes an eruption appears. In the early stage of the disease the patient is mentally dull, the pulse is rapid and there is malaise; the spleen and glands become enlarged. The patient may recover, or the disease become chronic.

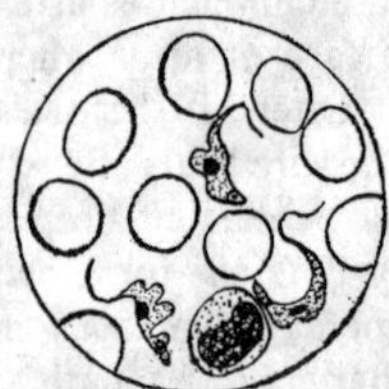

Fig. 27. *TRYPANOSOMES OF SLEEPING SICKNESS, with red cells in the blood. These organisms are conveyed by tsetse flies to man.*

SECOND STAGE. After a variable period of from three months to three years, if recovery does not follow, stage two develops, with increasing weakness, fatigue, fever, tremors, slow speech, uncertain shuffling gait, neuralgia and cramps, apathy, melancholy or irritability, and vacancy of facial expression; memory and intelligence are impaired. With treatment the patient may recover from *T. gambiense* infection even at this stage.

THIRD STAGE. In stage three, however, the patient sinks into a lethargic or paralytic condition, sometimes with convulsions or delirium, and is unable to speak or stand. The temperature is low, and the body is emaciated. Death generally occurs within eighteen months, from meningitis or coma.

In *T. gambiense* infections, the outlook is hopeful if treatment is given before the nervous system is involved. *T. rhodesiense* causes a far more virulent infection, and most cases end fatally once the nervous system is attacked.

Treatment. Preventive measures to secure protection against tsetse flies are essential but difficult.

Suramin is used as a preventive against the disease and the effect lasts for about three months; it is also used for the cure of early cases: Tryparsamide, an arsenical drug, which penetrates into nervous tissue, is of most value in advanced stages especially when the central nervous system is attacked. If the disease is due to *Trypanosoma rhodesiense*, tryparsamide is less effective and is used with suramin. For patients intolerant of an arsenical drug, pentamidine or stilbamidine are used intramuscularly but they are both only fully satisfactory in the early stages of the disease. Pentamidine is also useful for large-scale prophylaxis where people are exposed to the bites of tsetse flies.

Arsenical drugs such as tryparsamide may cause damage to the optic nerve, with disturbance of vision, while suramin may have an injurious effect on the kidneys. The spinal fluid should be examined at regular intervals during treatment.

The melarsoprol drugs are most useful when trypanosomes become resistant to suramin or tryparsamide, or in cases of relapse.

IV. Diseases Due to Rickettsias

The rickettsias are minute micro-organisms living in the tissues of infected lice, fleas, ticks and mites. They are transmitted to man through the bites of these insects, and are the agents causing typhus and several other typhus-like fevers.

Typhus Fevers

(*Gaol Fever: Spotted Fever*)

Epidemic typhus is liable to occur in huge epidemics. It is due to *Rickettsia prowazeki* conveyed by lice. War, poverty and dirt favor its spread which may be extremely rapid.

Endemic typhus is less severe than the epidemic form. It is due to *R. mooseri* which is conveyed by fleas, and occasionally by lice. The typhus fevers are most common in the Far East, north Africa and around the Mediterranean.

TRENCH FEVER, which was first recognized during the First World War, is a mild form of typhus in which there is much pain in the shins; it is a louse-borne rickettsial disease.

The incubation period of typhus is from five to fourteen days.

Symptoms. The onset is very abrupt with chills, pains in the back and legs, severe headache, nausea and vomiting and high temperature. The patient is prostrated but cannot sleep. His expression is vacant and the face is flushed, while the pulse increases in rapidity. After four days he becomes more restless and delirious, and a rash appears, starting in the armpits and wrists and spreading to the abdomen, chest and limbs; it is mottled and dusky, with spots of irregular size and shape. In delirium the patient may be restless and violent, or comatose. The tongue is brown and dry. In the second week there is extreme prostration, incoherence, muscular tremors, and increasing coma. The heart becomes weak, and the rash darkens. Hiccup may develop and is a grave sign.

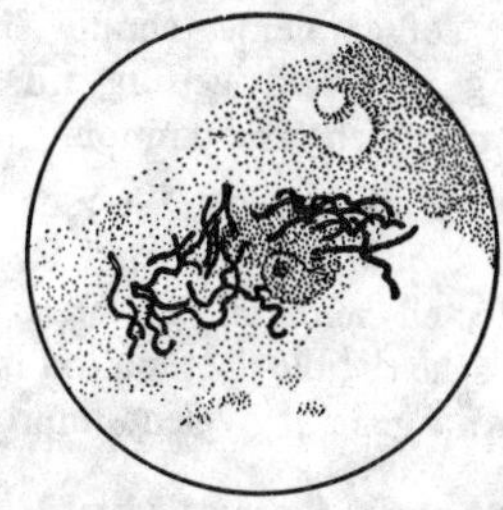

Fig. 28. *RICKETTSIAS which cause typhus fevers are smaller than bacteria, and sometimes join into thread-like chains.*

In unfavorable cases death may occur in coma. In more favorable cases the crisis occurs about the fourteenth day and, after sleeping, the patient wakes, very weak, but relieved of his symptoms. Convalescence is then short. In some epidemics the disease tends to be mild, whereas in others it is fatal in two or three days.

COMPLICATIONS are uncommon, but occasionally nephritis, gangrene, or venous thrombosis develop.

Treatment. The antibiotic drugs have proved of great value in reducing the duration of the fever. The tetracyclines or chloramphenicol will usually cause the fever to subside in two or three days.

General treatment is as for other severe fevers (p.264). The diet must be very light but stimulating (see p. 59). Alcohol with water may be given freely. During convalescence exertion must be restricted for some time.

PROTECTIVE MEASURES. Dicophane (DDT) is the most effective insecticide against lice and fleas. It has proved highly effective in delousing whole communities living in overcrowded verminous conditions. Typhus Vaccine is now less used than formerly owing to the effectiveness and widespread use of DDT and of tetracycline.

Q Fever

This is a rickettsial disease and is so named because it was first noticed in Queensland in 1937, among abattoir workers and was called Query fever.

Infection occurs from sheep and cattle through drinking infected milk or through breathing dust containing the infected fæces of ticks harboring the rickettsias.

Symptoms are those of the pneumonias, with headache and fever. Chest X-ray shows a pneumonic type of opacity.

Treatment is by use of the tetracyclines; headaches and cough are treated symptomatically.

Scrub Typhus

This form of typhus, due to *Rickettsia orientalis*, is conveyed by mites living on rats and mice in scrubby woodland and grass in the Far East. It caused much disablement among troops in Burma and the S.W. Pacific during the Second World War. At the site of the bite a sloughing sore appears and this develops into an ulcer. The lymphatic glands swell and a pimply rash appears by about the fifth day. In many cases the blood pressure falls and the heart beats increase in rapidity. Inflammation of the lung may occur.

Treatment. As for typhus fevers, although Typhus Vaccine is of no value. Dibutyl phthalate rubbed into the inner surface of clothing is a highly effective protection against mites.

V. Diseases Due to Spirochætes

Leptospirosis

(*Spirochetal Jaundice: Weil's Disease*)

This disease is due to infection with the parasite *Leptospira icterohemorrhagiae*, which is transmitted by rats. It occurs in local epidemics, causing jaundice, fever, swelling of the liver, hemorrhages, and sometimes inflammation of the kidneys. The patient is suddenly prostrated with chills, headache, and pains in the muscles. The appetite fails and there is vomiting and constipation. The jaundice develops about the fourth day and increases. The liver is enlarged and is very tender. Bleeding may occur from the lungs, stomach, nose, or anus, and bile is present in the urine for some weeks. The fever subsides in about two weeks, and the patient's condition then improves. Occasionally the typical jaundice is absent. Various complications may occur and the mortality is about 15 per cent.

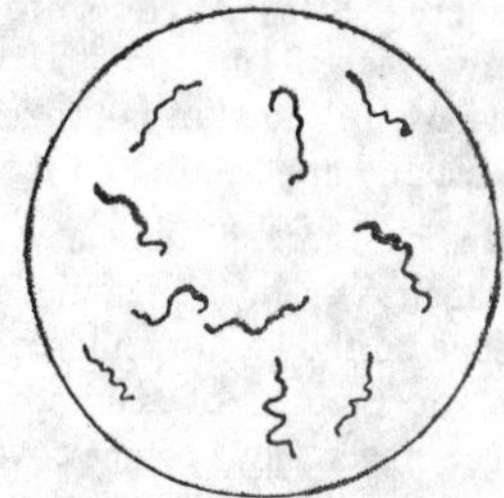

Fig. 29. *LEPTOSPIRAE which cause spirochetal jaundice.*

Treatment is mainly directed towards relieving fever and malaise. Fruit juices such as orange or lemon with glucose should be given freely. The urine and feces should be disinfected, and food protected from rats. Attendants must disinfect their hands thoroughly, and wear gloves if their skin is abraded to prevent entry of the parasite.

If the disease is diagnosed within 7 days of onset, penicillin is valuable, but it is useless later. It is given in maximum doses. A tetracycline may be substituted.

Relapsing Fever

(*African Tick Fever*)

This is an acute fever with alternating bouts of fever and normal temperature. It occurs in Europe, India, Ireland, and Africa, and is spread by lice or by ticks. Fever develops about a week after infection, with rigors, headache, sweating, pains in the bones, vomiting, giddiness, and sometimes jaundice. The crisis occurs after five or seven days, and in unfavorable cases debilitated patients may succumb. In other cases the patient improves rapidly but relapses after another fourteen days, the symptoms then returning in milder form. Convalescence is slow, and occasionally complications such as meningitis, paralysis, eye symptoms, or convulsions may develop. In most cases (98 per cent) the outlook is favorable if the patient is carefully nursed in hygienic surroundings, and receives two courses of tetracycline.

Prevention. Use gamma benzene hexachloride or DDT to kill the lice (see p. 471) in the louse-borne form or the African ticks in the tick-borne form.

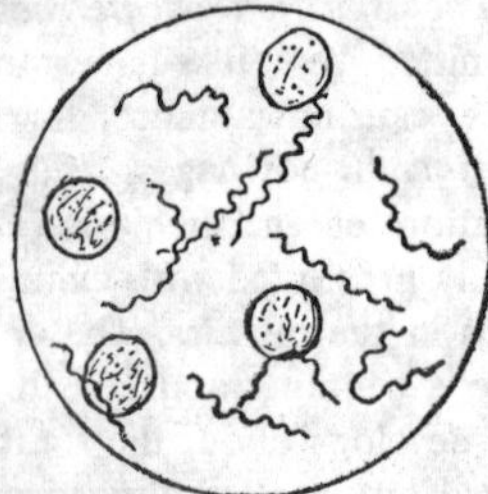

Fig. 30. *SPIROCHETA RECURRENTIS* (*or BORRELIA*) *of African tick fever, with red blood cells.*

Yaws

The spirochete, *Treponema pertenue,* which affects both children and, to a lesser extent, adults in tropical countries, is very similar to the organism causing syphilis, but yaws is not a venereal disease. The spirochetes are commonly picked up on the bare feet, especially where the skin is broken, and the papules usually appear first on the legs.

Symptoms. There is only a mild general malaise at first when the papules make their appearance on the legs of children, breasts of mothers, or mouths of babies, but as the lesions get bigger they become covered with a yellow scab known as the 'mother yaw.' The secondary stage occurs, three to four weeks after the first lesions appear, as an acute fever with headache and joint pains. The skin dries and peels off in patches, then yellowish papules develop becoming red and raspberry-like. These secondary lesions may heal without treatment but often recur for two or three years. Lymph glands and joints are often swollen. The third stage, which may follow the second within a few months but may lie latent for years, is characterized by widespread ulceration of skin and bone tissues and may often leave the sufferer deformed.

Treatment. Penicillin is most effective. If given early in the disease, a single injection of 1,200,000 units of PAM (procaine benzylpenicillin with 2 per cent aluminium monostearate), or half that dose for children, will effect cure in most cases. Tetracycline also produces a high percentage of cures.

Since yaws is often endemic among undernourished tropical populations, the general treatment of patients should include a nourishing diet and getting rid of worm infestations which are common.

Preventive Treatment. Wounds, cuts and scratches should be protected from flies or from infected material. In areas of heavy infection the whole population should be treated, and general hygiene improved.

VI. Diseases Caused by Viruses or Unknown Agents

Acute Colds

(*The Common Cold: Acute Rhinitis: Coryza*)

The common cold typically consists of acute inflammation of the membrane lining the nose and upper air passages. It is a widespread affliction of temperate countries and is especially liable to occur at times of seasonal change, as in early winter and spring. Some individuals are much more susceptible than others, and children are especially apt to develop frequent colds, often in succession.

The inflammation is due to a virus, but secondary infection with bacteria often follows.

Symptoms. The typical symptoms are sudden chill, headache, malaise, sneezing, and loss of appetite with a slight rise of temperature. The nose becomes congested and obstructed, so that nasal breathing is impossible; a watery discharge develops which gradually becomes thick and purulent.

The inflammation often spreads to the nasopharynx and tonsils, causing soreness of the throat and difficulty in swallowing. If the larynx is affected the voice becomes hoarse and there may be noises in the ears, or deafness. The eyes water and there are pains round the jaws, and loss of taste and smell. If the infection spreads downwards to the chest, laryngitis or bronchitis may develop, with hoarseness, soreness behind the breastbone, and cough.

Treatment. The patient shoud endeavor to avoid spreading the infection to other people by remaining in a warm well-ventilated room for twenty-four to forty-eight hours at home, preferably in bed.

Aspirin, *or* phenacetin and caffeine tablets, 1 to 2, taken at night with milk to induce sweating, often give relief. A hot bath should be taken in the early stages if the patient's health permits. A nasal spray (go easy with ephedrine) will help to clear the nose and ease breathing. A dose of Epsom salts or some laxative should be used to prevent constipation. Simple lozenges may be sucked if the threat is sore.

In cases of frequent recurrence a mixed or anti-catarrh vaccine may be found to confer some protection. Investigation of the nasal sinuses may be needed for the treatment of residual infections. Antihistamine drugs may reduce congestion. Vitamin C is of value especially in the form of fresh orange juice or ascorbic acid tablets.

Sufferers from frequent colds should pay attention to their general habits, and endeavor to take plenty of exercise in the fresh air, to avoid close stuffy atmospheres in rooms or offices, to eat fruit, vegetables, and dairy products freely, to avoid constipation and to get plenty of sleep. Excessive or heavy clothing is inadvisable, but wool or porous garments should be worn next to the skin in cold weather, and the feet should be well shod.

Adenovirus Infections

This is the term given to the contagious form of upper respiratory tract infection commonly seen where people live in close contact with each other, e.g. soldiers, or people in an institution. (See Fig. 13, p. 333.)

Mild cases are indistinguishable from those of the common cold, but severe cases show rhinitis and tonsillar and pharyngeal inflammation. There is often a degree of conjunctivitis present.

Treatment is symptomatic and no antibiotics are available to influence the course of the disease. The prognosis is excellent and there are no after-effects.

Chickenpox

(*Varicella*)

Chickenpox is a highly contagious disease, associated with mild fever and a blister-like eruption, called blebs, over the body, often developing in successive crops. Both children and adults are susceptible but the disease is most common in children, though in adults the disease is more severe. It appears to be related to shingles (herpes zoster) (see Diseases of the Nervous System, p. 427).

Symptoms. The disease appears usually from two to three weeks after exposure to infection. At first a mild fever and feeling of tiredness may cause the patient to stay indoors, although intense pain in the head, back and legs, with high temperature, vomiting and even delirium are not uncommon.

The eruption usually appears in one to three days and consists of small watery blisters averaging one-eighth of an inch in size. They are most numerous over the chest and trunk; a few may appear over the face and forehead, and even in the roof of the mouth. They do not have the so-called 'shotty' feeling when pressed under the finger as noted in smallpox, neither is the red blush around them so marked.

Unless the scabs are scratched off by the finger nails, or the case is very severe, very few scars will remain.

Treatment. The treatment consists in a mild diet for a few days, keeping the patient indoors to avoid exposure to cold or wet. When the eruption is severe the patient should stay in bed. Some simple medicine such as aspirin in doses of half a teaspoonful in water may be given every three hours to allay fever, and to keep the kidneys working properly. A cooling dusting-powder, olive oil, or calamine lotion may be used on the skin to reduce irritation. The blebs should not be scratched, or scars may remain, and the scabs should be allowed to separate naturally. The patient is infectious for about one month, or until all the scabs have disappeared.

Dengue

Dengue is a fever of hot countries, due to a virus conveyed by mosquitoes. At the onset there are chills, headache, severe pains in the eyes and muscles, swelling and flushing of the face and soreness of the mouth, with high fever. Because of the severe joint pains and backache, it is often known as break-bone fever. After two or three days' remission the fever and pains recur, and there is usually a rash with red patches which develop on the hands, back, thighs and legs; peeling of the skin follows as in scarlet fever. Convalescence is often prolonged from weakness, but the death rate is very low.

Treatment is symptomatic, and the pains may require alleviation by aspirin, methadone, or pethidine.

Prevention consists of anti-mosquito measures similar to those used in malaria.

Encephalitis Lethargica

(*Sleeping Sickness*)

Sleeping sickness is a disease of comparatively recent recognition. It became pandemic in America and Europe from about 1917 to 1926, and has since become rare.

There are several types of the disease. The St. Louis type is endemic in America. The virus is unknown, but the disease is characteristic, causing fever, lethargy and paralysis of the eye muscles with double vision. Infection probably takes place through the mouth and nose. See also p. 427.

The onset is often gradual and insidious, but sometimes acute delirium may be the first symptom. The condition often resembles influenza in the early stages, and hiccup is a common symptom. In severe cases mania or delirium is seen, or lethargy and coma; muscular pains, rigidity of the limbs, or convulsions may develop.

Later, in cases which recover, tremors and purposeless movements may indicate the true condition and the patient's face finally becomes mask-like and expressionless (parkinsonism). A drooping posture and the shuffling gait are characteristic.

The diagnosis is often difficult; about 33 per cent of cases are fatal. Complete recovery is rare, most cases ending in chronic invalidism, and the disease often runs on for months or years. There is no specific treatment. Isolation and careful nursing are essential. Hyoscine, artane and benadryl relieve tremors and stiffness of limbs.

German Measles

(*Rubella: Rose Measles*)

This is a mild acute infection with a rose-colored rash which develops at the onset of the disease. There are enlarged tender glands in the neck and sometimes in the axillae and groins, and slight malaise. The disease is very infectious and spreads by direct contact. The quarantine period is twenty-one days, and the incubation period fourteen to twenty-one days. There may be headache and slight fever, and some inflammation and watering of the eyes.

The rash breaks out first behind the ears and on the face and spreads first to the trunk and then to the limbs; it then usually disappears after two days.

In pregnant women who have not had the disease an attack of German measles during the first sixteen weeks of pregnancy may cause permanent defects in the baby. The possible defects are cataract, deafness, heart malformations, and mental retardation. Some doctors therefore consider that all girls should be allowed to have the illness in childhood when their blood will make preventive antibodies for life. It is a controversial point as to whether an abortion should be advised for women in early pregnancy who develop German measles.

A live attenuated vaccine has been available for immunization since early in 1970.

Treatment. The patient should be kept in bed while the temperature is raised, with a light diet, laxatives, and cooling drinks; other measures are symptomatic. Occasionally a more severe type of the disease occurs in epidemics, with higher fever and more constitutional disturbance, and in such cases more careful nursing is required.

Human Normal Immunoglobulin is used as a prophylactic in women exposed to the disease during the first four months of pregnancy.

Glandular Fever

This disease generally affects children and causes considerable swelling of the lymphatic glands in the neck and other regions. It is probably more common than is generally realized, and may occur in epidemics. The temperature rises suddenly to 39·4° C (103° F), and the glands of the neck swell but are not generally painful. If the abdominal glands, however, are involved they may cause considerable pain. The tonsils may be enlarged, and there is then pain on swallowing. The disease lasts for two to five weeks before subsiding. Occasionally blood is passed in the urine, but is not a serious sign. The glandular swelling of the neck may persist for some months and may be mistaken for tuberculosis involvement. A specific test may be made to confirm the diagnosis. See also Toxoplasmosis, p. 280.

Treatment must be directed towards the patient's general health and comfort. Symptomatic treatment may require the use of penicillin for a few days. Convalescence is generally slow, with debility continuing for some months. Iron tonics should be prescribed when there is anemia.

Influenza

Influenza is a very acute infectious virus disease which primarily attacks the air passages, but is accompanied by general symptoms and fever, and may give rise to serious complications. It often occurs in epidemics in the winter months, being spread by droplet infection through sneezing and coughing.

Three main types of virus are recognized: A, B and C. Major epidemics are usually due to A (Asian type) and recur every two or three winters. Minor epidemics are caused by the B type, and occur at 2- to 6-year intervals. Gastric 'flu is a misnomer and has nothing to do with influenza.

Symptoms generally develop within from one to three days after infection and are very variable.

The onset is generally sudden with fever, headache, vertigo, pains in the back and muscles, chills and collapse. In the majority of outbreaks the respiratory type of infection, with bronchitis, a running of the eyes and nose, and sore throat, is the commonest form of the disease. In elderly persons the heart is liable to be affected. The feverish stage generally lasts about five days or more.

Prevention. Fresh air, avoidance of crowds, general attention to health, and a nourishing diet, reduce the likelihood of influenzal infection. Asian influenza (1957) is still the prevalent virus and a vaccine given in autumn to persons at risk (nurses; heart cases) will prevent much of the disease, but immunity does not last long.

Treatment. The patient should be kept isolated in bed in a warm but well-ventilated room from the start, and not be allowed up until the temperature has been normal for at least three days and the symptoms have abated. The diet should be mainly liquid in the early stages. Aspirin, phenacetin and caffeine tablets may be given for feverishness and headache. The bowels should be opened with a laxative. The cough may be treated as recommended for acute bronchitis. Codeine phosphate syrup is a good sedative when the cough is troublesome. With cardiac weakness supportive measures should be used. In these cases glucose drinks, broth and other fluids should be given until vomiting subsides.

Pneumonia is a fairly common complication, especially in cases in which insufficient care is taken in the early stages, and in elderly or debilitated persons. When it develops oxygen may be required, and penicillin plus streptomycin (or erythromycin) are given to combat secondary infection. A combination of antibiotics should prevent further complications such as pleurisy, empyema or sinusitis. Nursing in a humid atmosphere may be advisable to ease the damaged bronchial tract lining.

Convalescence. Anyone over the age of 35 should rest in bed for three days after the temperature has returned to normal, because of the possible toxic effect on the heart muscle. Great care should also be taken for two or three weeks to avoid chill or fatigue; depression is a common symptom for which tonics should be given.

Measles
(*Morbilli*)

Measles is an acute and very infectious virus disease, common in children, and accompanied by a generalized rash, catarrh of the air passages, and fever. It often occurs in epidemics.

The incubation period is generally about ten days, but varies from seven to eighteen days. The infectivity of the patient ceases two weeks after the rash appears, unless there are complications.

Child contacts who have not had measles should not be sent to school for three weeks after the onset of a case in the house.

Injection treatment with gamma globulin is used for prevention, being especially advisable in the case of young infants. Active immunization with live attenuated virus vaccine is now included in many immunization programs for babies, being given early in the child's second year.

Symptoms. The disease sets in with the symptoms of a severe cold, namely chills, succeeded by fever, listlessness, languor, drowsiness and pains in the head, back and limbs. There is a fast pulse with sore throat, thirst, nausea, vomiting, frequent dry cough, and high-colored urine. These symptoms increase in intensity for four days. The temperature is about 38° to 39° C (101° to 102° F). On the third day the eyes become puffy and inflamed, the child cannot bear the light, and there are profuse tears. The nose discharges much watery secretion, and sneezing is frequent. The larynx and air passages become inflamed, and hoarseness, soreness of the chest, and cough develop. Small white spots (Koplik's spots, Fig. 31) are often found in the mouth. During this stage the child is often very irritable.

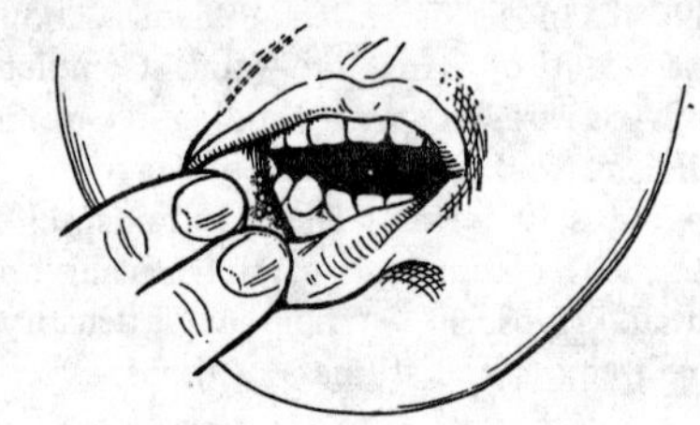

Fig. 31. *KOPLIK'S SPOTS. These small white spots are seen on the inside of the mouth very early in measles.*

The redness of the skin and eruption appear about the fourth day and cause heat and itching, with rise of temperature to about 40° C (104° F). The rash is characterized by a patchy redness which, on close inspection, is found to consist of numberless minute dusky red points and pimples, collected into irregular patches in the shape of a half or quarter moon. They appear first behind the ears, on the forehead and front of the neck, then upon the cheeks and around the nose and mouth. The rash spreads rapidly to the body and arms, and extends to the legs. The color of the skin, when the inflammation is at its height, is a bright raspberry red.

The decline of the rash takes place in the same order in which it appears. The coryza, the hoarseness and the cough abate about the seventh day. When the rash disappears the skin peels off in the form of branny scales.

Complications. These are fairly common, especially in severe epidemics, or when insufficient care is taken in the early stage. Bronchopneumonia, otitis media, laryngitis, stomatitis, and mastoid infection may occur.

Treatment. Treatment is aimed at (1) preventing spread of infection, (2) relieving symptoms, and (3) avoiding complications. Serum treatment has been used in epidemics to limit the spread of the disease.

The patient must be isolated and put in a room with a temperature of about 18° C (65° F). When the disease is mild and regular in its course, little will be required except rest in bed, light diet, cooling drinks, with some mild sedative or expectorant mixture to relieve the cough. Sponging with tepid water, if done frequently, moderates the fever and adds to the comfort of the patient. Direct light should be screened from the eyes. The mouth should be cleansed twice daily and a mild laxative given. The eyes may be bathed with a warm saline solution. Tissues used for discharges must be burned.

During the first stages of the disease, if the onset has not been severe, nothing further will be necessary than the precautions already advised.

If at any stage of the disease there should be pain in any part of the chest, which is made worse by coughing or by taking a full breath, bronchopneumonia may have developed and an antibiotic is indicated. Laryngitis arising late in the illness may indicate secondary diphtheritic infection and antitoxin is indicated.

In cases without complications, the child may get up in a moderately warm room about the sixth to seventh day of the illness. He should be out of isolation on the tenth day.

Mumps
(*Epidemic Parotitis*)

Mumps is due to a virus which infects the salivary glands. The patient is infectious until the swelling of the glands subsides. The disease usually affects children, and often occurs in epidemics in winter and spring.

The incubation period is about eighteen days. Contacts should be watched for signs of the disease from the twelfth to twenty-fourth day after exposure.

Symptoms. The first symptoms are soreness and stiffness in the side of the neck. Soon a swelling of the parotid gland behind the jaw is apparent on one side (Fig. 32). It is painful and continues to increase for four or five days, sometimes becoming very large and making it difficult to swallow or to open the mouth. After the fourth or fifth day the swelling subsides, and disappears in from seven to ten days, while the opposite side may then become swollen.

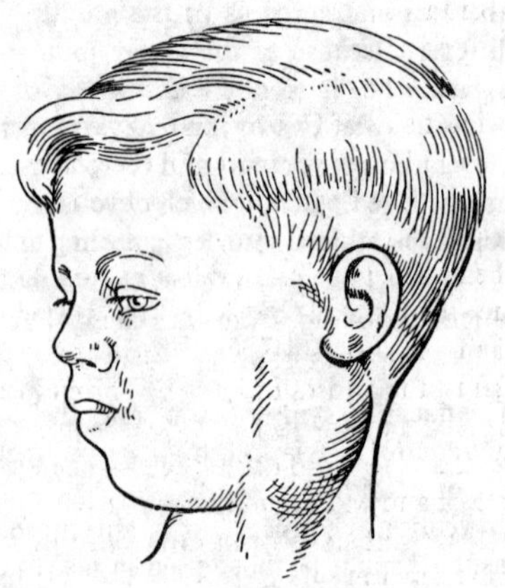

Fig. 32. *MUMPS. The salivary glands behind the jaw on one side are usually the first to be attacked, and a lop-sided swelling develops, which makes it difficult for the child to swallow.*

Both glands seldom swell at the same time, but sometimes the later swelling appears before the first has subsided, and occasionally the swelling is confined to one side.

In severe cases fever occurs, with dry skin, quick pulse, furred tongue, constipated bowels, and scanty and high-colored urine. In males over 12 years of age the testes may become swollen and painful. Occasionally the ears become inflamed.

Treatment. In mild cases very little treatment is required. The patient should be kept in bed for ten days at least and be given mild laxatives. Keep the face and neck warm, avoid exposure to cold and damp, and give a semi-solid diet of jellies, milk foods and cereals, purées and fish. If the case is severe, and other glands swell, the patient must be kept in bed longer and cooling lotions used; sweating should also be induced by aspirin, 300 to 900 milligrams every four hours.

Children should not return to school until at least seven days after the last swelling has subsided.

ORCHITIS. Treatment of this complication in youths and men is aided by giving prednisolone for three to four days to reduce the swelling of the testes. The scrotum should be lightly wrapped in cotton wool and the inflamed parts supported in a suspensory bandage or on a small pillow between the thighs. For associated abdominal pain, hot compresses should be applied to the painful area, and fat excluded from the diet. Recovery from orchitis is the rule.

Pneumonias: Virus and Rickettsial

There are several groups of infecting organisms for these pneumonias. They are:

viruses of influenza and measles,
psittacosis-ornithosis viruses,
adenoviruses,
repiratory syncytial (RS) viruses,
rickettsias of Q fever, the *Coxiella burneti*,
and other as yet unidentified viruses.

In patients suffering from influenza or from measles, the virus rarely causes a pneumonia; when such patients develop pneumonia it is due to bacteria complicating the disease. There is no specific treatment available against the viruses of influenza or measles but the secondary bacterial infection can be treated with antibiotics. See under influenza, p. 283, and under measles, p. 284.

The psittacosis-ornithosis viruses rarely cause pneumonia but like the psittacosis fever itself, it responds well to tetracycline (see below).

Pneumonia due to infection with adenoviruses (see Fig. 13, p. 333) is usually benign and, like the general respiratory infection which is described on p. 282, drug therapy provides little improvement.

Q fever is essentially a form of pneumonia with all the attendant symptoms. See p. 281. Tetracycline is the antibiotic of choice.

Poliomyelitis

(*Infantile Paralysis*)

See under Diseases of the Nervous System, p. 425.

Psittacosis

(*Ornithosis*)

This is a disease caused by viruses of the psittacosis-ornithosis group. It is endemic among birds, particularly parrots and budgerigars. Men most likely to become infected are those whose occupations bring them into contact with birds.

The incubation period is about seven days or longer.

Symptoms of the disease are not well defined. Fever, headaches, and malaise come on several days before the chest symptoms of coughing and breathlessness occur. X-rays show typical pneumonic-type shadows. Diagnosis can be made by special blood tests.

Treatment. The disease does not respond to penicillin but often the tetracyclines are quite successful. Convalescence may be slow and tedious.

Rabies

(*Hydrophobia*)

(See also Diseases of the Nervous System, p. 427.)

The bite of the mad rabid dog, or mad wolf, or other hydrophobic animal is one of the most dangerous wounds because, once the disease is established, it always ends fatally. Fortunately the human subject is not as susceptible to rabies as are some animals.

Symptoms. The interval between the bite and the appearance of the disease varies from twelve days to two months. The wound heals like any other animal bite. After a time, unless anti-rabic inoculations are given, the scar becomes irritable and begins to have lancinating pains which, if a limb has been bitten, run up towards the body. Sometimes the part feels cold, stiff or numb, or it may become red, swollen, or livid, and occasionally opens and discharges pus.

The patient feels a strange anxiety, is depressed and fearful, and has a desire for solitude, with disturbed sleep and spasmodic twitches. The pulse is fast and the nervous system is very excitable. The senses are more acute than normally; trifling noises produce agitation, and the eyes are so disturbed by light that the patient sometimes hides himself in a dark place. The appetite is lost, the voice is husky, and there is some difficulty in swallowing. This is the first stage.

Thirst develops and the patient attempts to drink, but the moment water approaches his mouth, a spasmodic shudder comes over him; he pushes it back with horror. Thenceforward he can swallow no fluids; he complains of pain and stiffness about his neck and is thrown into convulsions by the sight of water or even the sound of liquids, or by draughts of air, or bright lights. His throat is full of viscid saliva which he tries to swallow, and he becomes breathless. Between convulsions, in which he struggles and sometimes strives to bite his attendants, and comparative stillness, during which he suffers great depression of spirits, he passes three or four days, and then dies either paralyzed, or unconscious with heart failure.

Treatment. Immediate drainage of the wound by incision so that bleeding occurs, followed by cauterization with pure carbolic acid is essential within an hour of the injury being received, and the anti-rabic inoculation treatment should then be given. Lacerated wounds on the face are generally the most dangerous.

The Pasteur preventive inoculation treatment is now given in all cases in which it can be procured. The vaccine can be sent by mail or air. Many countries now produce anti-rabic vaccines but they vary greatly in strength and method of preparation.

The immunity lasts for three months—long enough to prevent development of the disease after the bite.

Rheumatic Fever

This is a very painful affection, involving various joints, and generally affecting the heart. The cause is not exactly known, although it is thought to be a form of streptococcal infection. The disease often develops after exposure to wet and cold, when living conditions are unhygienic or damp, after tonsillitis, or with septic conditions of the mouth such as decayed teeth or pyorrhea. The disease is somewhat different in adults and children, and is most common in adults between 15 and 35 years. There is probably an inherited tendency to the disease.

Symptoms. There may be an attack of tonsillitis or sore throat before the disease starts. The principal characteristics are: sudden onset with high fever, with a soft rapid pulse; furred tongue; profuse sweat, which has a sour smell and seems to increase the weakness without relieving the pain; scanty and high-colored urine with brick-dust sediment; and swelling of the joints, with redness, great tenderness and severe pain, which is particularly agonizing when the patient attempts to move. There is also loss of appetite, vomiting, constipation, and there may be sleeplessness from pain.

This affection often changes suddenly from one part of the body to another, or from one set of joints to another, several joints often being affected at once. The joints most commonly affected are the knees, ankles, wrists, elbows, and shoulders; the spine, jaw and fingers are only rarely attacked. The affected joints are hot, swollen, red and very painful on movement.

Rheumatic fever causes inflammation of the heart muscle (rheumatic carditis) and often attacks the lining of the valves of the heart (endocarditis), causing incompetence or obstruction, mitral stenosis being a common result. The heart muscle itself also suffers from increased strain which may ultimately prove fatal. In any case the heart is liable to suffer permanent damage.

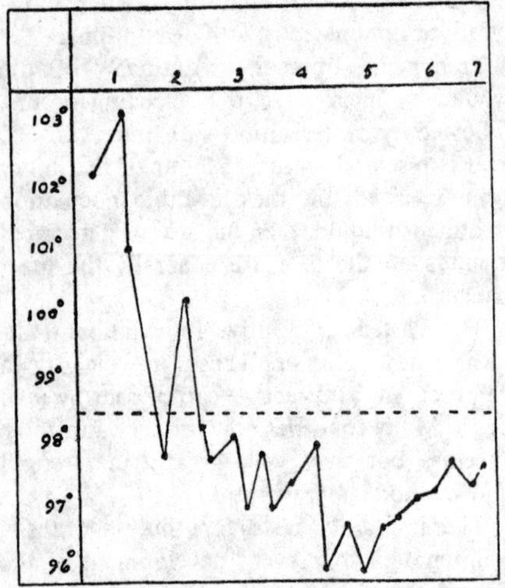

Fig. 33. *TEMPERATURE CHART IN ACUTE RHEUMATISM. The rapid fall in temperature is due to the use of sodium salicylate.*

The course is variable and the affection may subside quickly or may persist for weeks or months. Recurrent attacks are common, with increasing damage to the heart. (See pp. 297 and 298.)

The **complications** of rheumatic fever involve lung inflammation (pneumonia and pleurisy), chorea, rashes, rheumatic nodules especially on the elbows, wrists, shoulder-blades and spine, and permanent injury to the valves of the heart, or dilatation of the heart muscle. The immediate mortality from rheumatic fever is low, but the indirect eventual mortality from heart injury is high. In children the expectation of recurrence is 25 per cent, while in young adults it is less than 4 per cent.

Rheumatic fever in children is more insidious than in adults, since the joint swellings and pain are often mild and are not noticed.

Treatment. General Care. The patient should preferably be nursed in hospital and must be kept recumbent, resting in bed for a prolonged period, and for at least a month after the temperature becomes normal. About two months is a minimum period of rest, which must be extended to six or eight months if the heart is affected. A laxative should be given at the onset. A light diet of milk and cereals, with fluids and lemonade is advised for two weeks, and good nursing is essential, the patient being kept between blankets, and disturbed as little as possible.

Once the fever and the swelling in the joints are eased a good general diet should be given with ample fresh fruit and vegetables, and average helpings of meat or fish: up to two pints of milk daily is usually given.

For relief of pain locally in the joints, a liniment of wintergreen oil may be applied. (This preparation is a *poison*, and must be kept from the reach of children.) The joints may be loosely wrapped in warm cotton, and lightly bandaged in position.

Drug Treatment. As it is thought that the disease is due to the sensitivity of the patient to the toxins of the streptococcus organism which causes the sore throat and tonsillitis, the patient is put on penicillin injections at first and then maintained on penicillin tablets for weeks or months according to the individual case. Removal of tonsils is seldom a problem.

Salicylic acid and its salts, the salicylates, or aspirin, is the specific treatment; when given at the commencement of an attack, salicylates often arrest the course of the malady. This drug exerts such a beneficial influence that it is recognized as a specific. From 1.2 to 2 grams of sodium salicylate (aspirin added if gastric trouble) should be given every two to three hours to adults until relief is obtained and temperature falls. This usually takes place in from twelve to thirty-six hours. The dosage of the salicylate preparation may then be reduced to about half the above amounts. In most cases the fever and swelling will abate within the above time; if not entirely arrested, the disease is very much shortened. Vertigo, headache, or ringing in the ears indicate that the salicylate administration should be reduced. Paracetamol tablets may be needed if the pain is very severe at night.

Convalescence. After the long period of rest in bed, return to activity must be gradual. It is usually best for a child to go for a while to a convalescent home, preferably the sanatorium type, where he will have adequate supervision.

If there is obvious heart damage the child must never engage in strenuous sports and should be educated for a sedentary job. On the other hand undue fuss and care may create a neurosis. Choice of occupation should be guided by the doctor.

Sandfly Fever

(Phlebotomus Fever)

On the Mediterranean coast a fever called sandfly fever develops as a result of bites by sandflies. It runs a very short course, lasting for three days.

Symptoms are a severe headache behind the eyes, very flushed face and red eyes, and muscular pains. The pulse is slow.

There is no rash, no complications follow and the disease is never fatal.

Prevention is by clearing away rubbish, using insect sprays to kill sandflies, and using netting on windows and doors.

Sarcoidosis

Sarcoidosis is an uncommon diffuse systemic disease which may affect almost every organ of the body, but the exact cause is not yet known. It is believed to be an atypical reaction to tuberculosis which it resembles, except that it does not lead to the soft ulceration known as 'caseation' characteristic of tuberculous disease.

In most cases the disease first shows itself as swellings or nodules in the lymphatic glands, the lungs, the skin or the eye, but is often more widespread in other organs without obvious symptoms. Leprosy, chronic brucellosis, and some fungus infections give rise to similar nodules, and occasionally tuberculous bacilli, with a low infective power, have been found in sarcoid skin lesions. Active tuberculosis sometimes develops in the later stages of seriously affected patients.

Sarcoidosis may develop at any age, but most commonly occurs in young adults.

Signs and Symptoms. The nodules may be sparsely scattered, or generalized and widespread. The patient may not feel ill, and the disease may only be discovered by a routine X-ray examination of the lungs. In other cases there may be a high temperature with enlargement of the liver or spleen.

The course of the disease has sometimes been considered as moderately benign, with about 25 per cent of cases showing a slow regression of symptoms over months or years, though disabling scars may remain. Other patients show exacerbations and periods of improvement over a long period, or there may be a sudden rapid progression after apparent arrest of the disease.

The Lymph Glands. The commonest sign is enlargement of lymph glands, particularly in the chest, usually only one group or scattered nodes being affected. The glands are firm, non-adherent, and are not tender; swelling may subside completely or persist after acute exacerbations.

Lungs. The symptoms are generally mild, with only slight breathlessness on exertion and slight cough without expectoration of sputum. The disease may subside gradually, or the patient may remain relatively free from symptoms until some acute flare-up develops. After several years, affected lungs may become scarred and fibrous, with resulting shortness of breath, and eventual failure of the right side of the heart. The outlook for pulmonary sarcoidosis is variable: in about a third the disease regresses, in another third fibrosis of the lung tissue follows, and the remainder deteriorate.

Skin Lesions. When skin nodules occur, they generally appear on the face, the chest, abdomen, or extensor sides of the hands and feet. At first they are bluish-red, later fading to a yellowish-brown, without ulceration. The so-called chilblain-lupus (lupus pernio) develops in bluish-red raised patches on the face, nose and ears, or the backs of the hands and fingers; these plaques sometimes ulcerate and leave disfiguring scars.

The Eyes. The eyelids or any part of the eye may be involved, with the possibility of eventual blindness.

The Bones. The bone marrow shows the first signs of involvement in about 15 per cent of cases. Rarefaction of the finger and toe bones is usually painless.

THE LIVER AND OTHER ORGANS. Some enlargement of the liver and spleen occurs in about 33 per cent of cases at some stage of the disease. In a few cases the parotid gland, the facial or other nerves, the heart muscle, the brain and meningeal membrane, the pituitary gland, or the kidneys are affected.

GENERAL SYMPTOMS. These are not very marked or serious in the earliest stages. There is sometimes slight malaise with mild fever, fatigue, a little loss in weight, weakness, loss of appetite, and vague pains in the arms and legs.

Diagnosis. This is made by microscopical examination of a portion of lymph gland, skin nodule, or other tissue, or by X-ray examination of the chest, and the disease must be distinguished from miliary tuberculosis, Hodgkin's disease, and cancer of the lung.

Treatment. So far there is no specific treatment known for the cure of sarcoidosis. Arsenic and X-ray irradiation have been tried but are not used nowadays. Streptomycin has been given a trial, without much effect. Calciferol has led to some improvement in a few cases but is not always well tolerated, and the dosage needs to be carefully controlled.

When acute symptoms are present, rest in bed, with careful attention to the general condition, and supportive measures are required. Cortisone and prednisolone have been used to suppress the worst symptoms but they do not cure the disease. Complications such as tuberculosis or heart failure, which develop in the long-standing cases, must be given the necessary care when they appear. Sarcoidosis which involves the hilar lymphatic glands of the chest usually subsides spontaneously within twelve months but when the lung is involved, the outlook is not so good.

In subacute cases, with eye involvement, skin nodules, erythema nodosum, and parotid and lymph gland enlargement, remissions are common; recurrence after corticosteroid treatment is rare. In more chronic cases, remissions are much less common, and relapses generally follow corticosteroid administration. So far it has not been proved that steroids will prevent the progression of symptoms except in subacute iridocyclitis.

Since sarcoidosis is possibly related to tuberculosis, anti-tuberculosis chemotherapy may also be prescribed: PAS 5.0 grams and isoniazid 0.1 gram should be used in combination and taken by mouth twice daily.

Hormone therapy is also useful when sarcoidosis involves the eyes, lungs or heart, or when fever is prolonged.

Smallpox

(*Variola*)

Smallpox is an infectious virus disease characterized by a rash with blebs and pustules which leave severe pocks, or pits, associated with fever. Two types are now recognized: variola major and the much milder form, variola minor; in the former type the death rate is about 20 per cent, whereas in the latter it is only about 0·2 per cent. Vaccination is effective against both forms.

Smallpox is a notifiable disease. Contacts should be in quarantine for sixteen days and every member of the household vaccinated.

The fever precedes the eruption by three or four days, diminishing when the eruption is developed, and recurring when it has reached its height. The period between exposure and the attack of the disease, called incubation, is from ten to fourteen days, usually twelve days, being shorter in severe cases and longer in milder forms. One attack usually confers immunity.

Symptoms. The disease begins suddenly with languor and lassitude, shivering, and pains in the head and loins; with hot skin, quickened pulse and breathing; with thirst, loss of appetite, sore throat and furred tongue; with nausea, vomiting, constipation, restlessness and prostration. In children convulsions are common. To these symptoms sometimes succeed difficult breathing, cough, drowsiness and even delirium. The tongue, white at first, soon becomes red at the tip and over the whole surface. The fever is highest during the night. The constitutional symptoms are more severe before the initial eruption, which may resemble measles or scarlet fever, but subside when the true rash is developed, usually about the fourth day. Fever then recurs as 'secondary fever' about the eighth day.

The eruption is at first in the shape of small red points, which are hard to the touch and shaped like a cone; within a few hours they feel 'shotty', and after about five days form blebs, which are pitted in the center. They are most numerous on the face, scalp, hands, feet and shoulders. Itching is severe and the skin is painful. The blebs then become dome-shaped pustules with reddened areas around. About the tenth day the pustules break and after discharging pus form scabs before healing. Scabs may remain for four weeks and when they fall off they leave behind small permanent scars.

In severe attacks or unfavorable cases the patient passes into the typhoid state in about eight days, with extreme prostration, and may die in about fourteen days.

When the rash is confluent the early symptoms are more severe than when the spots are discrete, and the pustules which form may develop into abscesses. The skin is much swollen and the eyes close. Complications are more common in the confluent type. In hemorrhagic smallpox, which is fatal, hemorrhage occurs in the pustules.

Complications. Bronchitis and bronchopneumonia commonly occur. The pustules may involve the eyes or larynx, and on the face may cause unsightly pocks or scars. Nephritis and septicemia may also develop as complications.

Treatment. Cases of suspected or diagnosed smallpox should be removed at once to a special hospital.

There is, as yet, no known specific curative treatment, but penicillin should be given early to diminish pus formation. The ordinary uncomplicated form of smallpox requires careful symptomatic treatment. Confinement in bed, a fluid diet as well as cooling drinks and ice to suck, a cool and even temperature, frequent change of linen and sponging the body with cool water are required, and a daily bath of weak potassium permanganate may be given. The hair should be cut short. Pain in the early stages may require sedatives or morphine. When the fever of invasion is past, and the eruption is fully developed and secondary fever has occurred, some mild laxative should be given to keep the bowels open. Calamine lotion will allay skin irritation. Doses of chloral hydrate will also relieve itching and assist sleep.

Should the patient at this period appear to be sinking, a more generous diet and a little wine and brandy may be allowed. If the brain is affected and delirium develops, apply cold ice-cloths or iced boric compresses to the head, or an ice-bag behind the ears. An antiseptic dusting-powder or calamine lotion will relieve irritation.

Gargles will be needed frequently for the inflammation of the mouth and throat. Tepid sponging may be beneficial in both the primary and secondary fever. Thin starch and linseed compresses, or painting with 1 per cent solution of potassium permanganate, applied to the face, help to arrest pus formation, and prevent the unsightly scars which so often cover the face of persons who have suffered from smallpox. Frequent steam inhalations will relieve the laryngitis and bronchitis. The fluids given in the early stages should be supplemented with semi-solids such as jellies, soft cereals, custards, etc., when the rash has developed. Fruit juice and glucose drinks may be given freely.

Continuous warm baths are valuable to hasten separation of scabs. The eyes must be especially cared for by bathing with boracic lotion, and applying vaseline to the lids. Boils and abscesses require surgical treatment.

Isolation must be continued until all crusts have separated, the patient being kept in bed. Several months may elapse before normal activities can be resumed.

Prevention. A thiocarbazone drug is useful in the prophylaxis of variola infections. Doses are given to contacts in epidemics for three successive days. But it has no capacity to influence the disease once the rash begins to appear. Vaccination is much more effective.

IMMUNIZATION. Vaccination to give persons immunity against the attack of the smallpox virus has been used since 1798 when Jenner inoculated vaccinia (cowpox) into human beings. Vaccination is the only known safeguard and all children should be vaccinated, soon after four months of age if possible. There is a very slight risk of encephalitis if it is undertaken in adults.

Smallpox vaccination is usually placed on the outer upper part of the left arm, but the outer thigh or leg may be used. About three days after inoculation with the calf lymph, a small spot develops at the site, reaching its height about the eighth day when it is pustular. The pustule dries within a couple of days and a week or so later the scab falls off leaving a small scar. See also p. 266. For vaccinia reaction in pregnancy, see p.505.

REVACCINATION should be carried out after three years because most people have lost their immunity by then. Further revaccination should be done every five years.

If vaccination does not 'take,' it should be tried three times, using fresh lymph and/or a fresh site. Vaccination performed in the first four days of incubation, after a person has been exposed to smallpox, will usually protect him. If vaccination has been performed at any time during life, the chance of contracting smallpox is very small, and if it does occur, the disease will be mild.

Varioloid

(*Modified Smallpox*)

Varioloid, or modified smallpox, occurs in vaccinated people, and begins with symptoms similar to those of smallpox but subsiding more quickly when the rash develops. These symptoms include feverishness, nausea, vomiting, pains in the loins and head, and a quickened pulse. The eruption appears on the third or fourth day, and resembles that of smallpox. It reaches its height the fourth or fifth day, and then declines without any secondary fever. The pustules dry up and form brown scabs which fall off in a few days, and leave slight pits, and a few red or purple spots. Within five years of vaccination the disease is very seldom severe.

Yellow Fever

Yellow fever is an endemic virus infection spread by mosquitoes and is particularly prevalent in West Africa, the West Indies, and North and South America. The patient becomes severely jaundiced and has hemorrhages, especially from the stomach, which causes a black vomit. The onset is sudden after a short incubation period; there are three stages to the disease; (1) with continued fever, severe headache, pains in the back, and commencing jaundice; (2) a period of remission which may pass on into convalescence in mild cases, or may end in death after vomiting of blood and suppression of urine; (3) the secondary fever, the critical stage in most cases, with prostration, abdominal pain and vomiting. In favorable cases the patient improves after about a week, but may die if the vomiting and jaundice are severe. The mortality rate in white people is about 10 to 15 per cent.

Treatment consists in careful nursing, cold bland fluids by mouth, no food for three to four days and alkaline drinks of sodium bicarbonate and dextrose. Ice may be sucked, and cold sponging is used to allay high fever. Stimulants may be needed if heart failure threatens, or vomiting is severe.

Prevention. Preventive treatment consists in isolation of infected persons and anti-mosquito measures.

One subcutaneous dose of Yellow Fever Vaccine confers immunity for several years. For a person going abroad inoculation against yellow fever should be given four days before smallpox vaccination, otherwise a twenty-one-day interval may be needed.

Other Virus Diseases

There are many rare diseases coming to light today which are believed to be caused by viruses. Sometimes these are demonstrated, as in cat-scratch fever and those alimentary upsets caused by various enteroviruses. However, many diseases have as yet no proven etiology and their cause is often laid at the door of the virus. It is in this field especially that important advances of the future are to be made in the research laboratories of great institutions.

The great hope is that one day an antivirus antibiotic will be found. As yet only a few substances, e.g. interferons, have been found to have any inhibiting effect whatsoever, but many investigators have high hopes of success.

TABLE SHOWING THE DIFFERENCES BETWEEN SMALLPOX, VARIOLOID, AND CHICKENPOX

SMALLPOX

First. Period between exposure and onset of disease is from seven to sixteen days; the disease usually develops in ten or twelve days.

Second. Fever and temperature are high (103° F), but diminish after the rash appears.

Third. The rash appears on third or fourth day and is seen first on the forehead or some part of the face, and wrists, then to the arms and trunk. The rash is always more pronounced on the limbs than trunk. No rash in axillae.

Fourth. The eruption first consists of bright red pimples, then umbilicated watery blisters which become dome-shaped pustules. These rupture on the tenth day, exude pus, and then dry up. There may also be various initial rashes, resembling measles, chickenpox or urticaria.

Fifth. The tongue is coated and swollen.

Sixth. The eyelids are swollen and the eyes closed.

Seventh. Sore throat is often present. Delirium and convulsions may occur.

Eighth. Secondary fever develops after about eight days.

Ninth. Vision may be affected but by modern treatment this can usually be avoided. Confluent, hæmorrhagic and other less common types of smallpox also occur.

VARIOLOID

This modified form of smallpox occurs in vaccinated persons.

First. Period of incubation more irregular than Smallpox; may be ten to twenty days—average twelve days. Initial symptoms severe.

Second. Fever high until rash is well developed and then greater and more rapid improvement occurs than in Smallpox.

Third. Eruption appears on third or fourth day, and fever declines.

Fourth. Rash consists of pimples, vesicles and pustules of shorter duration: similar distribution to Smallpox. Pitting is rare.

Fifth. Tongue coated and swollen.

Sixth. No nasal or ocular symptoms as a rule.

Seventh. Slight sore throat. Delirium and severity of symptoms often marked at beginning but subside more quickly.

Eighth. No secondary fever, as in Smallpox.

Ninth. During convalescence, the patient often shows considerable weakness and anemia.

CHICKENPOX

First. Incubation period is from ten to twenty-one days, generally fourteen days.

Second. Very slight fever: 99° to 101° F for three or four days.

Third. Eruption appears on first or second day, on the palate, then on the trunk, and spreads slightly to limbs. Successive crops of spots often develop. Face not often severely affected. The rash is more pronounced on the trunk than the limbs and occurs under the axillae.

Fourth. Eruption consists of rose-colored spots changing to blebs in a few hours. No umbilication as in Smallpox. Spots always separate. Pustules form in forty-eight hours, which later form scabs.

Fifth. Eruption lasts about four weeks. Scabs gradually fall off, sometimes leaving small scars or slight pits.

Sixth. May be spots on palate, and scalp.

Seventh. Spots, vesicles and pustules present at same time, owing to successive crops of spots, usually on first, second and third days.

Eighth. Throat is not sore.

Ninth. The fever subsides after the third or fourth day and there is no secondary fever.

VENEREAL DISEASES

The venereal diseases often lead to much tragedy and mental suffering in the lives of the unfortunate persons who contract these forms of infection. In the early stage, when the disease might be quickly cured, the patient is often afraid to seek medical advice or treatment because he dreads that his suspicions as to the true nature of his complaint may be confirmed. He probably does not realize that the disease is much more easily cured if he is treated before the local infection has extended more widely. During this time it is possible that he may pass the disease on to another innocent person, thus often causing incalculable misery and anxiety to others.

These diseases can only be communicated by bodily contact as the organisms which cause them can only live at body temperatures; this means that they are practically always contracted during sexual intercourse, and that stories about lavatory seats are usually excuses.

A doctor, when he sees a patient with venereal disease, will treat the matter with the strictest confidence, and will not divulge the nature of the complaint even to the nearest relative. The patient may also fear that the medical adviser will condemn him as a sinful person, but in reality any doctor will be only too ready to help him. He will do all he can to prevent the tragic consequences which are only too likely to follow these diseases when they are neglected, to prevent possible spread of the infection to other innocent persons, and to ensure that any child who may be born to either a man or a woman who has had syphilis will not inherit the terrible disease from its parent.

SYPHILIS

(*Lues: The Pox: Bad Blood*)

The word syphilis comes from the Greek word meaning 'filthy.' The disease had a very early origin and was known among the Jews of the Old Testament.

It is commonly believed that syphilis was introduced into Europe when the first expedition of Christopher Columbus returned from America to Spain in 1493. The disease was spread rapidly through Europe when the names of most of the French royal family could be added to its 'roll of horror.'

Owing to its terrible late effects in giving rise to general paralysis and insanity with complete dementia, syphilis has always been regarded with fear and revulsion; but thanks to the advances of modern knowledge and new methods of treatment, the rapid spread of the disease can largely be controlled. The individual patient can now in most cases be cured with more certainty than in many other infectious diseases, for example tuberculosis or leprosy, which still take a heavy toll of human life.

In this century great advances have been made in the conquest of syphilis. The Wassermann test, the discovery of compounds of arsenic and bismuth for treatment, and the introduction of penicillin and other antibiotics have revolutionized the outlook in cases of syphilis provided treatment is started early.

Cause. Syphilis is a specific infective disease which may be acquired, or which may be inherited from a syphilitic parent. This disease, with all its train of symptoms, is caused by a minute, spiral-shaped motile germ which, in acquired cases, gains entrance to the body through the skin or mucous membranes. It is usually passed from person to person during sexual intercourse. In hereditary syphilis the germ passes through the mother's womb and the placenta into the blood of the developing child.

The micro-organism of syphilis (Fig. 1) is the *Treponema pallidum* and it is found in the sore at the site of the primary infection, in the blood, and in different organs of the infected patient. By bacteriological methods it is now possible to test the blood serum to demonstrate syphilitic infection; this test is called the Wassermann reaction.

Acquired Syphilis

Course. In this form of the disease the primary sore, or chancre, develops after some weeks at the point of infection, usually on the tip of the penis, or on the labia in women. If the patient is not treated by a doctor, or only has inadequate treatment, the primary sore is followed by the secondary rash, and then by a dormant stage until the late or tertiary symptoms develop. These tertiary manifestations may appear in the form of disease of the skin, or of the mucous membrane of the mouth or throat, or they may involve the blood vessels, the bones, brain, or abdominal organs, and the disease may end with foul ulcers or with general paralysis and insanity, or in other tragic ways.

Symptoms. Since syphilis is generally acquired through promiscuous sexual intercourse with an infected person, the primary sore develops on the external sexual organs after a varying incubation period of ten days to eight weeks, the usual time being about three weeks. In cases where infection has occurred through the lips or mouth from kissing, the sore develops in this area where the micro-organisms actually gain entrance.

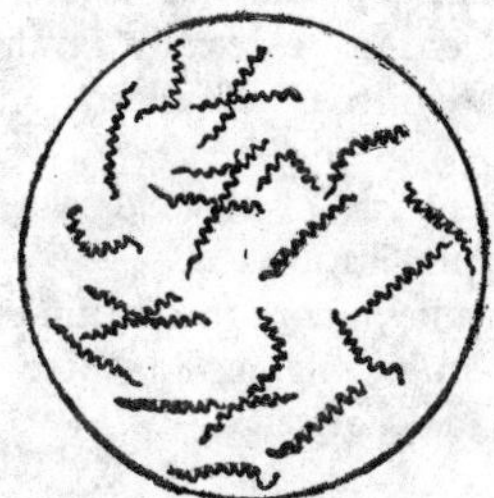

Fig. 1. *TREPONEMA OF SYPHILIS. The spiral or wave-like shape of this micro-organism enables it to rotate with great energy and rapidity.*

The Primary Stage. This consists of the characteristic hard sore which appears first as a small red patch on the glans of the penis in a man; or in a woman on the inner side of one of the lips of the vulva, on the clitoris, or on the neck of the womb. Hard, enlarged glands can generally be felt in the groin, but these do not form abscesses. The typical sore has a hard grayish base and hard edges; this sore is painless, with little discharge.

The chancre usually heals after a variable period, even without treatment; but occasionally spreading ulceration follows which may cause considerable destruction of the parts.

The Wassermann blood test is not of any value in diagnosis until about two to six weeks have elapsed after the appearance of the primary sore.

The Secondary Stage. This usually follows about six to eight weeks after the first infection and may last for about two years. The symptoms vary in severity, being more marked in debilitated or untreated persons, or they may be very slight in others.

There are usually some constitutional disturbances, with malaise, fever, anemia, sore throat, loss of hair, headache, and sleeplessness. Various types of rash develop; the commonest consists of flat or raised roundish red patches; in other cases pustular spots, scaly patches, blebs, or ulcers with crusts are seen. In general the spots, or syphilides, are rose-colored or have a brownish tint; there may be only a few but they tend to be symmetrically distributed and they do not cause pain nor do they itch.

In the throat the tonsils are swollen, with small gray ulcers, and the whole lining of the mouth and the tongue are inflamed, while there may also be hoarseness from inflammation of the larynx.

Flat gray ulcerated patches are seen at the angles of the lips or inside the mouth, on the uvula, soft palate, cheeks, or tongue.

Warty gray patches (condylomata) form about the anus or vulva, or on the toes, or beneath the breasts in women.

The lymphatic glands all over the body are enlarged.

In the eyes, iritis (or inflammation of the iris) is common, and retinitis (or inflammation of the nerve layer at the back of the eye) also occurs.

In the bones, the tibia may develop painful nodes (periostitis), while 'wandering pains' may be felt, especially at night. Arthritis sometimes occurs, especially in the knees. The nails are brittle, with ulceration around the bases.

Acute nephritis of the kidneys is a less common complication.

In pregnancy, abortion sometimes occurs.

The blood vessels may become diseased with resultant gangrene.

The Tertiary Stage. This may be delayed for some time after the primary stage, usually beginning within two to ten years, although up to thirty years may intervene.

Chronic inflammation may affect any part of the body.

The gumma, which is the typical tertiary manifestation, is a hard painless swelling that may form in any part or organ of the body. Gummata are often seen in the skin, muscles, or mucous membrane. When a gumma is near the surface the center part may soften, leaving a whitish ulcer, which is circular, with steep walls and a punched-out appearance, and there is often a foul discharge. Gummata usually heal quickly when anti-syphilitic treatment is given, except when they are formed in the brain. They may be absorbed or, when ulceration has occurred, leave a thin 'tissue paper' scar after healing. Gummata tend to recur readily, and when they develop in sites such as the larynx or rectum they may cause severe deformities and interference with the use of the part.

In the skin, syphilitic ulcers, tubercular syphilides, syphilitic lupus and other skin eruptions are seen. The nose, palate and larynx are often partially destroyed by ulceration and deformity.

The internal organs, especially the brain blood vessels, aorta (which is liable to be the site of an aneurysm), the liver, testes and bones are often diseased in late syphilis.

In the condition called leukoplakia the tongue is covered with thick whitened patches and fissures, which may later develop into cancer.

TABES DORSALIS (locomotor ataxia) and GENERAL PARALYSIS OF THE INSANE are late results of tertiary syphilis (see Diseases of the Nervous System). Blindness resulting from disease of the optic nerves may also develop.

Treatment

PENICILLIN. The treatment of syphilis has progressed greatly since the introduction of penicillin.

In early cases it is now possible to overcome the infection with procaine penicillin injections given daily for ten days in sero-negative cases. Although stay in hospital is unnecessary, sexual intercourse must not be allowed for six months in case of relapse. Blood tests are required every three months for at least two years before cure is quite certain, but results are very good provided the patient seeks medical help early.

In later cases results are not so rapid or favorable, and patients with advanced syphilis require careful prolonged treatment which cannot be given in such an intensive course as in early cases. When the heart or nervous system is affected intensive treatment is dangerous.

In pregnancy it is very important that treatment be given early to prevent the disease being transmitted to the child.

ARSENIC PREPARATIONS. Various compounds of arsenic are used, including neoarsphenamine, oxophenarsine, tryparsamide. acetarsol, etc. It is necessary to give these medications by injection at regular intervals. During treatment the patient should avoid alcohol.

BISMUTH is still considered to be of value especially in late syphilis. It is given by intramuscular injection at intervals of 5 to 7 days for 10 to 12 weeks. It is particularly useful for patients who have become resistant to penicillin, because it can provide a cure, though a slower one, and is often given in combination with penicillin.

MERCURY, an early remedy for the disease, is now seldom employed.

POTASSIUM IODIDE is also used in advanced cases, especially when gummata have developed, since it assists in the disappearance of these swellings, but this drug must be used carefully when the breast is affected.

Congenital Syphilis

A child may inherit syphilis from either of its parents. If the mother suffers from syphilis during pregnancy and does not receive proper treatment, the infant is often stillborn, or the mother may have a miscarriage before full-term; if the child does survive it will show various manifestations or stigmata. In the same way, if a syphilitic father infects the mother at the time of conception or during pregnancy, the child will also be affected.

Syphilis is commonly passed on to the developing fetus during the later part of pregnancy. If the mother, however, undergoes treatment for syphilis before this time the child generally escapes inheriting the disease, showing the importance of early treatment in expectant mothers who are infected with syphilis.

Signs in the Child. Nearly all children who inherit syphilis show signs of the disease within the first year. The child may be apparently healthy at birth, and may not show any evidence of the disease for a few weeks.

RASH. If a child has a rash of syphilitic blebs or blisters (syphilitic pemphigus) at birth, it usually dies.

The commonest type of rash is an eruption of red spots which appear about a month after birth; these spots are most abundant on the face, buttocks, palms and soles, and the nails and hair may be shed about this time. The patchy rash often ulcerates, and leaves conspicuous scars, especially near the corners of the mouth.

NOSE AND TEETH. The nose and larynx are very often affected, causing the well-known 'snuffles,' with chronic nasal catarrh, and a varying amount of discharge which sometimes contains blood and is very contagious. The bones of the nose may be eroded and destroyed, so that the bridge becomes very flattened, producing a permanent 'saddle-nose;' or the palate may be perforated. The child has a hoarse cry, and the first teeth are often cut early but are poorly formed. The permanent teeth which appear later are typically deformed, especially in the front; the incisors are small, widely spaced, and are peg-shaped, with a notch in the lower biting edge, the so-called 'Hutchinson's teeth.'

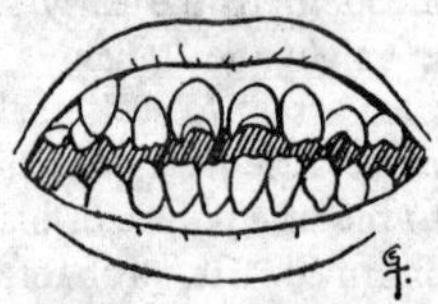

Fig. 2. *HUTCHINSON'S TEETH. The central incisors of the permanent teeth in a case of congenital syphilis are usually small and have a peg-shaped crescentic notch.*

EYE diseases in syphilitic babies are common and often lead to blindness (see also Interstitial Keratitis, p. 322).

OTHER AFFECTIONS, such as deafness, or disease of the testes, bones and joints or other structures, are common.

The syphilitic child is anemic, marasmic or wasted, with a wizened 'cafe-au-lait' colored skin.

Idiocy, different forms of paralysis, hydrocephalus (water on the brain) and general paralysis of the insane may also be caused by hereditary syphilis.

Treatment. As with acquired syphilis the specific drug treatment for infants and children suffering from the congenital form consists of penicillin, usually given by injection. Bismuth is also used in minute doses. Treatment is prolonged though not intensive, and several courses may be necessary.

It is now established that the popular belief that syphilis is inherited into the third generation is not valid. Almost invariably a congenitally syphilitic mother or father produces healthy children.

For reducing inflammation of the eye in interstitial keratitis, hydrocortisone ointment (one per cent) is very valuable, but it does not cure the underlying syphilis.

GONORRHEA

(*Clap: Blenorrhagia: A Dose*)

Gonorrhea is an infectious disease caused by the *Gonococcus* which is easily passed on to the partner in sexual intercourse. It is the second most common notifiable disease in the world today. The difficulties in eradicating it are:

its short period of incubation; its high transmissibility; cure provides no protection against reinfection; it is difficult to diagnose, especially in women who often show no outward symptoms; resistance to antibiotics of many strains of the gonococcus, especially in the less developed countries, with the result that treated patients are not cured.

The disease may also spread from the genital organs to other parts of the body, such as the rectum, the joints, the bladder and occasionally the heart or brain.

Unlike syphilis, gonorrhea causes somewhat different symptoms in men and in women, but, in general, the disease develops with a purulent discharge from the urethra (or water passage) in men, and a similar discharge from the neck of the womb and vulva occurs in women.

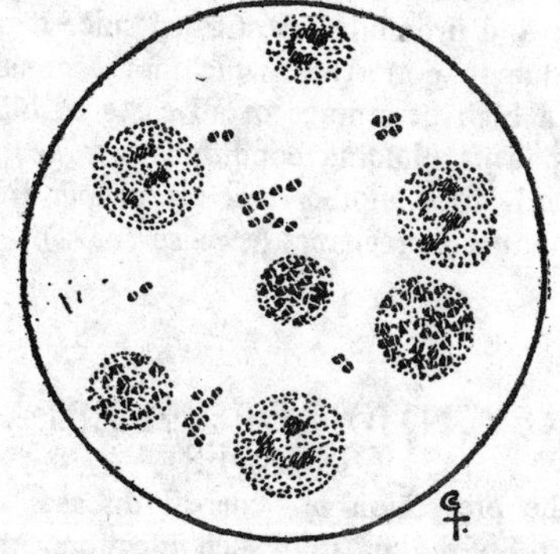

Fig. 3. *GONOCOCCI OF GONORRHEA. Some of the small paired cells of this diplococcus are shown free, and others lie within the scavenging white cells which have engulfed them and which will form pus.*

In acute and subacute stages a woman will probably be highly infectious and convey the disease to any man with whom she has intercourse, but in the later chronic stage infection is less liable to follow intercourse, and may only be conveyed intermittently. A woman is extremely likely to catch gonorrhea from an infected man.

THE GONOCOCCUS. The gonococcus is a minute kidney-shaped microbe which may often be seen lying within pus cells when these are examined under the microscope; it is a rather delicate organism and is fairly easily destroyed by cold, heat, or antiseptics. In the body, however, the gonococci penetrate the small glands below the surface of the lining membrane of the genital passages, and make the disease resistant to treatment.

Since about 1958, however, many strains of gonococcus have become resistant to the action of penicillin and other antibiotics and this makes cure of the disease a more difficult problem.

Gonorrhea in Men

In men, gonorrhea causes acute inflammation of the urethra, especially of the passage in the front part of the penis—that is, in the first six inches of the urethra; and treatment should always aim at preventing the inflammation spreading further back. It cannot be too strongly emphasized that no delay should be allowed before skilled medical treatment is sought, and that cases of venereal diseases must always be treated by a doctor.

Incubation and Symptoms. The earliest symptoms generally begin about three days after coitus with a woman who is the source of infection, although there may be slight irritation and soreness at the opening of the urethra on the second day. If treatment is sought at this early stage the disease can be aborted or cut short before it has spread down the passage, but a patient rarely attends to it until another day or more, when discharge has appeared. This discharge is at first thin but soon becomes thick, creamy and profuse, and the symptoms may rapidly become more severe, with discomfort in passing water, and inflammation and redness at the opening of the urethra. The patient is often disturbed by painful erections occurring at night. In many cases, however, there is little or no discomfort and the patient is not particularly anxious about the discharge. The condition continues for about three weeks and then in favorable cases may subside more or less completely. After six or eight weeks the infection becomes chronic and the creamy discharge becomes thin and watery, now being called 'gleet;' or it may disappear, but in the latter case the urine still contains threads of pus.

In many other cases, however, the inflammation does not subside so quickly. Even when the disease does not extend far up the urethra it persists in a less acute form for some weeks with slight discharge. In most cases after the third or fourth weeks the infection extends up the urethra and may spread to the prostate gland and to the seminal vesicles. There is much pain and frequency of passing water, and a little blood may be seen. When the disease runs this course the infection is liable to gain entrance into the bloodstream and then may involve the joints or other parts of the body.

The disease may finally subside or it may continue for months or years, with a slight discharge in the mornings.

The disease in men is thus very variable, and it is usually difficult to tell the patient how long infection is likely to last. Skilled treatment, however, shortens its course, and local treatment is very important.

The period of infection is prolonged by sexual intercourse and by alcohol.

Complications in the Male. Complications of gonorrhea may be caused by the irritating discharges, or by extension of the infection along the urethra. The disease may also be transferred to other parts of the body such as the eyes or rectum; or it may lead to general infection of the bloodstream, causing gonorrheal rheumatism, especially of the spine, inflammation of the eyes, or of the heart, especially the valves.

BALANITIS or inflammation of the prepuce. This condition may lead to phimosis or to gonorrheal warts on the foreskin.

The foreskin should be drawn back and any discharge must be washed off and the part well bathed. Repeat this treatment every three hours. If the foreskin cannot be drawn back, the penis must be bathed in warm saline for a quarter of an hour, and then cleansed by syringing under the prepuce.

PERI-URETHRAL ABSCESS. This may require aspiration, and the cavity is then filled with penicillin solution. Later, dilatation of the urethra is performed to prevent stricture.

EPIDIDYMITIS necessitates rest in bed, with a T-bandage to support the parts. Poultices or hot packs are beneficial, and penicillin or sulphadimidine are prescribed by a doctor.

ARTHRITIS. Acute gonorrheal inflammation of a joint may occur. The joint must be kept at rest with light splints or sandbags; an antibiotic and sedatives are prescribed by the medical attendant, and it may be necessary to inject penicillin solution into the joint. In chronic cases, the treatment consists in massage and exercises, with electrical treatment, and attention must be paid to any focus of gonorrheal infection in the genital or urinary organs.

INFECTION OF THE PROSTATE GLAND is common in all fairly advanced cases and leads to discomfort on passing the feces, the gland itself being swollen and tender. This inflammation may subside fairly quickly, but generally an abscess develops. Within a week or so there may then be complete inability to pass the urine, and a catheter (or rubber tube) has to be passed to relieve the distension of the bladder until the abscess breaks; it generally bursts into the urethra, but may sometimes break into the rectum or elsewhere. In acute cases the patient must rest in bed, and hot baths and compresses are useful.

Stricture. Stricture of the urethra is a late complication which can only be prevented by careful treatment. Probably 90 per cent of all cases of inflammatory urethral stricture are due to gonorrhea (see also p. 416).

Diagnosis. Acute gonorrhea in men is not difficult to diagnose, and is confirmed by microscopical examination of the discharge. In chronic cases, however, diagnosis is often very difficult, because the germs of the disease only appear periodically; but if time and trouble are taken the condition can generally be ascertained. Blood tests also may prove useful in diagnosis.

Treatment

PREVENTIVE. Gonorrhea is not generally contracted if a good quality sheath (or condom) is worn during coitus. The man should not touch the woman's sex organs before he puts the sheath on and he must handle it as little as possible after intercourse. The man

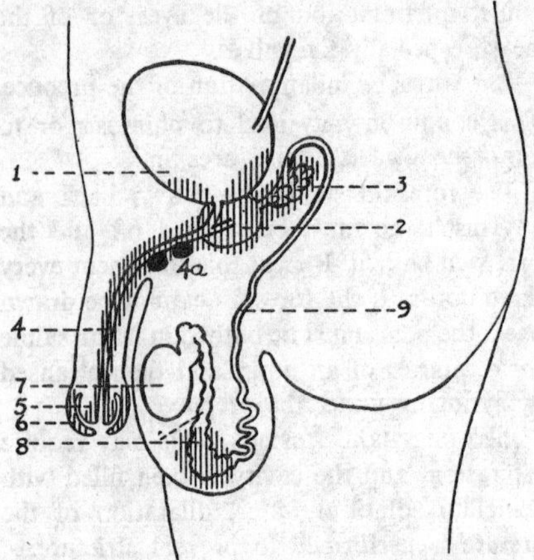

Fig. 4. *GONORRHEAL INFECTION OF MALE GENITAL TRACT (diagram of areas commonly involved). 1. Bladder. 2. Prostate gland. 3. Seminal vesicle. 4. Urethra. 4a. Peri-urethral abscess. 5. Glans penis. 6. Foreskin. 7. Testis. 8. Vas deferens. (In the bladder there is cystitis; in the prostate, prostatitis and prostatic abscess; in the urethra, urethritis; in the foreskin, balanitis; and in the epididymis, epididymitis.)*

should pass urine, and the genital parts must then be washed carefully with soap and water and as an added precaution the parts should be bathed with a 1 in 1,000 solution of mercury perchloride.

Curative. As soon as the laboratory has identified the diplococci in smears of the urethral discharge, the doctor should inject procaine penicillin and possibly benzylpenicillin and this should be repeated next day. Since many strains of the organism all over the world are becoming resistant to penicillin, tetracycline or erythromycin should be given if secretions still contain gonococci.

No alcohol should be taken for two weeks. No sexual intercourse until cure is established.

Gonorrhea in Women

In women, gonorrhea is most likely to infect the urethra and the canal of the neck (or cervix) of the womb. The outer parts, or vulva, also become irritated by the discharge which subsequently appears.

Symptoms. In the early stage there is some scalding during the passage of urine, with soreness, discomfort, and a sense of weight in the pelvis. In some cases the vulva becomes greatly inflamed with profuse discharge, but generally the symptoms are less severe and the discharge is not regarded as being very abnormal.

Complications in the Female

Bartholinian Abscess. Bartholin's glands in the vagina become inflamed and abscesses form. The fluid may be withdrawn by an aspirator and a penicillin solution injected. Chronic infection may necessitate surgical removal of the gland.

Cervical Erosion. Gonococcal infection sometimes causes acute erosion of the cervix which heals rapidly if treated with antibiotics but chronic erosions require cautery or excision.

Salpingitis. In neglected gonorrheal conditions, the sudden onset of acute abdominal pain usually indicates that the disease has spread up to the Fallopian tubes at the sides of the womb, causing fever and abdominal pain. The first attack may settle down in a few days, or it may develop into peritonitis, with suppuration or abscess formation in one or both tubes. Many cases of sterility in women are due to gonorrheal infection of the Fallopian tubes, which causes subsequent blockage so that the eggs cannot become fertilized or pass down from the ovaries into the womb.

It will therefore be seen that promiscuous intercourse holds very grave danger for women who, if they become infected with gonorrhea, may be deprived of the ability to bear children and of family happiness.

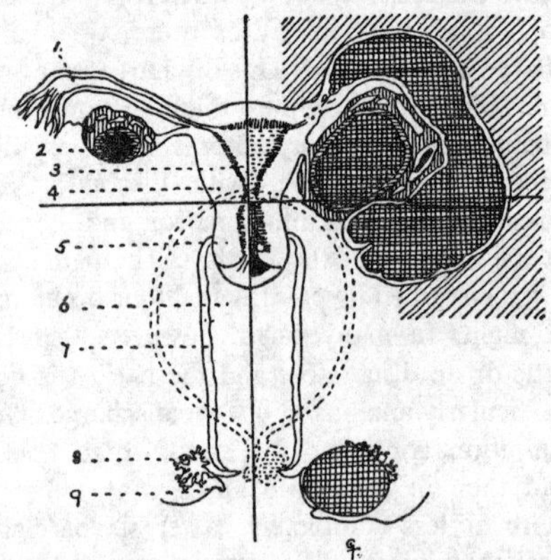

Fig. 5. *GONORRHEAL INFECTION OF THE FEMALE GENITAL TRACT (areas shaded on the unnumbered side are those commonly involved). 1. Fallopian tube. 2. Ovary and broad ligament. 3. Cavity of uterus (or womb). 4. Wall of uterus. 5. Cervix. 6. Cavity of vagina. 7. Wall of vagina. 8. Bartholin's gland in the vulva. 9. External labia.*

Pain in acute salpingitis is relieved by aspirin or other analgesics; morphine is sometimes required. The patient is nursed in a semi-recumbent position and antibiotics administered until the fever has gone. In severe chronic conditions hysterectomy may be necessary.

Proctitis. Rectal infection occurs in many cases in both men and women. Treatment is by penicillin injections plus proflavine suppositories.

Treatment. The treatment is in general the same as for men. A woman with recent gonorrheal infection should not take vigorous exercise, especially during the first menstrual period after infection. A penicillin or other antibiotic is given by a doctor, and the patient does not generally require to be kept in bed unless the disease extends to the Fallopian tubes and pelvis.

A surgical operation is sometimes necessary for the removal of the infected tubes, but this is not generally undertaken during the acute stage of inflammation.

Inflammation of the Vagina and Vulva in Girls

Gonorrheal infection of the vagina in young girls up to the age of puberty is often difficult to cure, and is liable to relapse. It is usually caught by direct contact such as may occur in sleeping with a grown-up person with gonorrhea, or from infected discharge on the fingers of an adult. Such cases in children must be treated with great care, and the child should be isolated and kept away from school and from other children.

Penicillin is the usual antibiotic used, and hot alkaline sitz baths twice daily are advised. Bismuth subgallate may be used as an external dusting-powder after bathing with dilute solution of potassium permanganate (1 in 10,000 parts).

Tests must be made before the child can be considered to be cured, or before she may be allowed to mix with other girls.

Ophthalmia Neonatorum

Any infant showing purulent or thick discharge from the eyes within three weeks after birth is notifiable by law. The case must be fully and promptly investigated since it may be due to gonorrhea which is responsible for a high percentage of all cases of blindness. This blinding condition may be prevented if the mother receives proper treatment during pregnancy (see also p. 321).

PREVENTION OF VENEREAL DISEASES

The prevention of venereal diseases and control of the spread of such infections are of immense importance to humanity. Every year unnecessary misery and untold suffering and loss of life occur as a result of these diseases which might have been prevented or avoided.

All possible means to reduce and limit the incidence of infection from syphilis or gonorrhea should therefore be taken. Young girls and young men should be instructed in the problems of sex and intercourse, with a frank warning of the dangers which attend illicit and casual relations, since in many cases the disease is caught or spread as a result of sheer ignorance.

Contacts. When a patient has contracted gonorrhea, any likely case of subsequent infection of another person should be investigated by the patient, the doctor, or a member of the clinic staff whenever possible.

An endeavor should also be made to discover the source of the disease contracted by the patient receiving treatment, and to prevent its spread.

CHANCROID

(Soft Sore)

A soft sore, or soft chancre, sometimes develops on the genital parts after promiscuous intercourse. The sore is not due to syphilitic infection but to the germ known as *Hemophilus Ducreyi.*

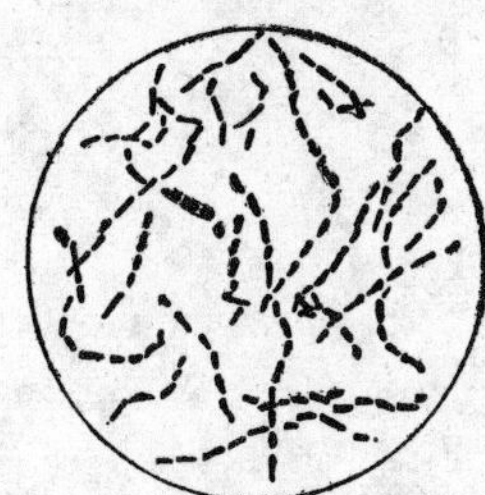

Fig. 6. *HEMOPHILUS DUCREYI, the short rod-shaped bacillus which causes chancroid, or soft sore.*

There may be one or more of these soft sores, and they are sometimes mistaken for the typical hard chancre of syphilis. Soft ulcers are also sometimes seen in the latter disease.

The incubation period of a soft sore is shorter than that of the chancre of syphilis; it generally develops within a week after intercourse. The discharge is contagious and may cause secondary ulcers, but if carefully treated it generally heals within two or three weeks. The glands of the groin swell and become tender, but as the sore heals they generally subside, although in a few cases suppuration may follow.

Treatment. Gauze dressings soaked in Eusol solution should be applied, and must be changed every four hours. If abscesses form in the glands of the groin, the pus may be drawn off by aspiration by a surgeon. The tetracyclines are effective in the cure of chancroid and may be prescribed by a doctor. Penicillin is of no value.

TRICHOMONIASIS

Leucorrhœa, or 'whites', is a fairly common complaint among women, but such cases often require to be investigated thoroughly to check on the presence of any infecting germs or bacteria.

In some cases an organism known as the *Trichomonas vaginalis* is responsible for the thin, white, irritating, vaginal discharge.

Treatment. When trichomonas is present in a case of vaginal discharge the condition may require a long period of treatment.

The doctor may prescribe tablets of metronidazole by mouth to be taken in a short intensive course. If the condition recurs, it indicates that the organism has passed during intercourse to the man's urethra where it causes him no trouble. To eliminate the organisms finally, it is advisable that both husband and wife take a short course of metronidazole tablets.

Treatment should be continued for as long as the doctor directs, until no more trichomonads can be found in the discharge.

DISEASES OF THE HEART AND BLOOD VESSELS

The amount of work accomplished by the heart is rarely appreciated, for its output amounts to something like ten tons of blood each day. For details regarding the normal functioning of the heart and the circulation of the blood, see section on Physiology, pp. 239 to 244.

The Symptoms of Heart Disease

The patient with heart disease may complain of many different symptoms. It should be emphasized, however, that each of the symptoms which is commonly found in heart disease may also be due to disease in other organs such as the lungs, the stomach, the kidneys, and the brain, the heart itself being normal. On the other hand, there may be no symptoms at all, and an abnormal heart may be found only on examination, for example, for life insurance. A complaint of one or more of the following symptoms should, however, direct attention to the heart.

Shortness of Breath, or Dyspnea. This is the most common, and perhaps the most important symptom of heart disease. It points to failure of the heart, early or late, although alone it is not evidence of heart failure unless other causes (such as lung diseases and anemias) have been excluded. The commonest type of breathlessness occurs on exertion, and it may occur long before the appearance of any other symptoms. If the patient becomes more breathless year by year, or month by month, by climbing the same hill, a gradual exhaustion of the heart's reserve may be presumed, in the absence of other causes.

PAROXYSMAL BREATHLESSNESS occurring at rest or during sleep, and causing the patient to awaken, is found in certain forms of heart disease. The patient wakes with a sense of oppression or suffocation, and sits by an open window seeking relief. The breathing is labored and wheezing, and distress may be very great. It is often accompanied by a cough with frothy and blood-tinged sputum. The attack may continue for a few hours, though it is often reckoned in minutes. It is commonly known as 'cardiac asthma.'

Palpitation. The patient is conscious of his heart beats, which he may describe as bumping, throbbing or fluttering in the chest, or he may be conscious of the heart missing a beat, or 'turning over.' The symptom is more common in excitable states of the nervous system than in true heart disease.

Pain in the Region of the Heart. Pain occurs frequently without much evidence of heart disease, and a diagnosis may have to rest on this symptom alone.

ANGINA PECTORIS. This may be a pain of extraordinary severity. It arises beneath the breast-bone, usually in its upper part, and is described as crushing or gripping in character, or as a sense of weight or tightness in the chest. Not uncommonly the patient refers to it as indigestion. It may pass towards the tip of the heart, and often to the neck, and down the inner aspect of the left arm as far as the elbow or the finger tips. The pain is usually so severe that the patient stops whatever he is doing, and stands motionless until it passes away in two or three minutes. The symptom is generally brought on by effort.

OTHER FORMS OF HEART PAIN. Pain in the region of the heart may be brought on by many other causes besides actual heart disease, and they should be carefully distinguished from the anginal type of pain just described.

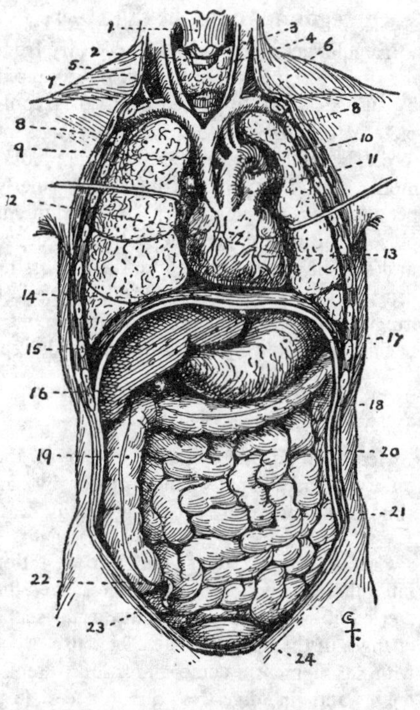

Fig. 1. *HEART AND LARGE BLOOD VESSELS IN RELATION TO OTHER IMPORTANT ORGANS.* 1. *Thyroid cartilage.* 2. *Thyroid gland.* 3. *Internal jugular vein.* 4. *Common carotid artery.* 5. *Trachea.* 6. *Subclavian vein.* 7. *Transverse cervical vein.* 8. *Lungs, retracted by hooks.* 9. *Superior vena cava.* 10. *Arch of aorta.* 11. *Pulmonary artery.* 12. *Heart.* 13. *Coronary blood vessels.* 14. *Diaphragm.* 15. *Liver.* 16. *Gall-bladder.* 17. *Stomach.* 18. *Transverse colon.* 19. *Ascending colon.* 20. *Descending colon.* 21. *Small intestine.* 22. *Cecum.* 23. *Appendix.* 24. *Bladder (urinary).*

Transient pain occurring over the tip of the heart is most usual in certain neurotic states, especially after fatigue. Aching and sharp pain occurs also in muscular rheumatism and neuralgia affecting the muscles and nerves of the chest. This is usually worse on movement of the affected part, and there may be some local tenderness.

The pain of pleurisy is generally severe and cutting in character, and is made worse by deep breathing.

Digestive Symptoms. Loss of appetite, nausea, and distension of the abdomen may be met with in heart failure. Pain may be felt in the right upper abdomen, and the liver may be tender.

Urinary Symptoms. A decrease in the quantity of urine passed, or oliguria, may be noticed in heart failure. The urine passed is highly colored, owing to its concentration. There may be complete suppression of urine, none at all being passed in very severe cases.

Nervous Symptoms. Fainting occurs when insufficient blood reaches the brain. It is generally seen in persons of nervous temperament, from emotional causes such as shock, fright, or unpleasant sights and smells. It is usually a harmless symptom and is not a characteristic feature of heart disease. In exceptional cases, however, it may be due to actual disease of the heart.

Dropsy or **Edema.** The patient may complain of swelling of the lowest parts of the body—that is, of the ankles and feet—towards the end of the day if he is up and about, and of the lower part of the back and the backs of the thighs if he is confined to bed. It is due to a collection of fluid in the tissues beneath the skin and its distribution is controlled by gravity. It is recognized by 'pitting' on pressure with the finger tips.

Cyanosis (Blueness of the fingers, toes, lips, and cheeks). This is seen particularly in disease of the mitral valve and in congenital diseases of the heart. It is also a feature of some chronic lung diseases. Blueness is increased by cold and exertion.

DISORDERS OF HEART FUNCTION

The heart may suffer from disturbances of function in the absence of real disease.

Palpitation

This symptom is more common in nervous states with anxiety than in actual heart disease. The patient is conscious of the heart's beat, though in severe cases there may be actual pain.

People who are affected by palpitations now and then during the course of their lives usually survive to old age.

Causes. The immediate cause of an attack is usually emotion but it may be due to excessive physical exertion. It is commonly associated with states of anxiety and neurasthenia. In women, it is more common at the monthly periods and during the change of life. In men, it may be particularly noticeable during adolescence, and in soldiers who are out of training and at the same time subject to emotional stress and strain, lack of sleep, etc. In such cases it is called the 'irritable heart of soldiers.' It is seen in certain cases of goiter in the neck, or Grave's disease, and is common in digestive disturbances, especially when attended by flatulent distension; this is often due to excessive indulgence in tea, coffee, alcohol, or smoking.

Treatment. Digestive disturbances should be corrected and the consumption of tea, coffee, or alcohol reduced. Excessive smoking should also be avoided. If palpitation is due to the change of life and associated with hot flushes, alternate monthly courses of stilbestrol 0·1 to 0·5 milligrams daily, may bring relief.

If these measures fail, sedatives should be tried, and are helpful in excitable or anxious patients. Phenobarbital, 15 to 30 milligrams, may be given twice daily.

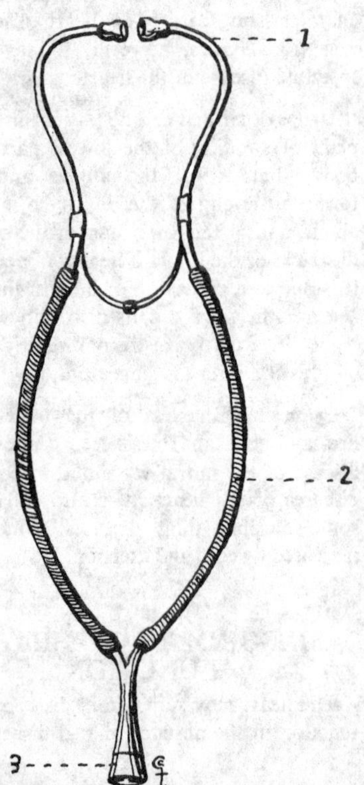

Fig. 2. *A STETHOSCOPE. An instrument for auscultation, whereby the sounds going on in the patient's body are made clearer*. 1. *Ear piece*. 2. *Rubber tube*. 3. *Chest piece*.

Abnormalities of Heart Rate

Increase in the Heart Rate
(*Tachycardia*)

A temporary increase in rate is the normal reaction to emotional excitement or physical exertion, while a more prolonged increase of heart rate is seen in various acute illnesses and during convalescence. Graves' disease (overactivity of the thyroid gland) and pulmonary tuberculosis are the commonest chronic diseases to be associated with a quick pulse. It occurs also after the excessive use of tea, coffee, alcohol and tobacco.

A special form of rapid heart beat is known as paroxysmal tachycardia. The attacks may last for a few hours to a few days, the rate of the heart beat being between 160 and 200 per minute. Any case of persistent tachycardia should be examined by a doctor.

Decrease in the Heart Rate
(*Bradycardia*)

This may occur in normal individuals, especially in athletic men and in elderly people. It is often seen during convalescence from acute illnesses, such as influenza, diphtheria, pneumonia and typhoid fever, and in jaundice. It is also a characteristic feature of underactivity of the thyroid gland which leads to the disease known as myxedema; and it is seen after the intensive use of digitalis.

Irregular Action of the Heart

Irregular action of the heart may vary from the simplest type of intermittent pulse caused by an occasional 'dropped beat,' to a complete irregularity both of rhythm and of force. Irregularities of this kind are commonly found in middle-aged and elderly people. The simpler types of intermittent pulse are often of no practical consequence and are simply due to gradual aging of the heart muscle. The more complex types of irregularity, such as auricular fibrillation, may be significant, however, of serious heart disease.

Intermission of the Pulse
(*Extrasystoles*)

Here the normal regular rhythm of the pulse is occasionally interrupted by an abnormally long pulse following a weak beat.

Causes. Extrasystoles, with the resulting intermittent pulse, are commonest over the age of 60, and are due to the usual senile changes in the heart muscle. They also occur with excitement, acute infections, septic teeth, and in digestive disturbances (e.g. heavy meals before retiring to bed), and after the excessive consumption of tea, coffee, alcohol or tobacco. Overdosage with digitalis is a not uncommon cause.

Symptoms. An individual who is subject to extrasystoles may be unconscious of their presence, or he may be aware of the long pause and complain that the heart stops, or he may feel a thud or shock in the heart. Extrasystoles are diminished by exertion and by any other condition which makes the heart beat faster.

Treatment. The most important step is to reassure the patient that an intermittent pulse is not a symptom of serious heart disease. Any obvious cause, however, should be corrected.

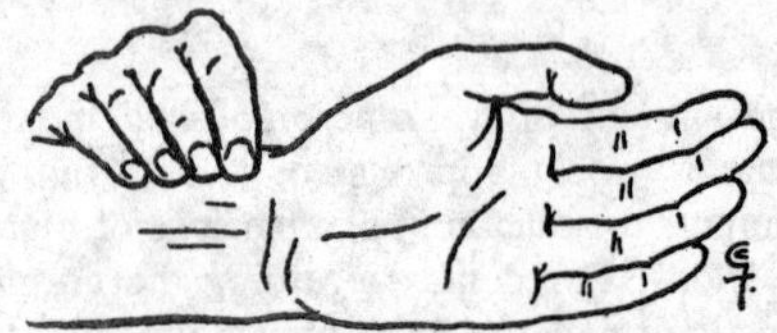

Fig. 3. *HOW TO FEEL THE PULSE AT THE WRIST. The patient should be seated or lying down for a few minutes before the pulse count is made.*

Auricular Fibrillation

In this disorder the heart rhythm is completely irregular, both in the spacing of the individual beats and in their force, the pulse at the wrist becoming small and irregular.

Causes. There are three main causes:

(1) Rheumatic fever, with resultant damage to the heart muscle and heart valves, especially mitral stenosis.

(2) Chronic heart disease from other causes such as high blood pressure and arteriosclerosis (hardening of the arteries).

(3) Hyperthyroidism (Graves' disease). The existence of auricular fibrillation indicates disease of the heart muscle.

Symptoms. There is frequently a sensation of fluttering in the chest and an awareness of the irregular action of the heart. It is accompanied also by shortness of breath on exertion, which causes a further increase of irregularity. If allowed to continue unchecked, it leads finally to heart failure.

Treatment. Digitalis must be used to reduce the rate of the heart, and to increase the force of the individual heart beats, thus improving the circulation as a whole.

Larger doses may be given at first, but as soon as the pulse has been reduced to between 70 and 80 per minute, a smaller dose should be given. The dose should be sufficient to control the heart, without causing symptoms of overdosage (loss of appetite, nausea, vomiting, diarrhea). These should lead to a temporary withdrawal of the drug and its resumption after a few days in smaller doses. The duration of digitalis treatment is often for life, and all patients taking digitalis should be examined at regular intervals.

In patients not well controlled by digitalis, propranolol (see p. 301) is often successful.

INFLAMMATION OF THE HEART
(*Carditis*)

Rheumatic Infection of the Heart in Childhood

Inflammation, usually of rheumatic origin, affects any or all of the three main parts of the heart—the inner lining or endocardium, the main muscle of the heart chambers or myocardium, and the outer sac or pericardium, which covers the heart. Rheumatic infection is the direct cause of most cases of heart disease under the age of 40.

In adult life a typical attack of rheumatism causes acute arthritis, with pain and swelling of the joints. In children, however, although the joint symptoms may be prominent, they may be vague or even absent, and

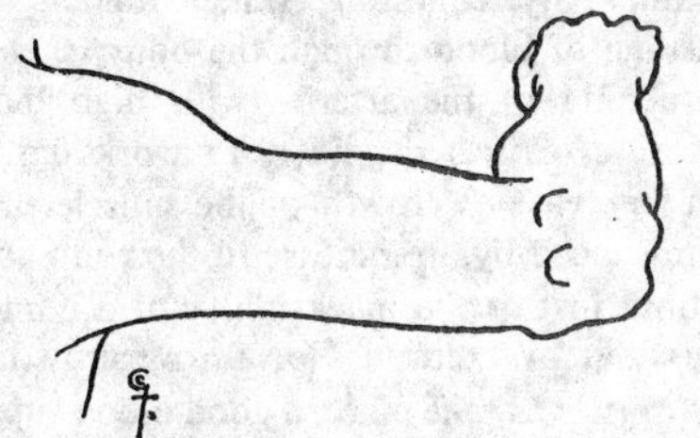

Fig. 4. *HARD NODULES in the elbows and knuckles are often found in cases of rheumatic fever.*

the rheumatism may appear in the form of various skin eruptions, pains in the legs, or 'growing pains,' 'rheumatic nodules' or small hard lumps the size of peas in the scalp and behind the knuckles and elbows, sore throat from tonsillitis, acid sweats, and chorea. Rheumatism in children is generally stealthy in onset, with complete absence of symptoms for a time. When they do appear, in the form of pallor, fatigue, loss of appetite and a failure to put on weight, they are apt to be mild, and apparently of no great significance so that they may be overlooked. In spite of this gradual onset, however, the heart damage is no less than in the highly feverish forms with typical painful swollen joints.

Any child with 'growing pains,' frequent sore throats, chorea, or rheumatic nodules behind the scalp and elbows should be protected from cold and damp, and the heart should be carefully examined.

Diseases of the Heart Lining
(*Endocarditis*)

Endocarditis is an inflammation of the lining membrane of the heart. In the great majority of cases the inflammation chiefly affects the valves, while some inflammation of the heart muscle (myocarditis) is generally also present.

Acute Endocarditis

ACUTE SIMPLE ENDOCARDITIS

Causes. Acute simple endocarditis occurs most commonly in childhood and adolescence, and in most cases is due to rheumatic infection, though it is occasionally caused by scarlet fever, pneumonia, typhoid fever and smallpox.

Symptoms. Besides the general symptoms of the main disease, usually rheumatism or rheumatic fever, there may be shortness of breath, palpitation and discomfort or pain in the heart, with an increase of fever, and a pulse rate quicker than normal.

The valves become swollen, and covered with small warty vegetations, and finally scarred, contracted and deformed.

Treatment. This aims at preventing as far as possible any permanent damage to the heart. Rest in bed for three months is essential, during which time the patient should not be allowed to do anything for himself; some further months of partial rest should follow, and a gradual attempt should be made at easy walking exercises. If at any stage any fresh symptoms appear, the amount of activity should be reduced. Children who have had an attack of acute endocarditis should be sent to a convalescent home with teaching facilities for six to eighteen months following the period of rest.

The diet should be mainly of milk, diluted with water or mineral water, and so long as there is fever, nothing should be added except peptonized milk or barley water. As the fever subsides, cereals, vegetable soups and chocolate may be added. Meat should be reserved for convalescence, and tea and coffee are best withheld.

At the outset of acute rheumatic endocarditis in an adult. 1 gram of sodium salicylate, made into a mixture which has been flavored with peppermint, should be given every 2 hours during the day and every 4 hours at night. As the symptoms subside, these quantities may be given less frequently. The dosage for a child of 12 years should be one-half of that for an adult.

Pencillin may be given in short courses if there is simultaneous infection of the tonsils.

ACUTE BACTERIAL ENDOCARDITIS; SUBACUTE BACTERIAL ENDOCARDITIS

Cause. The acute form is an uncommon but very serious disease of the heart. It is caused by a general blood infection with various micro-organisms—pneumococci, staphylococci, gonococci.

The subacute form usually follows an attack of rheumatism or other fever with endocarditis. After several years, the gradually increasing weakness of the damaged valves permits the invasion of bacteria—usually streptococci. Once infection develops in the vegetations of the heart valves, a condition of chronic blood poisoning results. Small pieces (emboli) of the vegetations may break off from the valves and, after being carried by the bloodstream, may block narrow blood vessels in the kidneys, spleen, retinae, brain, or limbs, with resultant pain, blindness, paralysis of one side, or sometimes brain hemorrhage.

Symptoms. In subacute bacterial endocarditis the onset may be sudden, with the general symptoms of an acute feverish illness and pains in the joints. The condition fails to respond, however, to treatment with sodium salicylate, and an irregular fever with repeated shivering fits (or rigors) occurs. More commonly, the onset is gradual, with slowly increasing weakness, sweats and anemia. The patient becomes increasingly anemic with a pale coffee-colored complexion, and continues to lose weight. Hemorrhages appear under the skin.

Treatment. General treatment consists of fresh air and good food, with extra vitamins and iron for the anemia. Penicillin is now used in high doses, and with this treatment the disease has a recovery rate of over 90 per cent.

Chronic Endocarditis

Chronic endocarditis is generally a sequel to the simple rheumatic type. There are, however, two other varieties, both of which are more common in men, and which appear in later life. The first of these is associated with arteriosclerosis, or hardening of the arteries. The second is the result of syphilis and generally begins in middle life.

MITRAL STENOSIS (narrowing of the mitral valve).

This, as already mentioned, is usually due to a previous attack of acute simple endo-

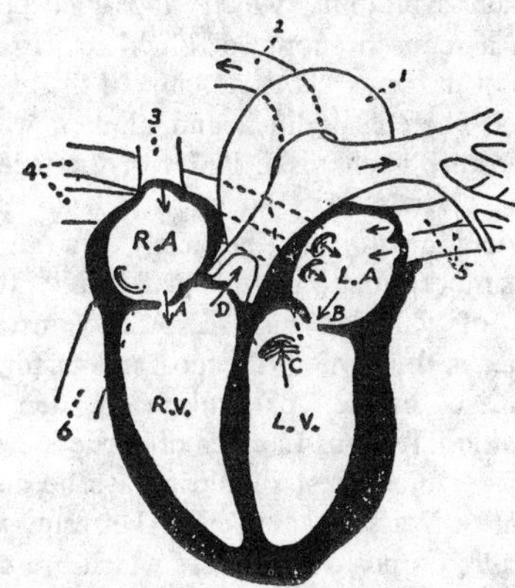

Fig. 5. *THE HEART.* 1. *Aorta.* 2. *Pulmonary artery.* 3. *Superior vena cava.* 4. *Right pulmonary veins.* 5. *Left pulmonary veins.* 6. *Inferior vena cava.* A. *Tricuspid valve.* B. *Mitral valve.* C. *Aortic valve.* D. *Pulmonary valve.* R.A. and L.A.: *Right and left auricles.* R.V. and L.V.: *Right and left ventricles.*

carditis. The two valve leaves become partly fused together, so that the opening is made much smaller. The blood is thus hindered in its passage onwards, and becomes congested in the organs behind the valve, that is, in the left auricle and the lungs; this causes shortness of breath on exertion, cough with blood-stained sputum, and bronchitis; there is usually an associated blueness of the cheeks, lips, tips of the ears and of the finger nails. Embolism is common.

MITRAL INCOMPETENCE (leaking of the mitral valve).

The most common cause of a damaged mitral valve is the weakening due to an attack of acute simple endocarditis. Incompetence of the mitral valve may also be due to a stretching of the valve after acute fevers, ànemia, disease of the aortic valve and high blood pressure. Regurgitation of the bloodstream may then occur backwards through the valvular opening because the valve fails to close. Incompetence of this type is known as functional.

In organic mitral incompetence there may be no symptoms. If present, they resemble those of mitral stenosis, which is generally also present.

AORTIC INCOMPETENCE (leaking of the aortic valve).

Aortic incompetence is most commonly found in middle or later life and in males. It is often due to a previous attack of acute simple endocarditis or rheumatic fever, although syphilis, which usually causes symptoms between 15 and 25 years after the primary syphilitic infection, is a fairly common cause.

Degeneration of the aortic valve in old age is usually associated with general hardening of the arteries. Rupture of a valve segment may very occasionally be caused by sudden physical overstrain.

Symptoms. The symptoms are often latent for many years, the commonest and the earliest being shortness of breath on exertion. Further symptoms which appear depend upon a reduced supply of blood to various parts of the body. Thus, anemia of the brain occurs. There is giddiness and faintness when the posture is changed. Pallor of the face is often associated with anemia.

Sudden death is another likely occurrence, and is more common in this than in any other form of valvular disease. Aortic incompetence is thus one of the most serious forms of heart disease, particularly if due to syphilitic infection. In cases of aortic incompetence a blood test should always be done (Kahn or Wassermann Test). The result will generally be positive in cases which are due to syphilis.

Surgical Treatment. Operative mortality is high but the prognosis, too, is grave. The damage in the stenosed aorta varies greatly in every case and consequently the results of operation vary.

Diseases of the Heart Muscle

(Myocarditis)

Acute Myocarditis

Causes. In most cases, inflammation of the heart muscle or acute myocarditis is caused by acute rheumatic infection, when it is usually associated with acute rheumatic endocarditis, and sometimes with pericarditis. Other causes a. diphtheria, influenza, pneumonia, smallpox and typhoid fever. The inflammation of the heart muscle may subside completely, the heart returning to normal, or there may be some permanent residual damage.

Symptoms. The onset may be gradual with vague symptoms, such as shortness of breath, palpitation and discomfort or pain in the heart. The pulse is fast and feeble.

In severe cases, with threatened heart failure, there may also be pallor, restlessness, faintness, vomiting without apparent cause, and coldness of the skin. Sudden death is particularly likely to occur in diphtheritic myocarditis, even when the patient may be considered to be convalescent.

Treatment. The treatment is the same as for acute simple endocarditis (p. 297), except that the period of convalescence is not so long. The patient should always be under medical supervision. In severe cases with collapse, the following measures should be adopted.

All pillows should be removed and the patient's head lowered, the foot of the bed being raised one to two feet. A firm binder should be applied to the abdomen and the patient kept warm and quiet.

Chronic Myocarditis

In fibrosis of the heart muscle, or chronic myocarditis, the heart muscle fibers are partly replaced by scar tissue, and the heart is consequently weakened. It is more common in men in late middle life and old age, and usually follows acute rheumatic disease. When it is due to arteriosclerosis it is known as senile heart.

Symptoms. These are gradual in onset, and usually appear first on exertion (tired heart). The most common are shortness of breath and fatigue, and occasionally there is palpitation and discomfort or pain in the heart. The pulse is fast, and there is usually some enlargement of the heart.

Chronic myocardial disease is overlooked more frequently than any other disorder of the heart. Examination by X-ray and by electrocardiogram may be of great value in diagnosis. The disease tends to be progressive and generally leads to congestive heart failure.

Treatment of the Senile Heart. It is important to remember that prolonged rest in bed for elderly people may lead to congestion of the bases of the lungs, with resultant infection and bouts of coughing. Complete rest should therefore be limited to the minimum period compatible with improvement. Diet in the aged presents its own problems, but in general the secret of success is to be found in moderation. All invalids and particularly elderly people should have their principal meal in the middle of the day. It should be as dry as possible, thus eliminating the tendency to flatulence.

A rest in the afternoon and a light meal in the evening will often be followed by a long night's rest. Hot milk, or a little diluted whisky taken some time before retiring may encourage sleep. Much insomnia and restlessness can be prevented by having the bed alongside an open window, and fresh air, as distinct from draughts, should be made freely available.

Enlargement of the Heart

Enlargement of the heart may be due to hypertrophy, or increase of its muscle, with thickening of its walls; or to enlargement and dilatation of its cavities; or, as is usually the case, to both of these conditions together.

HYPERTROPHY OF HEART MUSCLE. The presence of increased muscle shows that the heart is continuously working under an extra strain. Any condition which hinders the passage of blood through the body, such as hardening of the arteries with high blood pressure, causes the heart to work harder. The increase of growth of the muscle fibers is produced by an increase in their muscular action, just as the blacksmith's arm is more muscular by exertion. For an overgrowth of the muscle to take place, a good blood supply is essential. Thus it can occur more readily in young people than in the aged.

DILATATION, or enlargement of the heart cavities, may be acute or chronic.

Acute dilatation may occur in acute myocarditis from infectious diseases such as rheumatic fever, diphtheria, influenza, pneumonia, smallpox and typhoid. It may also occur in auricular fibrillation and, rarely, as

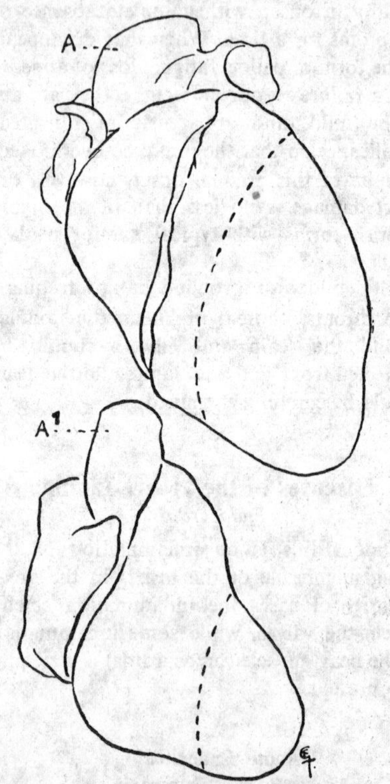

Fig. 6. *ENLARGED HEART COMPARED WITH A NORMAL-SIZED HEART.* A *is the aorta.*

a result of excessive physical exertion in persons who are out of training (primary heart strain).

Chronic dilatation is present together with hypertrophy in most cases of chronic heart disease, and may be compensatory in cases of chronic valvular disease, allowing the ventricles to accommodate a greater quantity of blood for expulsion with each heart beat. In cases of regurgitation through the heart valves, the dilatation thus allows an approximately normal quantity of blood to be passed onwards with each heart beat. Dilatation may also be associated with chronic heart failure, which brings about a lack of tone in the heart muscle. As the dilatation progresses, the amount of blood contained in the heart chambers becomes gradually increased, and the organ assumes a globular form.

Signs. When dilatation is associated with heart failure the pulse may be faster and weaker, and the blood pressure lower than normal. The enlargement of the heart may by recognized by X-ray examination.

For treatment, see Heart Failure (p. 299).

Diseases of the Heart Sac, or Pericardium

The heart sac encloses the heart, and consists of two membranous layers, which are movable one upon the other. The inner layer is closely applied to the outer surface of the heart.

Pericarditis, or inflammation of the heart sac, may be either acute or chronic.

Acute Pericarditis

This may be either dry, or accompanied by a liquid effusion between the outer and inner layers of the pericardium. In pericarditis with effusion, the liquid exudate, which may be clear, purulent or blood-stained, may actually distend the pericardial sac and produce pressure upon the heart and the surrounding structures.

Causes. Acute pericarditis occurs most commonly in young adults, and is generally due to rheumatic infection. Other less common causes are acute infectious diseases such as pneumonia, septic infections, and occasionally gonorrhea. It may occur also towards the end of chronic diseases such as Bright's disease and tuberculosis.

Symptoms. In acute dry pericarditis the symptoms may be slight or absent, but usually there is some fever and pain in the chest. The pain may be felt over the heart, or referred to the left shoulder, the left shoulder-blade, the neck or the upper abdomen. It may be made worse by deep breathing or coughing, or by pressure between the ribs over the heart. The pulse is generally rapid.

In pericarditis with effusion, the symptoms usually become worse when the effusion actually appears. Restlessness and sleeplessness, or mild delirium, with faintness, shortness of breath, an irritating cough and difficulty in swallowing may make their appearance. In children there may be actual bulging of the region over the heart.

If pus is present in the fluid the heart rate is very fast, and there is high fever and increasing pallor and collapse.

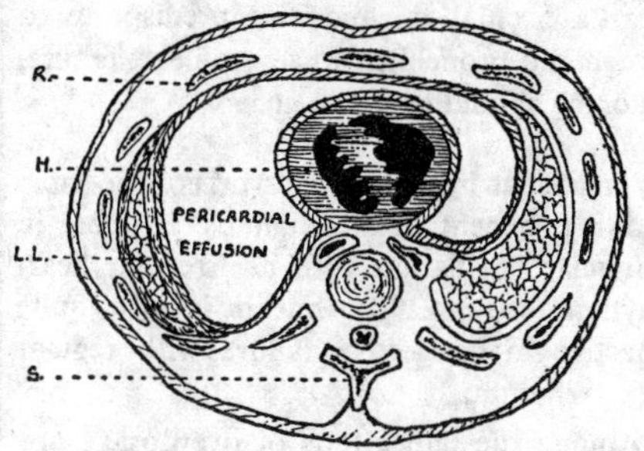

Fig. 7. *CROSS SECTION OF THE CHEST TO SHOW THE EFFECT OF PERICARDIAL EFFUSION. The pericardial sac of the heart* (H) *is distended with fluid to the extent that it reduces the size of the left lung* (L.L.) *by compressing it against the rib* (R) *cage.* S. *Spine.*

Treatment. All cases of pericarditis should be under a doctor's care. The general treatment is the same as for acute simple endocarditis (see p. 297), and of any other disease which may be present. In pericarditis with effusion, removal of the fluid is seldom necessary in rheumatic cases, since it usually becomes absorbed. It is carried out by a doctor by the insertion of a needle attached to a syringe.

HEART FAILURE

The real cause of heart failure lies in the heart muscle. It is due to changes which make it unable to carry on the proper circulation of the blood. These changes may follow valvular disease, disturbances of the heart rate as in auricular fibrillation, or diseases of the blood vessels associated with high blood pressure.

Left Ventricular Failure. This is liable to occur as a result of the increased work which the left ventricle has to do in cases of arteriosclerosis with high blood pressure, in diseases of the aortic valve, and disease of the blood vessels of the heart muscle. In left-sided failure the chief effects are upon the lungs, such as attacks of paroxysmal breathlessness or 'cardiac asthma,' often associated with copious frothy or blood-stained sputum. Left ventricular failure may be sudden in onset, and death may occur rapidly in severe cases.

Right Ventricular Failure. Right-sided heart failure is usually more gradual and occurs especially in mitral stenosis, which leads to congestion of the lungs, and in chronic lung diseases. These conditions cause extra work for the right ventricle, which, as it begins to fail leads to congestive heart failure. Congestion is apparent in several ways—in distension of the veins of the neck, in the enlarged tender liver associated with loss of appetite and nausea, in impairment of the kidney function, with scanty urine, and in dropsy, with swelling of the ankles.

Symptoms. The onset may be gradual or sudden and is shown by certain symptoms which appear on exertion. These symptoms occur as the result of less and less effort until some or all of them are present during rest. (See p. 295 at the beginning of this section).

Treatment. Both types of failure may disappear with treatment; the cause, however, remains, and the failure will recur later.

Rest. The most important question is that of rest. In cases of slight heart failure with shortness of breath, palpitation and fatigue on moderate exertion, partial rest is usually sufficient. In moderate failure with slight dropsy of the legs and a fast pulse at rest, the patient should remain in bed for at least three weeks. In severe heart failure with shortness of breath and palpitation on slight exertion with a considerable degree of dropsy of the legs, and with attacks of cardiac asthma, rest in bed is required for at least six weeks.

In all cases when a patient has had a long period of rest in bed, it should be followed by a period of partial rest (lifting to a couch or wheel chair for 15 to 30 minutes, with only a very gradual return to moderate activity). Climbing stairs should be avoided for several weeks.

Mode of Life. When some degree of activity has been resumed, it is important to live within the limits of the heart's strength, and the chief object of treatment is to prevent the recurrence of heart failure. The usual habits should not be too much restricted since the patient may become introspective and depressed. Every patient with early heart failure should be in bed for at least nine hours each night, and allow at least an hour for the midday meal. He should have one quiet day a week. With more severe degrees of impairment he should be in bed for 10 to 12 hours each night, resting for one or twoh ours after the midday meal, and should stay in bed for one day each week.

Excitement, worry, and all forms of emotional strain and exhausting activity should be avoided.

Exercise. Unnecessary tasks must be avoided, together with undue exertion. On the other hand, it is wise to take a moderate amount of exercise (walking on level ground, or a leisurely game of golf), short of producing symptoms, and always allowing for some reserve of strength. Sudden effort should be avoided, such as walking up hills or against a strong wind.

Massage. Massage is often useful for those who have not the opportunity for ordinary exercise, while simple passive movements of the limbs and light massage are beneficial in the early stages. In cases with dropsy, massage is often followed by an increased output of urine and a reduction in the amount of fluid in the limbs. It may be given for half an hour two or three times a week.

Diet. Moderation and temperance should be the chief rules of diet. Since most cases of heart disease are chronic, severe dietary restrictions are as unwise as excesses. Elderly patients with chronic heart disease are often improperly nourished, either because of dietary fads or because of unwise advice.

FLUIDS. In general the daily intake of fluids should be somewhat restricted. The meals should be as dry as the patient will take them, a sufficient amount of fluid (3 to 4 pints a day) being taken between meals, and consisting of weak tea, milk, fruit juices, aerated waters, barley water, or plain water.

MEALS. The three main meals of the day should be evenly balanced, since a large meal is likely to embarrass the heart. Meals should consist chiefly of the following articles of diet:

Fresh meat (beef, veal, lamb) in moderation, fresh fish, poultry, game (not high) and rabbit; but *no meat fat.*

Vegetables and vegetable soups and purées; salads with tomatoes; fruit (if possible fresh) and fruit juices (orange, grape-fruit, blackcurrant, or pineapple juice). Blackcurrant syrup is valuable because of high content of vitamin C.

Eggs, milk, cream cheese and butter (unsalted); margarine.

Biscuits, sandwiches of potted meat, thin toast, cereals.

The following articles should be taken only sparingly:

Salt. Sugar and sugared food. Bread and starchy foods. These are apt to produce flatulence with embarrassment of the heart and palpitation, and should be limited when a reduction of weight is desirable.

Tea and coffee should be unsweetened and weak, and should not be drunk late at night as they tend to delay sleep. Alcohol is usually best avoided, but a little whisky at bedtime may help to promote sleep.

The following articles should be avoided altogether:

Condiments and spices; twice cooked meats; salted and preserved meat and meat extracts; shellfish and smoked fish; cakes or pastries containing baking soda. Sauces, gravies and consommés have little food value and are best omitted.

DIET IN SEVERE HEART FAILURE

In severe heart failure with vomiting which is not due to overdosage with digitalis, milk is the best food.

In the absence of vomiting, light solids agree better than fluid foods, being less likely to cause flatulence. In extreme cases, only very small quantities should be allowed at a time, at fairly frequent intervals, with 5 small meals a day. Biscuits, small thin sandwiches of potted meat or small quantities of milk are often all that can be easily digested but as the condition improves, soft boiled eggs, cream soup, vegetable purées, orange juice, jellies and ice-cream should gradually be added. Glucose may also be given.

TOBACCO. This should be used in moderation, since excessive smoking affects the heart's circulation, and also predisposes to cough and bronchitis. In severe heart failure, smoking should be given up.

Treatment by Drugs. DIGITALIS. The most striking benefit from digitalis is seen in auricular fibrillation with its irregular heart rhythm (see p. 296), but it is also quite effective in congestive failure with regular heart rhythm.

Among the indications of overdosage are headache, which is followed in definite sequence by loss of appetite, nausea, vomiting and diarrhea, and occasionally by mental confusion, usually associated with 'coupling' of the pulse beats. It should be noted, however, that vomiting is not uncommon in heart failure quite apart from overdosage with digitalis, but usually the occurrence of the above symptoms is an indication to stop the drug for a few days and, when it is resumed, to give a smaller dose. The pulse rate should also be carefully recorded daily in digitalis intoxication and the drug withheld when the pulse rate falls below 60 per minute.

The secret of success with digitalis is to be found in the use of the drug in short intermittent courses of a few days' duration. It should be taken regularly day by day until the first appearance of headache or nausea is noted. It is then stopped for two or three days and a further course begun. A convenient rule is to omit all digitalis on two days, say Saturday and Sunday, of each week. All persons who are taking digitalis should be examined by a doctor at regular intervals.

OXYGEN. This may be needed in acute heart failure, especially with blueness of the lips and cheeks and marked shortness of breath, and in cases due to pneumonia. It should be given continuously through a nasal catheter, by a disposable plastic mask.

DIURETICS: TREATMENT OF DROPSY. If, in congestive failure the response to restriction of fluid intake, rest and digitalis is not sufficiently quick or adequate, diuretics, or kidney stimulants, are required to assist the removal of fluid from the water-logged tissues by way of the kidneys.

The newer diuretics have the advantage of being in tablet form, to be taken by the mouth. One to three tablets are taken early in the day, in divided doses, on two to five days in each week. Chlorthalidone (hygroton) has a longer-acting effect and two or three doses a week will provide complete therapeutic control of edema in most cases.

In severe cases of dropsy, they may be combined with injections of the mercurial diuretics. These diuretics are advisedly given first thing in the morning to avoid disturbances of sleep the following night. A profuse secretion of urine usually begins within two hours, and continues for 24 to 48 hours; as much as 10 to 20 pints of urine may be passed. It is important to restrict the daily intake of fluid to 1.2 liters (2 pints). It is wise to weigh the patient at weekly intervals, as a steady reduction of weight shows the efficacy of the treatment. A rest period of several weeks is generally advisable after 6 injections of mercurial diuretics.

This treatment must only be given under medical supervision, and may give rise to symptoms of mercurial poisoning if carried to excess, with inflammation of the mouth and bowel.

LAXATIVES: TREATMENT OF CONSTIPATION. Vigorous purgation is not to be recommended as a routine measure because of its weakening effect, and its tendency to produce digestive disturbances. Frequent use of the bedpan, moreover, is exhausting. In the acute stage of congestive failure, however, a dose of calomel in the evening, followed by a saline purgative such as Epsom or Glauber's Salts the next morning, is of benefit.

It is important to avoid straining, and the continued use of mild laxatives may be necessary.

SEDATIVES: TREATMENT OF RESTLESSNESS AND SLEEPLESSNESS. If the patient is excitable, sedatives may be prescribed. No sedatives should be given except on a doctor's advice.

In heart failure, sleep is often impossible without sedatives; 300 to 600 milligrams of chloral hydrate may be given in water by mouth, and the dose repeated in 2 to 4 hours if necessary.

Whisky is a good soporific for the elderly, especially if the patient is accustomed to it; as an alternative, paraldehyde (1 to 2 teaspoonfuls) may be given with chipped ice or brandy.

SEDATIVES: TREATMENT OF CARDIAC ASTHMA. For attacks of breathlessness at night the patient should sit upright in bed, supported by high pillows or a bed rest, and should be given a drink of smelling salts in water. More severe attacks require the injection (by a doctor) of 15 milligrams of morphine and 0·5 mg of atropine, or injection of aminophylline intravenously, and, if necessary, the withdrawal of 300 to 600 milliliters of blood by venesection.

Blood-letting (Venesection). This is occasionally used in heart failure due to high blood pressure with congestion of the lungs, and in cases with distended neck veins and an enlarged liver. It is performed by removing 300 to 600 milliliters of blood from one of the veins in front of the elbow.

Spa Treatment. Patients under 70 years of age often derive great benefit from a stay at one of the spas, under medical supervision. A mild climate is essential; altitudes of more than 5,000 feet should be avoided. Spa treatment is particularly beneficial for those who have indulged in excesses of various kinds, for the obese, and for those who are also suffering from chronic bronchitis.

HEART PAIN

The symptom of discomfort or pain in the region of the heart may be of three main types according to the origin, distribution, severity and duration.

1. Pain over the heart, or precordial pain.
2. True angina pectoris.
3. Myocardial infarction, or scarring of the heart muscle from clotting of blood in the arteries supplying the heart muscle (coronary thrombosis).

Pain over the Heart

Discomfort or pain in the region of the heart itself is in most cases not due to heart disease. It is common in neurasthenia and emotional states, and in digestive disorders with flatulence of the stomach and bowels, or disease of the gall-bladder. It may also be produced by over-indulgence in tobacco.

There is usually a dull aching sensation which is much more commonly due to emotional stress than to physical exertion. A well-known heart specialist in Vienna used to describe this type of patient as a 'Heart patient who has nothing the matter with the heart.' The symptom is usually of no serious significance, and treatment should be directed to the underlying cause, whether it be an 'affair of the heart' which has gone wrong, or simply indigestion.

Angina Pectoris

True angina pectoris is a transitory attack of paroxysmal pain in the chest, of two to three minutes' duration, usually felt beneath the upper part of the breastbone; it is produced by physical exertion, and relieved by rest and by nitrite drugs.

Causes of Anginal Pain. Any muscle which is exercised without an adequate circulation of blood through its fibers may give rise to intolerable pain from cramp. The heart, like any other muscle, has a blood supply of its own, and any condition which leads to a poor blood supply is apt to result in an attack of pain in the heart. If the reduction of the blood supply is brief, an attack of angina pectoris may occur.

PREDISPOSING CAUSES. Any condition which produces a narrowing of the arteries of the heart may predispose to attacks of angina pectoris.

1. Arteriosclerosis. The most common cause is arteriosclerosis, or hardening of the walls of the blood vessels. This may be considered a more or less normal event in advancing years and only if it is severe will symptoms be produced. Severe degrees of vessel changes may be due to hereditary tendencies, or the result of repeated attacks of rheumatism, but in most cases they are aggravated by the strain of modern life.

2. Syphilis. In syphilitic disease of the heart there are often attacks of heart pain which may occur at rest, or in bed at night. It is a cause of angina pectoris in patients under the age of 40.

3. Attacks of angina pectoris may occur in anemia and in exophthalmic goiter.

The symptom is rare in heart failure and in auricular fibrillation.

EXCITING CAUSES OF ANGINA PECTORIS. Even though any of the above conditions may be present in marked degree, the circulation will at first be adequate while the patient is resting or undertaking only slight exertion; it becomes insufficient only on strenuous effort. As the condition progresses, the attacks are more easily noticed, and they become more frequent and last longer. They may even follow emotional excitement. Finally, attacks may occur without any obvious cause, especially when the patient is tired. The average age of onset is 55, and men are more frequently affected than women.

Symptoms. The outstanding symptom is paroxysmal pain, of sudden onset, increasing rapidly in severity, and subsiding more gradually; different attacks, however, show great variation in severity. The pain is felt in the front of the chest, usually behind the upper part of the breast-bone, but it may occur in the upper abdomen.

It may extend to the left shoulder and

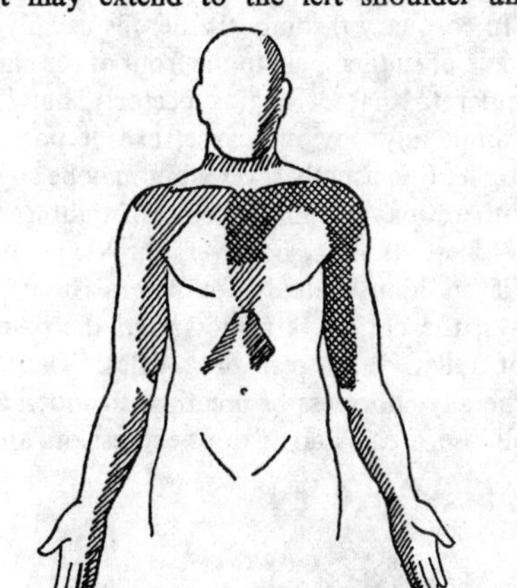

Fig. 8. *ANGINA PECTORIS, showing distribution of pain; cross-hatching shows areas most commonly affected.*

armpit, and often down the left arm to the elbow, occasionally as far as the fingers; or it may pass up to the left side of the neck and jaw. It often leads to a sense of pressure or constriction, as if the chest were held in a vice, and a burning sensation in the chest.

With the onset of the pain, the patient stands motionless, pale and perspiring. There may be great anxiety, and sometimes a sense of impending death. With rest, the attack passes after a short time. It is often followed by nausea, a considerable quantity of wind being brought up, and a large quantity of pale urine passed. There may be tingling and numbness of the left arm afterwards.

Diagnosis. Any form of pain in the chest, arm, or neck which comes on only after exertion should be suspected as arising in the heart. Angina pectoris should be distinguished from the following conditions:

1. Coronary thrombosis, or clot in a blood vessel of the heart. Here the pain lasts for longer than half an hour (see below).
2. Indigestion. Angina pectoris is often mistaken for indigestion, since the attacks often occur during activity after a meal.
3. Colic from gallstones, which may cause pain in the upper abdomen or lower chest.
4. Acute pleurisy, with severe cutting pain in the chest during breathing and coughing.
5. Neuralgia of the chest wall.

Treatment of an Attack. The patient must cease to move as soon as an attack begins, and remain still for several minutes after it subsides. After a severe attack the patient should always rest for an hour or two.

The traditional remedies are the nitrites. Amyl nitrite, 0·2 to 0·3 milliliters in glass capsules covered with silk, is inhaled after a capsule is crushed in a handkerchief. It has a rapid but rather short action.

A more suitable preparation is glyceryl trinitrate (nitroglycerin), 0·5 to 1 milligram. The tablets should be chewed or placed beneath the tongue and allowed to dissolve in the mouth. It may be necessary to repeat the dose. These tablets are apt to deteriorate in air and therefore only small quantities should be prescribed at a time.

Patients who suffer from angina pectoris should always carry with them one of these remedies for use as required. The effect of these drugs may be considerably increased by half a teaspoonful of smelling salts in water, or a tablespoonful of brandy, and by the application of heat over the front of the chest. Oxygen is also helpful, and windows should be opened. If these measures fail, morphine will probably be given by a doctor.

Propranolol, a newer cardiac depressant drug, reduces the drive on the heart and lowers blood pressure (see Fig. 9). It often reduces the frequency of anginal attacks and the number of glyceryl trinitrate tablets needed.

Long-term Management. A patient with angina pectoris must carefully readjust his habits. He must realize that he cannot expect the heart to do the same work at 55 as at 20.

ACTIVITY AND REST. All work should be done with the least expenditure of energy, and there should be no unnecessary hurry. Any activity which brings on an attack must be avoided. In milder cases, some exercise

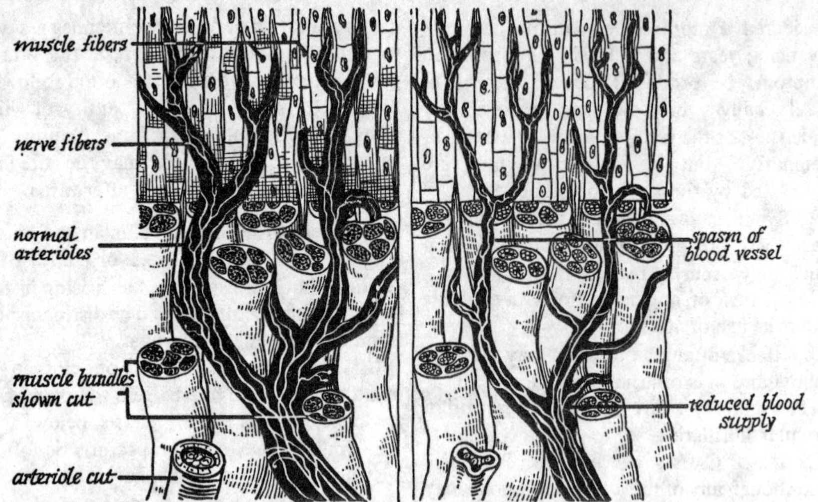

Fig. 9. *ANGINA PECTORIS.* Left: *normal heart muscle with normal blood vessels interlacing the muscle fibers* Right: *Spasm of angina causing constriction of the blood vessels, thereby reducing the blood supply, and the nutrients it carries, to the heart muscle fibers.*

may be advisable, though the more vigorous forms should not be undertaken. Walking on the level, mild physical exercises and massage are the safest, while light gardening, or golf may be indulged in if not followed by symptoms. Sufficent rest and sleep must be secured (see treatment of heart failure, p. 299), while cold rooms, cold sheets at night, and very hot or cold baths must be avoided.

Excessive smoking is harmful, and 5 to 10 cigarettes or their equivalent should be sufficient for the day, and are best indulged in, without inhaling, after meals.

Diet and Weight. Diet should follow the main principles set down on p. 300, while alcohol, in strict moderation, may be helpful. Constipation should be attended to and obesity treated. Reduction of overweight, however, should be gradual, and at the rate of not more than one pound per week. The loss of superfluous weight greatly eases the burden imposed on the heart, and may lead to striking improvement in the exercise tolerance without the use of any drugs.

Associated Disorders. Anemia should be treated, as even mild degrees may increase the likelihood of an attack. Other predisposing causes such as high blood pressure, syphilis, decayed teeth or infected nasal sinuses will require cautious and judicious treatment.

If these rules are kept, patients may live for many years without further attacks, but in the more severe cases, several weeks or months of complete or partial rest may be necessary, if possible with a complete change in a moderate climate. If retirement is necessary, the patient should have some hobby, such as photography or light gardening to compensate for the sudden change to an inactive life.

Myocardial Infarction

(*Coronary Thrombosis*)

This is a much more serious condition than uncomplicated angina pectoris, and it causes the majority of 'heart attacks.' It is not infrequently followed by sudden death (in one case out of three) in middle life and later. The blood supply to part of the heart muscle is completely cut off, usually by a clot of blood in one of the blood vessels supplying the heart muscle, so that part of the heart wall becomes permanently damaged. If recovery follows, the damaged portion of heart muscle, or 'infarct,' will gradually be replaced by scar tissue. On the other hand, the attack may lead to sudden death; in rare cases, the softened heart muscle may rupture.

Symptoms. Like angina pectoris, coronary thrombosis is more common in men than in women, and in half the cases attacks of angina pectoris will have occurred previously.

In coronary thrombosis there is usually an attack of sudden pain in the front of the chest, similar to that of angina pectoris, but it is without any obvious cause, except possibly fatigue. It is usually severe, but may be slight, or there may be only a sense of tightness in the chest. It lasts, however, for longer than half an hour, usually for several hours or days; the patient is restless, and the pain is not relieved by rest or nitrites. There is generally shortness of breath with shock and collapse, a pale and anxious expression, and a

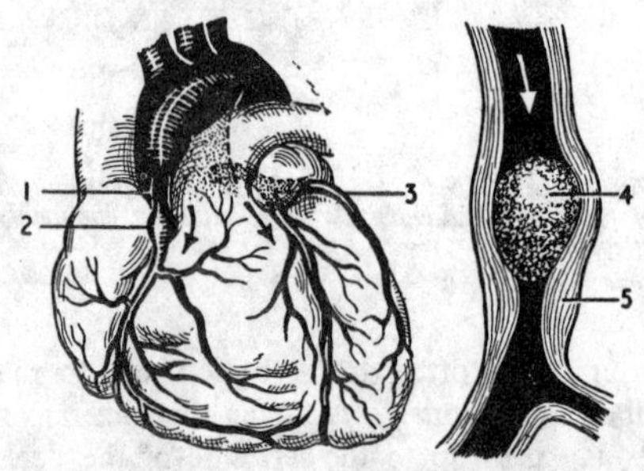

Fig. 10. *CORONARY THROMBOSIS.* 1. *Right coronary artery.* 2. *A blood clot impeding the flow of blood causes infarct in the portion of heart muscle fed by the artery.* 3. *Normal left coronary artery.* 4. *A thrombus (blood clot) becomes lodged in an arteriole because the diseased thickened wall(5) is too narrow for it to pass.*

cold clammy skin. The pulse is weak or imperceptible, fast, and often irregular. There may be slight fever during the first 24 hours, while flatulence, nausea and vomiting, with distension of the abdomen, are fairly common. An electrocardiographic tracing is helpful in diagnosis.

Treatment. Rest, morphine and oxygen are essential at the outset of an attack.

Anticoagulants are now commonly given if the circumstances are favorable. The patient should be either admitted to a hospital or clinic, or should be nursed within easy reach of one, in order that facilities for estimating the coagulation time of the blood may be close at hand.

Heparin is given at the outset, by intravenous injection, followed by oral anticoagulants. Treatment is continued for two to four weeks, and during this period the greatest care must be taken with shaving, etc., as the smallest cuts are apt to bleed profusely. Overdosage with anticoagulants may result in spontaneous hemorrhage; the blood usually appears in the urine. If this occurs, vitamin K_1 should be given immediately. Every patient who is receiving an anticoagulant drug, especially if it is for long-term treatment, should carry a card stating that he is on anticoagulant therapy, and giving his blood group, together with the address and telephone number of the hospital or clinic which is supervising the treatment.

Rest. A period of three weeks' complete rest is essential, followed by a similar period of partial rest. The first two weeks after an attack are particularly dangerous. The patient will require to be lifted in bed for changing linen and attention to the bowels. The bowels need not be moved for the first 48 hours, and for some weeks it will be sufficient if they are opened every other day by means of an enema. Pain may be lessened by the application of a hot-water bottle to the chest; when severe, large doses of morphine are given.

Diet. The diet for the first week should be fluid or semi-fluid and, if no food is taken for the first 36 hours, no harm will be done. Glucose should be given. (See diet in severe heart failure, p. 300.)

Convalescence. After three weeks the patient may be moved to a couch for a period of 20 minutes, at first every other day. If there are no new symptoms, sitting up may gradually be increased until 2 or 3 one-hour periods during the day are tolerated without fatigue. After two weeks of partial sitting up, a few steps may be taken and light massage may be tried.

The first effort at return to work, in six to seven weeks after the attack, should be limited to about two hours a day, and the increase to a full day gradually accomplished over a period of several weeks.

Only time can answer the question of the ultimate outlook, and there is always the possibility of recurrence and sudden death if reasonable discretion is not used, The patient must live, therefore within the limits of his diminished strength and keep something in reserve. At least eight hours should be spent each night in bed

DISEASES OF THE BLOOD VESSELS

Aneurysm of the Aorta

An aneurysm is a dilatation of an artery, usually a large one, and the vessel most commonly affected is the aorta, particularly in those parts which are nearest to the heart.

Causes. Aneurysm is five times more common in men than in women, and the commonest cause is syphilis, particularly in patients under 40 years of age. Syphilitic disease of the aorta begins a few months after the first infection, but only becomes advanced after 10 to 15 years have elapsed. There is a gradual weakening and stretching of the wall, and the vessel may become dilated like a spindle, or there may be a local bulging of its wall. The disease also affects the smaller blood vessels of the heart, with the frequent development of angina pectoris.

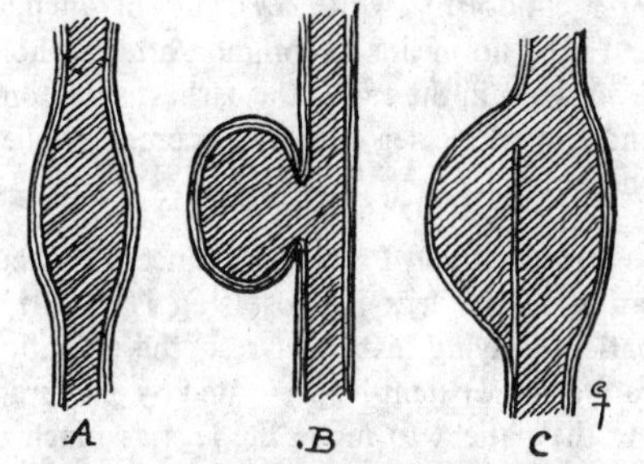

Fig. 11. *DIFFERENT TYPES OF ANEURYSM.* A. *Fusiform aneurysm.* B. *Sacculated aneurysm.* C. *Dissecting aneurysm.*

Dilatation of the aorta is occasionally due to arteriosclerosis, or hardening of the aorta wall, associated with long-continued physical strain.

Symptoms. These appear 10 to 20 years after the first syphilitic infection. They are due mainly to the effects of pressure on the various organs in the chest. The two earliest and most important symptoms are pain in the chest and shortness of breath.

Pain may vary from discomfort to a chronic boring pain in the front of the chest. Occasionally it extends to the neck and arms. It may come on spontaneously, apart from physical exertion, especially on lying down; or it may occur only on exertion, without, however, disappearing on resting. It lasts longer than true angina pectoris, and is more liable to occur at night. There may, however, also be true attacks of angina of effort. In the later stages the pain becomes more widespread, and may be very persistent.

Shortness of breath, both on exertion and in paroxysmal attacks at rest, is an important early symptom. A brassy cough may be due to pressure on the bronchial tubes.

Other symptoms, such as difficulty in swallowing, enlargement of the veins of the head, neck, and arms, and hoarseness, are mainly due to pressure of the aneurysm on surrounding structures.

Sudden death is by no means rare, being usually due to bursting of the aneurysm, with resultant hemorrhage. Death may also occur from gradually increasing heart failure.

Diagnosis. Syphilis of the aorta is a serious disease, the outlook depending on an early diagnosis, and appropriate treatment. Unfortunately there is a long latent period of 10 to 20 years without serious symptoms, so that these are usually a sign of advanced disease. An important measure in diagnosis is X-ray examination of the chest. A blood test for syphilis is generally positive in the early stages, but may be negative later.

Treatment. General measures should conform to the treatment of heart failure. Especially important are adequate rest, and the avoidance of sudden physical strain. Alcohol must be strictly limited.

Specific treatment for syphilis must be given with great caution. Potassium iodide 300 milligrams with water is prescribed three times daily, gradually increasing to as much as 1·2 grams three times daily. It is particularly effective in relieving pain. After some months of preliminary treatment bismuth and salvarsan are given under skilled medical supervision. Penicillin, combined with the above-mentioned treatments, is usually found to increase their effectiveness. Penicillin alone, beginning with low doses and gradually increasing them if there are no contraindications, has proved of value in a number of cases.

Arteriosclerosis

Arteriosclerosis is a diseased condition of the walls of the arteries, which become weakened, hard, and twisted.

Causes. While the actual cause is unknown, it is more common with advancing age, and is a noticeable feature of the strain of modern life. It is more common in men than in women. It is probable that heredity is a factor in its development, while overeating and heavy smoking may also be responsible.

Symptoms and Complications. It has been well said that a man is only as old as his arteries, and that long life is a question of the blood vessels. Certainly arteriosclerosis is a very common disorder, and it is a widespread process which tends to interfere with the nutrition of the body. It is usually most marked in the aorta.

Disease of the arteries of the heart and brain is especially common, causing attacks of angina pectoris, coronary thrombosis, and senile mental disorder. If an artery to the brain becomes blocked, or if it ruptures, a stroke due to cerebral thrombosis or hemorrhage will follow. Other internal vessels which are often involved are those of the pancreas, resulting in diabetes, and of the kidneys, resulting in high blood pressure. The arteries of the limbs are usually affected later, and if they are near the surface, they may be felt as semi-rigid twisted vessels.

When the arteries of the legs are affected, cramp or severe pain may occur in the feet and calves of one or both limbs after walking. In the earlier stages, fatigue develops in the muscles, with numbness and tingling or 'pins and needles;' later, attacks of acute pain occur in the legs after walking for a certain distance (intermittent claudication). In the later stages, ulcers of the toes and ankles may develop, or actual gangrene.

Treatment. General treatment consists in the treatment of the symptoms and complications mentioned above (see angina pectoris, cerebral thrombosis, diabetes, high blood pressure, etc.). It is important to avoid overeating and excess of alcohol. Smoking should be reduced; more than 10 cigarettes a day is excessive; with severe symptoms it is best omitted altogether.

Special points in the treatment of arteriosclerosis of the legs, with cramp on exertion (intermittent claudication).

EXERCISE should be limited, and the patient advised to walk slowly and to avoid hurrying, climbing hills, and going out in cold weather. The greatest care must be taken in removing corns and cutting the toenails, since the slightest injury may develop into an intractable ulcer. Strong antiseptics, such as iodine and carbolic, should not be applied to abrasions, as they may cause damage. A warm solution of boric acid should be used instead.

The circulation in the legs may temporarily be helped by certain exercises:

A. Lying flat in bed, the patient raises the leg about 60 degrees above the horizontal, allowing it to remain until the limb is pale, that is in ½ to 3 minutes. The patient then allows the foot to hang over the edge of the bed until the leg becomes warm and red, that is in 2 to 5 minutes. The leg is then laid flat on the bed for 3 to 5 minutes and the exercise repeated (Buerger's Exercises).

B. The legs are hung over the edge of the bed, and the feet are exercised by bending and stretching the ankles, turning the feet inwards and outwards and spreading and closing the toes.

Exercises of this type should be carried out two or three times daily for as long as possible, up to an hour, without producing undue fatigue or pain. An improved color and increased warmth in the limb will often follow.

It is often possible by treatment of this

kind to avoid the more serious complications such as ulceration and gangrene. In certain carefully chosen cases the operation of sympathectomy is occasionally helpful.

Diseases of the Veins

Phlebitis—Inflammation of the Veins

Causes. This is usually associated with thrombosis (clotting of blood in the veins) and may follow a variety of conditions: injury to the veins; certain diseases, such as gout and typhoid fever, and occasionally pneumonia and influenza; after operations on the lower abdomen, and after childbirth. It may attack any vein, but is most common in the veins of the legs.

Symptoms. There is pain and tenderness in the course of the affected vein, which may be felt as a hard cord. The overlying skin may become reddened, and the limb is usually somewhat swollen.

Treatment. Patients with phlebitis should be put to bed, and the affected limb rested absolutely, in severe cases, for a period of four to six weeks. All sudden movement must be avoided. The leg should be elevated and kept in position between sandbags.

In all cases of phlebitis, food containing much lime salts, such as milk, should be limited. Lemon or orange juice should be given freely as a sweetened drink, as it may help to prevent further clotting, and potassium citrate, in doses of 1 gram in water, should be taken three or four times daily for the same reason. Anticoagulants may be used in suitable cases (see treatment of coronary thrombosis). Antibiotics such as penicillin or a tetracycline are often given with good effect. Laxatives should be given freely.

At the end of the period of absolute rest (4 to 6 weeks, as a rule) gentle massage and passive movements may be started.

Varicose Veins

Varicose veins of the leg is one of the commonest of all diseases. The cause lies in a defect in the valvular mechanism of the leg veins, and the increased pressure to which the veins are exposed by the assumption of the erect posture.

Symptoms. A sense of fullness and a tired feeling in the lower leg are the most common symptoms.

Treatment. The elastic stocking has a definite place in the treatment of varicose veins, especially in the aged. In active healthy persons small groups of varicose veins may be treated by the injection of ethanolamine oleate. The more severe conditions are best dealt with by operation, which consists of ligaturing the main superficial vein at the upper end of the thigh, followed by removal of the affected veins by 'stripping.'

Complications of Varicose Veins

1. RUPTURE, WITH HEMORRHAGE. In the case of hemorrhage from a varicose vein, the patient should lie down, with the affected leg raised well above the level of the heart, in which position the bleeding will soon stop. A small pad of gauze placed over the bleeding point, and held firmly in position with adhesive strapping will control all further bleeding.

2. VARICOSE ECZEMA. The nutrition of the skin of the lower leg in an individual with long-standing varicose veins is greatly interfered with. Since the congestion in the veins tends to cause itching, the skin is commonly scratched, and a moist dermatitis which becomes septic is consequently liable to arise. In this way, the well-known eczema of the leg is produced. The skin involved is usually scaly, roughened and pigmented, often showing excoriations where the patient has scratched it. Eradication of the varicose veins, or the application of a zinc paste bandage usually alleviates the condition.

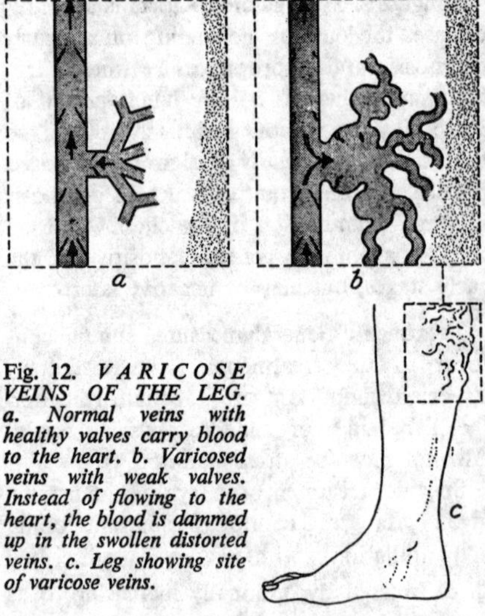

Fig. 12. *VARICOSE VEINS OF THE LEG. a. Normal veins with healthy valves carry blood to the heart. b. Varicosed veins with weak valves. Instead of flowing to the heart, the blood is dammed up in the swollen distorted veins. c. Leg showing site of varicose veins.*

3. VARICOSE ULCER. One of the most common sequels of untreated varicose veins of long standing is the appearance of an ulcer on the inner side of the lower leg, just above the ankle.

The direct cause of the ulcer is usually an injury which produces a break in the skin, and because of the interference in nutrition which is due to poor circulation, the injury does not heal and becomes a chronic ulcer.

Treatment of Varicose Ulcer. The basis of treatment lies in eradication of the varicose veins. Frequently a vein may be found feeding directly into the ulcer. Injection of ethanolamine oleate solution into this vein close to the ulcer area will often produce a dramatic cure. In the elderly, it may be necessary to resort to the application of a zinc ichthyol gelatin paste bandage. It may require renewal every two to four weeks. In long-standing chronic ulcers, it may be necessary to put the patient to bed, elevate the leg, and apply warm boric acid compresses as a preliminary to the above treatment. Obesity should be treated if it exists.

THROMBOSIS AND EMBOLISM

Thrombosis

This is the name applied to the clotting of blood within living blood vessels, whether in the heart, veins, or arteries. It is apt to occur in arteriosclerosis after injury to the lining membranes of a vessel or cavity of the heart, and if there is for any reason a slowing of the bloodstream within the vessels, as when a patient is resting in bed after an abdominal operation or after a confinement.

Femoral Thrombosis, or clotting in the main vein of the thigh. This is perhaps the commonest form of thrombosis, and usually appears in the left thigh. It frequently occurs after childbirth (white leg) and in anemia, and is by no means uncommon after typhoid fever. Pain in the calf is the earliest symptom, and the whole leg rapidly becomes swollen and painful.

Treatment and Prevention. Since the circulation in the legs is most sluggish while a patient is lying in bed at rest, the condition can to some extent be prevented by encouraging the patient to move the legs as much as possible. Once the condition has developed, the treatment is as for phlebitis (see above). Complete rest for at least 6 weeks is essential as a precaution against embolism into the lungs (see p. 305).

Cardiac Thrombosis, or clotting in the cavities of the heart. This is also one of the commonest and most important forms of thrombosis. It occurs especially in the left auricle, when it has become extremely dilated as a result of narrowing of the mitral valve, or of auricular fibrillation. Portions of the clot may break away from the thrombus, and may be carried by way of the left ventricle and aorta into the general circulation with resulting embolism (see p. 305). Portions of clot which form in the right auricle in heart failure may likewise break away and pass by way of the right ventricle and pulmonary artery into the lungs (pulmonary embolism).

Coronary Thrombosis, or clotting in the arteries of the heart, is likewise a very important condition, since it is a frequent cause of sudden death and of serious cardiac disability. It has already been discussed (p. 302).

Cerebral Thrombosis, or clotting in the small arteries of the brain. This is a common cause of 'strokes,' and is especially apt to occur when the arteries of the brain have become narrowed and hardened from arteriosclerosis.

Embolism

This is the chief complication of thrombosis, and is the process whereby a portion of clot becomes detached and is carried from one part of the circulation to another; it becomes impacted when it arrives at a vessel too narrow for its further progress.

Embolism of the Lung. (Pulmonary embolism). Emboli are not uncommonly detached from clots in the veins of the pelvis or leg (femoral thrombosis), especially after abdominal operations or after childbirth. About the tenth day after an apparently successful abdominal operation or an uneventful confinement, an embolus may occur in the lungs with appalling suddenness, leading either to death, or to sudden pain in the chest with cough and blood-stained sputum.

Treatment. Embolism can only be avoided in cases of femoral thrombosis by insistence on rest for the leg for a minimum period of six weeks. Tying, or ligature, of the vein of the leg may be necessary in order to prevent further emboli from becoming detached.

Embolism of the Systemic Arteries. As mentioned above, emboli are commonly derived from clots which may form in the dilated left auricle of the heart in cases of mitral stenosis. They pass by way of the left ventricle and aorta into the systemic circulation and are liable to become arrested in any of the following situations:

1. In the arteries of the brain, the patient being seized with instantaneous paralysis of one side of the body.
2. In the arteries of the spleen, giving rise to sudden pain in the left side, beneath the lowest ribs; there is enlargement of the spleen which becomes very tender.
3. In the arteries of the kidney, with sudden pain in the back, and the appearance of blood in the urine.
4. In the arteries of the intestine. The patient is seized with sudden violent abdominal pain and distension, with complete intestinal obstruction, and gangrene of the small intestine. Operation should be undertaken immediately, but recovery is very rare.
5. In the main artery of a limb. There is acute pain in the limb, followed by numbness and loss of power, and finally by gangrene.

HIGH BLOOD PRESSURE
(*Hypertension*)

Blood pressure rises in all the arteries at each beat of the heart and falls between each beat. This pressure is measured by an instrument called a sphygmomanometer (or manometer) connected to an inflatable rubber armband. For details of its use (and illustration) see Blood Pressure, p. 243.

Systolic pressure is the strongest force produced by the heart beat or contraction.

Diastolic pressure is the lowest force produced during relaxation of the heart muscle between contractions.

The diastolic measurement is by far the more important of the two in cases of high blood pressure, as it indicates the state of the arteries and of the amount of peripheral resistance which has to be overcome. The rise of systolic pressure which usually accompanies it is simply an indication of the compensatory increase in the force of the heart beat required to overcome this resistance. A raised systolic pressure with a normal diastolic pressure is of relatively slight importance. Readings should always be taken after ten minutes' rest.

Normal Pressure. The normal blood pressure in a young healthy adult lies between $\frac{110-130 \text{ Systolic}}{60-80 \text{ Diastolic}}$ millimeters of mercury.

Maximum normal values are $\frac{150 \text{ Systolic}}{90 \text{ Diastolic}}$

High Blood Pressure. Persistent readings above $\frac{160 \text{ Systolic}}{90 \text{ Diastolic}}$ in adults or above $\frac{170 \text{ Systolic}}{100 \text{ Diastolic}}$ in the elderly, should be considered to be abnormal. They may reach $\frac{260}{140}$ in the advanced stages of the complaint.

Hypertension

Causes. The causes of hypertension are obscure, since there are many predisposing factors involved. The one indispensable precursor to the condition, and the earliest physical change to take place in the system, is a narrowing of the caliber of the smaller peripheral arteries, due at first to spasm, which is in turn succeeded by permanent fibrotic thickening of their walls resulting in an increased resistance to the passage of blood through them.

Among the more important predisposing factors to this increased peripheral resistance are the following:

HEREDITY. The patient may have an inherited constitutional tendency, with a high familial incidence of the complaint.

NERVOUS FACTORS. Prolonged mental and emotional fatigue. The typical 'hypertensive personality' is usually active, ambitious, aggressive and enthusiastic, resenting delay and inactivity, but his mind is restless and he has a short explosive temper. An exaggerated sense of responsibility and habitual worrying are the most significant and constant traits. These factors of anxiety and continuous exposure to mental and emotional stress and strain contribute to psychological fatigue which is an important factor in the perpetuation and progression of the complaint.

DISORDERS OF NUTRITION, from habitual overeating. Hypertension is frequently associated with obesity, with the excessive consumption of carbohydrates, fats and condiments, and with chronic alcoholism.

CHRONIC TOXEMIA, OR POISONING. Excessive smoking over a long period of years may result in chronic nicotine poisoning which leads to increased constriction of the smaller arteries and resultant hypertension.

TOXEMIA may likewise be due to prolonged focal infection, e.g. a dental abscess neglected over a period of years, or chronically infected tonsils.

DISTURBANCES OF ENDOCRINE BALANCE. Hypertension is common at the menopause. It is common in diabetes from disorder of the pancreas, and of the thyroid in myxedema; and in certain disorders of the pituitary gland of the brain, and of the adrenal gland.

CHRONIC KIDNEY DISEASE. A few cases are associated with marked arteriosclerosis of the kidneys. Progressive damage to the kidney appears to cause a liberation into the system of some poisonous waste product which has the effect of increasing the constriction of the smaller arteries of the body still more, thus progressively perpetuating the disorder. The symptoms are apt to be severe and the course of the disease rapid, death often taking place within two years of the onset of symptoms. It is known as 'malignant hypertension.'

Symptoms. It is a progressive disease, but usually the rate of progress is slow. There may be no symptoms for several years after its onset, so that when they first appear the condition may be well advanced. In many cases it is discovered accidentally during this preliminary asymptomatic period, as for example, during an examination for life insurance.

EARLY SYMPTOMS. The earlier symptoms are due to impairment of the blood supply, with consequent deficient oxygenation, of the functioning tissue cells. They are chiefly of a neurological nature: e.g. insomnia; early fatigue, especially on mental effort; impairment of memory; mental irritability and garrulousness; diminished emotional control, with shortness of temper and explosive outbursts of anger; attacks of giddiness; a feeling of fulness, with frequent flushing and throbbing of the head, and actual headache of a dull and throbbing character, chiefly felt at the back of the head, and especially in the morning.

With a permanently increased resistance to the passage of the bloodstream, the left ventricle begins to hypertrophy (enlarge by thickening its walls) by way of compensation, and for a time there will still be no particular symptoms referable to the heart. This is a remarkable fact, considering that the output of the normal heart in a normal system is no less than 10 tons of blood a day, and that a rise of diastolic pressure from 70 to only 105 millimeters of mercury increases the work of the heart by at least fifty per cent. It is, in fact, surprising how long the heart can support a raised blood pressure without showing symptoms of cardiac strain.

HEART SYMPTOMS. Gradually, however, dilatation of the left ventricle begins to succeed hypertrophy, and the later and major symptoms of hypertension then begin to appear. They are chiefly cardiac in origin, and are an indication of the greatly increased burden which the ventricle is called upon to bear.

Consciousness of the heart's action (palpitation) with discomfort in the chest on exertion, and possibly attacks of angina pectoris are often associated with numbness, tingling and cramps in the leg muscles on walking (attacks of intermittent claudication, or angina of the legs). Shortness of breath is induced by less and less exertion.

These symptoms are frequently put down by the patient to smoking, fatigue, lack of exercise or, most commonly, to indigestion, but rarely to the true cause, namely increasing age and tiredness of the heart.

Associated with these cardinal symptoms may be found a florid, plethoric complexion and increased pulse rate, with thickened arteries at the wrist, in the arm, and in the temple, their texture resembling that of whipcord.

From this point onwards, the complaint passes almost imperceptibly into the third stage of frank cardiac decompensation from left-sided heart failure, with its attendant symptoms of congestion of the lungs and cough. Gradually the right side of the heart begins to fail as well, with the additional symptoms of cyanosis, engorgement of the neck veins, enlarged and tender liver and dropsy of the legs.

This phase of decompensation may persist for many years or, on the other hand, it may be brief. Of especially serious significance are attacks of 'cardiac asthma' (nocturnal shortness of breath) and edema of the lungs, while an attack of coronary thrombosis, liable to occur at any time, may prove fatal.

From time to time during the course of the disease, relief may be obtained from symptoms by attacks of nose-bleeding (epistaxis), from spontaneous rupture of a vessel in the nose. There need be no particular hurry to arrest it, since it acts as a sort of safety valve, and is usually beneficial. Occasionally it may take place from a vessel in the stomach, when the blood is vomited up (hematemesis).

In the later stages, hemorrhage of a more serious nature may occur from the degenerated arteries of the retina causing a clot of blood to appear in the eyeball, with consequent blurring of vision. Of still more serious significance is hemorrhage from the degenerated arteries of the brain, causing an apoplectic attack or 'stroke,' a by no means uncommon sequel to this complaint. Often there will be one or more preliminary apoplexies which may be completely or partially recovered from, leaving perhaps a paralyzed limb or half of the body, only to be followed by a major attack of cerebral hemorrhage with a fatal outcome.

Symptoms of 'Malignant Hypertension.' The emphasis of the disease process falls on the kidneys rather than on the heart, with some resultant modification of the general picture.

Depletion of the reserve of the kidney is apt to be without symptoms until the later stage but, as mentioned above, once symptoms have appeared, it tends to run a far more rapid course than the relatively benign type of hypertension already considered. Symptoms of uremia (decompensation of the kidneys) are apt to appear with apparent suddenness, and death frequently takes place within two years of the onset of symptoms. The blood pressure, especially the diastolic, is usually higher than in the benign type.

Among the more striking features are: quantities of pale weak urine, nocturnal micturition, albumen in the urine; pallor, poor appetite and loss of weight (in contrast to the frequently florid complexion and obesity of the subject of the benign type of hypertension), marked nervous symptoms, especially extreme lassitude and severe headache, and an early tendency to hemorrhage from the arteries of the retina. Death usually takes place from uremia or from cerebral hemorrhage.

Treatment of the Cause

Since the constitutional susceptibility of the patient is a major factor in hypertension, a complete cure cannot be expected to follow any form of treatment. On the other hand, neglect of treatment leads inevitably to degenerative changes in the tissues and increasing risks of a major catastrophe, such as a stroke. Early and persistent management is therefore indicated in all cases.

A reduction of the diastolic pressure is a guide to the extent and duration of the vascular relaxation. It is, however, important that there should be no rapid reduction of blood pressure, as it may lead to an attack of coronary thrombosis. The more gradual the fall the more lasting are the results.

CORRECTION OF MENTAL AND EMOTIONAL FATIGUE. Since this is the most important predisposing factor, in no complaint is a high degree of individualization of management more necessary than in hypertension. It is necessary to treat not only the disease, but also the whole complex individual personality of the patient. He must try to cultivate the art of relaxation, both physical and mental, avoiding as far as possible all causes of mental and emotional stress. These can often be eliminated by reasonable discussion, and it may be pointed out to him that while it will be wise for him to be concerned about his affairs, it is useless to worry about them. To worry is merely to set out on the high road for chronic invalidism. While his condition should be explained to him, and the reasons given for any measures and restrictions to be adopted, he should not be told the actual height of his blood pressure in figures. Nor is an alarmist attitude on the part of those about him either wise or necessary. The settling of emotional conflicts and the adoption of a calm philosophic outlook can do much to relieve the wear and tear on the circulatory system. Reassurance and encouragement should be the keynote of the approach by physician and family.

CORRECTION OF OVEREATING AND OBESITY. Moderation and temperance should be the basic rules, but since it is a chronic disorder requiring continuous management for many years, no very radical or abrupt alteration should be made in the eating habits. Too little food is as bad as unlimited excess. Condiments especially should be avoided, and alcohol taken only in moderation.

Gross obesity, however, is antagonistic to a long life, since it increases the work of an already overtaxed heart. Weight reduction at the rate of not more than one or two pounds a week should be aimed at, and it is often accompanied by an appreciable fall of arterial tension, and a decided increase in the sense of well-being.

Weight reduction programs should be individualized and specific. Bread, pastry and candy are the chief foods to avoid. Weekly weighings are a good guide to progress, and may be more important than repeated blood-pressure readings.

In general, the dietary measures outlined for the treatment of heart failure should be followed (see p. 300), avoiding overeating and overdrinking; at the same time nothing approaching starvation or semi-starvation should be contemplated. A diet which is largely lato-vegetarian in character and which includes all the vitamins and not more than one meal a day is probably all that is essential. Glucose is of value.

CORRECTION OF CHRONIC TOXEMIA. Excessive smoking is harmful, but there should be no abrupt stopping of tobacco; as with diet, moderation should be the keynote. Chronic infections, such as dental abscesses and grossly infected tonsils should be treated if they exist.

CONTROL OF GLANDULAR DISORDERS. For cases associated with the change of life, with hot flushes and their associated disorders, ovarian extracts will be found beneficial, daily for 3 weeks at a time, immediately after the monthly periods until the flushes are controlled. Cases associated with myxedema may require treatment with thyroxine daily. Diabetes should be controlled with dieting and if necessary with insulin or one of the oral antidiabetic drugs.

General Management

In no other malady, except perhaps in the related condition of angina pectoris is the mode of life of such great importance, and of the measures to be prescribed, an adequate amount of rest must take precedence over all others. Each patient with well-developed hypertension should be in bed for at least 10 hours each night. He should rest physically and mentally for at least half an hour after the midday meal, and have a quiet day each week. If the blood pressure is more pronounced he should be in bed for at least 12 hours, rest for at least an hour after lunch, and stay in bed on one day a week. (See treatment of Heart Failure, p. 299.)

For exercise, walking in the open air, riding a non-pulling horse, golf and mild cycling are suitable in moderation. Massage has the same effect as exercise, but without the accompanying fatigue.

Baths should be neither very hot nor very cold. A cold plunge may produce a serious contraction of the smaller arteries, just as sudden changes of external temperature may be dangerous, and should be guarded against by suitable clothing. Patients often derive much benefit from periodical courses of treatment at a spa, with baths and gentle massage, together with the change of air, regular mode of life, careful dieting, and graduated rest.

Treatment by Drugs

LAXATIVES. A regular and easy action of the bowels is important in order to prevent congestion of the liver. It may be promoted by a saline laxative in the morning—Epsom salts, or a teaspoonful of confection of senna may be taken at bedtime.

SEDATIVES. Where there is emotional tension and the patient is obviously nervous, 300 mg of chloral hydrate may be taken in a simple mixture in the morning and at night; or a tablet of phenobarbital (15 to 100 mg) may be taken at bedtime. The phenobarbital preparations can be obtained only with a doctor's prescription.

ARTERIAL DILATORS. Relaxation of the smaller arteries (where spasmodic contraction is initially responsible for raising the blood pressure) may be secured in mild cases by preparations of rauwolfia.

Treatment of Associated Disorders

ANEMIA. It is frequently found that the blood pressure falls as the percentage of hemoglobin (red coloring matter in the blood) rises. Anemia is treated by taking one of the many available iron preparations two or three times daily, with water, immediately after meals.

HEADACHE. This may be treated by cold compresses and the application of a menthol stick. A tablet containing aspirin, phenacetin and caffeine, e.g. APC Tablets, taken with a cup of tea is often effective.

Venesection (Blood-letting). This may be of value in the full-blooded plethoric type of patient, especially if there are head symptoms and an associated distension of the right side of the heart, engorged neck veins, enlarged tender liver, etc.; 400 to 600 milliliters of blood should be withdrawn and the operation may be repeated with advantage at intervals of four to six months.

LOW BLOOD PRESSURE

(Hypotension)

In hypotension the systolic blood pressure is persistently below 110 mm. of mercury in adult males, and 105 in adult females.

Causes. In certain quite healthy individuals the blood pressure is persistently below the level mentioned, i.e. it is constitutional. As a feature of underlying ill health, however, it may occur in a variety of disorders.

ACUTE CONDITIONS. In shock and collapse following injury, hypotension is frequently associated with severe hemorrhage; it also occurs in acute coronary thrombosis, in certain acute infectious diseases, e.g. diphtheria, and in the period of convalescence following an attack of influenza (post-influenzal depression).

CHRONIC CONDITIONS. A moderate degree of anemia is extremely frequent in patients with hypotension. In pulmonary tuberculosis, chronic myocarditis (disease of the heart muscle), and in certain chronic wasting diseases, e.g. prolonged starvation or malnutrition, cancer and Addison's disease, there is often long-standing low blood pressure.

Symptoms. The most characteristic symptom is a constant sense of fatigue which is aggravated by physical and mental exertion and by constant standing. Other symptoms are giddiness and faintness, especially on a change of position, and a tendency to mental depression and headache. There is frequently coldness of the hands and feet.

Treatment

TREATMENT OF THE CAUSE. Blood transfusion is given for severe hemorrhage associated with shock; serum for diphtheria; iron for anemia; and cortisone for Addison's disease.

REST AND EXERCISE. Acute cases require rest in bed. This should be prolonged according to age after acute infectious illnesses: in influenza, one day of convalescence is usually required for each 5 years of age; thus a man of 50 years requires 10 days of convalescence after the temperature has fallen to normal. Rest should further be required after effort and after meals.

Both physical and mental overexertion should be avoided, but in the constitutional type of hypotension without any definite underlying disease, there should be encouragement towards outdoor physical exercise, rather than to excessive mental activity. This will gradually contribute to a greater sense of well-being, and such activities as walking, fishing, horseback riding and non-strenuous golf are excellent for the purpose. The program of exercise should be systematic and continued, since sporadic bouts of activity interspersed with long periods of sedentary living may do more harm than good. Once the appetite has returned, a course of massage is excellent for toning up the system.

DIET. Many patients with hypotension are habitually underweight, and an ample diet with extra milk, eggs and meat, together with a liberal intake of all the vitamins from such foods as fresh fruit and vegetables.

ABDOMINAL SUPPORTS. In cases in which sudden changes of position induce faintness or palpitation, the application of an abdominal belt or binder may be very valuable.

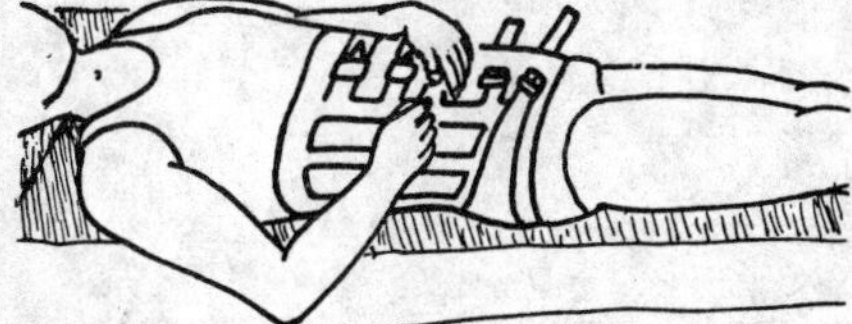

Fig. 13. *AN ABDOMINAL SUPPORT for a patient with hypotension. The support should be put on while the patient is lying down so that the abdominal organs are in their right positions.*

Binders and belts should only be applied with the patient in the recumbent position, e.g. before rising in the morning.

VASOMOTOR DISORDERS

Raynaud's Disease

In this condition, which is most common in girls and women between puberty and middle age, there are attacks of pallor and spasm, or contraction, of the blood vessels of the lower ends of the limbs, the hands especially being affected. During an attack, the hands or feet become cold and turn either white or blue, so that the parts become 'dead' and numb, or there may be pain or tingling. The attack may last for a few minutes or for some hours, and is due to spasm of the arteries of the fingers, precipitated by exposure to cold. The parts are very tender and, as the circulation returns, the previously discolored area becomes red, swollen, hot and painful; one or all the fingers may be affected, commonly the middle and ring fingers. In very severe attacks gangrene or local ulceration sometimes develops. In less serious cases there is a gradual return to normal but the attacks are recurrent, especially in cold weather. When warmth is applied the parts quickly regain their normal color. In some cases there is a hereditary factor but the exact cause is not known. Emotional disturbances may induce an attack. Occasionally the ears, nose or other parts are similarly affected.

Treatment. The avoidance of cold in any form is most important. The condition may be prevented to some extent by warm clothes, and a high-protein diet with extra fat, calcium and vitamins; many patients are helped by stopping smoking. In cold weather the hands and feet should always be washed in warm water. During attacks the parts should be kept warm in woolen coverings; gloves should be loose and long, overlapping the sleeves. For the feet two pairs of stockings should be worn, and bedsocks at night.

Minor injuries should be avoided, and when they occur should be treated at once.

A surgical procedure known as sympathectomy, which consists of division of the sympathetic nerves to the part, is indicated when the attacks are very distressing or interfere with work; this operation may give good results for a time, but symptoms often return again.

Erythrocyanosis

Erythrocyanosis is a circulatory disorder seen in girls and young women. The feet and legs are cold, and the backs of the legs, especially in the lower part, are bluish-red and swollen. Chilblains of the feet are often also present as well. The affected parts are painful and 'burning' when the legs are warmed. Generally the condition is only present in the colder months, during which period warm woolen stockings and stout shoes should be worn. No tight garters should be allowed. Active exercises such as skipping and walking, or massage, are usually helpful, while vitamin D may be prescribed by a doctor.

In very severe cases the operation of lumbar sympathectomy, with division of the sympathetic nerves to the legs, may be performed, and this often gives relief.

Thrombo-angiitis Obliterans

(Buerger's Disease)

In its early stages thrombo-angiitis obliterans is thought to be a vasospastic disorder (with spasm of the arteries), affecting the legs. This disease generally occurs in men (99 per cent of cases) and may develop between the ages of about twenty and sixty years, usually occurring at about thirty. In older patients there is generally also some disease of the arterial walls.

The cause of Buerger's disease is unknown, but prolonged exposure to cold or heavy smoking may be predisposing factors.

In the early stages coldness and pallor of the feet and the lower part of the legs are noted, with intermittent claudication which is a cramp of the leg muscles occurring after walking. (See Diseases of the Heart and Blood Vessels, p. 303). The pain gradually develops after walking quite short distances, or even during resting periods, and usually both legs become involved. The sufferer generally obtains most relief by letting his legs hang down over the side of the bed, but the constant attacks of pain often prevent sleep and the patient becomes very depressed and exhausted.

The feet are cold and dead white or dusky blue during attacks of pain, but assume a more reddish color when allowed to hang down. Later, phlebitis or gangrene is likely to develop.

Treatment. In the early stages rest is the chief aim, and prolonged standing or walking must be given up. There must also be complete abstinence from smoking. Cold must be avoided, and there must be no constriction of the legs or feet by garters or tight shoes. When intermittent claudication develops, postural exercises are used (see Diseases of the Heart, p. 303). The pain may be relieved by aspirin.

Surgical division of the sympathetic nerves to the lower limbs is carried out to produce dilatation of the blood vessels although this mainly helps the blood vessels supplying the skin rather than those to the muscle. This method is more successful in young patients. The procedure is known as sympathectomy.

When gangrene develops the outlook is not good, but even in these cases the frequency of the attacks of pain can be diminished. Occasionally amputation may be necessary in advanced cases.

CIRCULATORY DISORDERS DUE TO COLD

Chilblains

This common disorder is found in persons, usually children and old people, with a sluggish circulation in the hands and feet. Chilblains are brought on by exposure to cold, especially when it is associated with dampness, and occur chiefly on the fingers, toes and lower parts of the legs, and are intensely irritating. They are apt to ulcerate, producing indolent sores.

Treatment. The most effective method of prevention lies in keeping the extremities warm. Gloves should be loose and long; two pairs of stockings should be worn, especially in winter, and bedsocks at night. Always wash hands in warm water in cold weather. Regular exercise should be taken in the open air; walking is particularly suitable. Stout footwear should be worn in wet weather.

The diet should provide an adequate intake of calcium and vitamins, as supplied by a pint of milk and a daily helping of fresh fruit, salad and green vegetables. Vitamin D may be taken in the form of cod-liver oil and malt, or capsules of halibut-liver oil. For obese patients with chilly hands and feet, 15 to 30 mg of dried thyroid may be taken under medical advice three times daily throughout the winter. Anemia should be corrected by iron. During the winter, ultraviolet light baths (artificial sunlight) may be of value.

Irritation may be minimized by a paint of compound benzoin tincture. If ulceration is present, balsam of Peru may be applied and covered with a loose dressing.

Frostbite

This occurs when the limb is cooled to or is below the freezing point of water. It is most apt to attack those points which are unclothed, such as the fingers and toes, ears and tip of the nose. Frostbite may occur even at temperatures just above freezing point, when the skin is wet and is being cooled by a strong wind.

Symptoms. The affected skin becomes numb, dead white and hard; on thawing it becomes painful, bluish-red and swollen.

Treatment. Frostbite may be prevented by the provision of suitable clothing and by constant activity, the avoidance of direct contact with metallic objects, and by the minimum of exposure during urination and defæcation.

Small areas may be treated by covering them with a warm hand. In more developed cases the affected part should be kept completely at rest and the thawing process should be as slow as possible. The extremity is elevated and exposed to a cool draught while the rest of the body is kept warm.

After thawing, the parts must be warmed gradually. On no account should massage or artificial warmth be applied directly to the affected part. Blisters are best left untouched and unopened.

See also Disorders and Diseases of the Skin, p.467.

Immersion Foot, Trench Foot, and Shelter Foot

Immersion foot is a condition brought on by immersion of the legs and feet for several hours or days in cold sea water, and is common among shipwrecked seamen in waterlogged boats and airmen in rubber dinghies. Trench foot is a similar condition which affects soldiers who are occupying waterlogged trenches in cold weather.

In these conditions the feet are cold, swollen, discolored and numb. The stage of reaction, or flushing, follows some hours or days after rescue or removal from the causal circumstances, and lasts for six to ten weeks. The feet become swollen, red, hot and intensely painful. Blisters, ulcers and gangrene may develop, and the nails may be lost.

Treatment. This should begin as soon as possible after rescue. On no account should the patient be allowed to walk, and massage or rubbing in any form must be avoided. The essence of successful treatment of the stage of reaction is to be extremely gentle and to keep the feet cool and absolutely clean. The rest of the body should be kept warm by blankets, but the feet should be elevated, to reduce swelling, and exposed to cool air; if necessary they may be cooled by an electric fan. On no account should the affected parts be warmed rapidly by the application of heat in any form. Open sores, blisters and areas of gangrene should be kept dry and powdered with antibiotics.

DISORDERS DUE TO ALLERGY

Angioneurotic Edema

(Urticaria)

Angioneurotic edema is characterized by sudden weals or swellings of the skin or mucous membranes. It may occur at any age and sometimes affects various members of the same family. In most cases the eruption is due to intolerance to some foodstuff, but heat or cold, emotional disturbances, or handling certain plants occasionally cause this allergic response. Before the swelling is seen there is heat and intense irritation, and then whitish or red swellings develop, especially on the hands, face, feet, mouth or throat, and headache or indigestion may be complained of. In severe cases large areas of the body may be involved. When the disorder affects the throat there may be difficulty in breathing, while there may be joint pains or gastric disturbances. In less severe cases the attacks may be very brief or last for a few hours, the swellings then disappearing quite suddenly. Less commonly hives may persist for some weeks.

Treatment. The general health must be attended to, and fatigue avoided. Foods known to induce hives such as porridge, shellfish, eggs, strawberries, chocolate, and so forth should not be taken. Constipation should be corrected, and a weekly dose of Epsom salts may reduce the frequency of attacks.

When an attack has already developed an injection of adrenaline solution given by a doctor will cut it short and relieve the irritation. Ephedrine tablets, benadryl and other antihistamine drugs are extremely effective but some persons respond better to one than to the others: they should only be taken under medical supervision.

In some persons aspirin, or similar preparations will cause swelling around the eyes and face which is of a similar nature. These drugs should not be taken by persons who are sensitive to them.

Locally, calamine lotion, or coal tar and lead lotion may be applied as a cooling application. Warm alkaline baths containing sodium bicarbonate, or bran baths, also give relief. (See also Allergy, p. 482.)

Vasomotor Rhinitis

See Diseases of the Ear, Nose and Throat, p. 332, and Hay Fever in the Allergy section.

DISEASES OF THE BLOOD AND SPLEEN

The Blood

Composition of the Blood. When examined under the microscope human blood is found to consist of a pale yellow fluid which is called the blood plasma, and two kinds of corpuscles, the red and white cells, together with the platelets which assist clotting.

THE RED CELLS, or erythrocytes, are about a thousand times more numerous than the white leucocytes. On an average the human body contains about ten to twelve pints of blood, about one-eleventh of the body weight. In certain diseases the number of the red cells may be found to be decreased, as in the various froms of anemia, or their contents may be affected, or their shape may vary from the normal biconcave disc-like form.

THE WHITE CELLS, or leucocytes, become greatly increased in numbers in inflammatory diseases, fevers, cancer, and some blood diseases.

HEMOGLOBIN. The red cells contain an iron compound, hemoglobin, which carries the oxygen from the lungs to all parts of the body; in anemia the total hemoglobin is deficient.

For a more detailed description of normal blood, its cells, and plasma, see Physiology, p. 239.

Testing the Quality and Quantity of Blood

The Color Index is a measure of the amount of hemoglobin in each red cell, and is calculated as follows:

$$\frac{\text{Percentage of hemoglobin}}{100} \times \frac{5{,}000{,}000}{\text{Number of red cells}}$$

The normal number of red cells is taken to be 5,000,000 per cubic millimeter of blood. In an imaginary case of anemia, the hemoglobin is 35 per cent, the red cells are only 4,000,000; by a simple calculation,

$$\frac{35}{100} \times \frac{5{,}000{,}000}{4{,}000{,}000} = 0{\cdot}43$$

In health the color index is reckoned as 1, and in the above case of anemia it will be seen that it is much lower than normal.

Blood Counts. When a blood count of a patient is made, this is to estimate the total numbers of red and white cells, and the different types of each which may be present in a cubic millimeter (a very small drop) of blood. The examination and counting of the cells is carried out by means of a microscope. The percentage of hemoglobin and the color index are also estimated.

Cell Appearance. In various disorders such as anemias, infectious and inflammatory conditions and so forth, the red cells and the white cells often present unusual appearances which are characteristic of these diseases, and these abnormal types of cells thus help to confirm the diagnosis.

Clotting. While the blood remains in circulation in the body it is a fluid, but after bleeding occurs the shed blood undergoes certain changes while a clot is formed. The natural process of clotting helps to arrest bleeding, and is thus a protective process. When blood is clotting it becomes transformed into a jelly, which floats in a fluid; the jelly portion becomes more solid in consistency, and finally hardens.

The time taken for normal blood to clot is about five minutes. The process is described in Physiology, p. 240.

The Blood Volume, or Quantity of Blood in the Body. In the normal volume of about twelve pints of blood, about 42 per cent of the whole bulk consists of cells, and the remainder is the blood plasma.

In anemia the volume is less, while in leukemia it is somewhat increased. In pregnancy, the total amount of blood is increased to supply the developing child.

When the volume of the blood is suddenly diminished as in hemorrhage or shock, certain typical symptoms develop, including collapse, faintness, air-hunger, pallor, breathlessness, sweating and thirst.

The Sedimentation Rate. This test consists in measuring the rate of fall of the blood corpuscles in a vertical column of blood at 65° F. The test is used in the diagnosis of various diseases, an increased rate being found in most infectious conditions. In a healthy person the rate is about 5 millimeters an hour, while in acute rheumatism it may be as much as 80 to 100 millimeters an hour. If this test is carried out once a week it provides a useful guide to the patient's progress, and it is also a useful test in diagnosis.

DISEASES AFFECTING THE RED BLOOD CELLS

Anemia

This consists in any condition of the blood in which there is a decrease in the normal number of red cells, or of their hemoglobin, or in both together. In anemic conditions the blood can carry less oxygen around the body, and is slower in removing the waste substances such as carbon dioxide from the different tissues and organs.

The red cells are formed in the bone marrow of the long bones; their growth is aided by the action of an enzyme substance, called hemopoietin, formed in the gastric juice of the stomach. If either this supply of enzyme to the bone marrow is lacking, or the amount of iron absorbed by the body is insufficient for the manufacture of hemoglobin and red cells, two different types of anemia may be produced. In anemia due to lack of hemopoietin the red cells are large, whereas in iron deficiency the red cells are small.

Abnormal Cells

NORMOCYTES. The red cells are more or less normal in size and shape, and in their hemoglobin content, but the total number of cells is diminished.

MEGALOCYTES. The red cells are large and well filled with hemoglobin, but there are fewer of these cells than in normal blood.

MICROCYTES. The red cells are smaller and contain less hemoglobin than in normal blood.

Types of Anemia

There are many causes of the different types of anemias, and for general interest these may be grouped as shown below.

1. Anemias due to Deficiency of Factors required in Normal Blood Formation:

(a) IRON DEFICIENCY (the most common form)
  Nutritional anemia, chlorosis, anemia of pregnancy, etc.
  Anemia in infancy and childhood
  Anemia after hemorrhage

(b) DEFICIENCY OF THE ANTI-ANEMIA LIVER AND STOMACH FACTOR
  Pernicious anemia
  Megalocytic anemia of pregnancy
  Anemia due to gastro-intestinal conditions such as sprue, etc.

(c) VITAMIN C DEFICIENCY
  Anemia of scurvy

(d) THYROID GLAND HORMONE DEFICIENCY
  Anemia of myxedema

2. Anemia due to Blood Destruction
- Various hemolytic anemias, as from poisons, infections, toxins of disease, or abnormal red blood cells
- Anemias due to unknown causes

3. Anemias due to Inactivity of the Bone Marrow

4. Miscellaneous Blood Diseases, including
- Splenic anemia
- Hemorrhagic diseases: purpura and hemophilia
- Leukemias
- Hodgkin's disease, lymphosarcoma, etc.

Symptoms of Anemia. Anemia is most common in girls and young women, but owing to the more healthy pastimes of modern girls, it is less common than formerly.

Certain symptoms are common in all types of severe anemia. The skin is pale and waxy, and the lining membrane of the mouth and eyes is also seen to be pale and bloodless. The anemic person is tired and weak, and often suffers from headaches, giddiness, and fainting attacks and becomes breathless on exertion, with palpitation of the heart. Later there may be indigestion, constipation, menstrual disorders, swelling of the feet and ankles, and other systemic changes may develop, such as degenerative disease of the nervous system. The anemic subject is also especially likely to contract infective diseases such as tuberculosis, pneumonia, rheumatic fever, etc.

Prevention and General Treatment of Anemia. The possibility of anemia developing as a result of malnutrition should be more widely recognized, especially in growing children, during adolescence and pregnancy, or after prolonged illness. Anemia cannot be adequately treated unless the actual type of anemia present is known, and a blood count (see p. 311) carried out by a pathologist is generally advisable to enable the condition to be properly assessed. Examination of the bone marrow is also sometimes required.

Symptomatic types of anemia generally subside naturally if the cause is discovered and removed.

REST. Patients who are very anemic should be kept in bed. Fresh air and sunshine are also beneficial.

IRON. Iron is valuable in many types of anemia, but different preparations of iron vary a good deal in their activity. The following are generally useful for adults:

Ferric ammonium citrate, 1.3 to 2 grams or even 3 grams, three times a day, after meals, in water, taken through a straw to avoid discoloration of the teeth.

Ferrous sulphate tablets, 1 (200 mg) three times a day after meals.

Full doses at the beginning of treatment may cause dyspepsia or diarrhea, and the initial doses may be about one-third of the amounts stated above, the dose being increased gradually. Dyspepsia may also be a symptom of the anemia itself, and may be improved by persisting with iron therapy. Iron treatment should in most cases be continued for at least one month.

Maintenance treatment is often required afterwards, especially for women who menstruate, and in whom the iron reserve is thus reduced.

DIET. For severely anemic patients the diet must be light and very digestible, food such as milk, jellies, fish, eggs, fruit, vegetable purées, bread and butter, being given every two or three hours. As improvement occurs the diet may be increased to provide meat, chicken, vegetables and raw fruit, and should contain 10 to 15 milligrams of iron daily. Eggs, oatmeal, lentils, split peas, corned beef, brown bread, liver, rabbit and herring, and green vegetables have a high content of iron. Oatmeal may be used in many ways and contains 1.2 milligrams of iron per ounce, while raw beef contains 1.1 milligrams per ounce. Raw lentils contain 2.2 milligrams per ounce.

OTHER MEDICATION. Vitamin C is an essential factor in the formation of red blood cells, and many cases of iron-deficiency anemia respond well to vitamin C administration, either in the form of fresh lemon, orange or blackcurrant juice, or as ascorbic acid tablets.

Liver and hog's stomach extracts are now seldom used in pernicious anemia for patients who do not respond well to hydroxocobalamin injections.

Folic acid is required in the megaloblastic anemia of pregnancy and that of celiac disease. It is often given combined with iron in one tablet.

Anemia due to Hemorrhage

Bleeding, or hemorrhage, may either cause a rapid loss of much blood, as in gastric ulceration, abortion, consumption, or injuries, or there may be smaller repeated losses such as occur in an excessive menstrual flow, piles, or recurrent nose bleeds. The loss of a pint of blood does not lead to symptoms of anemia in a healthy adult; two pints, however, amounts to a considerable hemorrhage, while if three pints or more (2 liters) are lost rapidly, death may follow unless restorative treatment is available.

Treatment. In serious sudden hemorrhage the bleeding must be arrested as soon as possible, the method depending on the part involved. The patient must be kept between blankets, as warm and quiet as possible in bed, with the head low; in serious cases the foot of the bed may be slightly raised. A transfusion of blood, plasma, or saline solution may be necessary, and fluids must be given by mouth. Morphine may be given by a doctor to relieve restlessness, and oxygen may be ordered.

Chronic loss of blood causing anemia may be due to various causes. In men there is often some internal bleeding from the alimentary tract, as from varicose veins in the throat, gastric or duodenal ulcer, malignant growths of the intestine, or hemorrhoids. Other common causes are repeated nosebleeds, blood diseases such as hemophilia, scurvy or purpura, and, in women, bleeding from the womb in cases of fibroids, growths or glandular disorders with menstrual disturbance.

A careful general examination should always be made in such cases, and any necessary treatment be given to arrest the bleeding. Iron should be given in full doses, and a careful watch kept on the blood counts.

Pernicious Anemia
(Addison's Anemia)

In pernicious anemia an enzyme called hemopoietin is lacking in the digestive juice in the stomach. The number of red cells is often reduced to below 2,000,000 per cubic millimeter of blood.

Symptoms. The onset of the anemia is slow, but there is increasing weakness and breathlessness, and the skin becomes pale and of a peculiar lemon-yellow tinge; bleeding from the nose sometimes occurs. The tongue is often sore, red and smooth, especially at the sides and tip, and dyspepsia is generally present owing to lack of the gastric hydrochloric acid. The patient may suddenly have a severe relapse, with collapse, or weakness, palpitations and breathlessness.

In the later stages of neglected cases, there are numbness and tingling in the limbs, due to disease of the spinal cord called 'subacute combined degeneration,' which may finally cause difficulty in movements of the hands, or in walking. Middle-aged and elderly persons are most liable to be affected by the disease, and medical advice is often not sought until the condition is fairly far advanced; the patient may have taken iron tonics from which he derives no benefit.

When the blood count is taken, the hemoglobin is sometimes only 40 per cent, while the color index is higher than normal, often being about 1·3 before treatment is given because the red cells are larger than usual.

The disease can generally be fairly easily diagnosed by the above symptoms before the spinal cord is affected, and microscopic examination of the blood will confirm the deficiency of the red cells. The absence of hydrochloric acid in the stomach is also characteristic.

Treatment. Diet, rest, and careful observation are required, especially when serious cases are seen for the first time. Although the disease is usually fatal if neglected, it responds rapidly to hydroxocobalamin, the active principle of liver extracts. Only minute amounts are necessary and these are given intramuscularly, at first weekly and later every two to four weeks according to the individual need. Treatment is life-long.

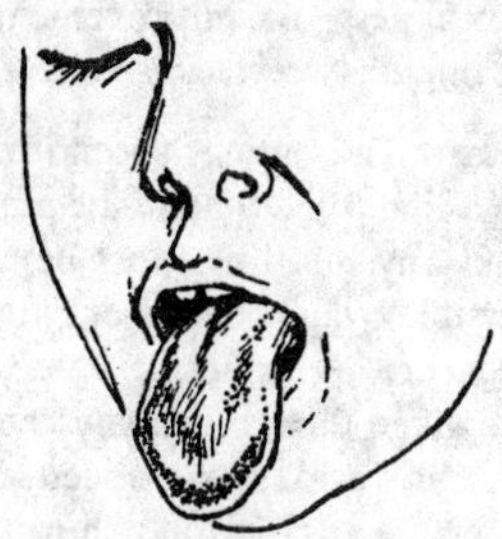

Fig. 1. *PERNICIOUS ANEMIA. The tip and sides of the tongue are characteristically red, smooth and sore.*

An important supportive treatment is an adequate intake of ascorbic acid (vitamin C) 50 milligrams three times a day for the first fortnight of treatment. The vitamin aids the blood response to hydroxocobalamin. Iron tablets must also be given.

In severe cases a blood transfusion is given, or when serious relapses occur, and the patient must be kept resting in bed. The mouth should be cleansed several times daily, by mouth-washes, and any decayed teeth should be attended to.

DIET. The food provided for the patient must be easily digestible and nourishing, with milk, eggs, bouillon, meat juice, or raw beef finely minced. As the patient improves a liberal mixed diet should be given.

In untreated cases the disease is generally fatal within two years; during this time, however, periodic improvement or 'remissions' are characteristic, but these are followed by more severe relapses.

Subacute Combined Degeneration of the Spinal Cord

This disease of the cord is one of the main complications likely to occur in pernicious anemia, but seldom develops when the blood level is kept within normal limits by means of hydroxocobalamin treatment. The patient's symptoms, however, cannot be used as a guide to his progress. Often he appears greatly improved within a few days but the red cells of the blood increase more slowly. It is in this type of case that spinal cord degeneration is likely to develop.

Blood counts should therefore be taken every three months, and if the red cells fall below 4,500,000 per cubic millimeter in women, or 5,000,000 in men, the dosage of hydroxocobalamin must be increased.

Such intensive treatment needs to be given for nine to twelve months after the blood count has become normal. So that seriously incapacitated persons may return to useful life, remedial exercises should be undertaken as soon as the patients are able to cope with them.

The use of hog's stomach preparations has declined chiefly because of the ease of administration of hydroxocobalamin instead of the massive doses required by the older treatment.

Anemia with Iron Deficiency

In this the lack of iron in the red blood cells may be caused by an insufficient supply in the diet, or by failure of absorption during digestion. The average daily intake of iron is slightly in excess of the body's requirements but a poor diet continued over a long period can easily lead to iron deficiency. It can readily be corrected by taking an iron mixture or tablets, with a full nourishing diet containing green vegetables, as well as plenty of fresh air, exercise and sunshine. Plenty of rest and time for sleep are also necessary.

Anemia due to iron deficiency is also common in pregnancy, and in women whose menstrual flow is profuse.

Anemia occurring with other diseases such as Bright's disease, cancer, infections, or general malnutrition should also be treated.

In anemia due to iron deficiency the diet should contain a liberal supply of liver, meat, green vegetables and beans. About 20 milligrams of iron is required daily by women before the menopause, but after the climacteric about 10 milligrams daily is sufficient; during pregnancy the requirement is even higher. When anemia occurs in pregnancy (and it is often present among the poorer classes) iron should be taken by mouth for the whole time and at least one month after the confinement as far as possible, to assist in maintaining the patient's general strength. When iron causes indigestion if taken by mouth, it can be given by injection.

General Treatment. The patient must rest, avoid chills, and be given a nourishing diet, with fresh air and sunshine. When the hemoglobin is less than 40 per cent, rest in bed is advisable.

The anemic patient often suffers from a poor appetite, a sense of weight and discomfort in the abdomen, nausea, flatulence, and constipation. The administration of iron preparations by mouth generally relieves these symptoms within about a fortnight.

When there is much dyspepsia a teaspoonful of aluminium hydroxide mixture should be taken after meals.

Vitamin C, taken in the form of fresh fruit or as ascorbic acid tablets, is an essential factor for the formation of red blood cells.

The tongue is sometimes sore and glazed or there may be painful cracks, but generally it improves when iron is given, especially if vitamin B or yeast tablets are prescribed in addition. Numbness and tingling of the limbs also generally disappear when iron and yeast or vitamin B are administered.

Iron Treatment. It may be pointed out that larger doses of iron than were formerly prescribed are now recognized as being necessary in most cases.

Iron preparations should always be taken *after* meals, with a drink of water.

The following preparations are recommended:

(Doses quoted are for adult patients)

1. Ferric ammonium citrate, 2 grams three times a day.
2. Ferrous sulphate or ferrous gluconate tablets, 1 three times a day.

In infants of the poorer classes mild degrees of anemia are common between the ages of six and eighteen months and in such cases the infant is pale, tires easily, and fails to thrive. Iron may be prescribed in the form of ferric ammonium citrate, 100 to 200 milligrams diluted in water sweetened with a little glycerin, given three times a day for a child aged three to six months; for children of six to eighteen months 200 to 300 milligrams may be given. Ferrous sulphate tablets are also a suitable iron preparation for children.

FOODS RICH IN IRON

Food	*Milligrams of Iron per ounce*
Meats, Fish, Eggs	
Ox liver, raw	3·9
Beef, raw	1·1
Corned beef	3·1
Rabbit	0·5
Herring	0·5
Egg	0·9
Cereals, etc.	
Oatmeal	1·2
White bread, 70% extraction	0·2
Rice	0·1
Golden Syrup	0·4
Vegetables	
Lentils, raw	2·2
Split peas	1·3
Cabbage, raw	0·3
Leeks, raw	0·4
Potato, raw	0·2
Carrot, raw	0·2
Onion, apple, orange	0·1

Hemolytic Anemias

These anemias are due to the destruction of a great number of circulating red blood cells. The cause of the destruction may be due to (1) hereditary factors as in acholuric jaundice, sickle-cell anemia, or Cooley's anemia, (2) toxins produced by severe infections, chemicals, or allergens, and (3) incompatible blood transfusions and those of unknown origin.

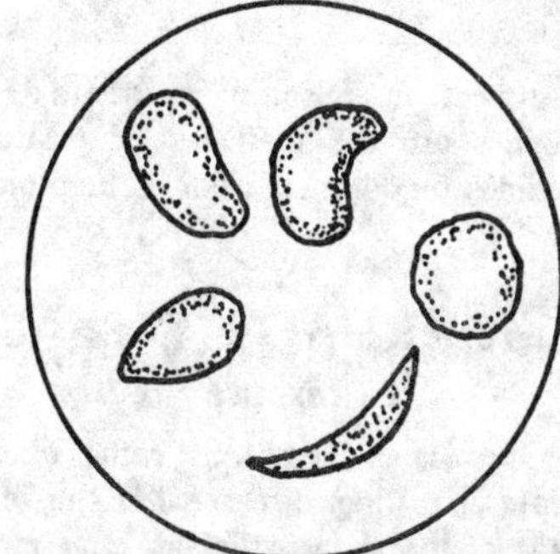

Fig. 2. *SICKLE CELLS. These mis-shapen red blood cells, roughly resembling curved sickles, are seen in an inherited form of hemolytic anemia found in some negroes.*

In these cases blood transfusion is often required to bring the level of the hemoglobin nearer normal. Sometimes surgery to remove the spleen is indicated.

Polycythemia

(*Erythremia: Osler's Disease*)

This condition is the reverse of anemia in that the red cells are increased in number and the blood becomes thicker; it is a rare disease and may occur in persons living in high altitudes, in congenital heart disease, in chronic lung disease, or in certain types of poisoning.

Treatment. In some cases blood-letting (venesection) is carried out to relieve the condition, but the relief given is transitory.

RADIOTHERAPY. Irradiation by X-rays of the whole of the patient's body is often used (the 'bath' treatment). It may be several weeks before there is a reduction in the number of red cells.

RADIOACTIVE PHOSPHORUS. An isotope of phosphorus (^{32}P), in the form of a clear colorless solution, may be given by mouth or by injection. As phosphorus is deposited in bone, the isotope effectively reduces the overactive blood-cell production going on in the bone marrow. Remissions may last for four months to two years. An interval of at least three months is essential between doses. The treatment is only available in hospital.

Agranulocytosis

Agranulocytosis is a rare disease and is the term given when there is a virtual absence of leucocytes in the blood. This is due to obstruction or suppression of the bone marrow which produces the leucocytes. The most common cause is poisoning of the marrow by certain drugs or heavy metals such as gold, arsenic, and mercury.

Symptoms usually begin with ulcers in the mouth and infective spots over the body since there are few or no leucocytes to fight infection.

Treatment in hospital is essential, and antibiotics are the mainstay of treatment. Sometimes blood transfusion is helpful.

HEMORRHAGIC DISEASES

Purpura

Purpura is a symptom rather than a separate or distinct disease; it is shown as a leakage of blood into the skin and mucous membranes and elsewhere, with the formation of small purpuric patches of various sizes in the skin, which are of a bluish-red color; the larger areas resemble bruises.

There are two main types of purpura: the primary form, and the secondary.

Primary Purpura

The primary form develops without any apparent underlying cause, and the symptoms are very variable. There is apparently some alteration, in the walls of the small capillary blood vessels, which allows the blood plasma and the blood cells to escape through into the tissues. The blood platelets are generally fewer in number than normal, and this also increases the tendency to bleeding, since the blood does not clot so easily.

The condition may be hereditary, or may develop later in life; women are rather more often affected than men. There is considerable bruising of the skin after very slight injuries, and severe loss of blood follows slight abrasions or the extraction of teeth. Anemia is common when the hemorrhages are frequent or severe, but is also often present in minor degrees as a chronic symptom.

The loss of the blood plasma from the blood vessels is likely to give rise to surface weals and swelling similar to those seen in nettlerash; joint swellings with pain are also common, and there may be attacks of abdominal pain.

Since the condition is constitutional the disease is apt to be chronic; it may tend to become worse or there may be periods of improvement. When once the primary form of purpura has shown itself, attacks are liable to occur at intervals of any length of time. These attacks may always be of the same type in any individual patient, that is there may be a purpuric rash with nose-bleeds, or they may vary from time to time. A single attack may prove rapidly fatal, or there may be a succession of slight purpuric symptoms throughout life. The commonest age for the condition to show itself is from five to fifteen years.

PURPURA SIMPLEX is the mildest form, and is usually seen in children. Purpuric spots develop, generally on the legs, and may appear in clusters. Diarrhea is often present, with slight fever, and sometimes there are joint pains. The attack lasts for several weeks.

PURPURA RHEUMATICA generally affects young men. At the onset the throat is sore, with a moderate rise of temperature. A purpuric rash develops, and there may be an urticarial eruption. Many of the joints become swollen and painful, and relapses are commonly seen at the same time each year. Each attack lasts for months but is seldom fatal, and there does not appear to be any connection with acute rheumatism.

In HENOCH'S PURPURA there is the typical purpuric rash with abdominal colic, vomiting, and diarrhea or constipation. Blood may be passed in the stools which look tarry. The condition may resemble acute appendicitis. Joint pains and relapses are common, and occasionally nephritis develops, with a high death-rate.

In HEMORRHAGIC PURPURA, which is usually seen in girls, the onset is abrupt after a few days of slight malaise. There is a severe purpuric rash with hemorrhages from the nose, gums and other parts, and fever, joint pains, and vomiting; nephritis may develop, and the anemia becomes more pronounced. Death may occur within a few days from general weakness, or improvement may set in within one or two weeks.

Treatment. The patient should rest in bed, and have a light diet. The limbs must be kept warm, and any bleeding must be checked as far as possible by adrenaline or cauterization, etc. Drugs are of doubtful value, but iron tonics are given during convalescence.

Blood transfusions are given in serious conditions. The cortisone hormones will produce remissions in many cases, especially if given in conjunction with blood transfusion. In severe cases in adults the spleen may have to be removed.

The condition often improves as the patient gets older.

Secondary Purpura

Secondary purpura is also called symptomatic purpura since it occurs in association with various other diseases, especially the acute fevers such as typhus, smallpox, cerebrospinal meningitis and scarlet fever; it is less common in measles and typhoid fever.

Purpura is also seen in septic conditions such as septicemia (blood poisoning) and infective endocarditis, in leukemia, nephritis, cancer, tuberculosis, old age, scurvy, jaundice, and nervous disorders, and also as a local condition after tight bandaging or other states of congestion.

Treatment is that required for the underlying disease, with the various measures used for primary purpura.

Hemophilia

In this familial disease there is a dangerous tendency to persistent bleeding, and when an accident or operation involving loss of blood occurs there is extreme danger to life, since the bleeding is difficult to control owing to failure or great delay in clotting. The condition only affects males, but is handed down through the family by the female line. Daughters of hemophiliac fathers should not bear children if they marry; mortality is high among hemophiliacs however great the care that is taken.

Hemophiliacs must strenuously avoid all risk of loss of blood, as from dental extractions or minor abrasions. If bleeding occurs, the application of normal fresh human blood to the bleeding area may arrest the flow. Blood transfusions may sometimes be required.

BLOOD TRANSFUSION

It seems appropriate to give here a brief account of the treatment process whereby whole blood is taken from a human donor and given to a sick person in need of it.

Blood Groups. In 1900 Landsteiner discovered that the red blood cells in different human beings are not identical, and that the blood serum of some persons will agglutinate (or clot) and destroy the red cells of other people.

There are now known to be four main blood groups which are called AB, A, B, and O (or 1, 2, 3, and 4). Group AB, or 1, is the *universal recipient* group, and can receive blood from donors in any of the other three groups, since the blood will mix and not clot. Group O is the *universal donor* group. In the actual practice of giving transfusions, blood from a donor in the same group as the recipient, or from Group O, is generally used. The compatibility of donor and recipient should always be tested before a transfusion is carried out, even when the blood is taken from a universal donor, or from a donor of the same group as the recipient.

Fuller details concerning the blood groups, and the Rhesus factor, are given in the section on Physiology, p. 239.

Technique. The donor lies recumbent. A 'cuff' or tourniquet is put on his arm. A vein on the inner fold of the elbow is selected, the skin area sterilized, and the vein punctured with a sterilized needle attached to the sterilized collecting apparatus. In the sterile jar or bottle is sodium citrate to prevent coagulation. About one pint of blood is usually taken from the donor. He then rests for fifteen to twenty minutes.

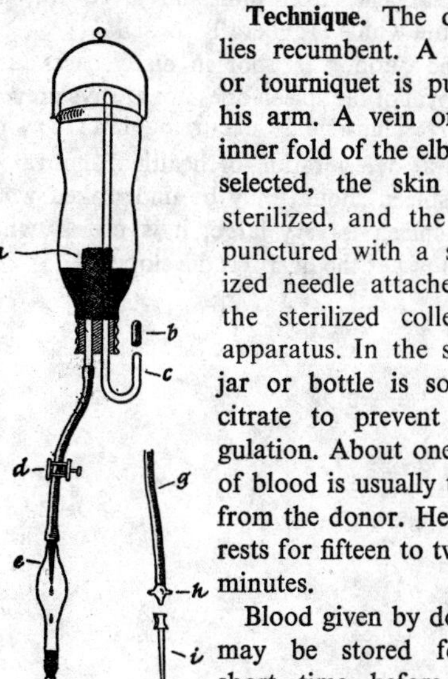

Fig. 3. *SKETCH OF BLOOD TRANSFUSION APPARATUS. (a) Wire gauze filter; (b) rubber cap; (c) inlet tube; (d) clip to control flow; (e) glass dripper; (f) (g) length of rubber tubing; (h) record fitting; (i) needle.*

Blood given by donors may be stored for a short time before use. Such blood banks are maintained in hospitals.

For the administration of blood, the 'continuous drip' method is used, about one to three pints being slowly run into the vein; a pint is transfused in about forty-five minutes. For emergencies there are plastic disposable sets, and blood in plastic bags.

Blood plasma, gum saline, and other solutions are also used for transfusion purposes when properly matched whole blood is not available, or in emergencies.

The main uses for transfusion are in accidents or severe wounds, for shock or hemorrhage, in surgery (before or after major operations), in childbirth, severe anemias, septicemia, and hemophilia.

DISEASES AFFECTING THE WHITE BLOOD CELLS

There are two main types of white cells in the blood, the leucocyte and the lymphocyte; the first grow in the bone marrow while the latter are formed in the lymph glands and spleen. In every cubic millimeter (a very small drop) of blood there are normally about 7,000 white cells, of which about 70 per cent are leucocytes and 30 per cent are lymphocytes. If there are fewer white cells than normal there is *leucopenia*, and if more than about 9,000 there is *leucocytosis*.

The white cells may be reduced in various conditions which affect the bone marrow, such as splenic anemia, pernicious anemia and tuberculosis, while leucocytosis occurs in infective diseases and inflammatory disorders, whooping-cough, glandular fever, after hemorrhage or injuries, in intoxications such as uremia, diabetic coma, gout, and poisoning, and in cases of leukemia and cancer.

Leukemia

Leukemia is a disease of the blood in which enormous numbers of partly developed white cells are formed, owing to disturbances in the work of the bone marrow, lymph glands or spleen. In *myeloid leukemia* the bone marrow's output of white cells is at fault, whereas in *lymphatic leukemia* the activity of the lymph glands and spleen seems to be uncontrolled. The white cells may be increased up to as much as 10,000 to 400,000 per cubic millimeter of blood, compared with a normal level of 7,000.

Both the myeloid form and the lymphatic form of the disease may occur as either an acute or a chronic condition. There is little difference in symptoms between the two acute types and the two chronic types of leukemia; the outlook is very grave in all cases of leukemia, and the chronic form is always fatal eventually.

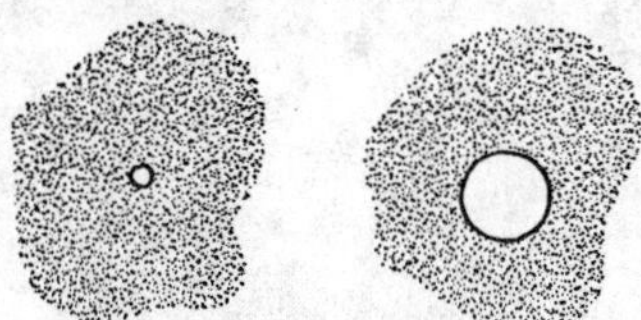
Fig. 4. *PROPORTION OF RED AND WHITE CELLS. In the drop of normal blood on the left, the gray portion indicates the area occupied by red cells, the white portion that of white cells. On the right, the greatly increased proportion of white cells indicates a state of leukæmia.*

Acute Leukemia

In acute leukemia the total white cell count is sometimes little changed, but many abnormal cells are present. The disease is very rapid in onset, being ushered in with vomiting, headache, small or large hemorrhages into the skin and from the gums, nose, womb and alimentary tract. The patient quickly becomes anemic, because accompanying the great increase in the white cells, the red cells become considerably reduced in number. The gums are spongy and the teeth loosen, the breath being very foul owing to the inflammation of the gums. The temperature is usually about 37·5°–39° C (100°–102° F). The course of this disease is usually very rapid; the patient may die in a few days, and in any case seldom lives for more than a few months. Occasionally the symptoms subside, and the condition becomes more like that seen in chronic leukemia.

Treatment. No medical treatment is known to be of much value in this disease. The patient must be kept in bed, and usually can only take fluids by mouth. The mouth must be carefully and frequently cleansed with weak disinfectants. Cortisone or prednisone is administered to patients in high fever and with severe anemia since it produces quick beneficial results, and when the patient shows resistance to the hormone, mercaptopurine tablets are given. Mercaptopurine administration is particularly helpful for children. An enzyme, L-asparaginase, has been found to be therapeutically active in leukemia if given together with other drugs.

Small doses of the tincture of iodine may relieve vomiting in the last stages, and morphine may be ordered by the doctor.

Chronic Leukemia

The cause of the disease is not known. It is important to make an accurate diagnosis between the acute and the chronic types of leukemia since more effective treatment is available for the chronic form. Chronic leukemia is commoner in men than in women and the symptoms are slow and insidious. The patient becomes anemic, breathless, and weak, and he may notice that the abdomen is becoming larger, owing to a great increase in the size of the spleen. There may be various hemorrhages as in the acute disease. The glands of the armpits, neck and groins are often enlarged. A complete blood examination must be carried out to confirm the diagnosis in a suspected case.

Treatment. The patient need not as a general rule be confined entirely to bed, although he must lead a quiet life, with daily rest periods. In the later stages the patient is generally bedridden. All forms of infection, such as colds or influenza, must be avoided. The disease is invariably fatal although the patient often lives several years (sometimes for eight to ten years), if treatment by X-rays, by such drugs as busulphan and the nitrogen mustards, or urethane, is given. Blood transfusion is often beneficial when the anemia is severe, and iron tonics should be given.

The diet should be varied and nourishing, and contain a liberal supply of fats, bacon and cereals. When the appetite is poor, a tonic may be ordered.

DISEASES OF THE SPLEEN

The spleen is a solid organ lying in the upper left part of the abdomen below the diaphragm (see p. 230). It consists largely of lymphatic tissue, and few diseases affect the spleen alone; on the other hand this organ often undergoes changes in many systemic disorders. It can be removed by surgical

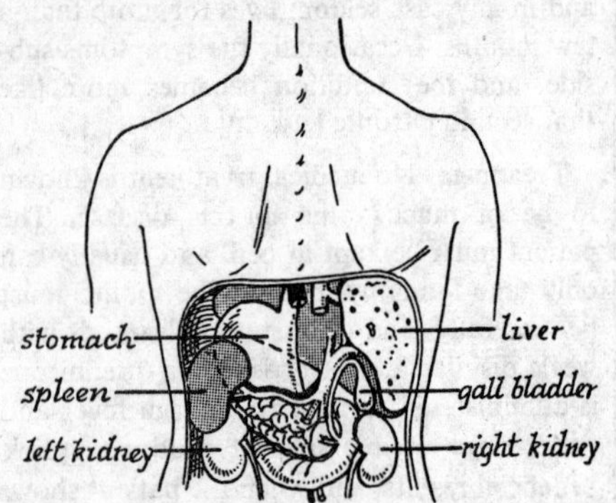

Fig. 5. *THE SPLEEN. Back view of viscera of mid-trunk showing the position of the spleen in relation to the stomach and kidneys.*

operation without causing permanent damage to health. (See also p. 381.)

The spleen may be completely absent, or may consist of several small 'spleniculi' scattered about the abdomen.

Floating Spleen

Floating spleen occurs in women, either when there is a general dropping of the other abdominal organs (visceroptosis), or when the spleen is enlarged or displaced as a result of disease or injury.

Symptoms may be very indefinite, but there may be pain from the surrounding adhesions or as a result of pressure on other organs. Sudden twisting may also occur, with severe pain such as occurs in twisting of an ovarian cyst.

Treatment. If the displacement causes much discomfort or other complications, surgical removal of the spleen is advisable.

Abscess of the Spleen

Abscess of the spleen is sometimes a complication of typhoid fever, phlebitis and other acute infections. The condition is not easily diagnosed, and consequently peritonitis may follow rupture of the abscess.

Rupture of the Spleen

Rupture of the spleen sometimes follows injuries in normal persons, but is more often a sequel when the organ is diseased or enlarged. Spontaneous rupture may occur in typhoid fever or malaria, leukemia, and other diseases in which the spleen becomes enlarged.

Symptoms. The sudden severe hemorrhage into the abdominal cavity causes pain and collapse. If the patient rapidly loses consciousness the condition may be very difficult to diagnose.

Treatment. Immediate surgical treatment is indicated, to prevent death from hemorrhage.

Banti's Disease

(*Splenic Anemia*)

This is an uncommon disease, with anemia and enormous swelling of the spleen; the disease may last up to about ten years. In the last stages, if the patient has not been successfully treated, there are cirrhosis of the liver, jaundice and edema. Hemorrhage from the stomach is also a common symptom.

Treatment. Iron must be given for the anemia which is generally present.

The outlook is poor in many cases, and removal of the spleen does not always prevent severe hemorrhage occurring later on, or general deterioration of health. Removal of the spleen should only be undertaken when the spleen is very large; it is useless when cirrhosis of the liver has developed.

DISEASES OF THE LYMPHATIC SYSTEM

The various diseases of the lymphatic structures generally accompany diseases in other tissues of the body, especially in conditions such as inflammation or certain fevers, or malignant disease.

Obstruction of the lymphatic vessels may be due to tumors. inflammation, or may occur as a result of injuries.

Acute Lymphangitis

This disease, which is comparatively common, is to be seen in association with septic condition of the fingers, hand, foot, or other parts of the limb. It is shown by the appearance of red lines in the skin passing from the point or area of infection to the nearest group of lymphatic glands. The patient feels ill, with shivering and fever, headache, and loss of appetite. The inflamed parts are very tender and, if untreated, the patient may die from septicemia.

Treatment. The original abrasion or abscess must be drained, and hot compresses applied. Antibiotic treatment is commonly used now to arrest the disease, but must be supervised by a physician. Complete rest and elevation of the part (a sling being used if the arm is affected) are required. Ichthyol ointment may be used along the inflamed area to reduce the inflammation. When the neighboring glands become involved they also should be compressed, except in the armpit, and often require surgical treatment when abscesses develop.

Glandular Fever
(*Infectious Mononucleosis*)

This is an illness probably caused by a virus, but although spread from person to

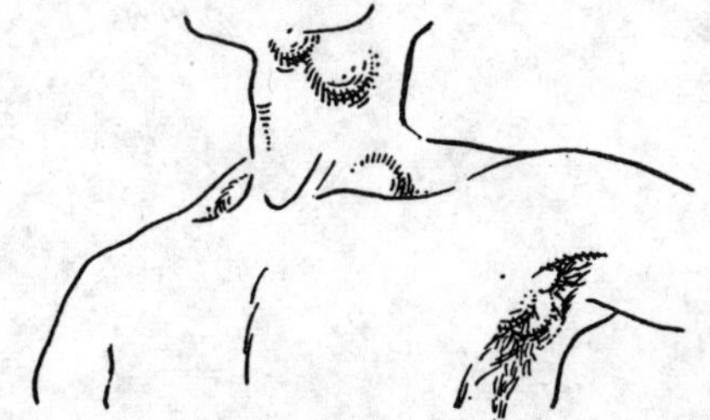

Fig. 1. *GLANDULAR FEVER. The most commonly affected groups of glands are those in the neck and in the armpit.*

person directly, it is not very infectious. It usually occurs in epidemics and affects children and teenagers. See also p. 283.

An influenza-like illness starts with a high temperature and, early in the disease, the lymph glands become swollen and tender. The group of glands in the neck are especially affected, and occasionally the groin and armpit glands and even the tonsils themselves. The illness may last two weeks or more, and recurrences may occur.

A more unpleasant form of glandular fever occurs in young adults, where the throat and tonsils are affected early with much pain and inflammation. This type of the disease may resolve in three to four weeks.

Treatment. The treatment consists in keeping the patient comfortable, for the disease process will burn out in time. Rest in bed is essential when the temperature is raised, and warm gargles, e.g. 1 teaspoonful of salt in a glass of warm water, give much relief if performed every four hours. Aspirin or its equivalent make the illness more bearable and the patient should be encouraged to take plenty of fluids even at the expense of the more solid parts of the diet.

Convalescence may be long, and the patient is often tired and debilitated for some months after this illness although serious complications following it are rare.

Lymphadenitis

Lymphadenitis, or local inflammation of the lymph glands, is due to drainage of infection from other tissues or organs. The glands of the neck are thus often seen to be swollen and tender when the tonsils are infected, or in cases of inflammation of the scalp or ear, or abscess of the teeth.

Tuberculous Adenitis, due to tuberculosis of the glands of the neck, is a serious condition met with in children; the abdominal glands may also be affected by tuberculosis. In the neck, streptomycin and other anti-tuberculous injections are now used to check the infection, but if the glands are not reduced in about eight weeks they should be treated surgically to prevent spread elsewhere. General and nutritional treatment is also required.

The glands at the root of any limb may be swollen as a result of infection in the area that they drain, while those of the armpit may be affected by breast infections.

General Acute Lymphadenitis is enlargement of lymphatic glands throughout the body and occurs in many acute infective diseases such as German measles, measles, and scarlet fever. It generally subsides without suppuration of the glands.

Lymphogranuloma Inguinale

This lymphatic disease of the genital organs is caused by a virus which may be transmitted during sexual intercourse (hence its other name, lymphogranuloma venereum). Fifty years ago it was mainly found in West Africa and South America, but now it is seen in any seaport in the world.

A small painless ulcer (or bubo) occurs on the genitals two weeks after infection, and this rapidly heals leaving a large group of affected glands. In the male these are always found in the groin, and in affected females the glands around the rectum often become involved.

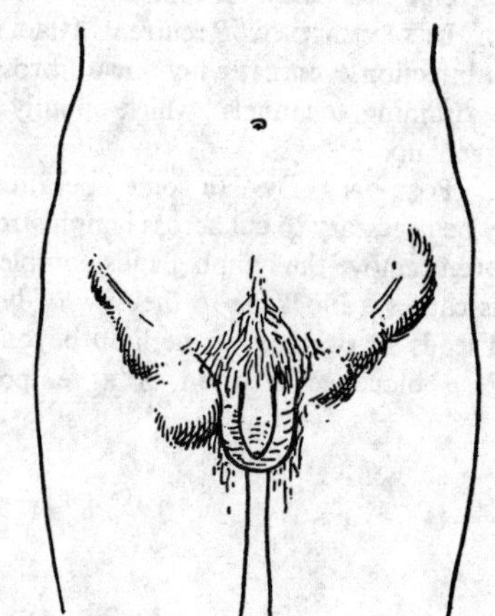

Fig. 2. *LYMPHOGRANULOMA INGUINALE. The characteristic painless buboes, in the male, are always confined to the groin.*

When the groin glands are affected a painless abscess slowly develops over several months, which may discharge pus through a chronic sinus, or it may remain as a closed pus cavity for years before discharging, but once established it is very difficult to cure. If the rectal lymph tissues become affected a stricture of the rectum follows which leads to increasing constipation and obstruction of the large bowel.

Treatment is difficult but if the patient seeks medical advice in the early stages some of the antibiotics, particularly chloramphenicol and tetracycline, may help. Surgical treatment may be required for the established abscesses.

Cystic Hygroma

A cyst occurring in the lymph glands of the neck in babies may be noticed soon after birth or may not be obvious until the child is a few months old. The swelling gets bigger and, although it may reach a large and frightening size, it rarely causes serious harm to the infant if treated properly.

Treatment. The best treatment at present is to inject the cyst to reduce its size and later to remove it surgically, although certain cystic hygromata respond well to X-ray treatment.

Lymphedema

Lymphedema is a diffuse swelling of a part, usually a limb, which is due to the damming back of lymph in the tissues. At first the space between the cells is filled with translucent fluid but gradually fibrosis occurs in this fluid and it 'sets,' thus causing further obstruction and making the swelling permanent.

Causes. Many conditions cause this disability, and the leg is more commonly affected than the arm.

1. CONGENITAL. There may be an absence of lymphatic ducts draining the limb, or the communications between the surface and deep channels may be missing.

2. INFLAMMATORY. Recurrent attacks of skin infection eventually lay down fibrosis in the draining channels which finally get clogged up.

3. POST-OPERATIVE. In some operations it may be necessary to cut across lymph streams or even remove the lymph glands completely. This causes a blockage to the flow of lymph and leads to swelling of the limb beyond it; such a blockage is often of a temporary nature and new lymph channels grow across the scar in time.

4. BLOCKAGE OF THE LYMPH GLANDS. The glands themselves in the groin or armpit may become blocked. In Africa, certain parasitic worms (filariae) and their larvae which are carried by a mosquito, invade the glands and cause a brisk fibrous reaction. In consequence gross swelling of the leg and genitalia may occur, causing elephantiasis (see Filariasis, p. 388).

In more temperate climates the lymph glands may be invaded by cancerous cells and give rise to obstruction.

Treatment. Lymphedema arising from any of these causes can be considerably lessened and the patient made more comfortable by raising the limb. If the leg is involved, the patient should rest flat with the affected leg on pillows, while the arm may be similarly carried on pillows or in a sling.

Surgery may be required to remove gross obstructions.

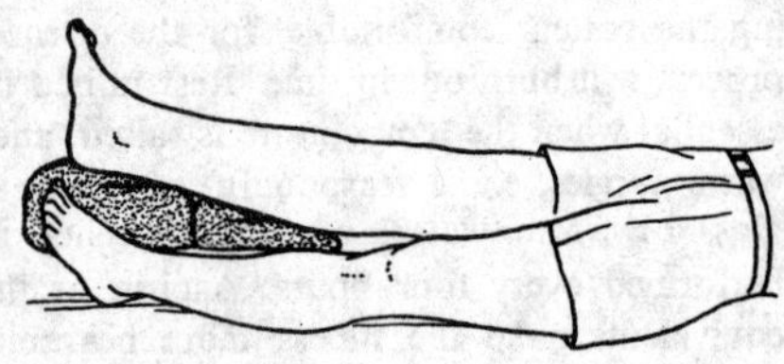

Fig. 3. LYMPHEDEMA. The swollen leg should be rested upon a pillow to ease the limb and to aid return of lymph to the body.

Hodgkin's Disease

(Lymphadenoma)

In Hodgkin's disease, there is enlargement of the lymph glands and spleen, with increasing anemia. The disease is more common in young men and is due to a malignant proliferation of lymphoid tissue cells.

In the beginning the glandular swelling is painless, and is especially noted in the neck, and the glands do not tend to break down. The patient becomes increasingly weak and loses weight. After a long interval of months to years, perhaps up to four years, the disease slowly progresses, and the glands may become enormous, with increasing anemia and attacks of fever. The enlarged glands may cause pressure on various organs. Death generally occurs from exhaustion or some other malady since, although the disease may be arrested for a time by X-ray irradiation, radium, nitrogen mustard, or chlorambucil, recurrence is usually inevitable.

Some patients, however, seem to get a benign form of the condition and may survive twenty years or more.

Tumors of Lymphatic Glands

Tumors of the lymphatic glands are often secondary to malignant growths in other organs. However, such tumors may occur primarily in the lymphatic system and are known as lymphosarcomata. They may be localized to one group of glands or may be generalized throughout the body.

Treatment of both types is difficult and may be given by surgery or by radiotherapy. The outlook for the localized group is much better than when the condition is generalized.

DISEASES OF THE EYE

THE EYE

The eye is the organ of sight, and it is wonderfully constructed for the perception of light, color and form, and for seeing near and distant objects and scenes. Its structure is described on p.233. Since the eye is a somewhat complex organ composed of various different parts and tissues, if any of these parts become diseased or injured, vision may be impaired. Good eyesight is also dependent on good general health, and various general diseases such as diabetes mellitus, high blood pressure, chronic nephritis, and so forth, may affect vision by interfering with the nutrition of the eye.

Cataract is a common complication of diabetes, while optic neuritis often develops in the later stages of chronic nephritis.

Common Affections of the Eyes. Disorders of the eyes may be accompanied by obvious signs, or the patient may only complain of particular symptoms with no apparent changes in the eye or surrounding structures. In most cases a systematic examination is generally necessary.

Examination of the Eye. The general health must be considered in relation to many eye diseases, and the examination of the eye should include inspection of the eyelids, the orbit, the lachrymal apparatus, the conjunctiva and sclera, the external muscles, the cornea over the iris and pupil, the anterior chamber in front of the lens, the lens itself, and the posterior chamber behind the lens, with the vitreous humor. A refraction examination, and examination of the retina and optic nerve by means of an ophthalmoscope, are often required, and finally tests of vision and color sense may be necessary. A general examination of this type should, of course, only be carried out by an ophthalmic surgeon.

The ordinary observer, however, can see if the lids and eyelashes appear normal, or if there is dislike of light, or spasm of the lids, or any discharge; he can also note if the conjunctiva (or white of the eye and lining of the lids) is red and apparently inflamed; and if so, whether the whole conjunctiva is affected or only the zone surrounding the iris, which may indicate iritis. The cornea over the pupil may be hazy or show opacities, or the chamber in front of the iris may contain pus or blood. The shape of the pupil may be abnormal owing to adhesions of the iris, or to an iridectomy operation; or the pupil may fail to react to light or to accommodation of sight to near and far obects. There, may be tremor of the eyeball, as in nystagmus; or the tension of the eyeball may be raised, making it harder to the feel than normal, as in glaucoma.

Any disorder of the eyes is liable to give rise to serious effects, and should never be neglected. Medical advice should be sought as soon as possible.

Care of the Eyes. Many people with normal eyes and good sight begin to suffer from gradual failure of the power of accommodation at about the age of forty-five years. In order to preserve the gift of good sight as long as possible, particular care of the eyes should be taken by paying attention to the general health, with a moderate and adequate diet, moderation in smoking and the use of alcohol, regular exercise, and care in the use of the eyes themselves. This care includes the use of a good light for reading or close work, with avoidance of glare; a direct light should not be placed in front of the eyes, but should be behind and above the left shoulder. Small print should be avoided. The eyes may be bathed daily in warm or tepid salt solution (1 teaspoonful of common salt to 1 pint of boiled water).

SIMPLE EXERCISES for the eyes are beneficial and may be carried out in bed in the mornings. The head should be kept still, and the eyes are turned as far as possible to the left side, then to the right, then up and down, each movement being made steadily three or four times. Try to avoid staring during ordinary work or occupations, and remember that blinking is beneficial to the eyes, and also that the eyes and lids should never be rubbed.

Children's Eyes. Great care should be taken of children's eyes, which are immature, like other organs of the body. The normal growth of the eye may easily be affected by too prolonged or irregular stimulation. Short sight, squint, eye-strain and fatigue may be caused by habitual use of a poor light, or by too prolonged close work.

EYE-STRAIN may be indicated by a constant tendency to frown, by twitching of the face, excessive blinking, or persistent rubbing of the eyes, or headaches.

Suitable exercises or glasses may remedy these defects in the early stages, and this does not necessarily mean that glasses will always have to be worn. A child may be considered stupid or slow when in reality he cannot see very well or without undue effort.

Children should always sleep in a darkened room, so that the eyes may be properly rested.

Blepharitis (inflammation of the lid margins) and conjunctivitis are common disorders in children; they should not be neglected, and may be associated with imperfect sight.

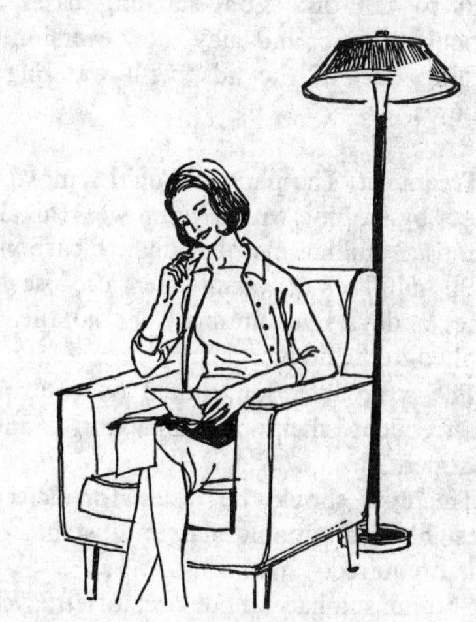

Fig. 1. *CARE OF THE EYES. For reading or close work, direct light should not be placed in front of the eyes, but should be behind and above the left shoulder.*

DISEASES OF THE EYELIDS

Sty

A sty is a small abscess or pustule at the edge of the lid, occurring in a sebaceous gland of a hair follicle. It often develops in people who are run down, or who are in poor general health, and in such cases sties tend to be recurrent.

The eyelash at the inflamed point should be pulled out with small forceps. The eyelids should be frequently bathed with hot lotions or a small hot boric acid compress may be applied and renewed frequently until the sty points or breaks. Some sties need to be gently incised by a doctor, but often when the lash is extracted the pus is discharged from the follicle. Eye ointment should be applied to the edges of the lids until healing is complete. In recurrent cases penicillin treatment is sometimes advised. The general health must be attended to, with a nourishing diet and fresh air; iron tonics and cod-liver oil are beneficial in such cases. In children, sties are sometimes associated with defective eyesight, and the eyes should be tested in case glasses are required.

Blepharitis

Blepharitis is an inflammatory condition of the edges of the eyelids, and affects the follicles of the eyelashes and the conjunctiva lining the eyelids. Blepharitis is common among school children and is often associated with poor eyesight.

The inflammation may be acute or chronic, and is common after some acute fevers, such as measles and scarlet fever. In most cases the condition is linked with dandruff of the scalp in seborrheic patients.

The lids are sore and reddened, and often show a slight discharge or small crusted ulcers along the margins where the lashes tend to fall out. Long-standing cases are difficult to cure, and may show eversion (or turning out) of the lids, with watering of the eyes.

Treatment. The patient should remove the crusts by bathing with a warm weak alkaline lotions (3 milligrams of sodium bicarbonate to 30 milliliters of warm water) used several times a day. Eye ointment should then be applied to the lid margins.

The scalp infection should be controlled by frequent shampoos and anti-dandruff treatment.

The eyes should be tested for defective eyesight, and suitable glasses must be worn when required.

Sodium sulphacetamide or chlortetracycline eye ointment is prescribed in many cases, with rapid and successful results. Sometimes these antibiotics may be combined with cortisone with good effect.

Meibomian Cysts
(*Chalazion: Tarsal Cyst*)

Rounded swellings, called meibomian cysts, about the size of a pea sometimes develop in the glands of the eyelids. They are commonest in the upper lids in young adults and often tend to recur. These cysts may begin by being acutely inflamed, or they may persist for a long time and finally become absorbed, or they may end by becoming inflamed. In the inflammatory stage they often cause much pain, since the abscess does not break easily.

Treatment by a surgeon consists in turning out the lid, and the entire cyst is removed under a local anesthetic.

Inversion of the Lids
(*Entropion*)

Turning in of the lids may be due to scarring of the conjunctiva or the skin of the face with subsequent deformity of the lid, and is generally caused by trachoma or burns of the face, either thermal or chemical. The upper lid is most commonly affected, and the eyelashes turn inwards and constantly irritate the globe of the eye.

Sometimes old people get an entropion if the muscles of the lids go into spasm. This may happen for a short while after eye operations.

Eversion of the Lids
(*Ectropion*)

This generally affects the lower lid, and leads to constant watering of the eye. Old people with chronic inflammation of the conjunctiva may suffer from this condition, or it may be seen as a result of scar formation after burns, injuries, or rodent ulcer. Occasionally, damage to the nerves of the eyelid after a stroke may cause an ectropion.

Surgical treatment generally relieves these deformities of the lids, while astringent eyedrops reduce the watering, and antibiotic drops the infection.

Ptosis

Ptosis, or drooping of the upper lid, is due to weakness or paralysis of the muscle which raises the lid, and the condition may be partial or complete. Where the lid cannot be raised at all, sight is obscured unless the head is thrown back, and the forehead muscles may be used to raise the eyebrow.

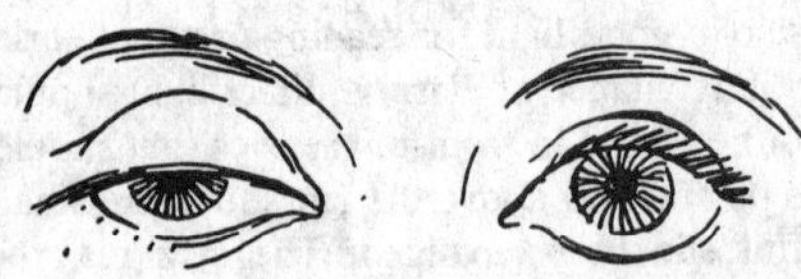

Fig. 2. *PTOSIS. Dropping of the upper lid is due to weakness or paralysis of the muscle which raises the lid.*

Ptosis may be due to hereditary weakness or absence of the muscle. These cases are best dealt with surgically, with good results. Ptosis, however, may be acquired as a result of some disease such as trachoma, or tertiary syphilis, or hysteria, which requires appropriate treatment.

LACHRYMAL DISEASES

Watering of the Eyes

In normal conditions of the eyes, tears leave the ducts of the lachrymal gland beneath the upper lid, and pass across the eye down into the lachrymal sac and its duct into the nose. Any disorder of muscles of the lids or of the duct will obstruct the drainage into the nose and the tears will flow over the lower lid, causing constant watering of the eye, and sometimes soreness of the skin below the lid.

This condition of *epiphora* may follow facial paralysis with dropping of the lower eyelid; or chronic blepharitis, or turning-out of the lower lid may be responsible—but the commonest cause is chronic inflammation of the nasal duct, with obstruction. Syphilitic disease of the nose, or injuries, etc., may lead to obstruction of the lachrymal duct. In some cases the lachrymal sac is dilated, forming a mucocele.

Treatment. When blepharitis or conjunctivitis is present, astringent lotions should be used to bathe the eye; zinc sulphate solution, 0·25 per cent, may be used for several days but this solution may cause slight irritation of the eye if used for too long. The lachrymal ducts may be syringed by a doctor and this may relieve any obstruction.

Surgical treatment may be required when the lower lid is turned outwards, and in some cases in adults the lachrymal sac can be removed and a by-pass made.

DISEASES OF THE CONJUNCTIVA

Conjunctivitus is inflammation of the conjunctiva which lines the eyelids and covers the eyeballs. There is redness of the conjunctiva, with increased watering of the eye, or discharge.

Causes. The inflammation may be short-lived, as in the irritation caused by a small foreign body or piece of grit in the eye; or it may be chronic, as a result of eye-strain with defective eyesight, or from general ill-health or gout, lachrymal diseases, occupation in a dusty or gritty atmosphere or in bright light, or exposure to smoke, fumes, or other irritants. Septic teeth or nasal disorders may also give rise to conjunctivitis.

The cause must be discovered and, whenever possible, removed and the general conditions of life must be improved as far as possible.

Local Treatment consists in the use of warm saline or weak sodium bicarbonate solution to clear away any discharge which is on the eyelids. Penicillin drops or sulphacetamide may be ordered by a doctor. The secretion formed in conjunctivitis may be watery, mucoid, or purulent.

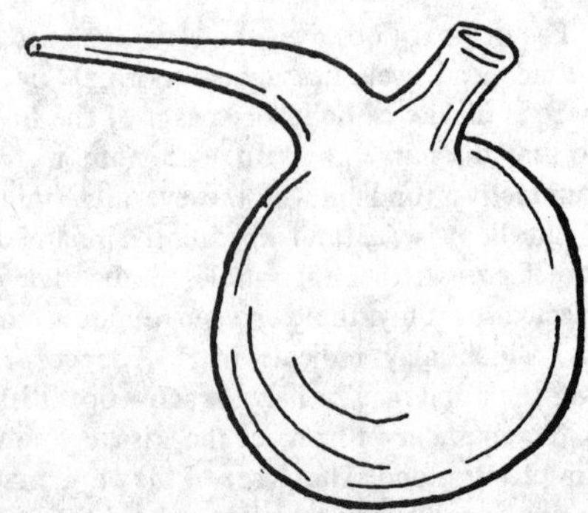

Fig. 3. *UNDINE OR GLASS FLASK. This type of flask is sometimes used for irrigating the eye.*

Acute Catarrhal Conjunctivitis

In this condition the congestion or inflammation of the eyes is moderately severe, and there is a mucous discharge which may make the lids adhere to each other. The disorder is often due to a 'cold in the eye' from cold winds, or from some catarrhal infection, and is commonly seen in the early stages of measles. Pain, swelling and dislike of light are generally present in varying degrees, and the eye may feel gritty or rough.

Pink Eye

A severe form of pink eye may cause a purulent discharge; the disease is very contagious and an epidemic may spread rapidly, especially in schoolchildren. Occasionally corneal ulcers are formed; this type of conjunctivitis is commonly caused by Koch-Weeks' bacillus, and is known as 'pink eye.'

From the closed lids, gently wipe off the discharge with a tissue dipped in saline solution. Medical advice should be sought early so that antibiotic eye-drops may be used as soon as possible. These must be instilled every two or three hours to be of value.

Yellow mercuric oxide ointment is smeared along the edges of the lids to prevent them sticking together and retaining the discharge. The eye should not be bandaged for the same reason; if the eye is very sensitive to light an eye-shade may be worn.

Towels, face-cloths, handkerchiefs, etc., must be kept separate to avoid spread of the infection.

Angular Conjunctivitis

Angular conjunctivitis is a mild and rather chronic inflammation of the corners of the eyes, causing redness of the lids and mainly affecting adults. Zinc sulphate eye lotion, 0·5 per cent, should be used for a few days for bathing the eyelids in this condition.

Gonorrheal Conjunctivitis

Gonorrheal infection of the eyes occurs in two types of cases, (a) in adults and (b) as ophthalmia neonatorum in newly born infants. A few cases of purulent ophthalmia are not gonococcal in origin.

Ophthalmia neonatorum is a preventable infection which develops in newly born infants as a result of contagion with gonorrheal discharge in the mother, or from other infections. Want of care at birth in gonorrheal cases used to cause about 30 per cent of all cases of blindness in children. Today only a quarter of the cases are of gonorrheal origin, and can be cured. The discharge is usually noticed on the third day or very soon after birth, and both eyes are generally affected. Within the first four weeks after birth any discharge in an infant's eyes, even if it is a watery discharge, should be examined by a doctor.

In gonnorheal conjunctivitis the discharge is at first watery, but soon becomes thick and purulent. The lids become red and enormously swollen, and the edges stick together or turn outwards; thick yellow pus exudes and the lining membrane is red and congested. There is great danger of ulceration of the cornea (transparent part of the eye in front of the iris and pupil) if the condition is neglected or improperly treated.

Preventive Treatment. As soon as the infant is born, cleanse each eye with separate pieces of clean cotton dipped in normal saline; burn the cotton after use. Wash the eyelids with normal saline and gently irrigate the lids. In doubtful cases instil a drop of silver nitrate solution, 1 per cent, into each eye. Do not let the bath water touch the child's eyes or lids; use separate water and a clean towel for the face. Repeat the cleansing of the eyes after 8 to 12 hours. In cases of uncertainty, a pathologist should examine the discharge from the mother's vagina. The infant's eyes must be carefully watched during the whole of the puerperium, and early treatment with antibiotics can be started.

Curative Treatment. When gonorrheal ophthalmia develops, highly skilled nursing in hospital is required. Penicillin is a curative agent if used properly. The eyes must be cleansed every hour and frequently irrigated, and the edges of the eyelids must be greased to prevent them from adhering. Sulphacetamide sodium eye-drops, 10 to 20 per cent, are used four-hourly, and antibiotics are given by injection or by mouth.

If the cornea over the pupil ulcerates, atropine drops, 1 per cent, should be used, and cauterization of the cornea is sometimes carried out.

If only one eye is affected, the child must lie on the affected side for drainage and wear an eye-shield. Treatment must be continued for a month after the discharge has ceased.

GONORRHEAL CONJUNCTIVITIS IN ADULTS. As the infection is often carried by the fingers to the eyes, often one eye is involved within a few hours. There is great pain and the lids swell enormously. If the cornea becomes infected, vision is impaired.

Penicillin injections should be given at once to clear the bloodstream of the cocci; this is repeated for four or five days. The conjunctival sac requires irrigation with warm 1 per cent saline solution and penicillin eye-drops every hour for 24 hours then sulphacetamide drops every four hours.

Phlyctenular Conjunctivitis

Phlyctenular conjunctivitis is a disorder commonly seen in weakly anemic children; in unhygienic conditions. A yellow pustule is formed on the side of the eyeball, which develops into an ulcer. There is watering of the eye, intense dislike of light, and generally spasm of the lids.

Treatment includes attention to the general health with a nourishing diet, cod-liver oil, plenty of rest, sunlight, and fresh air. Warm saline solution may be used to cleanse the eye. Antihistamine eyedrops and hydrocortisone preparations cause a rapid response.

If the cornea is affected, atropine should also be used, and the patient must rest the eye; a sterile pad with an eye-shade or smoked glasses are advisable.

Follicular Conjunctivitis

Follicular conjunctivitis is a condition commonly seen in weakly anemic children; small swollen follicles occur on the conjunctiva, and predispose to attacks of conjunctivitis. Adenoids and enlarged tonsils are often also present. The general health requires attention and chlortetracycline 1 per cent ointment placed inside the lower lid at night.

Trachoma

(*Egyptian Ophthalmia*)

Trachoma is a chronic specific viral conjunctivitis, and the disease is prevalent in the Middle East.

Symptoms. The disease tends to be chronic, and the onset is often insidious. The lids become everted, with sensitivity to light, watering and discharge; this is not usually profuse but is contagious. The edges of the lids are swollen and mauve in tint, the upper lid being most involved. On the inner surface the conjunctiva is seen to be granular; the eye feels gritty, and later this leads to conjunctivitis and scarring of the cornea from irritation and friction.

Treatment. General hygienic treatment and tonics are required. The cure will not be rapid. The patient must be kept in bed, in a dark room, with the head elevated. The eyes should be frequently and gently bathed with warm saline solution.

It is a disease of long duration and ought to be treated by an eye specialist, since iritis, scarring of the cornea and deformity of the lids may be produced. Some of the newer antibiotics may be useful.

CORNEAL ULCERS

Normally the cornea, or the transparent part of the eye in front of the pupil, is clear and reflects light; when it becomes inflamed, as in keratitis, the surface is dull and non-reflective, and blood vessels may be seen passing into it. The cornea is highly sensitive and any inflammation or injury causes much pain, with watering of the eyes, dislike of light and spasm of the eyelids. When the cornea becomes cloudy, sight is also impaired.

Ulceration or injury of the cornea, even when quite slight, can be clearly shown by the use of a stain called fluorescein; a drop instilled into the eye stains a corneal abrasion bright green.

Inflammation of the cornea may be of two kinds:

(1) SUPPURATING, in cases of ulceration from infection, injury, or loss of the nerve supply.

(2) NON-SUPPURATING, as in interstitial keratitis, and other forms of inflammation such as pannus, sclerosis and deep keratitis.

Infection and injury are the commonest causes of corneal ulcers which damage the surface and allow the entrance of harmful bacteria. The cornea is also likely to be affected by inflammatory conditions of the conjunctiva. These ulcers vary in size, shape and extent; they may heal rapidly, or they may spread and erode the deeper layers until they cause perforation of the eye. Ulcers can be seen by the naked eye as small grayish-white patches or specks on the clear background of the cornea.

A scar may be left on the cornea when the ulcer has been deep, and this will interfere with vision.

Behind the cornea lies the acqueous humor of the front compartment of the eye and the lens. If a corneal ulcer erodes through the cornea it perforates into the cavity of the globe and allows the aqueous fluid to drain out. The lens and the iris may be pushed forwards into the wound.

Hypopyon Ulcer

When deep corneal ulcers occur, especially after injuries in elderly and debilitated persons, a collection of pus (*hypopyon*) may be seen lying in the space between the cornea and the iris.

Treatment. Cauterization is often required to prevent perforation of the cornea, since this type of ulcer tends to spread and erode; or the ulcer may be incised to drain out the pus. Perchloride of mercury lotion, 1 in 5,000, should be used for frequent bathing, atropine drops then being used daily until healing occurs. Penicillin is now also used in these cases.

Chronic Phlyctenular Ulcers

Chronic phlyctenular ulcers are the most common type of corneal ulcers, and are seen in ill-nourished and weakly children; the ulcers are gutter-like and sodden.

Treatment. The child's general health and mode of life require urgent attention. Hydrocortisone eye-drops, or atropine sulphate eye-drops are instilled into the eye, and a protective dressing and bandage used to keep the eye at rest. The ulcer may heal more rapidly if lightly cauterized by a surgeon.

Dendritic Ulcers

Dendritic ulcers are the fairly common surface ulcerations of the cornea, with a grayish branching appearance. They should be cleaned with alcohol very carefully applied by a doctor and tetracycline ointment applied locally daily for two weeks.

Secondary Ulceration of the Cornea

This may follow purulent ophthalmia or glaucoma, or may be caused by severe acne of the face, shingles, or the eruptive fevers. Exposure of the eyes in cases of Graves' disease, or in prolonged coma in typhoid fever or meningitis when the lids remain open, may lead to irritation by dust particles, with ulceration of the cornea.

Treatment of corneal ulcers must include regular cleansing of the eye and ulcer, the relief of pain, and attention to the general health. The eyes must be kept at rest to assist healing. They should be bathed three or four times daily with warm boracic lotion, and 1 drop of 1 per cent atropine instilled, except in cases of glaucoma. A sterile pad of gauze and cotton is then used to protect the eye, being kept in place with a light bandage. Antibiotic eye-drops may be prescribed by a doctor.

BURNS OF THE EYES

Burns of the eyes are not uncommon accidents; they may be due to flames, hot vapors, or gases, or to corrosives such as lime and strong acids or alkalis.

Burns from Fire or Heat

In burns from fire or heat it is always important to discover at once if the eyeball has escaped injury. The eyes should be bathed as soon as possible in warm normal saline solution, and castor oil or olive oil drops are then instilled; the lids should be smeared with vaseline. If there is much discharge, bathing with saline solution should be continued and medical advice sought.

If there is much swelling of the lids, frequent cold compresses give considerable relief.

Burns by Corrosive Substances

Burns by corrosive substances are often very serious. Burns due to quick-lime should not be treated by bathing, oil being instilled into the eyes as soon as possible. Cocaine solution is often required to relieve the pain and may be ordered by a doctor. Careful nursing attention is required during the healing period, to prevent adhesion between the eyeball and the lids.

INTERSTITIAL KERATITIS

Interstitial keratitis is a form of inflammation which is nearly always due to syphilis, usually of the congenital type; it occurs in children with congenital syphilis between six and sixteen years. The conjunctiva may be seen to be of a salmon-pink color; later, the cornea becomes dull or 'steamy,' looking like ground glass. The disease is chronic and affects both eyes; relapses are common.

The sight is much impaired in the active stage but later the cornea begins to clear and vision may return; in severe cases a triangular scar is left. Medical attention is essential.

The complications which may occur are iritis, inflammation of the choroid coat of the eye, and sometimes glaucoma. Corneal ulceration is rare. Short sight may follow iritis, owing to deformity of the cornea with forward bulging.

Treatment. General antisyphilitic treatment is required (see Venereal Diseases, p. 290).

Atropine drops are used to prevent iritis and adhesions unless glaucoma is present, while cortisone is given in the hope of cutting down the ultimate scarring.

When the attack is over, the resultant scars are amenable for replacement by corneal grafts.

Arcus Senilis. This condition is usually seen in elderly persons and is caused by a deposit of fat in the cornea, which forms two white crescentic lines in the upper and lower parts of the cornea; there is often a family tendency to its development, and there may also be some degenerative changes in the blood vessels of the body.

IRITIS

The iris is the colored ring which lies in front of the lens of the eye; in health it is continually contracting or dilating to admit more or less light to the eye.

Causes. The iris may become inflamed after injury, or as a result of wounds or operations on the eye, but it is also a common sequel to rheumatism, gonorrhea and syphilis.

Cases of iritis fall into three groups:

1. IRITIS SECONDARY TO EXTERNAL INFECTION, in which the inflammation is caused by the spread of the infection from the conjunctiva, by corneal ulcers, or by perforating wounds.

2. NON-SPECIFIC IRITIS. Most cases fall into this group where there is no obvious cause, and in turn syphilis, tuberculosis, bad teeth, allergies, and metabolic upsets have been blamed. Usually, however, investigation shows none of the above to be present.

3. IRIDO-CYCLITIS, or serous iritis, is a chronic disease of slow progress, occurring in persons with poor health. Small white points are formed on the cornea as a result of the inflammatory process.

Symptoms. In all forms of inflammation of the iris, the movements of the iris are impaired and there is the likelihood of the iris becoming adherent to the lens. It is very important to recognize cases of iritis at their onset, so that atropine may be used to dilate the pupil and prevent such adhesions.

In iritis the cornea looks muddy and the pupil sluggish or fixed; the conjunctiva is congested and there is pain and headache, with dislike of light.

Complications. If any case of iritis is neglected, blindness may follow or glaucoma may develop. Even with adequate treatment there may be some loss of sight, but in favorable cases recovery is nearly complete.

Treatment. In all cases atropine sulphate (as a 1 per cent solution) should be applied every 2 hours for about two days, and then less often if the adhesions soften. Alternatively an ointment containing 2 per cent each of atropine and cocaine may be used. Prednisone cuts down the inflammatory response and may be used in place of atropine.

The eye should be kept at rest by a shade, or the patient may stay in a dark room. The pain is relieved by atropine. Sedatives may also be required.

If finally many adhesions remain, an operation called iridectomy may be performed, in which a small part of the iris is removed.

General Treatment. Because the eye affection is usually part of a systemic infection, the patient needs rest in bed for some days, and a convalescence in fresh air.

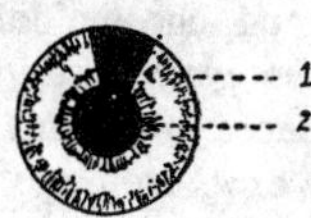

Fig. 4. *IRIDECTOMY. A portion* (1) *of the iris may be removed after iritis or in acute glaucoma. 2. The pupil.*

In syphilitic iritis, general antisyphilitic treatment is essential.

In rheumatic iritis, aspirin or sodium salicylate should be taken.

GLAUCOMA

In this disease there is an increase of pressure in the globe of the eye, due to imperfect drainage of fluid from the back part behind the lens into the chamber in front of the lens, where it is normally filtered off into the veins.

Glaucoma may be a primary or spontaneous disease, or it may follow other disease or occur as a complication after operations. Glaucoma is more common in elderly and long-sighted people, and occurs more often in women than in men.

A primary acute attack may be precipitated by eye-strain, or by anxiety, fatigue, cold, shock, insomnia, constipation, or alcoholic excesses.

Secondary glaucoma may be caused by injuries to the eye, especially when the lens is affected, or by iritis, tumors, or other ocular disorders.

Glaucoma may also occur in acute or chronic forms.

Symptoms. In acute glaucoma the attack begins abruptly with severe pain in and around the eye, and vision is reduced considerably. The patient often sees flashes of light, or a halo or colored ring around a candle flame; in very acute cases there may be nausea or vomiting. The eye may appear 'steamy' and red with swelling of the conjunctiva.

It is essential that the disease should be diagnosed early, as otherwise blindness or serious and permanent impairment of sight may follow. Atropine must never be used in these cases or in doubtful cases of glaucoma, since it dilates the pupil and reduces the drainage of the eye still more, thus further increasing the pressure inside the eye; this increase of pressure damages the retina and optic nerve at the back of the eye, which are the nerve elements essential for sight.

Treatment. The operation known as *iridectomy* is often essential to lower the pressure inside the globe of the eye, and must be performed without delay in urgent cases. Physostigmine, in a 1 to 2 per cent solution, is used to contract the pupil; morphine may be of use in promoting sleep, and saline purgatives should be given. Hot compresses over the eye also give relief.

When the operation is performed early the results are very good but, in late cases when vision has been lost for some time, surgical treatment will not restore the sight although it may help to relieve the pain.

CATARACT

In all elderly persons the lens of the eye gradually becomes harder, less elastic, and somewhat yellow; when these senile or degenerative changes take place and cause part or total loss of transparency of the lens, the condition called cataract is present. Often the cause is not known, but certain recognized diseases, such as diabetes mellitus, are liable to give rise to cataract; injuries, accidents, or foreign bodies in the eye may also be responsible, and the condition is commoner in people over sixty years of age, although cataract is sometimes seen in younger persons.

It is important for the specialist to recognize the different types of cataract since the outlook varies, some cataracts advancing to complete opacity of the whole lens, while others remain more or less in the same state. The urine should always be tested for sugar and albumin to detect diabetes or disease of the kidneys.

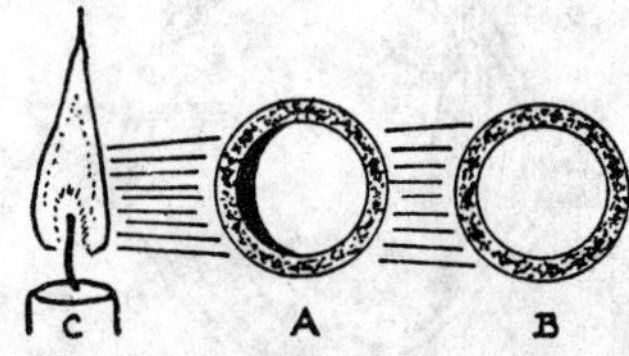

Fig. 5. *A TEST FOR CATARACT. To test for maturity of a cataract, a candle test is used. C.Lighted candle. A.Immature cataract, with a layer of healthy lens fibers behind the iris, which throws a shadow on the lens. B.Complete opacity of lens in a mature cataract.*

If the opacity is in the center of the lens it is called a nuclear cataract, while at the edge it is said to be cortical. Nuclear cataracts generally develop in old people, producing the senile type, but they may be present during middle age.

Cataracts may be hard or soft; the hard type is senile, and the lens can be removed by means of an extraction operation. Soft cataracts may occur in children or people under thirty years, and are removed by 'needling' or suction.

Senile Cataract

Senile cataract generally develops in people after forty-five or fifty years of age, and is caused by shrinkage. This type of cataract causes dark spots and dimness of vision, especially for distant objects, or there may be double vision, when objects are seen double. Progress is variable and the cataract may take two or three years to mature or ripen when, it becomes milky-white. Central cataract is slower than the cortical type.

Cataract often affects both eyes, but usually develops in one eye before the other. In the early stages suitable glasses often improve the sight.

Treatment. Extraction of the lens by operation and the provision of suitable glasses is undertaken for mature cataracts. Only one eye should be operated on at a time, since occasionally iritis or some other complication may follow. When one eye is affected before the other, it is usual to postpone the operation while the patient still has fairly good sight in the second eye.

The cornea or transparent coat of the eye in front of the pupil usually heals quickly in successful cases, but skilled nursing is essential. Care must be taken when the patient is up and about to avoid knocks, or straining such as sneezing or coughing, which may open the wound or cause the vitreous humor of the eye to be squeezed out.

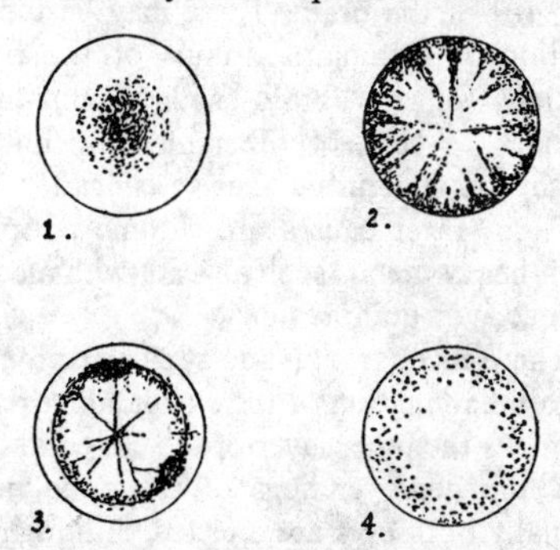

Fig. 6. *VARIOUS TYPES OF LENS CATARACTS. 1. Nuclear cataract. 2. Cortical cataract. 3. Cataract in a case of rickets. 4. Congenital 'dot' cataract.*

Diabetic Cataract

Diabetic cataract is a type of cataract similar to the senile cortical type, and always affects both eyes. It ripens quickly, but the possibility of surgical treatment depends on the patient's general health.

Cataract due to Lens Injury

Cataract due to injury of the lens may develop within a few days if a sharp instrument pierces the lens capsule, and iritis is likely to follow, for which atropine drops should be used three or four times a day as a preventive. Sometimes surgical treatment is required if there is much pain, but is generally avoided when possible.

Other types of cataract, such as the secondary type that may follow glaucoma, hereditary cataract, and cataract after gonorrheal inflammation in the eyes of infants, also occur.

'Needling' operations are used to break up soft cataracts; the lens capsule is torn. The softened lens becomes absorbed by the aqueous humor in the front part of the eye.

FLOATING SPECKS. Cataract is sometimes, though wrongly, suspected especially by a short-sighted person, when small floating spots, specks, threads, or chains of spots are sometimes seen to pass across the eye. These small particles are the remains of cellular fragments present during the development of the eye. When the eye is moved the spots or threads are jerked about and then slowly sink; they can often be perceived by looking at a white ceiling or light wall. They are not of serious import, and only opaque particles that can be detected by an ophthalmoscopic examination are likely to be a sign of any disorder of the eyes.

DISEASES OF THE OPTIC NERVE AND RETINA

Optic Neuritis

Optic neuritis, or inflammation of the optic disc, at the point where the optic nerve enters the back of the eyeball, is a symptom occurring in various conditions such as diseases of the kidneys, anemia, diabetes mellitus, high blood pressure, and certain diseases of the brain. These may be inflammation or meningitis, tumor of the brain, syphilis of the brain with gummata or tumors, abscess, or tuberculosis meningitis. Slight optic neuritis may occur after concussion; rarer causes are chronic poisoning with heavy metals such as lead, with alcohol, tobacco, or quinine.

There is congestion and swelling of the disc with inflammation of the surrounding retina, which is the inner layer of the eye containing the fine nerve endings of the optic nerve. Usually both eyes are affected, although this may occur at different times. There may be no pain or loss of sight, but usually this develops rapidly, causing blurring of vision, with sickness, pain and headache.

If optic neuritis progresses, it leads to optic atrophy or destruction of the optic nerve, which may also follow fractures of the skull.

In secondary syphilis, optic neuritis is liable to develop within six to eighteen months after the primary sore, if this is untreated.

Treatment. If syphilis is suspected, a Wassermann blood test must be carried out and antisyphilitic treatment given when this is indicated. The outlook is good in these cases if treatment is given early and carried out thoroughly.

When a tumor of the brain is suspected, it is often necessary to trephine (or drill) the skull to reduce the pressure, and save the eyesight.

In optic neuritis due to kidney disease the outlook is unfavorable, and cases often end fatally within eighteen months.

Inflammation of the Optic Nerve behind the Eyeball

Inflammation of the optic nerve behind the eyeball may develop in nicotine poisoning in heavy smokers who smoke strong dark tobacco over long periods. Loss of sight for green or red objects, or for yellow, occurs in this condition, while ordinary white light can still be seen.

If smoking and chewing tobacco are given up, the sight usually improves steadily.

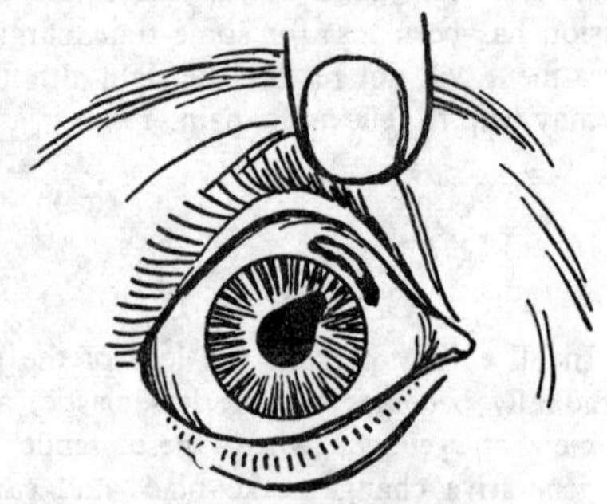

Fig. 7. *RUPTURE OF THE EYEBALL. Note the displacement of the lens towards the ruptured area.*

Detachment of the Retina

When a heavy blow falls upon a healthy eye it may cause bleeding into the retina, or nerve-layer, of the eye; while in short-sighted persons slight bruising, or even the strain caused by stooping down, may cause separation of the retina from the outer wall of the eyeball. There is sudden loss of sight, usually in the upper part of the eye, as though a curtain had half descended.

When the case is diagnosed the patient must lie absolutely quiet in bed, to allow the retina to settle back into place. Surgical treatment is often good for an acute attack, but recurrences may occur.

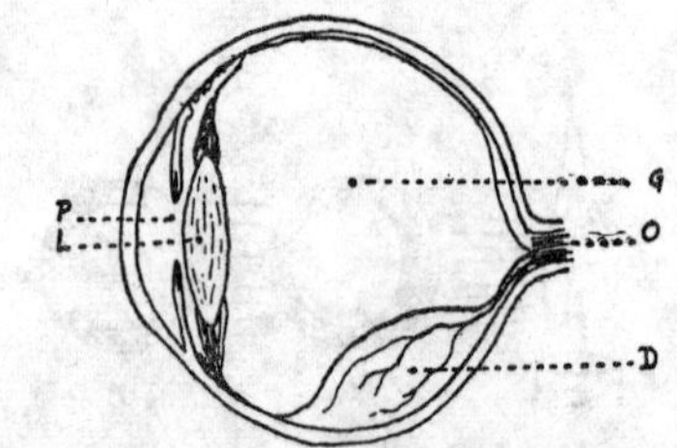

Fig. 8. *DETACHMENT OF THE RETINA OF THE EYE. P.Pupil. L.Lens. G.Cavity of eyeball. O.Optic nerve. D.Detached portion of retina, or nerve layer, separated from the globe.*

Tumors

There are various types of tumors of the orbit and eye which occur, but they are all relatively uncommon. They may affect the bony walls of the orbit, the optic nerve, retina, choroid or sclera, or rarely the iris. Tumors of the brain may affect the eyesight by pressure on the optic nerve.

BLINDNESS
(*Amblyopia*)

Blindness is a condition often considered to mean that there is no perception of light in either of a person's eyes, but actually those people whose eyesight is so poor that they cannot earn a living by ordinary work are usually accounted blind.

Many cases of blindness start in the first ten years of life as a result of gonorrheal ophthalmia, or from injuries.

There are three main causes of blindness. They are cataract (see p. 323), glaucoma (see p. 323), and senile degeneration of the macula. Other causes of blindness are the hysterical, usually found in young girls and accompanied by ptosis, and the rarer forms caused by tumors of the eye or brain, meningitis and chronic inflammatory conditions of the eyes. Occasionally, overindulgence in tobacco or alcohol may cause blindness, as can excessive use of certain drugs.

Treatment. Considering the three main causes, treatment gives very different results. Cataract can be remedied, while glaucoma can only be arrested, and macular degeneration progresses ruthlessly.

Night Blindness

This is probably caused by a hereditary defect which is due to a lack of sensitivity in the outer part of the retina. It was previously thought to be due to a deficiency of vitamin A but this is no longer considered to be true in many cases. Usually the condition cannot be improved.

COLOR-BLINDNESS

Most occupations do not require a very exact sense of color vision, but transport workers, signal and other similar types of workers are seriously handicapped if they suffer from a defective appreciation of color, and such a defect would prove dangerous to others. For work which requires a normal color vision, tests have been devised before such work is undertaken.

Color-blindness occurs more commonly in men but is inherited through the female line. About 8 per cent of all men are color-blind while only 0.4 per cent of women are.

Only a few people are color-blind to all colors; the lack of perception of red and green is the commonest defect, while blue and yellow color vision is also sometimes deficient. Most so-called color-blind people can only distinguish a small number of colors or shades, some colors being perceived as a grayish tint; such people rely on differences in the brightness of shades, rather than on differences of hue, to guess at colors they do not distinguish accurately, but this means of perception is easily diminished by fatigue, and becomes erroneous if mist, rain, smoke or other obscuring conditions are present.

Tests. Many tests for estimating color-vision have been devised, the best of these being a series of cards devised by Professor Ischihara in Japan. On the cards a group of numbers is printed in one shade on a background of a different color. The shades are so selected that the color-blind cannot distinguish the number from its background.

Color-blindness occurring later in life is rare and may be due to the effects of injury, disease, or old age on the lens, the retina or the optic nerve or brain, such as in optic neuritis or atrophy of the optic nerve, nicotine poisoning in heavy smokers, cataract, detached retina, or hysteria.

SQUINT

Squinting is deviation of the eyes so that their axes are not parallel. Two main types are recognized: the *paralytic* type, due to some fault in the external muscles controlling the movements of the eyeball; and the *non-paralytic* type, in which there is some interference with the control of these muscles.

In non-paralytic cases the two eyes move together, while in paralytic squint one-eyed movement is seen, but these types may overlap.

Paralytic Squint

There are many causes of paralytic squint. Some of these causes may be hereditary, or due to injury or hemorrhage into a muscle, nerve injuries or nerve diseases, brain disorders such as inflammation, meningitis, tuberculosis, syphilis, sleeping sickness, thrombosis, embolism, aneurysm of the blood vessels in the brain, arteriosclerosis, various poisons or toxins such as lead, alcohol, diphtheria or influenza, or general diseases such as syphilis, tumors, or other diseases affecting the brain.

Paralytic squint generally causes double vision, with giddiness or sometimes nausea, and more than one muscle of the eyeball may be affected, so that an accurate diagnosis must be made before treatment can be carried out. The squint may only be apparent when the patient tries to turn his eye in the direction of the paralyzed muscle.

Non-paralytic Squint

In non-paralytic squint the external muscles of the eyeball are not primarily paralyzed, but the axes of the two eyes are not parallel; only one eye is used, because the sight in the other eye is ignored or suppressed and the patient does not see double images. This condition is common in early childhood, but generally only becomes apparent between the ages of two and four years. When the patient looks straight forward the squint is obvious at once, and the defect remains whichever way he turns his eyes.

The eyes are normally used together, and can accommodate for near objects in binocular vision. The size, form and relative distance of objects can thus be judged, the images being fused in the brain. Binocular vision is not present at birth, but develops within a month. Babies, however, tend to squint easily as a result of wind or other small forms of irritation, and such squints in the first six months of life are usually not serious.

Causes. If the power of fusion is weak, or the external muscles of the eyeball do not act normally, however, squint may develop. Long-sightedness, severe short-sightedness, inequality of the eyes, corneal opacities, fevers, weakness of the eye muscles and other defects, or debilitating illnesses such as measles, may cause squint.

Varieties. In CONVERGENT SQUINT the squinting eye turns inwards.

In DIVERGENT SQUINT the eye turns outwards.

In ALTERNATING SQUINT either eye squints irregularly.

In CONCOMITANT SQUINT (non-paralytic or spasmodic squint), the two eyes move together, although the axes are not parallel.

In PARALYTIC SQUINT only one eye moves normally.

In OCCASIONAL SQUINT the defect only occurs at intervals.

Treatment. CONVERGENT SQUINT. Three lines of treatment may be adopted.

1. In most cases the defective sight must be remedied by the use of correct glasses.
2. Binocular vision may be aided by various exercises whereby the ability to use both eyes together may be developed and improved. This can only be done when the child is old enough to understand and takes part willingly.
3. The sight of the defective eye may be encouraged by using some form of occlusion of the better eye for a limited period, which makes the child use the weaker eye. In alternating squint this form of treatment is not used, since both eyes have about the same power of sight.

In a large number of cases when the angle of the squint is more than 15°, surgical treatment is required to straighten the eyes.

DIVERGENT SQUINT. An eye in which the sight has been lost often diverges, or turns outwards. Surgical treatment may be used to straighten the eye, but the defect often recurs. When associated with short-sightedness, glasses or surgical treatment may give correction.

LATENT SQUINT. With good binocular vision the eyes may maintain parallel axes in spite of some want of balance between the external eye muscles, and this condition, called *heterophoria*, may lead to considerable eye-strain. Treatment may be with prismatic glasses or even surgical treatment.

Nystagmus

Tremor or involuntary jerky movements of the eyes, called nystagmus, sometimes occurs; the eyes may be rapidly oscillated from side to side, or up and down. The patient is often unaware of the movements, and these are absent during sleep. Nystagmus is common in albinos, or may be present as a result of astigmatism of the eyes.

In adults it may be a sign of some form of brain disease, and the condition of 'miner's nystagmus' develops as a result of working in poor light with the consequent lack of development of a part of the sensitive lining of the eye.

THE EYE AS AN OPTICAL INSTRUMENT

The eye is often compared to a camera; the various parts of the eye, namely the cornea, the aqueous, the lens and the vitreous, normally focus rays of light entering the eye upon the retina (or nerve layer) at the back of the eye.

A normal eye is constructed so that parallel rays of light from an object more than 6 meters away pass through the lens of the eye and are focused on the retina without accommodation or effort being required. When objects are nearer than 6 meters the rays of light radiate outwards; in order to focus these divergent rays upon the retina, the eye 'accommodates,' or makes the lens more spherical, which causes the rays to converge and form a clear image.

Difficulty in Accommodation
(*Presbyopia*)

From about forty-five years of age onwards it is often no longer possible to read ordinary print at a comfortable distance, and glasses should be worn. These require to be changed at regular five-year intervals, between forty-five and sixty years.

Long-sightedness
(*Hypermetropia*)

In long-sightedness the eyeball is too short, and parallel rays of light are brought to a focus behind the retina. If the general health is poor, or in states of fatigue, the power of accommodation tends to diminish.

Short-sightedness
(*Myopia*)

In short-sightedness the eyeball is too long and parallel rays meet or focus in front of the retina. Defective vision for distant objects is the commonest symptom, and in all except mild cases print is held nearer to the eye than normal for reading.

Myopia is a disease which needs careful attention, since several complications are liable to affect the short-sighted eye, such as hemorrhage after slight injuries, detachment of the retina, and secondary cataract. Any severe illness or congestive conditions of the eye, such as eye-strain, tend to aggravate short-sightedness.

The rate of progress varies considerably in different people. Short-sightedness may develop about puberty and continue during adult life, but more commonly it develops earlier in childhood, and in cases of so-called 'malignant' myopia it tends to increase. The eyes are irritable and 'weak,' and conjunctivitis or inflammation of the lids are common symptoms.

Astigmatism

In astigmatism the curvature of the cornea or of the lens of the eye is not equal in all directions, and images of objects are distorted because the rays of light are not focused in a single point; a vertical line may be seen less clearly than a horizontal one. Astigmatism can be corrected by cylindrical lenses. Even slight astigmatism may cause severe headaches and should always be attended to.

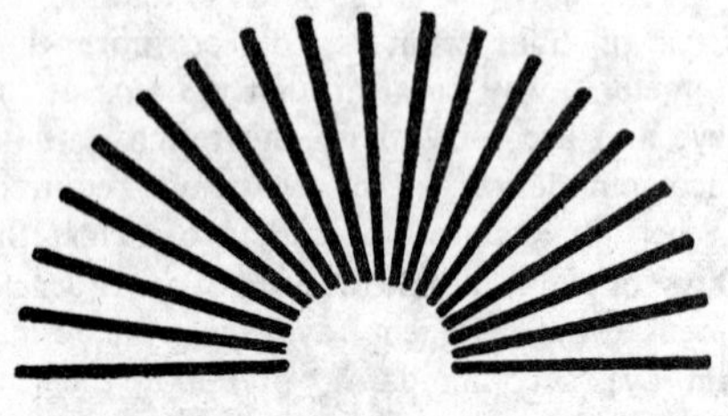

Fig. 9. *THE ASTIGMATIC FAN. In astigmatism one line is blurred or indistinct, owing to irregular curvature of the surface of the eye. The defect may be corrected by the use of a cylindrical lens.*

In other cases the sight of the two eyes is different, owing to a defect in only one eye, or to different defects in the two eyes.

Defective Eyesight

Defective eyesight can be tested by reading tests, and by the use of lenses in attempts to improve sight by their aid; or it may be tested by means of an instrument known as an ophthalmoscope.

In the case of short-sightedness a concave lens of correct strength is required, while in long-sighted persons a convex lens is used. These lenses alter the focusing point of the light rays (see Fig. 11).

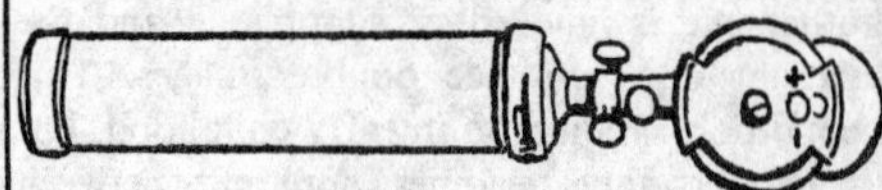

Fig. 10. *AN ELECTRIC OPHTHALMOSCOPE for illumination and examination of the interior of the eye.*

Muscle Balance

In normal people the eyes are perfectly balanced for sight, and there is no conscious effort required for binocular vision. In a large number of people, however, the muscle action or balance is not perfect and, although fusion prevents squint, the effort required causes headache over the eyes. Muscular imbalance is called *heterophoria.*

LENSES

Lenses manufactured by opticians are made from a standard glass called Crown Glass. This glass is light in weight and very hard; owing to this hardness the surface can be given a high polish, and a maximum amount of transparency is obtained. In its rough state the glass is cut into blanks, which are then ground by accurate machinery to the powers required by the prescription for the lenses. After this, the lens in making is smoothed by emery and finally polished. The shape of the lens required is then marked on the blank, and ground to the stated size. There are six different kinds or 'forms' of lenses used for spectacles. These 'forms' do not depend on the shape of the lens, but on the curvature of its surfaces.

The first lens illustrated (Fig. 11) is convex with equal convex curvatures on either surface (biconvex). The following one has one plane surface and all the convex curvature ground on its other surface (plano-convex). The third lens has a deep concave curve ground on its one surface, and a greater convex curve on its remaining surface (meniscus or toric convex form).

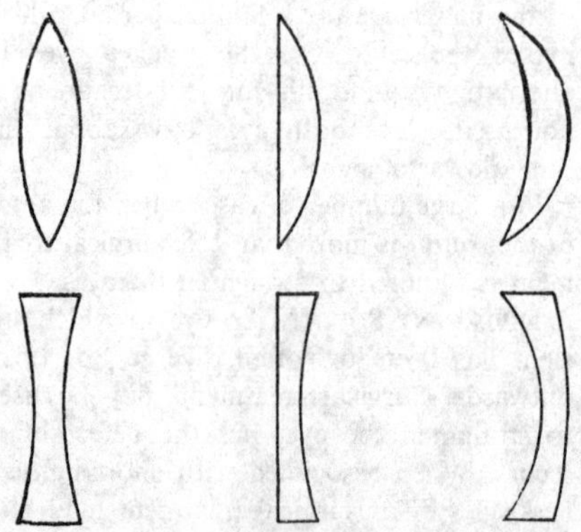

Fig. 11. *LENS SHAPES.* (Top) *Biconvex; plano-convex; and toric convex.* (Below) *Biconcave; plano-concave; and toric concave.*

Concave lenses are made on similar lines, Fig. 11 showing biconcave, plano-concave, and meniscus or toric concave. Cylindrical and prismatic lenses are also used. Lenses differ in strength according to the curvature; the flatter the curve, the weaker is the lens; and the greater the curve, the more powerful is the lens. The strength of lenses is measured by their focal length; a focal length of 1 meter is said to be that of a lens of 1 diopter.

The best form of lens is the meniscus or toric convex or concave. Owing to the special depth of their curves, a wider field of vision is obtained by the wearer, and distortion through the edges of the lens is minimal.

The plano-convex or concave forms of the lenses are very useful in many cases, and for practical purposes the ordinary biconvex and concave types are serviceable.

All these lenses can be made up in various shapes to suit the contour of the wearer's face, and also to serve different purposes. For distance wear, that is for seeing far objects, the round and oval shapes are best; and for reading or any close work, the partoscopic or clerical shape is often prescribed.

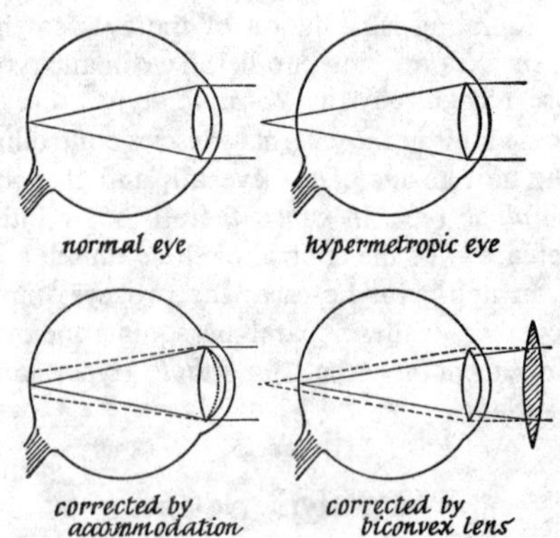

Fig. 12. *HOW FAR - SIGHT IS CORRECTED. Either by adjusting the lens through effort of accommodation, or by use of a biconvex lens.*

For persons who need glasses for distance and also a different pair for reading with, the bifocal or double-sight lens has proved to be extremely useful. Today only three kinds recommended by the optician—the cemented, bifocal, and the fused and solid types. The modern cemented form of bifocal consists of a very thin wafer of glass, either in the shape of a crescent or round, which is cemented by a transparent substance to the main lens. This wafer added to the lens gives the reading power to it. The fused bifocal owes its origin to the fact that flint glass fuses at a lower temperature than crown glass. From the rough blank of crown glass a groove is cut, and into this groove is placed a small piece of flint glass, and the combination is heated. Under the extreme heat the flint fuses with the crown glass. Owing to the flint glass being the denser of the two, the portion of the finished lens which contains the flint glass is stronger in power and is used for reading, while the remaining crown glass part is used for outdoor and distance vision.

The third and best type of bifocal is the solid, and when made up in a toric lens it is ideal. In this type the lens consists wholly of crown glass, the reading portion being ground on to the crown glass by very delicate machinery.

Sun glasses are manufactured by a special process. They have the property, in most cases, of absorbing the ultraviolet rays in light, and so eliminating the various disorders caused by these rays. The lenses are tinted in varying degrees, and vary from a very pale almost unnoticeable shade to a dark smoke-colored glass.

Contact Lenses

These are spectacle lenses which slip beneath the lids and are thus almost invisible externally. They are medically necessary in the rare condition of corneal irregularity, optically useful for extreme short-sightedness, and cosmetically convenient to a large number of other people.

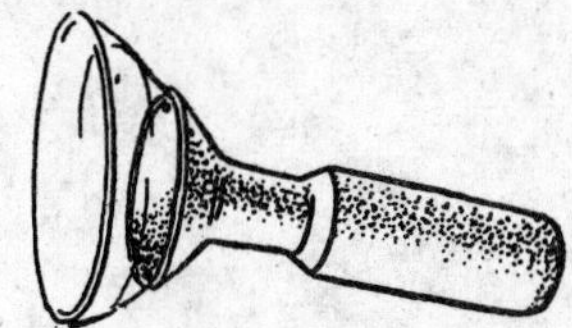

Fig. 13. *A CONTACT LENS held in position ready to be placed under the lid over the center of the eve.*

DISEASES OF THE EAR, NOSE AND THROAT

DISEASES AND AFFECTIONS OF THE EAR

Ear diseases are so common that in almost every family they require attention at one time or another. Deafness and other serious complications may result, so it is very important that disorders of the ear should receive early attention.

Examination of the Outer Ear and Drum

A simple metal tube (speculum) is used with a head mirror. A more elaborate instrument consists of an auroscope, containing an illuminating bulb.

In the healthy ear the lining of the outer passage (external auditory meatus) is smooth and dry. At the end of the passage the typanic membrane, or drum, may be seen, and this should be semi-transparent, dry, and grayish-white. Within this may be seen the handle of the malleus, coming from above downward and backward. This bone runs about half way across the drum, and divides it into an upper front, and a lower back part. This lower back portion, when viewed through the speculum, is more glistening than the upper and front part, and a bright cone of light is seen on its most rounded portion, which is just below and behind the point of the malleus.

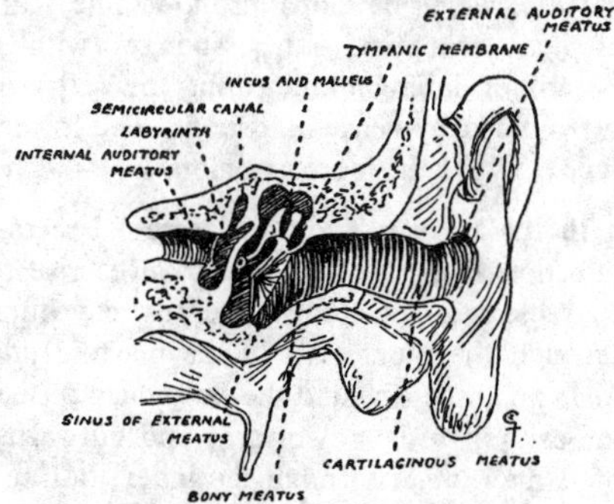

Fig. 1. *SECTION THROUGH THE OUTER, MIDDLE AND INNER EAR.*

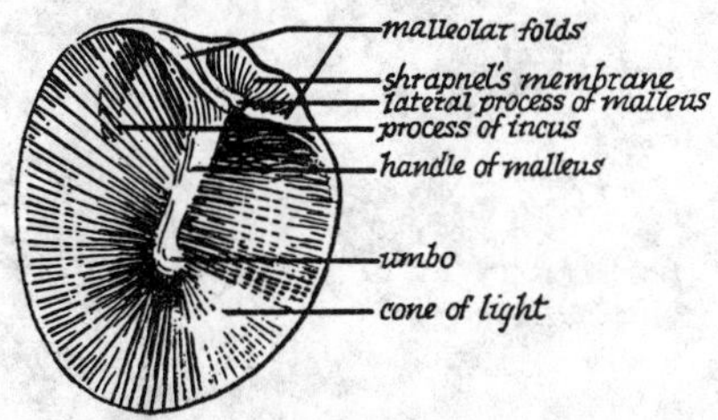

Fig. 2. *NORMAL RIGHT EAR DRUM. Part of the incus and malleus (bones of the inner ear) are seen through the membrane.*

Disorders of the Outer Ear

Bruising of the Outer Ear

Severe bruising of the outer ear occasionally occurs in football players or boxers, or as a result of blows. A large clot of blood may form under the skin, and should be removed by surgical puncture.

Eczema of the Outer Ear

Acute or chronic eczema often occurs on the outer auricle. Seborrheic dermatitis is fairly common in children, affecting the skin behind the ear, and on the folds of the ear; it should receive careful attention or it may spread into the passage of the ear. The skin is red and sore, and there may be fissures and cracks. Zinc oxide and ichthammol ointment may be used—or hydrocortisone cream may be prescribed by the doctor. When there is also seborrhea of the scalp this must be shampooed twice a week with soap or a medicated shampoo, which contains selenium sulphide.

Foreign Bodies in the Ear

Children sometimes push beads, buttons or other small objects into the passages of the ears.

If a fly or other insect gets into the ear, fill the ear with warm sweet oil, and it may then float out; the head should be held on one side for a short time, when the insect will rise to the surface. If any hard object is introduced into the ear, take the child to hospital or to a doctor, and do not attempt to remove it. With objects such as peas or seeds, water should *not* be used, or it may cause the substance to swell and become impacted.

Furunculosis

A furuncle or small boil in the passage of the ear may be followed by clusters of boils and gives rise to much pain while forming.

Treatment consists in the use of drops or a gauze pack soaked in 10 per cent ichthyol in glycerin, or magnesium sulphate paste, inserted into the passage of the ear. When the boil is quite ripe (and not before) it is occasionally incised to let out the pus; the passage should be syringed, and two or three drops of dilute alcohol (70 per cent) inserted to prevent further infection. In recurring furunculosis, the urine must be tested for sugar to exclude diabetes. The general health requires tonics and fresh air. Vaccine treatment is sometimes advised. The scalp must be kept clean with alcohol or shampoos.

Wax in the Ear

The ear sometimes becomes completely filled with wax mixed with hairs and flakes of skin; even a large collection of wax in the passage of the ear may not interfere with hearing, but sudden deafness may be noticed if water runs into the ear during washing, which makes the wax swell; in other cases there may be a more gradual loss of hearing.

Treatment. The ear should be gently syringed by a doctor, using warm water or boracic lotion, so as to clear out the whole mass. Four or five drops of almond oil or 8 per cent sodium bicarbonate ear-drops should be dropped into the ear three times the day before. The water should be at body temperature, and a little raw cotton should be loosely inserted after the syringing.

Earache
(*Otalgia*)

Pain may be felt in the ear from various causes. These include bruises of the outer ear from blows, which may give rise to much swelling and pain.

Decayed or unerupted teeth, infection of the passage of the ear, foreign bodies in the passage, wax, or a boil in the passage, or infection of the middle ear may all give rise to severe pain in the ear. Otitis media, described below, is the common cause of acute earache in children, particularly in the acute fevers, and it often affects both ears. The pain is very severe, and boring or throbbing in character.

Acute mastoid inflammation and arthritis of the joint of the lower jaw (or mandible) are other conditions which lead to pain in the ear, while diseases of the sinuses, pharynx, larynx, and the root of the tongue may also cause earache.

Neuralgia may give rise to very severe pain indeed, which occurs in sudden paroxysms; there is sometimes sensitivity of the scalp, and loss of taste on one side of the tongue, and occasionally facial paralysis or twitching spasms develop.

Investigation of any possible cause may require examination of the teeth (including X-ray examination), and of sinuses, pharynx, ears and larynx, since there may be some serious underlying condition which is not at first apparent.

Treatment will depend upon the cause and severity of the pain, and sedatives or analgesics may be ordered by a doctor.

In severe neuralgic cases with associated earache, an injection of alcohol by a surgeon made into the nerve may bring relief, and sedatives will be prescribed.

Acute Infection of the Middle Ear

(*Acute Otitis Media*)

This is a common complaint, especially in debilitated children suffering from malnutrition and living in unhygienic surroundings. The infection generally enters the ear from the pharynx through the Eustachian tube, and any chronic septic condition of the nose or throat is likely to spread to the ear. Adenoids are the most usual cause, but colds, decayed teeth, influenza and the acute fevers are also liable to give rise to middle ear infection. In summertime the infection sometimes results from bathing, and injuries to the drum from blows, or from attempts to remove wax, or from foreign bodies, occasionally lead to otitis media.

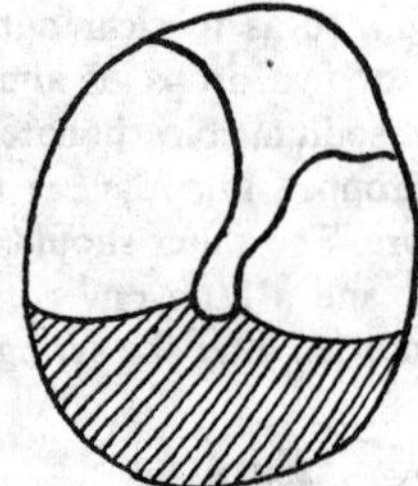

Fig. 3. *DIAGRAM SHOWING FLUID IN THE MIDDLE EAR, BEHIND THE DRUM.*

Symptoms. In the early stage the ear feels blocked, there is tinnitus (ringing in the ear), and the hearing is dulled; later, fluid is formed and the drum bulges and, as pus appears, the pain becomes more severe. Finally, unless treatment is given, the drum may burst, and pus run out through the outer passage of the ear; the mastoid antrum may also become infected

Pain is the chief symptom, felt deeply in the ear; it is severe and throbbing, and is worse at night. When the drum breaks after about forty-eight hours, the pain is relieved as the pus escapes, but sometimes the pain continues for a week or longer, as the drainage of pus may be inadequate, or complications may be setting in.

When there are repeated attacks of inflammation of the middle ear the discharge usually drains out of the old perforation of the drum, and pain may be slight or absent. The inflammation may become chronic, and a permanent perforation may remain. In severe chronic cases the ossicles of the middle ear may be destroyed. In scarlet fever or measles in children, fever and a discharging ear may be the only evidence of ear infection.

There is usually deafness during an acute attack, and noises in the ear are common, with popping and banging sounds until pus appears, when more crackling or bubbling noises are complained of. These may continue after the discharge has cleared up and the drum has healed.

Fever generally sets in in acute otitis media, but in adults the temperature is seldom above 37·8° C (100° F); in children it may be higher in the early stages. After the drum is opened the fever should quickly subside, and if it persists in a swinging or irregular course, mastoid infection must be suspected.

Treatment. To prevent the spread of the infection or the development of complications, penicillin or sulphonamides should be given as soon as the diagnosis is certain. If the patient is resistant or sensitive to penicillin, tetracyline or some other suitable antibiotic should be used. The antibiotic chosen must be given in sufficient dosage and for a suitable length of time—if this is not done, the infection will be 'masked' and the microorganisms not killed.

SURGERY. Unless perforation occurs naturally to release pus accumulating behind the red and bulging eardrum, early surgical treatment (paracentesis) may be required to open the drum and drain the middle ear, to limit the spread or consequences of infection, to relieve pain and to prevent undue damage to the drum from rupture which is likely to cause more scarring and deafness. Myringotomy (paracentesis) is indicated only in very severe infections when perforation is certain, or when the pain does not respond to palliative measures. The puncture of the drum should *not* be undertaken when the fluid in the middle ear is mucoid and there is little or no pain, fever, or general malaise. In these mild cases the fluid usually disappears of its own accord.

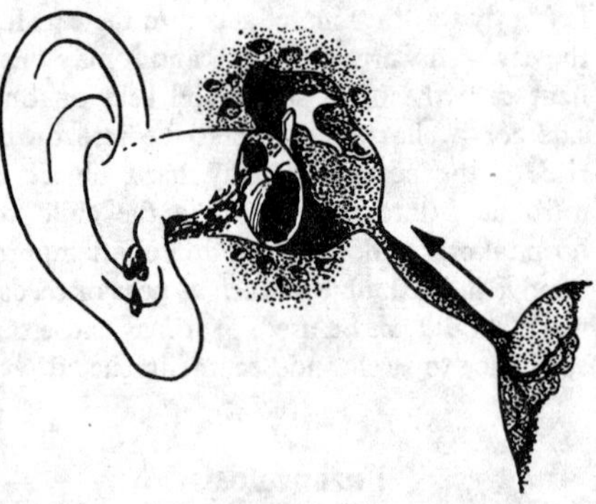

Fig. 4. *INFECTION OF THE MIDDLE EAR. The infection and inflammation has spread from the throat via the Eustachian tube (arrow) and the surrounding bone is also affected. Pus has perforated the drum and exudes from the outer canal.*

After puncture of the drum, the dressings must be changed carefully, with aseptic precautions. When the discharge is profuse the passage is gently syringed out with warm boracic lotion, but for the first two days it should be allowed to drain by itself. As the discharge clears up the passage is kept dry by mopping. The ear is covered with sterile gauze and the skin round the ear is protected with vaseline. When the discharge is very profuse the dressings may need to be changed every three hours in the daytime.

In most cases the pus drains out satisfactorily after the drum is opened, and the drum heals within two or three weeks.

Inflation of the Eustachian tube must always be done at the end of treatment if the hearing has not returned to normal.

Sometimes in severe infections the mastoid is involved, or the discharge from the middle ear persists with increasing deafness. In children in these cases the adenoids and tonsils are often infected and are responsible for the continued infection. They should be removed when the child has got over the ear trouble. An operation on the mastoid is used to clear up the mastoid infection.

General Treatment includes rest in bed in a warm room, with free administration of fluids. Aspirin or other analgesic is given to relieve pain, in doses appropriate to the patient's age. Steam inhalations of tincture of benzoin are useful.

Mastoiditis

The mastoid process is the bony prominence behind the ear, and infection of this part may follow inflammation of the middle ear, causing severe local or general symptoms. Within the mastoid process there is the antrum, which develops at about nine years of age, becoming either spongy (with a system of intercommunicating air cells) or surrounded by dense hard bone. The former type is by far the more common.

In the Spongy Type of Mastoid Process, infection from the middle ear gives rise to characteristic symptoms. The pus may burst through the outer wall of the mastoid and form an abscess behind the ear, which pushes the ear forwards, downwards and outwards; or it may break through the inner wall and track down the neck forming an abscess behind the sterno-mastoid muscle; or the pus may pass backwards or upwards through the roof of the antrum to form an abscess within the skull.

After the ear drum is opened in a case of acute infection of the middle ear, and when the discharge appears, the patient's condition should improve, but when the infection spreads backwards to the mastoid, persistent throbbing pain is felt, especially at night, and

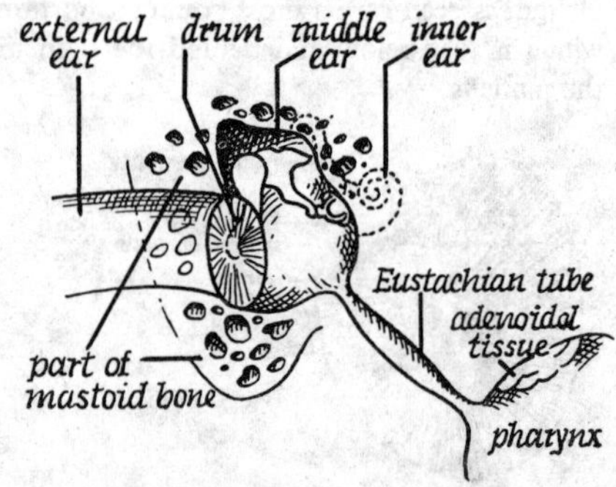

Fig. 5. *SECTION THROUGH THE MIDDLE EAR showing the mastoid process, the oval drum of the ear, and the Eustachian tube.*

the temperature is irregular. Tenderness over the mastoid is an important sign, and there is usually swelling, with displacement of the ear. Severe headache, drowsiness or irritability may be present, with slight vertigo, and occasionally paralysis of the face.

In a Dense or Hard Mastoid Process the early diagnosis of infection is more difficult. Fever in the evenings, occasional earache, sleeplessness, loss of appetite and headache suggest inflammation of the mastoid, but swelling over the bone is often absent or only appears later. The well of the passage of the ear or the drum may be swollen and bulging, and the discharge is often thick and profuse.

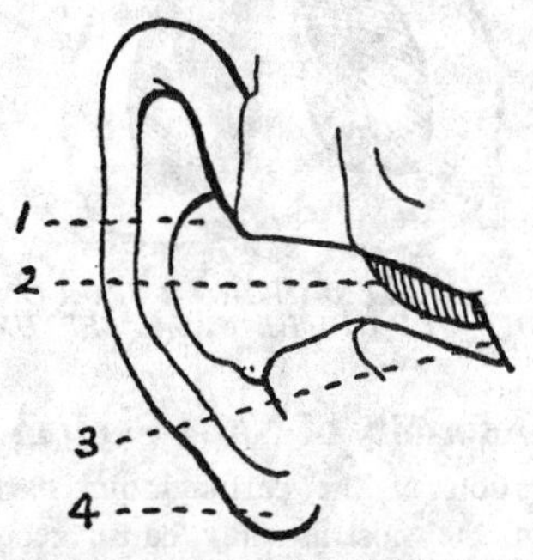

Fig. 6. *DIAGRAM SHOWING INFLAMMATORY SWELLING OF THE MEATUS IN ACUTE MASTOIDITIS. 1. The passage of the ear. 2. Inflammatory swelling near the drum. 3. The drum of tympanic membrane. 4. The lobe of the ear.*

X-ray examination is often of great help in diagnosis.

Surgical Treatment is required when fever persists after acute otitis media, without other complications, or when there is pain or tenderness over the mastoid; headache, giddiness, vomiting or persistent discharge after about four weeks of careful local treatment to the ear, also indicate the necessity of drainage of the mastoid.

Later signs may be swelling over the mastoid, the extension of inflammation into the neck, or signs of infection within the skull. The judicious use of antibiotics (with or without paracentesis) in otitis media has greatly reduced the incidence of acute mastoiditis.

Otosclerosis

Otosclerosis is a disease which affects young adults, especially women, and causes progressive deafness, which is often worse after pregnancy or illness. One of the small bones of the ear, the stapes, becomes fixed in spongy bone formation, and noises in the ear are often troublesome. The patient hears better in noisy surroundings such as in a train or a crowded hall.

For healthy patients surgical operation, removal of the stapes (*stapedectomy*), stape mobilization, or fenstration, can give improved hearing in about 50 per cent of suitable cases. The disease often runs in families.

Deafness

Deafness is unfortunately a common complaint, and in many cases it might have been prevented or rendered less serious if proper attention had been given to disorders of the ear, nose and throat, while they could be remedied. It is often, however, only when hearing is lost or seriously impaired that help and advice are sought. In children especially, deafness is apt to be difficult to detect in the early stages when it might be arrested, or the cause removed, and the child is then severely handicapped for the whole of his life.

The hearing apparatus of the ear has two distinct functions, that of the *conduction* of sound waves into the chambers of the ear, and the *perception* of these waves as sounds by the nerve of hearing and the brain. Sound waves are ordinarily conducted to the ear through the air, and thence into the middle and internal chambers of the ear by the special structures arranged for this purpose. (See Anatomy, p. 234.) If the outer passages of the ear are closed (as by wax) or if there is disease of the ear structures, some sound waves will be perceived by bone conduction, as occurs when a vibrating tuning fork is held in contact with the bones of the head, either on the forehead or behind the ear.

The main types of deafness are (1) *obstructive*, with disorders of the conducting apparatus of the ear, and (2) *nerve deafness*, with disease of the nerves of hearing.

Causes. The common causes of obstructive deafness are:

(*a*) Wax impacted in the ear,
(*b*) Foreign bodies (beads, etc.),
(*c*) Inflammatory conditions of the middle ear,
(*d*) Inflammation of the Eustachian tubes.

Obstructive Deafness is common, and often affects one side only. Catarrh of the Eustachian tube and middle ear often follows acute or chronic infections of the nose and throat, nasal obstruction or catarrh, adenoids, tonsillitis, and nasal deformity or sinus infection. The infection may spread through the pharynx to one or both of the Eustachian tubes, causing congestion, with a heavy dull sensation in one or both ears, with 'noises' (popping or cracking) in the ear and perhaps slight giddiness. If this catarrh persists the tubes become blocked, and there is catarrh of the middle ear with some deafness and possibly permanent damage to the sense of hearing. After a first acute attack of infection, hearing may often be restored by a specialist by means of Eustachian inflation. Measures should also be taken to prevent recurrence and to rectify infection in the nose and throat.

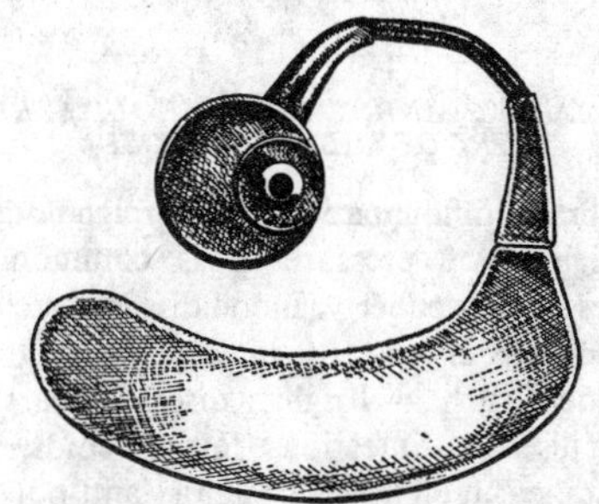

Fig. 7. *DEAF AID TO FIT BEHIND THE EAR. At this close level sounds are not muffled by clothing and there is no bulky attachment in the pocket.*

During the acute attack of catarrh, the patient should be kept warm in bed, with aspirin, three times a day for adults, and steam inhalations of tincture of benzoin (p.343).

Giddiness (vertigo) is sometimes due to obstructive deafness.

Chronic Catarrh of the Eustachian Tubes may follow repeated acute attacks, or it may be gradual and insidious. Noises in the ear (tinnitus) are common, with slowly increasing deafness. The degree of deafness varies considerably and hearing is usually best in a quiet place. In these cases treatment is less satisfactory, which shows how important it is to have adequate measures taken during acute attacks before the chronic stage sets in.

In Chronic Suppuration of the Middle Ear the amount of deafness produced is variable, depending on the degree of involvement of the bones of the ear and the amount of scarring produced.

Otosclerosis (see above) is an intractable cause of deafness which is sometimes hereditary.

Injury to the ear may cause deafness, especially when it causes fracture of bones around the ear; treatment is often ineffectual, but immediate measures consist in preventing infection. Loud sounds or blast may rupture the drum, with subsequent partial deafness, while continued loud noise may give rise to 'occupational' deafness; this should be prevented by the use of ear plugs.

Listening to loud 'pop' music through earphones to the point of ear pain will also lead to deafness.

Nerve Deafness in Old Age. Deafness in varying degrees is common. In the greater number of cases it is due to nerve deafness; the ear itself may be healthy but there is deterioration of the nerve conducting sounds to the brain.

Other occasional causes of loss of hearing are meningitis, mumps, alcohol, tobacco, quinine and certain other drugs, and syphilis.

Treatment. Lip-reading will sometimes be of service in cases of serious deafness if the patient can begin to learn early.

Deaf Aids. One of the electrical deaf aids which amplify sound, or a mechanical aid such as an ear trumpet, auricle or artificial drum (of oiled silk), may be used. These mechanical aids are seldom seen today but may be more acceptable to the elderly person who finds an electrical aid too difficult.

Electrical hearing aids, which used to be bulky and unsightly because of the large batteries used, are now being replaced by the transistor type—with a plug in the ear for air conduction or behind the ear for bone conduction.

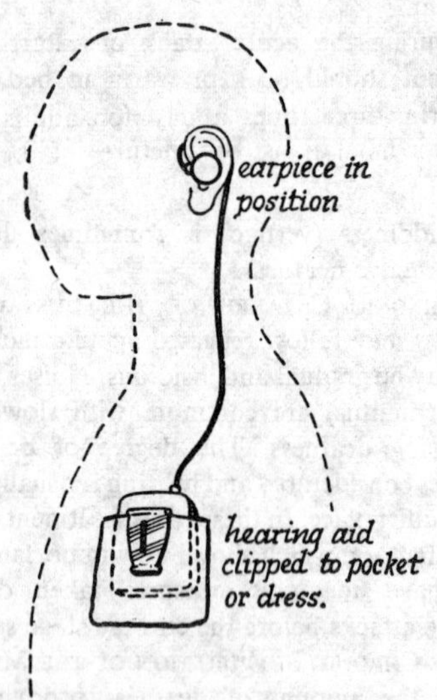

Fig. 8. *TRANSISTOR-TYPE DEAF AID showing how it is worn by a person who hears by air conduction.*

Menière's Disease

In this condition there is deafness and tinnitus accompanied by vertigo and sickness; various disorders may produce this combination of symptoms, such as bleeding into the internal ear, eighth nerve tumor, anemia, or high blood pressure with arterio-

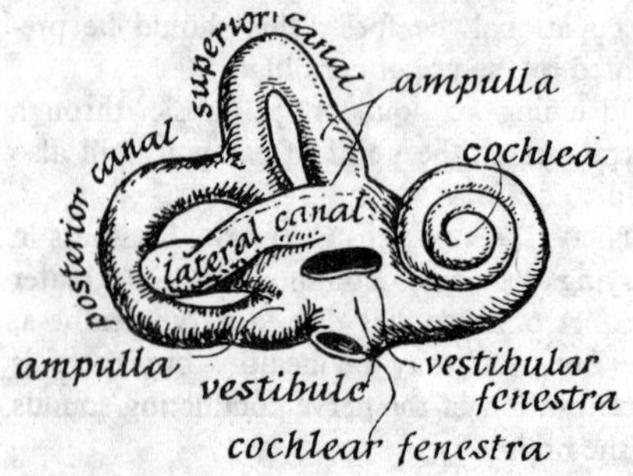

Fig. 9. *THE BONY LABYRINTH OF THE INTERNAL EAR. The cochlea is concerned with hearing, and the semi-circular canals assist the balance of the body.*

sclerosis. These conditions must be excluded before treatment is given.

Sedatives, such as phenobarbital which is prescribed by a doctor, often give relief, together with a salt-free diet. Operative treatment is justified in severe cases, but complete deafness in the affected ear results.

See also p. 423.

Tinnitus

Noises in the ear, or tinnitus, is a very common complaint and often accompanies other ear disorders. Mild cases cause little distress but severe cases often cause the sufferer extreme annoyance or nervous strain.

The treatment depends on the cause, if this can be found. Wax, decayed teeth, sinus infection or anemia are possible causes, but tinnitus may persist in spite of all measures for its eradication (see p. 423).

DISEASES OF THE NOSE AND THROAT

AFFECTIONS OF THE NOSE

Foreign Bodies

Small objects such as peas and beads are often pushed up the nostrils by young children. If retained, they will cause inflammation and discharge, and should be removed as soon as possible. This is generally done by a doctor. An attempt to dislodge and expel the object may be made by closing the mouth and opposite nostril and forcibly blowing down the obstructed side.

Nose Bleeding
(*Epistaxis*)

Nose bleeding is a fairly common complaint which may be troublesome.

Causes. It may follow injuries of the nasal bones or base or the skull, 'picking of the nose' in children with ulceration of the lining

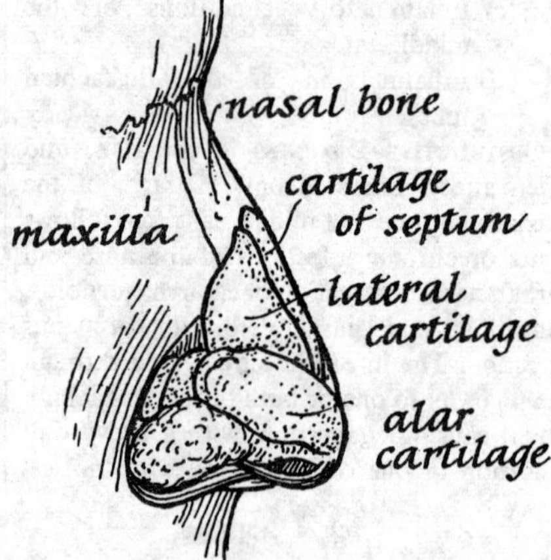

Fig. 10. *BONY AND CARTILAGINOUS STRUCTURE OF THE OUTER NOSE*

membrane, inflammation from foreign bodies, or high blood pressure. It is common in adolescents at puberty. Blood diseases such as purpura, scurvy, and hemophilia, kidney disorders such as Bright's disease, heart or lung diseases, infectious fevers, colds, influenza, nasal diphtheria, tumors and polypi, or changes in atmospheric pressure may also give rise to attacks of bleeding from the nose.

Treatment. In most cases the bleeding is from one side only. In some cases, as in high blood pressure, when the loss is not very severe or profuse, it may be unwise to check the bleeding immediately; when profuse or troublesome, however, measures must be taken promptly.

To control the hemorrhage, the patient should lie down with the head slightly raised. The blood should *not* be swallowed. The nostrils should be pinched tightly together for at least five minutes, when the bleeding usually stops.

Occasionally cautery is used for recurrent attacks.

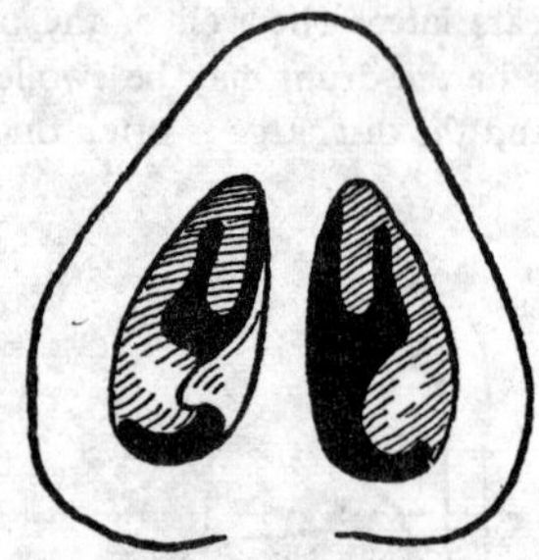

Fig. 11. *DIAGRAM SHOWING A SPUR ON THE RIGHT SIDE OF THE NASAL SEPTUM*

Deformity of Nasal Septum

Deviation of the cartilaginous partition between the nostrils may cause recurrent colds, obstruction of breathing, or paroxysmal sneezing. The condition is often due to injuries such as blows, or there may be a spur on the cartilage or bone of the septum.

When the deviation causes marked symptoms, surgical treatment often relieves the various secondary effects due to chronic obstruction, congestion, or infection. The obstruction may also cause frequent colds or sinusitis.

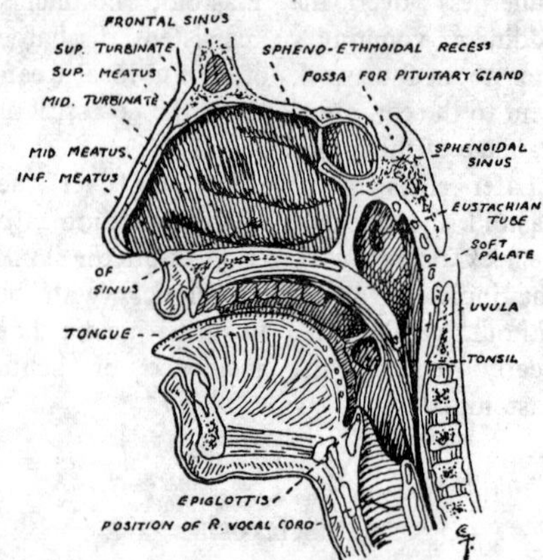

Fig. 12. *VERTICAL SECTION THROUGH THE NOSE, MOUTH, PHARYNX, AND LARYNX*

Acute Rhinitis
(*Acute Inflammation of the Nose*)

Acute inflammation of the nose is a common symptom in fevers such as measles, influenza, and whooping-cough; it also follows irritation of the nose from dust, fumes, or pollen, as in hay fever. The inflammation often spreads to the nasal sinuses or to the Eustachian tube of the ear, giving rise to headache, deafness, and loss of the sense of smell. Attacks of acute rhinitis should be avoided as far as possible, since frequently recurring attacks lead to congestion and thickening of the lining mucous membrane of the sinuses (the antrum and frontal sinuses of the forehead) and of the Eustachian tubes leading from the pharynx to the ear; this chronic state of congestion favors infection of the sinuses, and loss of hearing is likely to occur when the Eustachian tubes become partially blocked.

Treatment of the Acute Attack. Steam inhalations of tincture of benzoin or menthol in hot water usually give some relief and help to reduce the congestion so that nasal breathing is easier. Ephedrine hydrochloride (0·5 to 1 per cent) may be inserted into the nostrils (the patient lying on his back with neck extended) by means of a dropper, and this quickly reduces the congestion and obstruction.

The traditional treatment of a cold in the head is very helpful though not curative and it will usually enable the patient to get back to work earlier. Take a hot bath, then go to bed after having a hot lemon drink fortified with one or two tablespoonsful of whiskey. Certainly anyone suffering from an acute virus infection should be at home for 36 to 48 hours, remaining in a warm though ventilated room and taking

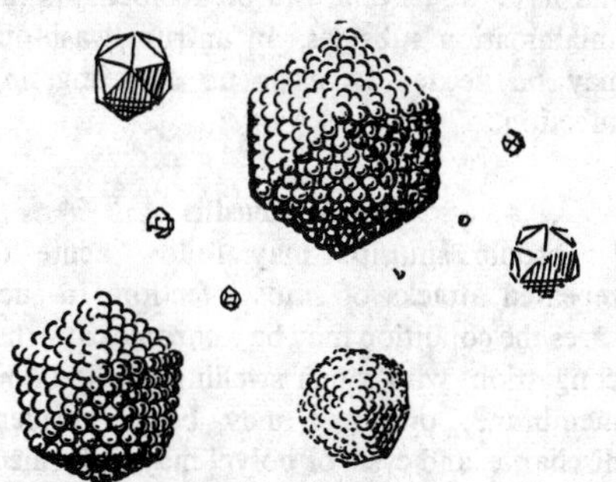

Fig. 13. *ADENOVIRUS. One of the micro-organisms causing the common cold in the head. Each 20-sided cell is only three-millionths of an inch in diameter, and can only be seen by an electron microscope.*

aspirin crushed in milk or water three or four times a day.

For severe nasal irritation as in hay fever, antihistamine drops or spray, are beneficial (see also Hay Fever, p. 334).

To maintain health and comfort in the nasal passages, proper drainage of secretion, a clear airway and a healthy condition of the mucous membrane are necessary.

Common Remedies. Sprays, drops, inhalations and ointments of various types are used. Care should be taken to avoid the use of any preparations which may prove irritating to the lining membrane; nasal powders and ointments are generally unsuitable. Drops are rather less effective than sprays produced by means of a nasal atomizer, but are simpler to use. Oily preparations should not be used in drops or lotions for sprays for young children, the elderly, or anyone with chest trouble, since the oil may be inhaled into the lungs and cause lung complications.

Medicated inhalations of steam containing menthol, oil of eucalyptus or pine, camphor, etc., are commonly used and effective.

Other forms of treatment include the use of caustic solutions, ionization, and cautery. The purpose of these forms of treatment is to reduce the bulk of the mucous membrane inside the nasal cavity so as to provide an adequate airway.

Prevention. Removal of infected tonsils or adenoids, and treatment of infected sinuses or nasal obstruction must be undertaken when necessary in recurrent cases.

Purulent Rhinitis

This condition is generally seen in acute fevers such as measles, or after severe colds in the head. In some cases, in children particularly, a small object such as a pea may have been pushed up the nostril and forgotten until the discharge draws attention to it.

The local treatment consists in nasal douches and medicated steam inhalations. Antibiotic treatment may be given if a sensitive organism is grown from a swab taken of the discharged pus.

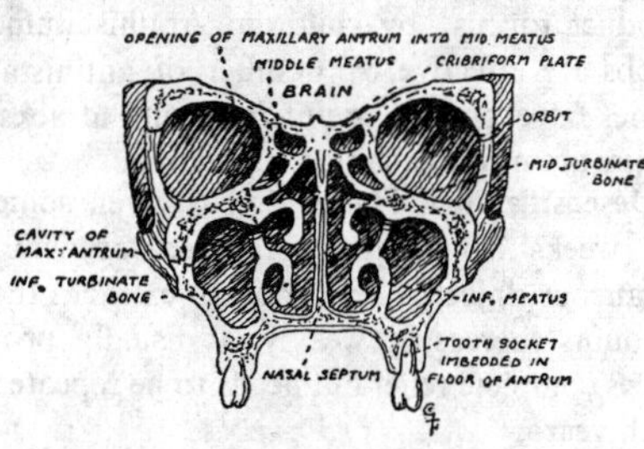

Fig. 14
CORONAL SECTION THROUGH THE NOSE

Chronic Rhinitis
(*Chronic Nasal Inflammation*)

In simple cases there is generally some underlying disease of the sinuses, or there may be enlarged adenoids. Less commonly the patient works in a dusty or irritating atmosphere. A deformity of the septum of the nose may be present, with swelling and thickening of the mucous membrane, and consequent obstruction to breathing. Simple cases often proceed to the following type when they are long-standing.

Hypertrophic or Congestive Rhinitis is a common form, in which the mucous membrane becomes much thickened, especially over the lower turbinate bone; in long-standing cases polypi develop, causing considerable obstruction, and there may also be a fairly profuse discharge of pus and mucus. In adults this condition is often associated with chronic sinusitis, pharyngitis, laryngitis, and deformity of the nasal septum, or follows frequent attacks of acute rhinitis.

In children, enlarged and infected tonsils and adenoids, and chronic infection of the maxillary antrum are common causes.

Symptoms. The main symptom is nasal obstruction, with dryness of the throat due to mouth-breathing; this is also increased by indulgence in smoking and alcoholic drinks. Occasionally there may be crusts in the nose.

Treatment should be directed towards removing any underlying causes, such as irritation from dust, living in stuffy rooms, or excessive smoking. Children should be taught to blow their noses regularly, and adults may use a cleansing spray. A vasoconstrictor spray such as mild silver protein with ephedrine will relieve congestion.

Surgical treatment is reserved for advanced cases, when cauterization and removal of part of the inferior turbinate bones, with strips of mucosa, may be undertaken.

Rhinitis Sicca

In this disease the lining membrane of the nose is dry, and crusts are often present. The condition usually develops in anemic and debilitated young girls who work in dusty atmospheres, or in hot dry atmospheres.

The patient's throat is dry, and sometimes nose bleeding occurs from separation of the crusts. There may be ulceration on the septum caused by frequent nose-picking.

The patient should avoid work in dusty or irritating atmospheres, or a protective mask should be worn, and the anemia should be corrected by iron tablets and tonics.

Atrophic Rhinitis and Ozena

This is a most unpleasant disease in which the mucous membrane of the nose becomes dry and shrunken, and extensive yellow crusts form which produce a foul smell, called ozena. The cause is unknown, but the disease sometimes runs in families, and women are most often affected. The disease sometimes starts in underfed children with tuberculosis or syphilis. Some cases appear to follow septic conditions of the nose and pharynx, sinus infection, adenoids, or nasal diphtheria. The condition may be diagnosed at once by the smell, of which, however, the patient is unaware. Both nostrils are full of crusts, and the membrane below is dry and glazed.

Treatment can only be palliative. The condition can be considerably improved by regular and careful daily spraying with warm normal saline to remove the crusts. The membrane is then painted with a 20 per cent solution of glucose in glycerin; this reduces the disagreeable smell, and sometimes a dilute mild alkaline solution is recommended as a spray. The general health should also be attended to, tonics being taken when required, and any underlying local infection such as sinusitis must be dealt with. A spray containing estradiol in oil is also helpful,

0.5 milliliters of a solution containing 5 milligrams per milliliter being used, at first daily, and later once a week or every two weeks.

Nasal Polypi

Polypi in the nose are common, and are usually small soft tumors which develop inside the nostrils; they are often multiple, and are generally due to allergic chronic congestion of the nasal mucous membrane, with nasal catarrh or sinus infection. They cause difficulty in breathing and nasal voice sounds, and there may be a thin discharge. The polyp should be removed by a surgeon, but tends to reappear. In cases of polypi with allergy, appropriate treatment must be given to the underlying cause (see under Allergy, p. 481).

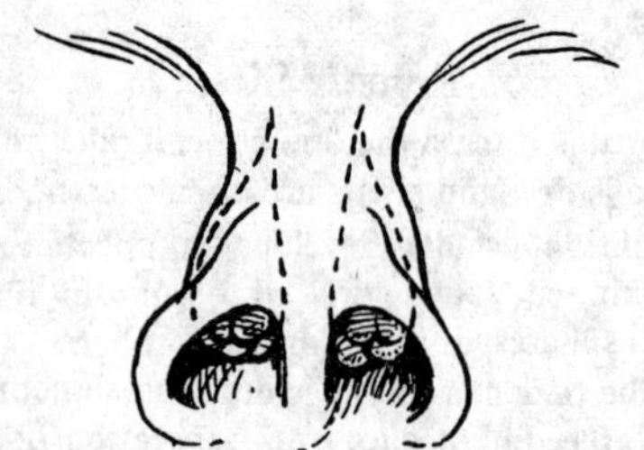

Fig. 15. *POLYPI IN THE NOSE. These small soft tumors develop in the nostrils and cause difficulty in breathing.*

Tumors of the Nose and Pharynx

All benign tumors are rare, except polypi. Cancerous tumors are occasionally seen, and the treatment is surgical or by irradiation with X-rays.

Nasal Catarrh

Nasal catarrh is a form of rhinitis, and consists in congestion of the lining of the nose, with swelling of the turbinate bones, and obstruction to breathing; it is a common and troublesome complaint. Mucus or mucopus is usually secreted, and drops down into the throat, much to the discomfort of the patient. The condition is often due to chronic infection of the sinuses, or to some allergic state, or to irritation.

Frequently the sufferer can only breathe with the mouth open. Upon rising in the morning a great effort is required to clear the head and the upper part of the throat. There is occasionally a feeling of pressure across the upper part of the nose which may give rise to headache, vertigo, and confusion. The sense of smell is frequently lost, and sometimes taste is diminished.

Treatment is as for rhinitis, with correction of nasal deformities and tonsil or sinus infection, and attention to the general health with exercise in the open air. The bedroom should be kept well ventilated. Excessive smoking or alcohol must be avoided.

Hay Fever

In certain individuals there is extreme sensitiveness to certain substances such as plant pollens, dust, feathers, face powders particularly those containing orris root, and other irritating particles. Such persons are said to be *allergic*, and hay fever is one of the allergic diseases. (See Allergy, p.483.)

When people who are thus sensitive breathe air containing the irritant (often a specific one in each case), it causes an attack of 'hay fever' with a sudden paroxysm of sneezing and the discharge of profuse watery secretion from the nose. The attack is often preceded by burning and irritation in the eyes, nose, or throat. Grass pollen is one of the commonest irritants, and hay fever is especially common in May, June and July. The specific irritant can often be identified in an individual case by skin tests which are carried out by a doctor.

Treatment includes avoidance of hay fever districts (country, fields, parks, etc.) when possible, or seasonal desensitization by injections, if the specific irritant can be discovered. Palliative treatment consists of the use of a nasal spray of adrenaline solution (1 : 10,000 parts) applied by means of an atomizer. A nasal spray of ephedrine (1 to 2 per cent) gives temporary relief. In adults Endrine may be instilled in drops into the nostrils, and there is a mild solution of this product for use by children. Antihistamine drops are effective. A number of antihistamines have proved useful for acute attacks; elixirs are now available for children.

Desensitization. The patient is given some ten weeks before the pollen season, subcutaneous injections of pollen extract, the amounts increasing weekly. It usually produces complete relief but needs to be repeated each year.

Sinusitis

Acute Sinusitis

The nasal accessary sinuses are the two frontal sinuses, the maxillary antra on each side of the nose, the ethmoidal and sphenoidal sinuses. These sinuses may become acutely infected as a result of nasal infection from a cold, acute fevers, or influenza, and the inflammation may be catarrhal or pus may be formed. Acute or recurrent sinusitis causes neuralgic pain, headache, feverishness, pain and tenderness over the bony cavity which becomes involved. During a common cold the lining membrane of the nose becomes swollen and congested, and a profuse watery or mucous discharge appears which later becomes thick and contains pus. The lining of the sinuses undergoes similar changes when the inflammation spreads into any of them; and the openings of the sinuses, which normally allow drainage, become blocked, giving rise to severe headache and pain. As the infection subsides, the sinuses gradually return to their normal condition.

In very virulent infections, or when there is some deformity of the septum of the nose

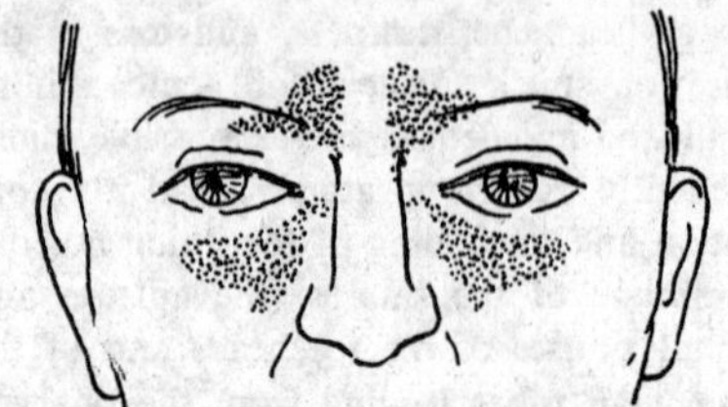

Fig. 16. *NASAL SINUSES. Shaded areas show the position of the nasal accessory sinuses in which sinusitis can develop.*

or enlargement of the turbinate bones, the catarrhal secretion may become purulent, the pus being blocked up in the sinus. The patient then has a high temperature, with chills and malaise. When the inflammation spreads to the Eustachian tubes deafness follows, and there may be pain in the ears and acute inflammation of the middle ear (otitis media).

Treatment. Most cases of acute sinus infection clear up with rest in bed and general care, and surgical treatment is avoided during the acute stage. Nasal sprays are used frequently. Steam inhalations with tincture of benzoin or menthol are valuable, and aspirin may be given, in four-hourly doses for adults.

In severe cases penicillin is injected if the organism is penicillin-sensitive. Systemic antibiotics are also given.

The nose should *not* be blown vigorously, and nasal douches are to be avoided. As the inflammation subsides, an antrum wash-out may be needed to clear up any lingering infection.

Chronic Sinusitis

Chronic sinusitis may follow acute or repeated attacks of sinus infection. In such cases the condition may be a chronic catarrhal congestion, with much swelling of the lining membrane; or there may be a purulent discharge, and cysts or polypi may be formed.

Chronic Antrum Infection

A chronic discharge from the nose or back of the nose is the commonest symptom, but in the latent intervals the discharge may be scanty. Neuralgic pain or pains round the jaws are common, and headache is likely to be persistent at intervals, although the position of the headache varies in different individuals. Obstruction to breathing, an unpleasant odor in the breath, and occasionally loss of smell are fairly common symptoms, and indigestion, fatigue, nausea, and failure of mental concentration are often complained of.

Surgical treatment, consisting in antrum wash-outs after surgical puncture, is sometimes necessary later on to drain the antrum, when the condition has been confirmed by X-ray investigation. The other method of 'displacement' has given good results, and sometimes does away with the necessity for more serious surgical treatment.

Chronic sinusitis should not be neglected, since it leads not only to headaches, frequent colds and difficulty in mental concentration, but may also give rise to bronchitis or other complications. Penicillin and sulphonamides are used to prevent or arrest suppuration.

Chronic Frontal Sinus Infection

The frontal sinuses lie above the eyes, in the bone over the ridge of the orbit. Chronic inflammation causes pain, especially in the morning; the amount of discharge varies, the nose is often stuffy on the affected side, and tenderness is felt on pressure.

Many cases clear up with the treatment described, or a doctor may order cocaine to be applied on small packs inserted into the nose. Occasionally, however, surgical treatment is necessary.

AFFECTIONS OF THE PHARYNX

Adenoids

Adenoid hypertrophy is an overgrowth of the soft tissue of the naso-pharynx behind the nose, which forms soft vegetations protruding from the roof and back wall of the pharynx. Adenoids are common in children living in unhygienic and crowded conditions, especially in cold damp areas. Adenoids are most likely to develop between the ages of three and twelve years of age; they may disappear naturally after the age of fifteen. The child often suffers also from infected and swollen tonsils.

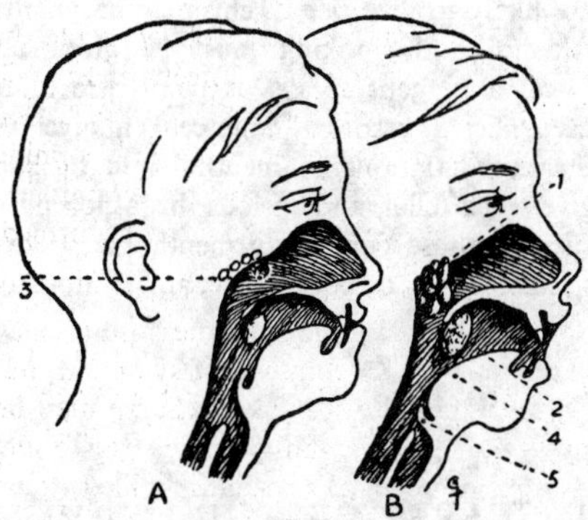

Fig. 17. *ADENOID OVERGROWTH. Nasal and oral passages (A) in a normal child; (B) in a child with adenoids and enlarged tonsils. (In B note the open lips in mouth breathing, and blocking of the Eustachian opening by adenoids.)* 1. *Adenoids.* 2. *Enlarged tonsils.* 3. *Eustachian tube to ear.* 4. *Tongue.* 5. *Epiglottis.*

Symptoms. The symptoms are characteristic, with mouth breathing, a nasal lifeless voice, and nasal discharge. There is usually a history of frequent colds. Chronic catarrh of the nose often affects the Eustachian tubes leading from the pharynx to the ear, causing obstruction and consequent deafness, and sometimes gives rise to an abscess of the middle ear, with discharge. The deafness is probably the cause of the mental dullness often found in this condition. Snoring and nightmares during sleep are common. Some children with adenoids suffer from bed-wetting, and there may be a tendency to coughs from downward extension of the catarrh. The chest is often flattened and poorly developed, and there may be curvature of the spine and a 'pot-belly.' The symptoms and appearance of the child generally make the diagnosis obvious, but a surgeon will examine the naso-pharynx with a mirror to confirm the presence of adenoids. X-rays are also sometimes used to aid in the diagnosis. Many children have some degree of adenoids, but these may not give rise to the above symptoms, or interfere with nasal breathing.

Treatment. Adenoids should be removed by a small surgical operation which is often combined with removal of the tonsils when these are also diseased. The child should be given a nourishing diet, with plenty of time for sleep in a well-ventilated bedroom. Clothing should be light but warm, and the bowels should be kept regular.

Tonsillitis

Acute Tonsillitis

Tonsillitis may be acute or chronic. The acute type of infection occurs as a result of colds or influenza, or may appear in epidemics of sore throat in the winter or spring months. The patient is feverish, with headache, malaise, a furred tongue and offensive breath, general muscular pains, the throat is sore, and the glands of the neck are swollen and tender; patches of coagulated discharge on the tonsils may give the appearance of ulceration. A throat swab should be taken for examination in case of diphtheria.

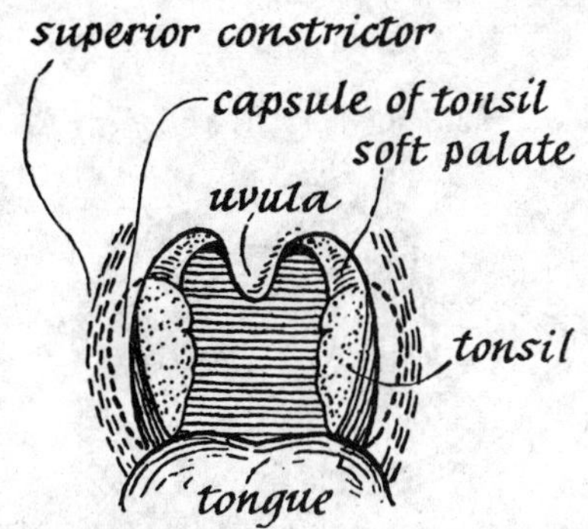

Fig. 18. *THE PHARYNX showing the position of the tonsils on either side.*

In Children attacks of tonsillitis tend to recur, and the glands in the neck become enlarged and tender. Between the attacks the swelling of both tonsils and the glands may subside, or there may be a thin layer of grayish pus on the tonsils.

The young child seldom complains of much sore throat, but the temperature is usually about 39° to 39·5° C (102° to 103° F). Infection by *Streptococci* in the mouth, throat or nose is generally the cause of enlarged glands of the neck in children, and when the tonsils are considered to be the source of the inflammation, surgical removal is often advisable. In children under three years of age removal of adenoids without removal of the tonsils is often sufficient to cure nasal obstruction.

When infection of the ears (otitis media) occurs in conjunction with inflamed tonsils, the aural condition may be improved by tonsillectomy (removal of the tonsils), which arrests the spread of the infection through the Eustachian tube from the pharynx to the middle ear. Attacks of acute rheumatism or acute nephritis in children may also be an indication for tonsillectomy. It should also be borne in mind that acute tonsillitis may herald an attack of scarlet fever, glandular fever, or some other acute fever.

In Adults the tonsils are seldom seen to be so grossly enlarged as in children, but they may show points of discharge. Recurrent sore throats generally follow tonsillar infection, giving rise to difficulty and pain in swallowing, a fairly high temperature, and tenderness of the glands of the neck.

Operative removal is generally required, but in some cases of chronic pharyngitis in men due to the abuse of tobacco and alcohol, surgical treatment fails to relieve the symptoms which are attributed to tonsil infection.

Quinsy and infections of the middle ear justify tonsillectomy to prevent future attacks of these conditions.

Treatment. The patient should be confined to bed, on a fluid or light diet, and the bowels must be kept open. Warm antiseptic gargles may be used, containing dilute peroxide of hydrogen, or phenol (1 in 80 parts).

Aspirin, or paracetamol tablets in appropriate doses are usually given by mouth.

Penicillin by injection or by mouth is invaluable in the early and acute stages in reducing the toxemia of the disease and shortening the course. These antibiotics must be given in full doses, otherwise a relapse may occur. Mild attacks should not be treated with antibiotics so that a natural immunity can be acquired.

Fluids such as glucose drinks and lemonade, barley water, weak tea, broths, and milk drinks should be given liberally. When the patient has a very high temperature, tepid sponging may be necessary.

Steam inhalations should be given when the larynx is also affected.

Complications. The commonest complication of acute tonsillitis is quinsy, but extension of the infection elsewhere, as to the ears or lymphatic glands of the neck, may follow.

Chronic Tonsillitis

Treatment. Chronic tonsillar infection may cause few local symptoms, but when these develop, gargles, and mouth washes are of little value. And, although penicillin may clear the superficial streptococci on the tonsils, there are usually residual pockets of them deep in the tissue.

Removal of these chronically infected tonsils is the only remedy.

Quinsy

(Peritonsillar Abscess)

Quinsy generally develops as a complication of acute tonsillitis by extension of the infection; an abscess develops near the tonsil, usually on one side only.

Symptoms. The abscess causes severe pain, difficulty in swallowing, and high temperature. The swollen tonsil bulges downwards and inwards, and there may be some spasm of the jaw muscles. The soft palate and uvula are swollen and congested, and the tonsil is often covered with pus. The glands of the neck on the affected side are swollen and very tender, and the neck may be stiff, with much pain on attempted movement. There may be so much difficulty in swallowing that the saliva is dribbled out of the mouth, and the patient looks and feels extremely ill.

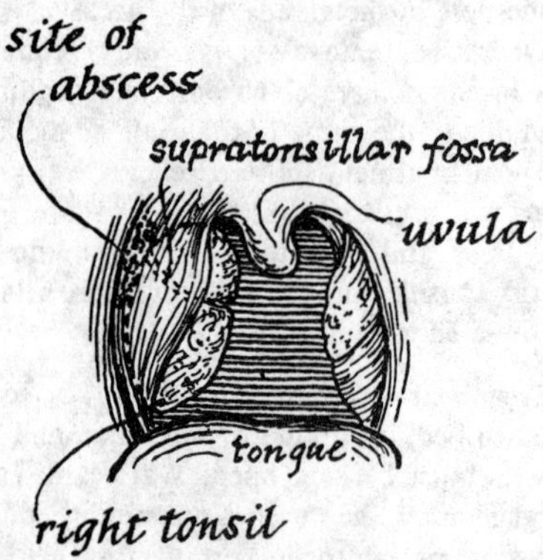

Fig. 19. *QUINSY. The peritonsillar abscess on the right side of the pharynx is an extension of the infection from the right tonsil.*

Treatment. In the early stages hot gargles are indicated to relieve the pain. Penicillin in large doses is given by a doctor and, if sleep is prevented by pain, a sedative and an analgesic may be ordered.

Early antibiotic treatment usually prevents the abscess pointing and breaking. In late or severe cases the pus is released through an incision made by a surgeon, after the throat has been sprayed with lignocaine. This gives rapid relief of the pain, and the abscess then usually subsides. Penicillin should be continued after incision.

Hot gargles and mouth washes assist healing, and afterwards iron tonics should be given.

Quinsy is very liable to recur unless the tonsils are removed when the patient has fully recovered from the first attack.

Elongation of the Uvula

The uvula is the small pendulous organ which hangs down from the arch of the palate, just over the root of the tongue. It is apt to become inflamed in acute or chronic pharyngitis, and becomes relaxed and elongated so that its lower extremity sometimes rests upon the tongue. This sometimes excites an incessant cough, which is worse on lying down, and there may be retching or vomiting.

Treatment. In some cases the condition may be relieved by astringent applications or an astringent gargle. Surgical treatment, however, is sometimes used in chronic cases, part of the uvula being cut off.

Pharyngitis

This consists of inflammation of the upper and back of the throat, or that part which can be seen when the mouth is opened widely.

Acute Septic Pharyngitis

This occurs in various degrees of severity, from acute swelling to ulceration or even gangrene, which may pass downwards to the larynx. In very severe cases the soft cellular structures of the neck are also involved, as in Ludwig's Angina, a form of the disease now seldom seen.

The ordinary acute form of inflammation is often associated with rhinitis or tonsillitis, and is due to similar infections. There is a sudden rise of temperature, with chills, pain in the throat, and soon swallowing is extremely difficult or impossible. The patient is often extremely pale, with a very fast pulse, and furred tongue. In very severe cases the outlook is grave, and death may follow as a result of bronchopneumonia, pleurisy or pericarditis.

Treatment. A doctor should be called; penicillin or other antibiotic treatment must be given early. The pain may be relieved by aspirin or other sedatives, and a laxative should be given. Mouth-washes and sprays of sodium bicarbonate (one teaspoonful to a pint of warm water) help to cleanse the mouth and pharynx.

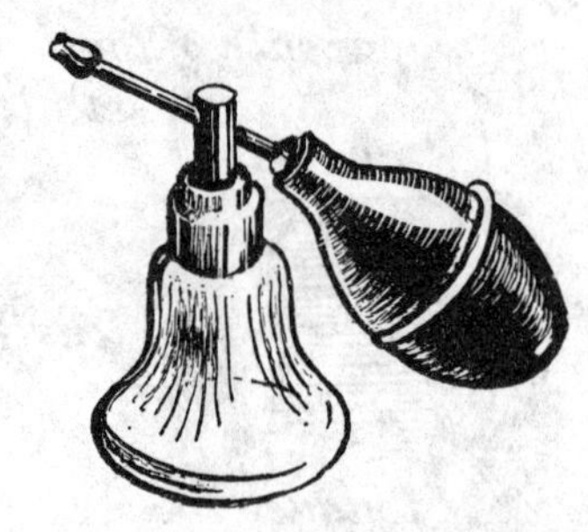

Fig. 20. *A THROAT SPRAY, with a vulcanite tip for the throat. It is used for watery solutions.*

Occasionally tracheotomy is required when the swelling spreads to the larynx.

Acute Simple Pharyngitis

This is often associated with rhinitis or tonsillitis, and is due to similar infections. For the local treatment steam inhalations of tincture of benzoin, or throat sprays, should be used. The patient is advised to remain indoors for a few days to prevent further spread of the infection. Frequent hot gargles also give relief but they are of little value against the infection in deeper tissues. The patient should not smoke during the acute attack. Lozenges containing menthol are soothing for the inflamed tissue.

Chronic Pharyngitis

This term covers various symptoms, and these may be due to several different causes. In general there is usually discomfort or a sense of roughness or slight soreness, usually worse in the mornings and not made worse by swallowing. Small quantities of mucus are frequently coughed up, and there is a slight huskiness or thickness of the voice which is improved when the throat is cleared by coughing. There is redness and small scattered granular swellings can be seen on the pharyngeal membrane. There is slight swelling of the palate and uvula.

Infection of the nasal sinuses, dental sepsis from decayed teeth or pyorrhea, chronic infection of the tonsils, or atrophic rhinitis are often present, while over-indulgence in tobacco and alcohol also lead to congestion of the pharynx.

Chronic pharyngitis is usually present in the late stages of syphilis, but the common form of chronic pharyngitis is most often seen in middle-aged men with gastric disturbances.

Treatment. Attention should be paid to the possible causes, and any necessary measures taken to remove septic conditions of the mouth, nose, or sinuses.

A glycerin and tannin paint should be applied to the pharynx. When a chronic cough is also present the chest should be thoroughly examined, since chronic bronchitis and other diseases of the lower air passages are likely to give rise to chronic pharyngitis. Alcohol and smoking must be given up. Local astringent sprays or paints are to be used, such as resorcin (5 per cent) in glycerin. Steam inhalations of menthol and benzoin give some relief, and various throat lozenges, such as those containing menthol or potassium chlorate, or benzocaine, are comforting.

DISEASES OF THE LARYNX

Diseases of the larynx may be divided into (1) acute and subacute inflammation; (2) chronic inflammation; (3) diphtheritic laryngitis; (4) acute edema; (5) spasms of the muscles (see Spasm of the Glottis); (6) paralysis of the vocal cords; and (7) new growths (cancer, papilloma, etc.).

Occasionally foreign bodies may be inhaled and become lodged in the trachea, larynx, or bronchi.

In inflammatory affections of the larynx there are characteristics which are common to each, with hoarseness or complete loss of voice, dryness and inflammation of the mucous membrane followed by exudation of secretion, and cough.

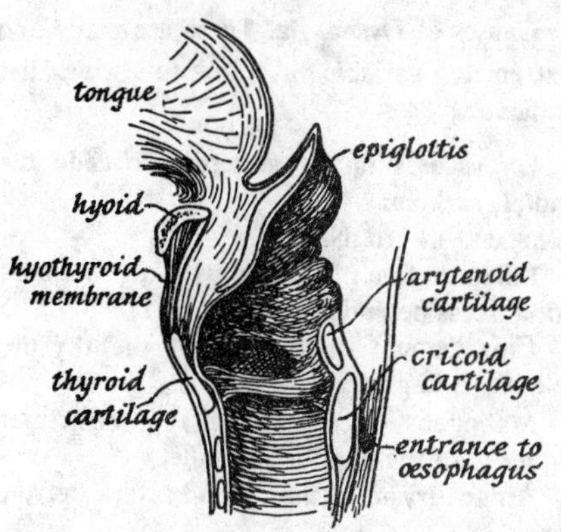

Fig. 21. *LARYNX AND LARYNGOPHARYNX. Vertical section showing the various structures around the larynx.*

Laryngitis

Several types of laryngitis or inflammation of the larynx are recognizable:

1. Acute catarrhal laryngitis, in which the membranes alone are commonly involved.
2. Acute edema or swelling of the larynx, in which the deeper tissues become inflamed and infiltrated.
3. Chronic laryngitis, in which the various types of inflammatory process become chronic.
4. Tuberculous and syphilitic laryngitis.

Acute Catarrhal Laryngitis

In moderately severe acute inflammation of the larynx the mucous membrane is congested, and later mucus is coughed up. This condition often follows a cold in the head or other infections of the air passages.

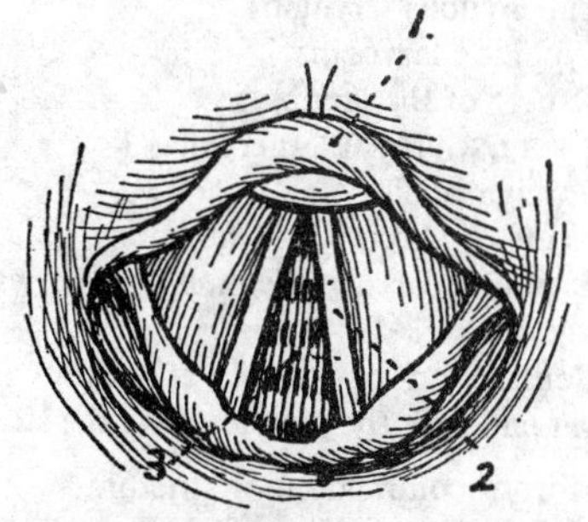

Fig. 22. *LARYNX AND PHARYNX. Horizontal view from the pharynx, looking down on the larynx.* 1. *Epiglottis.* 2. *The vocal cords.* 3. *Trachea.*

Acute catarrhal laryngitis is commonly seen in children, especially in the early stages of the infectious fevers; repeated attacks also occur in people with chronic septic conditions of the nose, mouth or throat, or with chronic bronchitis.

Symptoms. A tickling sensation in the larynx is followed by hoarseness, especially in the morning. Soon mucus is formed, with cough, and sometimes pain on swallowing. There is mild fever, and the glands of the neck may be tender. The disease usually lasts a few days, and seldom gives rise to complications.

Treatment. The patient should be kept warm in bed, and should rest the voice. Sprays, gargles, or throat paints are not generally effective, but medicated steam inhalations of tincture of benzoin or menthol usually give relief, and a steam kettle may be used in the room. Hot or cold compresses also help to relieve the discomfort in the throat.

Acute Edematous Laryngitis

Acute laryngitis is generally not severe, but sometimes a more severe form occurs, with much swelling of the larynx and occasionally this may end fatally. There is great difficulty in breathing, especially when this type of inflammation occurs in children. Acute septic pharyngitis or tonsillitis, measles or scarlet fever, swallowing corrosive substances, foreign bodies in the throat, or angioneurotic edema (see Allergy, p.4 82) may give rise to severe swelling of the larynx.

In these cases treatment is urgently required to relieve the difficulty in breathing, and tracheotomy may need to be performed. Steam inhalations generally assist in giving relief, and cold compresses to the neck, and an adrenaline spray may be used.

Chronic Laryngitis

In this condition there is chronic catarrh of the larynx, with congestion and hoarseness. Chronic laryngitis may follow repeated acute attacks, or there may be infection of the air passages, decayed teeth, infected tonsils, infection of the sinuses, chronic bronchitis, or tuberculosis of the lungs.

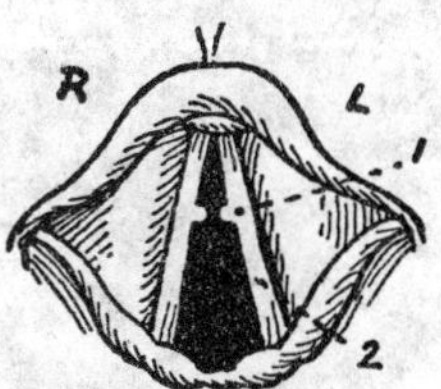

Fig. 23. *SINGER'S NODES ON THE VOCAL CORDS OF THE LARYNX.* 1. *Node.* 2. *Vocal cord.*

Public speakers, clergymen and singers also sometimes suffer from chronic laryngitis, from overstrain and faulty voice production. Singer's nodes consist in small nodules on the vocal cords which causes the voice to 'crack.'

Treatment depends on the cause, but complete rest of the voice is absolutely necessary, and septic conditions of the nose, mouth or throat must be attended to. Lessons in voice production are often valuable later, but local treatment is seldom very effective.

Croup in Children

Laryngeal diphtheria, acute laryngitis or bronchitis, an abscess behind the back wall of the pharynx, spasm of the glottis, papilloma of the larynx and foreign bodies may give rise to croup, which is a hoarse cough with difficulty in breathing. See also Spasm of the Larynx, below.

The exact diagnosis is not always easy at first, and treatment must be directed towards relieving the difficulty in breathing. Acute septic laryngitis is a serious condition which may be followed by bronchopneumonia and profound toxemia.

Spasm of the Larynx
(*Laryngismus Stridulus*)

The cause is not known, but repeated attacks of hoarseness and croup are seen in weakly or rickety children under two years of age. There is no fever, but the child becomes blue and there is a crowing sound during breathing. During an attack, the clothing round the neck should be loosened, the window opened, and cold water applied to the child's face and neck. Between the attacks the general health must be improved, with special measures for rickets.

Tuberculosis of the Larynx

The disease nearly always follows consumption of the lungs, through coughing up the infected sputum. In addition to the general symptoms of inflammation of the larynx there is usually hoarseness, but this may be absent if the vocal cords are not involved. The voice tires easily, or there may be periodic loss of voice, with dryness and irritability of the throat. Cough, pain on swallowing, and breathlessness develop later. These symptoms, together with sweating, loss in weight, irregular fever, morning nausea and malaise should lead at once to a thorough examination by a specialist.

Treatment. The general treatment is that for tuberculosis which is dealt with thoroughly in Diseases of the Chest, p. 352. The use of streptomycin and para-aminosalicylic acid (PAS), or isoniazid, usually clears symptoms within a few days, although the larynx usually takes a couple of months to return to its normal condition.

Local treatment to the larynx is not often effective, but the voice must be rested completely and the patient must make every endeavor to cooperate. Smoking and alcoholic drinks must be forbidden.

Sedatives may be needed to allay cough, fever, pain, diarrhea, and restlessness or anxiety. For anemia, benefit may follow the use of citrate of iron.

Paralysis of the Larynx

Paralysis of the larynx is an uncommon condition which may arise from injuries, wounds, aneurysm, tuberculosis or other

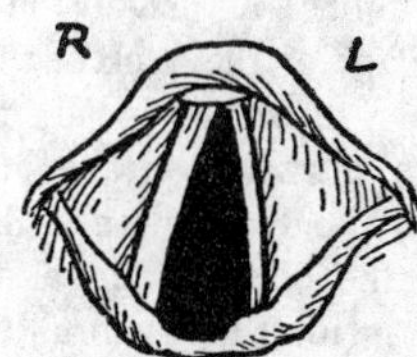

Fig. 24. *PARALYSIS OF LEFT VOCAL CORD of the larynx as seen on deep inspiration.*

disease of the glands of the neck, cancer of the esophagus, thyroid gland or other adjoining organs, affecting the laryngeal nerve.

Tumors of the Larynx

Benign Tumors

A PAPILLOMA is the commonest benign tumor affecting the larynx; it develops on the vocal cords and is generally seen in men or young children. Hoarseness is an early and constant symptom and sometimes cough and breathlessness are noted, but removal of the tumor is easily effected surgically. Papillomata, however, often tend to recur.

Other benign new growths are also met with, including fibrous, cartilaginous, cystic and muscular tumors.

Cancer

Cancer occurs moderately commonly in the larynx especially in men over forty-five years of age. The symptoms in the early stages are indefinite, but hoarseness is often persistent and should always be regarded as a danger signal in a middle-aged man when it persists for more than 3 to 4 weeks. He should be examined and kept under observation by a throat specialist. Later, blood-stained mucus is coughed up, and eventually the adjoining glands become invaded. The vocal cords ulcerate, and, if the patient is untreated, death occurs from septic absorption, pneumonia, hemorrhage, or obstruction to breathing. The treatment is surgical removal or irradiation, which should be undertaken as early as possible.

Intrinsic Cancer of the larynx usually develops in the vocal cords, and in this type of case the outlook is very hopeful if radiotherapy or surgical treatment is given early; the spread of the growth is fairly slow until the structures outside the larynx are invaded. This type of cancer is generally seen in men.

In growths in the vocal cords constant hoarseness is the only early symptom, and may continue for months before the patient considers he should consult a doctor. Later there may be breathlessness.

Treatment. If given early, radiotherapy or surgical treatment will give good results.

Extrinsic Cancer. Extrinsic growths arise in other parts of the larynx such as the epiglottis. In men this form of cancer is most likely to develop in the epiglottis or pharynx, while in women it usually involves the cricoid cartilage or the back of the pharynx. The extrinsic growths spread much more rapidly than growths on the vocal cords, invading the glands of the neck in the early stages, and the disease runs a much more rapid course, with a high mortality.

In extrinsic growths of the epiglottis or in the pharynx the main symptom is difficulty in swallowing, and voice changes are noticed when the larynx is involved.

Treatment. Radiotherapy and surgical treatment are used, but with less satisfactory results, in some cases, than in intrinsic cancer of the vocal cords.

Foreign Bodies in the Trachea or Larynx

Occasionally particles of food or other objects are swallowed 'the wrong way,' and these may lodge in the larynx. If there is choking, cyanosis (blueness), and breathlessness, a tracheotomy must be performed at once; with less severe symptoms, the particles may be removed by a surgeon with forceps after the patient's throat has been anesthetized. In the trachea or bronchi, beyond the larynx, the removal is very difficult, and requires a general anesthetic and extraction with the aid of an instrument known as a bronchoscope. Serious complications, such as delayed choking, lung abscesses, or pneumonia, may follow the entry of foreign bodies into the larynx or lower air passages.

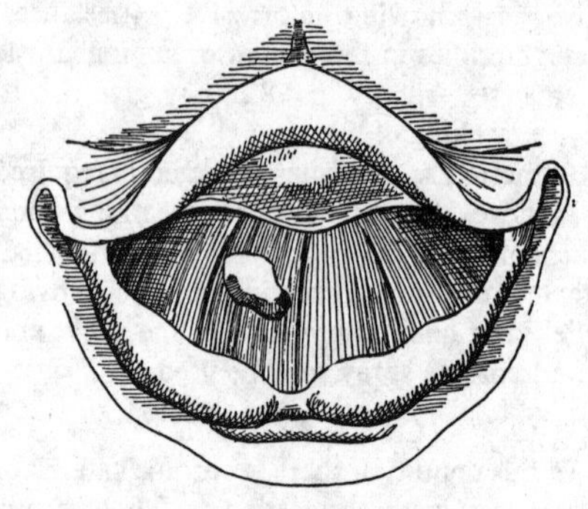

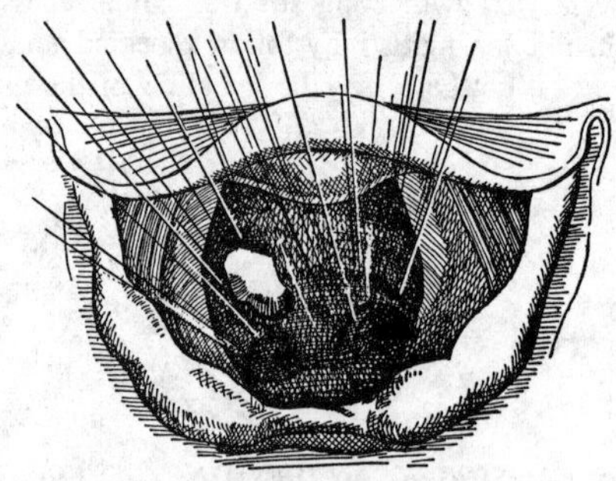

Fig. 25. *FOOD GOING THE WRONG WAY.* Above *a particle of food falls on the firmly closed vocal cords;* Below *the breath is forcibly expelled, the cords fly open and the irritating particle is coughed away.*

DISEASES OF THE ESOPHAGUS

Difficulty in Swallowing

(Dysphagia)

In cases of difficulty in swallowing, the mouth and pharynx, larynx, gullet, neck and chest must be carefully examined to find the cause, and the symptoms must be clearly described.

Causes of Dysphagia. These are many and extremely variable as the following list indicates.

1. Diseases in the structures outside the gullet, such as:

DISEASES IN THE NECK

Inflammation of the glands of the neck, or an abscess behind the gullet

Enlargement or tumors of the thyroid gland, as in goiter

Malignant disease (cancer) of structures other than the pharynx or gullet

An aneurysm of the carotid arteries of the neck

DISEASES AND DISORDERS IN THE CHEST

Enlarged glands in the chest

A goiter behind the sternum or breast-bone

Tumors and growths of the chest, lung, or spine

Backward dislocation of the inner end of the collar bone, causing pressure on the throat

Aneurysm of the aorta or its main branches

2. Affections in the pharynx or gullet itself

IN THE PHARYNX there may be:

Foreign bodies

Acute or chronic inflammation, or ulceration

Syphilitic infection

Contraction or narrowing of the pharynx as a result of scarring after ulceration

Malignant growths (cancer)

Paralysis

Hysteria

IN THE LARYNX there may be:

Acute or chronic inflammation (laryngitis)

Tuberculous laryngitis

Syphilitic laryngitis

Cancer of the larynx

IN THE ESOPHAGUS there may be:

Foreign bodies

Acute or chronic inflammation

A pouch (or diverticulum) in the wall of the gullet

Contraction or spasm, especially at the lower end near the junction with the stomach

Fibrous contraction, or stricture

Malignant growths (cancer)

Treatment. This will of necessity be as diverse as the many causes.

Malformations

Various defects in the structure of the gullet may occur, the commonest in adults being a *pouch*, or *diverticulum*, which usually develops near the upper end on the back wall, due to weakness of the muscles. Food tends to collect in the pouch and a swelling may be noticed, or the food may be regurgitated. The condition can be diagnosed by X-ray examination.

Treatment. Diverticulum is treated by surgical removal of the pouch.

Foreign Bodies

Objects such as dentures, coins, fish bones, or pieces of food may become lodged in the gullet. When this becomes blocked above the larynx death may follow almost immediately from suffocation.

When the objects become lodged for any length of time it may lead to ulceration, severe bleeding or even rupture (perforation) of the gullet, with inflammation of the surrounding parts.

Treatment. X-ray examination should be carried out to show the position of the object, which may then be removed by a surgical operation under a general anesthetic. An instrument known as an esophagoscope is used to examine the gullet. See Fig. 26.

Inflammation of the Esophagus

Inflammation may result from:

1. Acute catarrh of the gullet following specific fevers.
2. Injuries, as from foreign bodies, or swallowing corrosive substances, poisons or irritants;
3. Diphtheria or smallpox; or may be caused by cancer or local ulcerations.

Symptoms. The inflammation causes pain and difficulty in swallowing, which vary in severity according to the extent of the disease.

Treatment. The cause of the inflammation must be dealt with by a specialist.

The patient must be kept in bed, and should be given ice to suck, and olive oil, and bland fluids only, if he can swallow. When this is impossible, rectal feeding must be undertaken.

Varicose Veins of the Esophagus

These are sometimes present in cases of chronic heart disease, and cirrhosis of the liver. Rupture of a vein leads to severe bleeding which may be mistaken for vomiting of blood from the stomach (hematemesis).

Spasm of the Esophagus

(*Globus Hystericus*)

Spasm of part of the esophagus is sometimes seen in women as a hysterical condition, but it may also occur in cases of hypochondriasis. The patient complains of the feeling of a ball rising in the throat which makes swallowing difficult. When the patient's attention can be distracted, however, swallowing can be performed normally.

At first the attacks are quite short, but they may gradually become longer and more continuous. Food and liquids are regurgitated, and there is some loss of weight, although this is not usually serious.

Treatment. Psychological treatment should be given. Sometimes rubber bougies are used to relax and stretch the muscles of the gullet. Warm food is usually swallowed more easily than cold.

X-ray examination should always be carried out to exclude any serious lesion.

Cardiospasm

This is commonest in middle-aged women but may occur in either sex at any age; the lower end of the gullet becomes contracted and the muscle wall is much thickened, but the cause of the condition is not known.

Symptoms may develop suddenly or gradually, with difficulty in swallowing, regurgitation of food, and a heavy sensation in the lower part of the chest. There may be serious loss of weight if the spasm continues, but in some cases there are free intervals. The contraction can be demonstrated by X-ray examination after a barium meal, and the gullet may be examined by means of an esophagoscope.

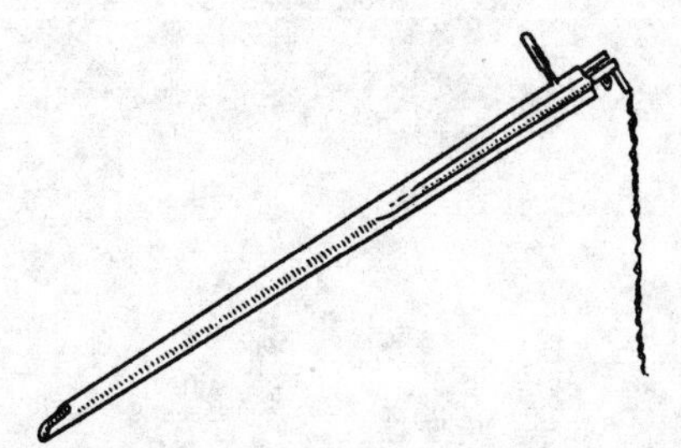

Fig. 26. *AN ESOPHAGOSCOPE for inspecting the inside of the gullet.*

Treatment consists in dilatation of the gullet either by surgical operation, or by passing weighted bougies down the throat of the patient.

Cancer of the Esophagus

This is most often found over the age of forty years, 80 per cent of cases occurring in men. The growth may develop at the upper end near the pharynx, in the middle of the gullet where it passes through the chest, or near the junction of the gullet with the stomach. The growth spreads round the wall of the gullet; secondary growths in other organs are uncommon, although the structures in the chest may be invaded, ultimately causing pneumonia or severe hemorrhage.

Symptoms. The patient has increasing difficulty in swallowing, which finally becomes extreme, and there is regurgitation of food with blood or mucus. The patient rapidly loses weight, but the amount of pain varies in different cases, and may even be absent. Hoarseness is noticed in a few cases, or there may be cough. When the growth develops at the upper end a swelling may sometimes be found in the neck, and the adjoining glands also become enlarged. X-ray examination usually indicates the diagnosis. Esophagoscopy is used to confirm it when a biopsy is taken.

Treatment. Dilation of the esophagus may be attempted by passing bougies of different types. Sometimes a silver tube is passed through the gullet and left in place for some weeks or months, to assist swallowing.

Radium is used for surface application or in the form of radon seeds which are inserted round the growth.

Surgical removal has been successfully undertaken in a few cases of cancer at the upper end of the gullet, but it must be diagnosed early if removal is to give good results.

GASTROSTOMY. In this operation an opening is made directly into the stomach, so that the patient can be fed through a tube when there is difficulty in swallowing. This form of treatment helps to prolong life, but death often takes place within six to twelve months of the operation.

DISEASES OF THE CHEST

The respiratory tract includes all those organs through which air passes from the atmosphere to the small air sacs (alveoli) of the lungs, as well as the structures which support those organs. It is divided into (1) the upper respiratory tract (nose, naso-pharynx and larynx), (2) the lower respiratory tract (trachea, bronchioles and alveoli), and (3) the supporting structures (pleura, ribs, and intercostal muscles). See also Anatomy of the lungs and respiratory organs, p.227.

Diseases of the upper respiratory tract are dealt with in the section on Ear, Nose and Throat Diseases, p.332.

SYMPTOMS OF RESPIRATORY DISEASE

Since many chest diseases are caused by the invasion of infecting micro-organisms, the general symptoms of infectious diseases—fever, sweating, emaciation or loss of weight, and debility—are commonly seen in addition to the symptoms specific to diseases affecting the respiratory organs. The specific symptoms are cough, difficulty in breathing, or shortness of breath (dyspnea), pain in the chest, and hemoptysis.

Cough. This is the most frequent and characteristic of all respiratory symptoms, and is often an expression of disease in the bronchial tubes or the lungs, e.g. bronchitis, bronchiectasis and asthma. As a rule, it indicates the presence of some irritating material in the air passages, and represents an automatic attempt to remove it. If the attempt is successful, expectoration of sputum results. A dry cough occurs when the lining of the bronchial tubes is congested, as in the early stages of acute bronchitis and pulmonary tuberculosis. A loose cough occurs when the exudate increases and lies free in the bronchial tubes; it is common in chronic bronchitis and bronchiectasis.

Cough may also result from such mechanical causes as a long uvula or an enlarged heart, and from the irritation of inhaled tobacco smoke (smoker's cough). In order, therefore, to estimate the significance of a cough in a heavy smoker, the effect of stopping all smoking should first be observed.

In some cases the cough may be nervous in origin.

Sputum. This varies in type and quantity, depending on the underlying disease and the amount of dust in the atmosphere. In certain chest diseases much useful information can be obtained from microscopic and bacteriological examination of the sputum. Unfortunately, owing to social customs which frown on spitting, the sputum is often swallowed rather than expectorated. This is to be deplored; the sputum should always be expectorated, if necessary into disposable tissues, a handkerchief, or a small container.

The appearance of sputum varies with different diseases. It commonly consists of muco-pus, which has a creamy-yellow gelatinous appearance.

Blood may be present in the sputum, especially in pulmonary tuberculosis. The sputum may be merely stained with blood, or it may consist entirely of blood. In pneumonia, the sputum often has a rusty appearance due to stale blood.

Large amounts of sputum ($\frac{1}{2}$ to 1 pint) may be produced in bronchiectasis, while its offensive smell is usually suggestive of this disease.

Shortness of Breath (Dyspnea, or difficult breathing). Owing to the disease process, carbon dioxide accumulates in the blood and the body attempts to correct this by increasing the frequency and depth of the respirations. This symptom is commonly seen in:

1. obstruction of the airway, as in asthma;
2. reduced elasticity of the lung tissue, as in inflammation, congestion, edema, and fibrosis;
3. limitation of movement of the diaphragm and chest wall, as in emphysema;
4. destruction of lung tissue, as in tuberculosis, bronchiectasis, and lung cancer.

Dyspnea is also a very important symptom of heart disease (see p. 295).

Pain in the Chest. Pain is not a very common symptom in diseases of the respiratory organs since lung tissue is insensitive, and pain in the chest is almost always due to some disorder in the structures surrounding the lungs. When the pleura is involved, however, pain may be a prominent symptom, and may be of a cutting, stabbing or tearing character, and sufficiently severe to prevent sleep. In pleurisy it is caused by the rubbing together of the inflamed surfaces of the pleural membranes, and is most commonly felt in the armpits and beneath the breasts.

There are, of course, many types of pain which occur in the chest which are not due to disease of the lungs or pleura, e.g. heart disease (angina pectoris), affections of the ribs and intercostal muscles (fibrositis and intercostal neuralgia), shingles, and certain diseases of the breast.

Hemoptysis (Coughing up of blood). Although blood in this case might be said to be the sputum, hemoptysis is such an important symptom that it should be specially mentioned. The blood, which comes from broken small blood vessels in the lung, may be mixed with sputum giving stained sputum, or it may be practically unaltered and bright red. It usually indicates the presence of a tumor, tuberculosis, or bronchiectasis.

INVESTIGATION OF RESPIRATORY DISEASES

The following six steps may be taken in investigating respiratory disease.

1. Detailed taking of the patient's medical history, with temperature records.
2. Physical examination.
3. Radiological, or X-ray, examination.
4. Bacteriological examination.
5. Examination, with special instruments and by special methods, of the larynx, trachea, bronchi, and pleura.
6. Blood (hematological) examination.

For most diseases of the respiratory tract, a reasonably accurate diagnosis can be made by the first two methods, i.e. by getting a detailed account of the history of the patient's illness, and by physical examination; but for tuberculosis and bronchogenic carcinoma, and for certain other diseases these are inadequate.

History Taking

Particular inquiry must always be made regarding the symptoms, their nature and duration, and their mode of onset. Inquiry should also be made regarding previous illnesses, especially tuberculosis, pneumonia, empyema, bronchitis, and asthma. In tuberculosis it is essential to enquire as to a family history of the disease and to check up on all contacts. Note should also be made of the patient's occupation.

Physical Examination

This must include a general examination, noting especially the temperature, pallor or flushed face, the type and character of the respiration, any cough—its duration, type and severity, the amount and nature of the sputum, cyanosis (blueness of the lips and fingers), and clubbing of the fingers. Enlargement of the lymph nodes in the armpits, wasting, and the presence of eye lesions should also be looked for.

Examination of the Chest

For examination of the chest, it is necessary for the patient to be stripped to the waist in a warm atmosphere and a good light. It is generally best carried out with the patient in the sitting position—preferably semi-reclining for examination of the front of the chest—unless it is essential for him to be lying down, as in pneumonia. As with the heart, the order of examination should be inspection, palpation, percussion and auscultation. Special investigations may be required in some cases.

Inspection is carried out to show the shape of the chest, the rate of respiration (normally 14 to 18 inspirations per minute), and the degree of movement of the chest wall, noting especially any inequality of movement between the two sides.

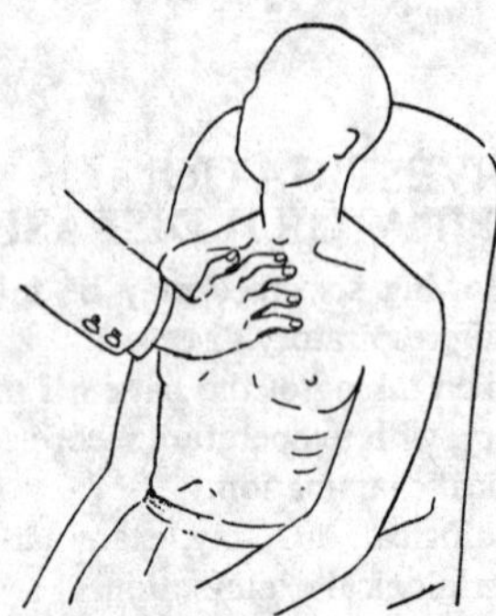

Fig. 1. *PALPATION. By feeling the contours of the patient's chest with the palm of his hand, the doctor is able to detect any abnormal hollows or prominences, pulsations, or tender spots.*

Palpation is made with the palm of the hand, which must be warm. It confirms the impressions gained from inspection, especially concerning the movements of the chest. It also helps to detect any abnormal areas of prominence or hollowing of the chest wall, together with areas of abnormal pulsation or tenderness, or an abnormal position of the apex beat of the heart.

Percussion is performed with the fingers. The middle finger of the left hand is pressed firmly on the surface of the chest, if possible between adjacent ribs, and is struck vertically

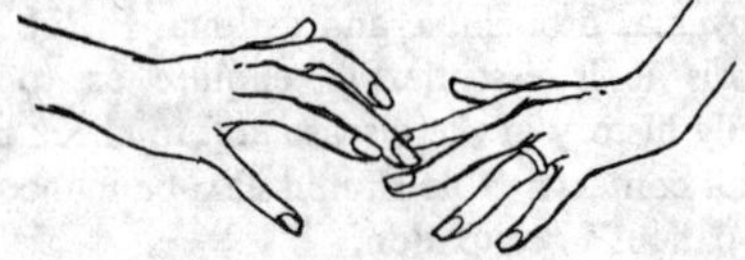

Fig. 2. *PERCUSSION. By striking the middle finger of the left hand (which is pressed on the patient's chest) with the middle finger of the right hand, the doctor is able to produce sounds from the chest which indicate the condition of the lungs.*

by the middle finger of the right hand, which acts as the instrument of percussion. Percussion is valuable for detecting changes in the character of the lung tissue, indicating whether these tissues contain more or less air than normal. It is of value also for distinguishing the normal air-containing lung from adjacent solid organs, such as the heart and liver, and from collections of fluid in the pleural cavity.

Auscultation is performed with the stethoscope. The presence or absence of breath sounds (the usual sound that air makes in the process of being breathed in and out) and any abnormality of the breath sounds may be ascertained.

Additional Breathing Sounds

STRIDOR. This is a noisy type of breathing heard when the main air passages are partially obstructed.

RHONCHI. These are dry musical sounds which are caused by the passage of air through bronchial tubes which are partially obstructed by phlegm or by congested mucous membrane. Just as the low notes of an organ come from the larger pipes, and the high notes from the smaller ones, so the low-pitched, or sonorous rhonchi are produced in the larger tubes, and the high-pitched or sibilant rhonchi in the smaller ones.

RÂLES. These are moist bubbling or crackling sounds, caused by the bubbling of air through a fluid medium such as mucus in the smaller air passages.

PLEURAL FRICTION. This is a grating or creaking sound such as may be produced by rubbing two pieces of wet leather together. It occurs in pleurisy when the roughened surfaces of the inflamed pleural membranes ride over one another during respiration.

Special Investigations

Certain special methods of examination may give fuller information than is possible to obtain by ordinary examination of the chest.

1. **X-ray Examination.** This should be employed in all doubtful cases of chest disease, and is particularly valuable for the early diagnosis of tuberculosis. An outline of the bronchial tree may also be obtained by X-ray examination after the injection of an opaque material into the bronchial tubes.

2. **Examination of the Sputum.** The patient should rinse his mouth with water before collecting the sputum, which should preferably be the first morning specimen. It should be expectorated straight into a sterilized cup (one which has been boiled). The specimen is then examined by special methods under the microscope, and may furnish valuable evidence in the diagnosis of pulmonary tuberculosis.

3. **Bronchoscopy.** By means of an illuminated instrument called a bronchoscope, passed through the mouth and larynx, the interior of the larger bronchial tubes may be examined by direct vision.

4. **Withdrawal of Fluid from the Pleural Cavity** (or Paracentesis). This is a useful measure in suspected pleural effusion, the chest wall being punctured and the fluid withdrawn, with aseptic precautions, through a surgical needle attached to a syringe.

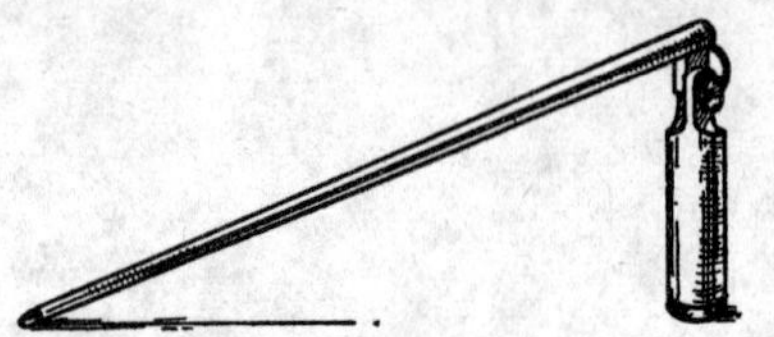

Fig. 3. *A BRONCHOSCOPE An illuminated instrument for inspecting the inside of the bronchi.*

GENERAL CARE IN CHEST DISEASES

The more general avoidance and prevention of acute respiratory infections, such as bronchitis and pneumonia resulting from the common cold and influenza, would help to reduce the high incidence of chronic respiratory disease. Education of people and instruction as to treatment of 'colds' and acute coryza would greatly reduce their incidence if precautionary measures were more widely applied.

People with colds should remain at home for the first forty-eight hours, as a social duty; failing this, they should avoid traveling in public conveyances or mixing with crowds in shops, theaters, clubs, and so forth. Elderly or delicate people with heart or chest diseases should avoid places of entertainment and crowded places during influenza epidemics, to reduce the risk of infection and possible serious complications. During the winter especially, everyone should try to avoid undue fatigue, and any unnecessary exposure to cold and wet, or fog.

Clothing should be sensible, with avoidance of over-clothing indoors. Sturdy shoes should be worn in cold and wet weather.

Smoking cigarettes, especially if accompanied by inhalation, irritates the lining of the respiratory tract. Those who smoke, therefore, tend to suffer from longer and more severe chest infections than non-smokers.

Lowered resistance is often responsible for respiratory infections, and the diet during the winter months should be adequate, and should include sufficient protein, minerals and vitamins; an extra pint of milk per day, with fresh fruit and vegetables will remedy any deficiency of these items. Inadequate sleep can also lower resistance to infection, so the full eight hours should be ensured, especially during the winter.

Obesity often predisposes to bronchitis, and overweight subjects should reduce their carbohydrate intake and include more protein in their diets.

DISEASES OF THE TRACHEA AND BRONCHI

Acute Infective Tracheitis

Infection of the trachea (windpipe) seldom occurs alone. It is usually caused by a downward extension of laryngeal infection or an upward extension of infection of the bronchi.

Acute Bronchitis

This very common disease consists of inflammation of the mucous membrance lining the bronchi. It is usually associated with disease of the trachea.

Causes. Several predisposing factors exist which make an individual prone to acute bronchitis. Although it occurs at all ages it is most common among the very young and the old. Mouth breathing facilitates infection and allows irritation by unfiltered and unwarmed air. Mouth breathing may be caused by the presence of nasal deformities such as a deflected septum, polypi, and adenoids. Damp, foggy, or dusty atmospheres, and pre-existing chronic respiratory disease also predispose to acute bronchitis.

The actual infection may be caused by downward extension of a common cold, by one of the infectious diseases such as measles, or by invasion of organisms from an upper respiratory tract infection when the patient's resistance is low, as in old age or in a debilitating disease.

Symptoms. An attack usually begins suddenly with aching in the limbs and a feeling of rawness behind the breast-bone. The temperature may rise to 37·8° C (100° F) in mild cases, or to 39·4° C (103° F) in severe cases, and it lasts for three or four days. Dyspnea and wheezing may be present.

Sputum is at first scanty and cough is ineffective and painful. Later, sputum is more profuse, yellow and muco-purulent, gradually becoming less until it is present only in the mornings. The cough and expectoration may continue altogether for six to ten days, or longer in old people.

The diagnosis is made chiefly by auscultation with the stethoscope, when rhonchi (dry sounds) may be heard all over both lungs.

Complications. Acute bronchitis may be followed by the more serious condition of bronchopneumonia, or it may lead to chronic bronchitis or bronchiectasis. Sometimes it may precipitate heart failure.

Treatment

Preventive. When coughs and colds are prevalent, it is wise to avoid as far as possible railway carriages, theaters, stuffy badly ventilated rooms, and other places where infection of this sort is easily passed on. Preventive inoculation by three injections of a stock vaccine at weekly intervals in the autumn, and subsequently once a month throughout the winter, is successful in a number of cases.

Of the Attack. However mild the attack, the patient should remain in bed until the temperature has been normal for two or three days. The bedroom should be well ventilated, without draughts, and kept at a temperature of 16° to 18° C (65° F). A stuffy atmosphere must be avoided, since it is a potent factor in maintaining an irritating cough. If the patient is not debilitated, and the temperature is scarcely raised, a hot bath may be allowed, provided the patient returns to bed immediately afterwards. Otherwise, tepid sponging of the whole body may be carried out morning and evening. The nightwear should be changed as often as necessary if sweating occurs.

While the temperature is raised, the diet should be an ordinary simple liquid diet suitable for feverish conditions. (See Invalid Cookery, p. 59.) Milk or one of the many invalid foods, weak tea, cocoa, broths, vegetable purees, cooked cereals, ice-cream, custard, jellies and eggs may be taken freely.

In the early stage when the cough is dry, the air of the bedroom may be moistened by means of a steam kettle at a distance of several feet from the patient. The steam may be medicated by the addition to the water of a few drops of oil of eucalyptus, or menthol. Medicated vapors may also be inhaled by the patient, either from a special inhaler, or from a jug with a towel over the head. For this purpose, compound tincture of benzoin may be used in the proportion of one teaspoonful to one pint of hot water which has been off the boil for a few minutes.

In the early stage, too, most patients complain of pain or discomfort behind the sternum but this will pass as the irritating dry cough loosens and the antibiotics begin to clear the system. In the meantime local application of heat to the area is most helpful. Compresses may be used but need to be changed often as they cool. It is suitable to use a half-filled rubber hot-water bottle covered with a piece of woolen cloth, or else an electric heating pad.

The patient and any visitors who call should not smoke.

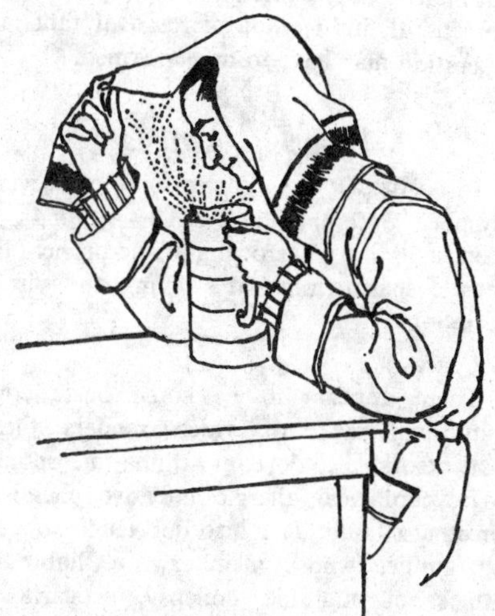

Fig. 4. *INHALING TINCTURE OF BENZOIN VAPOR. A simple but very effective remedy for the relief of nasal and chest stuffiness in acute bronchitis.*

Drugs. For Expectoration. It is by no means commonly realized how useful a hot drink may be in relieving painful spasm of the bronchial tubes and in loosening the phlegm. It is of little importance what the drinks are so long as they are hot and not tepid. Tea, coffee, cocoa, milk, hot lemon juice—all are useful, and a glassful should be taken every hour or two during the day.

Expectorant cough mixtures have been found to be of very little value and are much less frequently prescribed now.

For Breathlessness and Wheeze. Ephedrine hydrocholoride 30 to 60 milligrams by mouth will relieve spasm in mild cases but severe conditions it may be neccesary for the doctor to give an adrenaline or aminophylline injection

For Cough. To relieve the painful cough, give a sedative cough mixture, especially at night to permit sleep.

For Fever and Infection. In all cases when the temperature is 37·8° C (100° F), the doctor may prescribe antibiotics—a penicillin or a tetracyline being the more effective in bronchitis.

Sleeplessness. Before resorting to sleeping tablets or hypnotics, the following measures should be tried: sponging with tepid water, rearranging the bedclothes, getting the patient to pass water, and giving 5 grains of aspirin and a hot lemon drink, with or without whisky.

Convalescence. Although cure occurs when green or yellow pus is no longer seen in the sputum, even in a mild attack the patient is still rather exhausted and should not return to work until he is really fit.

However, after a severe attack of acute bronchitis or bronchopneumonia, it is advisable for the patient to have a holiday in the country or at the seaside with plenty of clean air and good food.

Chronic Bronchitis

Causes. Chronic bronchitis is commonest in middle life and advancing years, and is especially favored by disease of the heart, high blood pressure, kidney diseases, repeated attacks of acute bronchitis, constant exposure to irritants such as dust, tobacco smoke, molds or noxious gases, and to fog, damp, and sudden changes of atmospheric temperature. Chronic bronchitis affects males more than females, and there may be a familial tendency. It is also frequently associated with asthma and emphysema.

Symptoms. A patient with chronic bronchitis complains of cough and expectoration, together with shortness of breath on exertion, which is largely due to the accompanying emphysema. At first he notices that the breathlessness occurs only on going upstairs, or up a slope, but later it occurs even while walking on the level. During the warm weather he may be free from symptoms, and yet suffer for years from a winter cough. Once the disease is firmly established, it tends to remain chronic and to become progressively more severe.

The cough is paroxysmal and exhausting, and the sputum varies in quantity. Usually it is scanty, tenuous, mucoid, and may sometimes be streaked with blood. Alternatively, it may be profuse and watery. In acute flare-ups it may become purulent.

On auscultation with the stethoscope, numerous dry rhonchi (harsh sounds) may be heard all over the chest. In doubtful cases, the lungs should be X-rayed for possible tuberculous disease.

Treatment

Preventive. Young or old people who are subject to chronic bronchitis should live if possible in a warm and dry climate.

Exposure to wet and chill is dangerous at all times, and warm underclothing should be worn. Smoking is a factor of importance in maintaining a condition of chronic bronchitis, and striking benefit is often seen after it has been given up. Chronic bronchitics should avoid living in smoke-polluted and smog areas. The new measures to create smokeless zones are already proving effective in lowering the rate of serious complications in those with chronic bronchitis.

Associated disease, e.g. heart disease, high blood pressure or obesity will require appropriate treatment, and the measures which are adopted towards this end are often much more effective for the bronchitis than a cough mixture. Infection in the nose and throat (e.g. diseased tonsils) should also be dealt with. All possible measures should be taken to prevent attacks of the common cold (see pp. 282 and 342).

Medication. If the cough is troublesome one or two 5-ml spoonsful of codeine cough syrup may be taken, and this dose repeated, if necessary, four hours later. If the sputum is scanty and glutinous, medicated (menthol) steam inhalations or a dose of sodium chloride compound mixture in hot water may loosen it. Should much spasm be present, ephedrine hydrocloride may be prescribed.

A seven-day course of treatment with an antibiotic will usually stop an acute bronchitic flare-up in chronic cases, the antibiotic being given as soon as pus appears in the sputum. And postural drainage (see p. 346) will double the value of the antibiotic.

During the winter months a maintenance dose of tetracycline is sometimes given in severe cases.

Foreign Bodies in the Bronchial Tubes

In young children, the most common articles, or foreign bodies, which gain access to the bronchi by accidental inhalation are food particles, beads, bones, and coins. In an adult the usual article is a loose tooth or piece of a denture. Damage to the lung depends on the size of the article.

Symptoms. There is usually a rapid development of discomfort or pain in the front of the chest, together with a violent cough, which may lead to the expulsion of the foreign body from the chest. If a large bronchus becomes obstructed, the affected portion of the lung becomes collapsed, and the corresponding side of the chest shows less movement on respiration than the normal side.

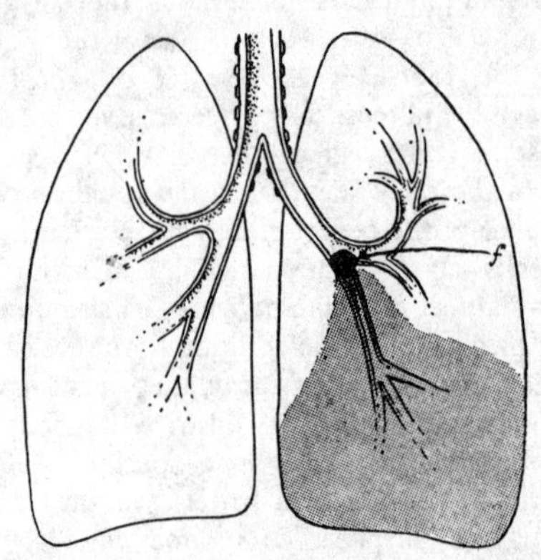

Fig. 5. *OBSTRUCTION IN LEFT LUNG. A swallowed foreign body* (f) *lodged in the bronchus of the left lung prevents air reaching a large area (shaded) of the lung, and renders it inert.*

Treatment. The foreign body *must* be dislodged and removed as soon as possible. If it has lodged in the larynx, death will be rapid unless the object is removed in a matter of seconds, or an immediate tracheotomy (slit made in the windpipe) is performed. An X-ray of the chest should be taken if it is suspected that the foreign body has passed into the bronchi.

Removal of the foreign body by a surgeon is usually accomplished by means of an illuminated bronchoscope (Fig. 3) introduced through the larynx, and a pair of special lung forceps. If this method of removal fails, an operation may have to be performed.

Bronchial Asthma

In asthma, the paroxysms of severe dyspnea accompanied by wheezing result from temporary narrowing of the bronchi by muscle spasm, mucosal swelling and viscid secretions.

Causes

There appears to be some basic constitutional make-up which renders these patients liable to develop asthma in response to psychological, allergic, infective, chemical or other stimuli. The disorder tends to run in families whose members are liable to attacks of migraine, epilepsy, urticaria or hysteria.

The first attack may occur at any age, but usually occurs before the age of twenty-five, and it may first appear in children when they cut their first teeth. The asthmatic patient tends to be emotional, highly strung, and intelligent.

1. The Psychological Factor. Probably the most important single factor in asthma is the psychological factor. Emotional strain and stress, nervous shock, worry, fatigue or excitement, which gives rise to a state of nervous tension, will precipitate an attack. If a child develops asthma, it will often be found that the mother herself is in a state of nervous tension which is unconsciously transmitted to the child.

One or more of the factors mentioned below may jointly operate with psychological disturbance in producing an attack.

2. Allergic Factors. Asthmatic attacks may occur as a result of hypersensitivity to certain foreign proteins. This type of the disorder usually starts in childhood or adolescence, and there may also be other allergic manifestations such as hay fever and hives. Most commonly the substances to which the patient is hypersensitive are:

(*a*) inhalants: dusts, molds, grass and flower pollens, feathers, animal hairs, and certain face powders;

(*b*) foodstuffs: wheat, eggs, milk, chocolate, beans, potatoes, pork products, beef, and shellfish;

(*c*) certain drugs or chemicals: e.g. aspirin. (See also Allergy).

3. Infection. Bacterial infection frequently accompanies asthma, especially in older persons, and the original attack of asthma may be directly related to some respiratory infection such as bronchitis or bronchopneumonia. In other cases the infection may appear as a complication of asthma. Either way, the infection always aggravates the asthma.

4. Reflex Factors. (*a*) Paroxysms in some cases may be caused by reflex stimulation of the vagus nerve, e.g. from inhalation of cold air, irritant gases or dust. (*b*) Attacks in other cases may be precipitated by gastric distension, flatulence, dyspepsia, or constipation.

5. Conditioned Reflex. As an example, a patient whose attacks may be precipitated by cat hairs might suffer an attack merely at the sight of a toy cat with simulated fur.

Symptoms. An attack of asthma often starts at night, but it may sometimes occur in the daytime. There are often certain premonitory indications that an attack will shortly develop, consisting of restlessness, irritability, depression, drowsiness, itching of the nose or chin, loss of appetite or flatulence for some hours beforehand. Usually, however, the patient wakes from sleep with a feeling of suffocation and tightness across the chest. In early attacks, great restlessness and anxiety occur, with increasing difficulty in breathing. The patient sits up in bed, or gets up to throw open the window, and fixes his arms to bring into action all the possible muscles of respiration. Breathing is slow and laborious, the phase of inspiration being short, and that of expiration greatly prolonged. Both phases are accompanied by loud wheezing sounds which can be heard at some distance from the patient, who is bluish or pale, with an anxious and distressed expression. The veins of the neck are engorged and prominent, and sweating may be considerable.

On listening to the chest with the stethoscope, inspiration is found to be short, while expiration is very prolonged, and accompanied by roaring (sonorous) and whistling (sibilant) rhonchi.

Later in the attack a cough develops, and is followed by the expectoration of small pellets of mucus. With the onset of expectoration the attack becomes less severe and finally subsides. The patient often passes a large quantity of pale urine, and may then sleep until morning.

An asthmatic attack may last from a few minutes to several hours. When it is very severe and prolonged, with few or no remissions, it is known as 'status asthmaticus,' as a result of which the patient may become extremely ill. More often the attacks recur each night at the same time for several weeks, after which they may disappear for a further period of weeks or months. Repeated attacks of asthma are liable to lead to emphysema.

Diagnosis. Spasmodic bronchial asthma must be distinguished from that due to heart failure (see 'cardiac asthma,' pp. 295 and 299).

Treatment

Of the Attack. The patient should be allowed to place himself in the most comfortable position, whether in a chair or in bed. The room should be well ventilated without being cold.

Drugs may be administered which have the effect of relaxing the contracted bronchial muscles, thus allowing the air to enter and leave the lungs freely.

In very mild cases a 20-milligram tablet of isoprenaline sulphate sucked slowly, or the inhalation of an oral spray of isoprenaline or of adrenaline solution may be sufficient to abort the attack.

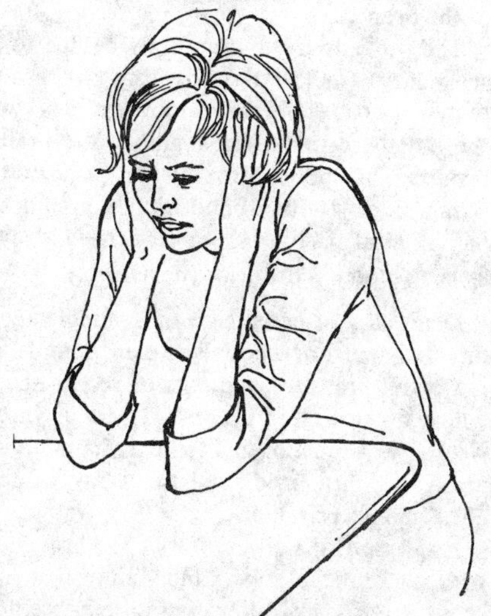

Fig. 6. *ASTHMATIC POSTURE. The sufferer may assume this characteristic posture, with shoulders hunched high in an endeavor to get easier breathing in the upper part of the lungs.*

In more severe cases a subcutaneous injection of 1 in 1,000 adrenaline solution may be given by the doctor, and intravenous injections of aminophylline usually relax the constricted bronchi. Other patients may, if the condition is intolerably chronic, be referred to a hospital for long-term treatment with corticosteroids.

If the patient shows signs of cyanosis, oxygen should be administered.

In *Status Asthmaticus* the attack must be treated as soon as possible. Injections of adrenaline or aminophylline will be given by the doctor, and corticosteroids if necessary.

If a chest infection, such as chronic bronchitis, is also present, an antibiotic (usually a tetracycline) will be given concurrently.

General Measures for relieving an attack of asthma include drinking a cup of strong coffee, and keeping in a quiet and warm atmosphere. If the attack has been severe and prolonged, the patient will be exhausted, and should stay in bed for twenty-four hours or longer. He should take a small, light, easily-digested snack or meal at two-hourly intervals, and large quantities of fluid, especially fruit juice sweetened with glucose.

Management Between the Attacks. Once the acute paroxysm has been relieved, the doctor is faced with the slower and usually long-term matter of finding what are the causes which set off an acute attack in his patient and how they can be reduced or eliminated. He must take into consideration the family background, the patient's medical history from infancy, his proneness to infections or to allergic reactions, his psychological make-up, and what triggered off the first attack of asthma.

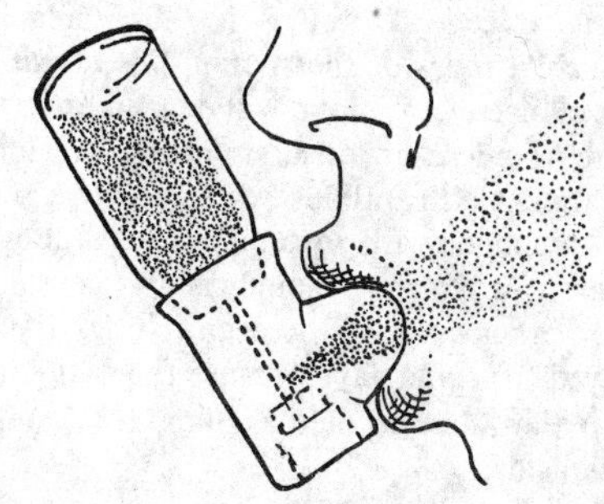

Fig. 7. *ASTHMA. For relief of an attack of asthma a measured dose is released from this pressurised container.*

Psychological Factors. All psychological factors which tend to precipitate a state of nervous tension must as far as possible be avoided, i.e. emotional stress, nervous strain, worry, fatigue, overwork and excitement. All of these tend to lead to exacerbations of asthma and, as with epilepsy, recurrent attacks of asthma bring about a steadily increasing instability of that part of the nervous system which controls the act of breathing, thus producing a vicious circle. In the case of children it is of the greatest importance that over-anxiety on the part of the mother should be corrected. Not only is the state of nervous tension unconsciously passed on to the child, but it leads to pampering, and making him wear excessive clothing. There should be no suggestion that the child is delicate and different from other children, and he must be encouraged to play with them in order to gain confidence. He must not be withdrawn from school for mild attacks, because he must not use his asthma as a means of avoiding his personal responsibilities.

When the disease starts in childhood or early adult life, it is often found to stop spontaneously or to be permanently relieved when some such psychological cause is discovered and removed.

A small dose of a sedative such as phenobarbital may be prescribed by the doctor to prevent an attack in anxious or emotional patients. To ward off frequent attacks, it may be beneficial to prescribe one 30-milligram ephedrine hydrochloride tablet three times daily, and a spray to use at the onset of an attack.

General Health. A natural and healthy mode of life must be followed. Exercise in the fresh air and sunshine are essential, but equally important is a sufficient amount of rest. The bedroom should be warm, but provided with a plentiful supply of fresh air. Constipation must be avoided.

Artificial sunlight is of great value for improving the general health, especially in winter.

Diet needs careful consideration. Any article of diet to which the patient is susceptible, or which may cause indigestion or flatulence, should be eliminated, and only the lightest of meals should be taken after midday. Asthmatics do best if they take a good breakfast and lunch, and a light evening meal. It is particularly important that they should take no food within an hour and a half of going to bed. Dextrose (glucose) is helpful in the asthma of childhood; give three teaspoonsful in lemonade or orange juice three times a day, with extra sugar, honey and sweets at meals.

Breathing Exercises. A large proportion of chronic asthmatics will derive great benefit also from a course of postural and breathing exercises.

Bronchiectasis

Bronchiectasis is a condition of permanent dilatation of one or more of the bronchial tubes; this is often secondary to some preceding disease of the bronchial tubes or lungs. The disease is usually due to repeated attacks of bronchopneumonia in childhood. It may also result from bronchitis, from unresolved pneumonia, and from obstruction of a bronchus by an inhaled foreign body. Bronchiectasis occurs sometimes in cases of tuberculosis which are associated with much fibrosis of the lungs. The disease may occur at any age, but is commonest between thirty and fifty years.

Symptoms. The onset is usually gradual. As the cavities become more and more dilated, more and more secretion tends to collect in them during the night.

COUGH AND SPUTUM. Periodically the cavities are emptied by coughing, which often occurs when the patient changes his position, e.g. bending forward or lying down. The cough is especially violent when the patient wakes up in the morning. It occurs in paroxysms, often with intervals of many hours between the bouts.

The coughing is associated with the expectoration of large quantities of sputum, sometimes 1 to 1½ pints in the twenty-four hours. It generally has a very offensive smell, and the patient's breath is also usually offensive.

HEMOPTYSIS (spitting of blood) is not uncommon. As the disease progresses, tiredness, loss of appetite and loss of weight occur, with bouts of fever. In well-developed cases there is usually well-marked clubbing of the fingers, of drum-stick character.

FEBRILE ILLNESS, which may at first be taken for influenza or pneumonia, occurs when infection develops in the dilated bronchi or the cavities. Dry pleurisy frequently accompanies this illness.

Diagnosis is usually confirmed by X-ray examination of the chest, particularly after the introduction into the bronchial tubes of an oil which is opaque to the rays. The iodized oil throws a shadow which serves to define the character and extent of the disease.

The sputum should be repeatedly sent for microscopical examination in order to exclude the possibility of tuberculosis, and bronchoscopy is often useful in the older patient for assessment of lung damage.

The chief complications of the disease are septic bronchopneumonia and abscess of the lung.

Treatment

1. **Preventive Treatment.** For patients suffering with chronic bronchitis, breathing exercises should be carried out regularly two or three times a day. The patient should guard against exposure to chill and infections and, when possible, should spend the winter months in a warm climate where there is a minimum risk of exposure to fog, cold and damp. A good and digestible diet is essential, and extra vitamins should be taken.

The mouth should be kept clean, and pyorrhea eliminated—if necessary by dental treatment. Septic tonsils may require removal and infection of the nasal sinuses, which is often present in cases of bronchiectasis, must receive adequate treatment.

2. **Postural Drainage.** Efficient emptying of the cavities of their secretions should be promoted by postural drainage. The body must be placed in the most favorable position for draining the sputum from the lower part of the chest. The patient should lie across the bed with the hands touching the floor. The head and shoulders are then slowly lowered to the level of the hands, with a resultant emptying of the chest by coughing. A basin should be placed on the floor to catch the sputum and also any vomited matter. This position should be adopted morning and night for about 15 minutes.

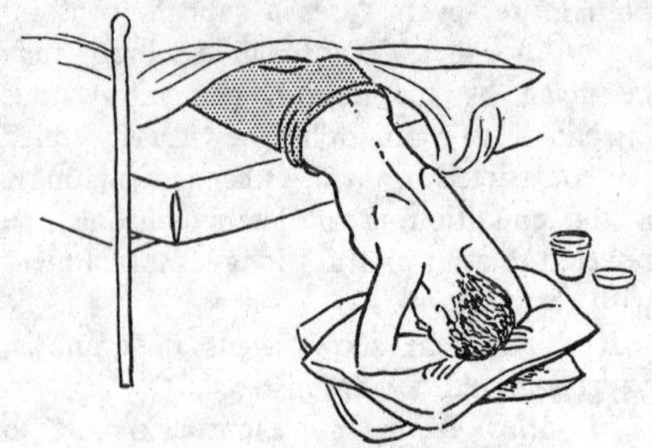

Fig. 8. *POSTURAL DRAINAGE. To clear the lower lobes of the lungs of secretions, the patient should lie across the bed with the body at an angle of about 45 degrees, as illustrated. The mattress should overhang the edge of the bed. See text for further details.*

If this is not effective in weak patients, the foot of the bed should be raised by at least 18 inches for 30 minutes thrice daily to allow continuous drainage. If regularly, persistently and efficiently carried out, the sputum should be reduced from several ounces to the merest trace in a few weeks.

If the sputum is thick, and if much bronchitis exists, it may be loosened by sipping hot drinks or inhaling steam medicated with tincture of benzoin (1 teaspoonful to 1 pint of hot water), before postural drainage begins (p. 343).

3. **Medication by Drugs.** This is necessary when infection occurs in the enlarged bronchial tubes or the sputum-filled cavities. The choice of antibiotic will depend upon the kind of micro-organism infecting the lung. Treatment with antibiotic drugs must be given in conjunction with postural drainage (above). Vitamin B tablets or supplements need to be given when any of these antibiotics is employed for some days because the antibiotics clear the intestine of the vitamin-B-forming organisms.

4. **Surgical Treatment** consists of the operation known as lobectomy, i.e. removal of one or more lobes of a lung in cases where the disease is confined to one side of the chest. It should be considered, however, only if the disease is extending, the sputum increasing, or the general health deteriorating in spite of efficient medical treatment, but it is only rarely performed in patients over forty.

INTRATHORACIC TUMORS

Tumors of the bronchus and lung may be either benign or malignant, and the latter may be described as being either primary, such as those arising directly in the bronchus or lung, or secondary, being spread from tumors in organs distant from the lung, such as the breast, uterus, or thyroid.

Bronchogenic Carcinoma
(Lung Cancer)

This is the commonest of all intrathoracic tumors. It occurs about eight times as often in males as in females, and most frequently between the ages of 40 and 60.

Causes. The breathing in of fumes and substances which irritate the bronchi is largely considered to be the initiating cause of the cancerous growth. Cigarette smoking is particularly suspect, especially for persons who smoke more than twenty cigarettes a day for many years: pipe and cigar smokers appear to run less risk. City and industrial town atmospheres may contain carcinogenic particles or fumes—and certainly the disease is more common there than in rural areas. Although as yet there is no direct evidence that lung cancer is precipitated by the following agents, they have all been suspected by investigators: dust, tar, gasoline or diesel fumes, asbestos particles, and fumes from making coal gas.

Symptoms. These are very variable and depend upon the site of the growth. The commonest site is one of the major bronchi.

The onset is usually insidious, with cough as the earliest symptom. The amount and character of the sputum depends on the degree of secondary infection, e.g. pneumonia, present. Small frequent coughings-up of blood (hemoptysis) is a common symptom but only rarely does massive hemoptysis occur. The breathing is not usually labored unless the tumor is obstructing a major bronchus and causing collapse. Such an obstruction may also give rise to a febrile illness resembling pneumonia or bronchitis. Pleuritic pain may be caused by obstruction of the bronchus.

The presenting symptom may be due to a secondary (metastatic) deposit, when a minute portion of the tumor spreads via the bloodstream to, for example, the brain, resulting in epileptiform fits or personality changes; or to the bone with consequent pathological fractures; or to the kidneys causing blood in the urine (hematuria).

Diagnosis. In every case of a middle-aged or elderly person, especially a man, complaining of respiratory symptoms of recent onset which do not clear up within two or three weeks, a bronchogenic carcinoma should always be suspected, and an X-ray of the chest should be taken.

Inspection of the interior of the bronchus with a bronchoscope, and removal of a scrap of tissue (biopsy) for microscopic examination is the only way in which the diagnosis can be established with certainty at an early and curable stage.

Course and Prognosis. Unless surgical treatment is practicable, the average period of survival after diagnosis is less than one year.

Treatment. In early cases the only curative treatment is removal of the entire lung (pneumonectomy), or of the lobe containing the tumor (lobectomy). Deep X-ray therapy is given as a palliative measure in those cases in which surgical removal of the tumor is not possible. This may relieve symptoms for a while and may prolong life.

Bronchial Adenoma

This is an uncommon tumor occurring in younger patients and affecting women as often as men. It is generally considered benign and the most common symptom is recurrent hemoptysis.

It is important to distinguish this tumour in the diagnosis of bronchogenic carcinoma.

Secondary Tumors in the Lung

Pulmonary secondary (metastatic) deposits may result from malignant disease anywhere in the body and, when these secondary deposits are found in the lung, a search should always be made for the site of the primary tumor.

DISEASES OF THE LUNGS

The Pneumonias

Inflammation of the lung tissue is known as pneumonia, and there are many types of this condition, some common, others rare.

The SPECIFIC pneumonias are caused by known bacteria and viruses which specifically attack lung tissue. The NON-SPECIFIC, or aspiration, pneumonias are due to organisms usually found in nose and throat infections but which invade the lungs, particularly when they are in a weak condition.

Details of the various forms of pneumonia and their treatment are given in the section on Fevers and Infectious Diseases, pp. 272-74.

Acute Edema of the Lungs

(Dropsy of the Lungs)

This condition is not primarily a disease of the lungs. It occurs most often as a complication of various forms of heart disease (especially when associated with high blood pressure), of Bright's disease, and occasionally of diabetes. The condition is sometimes know as 'cardiac asthma.' The air sacs of the lungs become filled with fluid so that the lungs become airless and unable to function (see p. 299).

Symptoms. The onset is usually sudden, and generally occurs at night. The patient wakes with intense shortness of breath and a sense of suffocation. He looks blue. Frothy fluid, often pink in color, soon begins to stream from the mouth and nose, being brought up in great gulps. The outlook is always very grave and, in severe cases, death may occur in a few hours.

Treatment. The patient should be propped up with pillows, oxygen is given if available and a doctor should be sent for immediately. The most effective treatment consists in withdrawal of half to one pint of blood from the forearm, to relieve the burden on the heart, and the subcutaneous injection of atropine and morphine. Intravenous injections of aminophylline may help.

Pulmonary Embolism

When a clot of blood is dislodged from some part of the body where thrombosis has occurred in the veins, it may be carried by the bloodstream through the heart to the lungs, where it obstructs one of the branches of the pulmonary artery. The clot, or 'embolus,' cuts off the blood supply to the corresponding part of the lung, and produces in *infarct*, a solid airless portion of lung. Pulmonary embolism results most commonly from clots dislodged in femoral thrombosis ('white leg,' see p. 304), or thrombosis following operations on the lower abdomen or pelvis.

Symptoms. If a large branch of the pulmonary artery is obstructed, immediate collapse occurs, followed often by death within a few minutes. If the embolus is smaller, there is sudden pain in the chest, with difficulty in breathing, followed in a few hours by cough and the expectoration of bloodstained sputum which persists for some days. The pain may continue for a few days owing to the development of pleurisy over the infarct, but if no further emboli are dislodged, progress is usually satisfactory.

Treatment. Immediately after obstruction has occurred it is necessary to treat the patient for shock, keeping him warm. A doctor should be sent for immediately. Anticoagulant drugs are given to break up the clot and to prevent further clots being formed. The patient will be under medical attention for many weeks.

Emphysema of the Lungs

(Enlargement of the Air Sacs)

Emphysema is a condition of overdistension of the air sacs of the lungs which leads to thinning of their walls and obliteration of their small capillary blood vessels. This disease is most often seen in middle and late adult life, and is commoner in men than in women. It is usually due to the strain of prolonged and repeated coughing induced by chronic bronchitis, bronchiectasis, asthma or whooping-cough.

Symptoms. Shortness of breath is the most characteristic and important symptom. At first it is present only on exertion, but in advanced cases it is constant and becomes very severe during attacks of bronchitis or asthma which commonly develop in the later stages of the disease, especially in the winter and in foggy weather. Cyanosis (blueness of the lips, cheeks, ears and nose) is common, and is often accompanied by clubbing of the finger tips. Cough is almost invariably present, and is due to the associated bronchitis, persons with emphysema being more susceptible to infection of the bronchial tubes than healthy people: the cough is usually worse in winter and in foggy weather.

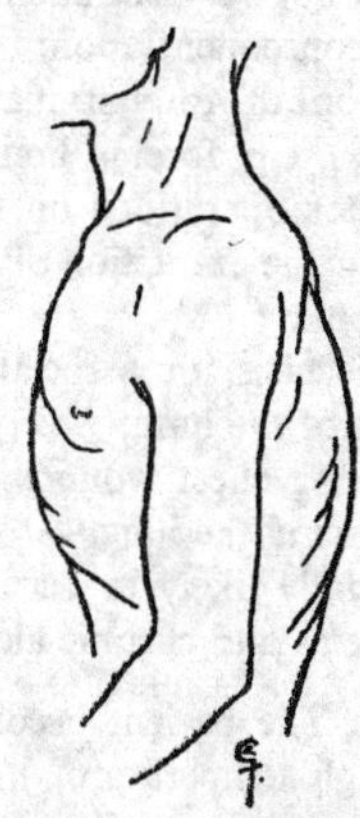

Fig. 9. *BARREL-SHAPED CHEST, showing elevation of the ribs in the front due to emphysema of the lungs.*

The chest is enlarged, particularly in the front to back diameter. The breast-bone protrudes forwards, the upper part of the backbone is rounded, and the ribs run forward in a more horizontal position than the normal. The general shape of the chest thus resembles that of a barrel, the chest as a whole being in the position of inspiration, and the respiratory movements being much restricted.

On listening with the stethoscope, the breath sounds are everywhere found to be weak, with a short inspiration, and greatly prolonged expiration.

Emphysema may exist for many years, and favors the onset of other lung diseases such as pneumonia. It places a great strain on the heart, which may eventually lead to heart failure.

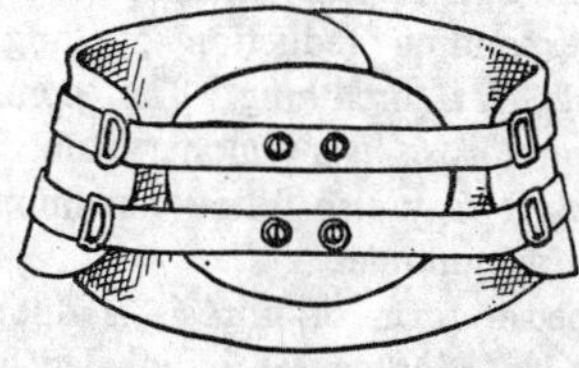

Fig. 10. *A SUPPORT FOR DIAPHRAGM BREATHING. Steel springs in the abdominal pad aid the emphysema patient to use his diaphragm for breathing.*

Treatment. Emphysema may be arrested, but it cannot be cured. When the disease is established the patient should take every precaution to guard against attacks of bronchitis. The diet should be simple and easy to digest; excess weight should be reduced by dieting. Some patients are benefited by a course of breathing exercises and by treatment in a special compressed air chamber. In other cases, respiration can be assisted by the use of a support for diaphragm breathing.

See also treatment of chronic bronchitis (p. 344) and asthma (p. 345).

Abscess of the Lung

An abscess of the lung, although a serious complaint, is not very common. It is due to an infection consequent upon:

1. inhalation of foreign material into a bronchus, e.g. foreign bodies, or blood clots after operations on the nose and throat or the extraction of teeth;
2. pneumonia;
3. bronchiectasis, or associated with new growths of the lung;
4. perforating chest wounds, or fractured ribs piercing the lung.

It is especially likely to occur in the subjects of diabetes and chronic alcoholism.

Symptoms. The patient becomes seriously ill with a high temperature, and chills and sweating are common. There is usually a cough with offensive purulent sputum, and hemoptysis sometimes occurs. Shortness of breath may be present, and acute pain develops in the chest if the pleura is involved.

X-ray examination of the chest should be carried out, and the sputum must be examined repeatedly to exclude tuberculosis.

Treatment. This is similar to the treatment of bronchiectasis (p. 346 Strict rest in bed is indicated for several weeks, with postural drainage and antibiotics, usually penicillin.

Surgical methods of treatment may be necessary if, in spite of medical measures, the patient does not make progress. Complete convalescence with a very gradual return to active life is often required in the surgical cases.

Fibrosis of the Lung

Fibrosis of the lung is a fairly common condition in the later years of life, being a late sequel of many acute and chronic diseases of the lung, when they give rise to large amounts of scar tissue in the lung and a corresponding reduction of lung tissue available for breathing. The commonest cause of fibrosis is pulmonary tuberculosis, although it may also follow pneumonia and bronchopneumonia.

A special form of fibrosis is due to the chronic irritation caused by inhaled particles of dust in certain occupations.

PNEUMOCONIOSIS is the term used for industrial fibrosis due to the dust of coal, silica, and asbestos, and the specific forms are:

1. ANTHRACOSIS, caused by inhalation of coal dust.

2. SILICOSIS, caused by inhalation of particles of silica by miners of quartz and slate, and by potters ('potter's asthma'). Goldminer's phthisis—the most serious form of

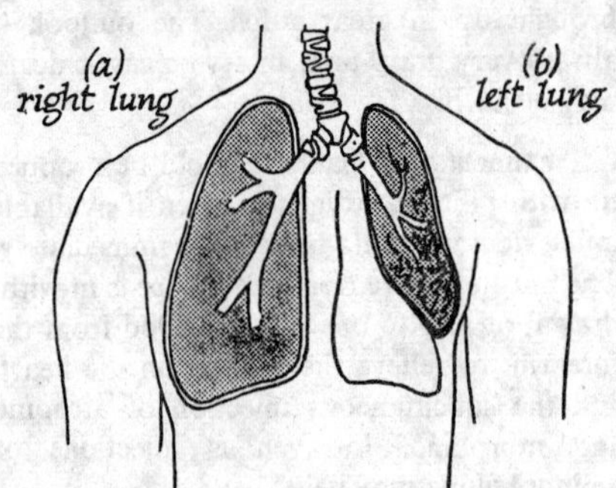

Fig. 11. *FIBROSIS OF LEFT LUNG. The right lung* (a) *is normal. The left lung* (b) *is contracted and fibrosed, permitting displacement of the heart and of the windpipe.*

pulmonary fibrosis—is especially prevalent in the South African gold mines, being due to inhalation of the fine dust caused by the rock drills.

3. ASBESTOSIS, which is occasionally found in those working in the manufacture of asbestos (which contains silicates) articles.

The lungs of persons living in the country are practically free from deposited matter, but in the lungs of city dwellers, a certain amount of carbon is always present. In coal miners, this occurs to such an extent that the lungs are black, without, however, producing much fibrosis, except in the miners of hard coal, or anthracite. In general it may be said that the harder and more gritty the particles, the more marked is the amount of fibrosis produced in the lung. In silicosis, particles of crystalline silica become deposited in the connective tissue of the lungs, leading to fibrosis (the formation of scar tissue) round the bronchial tubes and air sacs.

Certain forms of dust disease of the lung undoubtedly favor the development of tuberculosis, the determining factor being the presence in the dust of particles of silica. Thus, while miners of soft coal suffer less from tuberculosis of the lungs than all other males, workers in silica (quartz and slate workers, and gold miners) are extremely liable to develop this disease.

Symptoms. The onset is gradual, with bronchial irritation and cough, especially in the early mornings, and increasing shortness of breath and debility. The expectoration, which is at first scanty, generally becomes more abundant, and in course of time attacks of hemoptysis (coughing-up of blood) may occur, suggesting the possibility of tuberculosis. Loss of weight occurs later, tending to give the appearance of premature old age.

The most important complication is tuberculosis, which forms the end stage of many cases of silicosis. It may be suspected when fever, night sweats, coughing-up of blood, or loss of weight occur. Bronchiectasis (p. 345) is also very apt to develop. The course of fibrosis of the lung is always prolonged, and for many years the patient may be capable of light work. The condition, however, imposes a considerable amount of strain upon the heart, and heart failure eventually develops.

Examination by X-rays is helpful in the diagnosis of the condition, and sputum should be examined repeatedly for tubercle bacilli.

Treatment. Every means must be adopted to prevent the conditions which lead to the disease. Mines must be well ventilated, and respirators worn in dusty occupations. As soon as the condition is diagnosed in an industrial worker, the patient should be advised to change his occupation. All patients should be given good food and cod-liver oil, and require fresh air and (except when active tuberculosis is present) regular breathing exercises.

Fungus Infections of the Lung

Infection of lung tissue by a fungus is rare and hence more easily overlooked in diagnosis. See Fevers and Infectious Diseases, p. 278, for the first two infections.

Actinomycosis

Actinomycosis is a disease usually found in cattle but communicable to man.

Treatment. The infection responds to long-term (sometimes up to one year) treatment with penicillin or to tetracycline given in large doses.

Farmer's Lung

This is a dust disease caused by breathing in the dust from moldy grain or hay; the mold probably affects the lungs more by causing hypersensitivity than by direct infection of the lung tissue.

Moniliasis

After debilitating illnesses, or a bad attack of oral thrush, the fungus *Candida albicans* (also known as monilia) may be introduced into the respiratory tract. It causes a low-grade infection with much slow lung-tissue destruction.

Treatment. A prolonged course of nystatin is required, and measures must be taken to improve the patient's health with a good diet and vitamins.

DISEASES OF THE PLEURA

Each lung is enclosed by a layer of membrane called the pleura. This is continuous with another layer of the same membrane which lines the inner surface of the chest wall and the upper surface of the diaphragm. These two layers of the pleura, the outer and the inner, are normally in close contact with one another, being separated only by a small amount of fluid which lubricates the surfaces and allows them to glide smoothly over one another.

Any inflammation of the pleural membrane covering the lung and its reflection over the inner surface of the chest wall is known as pleurisy. If the process leads only to the deposit of a sticky mass of fibrin between the layers of the pleura, it is known as *dry pleurisy*. If fluid is poured out, separating the lungs from the chest wall and the diaphragm, the condition is known as *pleurisy with effusion*; and if pus appears in the fluid, it is known as *purulent pleurisy*, or *empyema*.

Acute Dry Pleurisy

Causes. The great majority of cases of fibrous or dry pleurisy are brought on by chill (exposure to sudden changes in the weather, cold winds, remaining in damp clothing, etc.). It is a common complication of many diseases of the lungs, especially of already existing pulmonary tuberculosis and lobar pneumonia. Sometimes it is caused by non-infective conditions such as bronchiectasis, growths of the lung and injuries of the chest wall such as gunshot wounds and fractured ribs.

The inflamed area is usually localized and, as a rule, both layers of the pleura become involved. The area of pleura affected becomes roughened and shaggy in appearance so that the two layers of the membrane rub harshly on one another.

Symptoms. The onset is usually sudden, with sharp stabbing pain in the side of the chest, but it may be referred to the abdomen or the shoulder. The pain is aggravated by deep breathing, coughing or sneezing, and even by movement. Cough is generally an early symptom, and it is usually short, dry, ineffective and distressing. The temperature is usually raised to 38° C (101° F). There is diminished movement on the affected side of the chest, and breathing may be shallow and rapid.

Diagnosis. Since pleurisy rarely occurs as a separate disease entity, the initial cause of the pleurisy must be looked for, and treated.

Treatment. However mild the attack may be, the patient should remain in bed until all fever and pain have disappeared. The diet should be fluid or semi-fluid at first, increasing rapidly to a light normal diet as the temperature subsides.

For the pain, hot-water bottles or hot applications generally give most relief. Care must be taken not to burn the patient. Strapping the affected side of the chest (in the same way as for a fractured rib) with wide adhesive bandage applied during expiration, helps to relieve the pain by limiting possible movement. The strips are applied from below upwards, each strip overlapping the preceding one.

Analgesics should be given to relieve the pain, especially when this is preventing sleep. Sedative cough mixtures should be given to relieve the pain produced by unproductive cough.

The temperature usually subsides in two or three days, the pain in the side disappears, and the convalescence is usually rapid unless an effusion appears. If a tuberculous patch of lung is discovered, it should be treated as for primary pulmonary tuberculosis (p.352). The patient should not be allowed to resume work, however, until he is fully restored to health.

Pleurisy with Effusion

When dry pleurisy complicating a case of pulmonary tuberculosis or of pneumonia does not clear, it progresses to the condition of pleural effusion. Sometimes the pleurisy is the initiating stage of tuberculosis. In pleurisy with effusion an exudation of fluid occurs and accumulates in the chest cavity between the two layers of pleural membrane. As the fluid increases in quantity, the lung becomes compressed upwards and inwards toward its root, and in this collapsed condition it resembles a bellows which has been closed, so that it is useless for purposes of respiration. The fluid in the pleural cavity is pale and clear and usually greenish-yellow or straw-colored; it may amount to as much as 5 or 6 pints in quantity.

Symptoms. The symptoms are at first those of dry pleurisy, but when the effusion develops the pain is often relieved, owing to the separation of the inflamed pleural surfaces. Shortness of breath results from the ineffectiveness of the collapsed lung.

There is very restricted movement of the chest on the affected side during breathing, because little or no air is entering the affected lung. The percussion note over the fluid is one of stony dullness and the breath sounds are usually absent on listening with the stethoscope.

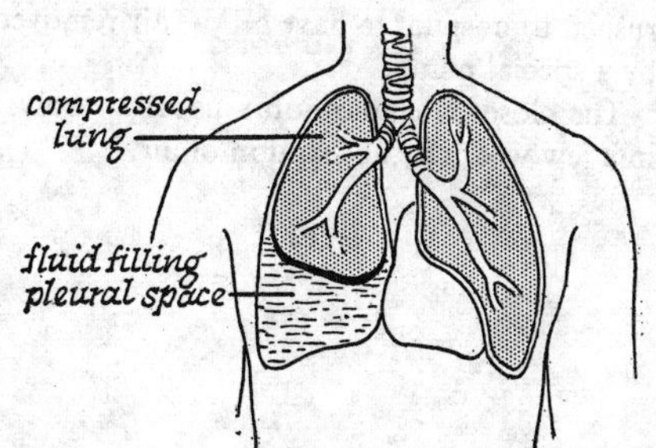

Fig. 12. *PLEURISY WITH EFFUSION ON THE RIGHT SIDE OF CHEST. The right lung is compressed upwards as fluid fills the lower part of the pleural space. Sometimes the trachea becomes pushed to the left.*

In effusions of moderate size the temperature usually falls in from seven to ten days and the fluid is spontaneously absorbed in the course of two to four weeks. In large effusions absorption may be much slower.

Treatment. The primary cause of the pleurisy should first be dealt with. If tuberculosis is suspected or present fluid is withdrawn from the lung two or three times and streptomycin instilled: and further tuberculosis treatment continued. Similar treatment is given using benzylpenicillin when the pleurisy is associated with pneumonia.

General Treatment. The patient should be kept in bed in a well-ventilated room until the temperature is normal.

Where the accumulation of fluid is causing distress, it may be removed by aspiration, after puncturing the chest wall between the ribs with a long needle attached to a syringe.

As soon as the patient is sufficiently fit, the lung should be made to re-expand by breathing exercises. Tonics and a nutritious diet with extra vitamins should be prescribed.

Empyema
(*Purulent Pleurisy*)

In this condition a pleural effusion becomes infected. It varies from a turbid watery fluid containing flakes of pus to a thick greenish or grayish exudate consisting of almost pure pus. It may collect locally between adhesions.

Empyema is most commonly due to extension of disease from the lungs, especially pneumonia. The organisms responsible for the formation of pus are usually pneumococci and streptococci.

Symptoms. The symptoms are generally masked by those of the primary disease of which it is the complication. In general the symptoms are similar to those of dry pleurisy, but are more severe, the patient appearing more profoundly ill with chills, sweats and shortness of breath. The temperature ranges to 39·5° C (103° F) or higher. The patient loses appetite, with subsequent loss of weight. Cough and sputum are usually related to the underlying lung condition. The fingers may also become clubbed. Unless the condition is treated, death may occur in a month or two.

An empyema should be suspected in any case of pneumonia when the fever persists beyond the normal course of 7 to 10 days. In any case in which it is suspected, three examinations will probably be undertaken by the doctor:

1. An X-ray examination of the chest.
2. An exploration of the chest with a needle and syringe.
3. A blood count, to find if there is an increase of white cells in the circulating blood.

Treatment. The most effective method of controlling infection in cases of empyema due to pneumococci, streptococci or staphylococci, is the direct introduction of penicillin solution into the infected cavity of the chest after withdrawal of the pleural fluid. If other bacteria are the causative agents, the doctor will use the appropriate antibiotics.

In cases which do not respond to this treatment, the pus will have to be drained away from the chest; this usually entails an operation. After operation and drainage, breathing exercises must be regularly performed.

Hydrothorax
(*Dropsy of the Pleural Cavity*)

This is a collection of sterile clear fluid in the pleural cavities, and is usually due to heart failure, or chronic kidney disease or severe anemia—especially pernicious anemia.

Symptoms. The only respiratory symptom is shortness of breath due to the size of the affection and the pressure it exerts on the lungs. There is usually no fever.

Treatment. This is the treatment of heart failure (see p. 299). Removal of the fluid by tapping the chest may give great relief.

Pneumothorax

(*Air in the Pleural Cavity*)

By pneumothorax is meant a collection of air between the layers of the pleura. It occurs spontaneously following a leakage of air from the bronchial tubes or lung tissue directly into the pleural cavity, in those diseases which weaken the bronchial walls or the lung tissue in the neighborhood of the pleural membrane which covers the lung. The cause of the air leakage is usually the rupture of (1) a small portion of air-distended lung tissue, especially if there is an adhesion of the pleura to the lung, (2) a focus of tuberculosis, or (3) a pulmonary abscess. (4) It may occasionally arise after injuries of the chest wall where a sharp fragment of fractured rib penetrates the pleura and lung.

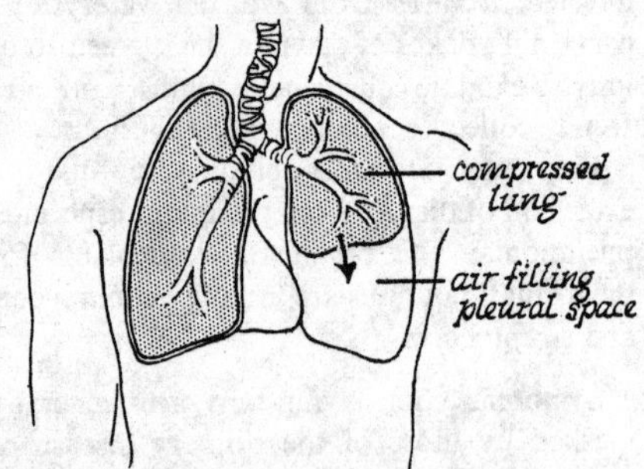

Fig. 13. *PNEUMOTHORAX ON THE LEFT SIDE OF CHEST. The left lung is compressed upwards as air leaks into the pleural space.*

There are two categories of pneumothorax:

1. The closed or benign condition in which the small ruptured hole seals off completely as the lung begins to collapse, and the air is gradually reabsorbed from the pleural cavity.
2. The tension pneumothorax in which the opening persists like a small valve. Pressure increases between the pleural layers and the lung collapses completely, compressing the opposite lung and the heart.

A pneumothorax may be produced artificially for the treatment of tuberculosis in order to rest the diseased lung tissue.

Symptoms. The onset of spontaneous pneumothorax is usually sudden, the patient being seized with severe pain in the chest, usually while coughing or when engaged in some heavy exertion. There is often a feeling of 'something having given way,' and at once great difficulty in breathing appears, with signs of collapse and a weak and rapid pulse. As a rule, in the closed type of pneumothorax, these acute symptoms subside in a few hours.

On examination of the chest, the affected side is seen to be almost entirely immovable, while the percussion note over the pneumothorax is like a drum, or tympanitic. On listening with the stethoscope the breath sounds are usually absent. In all doubtful cases an X-ray of the chest should be taken.

The outlook depends on the extent of the underlying disease. Thus, in cases with only slight disease, e.g. the rupture of a healed tuberculous nodule, the air is usually completely absorbed in a few weeks.

In the tension type, the symptoms increase with alarming rapidity and the labored breathing (dyspnea) worsens, the patient becoming bluish. Owing to the patient's lack of oxygen, it will be necessary to institute emergency treatment.

Treatment. The patient must be treated for shock, with warmth and hot drinks. He is usually unable to lie down because of the shortness of breath, and needs to be propped up in a comfortable position by means of pillows. A good supply of fresh air is essential. For the tension type of pneumothorax, an injection of morphine (15 mg) and inhalations of oxygen may need to be given by a doctor. When the pressure of air in the pleural cavity is very great, it may be necessary for the physician to introduce a trocar (a needle connected to rubber tubing with an under-water seal) through the chest wall in order to allow some of the air to escape, and so reduce the pressure. The patient is then rushed to hospital to have all the air removed by a special pump.

The closed pneumothorax usually resolves in a few weeks by absorption of air.

TUBERCULOSIS

Tuberculosis has been recognized from early times. Hippocrates, the father of medicine, in 380 B.C. advocated treating tuberculous patients with fresh air, good food and purgatives. Galen recommended plenty of milk and a dry climate. But it was not until 1882 that the infecting bacillus, *Mycobacterium tuberculosis*, was discovered and isolated by Robert Koch.

The lungs and lymphatic glands are most commonly infected by the bacillus, but the pleural, peritoneal and meningeal membranes, the intestinal tract, the bones, the kidneys, the adrenal glands, the reproductive organs and the skin may also become infected.

The tuberculosis bacillus exists in three main forms: (1) the human type; (2) the bovine type in cattle; (3) the avian type which affects domesticated and wild birds (swine can also become infected with it). Both the human and bovine types affect man. The avian type is transmitted to man only on very rare occasions.

Modes of Infection

The two main channels by which infection occurs are (1) by inhaling the bacilli, and (2) by swallowing infected food.

Air Infection. A patient with only moderately advanced pulmonary tuberculosis may in twenty-four hours expectorate no less than two to four billion tubercle bacilli. When a tuberculous patient has the germs in his phlegm, each time he coughs, sneezes, or even speaks loudly, a cloud of infectious material is sprayed into the air and these minute particles may be inhaled directly, or, after settling on a surface, may dry and become resuspended in dust. Thus the dust of house floors, places of entertainment, public vehicles and streets may become heavily infected by uncontrolled expectoration on the part of tuberculous individuals. Dried tubercle bacilli remain alive for several months if kept in the dark, but are killed if exposed to sunlight for an hour or two. Even the light of an ordinary room without sunlight will kill the germs in a few days. They are also rapidly killed by a solution of one part of carbolic acid in 20 parts of water.

CONTACTS. Since many tuberculous people, particularly elderly ones, may live for years with chronic cavities in their lungs, they may act as a reservoir of infection from which the germs are constantly fed into the house and the community at large, and this is one of the major factors in the spread of the disease.

Contaminated Foods and Milk. Since the tuberculosis germs are not destroyed by the stomach juice, infection through the gut is a common mode of production of tuberculosis in children, the main source of the bacilli being contaminated milk or dairy products such as cheese, butter, and ice-cream. Although the tonsils are rarely affected the tuberculosis germs from ingested foods may pass through them to infect the lymphatic glands of the neck.

Factors Predisposing to Tuberculosis

1. **Age.** Susceptibility is general; it is highest in children under three years, lowest from three to twelve years and intermediate thereafter. After the age of sixty, resistance often drops off again and such persons may have a chronic intractable form of the disease.

2. **Heredity.** Although the disease as such is not inherited from tuberculous parents, an increased susceptibility together with a decreased ability to resist its invasion, may be inherited by their children.

3. **Race.** Racial differences in susceptibility are noticeable, with a higher incidence in the Irish and Welsh than in the English, and aboriginal races have a greater susceptibility to tuberculosis than populations exposed to the disease for generations.

4. **Environment.** The undernourished and neglected are more susceptible to tuber-

culosis than the well fed and well cared for. There is a long-recognized association of the disease with poverty, with overcrowding and with poor housing conditions.

5. Debility. Debility and fatigue, whether the result of acute illnesses or an exhausting mode of life, increase a natural susceptibility when no hereditary weakness is present.

6. Influence of Other Diseases. The acute infectious diseases such as measles, whooping-cough and influenza, especially when complicated by bronchopneumonia, predispose to the development of pulmonary tuberculosis by lowering the resistance of the respiratory passages.

7. Occupations. Persons in occupations where they continuously inhale particles of silica, and so develop silicosis, are usually susceptible to develop tuberculosis. There is also increased risk among nurses, doctors and ancillary hospital staff in attendance upon persons suffering from tuberculosis.

8. Injury. Latent tuberculosis may, in a number of cases, be reactivated by injury to the infected organ. Tuberculosis of bones and joints can be affected seriously by incidental severe injury.

Changes in Tissues due to the Tubercle Bacillus

The tubercle bacilli may infect most of the tissues of the body and in so doing they set up a series of reactions. Of these, death of the tissue, tuberculous pneumonia and local multiplication of tissue tend to take place early in the disease, in any order or combination.

Tuberculous Pneumonia. When the bacilli reach a settling point in the lung, special protective cells in the tissues and from the blood begin to multiply and surround the invaders, destroying them as rapidly as possible. A generalized reaction of this sort in the whole or part of a lung is frequently the earliest reaction to infection and it may be referred to as exudative tuberculosis, or as tuberculous pneumonia.

Granulation Tissue. In some cases the central dead core of tissue may become surrounded by the protective cells to form microscopic tubercles which aggregate together and appear to the naked eye as grayish-white transculent nodules—known as tuberculosis granulation tissue.

Caseation. Eventually tuberculosis granulation tissue will either (1) be replaced by fibrous scar tissue, which is a repair process and which, if it continues, will arrest or cure the disease, or (2) the granulation tissue will die and caseation takes place, resulting in a semi-solid, white, cheesy mass called caseous material in which tuberculosis bacilli may be imprisoned. A caseous mass may remain

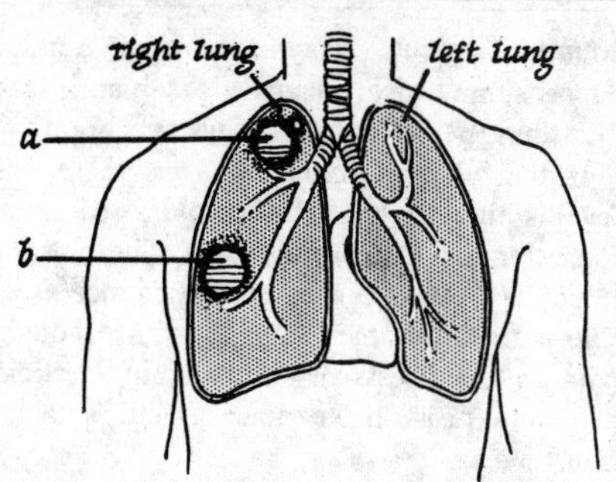

Fig. 14. *PULMONARY TUBERCULOSIS OF RIGHT LUNG, with large cavities* (a) *in the upper part of the right lobe, and* (b) *in the lower outer zone.*

unaltered for months or years, but softening of the mass frequently occurs and an abscess containing pus forms. This liquid pus is likely to be evacuated through a bronchus and expectorated as sputum, spreading the infection to other parts of the lungs and to the patient's surroundings.

Cavity Formation. The defect left after the evacuation of a caseous abscess is a tuberculous cavity and this may be no larger than a pea or may occupy a whole lobe of a lung. Such a cavity may remain open for years and on its walls—composed of tuberculosis granulation tissue—tubercle bacilli are able to grow luxuriantly.

Spontaneous healing of cavities does occur, but the cavity is a difficult lesion to heal. The chances of healing occurring, however, have been greatly increased since the introduction of the antituberculous drugs.

While cavitation may result from some caseous conditions, others may respond by fibrosis, calcification and ossification (bone formation) which are tissue reactions associated with healing.

SYMPTOMS

General Symptoms. Even though patients with advancing pulmonary tuberculosis may have no complaints referable to the lungs, they frequently have general symptoms of an indefinite character. Nervous irritability, excessive fatigue, vague abdominal discomfort, loss of appetite, loss of weight, and palpitations are common symptoms. Fever may be an early symptom and commonly occurs in the evening. The temperature usually falls in the early hours of the morning and there may be profound sweating (night sweats). In women the menstrual periods often stop.

Pulmonary Symptoms. Cough is usually present at some stage of the illness. Early in the disease the patient may expectorate little or no sputum, but if the disease advances the sputum may become profuse, purulent (containing pus), and in some cases contains blood.

Pulmonary tuberculosis may first become manifest by pain in the chest, and this is frequently associated with a pleural effusion (see p. 349), especially in young persons.

History of Exposure. Most persons with active pulmonary tuberculosis are unaware of how their infection started although the disease usually results from prolonged close contact with someone who has 'open' pulmonary disease. If pulmonary tuberculosis is suspected it is important for the patient to be carefully questioned regarding contact with persons known to have tuberculosis or undiagnosed lung symptoms.

The patient with a history of pleurisy with effusion in the past is more prone to pulmonary tuberculosis although it may appear several years after the effusion. Diabetes mellitus, too, definitely predisposes to tuberculosis.

Physical Examination

General Examination. In cases of pulmonary tuberculosis the patient must undergo a thorough general examination to identify other diseases which might influence the tuberculosis or which might affect the selection of appropriate treatment. Clubbing of the fingers and toes, a condition where the nails are curved like a parrot's beak, is

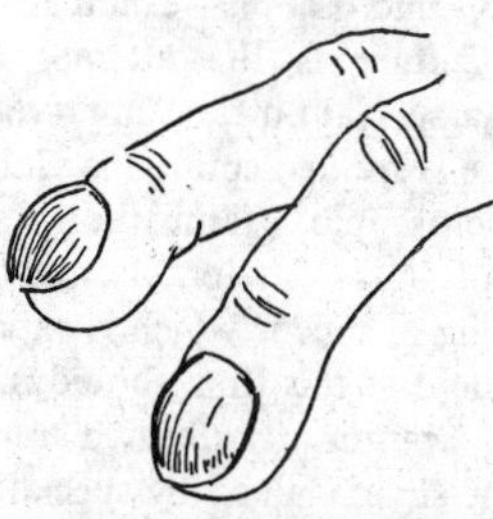

Fig. 15. *CLUBBED FINGER TIPS are frequently seen in cases of chronic pulmonary diseases, including tuberculosis. The soft terminal portions of the fingers become rather bulbous, and the nails excessively curved. The fingers illustrated are from a long-established case with severe nail curvature.*

usually evidence of long-standing pulmonary disease and is commonly found in association with bronchiectasis (see p. 345).

Examination of the Lungs. Physical examination of the chest supplements information revealed by X-rays.

In some cases a stethoscope may reveal nothing abnormal, in others it may produce evidence not detectable by X-ray examination. For example, there may be wheezing râles (moist sounds) which would imply obstruction of the bronchus; such sounds suggest the need for further investigation by special methods such as bronchoscopy.

Palpation with the fingers may reveal diseased lymph glands, especially those just above the collar-bone (clavicle). Palpation of the chest during quiet and forced breathing may also confirm other physical signs such as impaired chest expansion.

X-ray Examination of the Chest. A definite diagnosis of pulmonary tuberculosis cannot be made by X-ray examination alone. Physical examination and testing of sputum for tuberculosis bacilli are essential to confirm the X-ray indication. X-ray photographs reflect the gross changes in the tissues and they range from small, indefinite mottling of the lungs, giving a 'raw cotton' appearance most commonly seen in the upper third of the lung, to extensive areas of consolidation in one or both lungs. The chronic disease may be associated with scarring or calcification in the lungs or there may be calcification in the lymph nodes of the pleura.

Two or three X-ray photographs are usually taken at intervals of several weeks in order to compare the growth or regression of the mottled or dark areas.

The widespread use of mass-radiography, whereby hundreds of thousands of the population had routine check-ups of their lungs by X-ray filming, brought to light many unsuspected early cases of the disease.

Examination of the Sputum for Tubercle Bacilli. Accurate diagnosis of tuberculosis is dependent on the identification of the bacilli in the patient's sputum. Every effort should be made to secure sputum.

Stomach washings or laryngeal swabs may be examined where sputum is absent or does not reveal the presence of tubercle bacilli on microscopic examination and culture. (Culture is the attempt to grow bacilli on a special nutrient mixture on or in which some suspected sputum is placed.)

For microscopic examination, an early morning specimen is preferable, and the single isolated plug of mucus which is expectorated by the patient at this time should not escape attention. Sputum is smeared on a glass microscope slide, stained by special methods and examined under the microscope.

Examination of the Blood. Determination of the sedimentation rate (the rate at which the red blood cells settle out of the blood) gives information with respect to the patient's general health, since an elevated sedimentation rate is frequently found in active tuberculosis. A normal sedimentation rate, however, does not exclude the presence of active pulmonary tuberculosis.

As in other chronic infections, the hemoglobin and red cells of the blood may show a moderate reduction, indicating an ordinary secondary anemia. In tuberculosis an increase in the white blood cells may occur but has no diagnostic significance.

VARIETIES OF PULMONARY TUBERCULOSIS

It is important to recognize the particular type of tuberculosis from which a patient may be suffering, for upon this recognition both the treatment and the outlook depend.

Acute Miliary Tuberculosis (*Acute Phthisis: Galloping Consumption*)

This is caused by the widespread dissemination of tubercle bacilli which have become dislodged from some infected area. They are carried by means of the bloodstream to all parts of the body, but especially to the lungs, which become studded with countless minute gray tubercles. Similar deposits may also occur in the pleura, the intestines, peritoneum, kidneys and brain.

In the fully developed miliary disease, the fever is high, up to 40·7° C (105° F) with small remissions, and profuse sweats. The pulse is rapid, and the rate of breathing is increased. The patient becomes very ill, with a cough, pain in the chest, dry tongue, indigestion, profound prostration, anemia and emaciation.

The disease will run a rapid course to coma and death unless the patient is given antituberculous drug treatment as soon as his condition has been diagnosed, and he must be nursed in hospital. Drug treatment may have to be continued for at least a year, and corticosteroids may be of added help in seriously ill patients.

Acute Caseous Tuberculosis (*Acute Pneumonic Phthisis: Tuberculous Bronchopneumonia*)

This may occur as a terminal event in cases of old pulmonary tuberculosis. It may, however, have a sudden onset without any previous history of phthisis and resembles an attack of lobar pneumonia. There is a high temperature (103° to 105° F), with profuse night sweats, shortness of breath, severe cough, and profuse and often bloodstained sputum. Instead of the normal crisis of pneumonia, however, the fever and the signs in the chest persist for seven to ten days, and, unless antituberculous drug treatment is instituted, the disease usually terminates fatally in a few weeks to a few months.

Fibro-caseous Tuberculosis (*Consumption: Phthisis*)

This is the commonest variety of the disease, and the condition of the lung varies with the relative extent of the caseous destruction and the fibrotic repair changes. The earliest changes usually occur at the apex of the upper lobe of one lung. The apex of the lower lobe is next affected, and then the apex of the upper lobe of the opposite lung. Pleural adhesions are usually present over the oldest areas of disease.

If suitable drug treatment is not given, the patient may have episodes of ill health with pulmonary symptoms for a period of thirty to forty years. An exacerbation shows itself by increasing general debility, with loss of weight and strength, and chronic cough with expectoration which is most troublesome in the mornings. Hemoptysis is common, and occasionally massive bleeding. An open cavity, from which infected sputum is discharged, is common in this type of disease and is a potent cause of spreading the disease.

Fibroid Tuberculosis (*Chronic Consumption: Fibroid Phthisis*)

Fibrosis may spread as a process of repair throughout a lung in which caseation or cavity formation has occurred. The affected lobe, or the whole lung, then becomes firmer and contracted in size. The shrinkage may lead to bronchiectasis, especially in the lower lobes, and the pleura becomes much thickened and adherent to the lung, while the heart is drawn over towards the affected side.

Fibroid tuberculosis is fairly common in aging people in whom the active disease may undergo complete arrest. Shortness of breath becomes more pronounced, especially on exertion, and the effect on the heart and circulation results in increased sensitivity to cold, and to coldness of the hands and feet. The damaged bronchial tubes become susceptible to respiratory infections.

Many elderly patients with extensive fibroid disease are capable of attending to their work and businesses and should not be prevented from doing so. Their treatment consists largely in relieving the cough and the shortness of breath on exertion, and is very similar to that required for chronic bronchitis and for emphysema (see pp. 344 and 347).

Primary Tuberculosis in Childhood. Many children with primary pulmonary tuberculosis remain clinically well and their disease heals without treatment. A few develop spread of the disease to other parts of the body, such as the kidneys, bones, joints, and distant lymph glands. A still smaller number develop generalized miliary tuberculosis and meningitis.

The chief problem is that, in a few cases, live tubercle bacilli may remain in healed calcified lesions and constitute a threat to the child's future health.

PROGNOSIS

Having determined that tuberculosis is present, active and in need of treatment, having decided where the disease is localized and having developed some notion of the nature of the damage wrought, the physician then considers his patient as a whole person and estimates his power of recovery. Age, race, social and economic factors should each be given thoughtful consideration. The outlook is most serious in infants and it becomes less favorable in those over fifty years of age.

Poor physique and the presence of diabetes, chronic alcoholism or silicosis in patients with pulmonary tuberculosis are also factors which militate against recovery.

Few medical problems are so complicated and, in former decades, few diseases were so elusive and frustrating as tuberculosis. Today, there are few diseases which may be so successfully treated by so many and varied approaches when these are wisely combined.

TREATMENT OF ACTIVE TUBERCULOSIS

Activity is harmful and rest is beneficial in tuberculosis. This is a sound rule, the acceptance of which will simplify many decisions. Rest, as defined by the tuberculosis physician, can be a radical form of treatment and should be viewed as such by the patient despite the great sacrifices entailed.

A decision has also to be made as to whether hospital care is necessary or whether home care will be adequate. Some homes are utterly unsuited to any rest program, and these are by no means limited to the homes of the poor. It is unlikely that the mother of a family of young children can relax at home, yet she is the most reluctant of all to leave.

In Hospital. When available, hospital treatment should be recommended for the initial phases of treatment. Return to a more normal environment should be urged as soon as the home in question provides a better environment than the hospital for the person involved.

During the hospital phase of treatment the following objectives should be attained:

1. control of symptoms;
2. institution of the long-term medical treatment program;
3. instruction of the patient and his relatives;
4. modification of the home situation, if necessary and possible.

In addition efforts towards rehabilitation should be started.

The Rest Program

Rest in the hospital and the home will be required until the disease is no longer active. This may take up to nine months to attain. Patients who are critically ill and most others who have fever should remain in bed constantly.

If necessary, the lung may be immobilized by collapse therapy through (1) an artificial pneumothorax (introduction of air into the space surrounding the affected lung), (2) a pneumoperitoneum (introduction of air into the peritoneal cavity), or (3) a thoracoplasty, which is a plastic operation on the chest wall.

Rest plus Activity. When the infection has become quiescent, a program of gradually increasing physical activity is usually prescribed.

Patients in good condition, especially if there is no fever, can safely make a few trips to a nearby bathroom each day. Men should be encouraged to use electric razors in bed to prevent long periods of standing when shaving. Well-designed chairs which permit a semi-reclining position should be used in sheltered outdoor locations at an early stage of treatment.

When the sputum is no longer found to contain tubercle bacilli and all constitutional symptoms have disappeared, a modest schedule of graduated exercise may be permitted the patient who is under the protection of specific antibacterial drugs.

After maximum improvement has been attained, as judged by X-ray examinations of the chest, an exercise schedule may be devised which will gradually increase the time spent out of bed each day, so that within six months the patient is able to remain up for twelve hours a day. For the next year or more the patient should spend twelve hours out of every twenty-four hours in bed.

Climate and Air. That climate which is best for healthy persons is best for the person with tuberculosis. Extremes of heat and cold are undesirable and high altitudes must be avoided by those with any signs of breathlessness at rest or on exertion. In the industrial areas, where the air is polluted by fine particles of dust and gases such as sulphur dioxide, further damage to the lungs of a tuberculous patient will take place and whenever possible he should be moved to an area with cleaner air.

During convalescence there are great advantages in a mild climate and a pleasant environment with a resort atmosphere, particularly one which permits outdoor exercise throughout the year.

Nutrition. There is no special diet necessary for tuberculosis except a well-balanced and appetizing combination of foods. Vitamin supplements are often prescribed, particularly vitamins C, A and D.

A high protein and high calorie diet protects against the wasting effects of chronically active disease. This protection may be ensured by taking a good helping of meat (or poultry) and fish, an egg, and at least one, and preferably two, pints of milk (tuberculin-tested) in the course of the day.

Smoking. Even in healthy people, smoking reduces the efficiency of breathing by about 10 per cent and this is worsened in such diseases as pulmonary tuberculosis. In addition it appears that smoking encourages the breakdown of healed tuberculosis. Patients should be advised, therefore, to abstain from smoking.

Rehabilitation. Patients must be assisted as early as possible to procure advice and training for a life free from stresses, yet adequately productive. The need for rehabilitation is in direct proportion to the extent of injury caused by the disease, hence prompt diagnosis and thorough treatment should increase a patient's chance of resuming his former occupation.

Drug Treatment

Every patient with active tuberculous infection should receive chemotherapy or treatment with specific antituberculous drugs. Tests to find out the specific drugs to destroy the tuberculous bacilli (taken from the patient's sputum) should be performed, and such tests should be repeated in six months if the sputum still contains tubercle bacilli.

The main specific drugs now in use in the treatment of tuberculosis are streptomycin given by intramuscular injection, and isoniazid (INH) and aminosalicylic acid (PAS), both given by mouth.

Prompt treatment with these drugs is indicated as soon as the tests show the particular species of the infecting bacillus. When any one of the drugs mentioned is used alone, the tubercle bacilli frequently develop a resistance to it during treatment. In an effort to overcome this tendency, two and sometimes three drugs in combination are now employed.

Other antituberculous drugs such as pyrazinamide, ethionamide, capreomycin, and cycloserine are less satisfactory but are reserved for use in cases where the bacilli are resistant to the standard drugs.

Specific treatment should be continued so long as any evidence of improvement is seen and for a considerable time thereafter. A useful rule is that drug treatment should be continued for some twelve months after the last positive sputum culture, after the last improvement indicated on the X-ray plate, or the last sign that a cavity was present. The total duration of drug therapy will be at least eighteen to twenty-four months if this rule is followed.

Treatment of Symptoms

Cough. In early cases of the disease, cough is often no more than a bad habit which may be maintained by excessive talking, smoking, or exertion, and patients should be trained to control it as far as possible. Rest in fresh air which is free from dust is often all that is needed, and in such cases it is unnecessary and undesirable to give drugs to suppress it.

A dry unproductive cough, however, may exhaust the patient by being so frequent as to disturb sleep or so violent as to lead to vomiting; and violent coughing may lead to an extension of the disease. For a cough which causes disturbance of sleep, a hot drink should be taken at bedtime with, if necessary, a sedative cough mixture. For this disturbing cough the drug of choice is codeine.

Pain in the Chest. Severe pain in the chest in the course of pulmonary tuberculosis is usually due to pleurisy, or occasionally to spontaneous pneumothorax. For treatment, see Pleurisy, p. 349, and Pneumothorax, p. 350.

Fever. Rest in bed in the fresh air is the best means of lowering the temperature, and the rest must be absolute. If the fever is high and the patient is very uncomfortable, he should be sponged down with tepid water. Headache and discomfort may be relieved by a tablet containing:

Aspirin	225 mg
Phenacetin	150 mg
Caffeine	30 mg

but drugs should be avoided if possible.

Night Sweats. All windows should be widely opened at night. Sweating may be due to too many bedclothes, and these should be reduced. A change of nightclothes should be kept at the bedside.

Insomnia. Every effort should be made to procure for the patient a good night's rest by relieving cough and pain; if necessary, the physician may prescribe a suitable sedative to ensure sleep.

Hemoptysis (Coughing up Blood). Most patients dread this complication and whether it is slight or profuse the patient should be in bed at rest. If there is anything more than slight streaking of the sputum this information should be sent immediately to the doctor who may decide that an injection of morphine is necessary.

No solid food should be taken for some twenty-four hours after a severe hemoptysis, and feeding should subsequently be started with caution. The meals should be taken cold, and drinks may be iced.

Digestive Symptoms. Irritation of the stomach and intestines by swallowed sputum is sometimes responsible for dyspepsia and diarrhea, and for the more grave complication of tuberculous ulceration of the bowel. All patients must therefore be impressed with the importance of always expectorating sputum into a sputum cup or carton.

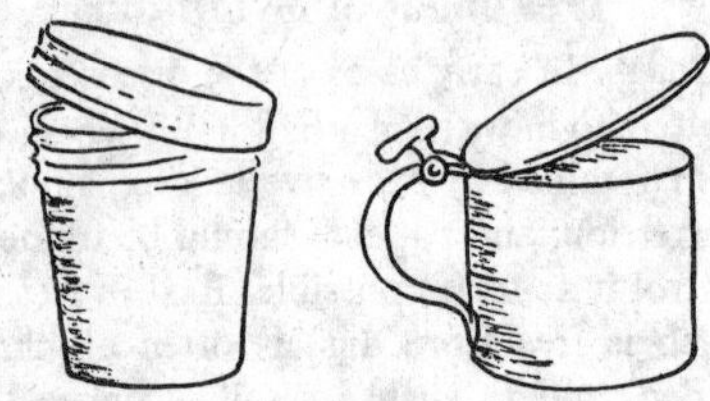

Fig. 16. *SPUTUM CONTAINERS. A waxed carton (with screw-on lid) which can be burned after use. An enamel mug which can be boiled to sterilize it after use.*

Constipation is common in tuberculosis, and may need correction by mild laxatives. Diarrhea may be controlled by a diet containing little roughage.

Surgical Treatment

Reversible forms of lung collapse (pneumothorax, pneumoperitoneum and phrenic nerve interruption) which are designed to rest the affected lung have largely been abandoned. Resection (removal by operation) of all or part of the affected lung is used increasingly in conditions of permanent and irreversible damage and this is usually undertaken within six to nine months from the start of specific treatment. Thoracoplasty is still used occasionally in selected cases.

TREATMENT IN PREGNANCY

Even if the disease is inactive in early pregnancy, it may be of significance both to the mother and prospective infant. Prenatal medical examinations should be performed on all pregnant women and the advisability of chest X-ray examination is usually recognized and advised soon after the third month of pregnancy. It is as a result of such an examination that active pulmonary tuberculosis may be discovered for the first time.

Active disease may be treated during pregnancy and it frequently becomes noncontagious before delivery. It is now generally agreed that pregnancy today has no deleterious effect on tuberculosis which has been diagnosed and that, with the present treatment regimes, active tuberculosis can be well controlled.

Patients with quiescent disease and those under observation who are not receiving specific drug treatment should be assessed at intervals during pregnancy and more particularly after the birth of the baby. Unrecognized or untreated pulmonary tuberculosis associated with pregnancy almost invariably results in a flare-up or extension of the disease.

Patients known to have active disease should be nursed in a sanatorium or in a chest unit in a general hospital where a visiting obstetrician is responsible for their prenatal care. The delivery of the baby should take place in a maternity unit or hospital where there are proper facilities for isolating an infectious tuberculous patient. For a woman with quiescent tuberculosis the delivery may be at home or in a maternity unit or hospital at the discretion of the obstetrician in charge.

Provided the physician is satisfied that the mother is non-infective and is anxious to feed her baby, breast feeding may be allowed.

PREVENTIVE TREATMENT

While the therapeutic treatment of tuberculosis is very important, it must be emphasized that preventive treatment is equally, if not more, important from the long-term point of view. The preventive measures to be recommended are as follows.

Public Health Education. The public must be made aware of the danger of tuberculosis, its mode of spread, and the methods of control. This health education can be given through the media of television, radio talks, films and film strips.

Improved Housing and Sanitation. Overcrowding, deficient ventilation, dampness, dirt and defective sanitation, which may occur both in slums and in suburban houses, should all be remedied, since they predispose to infection and favor its spread.

No Food Handling. No person who is known to be suffering from tuberculosis should be employed in any trade or occupation involving the making, supplying, or handling of any article of food.

A Safe Milk Supply must be ensured through pasteurization of milk and elimination of tuberculosis among dairy cattle.

Routine X-ray Examination is most important among groups that have a higher prevalence of tuberculosis than the general population. Such groups include nurses, medical students, patients and out-patients in general and mental hospitals, selected groups of industrial workers, e.g. those working in silica dust, and those who constitute a special hazard to others if infected, such as schoolteachers.

MASS RADIOGRAPHY has an important part to play in discovering undiagnosed cases of tuberculosis at large in the community; such persons do not know of the infection they are unwittingly spreading. The number of these cases is enormous.

Adequate Hospital Facilities for the isolation and treatment of active cases must be provided. During this stage of the disease the patient and his relatives must be taught a strict regime of personal hygiene for the patient.

PERSONAL HYGIENE OF PATIENTS. Great care must be taken in the disposal of the tuberculous sputum. It should be burned if possible, or otherwise emptied into a toilet after disinfection with carbolic, and the sputum cups or flasks should be sterilized by boiling. Waxed cartons with screw-on tops may also be used, and burned afterwards.

Nursing Services. Public health nursing services are essential for home supervision of patients and to encourage and arrange for examination of contacts.

Segregation of Children from patients suffering from tuberculosis. Tuberculous mothers should not nurse their infants, and the direct contact of all young children with tuberculous parents should be limited. It may be advisable for small children to attend a nursery.

When it is impossible to avoid having an open case of tuberculosis and a young child in the same house, it should usually be possible for the patient to have a separate sleeping room from which the child must be excluded, and to have separate towels and bedclothes, and separate utensils for eating.

DISEASES OF THE LIPS AND MOUTH

THE LIPS AND PALATE

Harelip

When a child has this somewhat common deformity he is born with a defect in the upper lip due to congenital non-union of the middle part of the lip with the outer parts, and the nostril on the affected side is broad and flat. There may be:

(a) A mere notch on one side in the red edge of the lip.

(b) A cleft on one side through the soft portion of the upper lip only (unilateral harelip, which is twice as common on the left side as on the right).

(c) A cleft through the lip and nostril which may be accompanied by cleft palate.

(d) Double or bilateral harelip, with an unattached piece of bone and a cleft palate, a variety seen in one-tenth of all cases. In the latter type of case the pieces of bone usually project and are either covered by skin or connected with the septum of the nose, protruding sometimes as far as the tip of the nose. When the cleft extends into the nose there is always a defect involving separation of the middle and lateral incisor teeth.

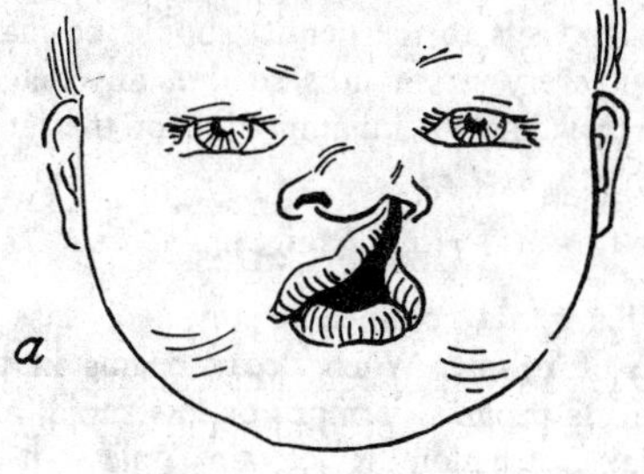

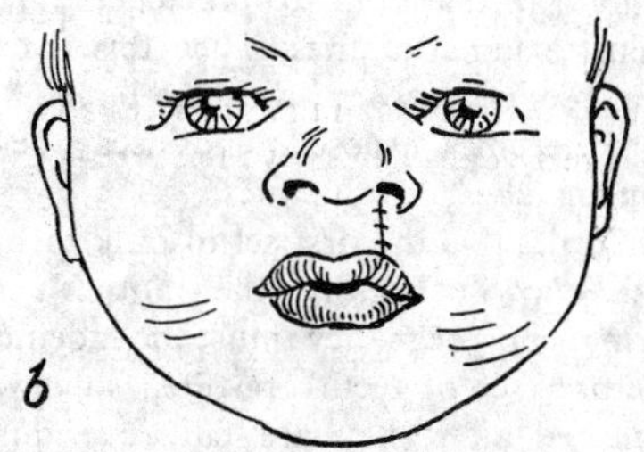

Fig. 1. *HARELIP is repaired before the baby's teeth appear. a. Shows the external appearance of an extensive harelip. b. The same deformity shortly after operation.*

Other deformities of the face, due to defects in development, are sometimes present, such as fissure of the cheek or eyelid, or cleft palate. A simple harelip does not greatly interfere with the infant's feeding, but in cases of double harelip or cleft palate there may be serious difficulty in swallowing, which may need early surgical attention to save the child's life.

Treatment. Only surgical treatment is of any value; in simple harelip the age for operation is from two to four months, before the teeth begin to appear. The general recuperative powers of the child should first be considered since, to obtain a good result, quick healing is necessary to prevent scarring.

If only the soft parts are involved, operation should be done as early as possible. If the child is weakly, or if the fissure is double and extends through the palate, then the operation ought to be postponed for some weeks after birth; from six weeks to three months is probably the best time for operating. Before operating it is very important to know that the child has not been exposed to any contagious fevers such as measles, or scarlet fever; this is one cause of failure in securing an inconspicuous scar. Others include continued crying by the child, and too much tension on the repair. Often the sutures are left in many days and the strain may be taken by a metal bow from one cheek to the other, which may be worn for several months. Infection is a common cause of serious failure in healing.

Breast feeding can usually be resumed in five days' time, the breast milk meanwhile having been expressed.

After the operation, if there is difficulty in breathing through the nostrils, rubber tubes introduced will be found a great aid and may prevent collapse of the nostrils.

Cleft Palate

In cleft palate there is a failure of union of the palate bones in the mid-line, so that the cavity of the mouth communicates with that of the nose. The cleft may only affect the uvula, or may involve both the hard and soft palates as well.

Cleft palate repair is done later than harelip, being often performed in two stages. The procedure is usually completed before the child starts to talk. It provides a roof to the mouth to aid articulation and mastication, and to prevent food passing up into the nasal cavities.

During the first few months an infant with a cleft palate must be spoon-fed, with the head well back, since regurgitation of fluids into the nose is likely to occur, and a child may die from undernourishment if feeding is carried out without due care. In untreated cases the voice is nasal in tone, and consonants cannot be pronounced properly.

The essential result to be aimed at after repair of a cleft palate is complete blocking of the nose from the mouth. Only by so doing can proper speech be achieved and food be stopped entering the nasal cavity. Often the soft palate is too short and food can escape at the back of the nose. Many children benefit from speech therapy, but this can only help those with good, mobile, soft palates and is no substitute for surgery.

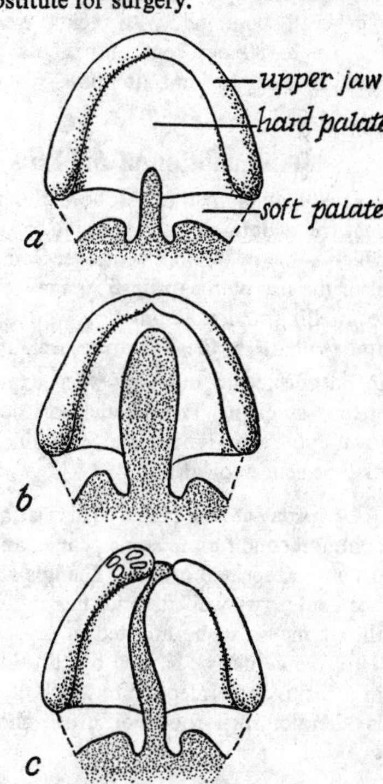

Fig. 2. *CLEFT PALATE. The cleavage varies in extent from case to case. a. Cleft soft palate. b. Both the soft and hard palates are cleft. c. Unilateral complete cleft through the hard and soft palates as well as the upper jaw.*

Ulcers of the Lips

Ulcers of the lips may be simple cracks due to cold, or colds in the head, or due to syphilitic or sometimes malignant ulceration (epithelioma), or occasionally due to tuberculous disease.

Small cracks and simple sores or 'cold' sores (herpes labialis) should be kept dry, and calamine cream or zinc paste applied. Cracks at the corners of the mouth may also be due to deficiency of vitamin B in the diet, particularly in old people who do not eat properly.

Tumors of the Lips

BENIGN TUMORS of the lips include nevi or birthmarks, warts and cysts. They may generally be dealt with by surgical methods, such as operative removal, or by cautery.

MALIGNANT TUMORS. Cancer of the lip is fairly common in elderly men, especially those who smoke clay pipes.

The lower lip at the corner of the mouth is the site at which the growth usually occurs. This may first develop as a hard crack, which slowly spreads and ulcerates, or there may be a hard nodule or a hard plaque of skin. Later the growth invades the glands of the neck; these become swollen and hard and may finally ulcerate through the skin. Death occurs from this form of ulceration, or from exhausting pain and infection, or sometimes following hemorrhage. Any hardened swelling of the lip should be examined by a doctor in case the growth is an early cancer.

Treatment of this type of growth, if given early, produces good results. Surgical removal is generally combined with radium treatment and up to 80 per cent of patients can be cured by early prompt attention.

Inflammation of the Lips

This may sometimes follow the use of dentifrice containing peppermint or salol, to which some people are sensitive. Sometimes, also, the use of cheap lipsticks may give rise to swelling and inflammation, with burning and tenderness; the lips are especially likely to be affected in this way when exposed to strong sunlight. The lipstick or dentifrice should be abandoned, and calamine lotion or ointment applied.

Urticaria of the Lips. This is a fairly common condition in some people, and often occurs in repeated attacks. The lips suddenly become very swollen, and the mouth and throat may also be affected in severe cases. The edema may be caused by certain foods, or aspirin, or an infection to which the person is allergic; such foods or drugs should be avoided.

Treatment. Antihistamine drugs may prove helpful and these will be recommended by the doctor. If stronger measures are needed, he may give adrenaline injections to reduce the swelling.

THE GUMS

Epulis

A simple epulis is a small smooth tumor of the jaw arising from a tooth socket. An epulis tends to spread and may sometimes ulcerate, and should be removed without delay.

Cancer of the gums which usually indicates involvement of the jaw, occasionally occurs, and should be dealt with by a surgeon. It may be caused by irritation from an ill-fitting denture, and any ulceration from such a source should never be neglected, since it may favor the development of malignant disease.

Pyorrhea Alveolaris
(*Gingivitis*)

This usually begins in early adult life, and is caused by infection and inflammation of the gums around the teeth and, if unchecked, the surrounding bone is also involved. Dental caries or retention of decomposed food particles which harbor infective organisms is often the cause.

Symptoms and Course. The infection often begins around the front teeth. Mouth-breathing, injury of the gums by toothpicks, stale or retained particles of food, irritation from tartar or long-continued neglect of the teeth are conditions favoring pyorrhea.

If the disease is discovered early, treatment is simple and more likely to be successful, but pyorrhea usually causes no pain until some complications have developed and is therefore often neglected until it is advanced.

The first sign is a bright red line along the edge of the gum, with shrinking of the gum between the teeth. In some cases the gums appear swollen and reddened, and pockets extend up between the teeth. The mucous membrane bleeds easily when picked or brushed, and pus can be squeezed out by

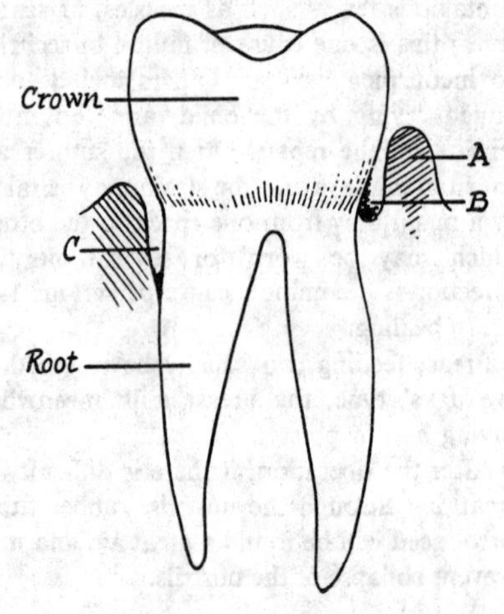

Fig. 3. PYORRHEA. *The infection causes the gums to swell and redden (A), then there is a loosening of the gums away from the teeth, leaving pockets (B) in which food debris lodges and decays. The gum shrinks back exposing the vulnerable root (C).*

pressure. In time, loosening of the gums from the tooth will occur, forming a pocket which enlarges until the root is exposed. This pocket favors retention and decomposition of food particles and the formation of foul-smelling pus which collects around the teeth. In time the teeth become loosened and fall out. Finally, root abscesses and destruction of bone may follow. An X-ray examination will reveal the extent of the condition.

In the last stages the gums are no longer swollen or inflamed, but shrink down so that the teeth appear to be long and widely spaced. Although the teeth may appear to be healthy, X-ray examination may show a root abscess or bone infection which may be responsible for disorders such as rheumatoid arthritis.

In the early stages removal of tartar and the use of astringents and antiseptics may arrest the condition, but generally treatment is prolonged and tedious.

Treatment. The treatment consists in scrupulous attention to cleanliness, healthy diet, with vitamins C and D, nasal breathing, and attention to the general health. The teeth must be well brushed twice daily and the mouth rinsed at night. Diluted hydrogen peroxide solution makes a cleansing mouth-wash.

Proper dental treatment should also be given, with cleaning and scaling of the roots, removing dead and bare bone, and cleaning out diseased pockets.

Gentle massage of the gums may help to harden them.

Anemia or constipation should be corrected by appropriate treatment, and antibiotics are occasionally useful.

TEETH

Decay and loss of the teeth are unfortunately common, even among young people. Comparatively few persons at the age of twenty have entirely sound teeth. The tendency to dental decay is no doubt to some extent inherited, but with regular and careful attention the teeth may be preserved in good condition until late in life. Parents should inculcate early in their children the habit of regular thorough cleaning of the teeth, and regular visits to the dentist should be made about every six months so that any defect, overcrowding, or inflammation of the gums may be corrected.

Dental Caries

This is not confined to any age, class or race of people. When decay begins in the teeth its progress is more or less rapid, and their destruction is certain unless it is arrested by proper treatment. The enamel is nature's fortification to protect the teeth against external injuries; when this is damaged, broken or worn away, the bone of the tooth becomes exposed, and decay begins immediately.

In order that the first set of milk or baby teeth may be healthy, the mother's diet during her pregnancy must be adequate. The first set of teeth are often somewhat neglected after they are cut, but during the first few years the permanent teeth are also developing and they may become defective before they appear.

The proper growth of the teeth requires full supplies of calcium and the vitamins A, D and C, and they will all be supplied if the diet contains milk, orange-juice and cod-liver oil.

Fluorine is essential for making strong enamel in early childhood. The minute quantity required comes from food and mainly drinking water.

Injury to the Enamel. Many sweets or much sugar are harmful to the teeth, especially when eaten between meals, since they favor bacterial growth in the mouth. Acids are injurious to the enamel; when taken as medicine they should be well diluted and, in some cases, drunk through a straw or tube, so that they do not come in contact with the teeth.

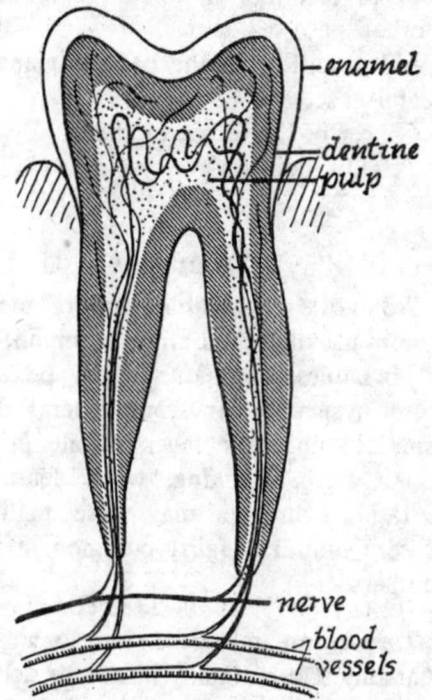

Fig. 4. *SECTION THROUGH A NORMAL TOOTH showing the enamel, dentine, and pulp, as well as the nerves and blood vessels which nourish it.*

Food lodged between the teeth, and in their depressions, is likely to cause extensive decay; sugar foods (less so glucose) expecially soon undergo fermentation which corrodes the enamel. The teeth, consequently, often begin to decay on the surfaces between adjoining teeth, and in depressions, where food particles are retained; this shows the necessity of cleansing the mouth and teeth often, particularly after meals.

Cheap tooth-powders, or those containing gritty particles, should be avoided. Smoking may cause chronic irritation of the tongue or pharynx, and this may be indirectly injurious to the teeth; smoking also blackens the teeth.

A crowded condition of the teeth in the mouth renders proper cleansing difficult and may lead to decay; in cases of irregular or crowded teeth in a child, the condition should be corrected early by a dentist.

TARTAR. Tartar is a calcareous or chalky substance which is deposited around the teeth; when not brushed away, it becomes discolored and in children it often becomes a dark green. It destroys the beauty of the teeth and, when near the gum margins, irritates the mucous membrane and may lead to pyorrhea (see p. 356). It causes the gums to become irritated, inflamed, swollen, tender and ulcerated, and the unhealthy condition of the mouth gives the breath a disagreeable smell. In all cases, tartar should be immediately and carefully removed, and an astringent and disinfectant mouth-wash should be applied to reduce the inflammation and swelling of the gums.

Toothache

In investigating a patient with toothache, the sensitivity of each tooth to tapping and to heat and cold should be tested; sensitive spots due to exposed dentine may be present, or there may be cavities or exposed pulp, and there may also be some swelling or tenderness of the gums. The possibility of referred pain from the nasal sinuses or other parts, or of neuralgia, should also be considered.

EXPOSED DENTINE (beneath the enamel) may give rise to sharp pain during brushing, or when cold, sour, or sweet foods are eaten. The sensitive spot should be treated by a dentist.

DENTAL DECAY, with acute inflammation of the pulp, requires dental treatment, but the pain can often be relieved for the time being.

UNERUPTED WISDOM TEETH may give rise to pain, especially if the tooth is impacted, or there is inflammation of the gum. The tooth may need to be extracted, but the pain may be relieved by hot mouth-washes.

DENTAL NEURALGIA may develop in some cases in which there is no actual malady of the teeth. A search should be made for any possible cause in the sinuses, throat, eyes, or ear. Sedative drugs, or electrotherapy may be of benefit. Occasionally an alcohol injection is given by a surgeon to relieve the pain.

Treatment

Temporary Treatment. Toothache may be relieved by placing a drop of oil of cloves upon a small piece of raw cotton, and inserting it into the cavity of the tooth. Do not let clove oil on the gums.

An alternative packing which may be used

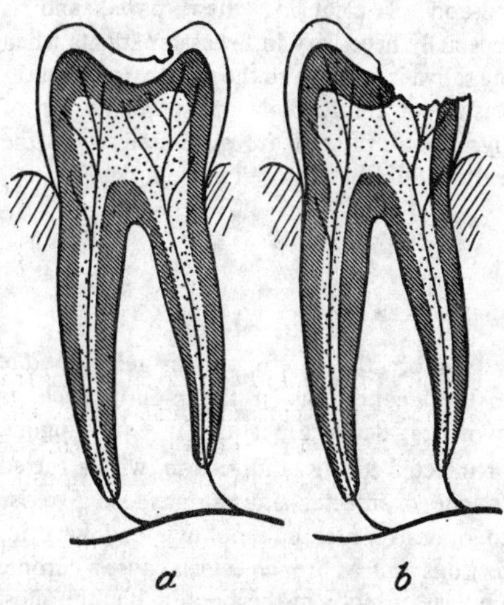

Fig. 5. *STAGES IN TOOTH DECAY.* (*a*) *shows a small carious cavity appearing on the enamel layer of the tooth.* (*b*) *Without dental treatment the cavity has extended right through to the sensitive pulp of the tooth and exposed the nerve.*

as a temporary anodyne is a paste made by mixing well together clove oil and zinc oxide. In lieu of the clove oil, eugenol may be preferred; it has a flavor and properties similar to those of clove oil.

Codeine compound tablets may relieve the pain due to decayed teeth or to unerupted wisdom teeth.

Pain of the face and jaw, when not caused by decaying teeth, may be relieved by hot external applications.

Extraction and Filling. For teeth too decayed to be saved by filling, extraction is necessary.

A tooth that is properly filled may be made serviceable and preserved for many years. When decay is extensive, the nerve may need to be destroyed before the cavity is filled; otherwise there may be sensitivity or severe pain. It is very important that teeth should be filled early, before the nerve needs to be destroyed.

Preventive Treatment. It is an important duty of parents to see that their children's teeth have early, regular, and careful attention. The sound formation and durability of the permanent teeth depend on the healthy condition and regular care of the first or temporary set. Probably the commonest single cause of tooth decay in the young today is eating sweets. The quantity consumed should be limited, and teeth should be cleaned to remove sugar from the crevices where it starts its mischief.

BRUSHING THE TEETH. The most important rule to be observed in the preservation of the teeth is to keep them perfectly clean, and never to allow any food debris to collect or remain around them. A decaying tooth should never be neglected. If tartar is present, it should be removed immediately. The teeth should be carefully and thoroughly brushed twice a day with warm water and a dentifrice; the type of tooth powder or paste used is not so important despite advertised claims.

Brushing has no injurious effects upon the teeth, and the parts of the teeth which are most exposed to the friction of a brush do not first begin to decay. This beginning of decay usually takes place in the depressed surfaces, and where the teeth touch each other. The brush should always be used in a thorough and effective manner, namely, down the upper gums and teeth, and up the lower gums and teeth.

TOOTHPICKS, made of quill or wood or ivory, may be used after meals, and all particles of food lodged between the teeth should be removed.

Long-term Neglect. The injurious effects of decayed teeth and an unclean mouth upon the general health are of more serious consequence than most people are aware. Rheumatism, rheumatoid arthritis, dyspepsia, and other general diseases may be worsened by decaying teeth and pyorrhea.

Alveolar Abscess

An alveolar abscess in the socket of a tooth may develop from a decayed tooth, causing severe pain, swelling and spasm of the jaw. The affected tooth should be removed to allow drainage of the abscess in the socket. Mouth-washes should be used frequently for a few days, and an antibiotic is often prescribed.

THE JAWS

Necrosis of the Jaws

The jaws occasionally undergo necrosis or destruction. This destruction can be the result of a dental abscess, fractures, acute fevers, mercury or phosphorus poisoning, syphilis, or tuberculosis. Hot mouth-washes and wet compresses should be used unless pus forms, when treatment must be surgical. Sulphonamides and penicillin may be used to arrest infection.

Mandibular Joint Pain

The mandibular joint may be affected by acute arthritis or by chronic osteo-arthritis Either disease causes pain on opening the jaws, a click on opening, and difficulty in mastication. If medical treatment fails, the upper part of the jaw bone is sometimes removed, and a 'false' joint is formed.

Locking or Clicking Jaw

Locking or clicking jaw sometimes occurs, with pain and a clicking noise on opening the mouth. The condition may cure itself spontaneously, but if it persists and causes much disability, the cartilage of the joint may be removed.

Jaw Tumors

Various kinds of tumors of the jaws are to be found; the commonest type is an epulis (see p. 356), which may be benign or locally malignant. These require surgical treatment.

Spasm of the Jaws

Spasm of the jaws is due to a variety of causes such as chronic arthritis, bony deformities or tumors, irritation from decayed teeth, tetanus (lockjaw), or hysteria.

THE MOUTH

Examination of the mouth often shows some unhealthy condition of the lining mucous membrane, or of the teeth, gums, tonsils, or tongue. Any such disorder requires treatment to prevent the general health being affected.

In local conditions such as thrush, only local treatment is usually required.

General diseases may, however, produce signs in the mouth, as ulceration in syphilis, or bleeding of the gums in scurvy, and soreness of the tongue in pernicious anemia. The main disease must receive the appropriate treatment, but local measures must not be neglected.

Some drugs, e.g. barbiturates, bromides, and sulphonamides, which cause skin rashes, also affect the mouth and give rise to swelling, redness, and tiny blisters in sensitive persons.

Mouth Care in General Diseases

The mouth requires careful attention in many different general disorders, especially in fevers, or cases of prolonged illness, in which the tongue becomes furred and sores develop round the lips. Sponging of the tongue and lips with pieces of gauze soaked in lemon juice, or simple rinsing with warm (boiled) water is generally found to be a satisfactory method of cleansing these parts, and is especially necessary in feverish patients when the saliva is scanty and the mouth dry. Mouth-washes of dilute hydrogen peroxide, or of glycerin of thymol are also used, while the teeth should be cleansed twice a day.

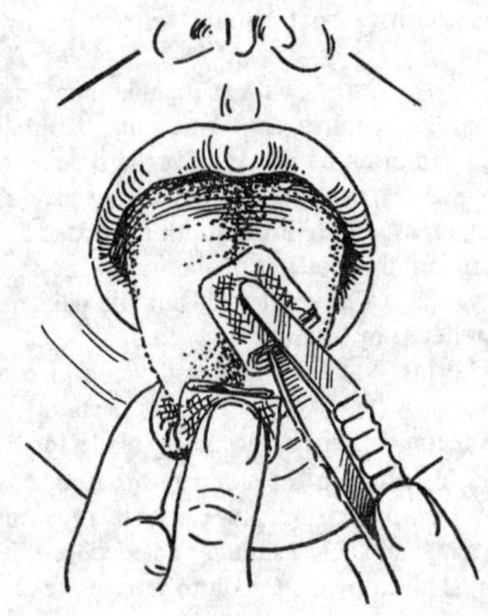

Fig. 6. *TONGUE IN FEVERS. The mouth is usually very dry and the tongue heavily furred. Sponge them with gauze soaked in lemon juice to relieve the patient.*

Foul Breath

Foul breath, or fetor oris, is generally due to local conditions in the mouth, such as pyorrhea, decayed teeth, Vincent's angina, or infected tonsils. Indigestion, with a furred tongue, or infected sinuses, may also give rise to offensive breath. Smoking, and lung infections such as bronchiectasis cause a chronic unpleasant odor in the breath, but the most offensive smell is noticed in cases of cancer of the stomach.

Treatment. The underlying disease or disorder must be treated. Temporary relief may be obtained by the use of mouth-washes as advised in Mouth Care.

Trismus—Inability to Open the Mouth

This may be due to various causes including the following:

Arthritis of the joint of the mandible, with fixation.

Bony deformities due to fractures or tumors.

Scars from burns, lupus, or operations.

Spasm of the muscles from irritation of decayed teeth, or of an unerupted wisdom tooth.

Inflammation of the parotid gland, or a dental abscess.

Cancer of the throat or cheek.

Tetanus (lockjaw).

Stomatitis

Stomatitis or inflammation of the lining membrane of the mouth is common, especially in babies and children. It may be catarrhal from dyspepsia, or from general debility, especially in acute fevers; while in adults, rough teeth, smoking, worn dentures, or irritation from food may cause small ulcers. A sore mouth is fairly common in nursing mothers.

Thrush, an infection due to a fungus, generally affects weakly infants or debilitated persons, or in some cases insufficient care is taken in keeping nipples and bottles clean. Special attention should be paid to the sterilization of nipples and other utensils which should be well washed each time after use, boiled once a day, and protected from flies and dust. Gentian violet 0·5 per cent may be used to paint the mouth, and the antibiotic nystatin may be given to prevent spread of the fungus to the bowel and lungs.

Catarrhal Stomatitis is seen in undernourished children, especially during teething, and in adults it may be caused by dyspepsia, highly seasoned foods, excessive smoking, specific fevers, or by pyorrhea or carious teeth. The gums and lips may be affected, or the whole inside of the mouth and the tongue may be inflamed, red and dry, with the tongue swollen. There is an unpleasant taste, especially on waking, and the breath is offensive.

The teeth and gums must be cleaned carefully and regularly twice daily, and a mouth-wash should be used after every meal. The bowels must be opened regularly.

Aphthous Stomatitis may occur in children or adults, often associated with some stress or digestive disturbance. It may be due to a herpes virus. Small red raised vesicles or blebs are seen in the mouth, which soon break and leave little gray ulcers with reddened edges. The mouth is sore, and the patient is often unwilling to eat. The lesions should be coated with a dental paste, after meals, or amethocaine tablets sucked.

Syphilitic Ulcers of the mouth sometimes

develop in the late tertiary stage; a primary sore is less common; either type require prompt appropriate anti-syphilitic treatment, which must be continued under medical supervision.

Vincent's Angina (also known as Vincent's Infection, Vincent's Stomatitis, Ulcerative Stomatitis, and Trench Mouth) occurs in debilitated persons or in minor epidemics in crowded communities, causing ulceration in the mouth and pharynx, with the formation of yellowish membrane over the ulcers. The infection often affects the gums, causing inflammation and receding of the gum margins. The glands of the neck are commonly swollen, and there is slight fever and general malaise. The breath is offensive and the tongue is coated. The condition is very infective and the patient should use separate eating utensils.

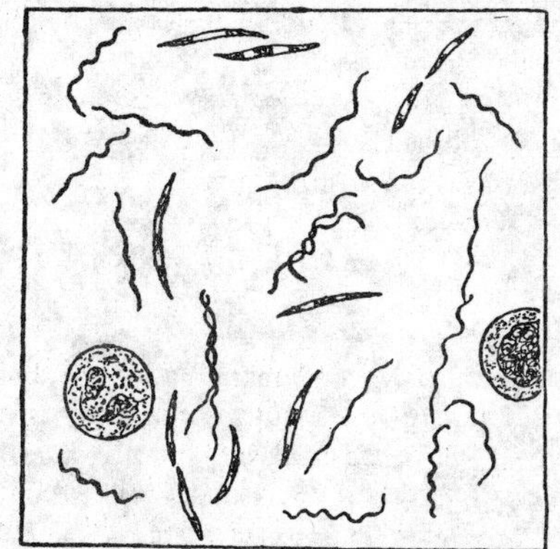

Fig. 7. *VINCENT'S ANGINA. This mouth disease is caused by an association of two organisms, a fusiform (spindle-shaped) bacillus and a spirochete (spiral-shaped organism). The larger round bodies are white blood cells.*

Mouth-washes of weak hydrogen peroxide should be used several times daily, and weak iodine may be painted round the affected areas. It is advisable to consult a doctor, who may prescribe penicillin and the local application of an arsenical solution.

THE TONGUE

In healthy persons the tongue is red, firm and moist. In ill health digestive disturbance, fever, or mouth breathing is likely to cause fur and dryness of the tongue. Fur forms most readily during sleep, particularly when the patient is on a milky diet. The tongue is especially likely to be dry in feverish conditions such as septicemia (blood poisoning), peritonitis, and typhoid fever, when it becomes brown and shaggy.

In diabetes the tongue is often large and red. In pernicious anemia it is red, sore and glazed at the tip; this soreness and redness may also be seen in other forms of anemia.

Tongue Tie

Tongue tie is a condition occasionally seen in young babies, and it may cause some difficulty in suckling. The membranous fold under the tongue is short, and the tongue cannot be protruded forward. It is sometimes necessary to make a small snip through the fold of the frenum, but it must not be too freely divided or the child will then tend to swallow its tongue. (See also Speech Therapy, p. 187.)

Inflammation of the Tongue

Inflammation of the tongue, or glossitis, may be associated with stomatitis of various types; it generally causes soreness, and there may be swelling of the whole tongue, with difficulty in speaking and swallowing. Patchy inflammation may be of a chronic nature, and often affects the sides and tip of the tongue; it is sometimes caused by smoking, dyspepsia, anemia, pyorrhea, dental sepsis, too hot or highly seasoned foods, or tertiary syphilis.

The tongue may show red patches or raised white areas which, if persistent for a prolonged period, may develop cracks, fissures and ulceration. This condition is called *leukoplakia,* which often precedes cancer of the tongue, and every possible means to reduce dental sepsis or irritation from teeth or any other source must be used. Any case of leukoplakia should be examined by a doctor, since it is also seen in cases of tertiary syphilis which must be treated. In other cases a doctor should keep the patient under observation.

Smoking, condiments, chewing of tobacco, alcohol and so forth must be abandoned, and mild antiseptic washes used daily.

'Smoker's patch' is a red area commonly seen on the front part of the tongue, the membrane being smooth, or covered by a yellowish crust.

Black Tongue

In this condition the back of the tongue is stained black; even persistent scraping cannot remove much of the discoloration which is due to the growth of a yeast-like substance. The condition is not serious. The infection often develops during treatment with penicillin lozenges when the usual flora of the mouth are killed. When the antibiotic is stopped, the yeast organisms disappear.

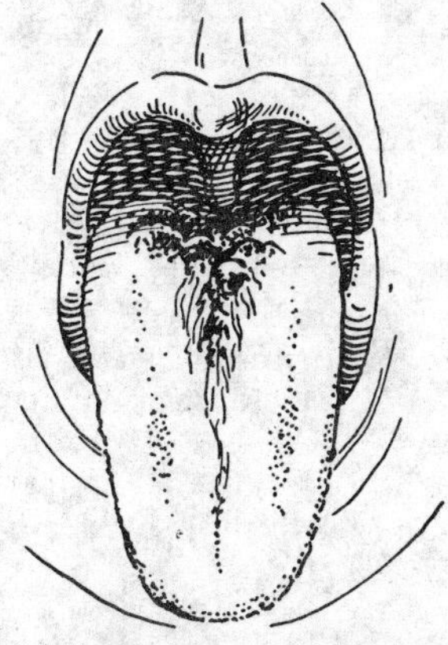

Fig. 8. *BLACK TONGUE indicates the invasion of the back of the tongue surface by a yeast-like organism. The organism grows after penicillin lozenges have killed all the normal organisms in the mouth.*

The furry discoloration can be partly removed by brushing the tongue twice daily with a toothbrush and swabbing with 10 per cent sodium bicarbonate solution.

Ulcers of the Tongue

Ulcers of the tongue are moderately common, especially dyspeptic ulcers which are small but painful and generally appear near the tip.

Dental ulcers are the result of irritation from broken or roughened teeth or dentures, and occur round the edges of the tongue. They should not be neglected, owing to the possibility of cancer if they become chronic. Other types of ulcers are less commonly seen, but include those due to syphilis or lupus.

In whooping-cough small ulcers sometimes appear on the frenum under the tongue, and are a diagnostic sign of this disease.

Cancer of the Tongue

Cancer of the tongue generally occurs in men over forty years of age; it often follows glossitis or chronic irritation from decayed or rough teeth, and excessive smoking or tobacco-chewing. The disease often starts at the side of the tongue, which is first hard or fissured, or there may be a raised warty patch or early ulceration. The breath becomes foul, with pain in the tongue and difficulty in movement as the growth progresses. The glands of the neck become enlarged, and the pain extends to the ear.

Treatment is either by surgical removal of the affected part or by radium irradiation. Any teeth which cause irritation should be removed.

THE SALIVARY GLANDS

Calculus

A calculus or stone sometimes develops in the salivary glands, causing periodic swelling with pain in the gland concerned; if not

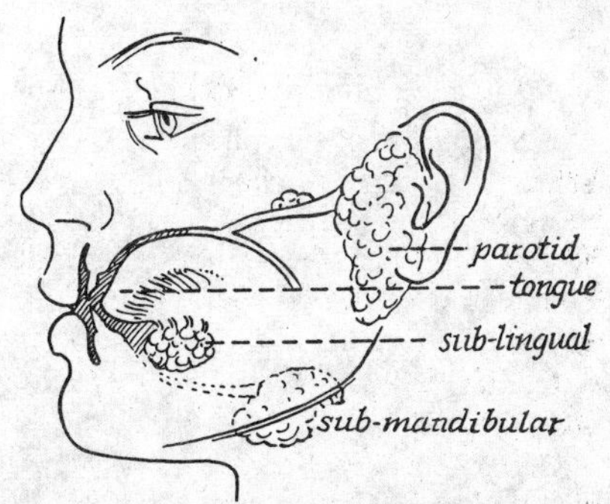

Fig. 9. *THE SALIVARY GLANDS. Section through the face showing the three groups of salivary glands: in front of the ear, under the tongue, and by the side of the lower jaw.*

treated, the gland may become permanently swollen, or an abscess may be formed. The stone, however, may be fairly easily removed by a surgeon.

Tumors

Various tumors may involve the parotid gland, cancer and the so-called mixed tumor being not uncommon. The treatment of these conditions is usually surgical to remove the whole of the diseased area.

Parotitis

The parotid gland may be inflamed in a mild degree, sometimes when there is infection in the mouth, but more usually when there is no apparent cause; in some cases cold or injury may be responsible. Occasionally the inflammation proceeds to suppuration, as in cases of typhoid or scarlet fever, or in pyemia, especially when the patient is debilitated and anemic.

Treatment. Many cases can be prevented by careful nursing, but surgical treatment may be needed. Penicillin injections may be given.

The parotid gland is usually the site of inflammation in mumps (see p. 284).

DISEASES OF THE DIGESTIVE SYSTEM

DISEASES OF THE STOMACH AND DUODENUM

Symptoms Associated with Diseases of the Stomach

Both abdominal pain and vomiting are common in diseases of the stomach, but it must be emphasized that dyspepsia may be a prominent symptom in diseases of other organs, e.g. gall-stones, pulmonary tuberculosis, anemia, and chronic appendicitis.

Pain. This is localized in the middle of the upper abdomen, and is usually due to the contractions of the stomach during the process of digestion. It is a common symptom in ulcer of the stomach, beginning characteristically when digestion is well started, that is half an hour to one and a half hours after meals. In cancer of the stomach the pain is normally much less constant or absent, and

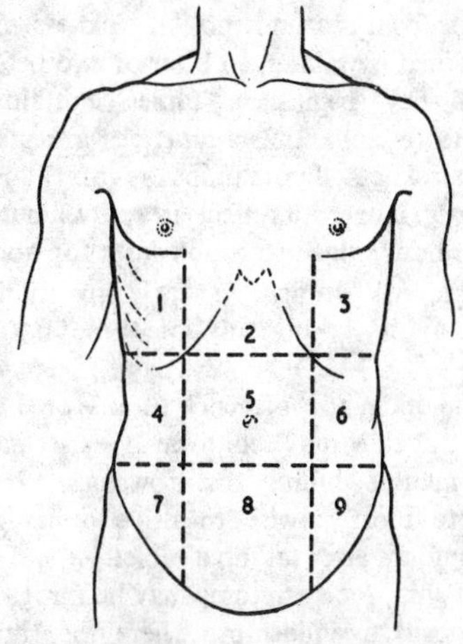

Fig. 1. *THE REGIONS OF THE ABDOMEN.* 1. *Right hypochondrial region.* 2. *Epigastrium.* 3. *Left hypochondrial region.* 4. *Right lumbar region.* 5. *The umbilical region.* 6. *Left lumbar region.* 7. *Right iliac fossa.* 8. *Hypogastrium.* 9. *Left iliac fossa.*

not so closely related to meals. Short of actual pain, sensations of discomfort, fulness or pressure may occur in less serious diseases of the stomach.

Vomiting. This is a common feature of serious diseases of the stomach, such as ulceration or cancer, and it generally occurs after the digestion has been in process for some time. It is usually preceded by nausea. Disease of the stomach should be suspected when abdominal pain is relieved by vomiting.

Vomiting of Blood (Hematemesis). This is an important symptom of stomach disease, and is most frequent in cases of gastric ulcer and cancer of the stomach. The amount of blood vomited may vary from an ounce to a pint or more.

Loss of Appetite. This may be caused by disturbances in many parts of the body, e.g. gall-stones, tuberculosis, anemia, and long-continued nervous and emotional tension. It is, however, particularly common in diseases of the stomach, e.g. gastritis and cancer.

Flatulence ('Wind'). The stomach or intestines may be distended with gas, the patient complaining of 'wind' or flatulence, which may be belched through the mouth, or passed by the rectum. It is common in many types of digestive disorder, but in most cases the gas is mainly swallowed air.

COMMON DISORDERS OF DIGESTION

Gastric Flatulence

Causes. The causes of gastric flatulence may be functional (that is without any actual disease of the organs of digestion) or organic (associated with disease). By far the commonest cause is the habit of swallowing air. It may be either swallowed while eating hurriedly, or swallowed unknowingly throughout the day. The patient usually feels discomfort in the stomach which he thinks he can disperse by belching. The attempt, however, proves unsuccessful, and results in the swallowing of air. After several attempts have been made without success, air being swallowed on each occasion, the stomach becomes distended with air which is noisily expelled. The severest cases of air swallowing occur independently of dyspepsia in patients (usually women) of a particularly nervous disposition.

The commonest and most persistent gastric flatulence due to organic disease is associated with disease of the gall-bladder, especially gall-stones. It is sometimes due to excessive fermentation of carbohydrate foods in the large intestine.

Symptoms. Wind in the stomach gives rise to a sensation of fulness in the upper central abdomen, which may extend under the left lower margin of the ribs. It causes the diaphragm to be pushed up, and may give rise to palpitation and attacks of shortness of breath. Severe distension of the stomach may actually simulate the pain of angina pectoris (see p. 301).

Treatment. When flatulence is due to air-swallowing, it is generally only necessary to explain to the patient the cause of the trouble in order to cure him. He should be told not to attempt to belch, and if he finds it very difficult to restrain himself, he should clench his teeth upon a cork, or separate them with a cigarette holder, as it is then difficult to swallow any more air. Relief can further be obtained by sipping a little hot water, preferably containing a pinch of bicarbonate of soda, or half a teaspoonful of aromatic spirits of ammonia in half a glass of water. Alternatively, a few drops of a carminative, such as oil of peppermint, may be taken on a lump of sugar.

In cases of carbohydrate fermentation, foods consisting largely of starch and cellulose—potatoes, peas, lentils, rice, carrots, and onions—should be avoided or only eaten occasionally.

Heartburn

Heartburn or pyrosis is a burning sensation felt behind the breast-bone usually a little while after a meal. It may be accompanied by regurgitation of the acid stomach contents into the mouth. Its site of origin is the lower end of the esophagus (gullet) and it is probably due to muscular contraction at this point, from the irritation of the regurgitating contents of the stomach. It is not normally associated with serious disease of the stomach, but is a common symptom of hiatus hernia of the stomach (p. 384), and is often experienced in the later months of pregnancy.

It usually responds to treatment with antacids such as compound powder of magnesium trisilicate.

Water-brash

Water-brash consists in the regurgitation into the mouth of a watery fluid, sometimes consisting of mucus, sometimes of saliva, and sometimes of both mixed together. It is not necessarily caused by any disease of the stomach, though it is strongly suggestive of a duodenal ulcer, being uncommon in other forms of chronic indigestion.

Symptoms. At a certain interval after a meal, an uncomfortable sensation of constriction is felt beneath the lower end of the breast-bone, accompanied usually by profuse salivation. Relief occurs in bringing up several mouthsful of clear fluid, which rises with little or no effort into the mouth from the esophagus where it has collected.

Treatment. The momentary discomfort

can be overcome by taking a little milk of magnesia, or an alkaline tablet of bisurated magnesia.

Nervous Dyspepsia

Causes. Many emotional patients suffer from indigestion as a result of an abnormally irritable nervous system with its associated lack of muscular tone. Depressing emotions, business or domestic worries, and long hours of physical and mental overwork, often associated with irregular or 'bolted' meals are frequent causes of the complaint.

Symptoms. The digestive symptoms are characterized by their extreme irregularity, the patient feeling very ill one day and comparatively well the next. The most constant complaint is of vague abdominal fulness or discomfort as soon as a small quantity of food has been taken. It is made worse by fatigue, worry and excitement, but rarely amounts to actual pain. Many patients complain of flatulence which is generally due to swallowing of air (see above). The appetite is poor so that an insufficient amount of food is taken; this leads to further depression of the nervous system, which reacts again on the digestion, so that a vicious circle is produced. Constipation is almost always present.

The stomach symptoms are generally associated with other symptoms, such as headache, backache, palpitations, and sleeplessness, while the loss of appetite leads to progressive loss of weight and strength, the patient being depressed and pessimistic, and paying great attention to his bodily functions and symptoms.

Treatment. A very thorough examination is necessary, in order to exclude the possibility of serious disease of the stomach. The general emotional disturbance first requires attention, by means of mental and physical rest. A drastic restriction of the diet is not necessary. In the earlier stages of treatment, a diet as for peptic ulcer may be prescribed (p. 365), increasing in the course of a few weeks to a normal varied diet, with some form of food or drink taken every 2½ hours or so. It is important that meals should be sufficient in quantity and appetizingly prepared, but they must be eaten slowly and properly masticated. A period of complete rest should be followed by graduated exercise and later by a holiday away from work. There should be a general atmosphere of optimism about the complaint and, with reassurance and encouragement, the dyspepsia will gradually disappear by itself.

Constipation may be relieved by small doses of senna, or milk of magnesia Any associated anemia should be treated by iron. Dental treatment should be given where necessary.

VOMITING AND ALLIED DISORDERS

Vomiting

Causes. Vomiting may occur in a great variety of conditions.

1. Reflex Vomiting. This may occur in various disorders of the stomach and bowels. The most common of all causes is an irritation of the lining of the stomach due to eating contaminated food or swallowing poisons. Over-distension with food and drink, especially if it occurs rapidly as when a big meal is bolted, has the same effect. Organic obstruction of the outlet of the stomach (pyloric stenosis), usually from a chronic gastric or duodenal ulcer in its neighborhood, is a not uncommon cause of persistent vomiting, and likewise intestinal obstruction from any cause, particularly cancerous growths of the bowel. Painful abdominal conditions, such as appendicitis, inflammation of the gall-bladder, gall-stones, and colic from stone in the kidney, are also common causes.

2. Toxic Vomiting. It may occur from poisons produced in the body, which give rise to vomiting by their irritant action on the lining of the stomach. These poisons may result from acute infections such as gastric influenza, pneumonia, or fevers such as scarlet fever, or chronic conditions, such as Graves' disease. Addison's disease, or Bright's disease with uremia.

3. Central Vomiting. This may occur from various nervous causes. Certain emotions, particularly those of disgust and fear may result in vomiting, especially in neurotic or highly strung individuals. The vomiting of migraine and the cyclical vomiting of children are also of nervous origin. Travel sickness is due to excessive stimulation by movement of certain structures in the internal ear. Certain diseases of the nervous system, such as tumors of the brain and meningitis, are frequently accompanied by vomiting, and it may also occur in concussion.

4. Pregnancy. Vomiting is a fairly constant symptom in the early months of pregnancy and usually occurs in the mornings.

Treatment. In vomiting due to swallowing poisonous substances, or eating tainted food the symptoms may be relieved by dilution of the stomach contents with a large draught of water, or still better, a drink of sodium bicarbonate, a level teaspoonful to a glassful of water. Such alkaline drinks may be repeated and, if relief is not obtained, complete evacuation by stomach washout will bring relief (see p. 39).

With severe vomiting, complete rest in bed, lying down with the head low, is advisable. No food should be taken for the time being, but water may, as a rule, be allowed freely. Iced drinks, especially effervescing drinks such as soda water, are often better retained. Champagne, especially when iced, has a deserved reputation, but care must be taken to see that it is taken only in moderation.

When vomiting persists in patients already debilitated by an exhausting illness, rectal injections of saline and glucose should be employed.

Local Applications to the upper abdomen are sometimes helpful: hot-water bottles or compresses will provide heat, ice-bags provide cold, and mustard plasters may be used in hysterical vomiting.

Motion Sickness

Causes. This is a disorder of the nervous system produced by unaccustomed stimulation of the eyes and of the organs of balance in the internal ear. There are also certain added factors which act by suggestion, such as apprehension from previous experience, cold, odor, dyspepsia, and the presence of others suffering from sickness. Small infants are immune from the affection, and old people are usually relatively immune. Children, however, are somewhat prone to car-sickness especially in well-sprung vehicles.

Treatment. To avoid motion sickness, a susceptible subject should, for two or three days before traveling, eat only a plain and simple diet, with extra sugar added, and avoid alcohol and overtiredness. He should take regular exercise and see that the bowels are well moved. It is wise to take a good wholesome meal about two hours before the journey.

Relief from sea and motion sickness may be obtained by taking, an hour or two before the journey begins, a tablet containing hyoscine or an antihistamine. As a remedy for seasickness Dramamine is an almost ideal drug. It exerts its effects in approximately half an hour, and protection lasts for about 4 hours. All women in early pregnancy should avoid taking any of these potent drugs.

While under the influence of any of these drugs, travelers may temporarily experience slight mental dulling or drowsiness. It is therefore most unwise to drive a car for several hours after taking a tablet.

On a ship, the symptoms may be mitigated by a position amidships, where the tilting movements are least, by lying on the back with the head low, and by keeping warm. In an airplane, ascents and descents should not be watched through the window.

During the attack it is essential to keep as warm and quiet as possible. Swallowing food should be insisted upon, and the administration of very small, perfectly dry meals, such as cold chicken and crackers, will often stop the vomiting and stimulate the appetite. Glucose or barley sugar can be taken by most people, and is a valuable and easily assimilated food. In a prolonged attack with serious loss of body fluids, water should be given by mouth, or 2 or 3 teaspoonsful of glucose dissolved in water. Iced brandy and water, iced champagne, or cherry brandy may be sipped, and an occasional dose of aromatic spirits of ammonia (15 to 20 drops in half a glass of water) may be effective. In a severe case the patient should always be brought on deck into the open air after four days in the cabin.

Hematemesis

(*Vomiting of Blood*)

Causes. Hematemesis results most frequently from a chronic ulcer of the stomach, and less frequently from a duodenal ulcer. It may occur in smaller quantities in cancer of the stomach, and from varicose veins of the esophagus (gullet) in alcoholic individuals with cirrhosis. It may be due to the swallowing and subsequent vomiting of blood which has come from the nose, mouth or lungs. Finally, it may occur (in susceptible individuals) from the taking of aspirin, especially if the tablets are swallowed whole and apart from meals.

Diagnosis. The amount of blood vomited may vary from a few ounces to several pints. *Hematemesis* must be distinguished from *Hemoptysis* (coughing of blood from the lungs); in the former, the blood is generally dark, partly clotted, and mixed with more or less food, whereas in the latter it is bright red, frothy, and unclotted. Hematemesis is always followed by the passage of dark tarry stools (melena). Hence it is important always to inspect the stools for several days after an attack.

Treatment. The most important factor in the treatment is rest, which must continue for at least three or four weeks. No undue haste should be displayed in moving a patient from the place in which the hemorrhage has occurred, and it is far better for him to lie quietly on the floor in his clothes until the preliminary period of shock has passed than that he should be hurriedly undressed and carried a long distance to his bed. Once in bed, he must be kept lying flat on his back with the head low, and must on no account be allowed to move himself. He should not leave the bed even to pass water, nothing being allowed to disturb his complete rest for 24 to 48 hours after the hemorrhage appears to have stopped. To keep him at rest and allay anxiety, an injection of morphine and sometimes atropine is usually given. The room is kept quiet and semi-darkened, and a hot-water bottle, carefully covered, is applied to the feet. The pulse rate is taken half-hourly or hourly, and the blood pressure measured by a doctor.

When vomiting ceases, feeding by mouth begins at once with two-hourly 200 ml feedings of skimmed milk; the diet is rapidly increased to puree foods by the third day. A useful addition to the diet is glucose, 1 kilogram of glucose being dissolved in 1.1 liters of boiling water (about 2 lbs to a quart). Flavored with the juice of two lemons, this makes a palatable drink, of which half a cupful may be given at a time between the feedings of milk.

Two-hourly feeding should be continued on the second and third days, the diet being varied with cereals, an egg beaten up in milk, with a buttered rusk, a slice of thin crustless white bread and butter, vegetable purée, custard, jelly, or junket, fruit purée, and an ounce of cream.

Feeds should be continued during the night when the patient is awake, and should consist of 200 ml of milk or of an egg beaten up in milk. An ounce of strained orange or tomato juice should be given three times a day.

No purgatives should be given, the bowels generally opening spontaneously on the third day. An enema, if it should be necessary, should not be given until after the fifth day.

BLOOD TRANSFUSION. Patients who have had a severe hemorrhage will have been transferred to hospital where the blood group will be checked and hemoglobin estimated. If the patient's pulse rate continues to be high and does not fall steadily and there are obviously further hemorrhages occuring or continuous bleeding, immediate blood transfusion is vitally necessary. This is particularly important for elderly patients who may need massive transfusion. Those under the age of 35 usually recover without transfusion.

GASTRITIS

Acute Gastritis

Causes. Acute inflammation of the stomach results from a severe irritation of the mucous lining of the stomach. This may result from 'chill,' especially in the tropics, or it may be due to errors of diet, such as the ingestion of a large quantity of indigestible food, or an excessive amount of concentrated alcohol, particularly spirits, such as whisky or gin. Food or drink which is already contaminated with the organisms of food poisoning is a fairly common cause. The symptoms of 'gastric influenza' are due to the acute gastritis produced by the toxin of influenza. Finally, the ingestion of irritant poisons such as arsenic, phosphorus, corrosive sublimate, and concentrated acids and alkalis will result in a chemical burn of the stomach wall which gives rise to a severe form of acute gastritis.

Symptoms. A sensation of fulness or discomfort is felt in the upper abdomen, and in severe cases there is acute pain. The appetite is lost and thirst is great. The tongue is covered with thick fur, and there is an unpleasant taste in the mouth. Vomiting, preceded by nausea, almost always occurs, and gives more or less relief to the discomfort and pain. Since the irritant usually acts on the bowel as well as on the stomach, the vomiting is often accompanied by diarrhea. There is also much general constitutional disturbance, with slight fever, headache and general prostration.

Treatment. The first measure is to remove the irritant cause as quickly and as safely as possible. Vomiting may be induced by drinking copious quantities of warm water in which sodium bicarbonate has been dissolved (1 level teaspoonful to the pint). This can be continued until the vomit is returned free from altered food. If the vomiting is very persistent, the stomach should be washed out through a stomach tube with sodium bicarbonate solution. If the effects of a known poison are recognized, or a clear history is obtained, the appropriate therapy (see Poisons and Antidotes, p. 39) should be given after the stomach has been washed out. To rid the bowel of the irritant, a dose of castor oil, 1 or 2 tablespoonsful, may be taken with advantage, but *not* if there is any suspicion of appendicitis. As an alternative, a dose of Epsom Salts, or a large dose of effervescent saline may be given.

REST. The next principle in treatment is to secure rest, both for the patient and for the inflamed stomach. In all but the slightest cases, rest in bed is advisable until the acute symptoms have subsided. Hot applications such as a covered hot-water bottle may be placed on the abdomen, unless the patient is in a state of shock when warm blankets are better.

Rest for the inflamed stomach is best secured by preliminary starvation for 24 to 48 hours. During this time, water alone should be allowed, in small amounts, at intervals of half to one hour.

DIET. When the acute symptoms have disappeared, barley water, rice water, sweetened arrowroot made with water (not with milk), or jelly preparations may be given. When such feedings are well tolerated, and the appetite is returning, a cautious advance may be made with milk diluted with water or mineral water, fruit juices, bouillon, chicken broth, eggs beaten up in milk, soft boiled or poached eggs, junkets, jellies, custards, or milk puddings. Fish, chicken, and meat are gradually added until a more or less ordinary diet may be taken at the end of the week.

Chronic Gastritis

Causes. Chronic gastritis is due to long-continued irritation of the stomach lining by mechanical or chemical means. It is often the sequel of repeated attacks of acute gastritis, but more usually the result of dietetic errors of long duration, from insufficient mastication, bolting of food, the excessive consumption of strong tea and coffee, pickles, condiments and over-indulgence in alcohol, especially of spirits taken on an empty stomach. Long-continued and excessive smoking on an empty stomach will also cause gastritis.

Persons who suffer from severe pyorrhea or infected tonsils may swallow large quantities of germ-laden mucus, and develop chronic gastritis as a result, while it is often seen as a secondary effect of chronic congestion of the stomach in people suffering from chronic bronchitis, heart disease, or cirrhosis of the liver.

Symptoms. The most common symptom is nausea, especially in the early morning, leading to loss of appetite. It is characteristic of alcoholic gastritis that the patient may be unable to eat any breakfast, although he has a good appetite for the remaining meals of the day. Early morning vomiting may occur if nausea is severe, the vomited matter consisting largely of mucus and swallowed saliva. The tongue is often furred, and the patient may complain of a bad taste in the mouth. A sense of fulness or pressure in the upper abdomen is not uncommon, but actual pain is rare; it follows immediately after meals, especially if they are rich and heavy. The patient suffering from chronic gastritis is liable to be irritable and depressed.

Treatment. Attention should be directed towards the cause, dental treatment being prescribed where necessary, and septic tonsils removed. Alcohol should be rigorously avoided, and smoking limited to a few cigarettes a day after meals. In severe cases the diet should be similar to that of gastric ulcer (p. 365), and in all cases attractive small meals should be provided regularly with short intervals between; half an hour's rest should be taken after meals.

The bowels should be kept active by taking stewed fruit from which seeds and skins have been separated, and honey. If necessary, a saline laxative may be taken.

In severe cases, the stomach may need to be washed out every morning for a time with a solution containing 1 to 4 teaspoonsful of hydrogen peroxide to a pint of warm water. Alternatively, a level teaspoonful of sodium bicarbonate in a glass of soda water first thing in the morning and again before meals throughout the day.

GASTRIC AND DUODENAL ULCERS

(*Peptic Ulcers*)

Causes. The mucous lining of the healthy stomach is always bathed in gastric juice which is composed chiefly of the digestive ferment pepsin, together with free hydrochloric acid. Normally these digestive juices act only on the food in the stomach. If the hydrochloric acid becomes either too strong or is made in too great a quantity, it may act on the stomach wall as well as on the food. A peptic or digestive ulcer is the result of local destruction of the mucous membrane and the underlying tissues of the stomach wall in the case of a gastric ulcer, while a duodenal ulcer occurs in the upper one and a half inches of the duodenum. Such an ulcer may be acute or, more commonly, it may be chronic and persist for years.

Gastric ulcers are more common in men than in women, while duodenal ulcers are three or four times more frequent in men.

About 10 per cent of all people have a tendency to secrete more and stronger hydrochloric acid than normal, and it is these who are most likely to develop a gastric or duodenal ulcer. This tendency is increased by excessive smoking. Emotional depression and anxiety are common causes of peptic ulcer in those who are predisposed, especially when associated with fatigue, while the bolting and imperfect mastication of coarse and highly seasoned food, and the swallowing of germs from infected teeth and tonsils may cause repeated injury to the mucous membrane, and in time cause an ulcer.

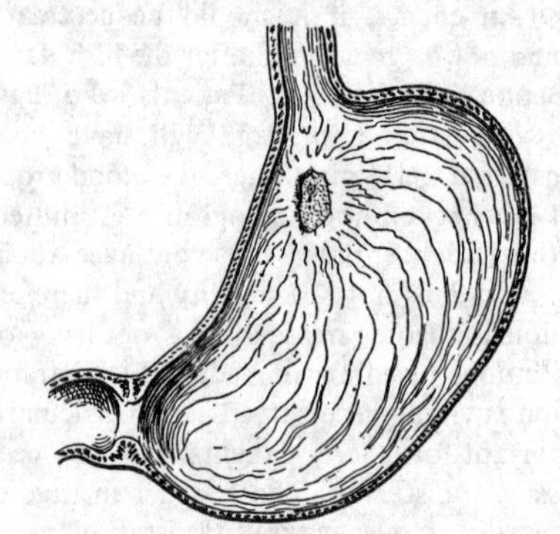

Fig. 2. *GASTRIC ULCER. Interior of the stomach showing a chronic gastric ulcer with erosion of the mucous membrane.*

Symptoms

In Gastric Ulcer, the onset is generally insidious, the symptoms first appearing after big or indigestible meals, and consisting of discomfort or fullness coming on between half an hour and two hours after meals. This discomfort is gradually replaced by pain, which is often burning in character and may be very severe; it is felt in the middle of the upper abdomen, rather nearer to the navel than to the lower end of the breast-bone. The pain generally disappears spontaneously after about an hour, and is also relieved by alkalis and by vomiting.

In Duodenal Ulcer, the symptoms are similar, but the pain occurs at a longer interval (two or three hours) after meals, and it often wakes the patient in the early part of the night, between 1 and 2 a.m. The pain is often associated with a feeling of hunger, and is more or less completely relieved by taking food; it is therefore commonly known as a 'hunger pain.'

In peptic ulcer, periods of hunger pain lasting some weeks or months tend to alternate with periods of more or less complete freedom from symptoms. These attacks tend to occur regularly for a few weeks every spring and autumn, and a history of such waves of remission and relapse over many years is almost diagnostic. Attacks are liable to be brought on suddenly by worry, exposure to cold, an acute infection of the breathing passages (tonsillitis, bronchitis, etc.), an indigestible meal, and by excessive smoking and drinking. With increasing pain, vomiting may develop, especially in gastric ulcer. It occurs at the height of a pain, a small quantity of acid fluid with a little digested food being brought up. Constipation is commonly present, but the appetite remains good, and the patient does not usually lose weight or strength.

A diagnosis of suspected peptic ulcer should be confirmed by X-ray examination after a barium meal (see p. 565).

Complications

Hemorrhage occurs in about 20 per cent of all cases of peptic ulcer. In gastric ulcer it shows itself in the vomiting of blood (hematemesis, p. 363), and in duodenal ulcer in the passing of black tarry stools (melena). A sudden large hemorrhage may be accompanied by faintness, pallor, thirst, restlessness. with 'air-hunger' and a small rapid pulse.

Perforation. This is the most serious complication of peptic ulcer, and is especially likely to occur in duodenal ulcer. It is marked by the sudden onset of severe upper abdominal pain which gradually becomes more diffuse and severe, with board-like rigidity of the abdominal muscles. It requires the earliest possible treatment by operation, without which it leads to general peritonitis, and may be fatal. The success of surgery, however, is remarkable, even after perforation of the stomach wall has existed for several hours.

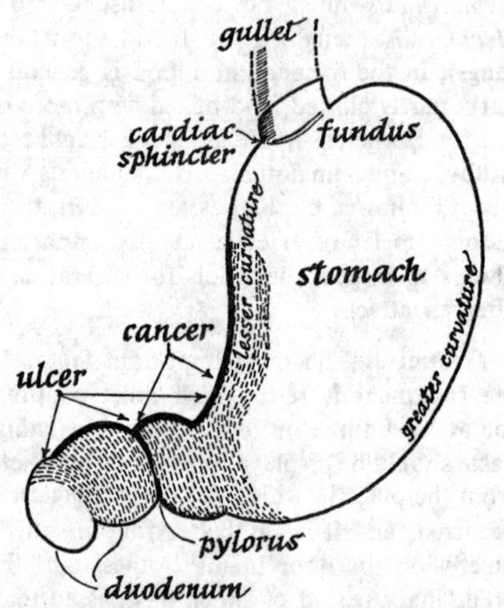

Fig. 3. *PEPTIC ULCER and CANCER. The shaded areas show the sites in the stomach and duodenum most commonly affected by peptic ulcer and by cancer.*

Obstruction of the digestive tract. Inflammatory swelling around a large ulcer, especially in the duodenum, may lead to intermittent spasmodic obstruction, the first symptom of which is generally vomiting. In time, actual scarring may cause persistent obstruction, the treatment of which is surgical.

Malignant Degeneration may occasionally occur in a large chronic gastric ulcer, and should be suspected if there is increased pain without remissions, and associated loss of appetite and vomiting.

Treatment of Peptic Ulcer

The healing of a chronic peptic ulcer is a long process, and strict treatment is necessary for at least six months in order to avoid breaking down of the ulcer before it is healed.

1. **Rest.** The most important factor in the promotion of healing is rest, both mental and physical. The patient should therefore be kept in bed for a period of four to six weeks, getting up only to have a bath and to move the bowels. Circumstances may sometimes shorten the full period of complete rest, but rest in bed is essential at first.

2. **Diet.** Next in importance is a suitable non-irritating diet.

HOURLY FEEDING SCHEDULE

(a) Every other hour from 8 a.m. to 10 p.m. 5 ounces of milk are given. This can be warm or cold, or flavored with tea. 600 milligrams of sodium citrate in a little water should be added to each milk feed.

(b) Every other hour from 9 a.m. to 9 p.m. give a 5-ounce feed of arrowroot, malted milk, junket, or custard. To any of these redcurrant or apple jelly can be added. At least two of these feeds should consist of a thick soup or semi-solid purée of potato, artichoke, cauliflower, or parsnip.

(c) A coddled egg, prepared by placing a fresh egg in boiling water, and allowing it to stand without further boiling for 5 to 8 minutes, or a boiled, scrambled or poached egg may be taken twice a day.

(d) Toast with butter, plain biscuit, thin bread and butter with honey, molasses, syrup or jelly, or a piece of sponge cake, may be eaten with any of the feeds.

(e) One ounce of cream should be added to the 11 a.m., 1 p.m. and 5 p.m. feedings, and ½ an ounce of olive oil should be taken before the 9 a.m., 2 p.m. and 7 p.m. feedings.

(f) An ounce of strained tomato or grapefruit juice should be taken with three of the remaining feedings.

(g) An additional feeding should be given each time the patient wakes during the night, and for this purpose he should always have some citrated milk at the bedside.

This strict diet should be continued for at least four weeks, and gradually be replaced by the following scheme.

TWO-HOURLY FEEDING SCHEDULE

On waking. A glass of milk.

Breakfast (8 a.m.). Orange juice or tomato juice, 1 ounce well diluted with water.
Strained cereal with milk.
1 egg, boiled, scrambled or poached, or grilled or steamed white fish.
2 thin slices of cold buttered toast. Honey or jelly.
Weak tea.

11 a.m. A glass of milk, malted milk.
Plain biscuit.

Lunch (1 p.m.). White fish (creamed or soufflé), or minced chicken or tender meat or tripe, or an omelet. Potato, mashed or purée.
Carefully sieved green vegetables, or carrot or turnip.
Fruit jelly or purée of fruit, or junket, egg custard or milk pudding, served with cream or milk.

3 p.m. A glass of milk and plain biscuit.

Tea (5 p.m.). Weak tea, freshly prepared.
2 thin slices of crisp buttered toast, or thin bread and butter, with honey, treacle, syrup or jelly.
Plain biscuit or sponge cake.

Dinner (7 p.m.). As at lunch.

Supper (9 p.m.). Glass of milk.
Plain biscuit.

During the night. A glass of milk should be kept at the bedside to be taken, if awake, during the night.

GENERAL DIRECTIONS. Two pints of milk should be taken daily and butter should be used freely. A tablespoonful of olive oil or cream should be taken in addition, a quarter of an hour before the four main meals. Extra vitamins should be supplied. The mouth should be washed out after each feeding.

3. **Alkalis.** These are prescribed in order to neutralize the excess acid in the stomach. A useful prescription is:

Calcium carbonate	..	2 parts
Heavy magnesium carbonate		2 parts
Bismuth carbonate	..	1 part

200 grams of the powder will be sufficient.

The dose is one teaspoonful or more in water or milk, half an hour after the four main meals, last thing at night, and when indigestion or heartburn is felt.

4. **Antispasmodics.** Where pain is persistent, especially at night, despite careful dieting and the use of antacids, antispasmodics may be taken to reduce the secretion of gastric juice and to relieve spasm of the pylorus.

5. **Constipation** can usually be prevented by the use of magnesia or a paraffin emulsion, such as agarol or petrolagar, but if the bowels are not opened on two consecutive days, a suppository or an enema should be given.

6. **Smoking** As smoking delays healing, it must be forbidden during the early stages of treatment (2 to 3 months).

7. **Teeth.** Diseased teeth must be attended to, and provision made for adequate mastication in future.

Post-ulcer Régime. *This continuation treatment should be followed permanently.*

It is futile to give a patient with a peptic ulcer a period of six months' strict treatment if steps are not taken to prevent the recurrence of the ulcer after it has healed. Therefore he must be given a régime which he must follow for the rest of his life. It must be explained that his recent illness is the result of a constitutional tendency, and that a recurrence is almost certain if he returns to the conditions of life which preceded its onset. However long he remains free from symptoms, he must keep to the new régime, as he will never outgrow the constitutional tendency.

It is quite easy to arrange for 2-hourly feedings in almost every civil occupation with the help of two or three pints of milk. A truck driver, farm laborer, or clerk can take the milk with him in a bottle, and have a drink as often as necessary, and tablets of Maalox® or Gelusil® can be taken at intervals in almost any circumstances.

Instructions to the patient which are to be followed permanently.

1. For the first six months. A meal or feeding of milk, plain biscuit, or chocolate should be taken at intervals of not more than two hours from waking to retiring, and again if awake during the night.

After six months of complete freedom from symptoms, a feeding should be taken in the middle of the morning, on going to bed, and again if awake during the night, in addition to breakfast, lunch, tea and dinner. Take plenty of milk, eggs, butter and cream, and a teaspoonful of olive oil before each meal.

2. Eat slowly, and chew very thoroughly. Adequate time must be allowed for meals. Rest for at least a quarter of an hour before and after the principal meals. Avoid taking a meal when tired; when there is not time for a proper meal, it is better to drink some milk, or eat some chocolate or biscuits, than to bolt some less digestible solid food.

3. Do not smoke more than six cigarettes or two pipes a day. They should be smoked *only* after meals. Do not smoke at all if you have any indigestion.

4. During periods of overwork, especially of mental stress, whenever possible one day or half day a week should be spent resting in bed or on a couch, or lying out of doors, on a strict 2-hourly diet. If you are much worried or are sleeping badly, ask your doctor for a sedative.

5. Special care should be taken to avoid chills. If you get a cold, sore throat, influenza or other infection remain in bed on a very light diet until you have completely recovered.

6. Magnesia may be taken for the bowels if necessary, but other laxatives should not be used.

7. Take no drugs or pills in tablet form. Take no aspirin, or tablet containing aspirin, as this is a common cause of hemorrhage in the stomach.

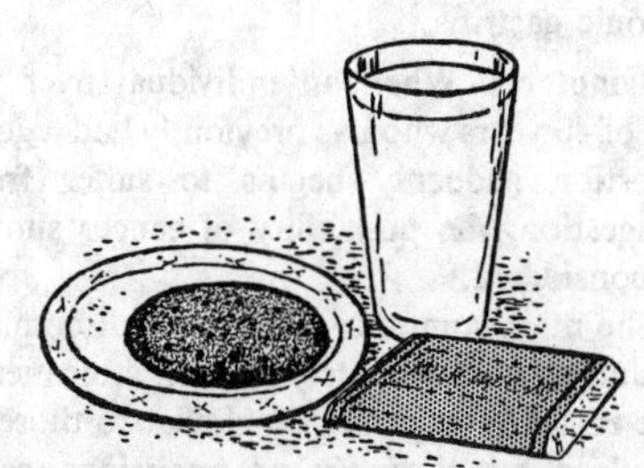

Fig. 4. *FOR THE ULCER PATIENT. Milk, plain biscuits and chocolate are sustaining foods for those suffering from peptic ulcer.*

8. If you have the slightest return of symptoms, go to bed on a strict diet at once. Consult your doctor, and do not wait for the symptoms to become serious.

9. *Avoid the following:*

(a) Alcohol. If desired later on, a small quantity of beer, light wine or diluted whisky may be taken with (but never before) meals.

Effervescing drinks and coffee (except the de-caffeinated varieties).

Strong tea.

(b) Seeds and skins of fruit (raw, cooked or in jam), raisins, currants, figs, ginger and lemon peel in puddings and cakes, nuts and all unripe fruit. An orange may be sucked but not eaten. Currants, raisins and figs are particularly undesirable.

(c) All raw vegetables (celery, tomatoes, radishes, cucumber and watercress), whether taken alone or in pickles and salad.

Spinach, stringy beans and hard peas and beans. Coarse green vegetables (cabbage, etc.) must be passed through a sieve and mixed with butter in the form of a purée.

(d) Coarse oatmeal. Wholemeal and new bread.

(e) Tough or twice-cooked meat; pork and game.

Clear and thick meat soup.

Salted meat or fish. Left over and fried dishes, especially fried fish.

Very ripe cheese and cooked cheese.

(f) Highly seasoned foods.

Mustard, pepper, vinegar, pickles. Excess of salt.

Lemon juice and sour fruit.

If in doubt about any food, remember that you must not eat anything which cannot be chewed into a soft pulpy mass.

Operation is required only rarely for peptic ulcer and in the following conditions:

1. at the earliest moment after perforation;
2. if there are symptoms of persistent obstruction to the emptying of the stomach, in spite of continued medical treatment; and
3. if there is reason to suspect malignancy, with persistent pain, bleeding, loss of appetite and vomiting.

CANCER OF THE STOMACH

Causes. Cancer or carcinoma of the stomach is commonest between the ages of 45 and 65, and is more common in men than in women. It may occasionally develop from a chronic gastric ulcer, or it may be a sequel of chronic gastritis.

Symptoms. When an individual over the age of 40 years who has previously had a good digestion suddenly begins to suffer from indigestion, the possibility of cancer should be considered.

The most common symptom is discomfort or dull pain immediately or soon after meals. The earliest symptoms are similar to those of an ulcer, but there are no remissions, as in the case of simple ulcer, and the pain is not relieved by taking food. The appetite is lost at an early stage. Flatulence is commonly present, the gas which is brought up being at first odorless, but subsequently foul.

Vomiting is generally present sooner or later; the vomited matter may contain blood, and often has the look of 'coffee grounds.'

The patient rapidly loses weight and strength, and anemia generally follows the constant oozing of blood from the ulcerated growth.

The condition may be diagnosed by an X-ray examination of the stomach by means of a barium test meal, and these investigations should always be performed if there is reason to suspect a malignant growth of the stomach. If neglected, it may lead to cancerous deposits elsewhere.

Treatment. In all cases in which there is no evidence of involvement of the liver or peritoneum by extension of the growth, an operation should be performed. With proper preparation and skillful surgery, many apparently inoperable growths can be completely removed.

Once a decision to operate has been taken, it is advisable that the patient's general condition be improved as far as will be possible. Blood transfusion should be given to counteract the anemia which is usually present and the loss of fluid through vomiting should be made good with water containing electrolytes.

In cases which are inoperable, medical treatment can only be palliative.

THE DIET should be as for gastric ulcer, (p. 365). Small feedings are best, and all food should be reduced to an easily digestible form by mincing or pounding of meat and fish, and by passing vegetables through a fine sieve. Raw eggs, beaten up in milk, oysters, and ice-cream will all find a useful place in the diet.

Parenteral feeding is quite unsatisfactory in these cases and attempts to use it only add to the discomfort of the patients.

MEDICATION. If there are any symptoms of obstruction to the outlet of the stomach, with persistent vomiting, lavage of the stomach may be required, a solution of bicarbonate of soda, 1 level teaspoonful to the pint of warm water, being used for the purpose. This is an important palliative measure which is far too seldom employed.

DISEASES OF THE INTESTINES

THE SMALL INTESTINE consists of the duodenum, a tube ten inches long connecting the stomach to the twenty-two feet of small intestine proper—jejunum and ileum (see Fig. 5).

THE LARGE INTESTINE, which extends from the cecum (in the right lower abdomen) to the rectum, is about five feet long.

For details of the normal functioning of the intestines, see section on Physiology, p. 249.

Examination of the Intestines

Palpation of the Abdomen with the hand may detect the presence of a lump or new growth in the intestine, while tenderness may be present in certain intestinal diseases, especially in appendicitis and diverticulitis.

X-ray Examination may enable the condition of the intestines as a whole to be visualized, by the use either of a barium meal by mouth, or of a barium enema by the rectum. It is of value especially in cases of obstruction of the large intestine and in diverticulitis (inflammation of the pelvic colon).

Sigmoidoscopy is used for the direct visual examination of the interior wall of the rectum and pelvic colon by the insertion via the rectum of an illuminated sigmoidoscope. It is of value when ulceration, as in amebic dysentery, diverticulitis or malignant disease of the colon, is suspected.

Examination of the Feces

A simple examination of the stools should not be omitted when a patient has symptoms of intestinal disease. The quantity, odor, color, consistency, and the presence or absence of abnormal constituents should be noted. In persons on a milk diet, the stools are very yellow in color, while in those taking much meat they are dark. When bile pigments do not reach the intestine, as in

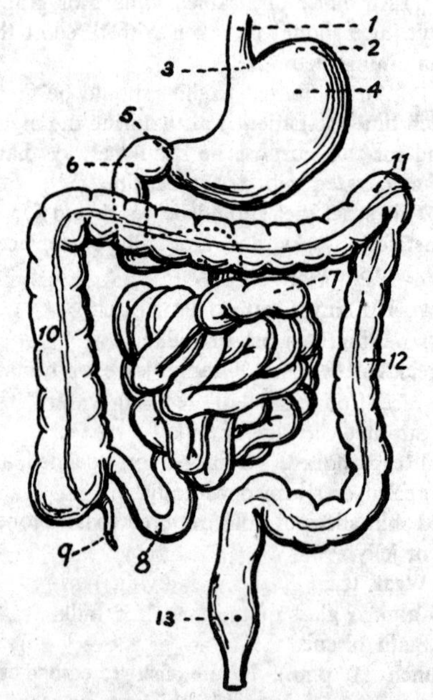

Fig. 5. *STOMACH AND INTESTINES.* 1. *Esophagus.* 2. *Fundus of stomach.* 3. *Cardiac sphincter.* 4. *Stomach.* 5. *Pyloric sphincter.* 6. *Duodenum.* 7. *Jejunum (small intestine).* 8. *Ileum (small intestine).* 9. *Appendix.* 10. *Ascending colon.* 11. *Transverse colon.* 12. *Descending colon.* 13. *Rectum.*

jaundice, the stools are pale or clay-colored.

Abnormal consituents are most easily recognized by microscopical examination.

Mucus. This occurs in two forms, as small flakes, intimately mixed with the feces, when it is usually due to inflammation or catarrh; or as jelly-like membranes coating the surface of hard fecal masses. The presence of mucus with constipated solid stools is not in itself a sign of disease, the mucus being secreted to protect the mucous membrane from the irritating effects of the hard masses as they pass along the bowel.

Blood. This may also be found in two different forms. Firstly as bright red blood derived from the intestine. The most usual cause is hemorrhoids, but it may also occur in cases of cancer or polyp of the lower bowel, and in dysentery. Secondly, as dark tarry-looking blood (melena) which usually originates from a bleeding gastric or duodenal ulcer, and which becomes partly digested in its passage through the intestines.

Occult blood, that is unobservable amounts only detectable by special tests of the feces, may be found in cases of intestinal tuberculosis and in any of the above disorders.

Pus indicates the presence of ulcerative colitis, or of malignant disease of the colon or rectum.

Excess of Fats. This is recognized by the pale, bulky and greasy nature of the stools, and generally indicates a failure of fat digestion through insufficiency of bile (as in obstructive jaundice) or of pancreatic juice.

Parasites. Many kinds of parasites may be found in the stools, the tapeworm, roundworm and threadworm are not uncommon. (See section on Intestinal Parasites, p. 385.)

FUNCTIONAL DISORDERS OF THE INTESTINES

Constipation, diarrhea, and pain (or colic) are the three most important symptoms caused by disorders of the intestines. Persistence of any of these symptoms should always be investigated, as they may be the result of serious organic disease.

Constipation

In the average person, evacuation of the bowels takes place once daily, but the event may occur twice daily, or only once in two days in persons of quite good health. For practical purposes an individual may be considered to be constipated if his bowels are not opened at least once every forty-eight hours.

Habitual constipation may be classified into two main types:

1. COLONIC CONSTIPATION, which is due either to sluggish action of the colon, or to spasm of the colon (spastic constipation).

2. DYSCHEZIA, a name applied by Hurst to distinguish those cases where the constipation is due to a loss of power to expel the contents of the rectum and pelvic colon. In persons of careless habits the feces frequently pass normally through the colon to the rectum, but owing to neglect of the urge to defecation, they accumulate and cause ballooning of the rectum, with loss of tone in its walls. A greater and greater amount of feces is therefore required to give the necessary stimulus for defecation. Dyschezia from inefficient defecation is the most common form of habitual constipation.

Causes. The causes of this disorder range from careless habit to serious organic diseases.

1. FAULTY HABITS. As mentioned above, dyschezia often originates in neglect to respond to the call to defecate owing to laziness, insanitary conditions of the toilet, or false modesty. Weakness of the muscles of defecation, and the assumption of an unsuitable posture during the act of defecation are subsidiary causes. Most people usually make an effort to move the bowels once a day, generally after breakfast. In modern conditions, the rush to school or to catch the morning train may interfere with the habit of regular defecation is broken the the sensation of the 'call to stool' once voluntarily suppressed may not easily return again throughout the day. Moreover, many schools and offices are inadequately provided with the necessary conveniences, and once the habit of regular defecation is broken the patient becomes constipated, and usually begins to take purgatives.

2. ERRORS OF DIET are often due to eating very concentrated foods, combined with an insufficient intake of fluid. Foods which are easily digested and which leave little residue, such as meat, fish, eggs and cheese, and especially a diet which is composed almost exclusively of milk, are often productive of troublesome constipation by failing to provide sufficient stimulus to the normal movements of the intestines.

3. DEFECTS IN NERVOUS CONTROL OF COLON. The influence of the mind in causing constipation is common enough knowledge. Some patients cannot move their bowels when nervous or worried or in unusual surroundings. Failure to move the bowels on the first day of a vacation is usually due to the unfamiliar lavatory, and perhaps to the unusual hour of getting up, such small changes being sufficient to upset the nervous control of defecation. Workers on alternate day and night shifts are likewise at a disadvantage and may become very worried about the failure of a previously regular habit.

The movements of the colon may be more consistently impaired by the loss of muscle tone which is apt to occur with sedentary habits, and in old age. Malnutrition, dropsy, or melancholia and depression are also associated with inactivity of the colon.

4. ORGANIC DISEASE OF COLON AND RECTUM. Intestinal obstruction from any cause, such as cancer of the colon, and painful affections of the rectum or anus, such as fissures, inflamed piles, etc., will give rise to constipation which tends to persist until the primary cause is removed.

Symptoms. Among the most common symptoms of constipation are loss of appetite, furred tongue, a bad taste in the mouth, flatulence, headaches, general mental and physical fatigue, irritability of temper, and pigmentation of the skin. Retention of hard masses of feces is a common cause of intestinal flatulence and colic, while accumulation and retention of feces in the rectum may lead to hemorrhoids, fissure of the anus and irritation of the skin around the anus (pruitus ani). Defecation may be painful if the feces are very hard.

Treatment of Faulty Habits. An effort to move the bowels should be made after breakfast, even when there is no desire to do so, and an urge to defecation at any other time should be obeyed at once. Sufficient time should be allowed for the act. For those who have little leisure in the morning, the evening may be a more suitable time.

The usual form of toilet is not well adapted for persons with weak abdominal muscles who need to do much straining. Help may be afforded by a footstool, nine to twelve inches lower than the seat, which allows an attitude more like the natural one of squatting. In severe cases the patient may squat over a bedpan placed on the floor.

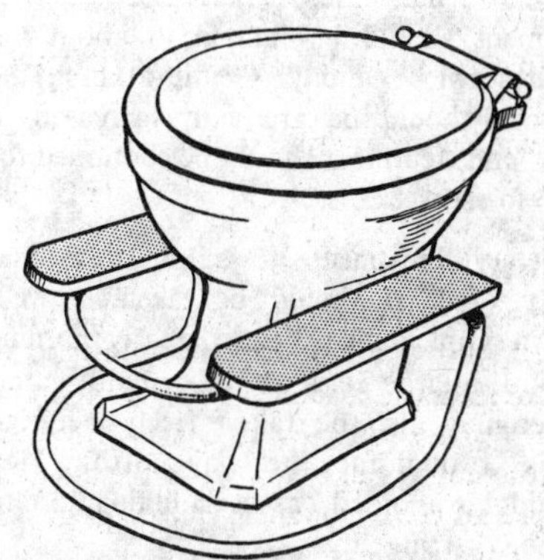

Fig. 6. *A POSTURE FOOTSTOOL for persons with weak abdominal muscles who suffer from\ constipation. The raised foot rests permit a posture nearer the natural one of squatting.*

Physical Treatment by exercises, massage, etc. Regular exercise in the open air is an effective means of preventing constipation, particularly for persons in sedentary occupations. Riding, rowing and gardening are especially suitable.

When outdoor exercise is impossible or insufficient, indoor exercises may be used for developing the abdominal muscles. They should be performed every morning and evening, and are particularly useful for women after child birth. The following exercises are useful:

Exercise I. The patient lies flat on the back on the floor with the hands by the side.

(a) The knees are drawn up to the chest, then straightened out at right angles to the trunk. With the knees kept stiff, the legs are slowly lowered until they touch the floor.

(b) Each leg in turn is slowly raised to a right angle with the body and slowly lowered again.

(c) The preceding exercise is repeated but with both legs together.

(d) The patient raises himself slowly into the sitting position without the use of the arms.

(e) From the sitting position, with the feet firmly on the floor, he sways himself backwards and forwards from the hips.

Exercise II. The patient is standing with the hands on the hips.

(a) Each leg is raised slowly until the knee touches the chin.

(b) The body is slowly rotated first in one direction, then in the other.

(c) The patient squats on his heels and then raises himself into the standing position again.

Abdominal Massage is also useful, and is most effective if applied by a trained masseur or masseuse. At first the duration of treatment should be limited to about ten minutes twice a day. Gentle at first, the massage should be gradually increased in force, and treatment should be continued for three to six weeks.

Dietary Treatment. It is important that plenty of fluid should be taken, a well-known simple remedy being the early morning drink of a large glass of hot or cold water. Water may also be taken freely between meals throughout the day. Strong tea should be avoided, as it contains tannin which is astringent.

It is important to see that sufficient food is taken, since constipation is often as much due to insufficient quantity as to unsuitable quality. The diet should contain an increased proportion of vegetable foods. Stewed prunes or figs at breakfast are valuable. Fresh, dried, stewed or canned fruit should be taken three times a day, and salad or green vegetables (lettuce, spinach, cabbage, cauliflower, onions or turnips) should be taken at lunch and dinner. Cereal and wholewheat bread are also useful, and sugar in the form of honey or molasses has mild laxative properties. An adequate amount of fat, butter, cream, margarine and olive oil, is of value; the olive oil may also be used as salad dressing or for cooking.

In constipation due to spastic colon, the diet prescribed for gastric ulcer (see pp. 365-66) containing only a small residue of indigestible matter, is more suitable.

Treatment by Medicinal Agents

(a) Occasional Constipation. For the treatment of occasional constipation which is liable to attack perfectly healthy individuals, especially after a change of habits or diet, a glycerin suppository may be inserted into the rectum. It should be followed the next morning by some saline laxative such as a teaspoonful of Epsom salts in water, or an effervescing saline preparation such as a Seidlitz powder. Other remedies valuable for occasional constipation are the vegetable laxatives such as cascara or senna.

(b) Habitual Constipation can be cured without drugs if proper treatment is started at a sufficiently early stage. In cases of inefficient emptying of the rectum, the indiscriminate use of purgatives will only cause colic. In diseases which are aggravated by co-existing constipation (neurasthenia and hypochondriasis, epilepsy, migraine, asthma, diabetes and Bright's disease) laxatives should be given regularly.

The stool produced by a laxative should be normal in appearance. The dose should be regulated so that one stool is passed every day, preferably shortly after breakfast. It should cause no discomfort and should not irritate the intestinal canal to cause mucus in the stools. It is therefore important to avoid the constant use of drastic purgatives.

Senna. An infusion of senna pods prepared by soaking the pods for six hours in cold water is one of the most generally useful preparations, since senna acts on the colon alone, and the dose can be regulated from day to day by the patient. An adult will usually need from six to twelve pods. An attempt should be made at intervals to reduce the number of pods one at a time until finally none may be required.

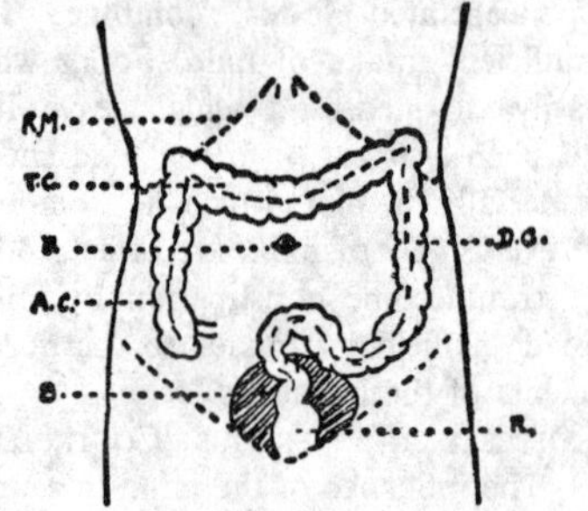

Fig. 7. *NORMAL COURSE OF COLON. R.M. Rib margin. T.C. Transverse colon. U. Umbilicus. D.C. Descending colon. A.C. Ascending colon. B. Bladder. R. Rectum.*

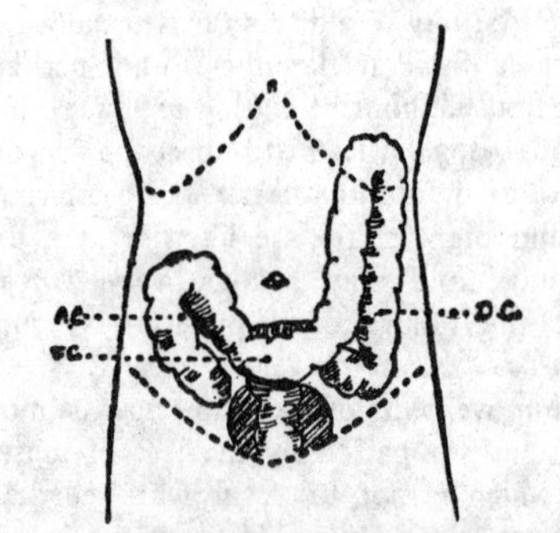

Fig. 8. *DROPPED COLON (Enteroptosis), a mechanical cause of constipation. A.C. Ascending colon. D.C. Descending colon. T.C. Transverse colon.*

Cascara. The virtues of cascara are so familiar that it is generally tried before medical advice is sought. It is often taken as tablets in the form of dry extract of cascara, but it usually acts more effectively when the liquid extract is used.

Lubricants. The various froms of mineral oil are household remedies for chronic constipation. The oil acts as a non-irritating lubricant, and is most serviceable in the slighter cases where the stools are particularly hard. Mineral oil (plain) should not be taken habitually (especially by children and nursing mothers since it prevents the absorption of vitamins by the lining of the intestine.

Mineral oil is often combined with agar-agar and, like plain oil, it is not absorbed. It remains in the bowel where it takes up a large amount of water, and increases the bulk of the feces.

Treatment by Enemas and Colonic Irrigations. The regular use of enemas and of continuous intestinal lavage with many pints of fluids is very harmful, and should be avoided in habitual constipation.

Enemas may, however, be used with advantage when the treatment of a case of constipation is first undertaken, in order that the lower bowel may be thoroughly emptied of any accumulation of hard feces. Soap and water solutions and saline washouts are among the simpler enemas for irrigating the rectum and colon. For softening very hard feces, olive oil or liquid paraffin may be used. Glycerin enemas or suppositories should only be used occasionally.

For the method of giving an enema, see Medical Procedures, p. 566.

Suppositories can be used. This preparation acts only on the large intestine and is particularly suitable for elderly persons.

Diarrhea

Diarrhea is a condition in which unformed loose or watery stools are passed, and are evacuated more often than normal, usually several times a day. The essential feature is the abnormally rapid passage of the intestinal contents through the bowel. It is not mere frequency of defecation, which may also occur in constipation.

Causes

Infection of the small intestine is by far the commonest cause of acute diarrhea, which is generally profuse and watery in type. It is generally due to the consumption of infected food or drink, e.g. decomposing and infected fish, or meat, or unwashed fruit, salads or vegetables, especially in tropical and semi-tropical climates. It may also occur as a result of rapid changes in the atmospheric temperature, leading to a chill to the surface of the body, and in this form is common among newcomers to the tropics, where hot days are apt to alternate with very cold nights, Similarly it may appear as a result of acute general infections such as abdominal influenza. (See also Food Poisoning, p. 42).

Infective diarrhea in newborn babies is usually only seen in institutions.

Diarrhea is also a constant symptom of acute inflammation of the large intestine (colon). Thus it is always present in ulcerative colitis and bacillary dysentery (which is common in tropical and semi-tropical climates) and is characterized by the presence of blood in the stools. Intestinal diarrhea may also occur in cancer of the colon.

MECHANICAL OVER-STIMULATION. A common cause of diarrhea is the habit of taking laxatives in excess of what is required. Mechanical over-stimulation of the intestine may also result from over-indulgence in green vegetables, salads and unripe fruits, and similar indiscretions of food and drink.

GASTRIC DIARRHEA may occur in cases where the gastric juice is deficient or absent (as in pernicious anemia and cancer of the stomach), so that undigested lumps of meat or vegetable leave the stomach and pass through the small intestine, where they act as irritants and are liable to undergo bacterial decomposition.

FATTY DIARRHEA. Deficient digestion of fat may give rise to fatty diarrhea in cases of jaundice, disease of the pancreas, sprue, and in tuberculosis of the abdominal lymph glands. In such cases the stools are pale in color and increased in bulk.

NERVOUS DIARRHEA. Diarrhea is a frequent manifestation of nervousness occurring as a result of emotional causes or chronic fatigue, where it is due to overexcitability of the nerves of the intestines. In certain individuals the bowels may be opened after every meal. Such diarrhea is chiefly troublesome because of the inconvenience it causes. Similarly, it is not uncommon for a fright or nervousness to cause the immediate passage of a semi-fluid stool.

Many people who have lived in the tropics and have suffered from attacks of diarrhea or dysentery continue to be liable to diarrhea for many years after they return to a temperate climate. Such patients have what may be described as a 'hair-trigger' colon, and they are particularly susceptible to chill.

Symptoms. The chief, and often the only symptom is the abnormally frequent passage of unformed stools. Colicky pain may be felt round the navel and, in severe cases, over the whole of the lower abdomen for a short time before the bowels are opened; it is generally relieved by the application of warmth. In severe and persistent cases there may be considerable loss of weight.

Diagnosis. Examination of the stools is of the greatest importance. In small intestine diarrhea (enteritis), the stools are watery, whereas in colitis they are semi-formed. The presence of blood, with or without pus, indicates ulceration from colitis or dysentery or from a malignant growth, provided that hemorrhoids can be excluded. Hemorrhage from a gastric or duodenal ulcer is recognized by the black tarry appearance (melena) of the stools.

PSEUDO-DIARRHEA. Certain forms of constipation may give rise to a condition known as pseudo-diarrhea. Thus a collection of hard feces in the rectum which is never completely evacuated may give rise to a secretion of clear mucus into the rectum, which is passed at intervals, either alone, or mixed with hard particles of feces. Likewise, a growth of the rectum or pelvic colon may cause faces to be partially retained above the growth while the fluid exuding from its surface may be evacuated at more or less frequent intervals.

Treatment of Acute Diarrhea

REST AND WARMTH. The patient should be kept warm and at rest in bed until the attack has subsided. Warmth may be applied to the abdomen by means of a hot bath or a hot-water bottle. For mild attacks temporary confinement to a warm room may be sufficient.

DIET. For severe cases no food should be given for 24 hours, but the patient may drink as much water, barley water or lemonade as he likes. Drinks should be neither too hot nor too cold, since either of these tends to increase the symptoms. If much collapsed, the patient may take a tablespoonful of brandy with an equal quantity of water every two hours.

At the end of 24 hours, sweetened arrowroot made with water (not with milk) may be given, but nothing else should be taken until the diarrhea has stopped. Next allowed are milk (diluted, if necessary, with an equal quantity of weak tea, water or lime water), junket, milk puddings (sago, tapioca or ground rice), egg custard, sweetened fruit juices, puree of potato, and bread and butter. No meat extract or meat soups, vegetables, fruits, nuts or brown bread should be taken until the condition is completely cured, when an ordinary diet can be resumed gradually.

MEDICINAL TREATMENT. If the diarrhea is due to food poisoning, the most valuable drug, and one which has stood the test of time, is castor oil in doses of 1 to 2 tablespoonsful for adults; it should be given, if available, within twelve hours of the onset of the attack. It may be disguised by brandy, milk, or warm malted milk, or taken in the form of gelatin capsules, each containing half a teaspoonful, the normal adult dose being from four to twelve capsules. In children, compound rhubarb powder (600 milligrams) is a valuable purgative for attacks of acute diarrhea.

In severe cases of infective diarrhea it is common to prescribe antibiotic preparations for 36 to 48 hours, followed, if necessary, by a kaolin preparation.

Treatment of Chronic Diarrhea

REST AND WARMTH. The successful treatment of chronic diarrhea depends upon the recognition of its cause, but in all cases recovery occurs most rapidly if the patient remains in bed for the first few days of treatment, the improvement being due to rest and warmth. It is important for him subsequently to avoid overexertion, and to keep the abdomen warm by means of a woolen binder, or an abdominal 'cholera belt,' the modern type of silk and wool being the best. Exposure to cold should be carefully avoided, and if the patient feels chilled at any time he should at once have a hot bath and go to bed. By this means a recurrence may be prevented. Patients who have recently suffered from chronic diarrhea should not go to the tropics, and should even avoid the Mediterranean, since even a slight intestinal upset is likely to have a more serious result than in the average individual.

DIET. Regulation of the diet calls for much care, and it is very important to avoid anything which will produce mechanical irritation of the bowel; the food should be thoroughly masticated, and articles such as new bread, hard cheese, tough meat, pickles and condiments should be avoided. Cooked green vegetables should be allowed only in the form of purees. The seeds and skins of fruit whether raw, cooked or in jams, and currants, raisins and lemon peel in puddings and cakes must be avoided. (See also diet for Gastric Ulcer, p. 365.) Boiled or steamed fish, eggs, junket, etc. may be given, but of meats, only tender lamb, veal, chicken, brains or tripe are suitable.

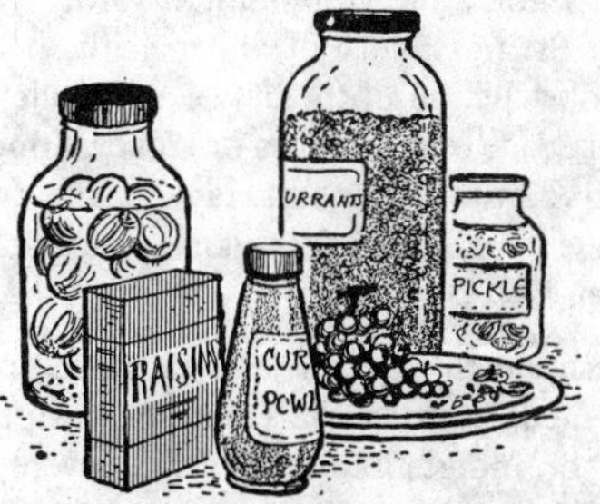

Fig. 9. *AVOID THESE FOODS in chronic diarrhœa. Pickles, raisins, currants, curries, and fruit seeds and skins.*

Fatty Diarrhea stops at once on a diet which is free of fat, cream, butter, etc.

Treatment of Nervous Diarrhea

This is more a social inconvenience than an actual disease, and is often not influenced by diet.

After meals or after some emotional disturbance, there is an urgent desire to defecate and loose stools are passed. This may occur so often that the patient fears to take part in social occasions such as traveling with friends or going to a concert.

The most effective drug is codeine since it has a constipating quality. It is taken in doses of 15 milligrams on waking and with meals. Somewhat larger doses may be required in certain cases. The patient should carry codeine phosphate tablets B.P. with him to use as necessary.

Intestinal Colic

(Stomach-ache)

By the term colic is meant a painful contraction of the intestines which gives rise to griping abdominal pains, often associated with considerable flatulent distension of the abdomen. It is a symptom found in many different affections of both the small and large intestine, the most common cause being the presence in the bowel of some irritating mass, e.g. indigestible food, especially unripe fruit, hard fecal masses in constipation, and intestinal worms. Flatulent colic (caused by intestinal gas) is often associated with severe constipation, and is apt to occur also in some individuals who are unable to digest starchy foods completely.

Symptoms. An attack of colic is generally felt in the region of the navel. It is usually relieved by pressure with the hands. Abrupt relief may follow the passage of gas by the anus.

Diagnosis. It is of the greatest importance to recognize the complaint in order to exclude the possibility of appendicitis, peritonitis, obstruction of the bowel, and colic from the passage of gall-stones or kidney stones. In children, the symptom may be due to the serious condition of intussusception of the bowel.

Treatment. Any obvious cause should be remedied, such as the eating of unripe raw fruit or indigestible foods, and severe constipation. A hot-water bottle should be applied to the abdomen, and in cases of severe colic, the safest practice is to attempt to empty the bowel by an enema. A large enema (1 to 2 pints) of soap and water, should be given; or 4 ounces of warmed olive oil or mineral oil may be introduced into the rectum and followed by an enema of salt and water (1 level teaspoonful to the pint).

In milder cases milk of magnesia may be given. It is important not to give castor oil if there is any suspicion of appendicitis, as it may cause an inflamed appendix to rupture, with resulting peritonitis.

Lead Colic

(Painter's Colic)

Lead colic is due to chronic lead poisoning, and was one of the most common of occupational risks. The lead is absorbed into the system chiefly by inhalation through the lungs, but it may be swallowed. Lead colic is often linked with lead neuropathy, usually in the form of wrist-drop of the right hand; there may also be a blue line along the gums, especially round infected or dirty teeth.

An acute attack of colic is usually preceded by several days of constipation. The pain is of a tearing nature and is situated round the navel.

Prevention of Lead Poisoning. The most important preventive measure consists in the elimination of dust and fumes containing lead in industries where lead is used. In addition to cleanliness in workrooms, the hands and face must be washed several times daily, and always before meals, and the teeth cleaned twice daily. No food or drink must be allowed in workrooms where lead is used. A diet high in calcium is a useful preventive measure, and in lead works it is customary for all workmen to be provided with a glass of milk each morning.

Treatment of an Attack of Lead Colic. Heat should be applied to the abdomen by hot-water bottles, and the bowels moved by an enema of olive oil or mineral oil (180 ml.), followed by warm water and salt (1 level teaspoonful of salt to the pint of water). A tablespoonful of magnesium sulphate in half a glass of water should be taken by mouth, followed by 2 cups of hot tea.

The doctor may give intravenously 10 milliliters of a 10 per cent solution of calcium gluconate. The diet should be rich in calcium (see p. 67) plus three pints of milk daily. This causes the lead to move into the bones and muscles.

Treatment of Lead Poisoning. Once the immediate colic has been relieved, the most effective treatment to rid the body of the lead is by the intravenous injection of sodium calcium edetate twice daily for up to five days.

ORGANIC DISEASES OF THE INTESTINES

Enteritis of Small Intestine

Acute enteritis forms an important part of the picture in most cases of acute food poisoning, and 'gastric influenza,' and gives rise to watery diarrhea. It is usually associated with acute gastritis (p. 363), when vomiting is associated with the diarrhea. The treatment is as for Acute Diarrhea (p. 369).

For the causes, diagnosis and treatment of chronic enteritis (chronic inflammation of the bowels), see Chronic Diarrhea, pp. 368-69.

Colitis of Large Intestine

Acute Colitis or inflammation of the colon occurs most frequently as a result of food poisoning, and is usually associated with acute gastritis and enteritis, the chief symptoms being diarrhea with frequent fluid and offensive stools. For treatment see Treatment of Acute Diarrhea, p. 369. For treatment of acute colitis due to dysentery see pp. 270 and 385.

Chronic Colitis is a more established condition and has several causes.

Causes. Chronic colitis may be the sequel to an attack of acute colitis, or the colitis due to some specific infection such as bacillary or amebic dysentery (pp. 270 and 385). The most usual cause, however, is the habitual use of purgatives, which are often taken even when constipation does not exist, and the habitual consumption of an undue amount of roughage in the diet.

Symptoms. There is discomfort and a sensation of fulness in the lower abdomen, which is usually somewhat distended and tender. The discomfort is generally worse after meals, and is relieved if the bowels are well opened. Diarrhea is usually present and the stools contain mucus and occasionally traces of blood. If blood is present the patient should be examined for hemorrhoids (piles), and if these do not exist further investigations should be undertaken to exclude the existence of chronic dysentery, ulcerative colitis or cancer of the colon. These investigations necessitate detailed examination of the stools, including microscopical examination and X-ray examination of the bowels by means of a barium enema.

Treatment. The teeth should be put into good order and the food thoroughly masticated. The diet should be as for gastric ulcer (p. 365). (See Treatment of Chronic Diarrhea, p. 369.)

Chronic Ulcerative Colitis

This is a special form of colitis in which there is a surface ulceration of the bowel wall. It is particularly important because of the serious state of ill health and emaciation to which it may lead.

Causes. It is a common disorder in England, and is almost entirely confined to adults between the ages of 20 and 40 years, women being affected more often than men. It is possible that some cases are the result of infection with dysentery bacteria or amoeba, the condition becoming chronic. On the other hand there is no doubt that the disease may appear soon after some acute mental or psychological disturbance, which suggests some disturbance of the nervous control of the bowel. Patients suffering from this complaint nearly all have unusual or abnormal personalities, being tense, sensitive, overconscientious, shy and timid, as well as having some superimposed emotional disturbance. Much of the abnormality is due to the disease itself and improves as the intestinal condition improves.

The disease usually runs a chronic course for many months, the symptoms being worse periodically. Relapses are especially liable to occur after worry and fatigue from mental or physical overwork, exposure to cold and damp, and with acute infections such as tonsillitis.

Symptoms. The onset is usually slow and insidious, the first symptoms being the passage of blood and mucus, usually with diarrhea. In the fully developed condition diarrhea is always present, and as many as twenty to forty stools, most of which are quite small, may be passed in the day. Blood, pus and

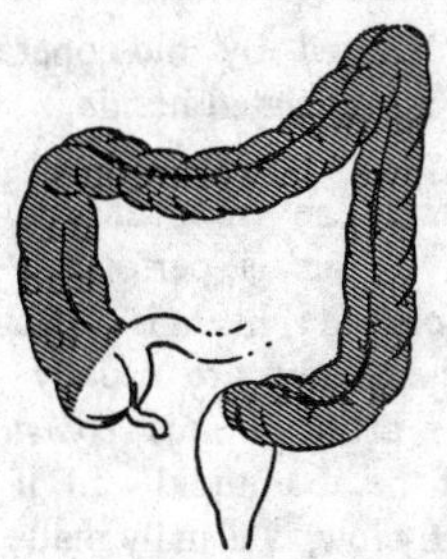

Fig. 10. *SITE OF ULCERATIVE COLITIS. The shaded area of the colon or large intestine indicates the portion of the bowel in which ulcerative colitis may occur.*

mucus are constantly passed, either alone, or with semi-fluid feces. The blood is bright red, and never produces the black tarry stools (melena) seen in hemorrhage from gastric and duodenal ulcers.

Discomfort is usually present in the lower abdomen and in the rectum, but actual pain or colic is rare; when it occurs, it disappears as soon as the bowels are opened, especially if gas is passed. The constant diarrhea leads, in time, to loss of weight and emaciation, and to the development of abscesses round the anus, while the loss of blood causes severe anemia. In the course of healing the bowel may become narrowed from scarring of the ulcers in its walls.

Diagnosis. The presence of blood, pus, and mucus in the stools indicates either ulcerative colitis or a growth of the pelvic colon or rectum. If the patient has been in the East, or in tropical climates the possibility of amoebic dysentery should be considered.

Treatment. The treatment of ulcerative colitis is bound to be very prolonged, requiring the utmost patience and perseverance both on the part of the patient and the physician. In the mildest cases several months of strict treatment in bed are required, while in more severe cases the patient may have to rest in bed under observation for a year or more. He should stay in bed so long as there is any raised temperature, and while more than two or three stools are passed in the twenty-four hours. After that he may be allowed a warm bath, and to lie on a couch during the day.

NUTRITION. Since ulcerative colitis is a wasting disease, patients who are very debilitated by the time they come for treatment will need replacement of water and electrolytes, often by parenteral infusions. Protein loss may be very high and only in extensive burns can it be so severe.

Patients with mild ulcerative colitis usually have quite a good appetite. Since the disease affects only the colon, digestion and assimilation of food remain largely unimpaired. For these reasons, a full diet of high caloric value should be given, and it is unnecessary to make any restrictions beyond the avoidance of seeds and skins in fruit, and fibers of vegetables. Milk, up to 5 pints a day, may be given hot or cold, with a variety of flavors, and fortified if necessary. Tender meat is allowed, and fruit and vegetables are best given in the form of strained juice and purees. (See diet for Gastric Ulcer, pp. 365-66.)

MEDICATION. For patients with intestinal gas, with distension of the abdomen and colicky pain, a tablespoonful of powdered charcoal or a charcoal tablet may be given two or three times a day. Codeine, 15 to 60 milligrams twice daily, will control bowel movements.

Since most patients with ulcerative colitis are anemic, ferrous sulphate tablets, 200 milligrams, should be taken three times a day after meals. Whatever the degree of anemia, repeated small blood transfusions are often beneficial. Vitamin supplements are also helpful.

Cortisone, or corticotrophin, greatly increases the chance of a remission and should be given in all cases except the mildest. Hydrocortisone sodium hemisuccinate, administered in a rectal drip, may have a rapidly beneficial effect.

Cortisone by mouth or by rectal drip may with advantage be given simultaneously with Asulfidine, a preparation combining the properties of a salicylate and a sulphonamide.

PSYCHOLOGICAL TREATMENT. Any patient who suffers from chronic diarrhea and has lost much weight will show personality changes, some becoming irritable and difficult and other depressed and apathetic. This is certainly so with ulcerative colitis patients.

In the acute stage, patients need much sympathy and confident attention and when in hospital are best in a unit where their disease receives special attention. Formal psychiatric therapy is not usually required.

SURGERY is successfully done by removing a much-diseased colon and providing an ileostomy.

After-treatment. Even after the disease appears to be cured, dietetic precautions must only be relaxed very slowly, and a body belt of silk and wool should always be worn round the abdomen. Purgative drugs should never be used, but the bowels kept regular by suitable diet and the use of mineral oil when required. With expert care approximately 75 per cent of sufferers from this disease may be rehabilitated.

Irritable Colon

(*Muco-membranous Colic*)

The outstanding features of this complaint are obstinate constipation frequently alternating with attacks of diarrhea, and the passage of large amounts of mucus with the stools. There is, however, no actual disease or inflammation of the colon. The condition is commoner in women than in men, especially in highly-strung and nervous individuals.

The mucus normally protects the lining of the bowel from irritation and provides natural lubrication for the fæces. In certain people with an unusually irritable nervous system, constipation may be associated with a painful spasm of the lower colon (spastic constipation) with excessive production of mucus. If the mucus, normally liquid, remains sufficiently long in the colon, it becomes coagulated, and forms a grayish-white membrane. This may be passed in long tube-shaped casts, or it may be rolled into balls. The membranes may be mistaken for tapeworms.

Symptoms. Pain, if it is frequent, usually occurs in the left lower abdomen, and the stools consist of hard small lumps covered with grayish membrane.

In milder forms, there may be recurring attacks of slight abdominal pain, associated with an upset of bowel habit, often diarrhea following a bout of constipation. Between attacks, the bowels tend to be constipated.

The attacks are nearly always due to emotional disturbances, and may occur at intervals of weeks or months. There is generally an anxiety neurosis, the patient being depressed, with irritability and peevishness. The condition is apt to be chronic, though complete recovery may suddenly occur at any stage.

Treatment. The most important part of the treatment is to encourage the patient to neglect slight symptoms and to think no more of the complaint. As these patients are always self-centered, it is important that they should not concentrate their attention on their bowels. They should lead as normal a life as possible, and take regular exercise in the open air.

Most patients with this complaint have treated their constipation by almost every purgative offered to the public. These must be forbidden, and permission given only for olive oil or mineral oil.

For severe spasm of the colon, with colicky pain in the left lower abdomen, belladonna is the most useful drug, and may be combined with small doses of phenobarbital.

This complaint should never be treated by colonic lavage or enemas, as they only serve to concentrate the patient's attention on the bowels.

Diverticular Disease

In about 10 per cent of men and women over the age of 45, and especially in obese persons with chronic disease of the gall-

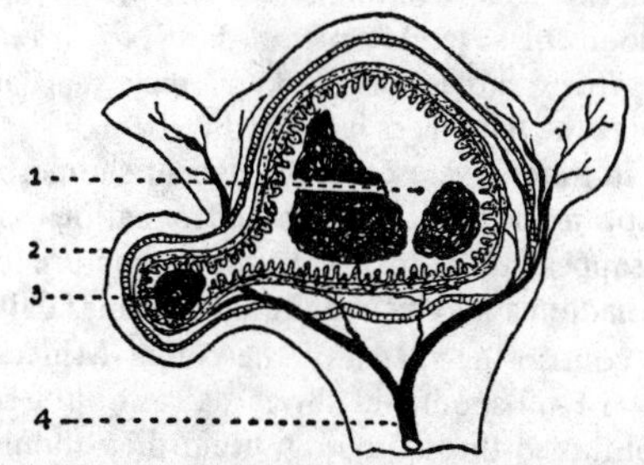

Fig. 11. *DEVELOPMENT OF AN INTESTINAL DIVERTICULUM. The cross section through the bowel shows how the diverticulum (or pouch) develops. 1. Cavity of intestine. 2. Diverticulum. 3. Fecal mass in diverticulum. 4. Artery supplying the colon.*

bladder, and in those who have habitually taken laxatives for many years, there develops in the lower or pelvic colon a number of small outward projections of the mucous membrane through the wall of the bowel. At first they are mere pouches, but later they become elongated and sac-like with a fairly definite neck, when they are known as diverticuli. Generally they give rise to no symptoms, but occasionally inflammation causes the condition which is known as *diverticulitis*.

Symptoms. The patient complains of discomfort in the lower abdomen, and later of attacks of colic in the left lower abdomen, which gradually increase in frequency and severity. The condition resembles an attack of left-sided appendicitis. The constipation, which in any case is habitual, may become

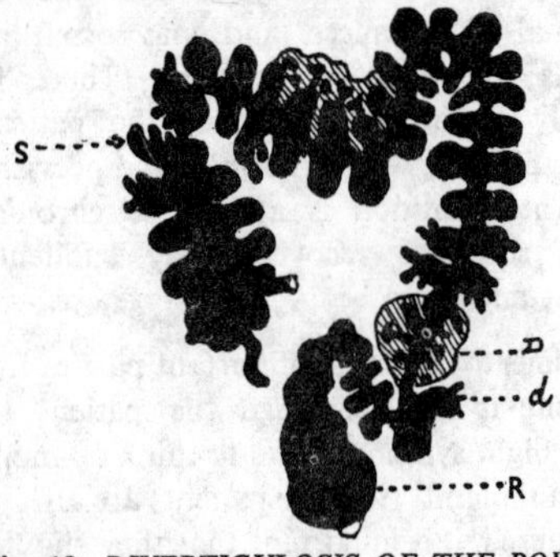

Fig. 12. *DIVERTICULOSIS OF THE BOWEL AS SEEN BY X-RAY. With the formation of pouches along the wall of the colon, strictures also occur, causing narrowing of the gut cavity. S. Site of a stricture in ascending colon. d. Diverticulum (or pouch). D. Inflammation (diverticulitis) with stricture. R. Rectum.*

even more severe, but the administration of laxatives actually increases the pain. The passage of bright red blood per rectum may occasionally accompany these attacks. The bladder is often irritable, the patient having to pass urine very frequently.

Diagnosis. The condition must be distinguished from cancer of the colon. In the latter disease, however, the stools usually contain pus and blood, which are not usually present in diverticular disease. The latter condition may be confirmed by X-ray examination after a barium enema.

Treatment. Irritation of the bowel must be avoided by adopting a bland diet. (See diet for Gastric Ulcer, pp. 365-66.) In mild cases the stools should be kept permanently soft by means of mineral oil, 1 to 2 5-ml spoonsful several times a day. No strong laxatives should be used, as they tend to force the fluid feces into the diverticuli.

In more severe cases the patient should be kept in bed until active inflammation has disappeared; 5 to 15 drops of tincture of belladonna may be required three times daily to control the spasm of the colon. Mineral oil 3 5-ml spoonsful thrice daily should be continued throughout. A fluid diet should be given at first and fresh lemon or blackcurrant drinks. Heat applied to the painful part will relieve much pain, and electric pad being most suitable.

Antibiotics, such as penicillin or erythromycin in combination, should be given for a week to ten days to clear the infection causing the inflammation and this may take some weeks to clear.

Surgery by resection of the affected segment of the colon has been very successful especially in cases in which severe internal bleeding has complicated the condition. A colostomy is sometimes made.

Cancer of the Colon

The small intestine is practically never affected by cancer, but the colon and the rectum are affected with equal frequency. The sigmoid colon is involved more commonly than other parts of the colon. The growth usually forms a ring round the bowel, causing a gradual narrowing of its lumen. Less commonly (though frequently in the rectum), it may develop into a fungating and ulcerating mass which projects from the wall into the cavity of the bowel. The growth is liable to extend to the peritoneum and liver, but such involvements are usually late complications.

Symptoms. Cancer of the colon is generally slow in growth compared with cancer in many other parts, and symptoms are therefore slow and insidious in onset. It is commonest between the ages of 40 and 65. The first symptom may be a feeling of vague discomfort in the lower abdomen, with slight attacks of colic when constipation becomes more severe; these attacks are rarely severe until the obstruction is almost complete, when there is much distension of the abdomen. Attacks of constipation often alternate with diarrhea, but in most cases the constipation becomes more and more severe until it ends in complete obstruction of the bowel by a hard mass of feces.

Bleeding from the growth nearly always occurs at some stage, and in the later stages the stools generally contain obvious blood, pus and mucus. The constant loss of blood leads to anemia.

Diagnosis. The possibility of cancer of the bowel should be considered whenever an individual over the age of 35, whose bowels have previously been regular, develops without change of diet or habits, either constipation or diarrhea or if blood appears persistently in the stools. In a few cases, a lump may be felt in the abdomen by the hand. The rectum should be examined with a gloved finger, when a growth which is sufficiently low down may be felt by the finger. Usually, however, the condition is diagnosed by X-ray examination after a barium enema or barium meal, followed if necessary by sigmoidoscopy.

It requires to be distinguished from diverticulitis, appendicitis, intestinal polyposis, amoebic dysentery, and from fecal impaction caused by old operational adhesions or strangulated hernia.

Treatment. The treatment is usually by operation. If this is performed sufficiently early, before the liver is affected by the growth, the results are usually quite satisfactory. An artificial anus (*colostomy*) at the left side of the abdominal wall, if the growth is sufficiently low, is usually made in order to drain the bowel. In unfavorable cases, it may be followed by surgical removal of the whole growth.

Acute Intestinal Obstruction

Intestinal obstruction is a condition in which the passage of the contents of the bowel is more or less suddenly obstructed. It is important that the condition should be recognized at the earliest possible moment because every hour's delay in relieving the obstruction (usually by operation) greatly increases the mortality.

Causes. 1. The commonest cause in adults is a narrowing of the bowel due to cancer of the colon, with resultant impaction of feces.

2. Strangulation of a loop of bowel by adhesions may be the result of old tuberculous or inflammatory disease, or the sequel to previous abdominal operations.

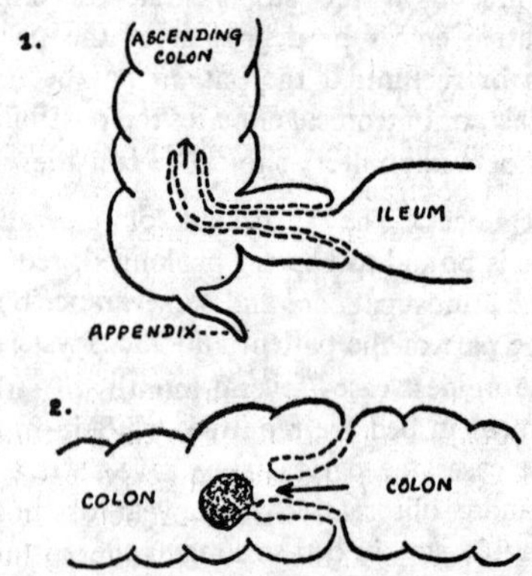

Fig. 13. *INTUSSUSCEPTION OF THE INTESTINES. 1. Ileum 'telescoped' into the ascending colon. 2. Portion of colon 'telescoped' into another portion due to tumor on the intestinal wall.*

3. Strangulation of a rupture at the usual hernial openings and internally. In some cases of small femoral hernia in obese persons it is easy to overlook this condition. (See Hernia, p. 384.

4. In infants under the age of 12 months, intussusception, or the telescoping of one section of bowel into the part immediately beyond it, sometimes causes intestinal obstruction.

5. A less common cause is known as *volvulus*, in which there is a twisting of a coil of bowel upon itself. It generally occurs late in life.

Complications. First, the contents of the bowel are retained and poisons are absorbed from the stagnant products. Secondly, the blood vessels supplying the affected bowel become blocked, leading to gangrene of the bowel and, if the condition is not relieved by operation, to perforation and peritonitis.

Symptoms. In all cases of acute intestinal obstruction, certain general symptoms are fairly constantly present, namely pain, vomiting, collapse and constipation.

PAIN is an early and severe symptom; a patient in perfectly good health may be seized with sudden abdominal pain which doubles him up. It is at first colicky, but soon becomes continuous, and may be felt over the whole abdomen.

VOMITING. This usually comes on about an hour after the pain, but it may be delayed for some hours. The higher the obstruction, the greater the vomiting, which soon becomes fecal in character.

COLLAPSE is early and severe, the patient being prostrated, anxious and restless, with a cold clammy skin. The pulse becomes small and rapid, the temperature is subnormal and the tongue dry.

CONSTIPATION. The bowel below the obstruction may empty itself shortly after the onset of the pain and vomiting, or an enema, if given, may have a positive result. Subsequently, however, constipation as a rule is complete.

Above the obstruction the intestinal contents accumulate and decompose forming gas. The abdomen becomes distended and the gas, which cannot escape downwards, is belched up. In the case of an acute obstruction by feces following partial chronic obstruction, the distended coils of bowel may be felt to contract under the hand and the outline of their movements may be seen (Visible peristalsis).

Diagnosis

PERITONITIS. Peritonitis may be secondary to the spread of infection, or to the perforation of an organ, and may quickly lead to paralysis of the bowel (paralytic ileus). It is often a source of difficulty in diagnosis, but the extreme tenderness and rigidity of the abdomen are characteristic.

ACUTE PANCREATITIS is usually associated with a history of gall-stones. Vomiting is a prominent symptom and upper abdominal pain is intense.

Rectal examination should be performed in every case of suspected intestinal obstruction.

Treatment. In no circumstances should purgatives be given in a case of suspected intestinal obstruction.

Two modes of treatment are used.

If the obstruction is mechanical (an adhesion, tumor, rupture strangulation) an operation will be needed quickly.

If the condition is due to a paralysis or non-movement of the bowel wall caused by peritonitis or a perforated peptic ulcer, careful management may be given in a hospital. The intestine must be cleared by gastric suction and fluids and electrolytes lost in vomiting and sweating must be replaced by parenteral infusion. Antibiotics will be required to kill infection from the peritoneum.

Appendicitis

The appendix arises at the junction of the small and large intestines in the right lower part of the abdomen. It is a small worm-like tube about three to six inches long.

Acute appendicitis, or inflammation of the appendix, is the most common acute abdominal emergency, occurring more frequently than all other abdominal emergencies put together. It may vary from a simple catarrh to a tense swelling of the whole organ which may become filled with pus. In such cases, if operation is not undertaken, gangrene or perforation of the appendix is likely to occur, leading to an abscess, or to peritonitis.

Symptoms. In acute attacks, which most commonly occur in children and young adults, the onset is generally sudden.

ABDOMINAL PAIN is usually a prominent symptom, the patient being seized with sudden and severe pain, usually felt at first round the navel, especially in children. It is not at first accompanied by local tenderness. Later the pain is felt in the lower right side of the abdomen.

GASTRIC AND INTESTINAL DISTURBANCES are almost always present. The tongue is furred and rapidly becomes dry. Vomiting is usually present, beginning within a few hours of the onset of the pain; it may occur once or twice and then cease, but nausea usually persists. Constipation is generally severe, though diarrhea may occasionally occur if the inflamed appendix happens to be close to the rectum.

RAISED TEMPERATURE is almost always present at some time during an attack, the rise often being to 38°–39° C (100°–102° F). It may be preceded by a shivering fit or chills.

THE PULSE RATE is moderately increased, often to 90 or more, especially in children.

LOCAL SIGNS. There is considerable stiffening of the abdominal muscles in the right lower abdomen. This rigidity, or 'guarding,' is often too great to allow much to be felt by deep pressure with the fingers. In addition, there is great tenderness. In some cases local rigidity is slight or absent, as when the appendix lies behind the cecum, in which case pain is felt in the right loin; or when the appendix passes directly downwards into the pelvis causing diarrhea and irritability of the bladder.

Course. When a correct diagnosis has been made, immediate operation should be undertaken. In the hands of a competent surgeon, operation in the early stages is one of almost complete safety, death being rare after operations which are undertaken within 36 hours. A further advantage of early operation is that drainage of the abdomen can usually be avoided, whereas in later operation, drainage by a tube is often necessary. It should be noted that the disease is apt to run a very rapid course in children and old people. The introduction of antibiotic drugs, however, has greatly reduced mortality due to associated peritonitis.

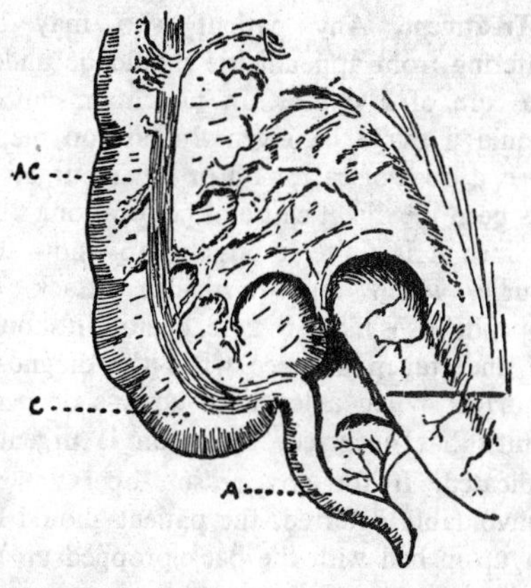

Fig. 14. *THE APPENDIX. AC Ascending colon. C. Cecum. A. Appendix, which may be from three to six inches in length.*

Sequels. If for any reason operation is delayed, the disease may take one of three possible courses:

1. IN MILD CATARRHAL CASES the inflammation tends to settle down after two or three days, and the appendix may return to an apparently normal condition. Successive attacks of appendicitis, however, tend to become more severe, and a patient who has had two attacks is almost certain to have further trouble.

2. ULCERATION OR GANGRENE of the appendix may occur, with later perforation, the symptoms persisting for longer than a week and becoming aggravated.

3. GENERALIZED PERITONITIS may occur, and is by far the commonest cause of death in this disease. *The great danger of appendicitis is that general peritonitis may occur from the beginning of the attack*, and its symptoms may be indistinguishable from that of the appendicitis itself.

Diagnosis. In the first few hours of the attack, when the only symptom is central abdominal pain, perhaps accompanied by nausea or slight vomiting, the attack may be mistaken for intestinal colic, gastritis, indigestion, or food poisoning. The only safe plan is to watch such cases very carefully. Some fever and localization in the right iliac fossa will soon develop if the case is one of appendicitis. Recurrent mild attacks of appendicitis in children are often diagnosed as 'bilious attacks.' Pneumonia in children often starts with abdominal pain.

When the pain has become localized in the right lower abdomen, it may have to be distinguished from disease of the lung (right-sided pneumonia), pleura, liver, gall-bladder, duodenum, pancreas, kidney, and cecum, while in females acute disease of the ovary or Fallopian tube on the right side may give rise to doubt as to whether the appendix is involved or not. A careful history and consideration of accompanying symptoms, together with examination of the chest, abdomen, rectum and urine should help to distinguish these various conditions from an attack of acute appendicitis.

Treatment. Any patient who may be suffering from appendicitis should be under the care of a doctor. In no circumstances should a purge be given. In far too many cases a dose of castor oil or other purgative has been the direct cause of perforation.

Since it is quite impossible to know the course which any particular attack of appendicitis is likely to take, operation should be undertaken at once when the diagnosis is made. When a localized abscess or peritonitis has occurred, operation is urgently indicated. If for any reason operation is unavoidably deferred, the patient should be sat up in bed with the back propped up by pillows (Fowler's position) and should be given nothing to drink. The mouth may be rinsed with water, which should not be swallowed. Water may be administered by the rectum, however, or saline solution may be given intravenously.

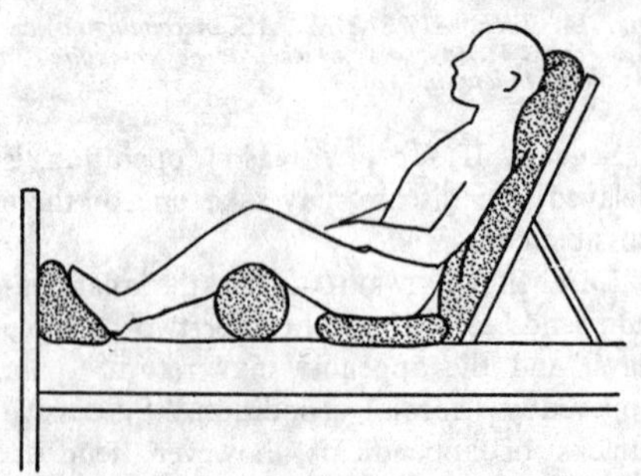

Fig. 15. *FOWLER'S POSITION. If an appendix operation has to be temporarily deferred, the patient is best placed in Fowler's position.*

Regional Enteritis

(Crohn's Disease)

This is a non-specific inflammatory condition, usually chronic, affecting mainly the terminal part of the small intestine (ileum) and ceasing at the ileo-cecal valve in the cecum. The bowel becomes thickened, with a narrow lumen, and the mucosal surface shows varying degrees of ulceration. The mesentery is thickened and contains numbers of enlarged lymph glands. The majority of cases appear in people under 40 years of age. The cause is unknown, though it often occurs in members of the same family, which suggests the possibility of a genetic or environmental predisposition.

Symptoms. In the acute phase the symptoms are almost identical with those of appendicitis, for which it is almost invariably mistaken. It is therefore rarely diagnosed before operation.

In chronic cases, the patients give a history of months or years of intermittent abdominal cramp and attacks of offensive diarrhea without blood. There is considerable loss of weight and anemia, often with intermittent attacks of fever. In some cases there may be symptoms of subacute intestinal obstruction.

Treatment. Rest in bed is essential, with a nutritious diet of low residue (see treatment of peptic ulcer, p. 364. There is no specific treatment and surgical intervention should be avoided in young subjects during the acute active stages. In general, surgery should be deferred until the disease has become quiescent, and should be restricted to the treatment of sequelae, such as intestinal obstruction or the formation of fistulae.

DISEASES OF THE RECTUM AND ANUS

The rectum is the last part of the alimentary canal. It is about six inches long, and it opens at the anus.

When necessary the rectum may be examined by a doctor by means of the first finger covered with a rubber glove, and lubricated with Vaseline. The patient should be lying on the left side with the knees well drawn up towards the chin. Examination is used to investigate the condition of the anus, the presence of hemorrhoids, contents of the rectum, the condition of the prostate gland, and especially the presence of any new growth in the rectum itself, or of any tumors in the surrounding parts which may press on the rectum.

Hemorrhoids

(Piles)

Piles are one of the commonest of all complaints. They are produced by congestion of the rectal mucous membrane containing the hemorrhoidal veins which become dilated, varicosed and enlarged.

Piles may be external, when they appear outside the anus, or internal, when they are concealed above the anal canal.

Causes. Piles are often caused by habitual straining in chronic constipation, or by persistent diarrhea especially from the abuse of purgatives; the same effect may be produced by strain resulting from a chronic cough, from heavy manual work, or from urinary obstruction due to enlargement of the prostate.

Any condition which leads to continual obstruction to the blood flow in the veins of the rectum may give rise to piles—e.g. pregnancy, fibroids or large ovarian cysts in women. Congestion of the liver from habitual overeating, alcoholism, or heart failure, is a not uncommon cause.

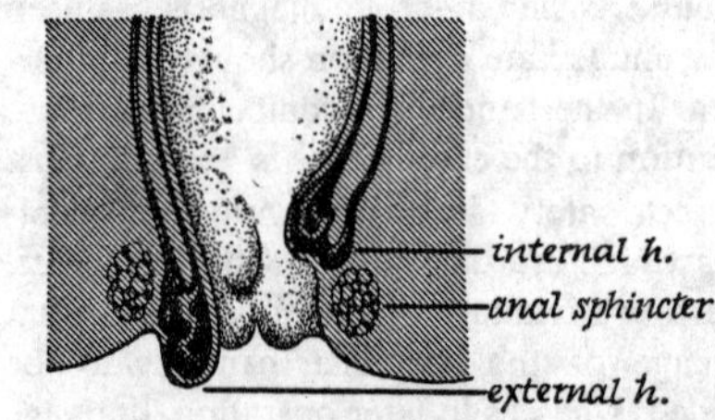

Fig. 16. *PILES. An early case of hemorrhoids, showing an internal hemorrhoid, and how a thrombosed vein protrudes beyond the anal sphincter to form external piles.*

Symptoms. The chief symptoms are bleeding on defecation, and prolapse, which is descent of the congested lining membrane of the rectum outside the anal canal. Pain is not common, but it may be produced by thrombosis, or clotting in the vein of a hemorrhoid. A thrombosed pile appears as an oval bluish swelling, tender and firm, near to the anus. Pain may also be caused by infection or the development of an abscess, while very severe pain is most likely to be due to an accompanying fissure of the anus (see p. 375). Pain from any cause is aggravated by sitting and walking and especially by defecation.

Course. Symptoms may at any time be slight or absent, but there may be periodical exacerbations, and there is usually slow progression over a period of years. Repeated bleeding may in time lead to the development of secondary anemia, sometimes of severe degree, while the prolapse becomes increasingly worse. Attacks of thrombosis are commonly associated with surface ulceration and infection, which in turn may lead to gangrene of the pile. There is, however, no tendency for hemorrhoids to lead to cancer.

Treatment. A regular natural action of the bowels should be encouraged by daily exercise, and by eating a reasonable amount of fresh fruit and vegetables and drinking plenty of water. If necessary, a mild laxative such as senna should be taken at night, or otherwise 2 x 5-ml. spoonsful once or twice daily of mineral. After the bowels have acted, the anus should be carefully cleaned with very soft toilet paper or moist raw cotton, and it should be washed with soap and water. A hemorrhoidal suppository should be inserted through the anus in the morning, if possible after the bowels have acted, and again in the evening. The insertion of a suppository should be immediately followed by the use of a hemorrhoidal ointment both inside and outside the anus.

Treatment of Chronic Thrombosed Piles

The treatment of prolapsed thrombosed, ulcerated or sloughing piles should be aimed at relief of the symptoms, and no type of operation should be undertaken until the condition is quiescent. The patient should be put to bed, and the anus shaved. Pressure should then be applied with the gloved finger and a moistened raw cotton swab, and an attempt made to replace the prolapsed piles inside the rectum. Moist antiseptic compresses are then firmly applied to the anus and kept in position by a T-bandage passing between the thighs. The compresses are prepared by soaking pads of raw cotton in a lotion of mercuric chloride 1 in 2,000. The compresses should be renewed every four hours. After each action of the bowels the parts should be inspected, cleaned and redressed. A sitz-bath in 5 inches of warm water at 43.3° C (110° F) may be taken for 5 minutes night and morning, and before the compress is reapplied a hemorrhoidal suppository may be inserted.

For cases which do not clear up with these measures, surgical treatment may be needed. Small uncomplicated internal piles may be treated by injection, but larger piles may require an operation.

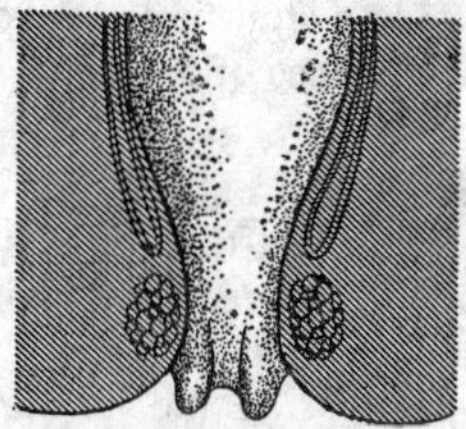

Fig. 17. *PROLAPSE OF RECTUM. A slight prolapse of the mucous membrane lining the rectum. In more severe cases, the lining may protrude for several inches.*

Prolapse of the Rectum

Causes. A protrusion of the mucous membrane of the rectum through the anal orifice is not uncommon in children between the ages of 1 and 3 years. It results usually from straining in diarrhea, whooping-cough or bronchitis, and is especially likely to occur if the child is poorly nourished.

In adults a moderate degree of prolapse is often associated with severe internal piles, and it may be aggravated by the straining due to chronic constipation. A more advanced form of prolapse, involving the whole thickness of the walls of the rectum, may occur particularly in women who have undergone several confinements.

Complications. The prolapsed rectum is liable to undergo the same inflammatory conditions as prolapsed hemorrhoids, namely congestion, thrombosis (clotting in the veins), and ulceration, while bleeding is often caused by friction.

Treatment. In children, attention to the general health and the training in regular bowel habits are important. Constipation can usually be overcome by giving plenty of water to drink. An attempt of defecation after breakfast must be persevered with until it becomes a regular habit. Laxatives such as milk of magnesia may be required at first. In difficult cases, a small olive oil or saline enema may be needed each day for a time, the enema being given with the child lying on the left side.

For prolapse in adults see Treatment of Hemorrhoids, p. 374. Temporary support with a sanitary napkin and T-bandage may be required, while in severe and persistent cases, surgical treatment may be necessary.

Cancer of the Rectum

Cancer of the rectum is one of the commonest forms of malignant disease, and amounts to between 8 and 12 per cent of all malignant tumors. It is nearly twice as common in men as in women, and it occurs most often between the ages of 50 and 60.

Cancer begins as a hard thickening in the wall of the rectum. This area gradually becomes ulcerated at its center, the ulcerated surface having a hard raised edge. The cancer extends circularly round the wall until eventually it passes round the entire circumference, so that symptoms of obstruction may develop.

Symptoms. The early symptoms may be very slight. A little bleeding at defecation is usually the earliest sign, often with a little discharge of mucus. Next there may be slight morning irritation of the rectum with possibly a feeling of incomplete defecation and failure to empty the rectum at one sitting. Increasing constipation may then be noticed, requiring gradually increasing doses of laxative. Later symptoms are alternating constipation and diarrhea with frequent calls to stool, and a feeling of pressure in the rectum. Symptoms of advanced disease include pain in the pelvis, and enlargement of the liver, together with general wasting and loss of weight.

Diagnosis. Everyone aged over 50 who has bleeding from the bowel or change of bowel habit must be considered as possibly suffering from cancer of the rectum. Highly suggestive signs are increasing constipation, or constipation followed by numerous stools, early morning diarrhea, and a frequent desire for stool, at which time the patient passes little except flatus, mucus and blood.

Growths low down in the rectum can usually be diagnosed by examining the rectum with a gloved finger, while those which are out of reach of the finger may often be located after examination by barium enema or by sigmoidoscopy.

Treatment. Surgical removal is the treatment of choice in the majority of cases and, with careful treatment beforehand, the operation is usually remarkably successful. An operation means, however, that a permanent colostomy or artificial anal opening will have to be made in the abdominal wall.

For inoperable cases, symptomatic treatment is given, relief of pain being the chief need. At first aspirin is sufficient, but in the late stages morphine, may have to be ordered by a doctor.

Fissure of the Anus

A painful fissure, crack or ulcer in the anal canal may cause a good deal of spasm, or tightening, of the anal muscle ring. It is generally found at the hind part of the anus, and is usually caused by stretching of the anal canal by large constipated stools.

Symptoms. The most typical symptom is severe pain on defecation. The pain is of a burning, cutting or tearing character, and it may last from a few minutes up to several hours. The onset of a throbbing or boring type of pain in a chronic fissure suggests infection, with the formation of an abscess.

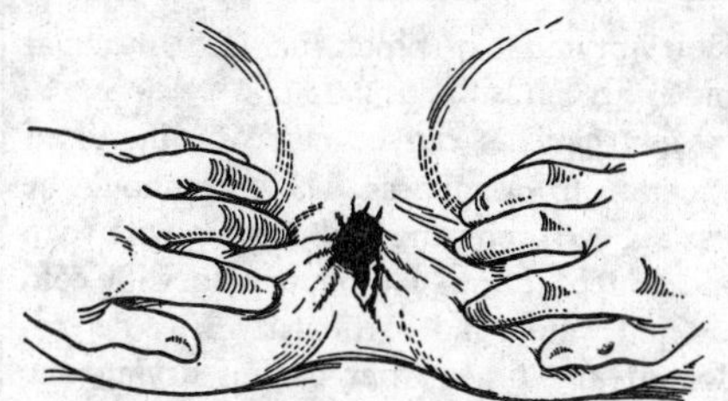

Fig. 18. *FISSURE OF ANUS. This crack or fissure is usually found at the hind part of the anus, and is often the consequence of overstretching the anal area in chronic constipation.*

Treatment. A small fissure of recent onset will usually heal with palliative treatment. Mineral oil should be given by mouth, and no violent exercise should be taken until the fissure is soundly healed. The application of 2% silver nitrate to the surface of the fissure stimulates healing and may be repeated on alternate days. The patient should insert a hemorrhoidal suppository into the rectum night and morning (see Treatment of Hemorrhoids, p. 374) followed by the application of a lubricating cream into the anal canal. A useful lubricant is zinc and castor oil cream, to which may be added benzocaine, 600 milligrams to 30 grams of ointment.

For the relief of pain the continuous application of compresses wrung out in hot witch hazel solution is extremely helpful, followed by the introduction of 60 milliliters of warm olive oil into the rectum by means of a rubber catheter.

For obstinate cases of fissure, treatment by operation may be required.

Pruritis Ani

(*Itching of the Anus*)

Causes. This is a very common complaint at any age. It occurs most frequently in summer and is often due to lack of cleanliness, especially associated with long anal hairs, hemorrhoids, thickened skin tabs round the anus, threadworms (a common cause) and lice. Other predisposing conditions are constipation with overloading of the rectum, diarrhea, and inflammation of the rectum with leakage of mucus, and leakage of mineral oil. A few chronic cases are due to overeating, alcoholism, diabetes, and allergy to certain foods or drugs. Leakage of highly acid, concentrated or infected urine, as in cystitis, or a vaginal discharge in women may also precipitate anal itching. Such a discharge usually occurs in vaginal infection with *Trichomonas* (see p. 293).

Symptom. The chief symptom is itching round the anus. It commonly follows defecation, and is also apt to occur at night.

Treatment. The first step should be removal of the cause—hemorrhoids, fissures, etc. being dealt with, and threadworms eradicated with viprynium or piperazine (see Intestinal and Other Parasites, p. 387.

Most patients can be cured by increased attention to cleanliness. The anus should be washed each morning and evening with soap and water, followed by sponging with cold or tepid water, and particularly after defecation at any time. After careful drying, the anus should be dusted with a powder containing zinc oxide 2 parts, starch 2 parts and boric acid 1 part.

At night a lotion such as the following should be applied:

Phenol	4 g
Zinc Oxide	8 g
Calamine	4 g
Glycerin	8 ml
Alcohol (90%)	8 ml
Rose Water	15 ml
Milk of Magnesia ..	to 120 ml

In acute cases, at night, a piece of gauze moistened with the lotion may be placed against the anus. A cream or lotion containing hydrocortisone or triamcinolone is sometimes prescribed.

Ointments should be avoided. Mineral oil should be discontinued, if in use, or reduced to a minimum. Highly seasoned foods, alcohol and coffee should be avoided. A light-weight cellular type of underclothing should be worn near to the skin, as wool can be extremely irritating, especially in hot weather. In cold weather, however, wool can be worn over cellular or cotton underclothing.

Very obstinate cases may need treatment by injections, and occasionally nerve-cutting operations are undertaken.

DISEASE OF THE LIVER AND THE GALL-BLADDER

The liver is able to suffer a remarkable degree of damage from injury or disease, to the extent of four-fifths of its bulk, before its function is much impaired, and it possesses a corresponding capacity for recovery unsurpassed by that of any other organ.

Projecting forwards from the under surface of the liver is the gall-bladder (see Fig. 20, p. 379), which, no less than ten times in every twenty-four hours, concentrates the bile formed by the liver. Partly digested food passing from the stomach stimulates the release of this bile to aid in the digestion of fats.

Bile is a bitter-tasting greenish liquid which consists of three main constituents:

1. Bile Salts, which play an important part in the digestion of fats and have an effect on the movements of the bowels.

2. Bile Pigment, which is derived from the coloring matter (hemoglobin) of the red blood cells. It is a waste product and gives feces their usual brown color.

3. Cholesterol. This is widely distributed in the body. Its presence in the bile suggests that it is a product of excretion. It enters into the formation of gall-stones.

For further details on the functioning of the liver and gall-bladder, see Physiology, p. 251.

Jaundice

Jaundice is the name given to a yellow coloration of the skin caused by excess of bile pigment in the blood. It is not a disease in itself, but a sign of some underlying disorder usually affecting the liver and/or the ducts connecting it with the gall-bladder and the duodenum.

Causes. All cases of jaundice can be classed in one of the three following groups:

Infective Jaundice. This is by far the commonest type, and is the result of damage to the liver by infection (see Acute Infective Hepatitis below). The cells become largely incapable of passing the bile pigment into the bile vessels, so that it is absorbed into the general circulation instead, while any which may be excreted into the biliary capillaries is obstructed by inflammatory swelling (cholangitis) and it is consequently absorbed into the bloodstream.

Toxic Jaundice results from damage to the liver by certain chemical poisons such as phosphorus, trinitrotoluene (affecting munition and airplane workers), arsenic (occasionally during the treatment of syphilis by injections of arsenic), and alcohol.

Obstructive Jaundice. This is due to blockage of the bile passages between the liver and the duodenum. The obstruction may be caused by gall-stones, usually in the common bile duct, or by pressure on the ducts from without, e.g. in cancer of the liver, of the pancreas or of the stomach. The bile continues for a time to be formed by the liver but, as it has no outlet, it is reabsorbed by the smaller blood vessels of the liver and passed into the circulation.

Hemolytic Jaundice. This is a less common type of jaundice in which the skin is colored a lemon-yellow rather than the bright greenish-yellow of common jaundice. It sometimes occurs in newborn babies for a few days after birth, and is also seen in pernicious anemia. It is due to an abnormality of the red blood cells, which are broken down more rapidly to form an excess of bile pigment which circulates round the system. Since there is no obstruction to the outflow of bile from the liver, there is no alteration in the color of the stools or urine (acholuric jaundice).

Jaundice associated with hemolytic disease of the newborn is related to incompatibility of the Rhesus blood types of mother and infant (see Physiology, p. 240).

Symptoms. The chief symptom is a yellowish discoloration of the skin and mucous membrane of the lips and palate. It appears first in the whites of the eyes, and then successively on the face, body and limbs. In cases of persistent obstructive jaundice such as in jaundice due to cancer, the pigment in the skin gradually changes from yellow to dark olive green.

The urine becomes stained with bile and is of a dark brownish color. The presence of bile in the urine can be confirmed by one of the following tests (see also p. 407).

Froth Test. A few milliliters of urine are shaken up in a test-tube. Yellow froth indicates the presence of bile pigments in the urine.

Iodine Test. A few milliliters of urine are placed in a glass test-tube, and on to the urine is slowly poured one milliliter of tincture of iodine. If bile is present, a greenish-blue color develops at the junction of the iodine with the urine.

Feces. The feces in jaundice are bulky and often offensive. When the obstruction is complete they are pale or clay-colored owing to an excess of the products of fat-digestion, which require the presence of bile acids in the intestine for their absorption into the system. This loss of fat via the stools may lead to considerable loss of weight.

Purpura. In obstructive jaundice the clotting time of the blood is considerably increased owing to lack of vitamin K in the blood. This important vitamin is soluble in fat, and thus, like the fat in the feces, it fails to be absorbed into the system in sufficient quantities when bile is absent from the intestine. This lack of clotting power in the blood may cause bleeding from the nose and gums, and a blotchy rash of the skin, known as purpura.

Pruritus and Irritability. The presence of bile salts in the blood may lead to a slowing of the pulse rate to 50 or 60 per minute, and to intense irritation of the skin (pruritus) which may seriously interfere with sleep. Since the functions of the liver are greatly deranged, mental depression and irritability are constant features of jaundice.

Diagnosis. Patients should be examined if possible in daylight, as it is very easy to miss the onset of jaundice if the examination is made in artificial light.

Age

Infancy. Transient hemolytic jaundice is common in the newly born.

Under 30. In youth and early adult life jaundice is usually due to infective hepatitis.

Over 30. Gall-stones are a common cause, especially in women.

Over 40. Cancer is the most common cause in both sexes.

Color

A pale lemon-yellow color is seen in hemolytic jaundice (e.g. pernicious anemia), and there is no bile in the urine.

A bright yellow color is seen in infective hepatitis and in toxic jaundice from poisoning by arsenic compounds, trinitrotoluene, etc.

A greenish-yellow color occurs in chronic and progressive obstructive jaundice, usually due to cancer of the liver or head of the pancreas.

DURATION

If short, it is usually due to infective hepatitis, or to the passage of a gall-stone.

PAIN

Absence of pain suggests infective hepatitis.

Attacks of pain suggest gall-stones.

Constant pain suggests cancer of the liver.

Treatment. Since jaundice is a symptom and not a disease in itself, the treatment of jaundice is the treatment of the underlying condition. For general points see treatment of infective hepatitis below. (See also treatment of cancer of the liver, of gall-stones, etc.—according to the cause.)

DISEASES OF THE LIVER

Acute Infective Hepatitis

(*Acute Viral Hepatitis*)

This was formerly known as catarrhal jaundice. It is an acute infective inflammation of the liver cells and bile ducts and is believed to be caused by a virus. In recent years many epidemic outbreaks have occurred. Epidemics tend to begin in the late summer. It affects the young far more than the elderly, and the incubation period is between three and five weeks, usually about a month.

For Spirochetal Jaundice, see p. 281.

Symptoms. Loss of appetite is the most frequent and outstanding early symptom. It is often accompanied by headaches and weakness, and occasionally by vomiting and diarrhea. The temperature is somewhat raised, the fever lasting for 1 to 7 days. It is present until the jaundice appears, when it subsides to normal. About the third day the urine becomes dark brown, the stools are pale, and the whites of the eyes become yellow, with gradually increasing jaundice all over the body. The liver is slightly enlarged and tender. The jaundice may last for a week, or it may be prolonged to two or three months, and convalescence may be protracted.

Treatment. There are certain general points in treatment which should also be followed in all disorders of the liver and gall-bladder.

1. REST IN BED and warmth, until the feces have regained their normal color and until the urine has been free from bile pigment for three consecutive days. If bile pigment reappears in the urine, the patient must immediately return to bed. This period of rest is necessary to protect the intact liver cells, and will take about three weeks in the average case. It should be followed by three weeks of strict convalescence.

2. DIET: (a) *Glucose.* The most important step in treatment is to give glucose, which is stored in the liver cells. In mild cases glucose may be given in solution in water with fruit juices, as in glucose lemonade, which is prepared as follows:

medicinal glucose 200 grams (or ½ lb),
water 1 liter (or 2 pints),
the thin rind of 2 lemons.

Mix together and boil for 5 minutes. Strain, and when cold, add the juice of 2 lemons.

Glucose may also be added to barley water, in the proportion of 1 to 2 tablespoonsful to a tumbler: it can be flavored with orange or lemon juice.

(b) *Fats* used to be considered harmful but this has not been proved by experiment and experience. In any case few patients in or after a feverish state like much greasiness with their food. So let the patient have what he fancies.

(c) *Proteins* should be given in adequate amounts, especially in the form of skimmed milk, which may be diluted with soda water, mineral water, barley water, etc. In general, a light diet should be given consisting of custards, junkets, jellies, meat extracts, together with honey and jam, and fruit in moderation. As the condition improves, a little thin bread, lightly spread with butter, in moderation. As the condition improves, a little thin bread, lightly scraped with butter, minced meat, lamb or chicken may be added.

(d) *Vitamin B.* This is a necessary addition to the diet and is best given in the form of brewer's yeast, two or three times daily.

3. DRUGS. A sufficient amount of epsom salts or other saline laxative should be taken each morning to keep the bowels well opened. Disprin or chloral hydrates may be prescribed for sleep, but barbiturates should be avoided.

Antibiotics are valueless since this is a viral infection.

4. PRURITUS (Itching). This may be treated by a starch or bran bath. The former is prepared by making 2 pounds of starch into a paste with cold water, and then running the hot water into the bath through the basin of starch. A bran bath is prepared by putting 2 to 4 pounds of bran in a loose muslin bag and tying it under the hot tap, the water being run into the bath through the bag, which should be squeezed at intervals.

After the bath, a lotion of carbolic acid (1 in 50), in calamine lotion should be dabbed on the skin.

5. HEMORRHAGE. The tendency to bleeding can be controlled by giving vitamin C and vitamin K by mouth, together with bile salts.

No person who has had viral hepatitis should become a blood donor.

After-treatment. This is extremely important. On no account should alcohol in any form be taken for six months after an attack, and hard physical exercise in the form of athletics or swimming must be forbidden for a similar period. It must be remembered that enlargement of the liver may persist for months after a patient feels perfectly well, and failure to observe these two important restrictions may easily cause a relapse.

Congestion of the Liver

(*Nutmeg Liver*)

This follows right-sided heart failure, which is often due to chronic lung disease. The liver becomes enlarged, firm and tender, its outer covering being stretched and giving rise to a feeling of fulness or weight in the right upper abdomen. Congestion of the liver leads in turn to congestion of the stomach and intestines, with loss of appetite, discomfort after food, flatulent distension of the stomach, and constipation. It is often associated with dropsy of the legs and of the abdomen (ascites).

Treatment. The treatment is that of heart failure (see p. 300), digitalis being especially valuable; it should be given in short courses. The ascites should be treated as outlined under Diuretics, p. 300. Mild purgation with Epsom salts also helps to relieve the congestion.

Cirrhosis of the Liver

(*Hobnail Liver*)

Causes. This is one of the most common of the chronic diseases of the liver. The liver hardens as a result of new fibrous tissue, and is at first larger than normal, but in the later stages it tends to contract and to show irregular projections on the surface which give it a 'hob-nailed' appearance.

Most patients with cirrhosis have indulged heavily in alcohol. It occurs in the type of individual who takes too much alcohol, too much food and too little exercise, its development being further favored by conditions such as amoebic dysentery, malaria, or syphilis

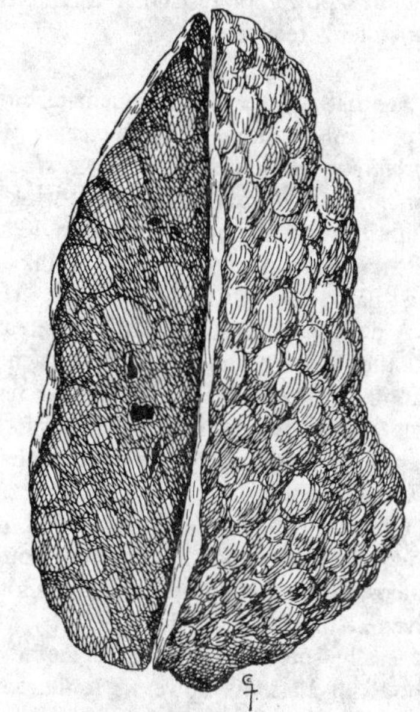

Fig. 19. *COARSE CIRRHOSIS OF THE LIVER. The nodules of new fibrous tissue which form on the surface have earned it the name of 'hobnail' liver.*

which also cause damage to the liver. While there is an undoubted relationship between cirrhosis and the excessive and prolonged use of alcohol, the disease may also appear in persons who have never touched any alcohol at all.

Symptoms. Cirrhosis of the liver is more common in men than in women. The early stages are long and quiet, the first symptoms appearing usually between the ages of 40 and 50. Early symptoms are 'liver attacks' with nausea on waking in the morning, vomiting of small amounts of mucus, and a lack of appetite for breakfast. Flatulence is a constant early symptom, with a sense of uncomfortable fullness in the upper abdomen after meals.

In the later stages of the disease, there is headache, irritability and drowsiness, and a general feeling of emptiness, with muscular weakness and loss of energy. Neuritis of the legs is common, characterized by muscular cramps and tender calves. The complexion is generally sallow and bloated, with dilated capillary blood vessels, especially over the nose and cheeks, and the tongue is flabby and furred. The liver is always very hard, and its irregular edge can sometimes be felt in the upper abdomen.

After some months, dilated veins appear on the abdominal wall and on the lower chest wall. Dilated varicose veins may also appear at the lower end of the esophagus or gullet. It is not uncommon for these to rupture, leading to vomiting of blood.

In the final stages of cirrhosis, fluid (ascites) appears in the peritoneal cavity. The patient's power of resistance to infection is appreciably reduced.

Treatment. The real treatment of cirrhosis is preventive, and in all cases *alcohol must be absolutely prohibited for the rest of the patient's life.* Some people can drink large quantities of alcohol with safety. Patients with cirrhosis cannot, and one drink is one too many.

A defeatest attitude towards the treatment of the disease, however, should not be adopted, since a damaged liver has remarkable powers of recovery and, in its early stages, cirrhosis of the liver is probably a reversible process.

Glucose lemonade should at first be the only drink allowed, and half a pound of glucose in two pints of lemonade should be given daily. When the patient, who is generally socially inclined, begins to move about his business however, tonic water or bitter lemon drinks (which contain sugar) are of great value.

The diet should be similar to that prescribed for gastric ulcer (p. 365) and should consist largely of milk and milk foods, eggs, fish, poultry, lean meat and liver, cereals, fruit and green vegetables. Vitamins B and C are useful: for C drink a glass of orange, lemon, grapefruit or tomato juice each day, or take ascorbic acid tablets (200 milligrams daily). In all cases highly seasoned food such as curries, pickles, vinegar, mustard, pepper, ripe cheese, and ginger must be permanently avoided.

The bowels should be kept open daily by Epsom salts.

Amoebic Abscess of the Liver

(Tropical Abscess)

Amoebic inflammation of the liver and amoebic abscess are always due to amoebic dysentery (see p. 385). It is not uncommon, therefore, for a tropical abscess to develop some considerable time after a patient has returned home from the tropics, apparently ently quite cured of any dysentery from which he may have suffered. It is ten times commoner in males than in females. Chronic alcoholism is an important predisposing factor.

A single abscess is usually present, but occasionally there are several. The cavity contains thick pinkish pus. When a liver abscess reaches the surface of the liver, adhesions form between the liver and adjoining structures, so that the contents of the abscess may burst into the stomach or bowel, or it may even open on to the outer surface of the abdomen. Inflammation of the lower lobe of the right lung may result when the liver abscess ruptures through the diaphragm.

Symptoms. A tropical abscess generally appears between the ages of 20 and 50. There is a sense of discomfort in the right upper abdomen, developing into severe pain, which may be felt in the right shoulder. In advanced cases the skin behind the right lower margin of the ribs may become puffy and swollen. There is at first a moderate rise of temperature, up to 39·4° C (103° F) in the evening, and sinking below normal in the early morning, the fall of temperature being accompanied by profuse sweating.

Diagnosis. Amoebic abscess may run a lengthy course, and may be unrecognized for a long time. The possibility of its existence should be considered, however, whenever an individual who has been in the tropics is suffering from deterioration of health with obscure abdominal symptoms, together with fever, chills and sweating. It is most commonly confused with malaria. Quinine, however, fails to influence the temperature, whereas the injection of emetine is followed by rapid improvement.

Treatment. The patient must remain in bed under the supervision of a doctor. Very rapid improvement follows the intramuscular injection of 60 milligrams of emetine hydrochloride in 1 milliliter of water (adult dose) on nine consecutive days, and the temperature may fall to normal within twenty-four hours. The patient must remain in bed, however, for the whole course of the injections, and for three days after, since the drug is very toxic. Further courses of 6 or more injections should be given three, six, and twelve months later in order to prevent recurrence.

In resistant cases, a course of chloroquine diphosphate, 0.5 gram daily by mouth for twenty days, may follow each course of emetine injections. It is considerably less toxic than emetine, and may be used as an alternative to emetine in patients with damaged heart muscle.

Once an abscess has actually formed, the most satisfactory treatment is evacuation by aspiration through a large needle attached to a syringe. It is only rarely that an operation is required for a liver abscess.

Cancer of the Liver

Malignant disease of the liver is usually secondary to cancer elsewhere in the body. In women it is a common sequel to cancer of the breast or uterus. The liver becomes enlarged, abnormally hard and irregular in shape. It occurs most frequently after the age of 50.

Symptoms. For a time the only symptoms are those due to the primary growth. When the liver becomes involved, the appetite is lost, and the loss of weight becomes more noticeable. Anemia develops and the patient becomes rapidly weaker.

Persistent pain is usually felt in the right upper abdomen, sometimes passing to the right shoulder and occasionally down the arm. Persistent jaundice is often present owing to pressure by the growth on the bile ducts in the liver. Ascites or fluid in the peritoneal cavity is also often present.

Diagnosis. A painful and irregular enlargement of the liver is most frequently due to a growth. If there is a primary growth elsewhere, or if a growth has been removed by operation within the last five years, the diagnosis can be made with certainty.

Treatment. Since the disease is always fatal, it is not usually justifiable to operate on the primary growth if it is known that the liver is involved. Medical treatment is purely palliative. The patient should be allowed to eat and drink exactly what he likes, and no restrictions should be made. In many cases, however, milk foods, jellies, soups, etc. are all that can be tolerated.

Whenever pain is felt, an injection of morphine or heroin should be ordered by a doctor, and the dose should be increased as the disease progresses. The bowels should be kept regular by purgatives such as senna or cascara, the dose of which generally requires to be increased as more morphine is given.

DISEASES OF THE GALL-BLADDER

Cholecystitis

(Inflammation of the Gall-bladder)

Inflammation of the gall-bladder is due to infection of its walls with micro-organisms.

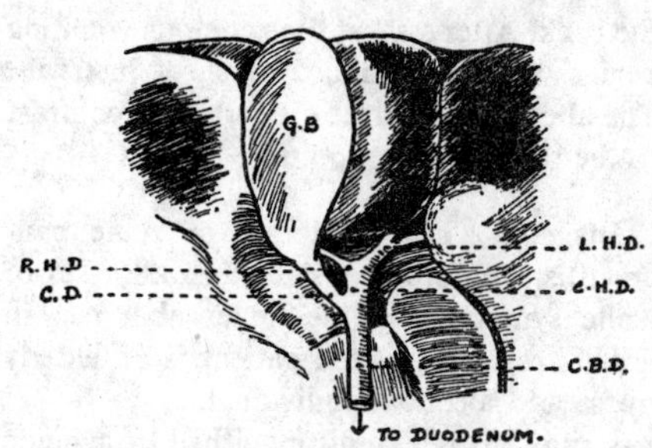

Fig. 20. *GALL-BLADDER AND BILE DUCTS (viewed from the under surface of the liver). G.B. Gall-bladder. R.H.D. Right hepatic duct. C.D. Cystic duct. L.H.D. Left hepatic duct C.B.D. Common bile duct.*

Most cases are probably due to an ascending infection from the duodenum by way of the common bile duct, the infecting organism being *Escherichia coli*, a normal inhabitant of the bowel. Cases often occur as a sequel to typhoid fever, and a few may result from streptococcal infection carried to the gall-bladder by the bloodstream and originating in an infected tooth, tonsil, or appendix.

Cholecystitis and gall-stones are much commoner in women than in men, particularly in women who are past the age of 50 and who have been pregnant. During pregnancy the gall-bladder empties more slowly and less completely than normally, leading to stagnation of its contents, with increased likelihood of infection.

It is not uncommon for symptoms to date from an attack of food poisoning or an acute infection of the stomach and duodenum.

Acute Cholecystitis

Symptoms. Acute and severe pain in the right upper abdomen is the most constant symptom. It often radiates to the lower point of the right shoulder blade, and occasionally to the right shoulder itself. It is sometimes made worse by lying on the left side. Fever is always present, and vomiting is a common symptom.

Treatment. The patient should be put to bed, and the bowels well opened by an enema. For vomiting, warm drinks of sodium bicarbonate solution may be given.

The pain may be alleviated by heat—an electric pad is quite suitable. But the pain is often so agonizing that morphine has to be given, usually with atropine. A careful watch has to be kept on the temperature, pulse, and blood conditions.

The diet for the first day or two should be restricted to bland fluids, such as glucose and lemonade, barley water, milk and mineral water, and weak tea added to the milk. After a day or two, the diet may be cautiously increased, junket, jelly, milk puddings, cereals, vegetables puree, fresh fruit and salads, steamed fish, or a little minced chicken being gradually added. All cooked fat and fried foods, bacon, eggs, red meat, kidneys, liver, sweetbreads and brain should be prohibited.

Penicillin and streptomycin are commonly given by injection and, with adequate treatment, mild cases usually subside in a few days. Since gall-stones are nearly always present in this complaint, recovery should be followed by X-ray examination of the gall-bladder, with a view to deciding on operation.

Chronic Cholecystitis

Symptoms. Chronic infection of the gall-bladder is a common cause of chronic dyspepsia. It is nearly always associated with gall-stones. The patient complains of loss of appetite, and of continual indigestion which is in striking contrast to the clock-like regularity of the pain in duodenal ulcer. Pain begins sometimes immediately after food, or it may be delayed for 2 or 3 hours. It is unaffected or only incompletely relieved by taking food and by alkalis, and it is often made worse by fatty foods. The indigestion is accompanied by a sensation of fullness and upper abdominal distension, with belching of wind. Nausea is common, and it is sometimes followed by vomiting, which gives much less relief than in ulcer. Constipation is generally present.

Tenderness of the gall-bladder is the most characteristic sign. The diagnosis can be confirmed by X-ray examination (*cholecystography*) after taking a special dye preparation by mouth.

Treatment. Since gall-stones are nearly always present, operation is the treatment of choice. Medical treatment may, however, be useful as a temporary expedient to allay distressing symptoms.

The diet is as for acute cholecystitis (see above). Fluids should be taken freely, and sipped slowly on an empty stomach half an hour before meals.

It is important to secure a regular drainage of the bile passages. This can be brought about by giving magnesium sulphate and olive oil by mouth, the oil being taken in tablespoonful doses twice daily before a meal.

Treatment by magnesium sulphate and olive oil should be carried out daily for several months; when all symptoms have disappeared it should be repeated periodically.

Regular exercise should be taken to increase the movements of the diaphragm which encourage a flow of bile. If open-air exercise cannot be tolerated, massage and deep breathing exercises may be carried out at home. Infection in the teeth and tonsils should receive attention.

Gall-stones

(Cholelithiasis)

Infection of the gall-bladder favors the formation of gall-stones, particularly if the flow of bile from the gall-bladder is less free than it should be, as during pregnancy and in obese people.

A starvation diet, low in fat, provides no stimulus for the gall-bladder to contract. As a result, the bile accumulates in the gall-bladder and undergoes progressive concentration which favors the formation of gall-stones.

Most gall-stones consist of cholesterol, bile pigments, and lime salts. The stones are solid, brown in color, and generally have facets, caused by the stones being impacted one against another.

Symptoms. Many older people go through life with gall-stones in the gall-bladder, and yet have no symptoms which may be attributed to them. But their development is preceded in many cases by a long period of continual irregular dyspepsia.

Sooner or later, many patients with gall-stones complain of short attacks of

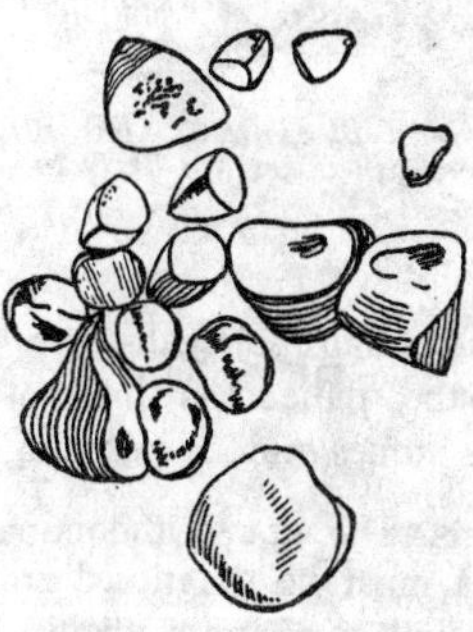

Fig. 21. *GALL-STONES. The stones are usually brownish in color and have facets due to pressure one on the other.*

severe pain which may occur at any time of the day or night, usually after indiscretions in diet, or after a long railway journey or a drive in a motor-car on a bad road. The pain appears in the right upper abdomen.

Occasionally there may be more severe attacks of typical gall-stone colic, often from impaction of a gall-stone in the neck of the gall-bladder. These attacks often occur in the night and begin extremely suddenly with severe (referred) pain in the right upper or middle abdomen, and frequently associated with pain at the lower angle of the right shoulder blade or in the right shoulder. The violent pain is accompanied by great restlessness and sweating, the patient often rolling about in agony. It is made worse by deep breathing and by movement, and is often aggravated by lying on the left side. Nausea almost always occurs, and is often followed by vomiting. Constipation is complete.

Some relief may be obtained by pressing on the abdomen, but the pain commonly disappears with absolute suddenness with the passage of the stone either onwards into the intestine or backwards into the gall-bladder. This sudden onset and sudden cessation are especially characteristic of gall-stone obstruction of the cystic duct. If a stone in passing onwards fails to reach the duodenum and becomes impacted in the common bile duct, jaundice occurs, and continues until the stone becomes dislodged.

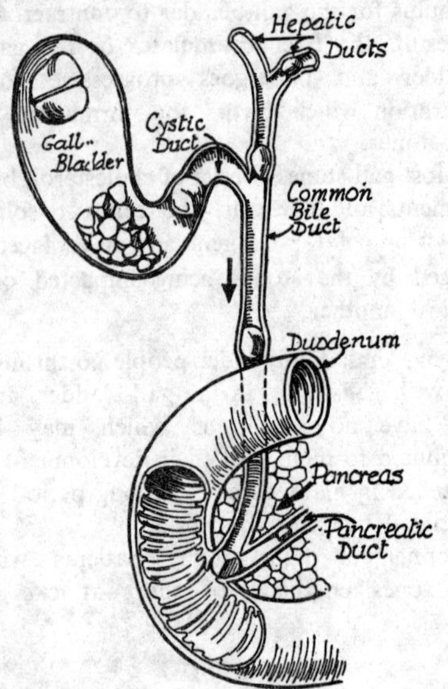

Fig. 22. *GALL-BLADDER AND BILE DUCTS showing where gall-stones are likely to lodge in the narrow ducts.*

Once an attack of gall-stone colic has occurred the patient is liable to further attacks, as stones seldom exist singly.

Diagnosis. The upper abdominal pain of gall-stones must be diagnosed from gastric and duodenal ulcer, appendicitis, and from disease of the coronary arteries of the heart,

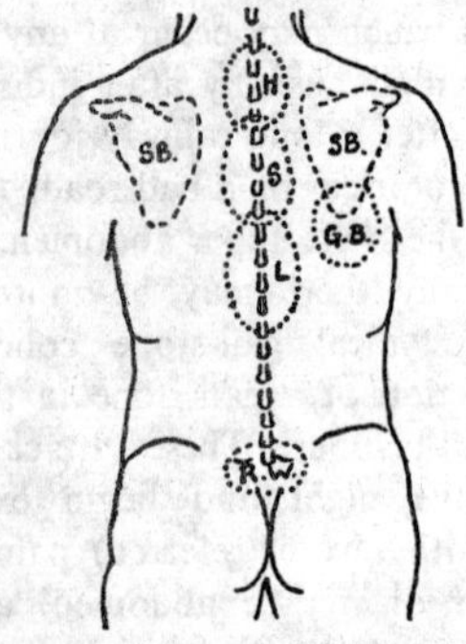

Fig. 23. *AREAS OF REFERRED PAIN over the spine and back in various diseases. H. In heart diseases. S. In stomach diseases. L. In liver diseases. R.W. In diseases of the rectum and womb. G.B. In diseases of the gall-bladder. S.B. Shoulder blades.*

which sometimes gives rise to pain in the upper middle abdomen. An attack of typical gall-stone colic must be distinguished from renal colic due to a kidney stone. X-ray examination may be necessary to distinguish these conditions.

Persistent jaundice from obstruction of the common bile duct by a gall-stone must be distinguished from jaundice due to cancer of the head of the pancreas, and operation may be necessary before the question can be finally decided.

Treatment. For the prevention of gall-stones, the early recognition of cholecystitis is essential, and treatment for this complaint should be thoroughly carried out (see p. 379).

Once gall-stones have formed in an infected gall-bladder, there are no known medical means of dissolving them.

During an attack of gall-stone colic, the pain should be controlled by the injection of morphine (15 mg), and atropine (1 mg) prescribed by a doctor. Slight attacks may be relieved by 1 gram of Dover's Powder taken by mouth, or by a tablet of nitro-glycerin (0·5 mg) placed under the tongue and allowed to dissolve in the mouth. A hot-water bottle should be applied to the abdomen.

If symptoms point definitely to the presence of gall-stones, and if repeated attacks of severe gall-stone colic have occurred, an operation should be undertaken, the gall-bladder and its contained stones being removed. This is at present the only certain cure for gall-stones.

In old patients and in those suffering from advanced disease of the heart or lungs, especially if they are practically free from symptoms, it is wisest to avoid operation.

DISEASES OF THE PANCREAS

The pancreas, or sweetbread, is a glandular organ lying behind the stomach and near the back wall of the abdomen. See also Physiology, p. 261.

Insulin is produced in the 'tail' part of the organ, and a deficiency of this hormone causes diabetes mellitus (see Fig. 24). The disease is described on p. 392.

Acute Pancreatitis

This disease is usually found in persons between 40 and 70 years of age, who in many cases have suffered from gall-stones. Obstruction of the mouth of the common bile

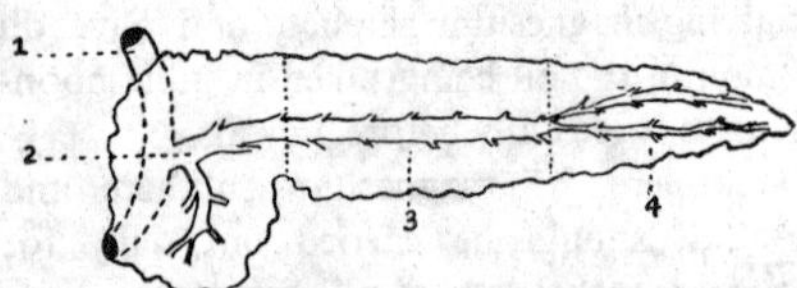

Fig. 24. *PANCREAS. Diagram showing the sites giving rise to various disorders of the pancreas. Obstruction by gall-stone in* (1) *the common bile duct, and* (2) *the pancreatic duct, causes jaundice. Disease of area* (3) *causes pain. Disorder of 'islets' in the 'tail,' where insulin is produced, causes diabetes mellitus.*

duct, or of the pancreatic duct itself, usually by a gall-stone, causes an increase in the pressure of secretion of the pancreas, and a release of enzymes which damage the cells of the gland.

Acute pancreatitis is also occasionally seen in influenza, typhoid fever and smallpox, and is a rare complication of mumps.

Symptoms. The disease when fully developed is remarkable for the intensity of the symptoms, and for their extraordinary suddenness. Without any warning, sudden agonizing pain is felt in the upper abdomen and across the back. After a short time copious vomiting begins, and is continued at short intervals. The abdomen becomes distended, in contrast to the rigidity in peritonitis.

Diagnosis. The possibility of acute pancreatitis should be considered in all cases of acute symptoms in the upper abdomen in adults, especially if the patient is an elderly obese and alcoholic individual.

It may have to be distinguished from acute cholecystitis (which may actually be present at the same time), perforated peptic ulcer, acute intestinal obstruction, coronary thrombosis, and acute appendicitis. Changes in the composition of the urine are of great importance, and may include blood, bile, sugar, acetone bodies and increased urinary diastase.

Treatment. Modern treatment tends to be conservative, and consists of intravenous therapy with saline and calcium gluconate for three to four days, and continuous gastric suction to relieve vomiting and distension. No food is taken by mouth during this period.

Operation should only be undertaken if there is uncertainty about the diagnosis, in the presence of acute cholecystitis or obstructive jaundice, and when there is spreading peritonitis.

Cancer of the Pancreas

Cancer of the pancreas is fairly common in persons over 50 years of age. It is twice as common in men as in women. The head of the pancreas is affected in over 60 per cent of cases, causing obstruction of the pancreatic duct and later of the common bile duct.

Symptoms. Jaundice is a very common symptom and it increases until it becomes an intense greenish tinge. Bile is completely absent from the feces, which are bulky and pale. The patient complains of a dull aching pain in the upper abdomen, passing to the back. There is rapid loss of weight, the disease being fatal within a few months to a year.

Treatment. Apart from operation, no treatment is known which has any effect upon its course.

Cystic Fibrosis of Pancreas

This disorder is genetically determined, the tissue of the pancreas being unable to function properly as it becomes fibrous and cystic. The nature of the defect is not understood but a child so born is unable to combat infections, especially staphylococci in the lungs. In many cases the infant dies of pulmonary sepsis by the age of fourteen months. If a child survives, his heart is so strained that death is usual about puberty.

Treatment. Most children have to be permanently on antibiotic therapy. Diet should be rich in protein, low in fat, and plenty of salt taken.

DISEASES OF THE SPLEEN

The spleen is an organ about the size of the palm of the hand, which lies in the left upper abdomen, tucked away under the left lower margin of the ribs. It is a composite organ and one of its functions is to act as a blood reservoir.

Rupture of the spleen may occur as a result of injury to the abdomen. It is commonest when the organ is diseased and enlarged, as in typhoid fever or malaria. It gives rise to severe internal hemorrhage, and requires immediate treatment by surgical operation.

Chronic Enlargement

An enlarged spleen can be felt as a smooth hard mass in the left upper abdomen projecting from below the left lower margin of the ribs. The whole spleen becomes dense and fibrous and occasionally attains an enormous size.

Enlargement of the spleen is a feature of many diseases, both in the tropics and in temperate climates. It is common in malaria, kala-azar, tuberculosis, syphilis, Hodgkin's disease, and in various types of anemia and blood diseases. Examination of the blood by special methods is usually necessary to discover the cause of enlargement in any particular case.

Treatment. This will vary according to the treatment of the fever or blood disorder that is causing the enlargement.

See also Diseases of the Blood and Spleen, p. 315.

DISEASES OF THE PERITONEUM

The peritoneum is an extensive membrane which lines the whole of the inside of the abdomen, enveloping all of the contained organs, and extending downwards in front of them as a double fold, or apron, known as the *omentum*. The whole peritoneal surface is almost equal in area to the skin surface of the body.

Acute Peritonitis

Causes. Acute peritonitis is due to bacterial infection, usually from the alimentary canal. The most common seat of the primary condition is an inflamed appendix. The infection passes through the damaged walls of the appendix, leading to the formation of peritoneal adhesions and possibly of an appendix abscess.

When the infection is particularly virulent, or the patient's resistance is unusually low, a spreading infection of the whole peritoneal cavity occurs, causing the coils of intestine to become glued together with a sticky exudate, and leading to acute general peritonitis. As well as infection due to a ruptured appendix, peritonitis may follow infection caused by perforation of stomach or duodenal ulcers, an infected gall-bladder, or perforating wounds of the abdomen, intestinal surgery, or septic abortions.

Primary pneumococcal peritonitis may occur in children, especially girls between the age of six and ten, from infection through the genital passages.

Other cases of primary peritonitis are seen in which there is no apparent infection of any abdominal organ. In such cases the organisms presumably reach the peritoneum by the bloodstream from an infected focus elsewhere in the body.

Symptoms. (See also Acute Appendicitis, p. 373).

Abdominal pain is the earliest and most constant symptom, usually central and in front; vomiting follows and generally the pain becomes more local, with tenderness and fever. If the infected organ is near the abdominal wall, the central pain may be absent, and local pain occurs at the outset. The patient lies immobile.

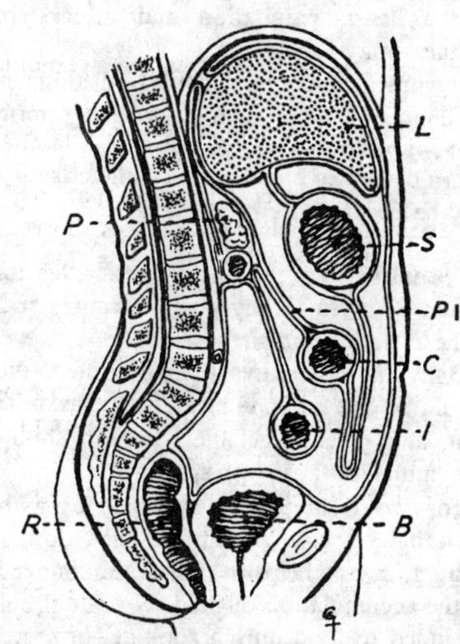

Fig. 25. *PERITONEUM. Vertical section indicating the relationship of the abdominal organs contained within the many folds of the peritoneum. L. Liver. P. Pancreas. S. Stomach. Pl. Peritoneum. C. Colon. I. Intestines. B. Bladder. R. Rectum.*

The pulse increases up to 100 or 120 per minute, and diminishes in volume, giving rise to the 'wiry' pulse of late peritonitis. The temperature begins to rise and the tongue becomes dry and furred. In the early stages, and especially in young and vigorous patients, the abdomen has an immovable board-like rigidity, and is extremely tender on pressure. The patient lies with his knees drawn up to relieve the abdominal tension and the movements of respiration are confined to the chest. Unless the condition is relieved by surgical operation, the paralyzed intestine gradually becomes dilated and the abdomen distended. Vomiting then becomes frequent, the vomited matter being exceedingly foul. The breath is offensive and the urine scanty.

Throughout the whole course of the disease the outstanding feature is the pain, which may at first be intermittent and colicky but soon becomes constant and agonizing, and is increased by the smallest movements. In old, fat, or feeble persons, whose muscles are poorly developed, pain and rigidity may be slight or absent, though the other features remain.

Treatment. The condition is always dangerous and must be diagnosed as soon as possible. Treatment must be directed at removing the cause, e.g. surgical removal of an infected appendix, or surgical treatment of a perforated peptic ulcer.

Until a definite diagnosis has been made and operation agreed to, no morphine or opium should be given in any form, since it masks the symptoms.

It is important also *that at no time previous to operation should any fluid or food be given by mouth*, as it will tend to leak away through any existing perforation in the abdomen, and thus cause a further spread of infection. The most that should be allowed is an occasional moistening of the tongue with a few drops of water. Above all, *no purgatives* (*castor oil, etc.*) *should be given*, as these have often caused the rupture of an already inflamed appendix. An enema, however, may be required to clear the lower bowel before operation is undertaken, and saline solution (1 level teaspoonful of salt to the pint of warm water) may be given by this route to combat the collapse and relieve thirst. The intestines meanwhile are rested by passing a Ryle's tube and aspirating the contents of the stomach at frequent intervals. In severely collapsed patients, fluid may be given intravenously.

Operation is followed by drainage of the peritoneal cavity with a tube. Both before and after operation the patient should be propped up in bed in a sitting position (Fowler's position, p. 374) to allow the infective material to gravitate downwards to the lower abdomen and pelvic cavity, where the peritoneum has a diminished absorptive surface and from where it can be removed more easily.

The outlook in acute peritonitis has been greatly improved by the use of antibiotics. Streptomycin and penicillin are commonly used together, both for prevention and for treatment, as the infection is usually a mixed one.

Tuberculous Peritonitis

Chronic tuberculous peritonitis is often associated with tuberculosis in other parts of the body, especially of the lungs. Most cases occur between the ages of 3 and 20 years. In children (who do not often have tuberculosis of the lungs) the drinking of tuberculous milk may lead to infection of the abdominal lymph glands, which in turn gives rise to infection of the peritoneum.

Symptoms. The onset is gradual. The general symptoms of ill health which are common to all types of tuberculosis are the first to appear. The patient loses weight and strength, the appetite is poor, and the temperature tends to become slightly raised at night. After a time there are symptoms of general abdominal discomfort, which are especially marked after exercise or hard work. Attacks of colic, together with either constipation or diarrhea may occur in the later stages.

Treatment. The most important prophylactic measures are the provision of a pure milk supply, and the removal of children from contact with adults suffering from active pulmonary tuberculosis.

OPEN AIR. When the disease has actually developed, the patient should be kept in bed completely at rest so long as his temperature is raised. Complete rest in bed may be necessary for several months and, whenever possible, the child should be nursed in an open-air hospital or sanatorium.

DIET. The diet should be as liberal and as nourishing as possible, with extra milk, cream, butter and eggs. Cod-liver oil or halibut-liver oil should also be given together with ascorbic acid (vitamin C).

MEDICATION. Diarrhea should be treated with a non-irritating fluid or semi-fluid diet, and by an intestinal sedative medicine containing kaolin (see Treatment of Diarrhea p. 369).

The standard treatment today is to combine and P.A.S. isoniazid.

OPERATION is only rarely indicated, though fluid may require to be withdrawn from a distended abdomen.

Cancer of the Peritoneum

Cancer of the peritoneum is nearly always secondary to cancer of one of the abdominal organs, especially the stomach or the ovary. The disease may also follow cancer of the breast.

Malignant peritonitis generally leads to ascites and may cause extensive peritoneal adhesions with possible obstruction of the intestine. The navel is often infiltrated with growth.

Treatment. This is purely palliative, and it is rare for a patient to survive for more than six months after the peritoneum becomes involved. Considerable relief may follow tapping of the abdomen for fluid.

MISCELLANEOUS CONDITIONS OF THE ABDOMINAL ORGANS

Ascites

(Dropsy of Abdominal Cavity)

Causes. Ascites, or the accumulation of free fluid in the peritoneal cavity, is not a disease in itself but a symptom of a large variety of pathological processes. It occurs in the later stages of cirrhosis of the liver, in heart failure when it may be associated with dropsy of the legs, and in disease of the kidney when it may be associated with dropsy of the skin. It is a common complication of malignant disease of the liver or peritoneum in adults and the aged, and of tuberculous peritonitis in children.

Symptoms. There is a sensation of tightness in the abdomen. As the fluid accumulates the abdomen becomes larger and larger, and its walls more and more stretched so that a man may find it impossible to fasten the top buttons of his trousers. At the same time the veins round the navel may become dilated. The rise in the pressure inside the abdomen causes obstruction to the return of the blood flow from the legs, with dropsy of the ankles, while pressure on the kidneys may lead to a decreased amount of urine. The diaphragm is pushed up towards the chest, and shortness of breath may follow the limited expansion of the lungs. Irregularity of the heart, palpitation and attacks of faintness may follow.

In women it may be difficult to distinguish the condition from a large ovarian tumor. It is important also to distinguish ascites from a distended bladder, and catheterization may be necessary.

Treatment. To prevent ascites, attention should be given to any possible causes such as heart failure or cirrhosis.

DIET. In most cases a high protein diet should be given, rich in meat, fish, eggs, milk, fruit, and green vegetables. Protein should be minimal for those with acute nephritis.

For two to three weeks at a time it may be advisable to give a salt-free diet, low in sodium, as this helps to reduce the tendency to the accumulation of fluid. No salt should be added to food during cooking, or served with a meal, and the following foods should be avoided: canned foods which have added salt (meats, vegetables, soups, and tomato juice), smoked, brine-cured and salty food (bacon, ham, sausages, smoked fish such as kippers, and pickles), meat extracts and sauces, shellfish, cheese and salted butter. Foods to which baking powder or baking soda has been added should also be avoided. No sodium-containing medicines such as sodium bicarbonate, soda mints, sodium sulphate, or sodium bromide should be taken at these times.

A sodium-free diet should not be persisted with for more than three consecutive weeks, as there is a danger of uremia developing if sodium is withheld for too long.

A dose of magnesium sulphate (Epsom salts) should be taken each morning.

DIURETICS. A considerable reduction in the amount of fluid may follow injection of one of the organic mercurial diuretics, of the type used in the treatment of heart failure. Although these diuretics are very effective, they should be used with caution in patients with nephritis; chlorothiazide or another non-mercurial diuretic may be of value through its relative absence of side-effects.

Patients who are being treated with any diuretic need to be under the careful observation of a doctor so that he may regularly check up on its effect on the balance of potassium and sodium in the blood plasma.

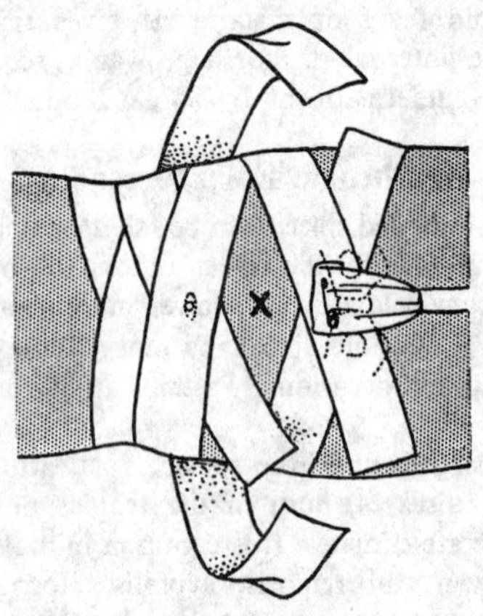

Fig. 26. PARACENTESIS. When fluid has accumulated in and distends the abdomen, and the condition is little improved with diuretic drugs, a puncture may be made at X and the fluid drained off. The many-tailed abdominal bandage is periodically tightened as the distension is reduced.

PARACENTESIS. If, in spite of these measures, the accumulation of fluid continues to cause discomfort, or seriously to interfere with breathing or digestion, the abdomen may be tapped by a physician. It is essential before this is done for the bladder to be emptied by catheterization and the tapping is usually performed in the mid-line of the abdomen, halfway between the navel and the pelvic bone. A many-tailed bandage is placed round the abdomen, with an opening over the site where the puncture is to be made, and it should be periodically tightened as the amount of fluid diminishes. The drainage may continue for a day or longer, and eleven to fifteen pints of fluid may be removed at a tapping. The operation may have to be repeated at intervals, but the number of tappings should be kept to the absolute minimum, since repeated tapping has the effect of depleting to an undesirable extent the patient's store of protein. See also Medical and Technical Procedures, p. 568.

Visceroptosis

(Dropping of the Abdominal Organs)

Causes. In visceroptosis, the abdominal organs lie at a lower level than usual in the abdominal cavity. The condition is usually due to a fall of pressure inside the abdomen caused by weakness of the abdominal and pelvic muscles, the normal tone of which maintains the abdominal organs in position. Weakness of the abdominal muscles tends to follow the stretching which takes place during pregnancy. After confinement a considerable fall occurs in the pressure inside the abdomen, and the stretched muscles are at first very lax. If the patient remains in bed for a sufficient time they gradually regain their tone, but otherwise they may become permanently weakened. Weakness of the abdominal muscles is also common in people who do not take sufficient exercise, and in those who have lost a considerable amount of weight for any reason.

Symptoms. There may be no symptoms at all but, when present, they occur only when the patient is standing up. The symptoms are worse in the later part of the day than in the morning, owing to the progressive relaxation of the abdominal muscles from fatigue. They disappear on lying down, and are relieved by pressure to the lower abdomen, which in the standing position can be noticed to bulge unduly.

The general effects of visceroptosis are of greater importance than those which are due to the dropping of the individual organs such as the stomach, intestines, liver, or kidney. They include a feeling of weakness and exhaustion, together with vague abdominal discomfort of a dragging nature, and often associated with chronic backache and flatulence. Constipation is common, and is due to the interference with the voluntary act of defecation by the weakness of the abdominal and pelvic muscles. The mental state is commonly one of depression or anxiety, with marked introspection concerning the state of the abdominal organs. In some cases the symptoms arise from an anxiety neurosis.

Diagnosis is usually made by X-ray examination of the abdominal organs (see Fig. 8, p. 368).

Treatment

PREVENTION. Much can be done to prevent the development of visceroptosis in women by proper management of the period following child birth. Early ambulation is now largely practiced, the patient getting up on the third or fourth day for gradually increasing periods daily to help her regain her strength more quickly. It must be emphasized, however, that early ambulation and early return to domestic duties are two very different things, and, although getting about early is wise, patients should not be discharged from hospital or nursing home, or allowed to return to their duties any earlier on account of it.

Many mothers, however, who have had difficult deliveries, or who are much debilitated by frequent childbearing, and who are very tired at the end of another pregnancy, are able to benefit from prolonged rest after delivery. In such cases they should get up only on the third day for the toilet and for a bath, but the patient should move about freely while in bed and should be encouraged to move her limbs. After the first five days, in all cases, exercises for the abdominal muscles should be regularly practiced (see p. 368). In debilitated patients most of the time during the first few days after getting up should be spent on a couch, and a return to full physical activity allowed only after three to six weeks.

FOR THE DEVELOPED CONDITION. Early to bed should be the rule, and an additional rest during the day may be helpful.

Exercises out of doors, daily breathing exercises and special remedial exercises to develop the muscles of the abdominal wall and pelvic floor are of great value. Those which are suitable for chronic constipation are equally suitable for visceroptosis (see p. 368). These exercises should be graduated, and should begin with the least strenuous. For weakness of the pelvic floor the patient should be instructed to perform the movement she would make if she were attempting to overcome an urgent desire to defecate. This exercise should be repeated about thirty times a day while lying down, and is of value in curing the associated constipation.

Abdominal massage is useful as a supplement to the exercises.

Abdominal supports. To prevent the overstretching of the abdominal muscles in the standing position, a support may be required for a time to press the abdominal contents upwards, backwards and inwards, but it should be discarded as soon as the abdominal muscles have regained their normal tone. It should be made specially for the individual patient, so that it fits closely to the pelvis below, and does not extend upwards beyond the navel.

An abdominal support should always be put on when the patient is lying down, and it should be worn all day except when exercises are being performed.

Diet. Since many patients with visceroptosis are exceedingly thin, a serious attempt should be made to increase their weight by a good nourishing diet. The best extra food is milk, and it may be taken plain or in made-up dishes. Cream and butter should be taken in as large amounts as possible. It is sometimes an advantage for fluids to be taken half an hour before the meals.

Medicinal Treatment. For the relief of constipation, simple lubricants will usually be sufficient, supplemented, if necessary, with a dose of milk of magnesia or health salts.

Operation. In no circumstances should any operation be performed for raising dropped organs, as it almost invariably happens that no satisfactory benefit results. Only in the event of a surgical emergency should an operation be resorted to.

Hernia

(Rupture)

By the term hernia is meant the protrusion beyond its normal position of some part or structure of one of the body cavities. When used without any special qualifications, the term is understood to mean an external abdominal (inguinal) hernia, or rupture. This type accounts for over 90 per cent of all hernias in men and 50 per cent of all hernias in women, in whom femoral hernia is much commoner than in men. Next in frequency come post-operation hernias, or hernias through weak operation scars in the abdominal wall. These account for nearly 10 per cent. Hernia of the navel (umbilical hernia) is not uncommon in infancy.

External Abdominal (Inguinal) Hernia

External abdominal hernia is a very common complaint especially amongst those engaged in strenuous occupations. In men, it is closely associated with the passage by which the testis in early life descends from the abdominal cavity into the scrotum, and in advanced forms of rupture the contents of the hernial sac may occupy one side of the scrotal sac. The contents of a hernia usually consists of folds of peritoneum (*omentum*) or small intestine, or both. A hernia may be wholly or partly reducible, or it may be irreducible, the contents being retained in the sac by reason of their bulk or by a constriction at the neck of the sac, or by adhesions between the contents and the wall of the sac.

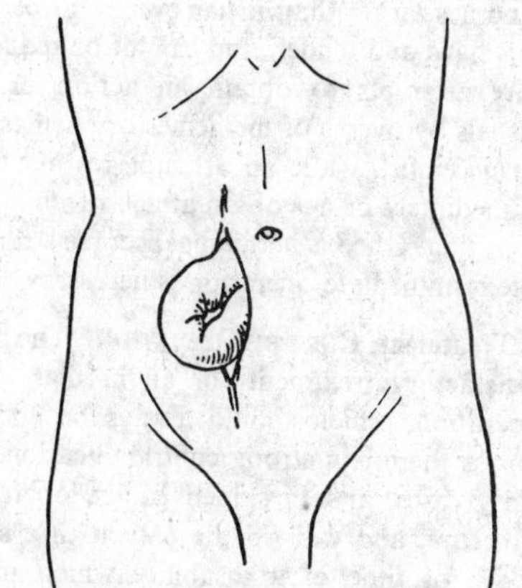

Fig. 27. *AN ABDOMINAL HERNIA. A loop of intestine protruding through a broken thin abdominal scar.*

Symptoms. As a rule the patient notices some slight discomfort which draws attention to the part in which an abnormal swelling is found. Such a swelling may be present only intermittently, and in the early stages it usually disappears when the patient lies down. Often there is a feeling of weakness or insecurity in the region of the groin.

Some hernias are present from birth. Others appear suddenly later in life, usually after some strain, while the remainder appear gradually and are first recognized as an unusual swelling or lump. Once it has appeared, a hernia tends to become progressively larger. Hernia is rarely associated with acute pain unless it becomes strangulated, but may give rise to constipation and dyspepsia or nausea.

An abdominal hernia forms an external swelling which is usually soft and compressible. When it can be reduced, i.e. returned to the abdomen, the process is sometimes accompanied by a gurgling of intestinal gas and liquid. The swelling gives an impulse on coughing which can be both seen and felt by the person examining the swelling.

Complications

OBSTRUCTION. A hernia may become obstructed in the sense that the contents of the bowel in the sac do not pass on. The condition may often be relieved by enemas assisted by manipulation of the hernia, after ensuring by catheterization that the bladder is empty.

STRANGULATION. If an obstructed hernia cannot be reduced, there is a risk that it may become strangulated, from increased bulk of the contents of the sac. Acute strangulation is due to congestion which leads to complete stagnation of the circulation in the contents of the sac, which, if not relieved by operation, results in gangrene of the bowel. It is one of the commonest causes of acute intestinal obstruction (see p. 372).

The onset is usually heralded by an attack of pain which is at first referred to the navel and is later felt in the hernia. The hernia becomes larger than it has ever been before. It is hard and tender, and cannot be reduced. Any attempts to obtain an action of the bowels by means of medicines or enemas are unsuccessful, while an attempt to take food immediately brings on an attack of colic and vomiting. Once a hernia has become strangulated, immediate operation is necessary.

Treatment. CURE BY OPERATION. The most satisfactory treatment for all hernias is by operation, which should always be advised unless there is a strong contraindication. In early cases, and in skilled hands, operation can cure, and will rid the patient in a short space of time of a disability which might otherwise last a lifetime and which may, with increasing years, become a danger.

Contraindications to operation are few, but it should not be undertaken before a persistent cough has been brought under control, or in cases of uncontrolled diabetes mellitus, or of great or increasing obesity.

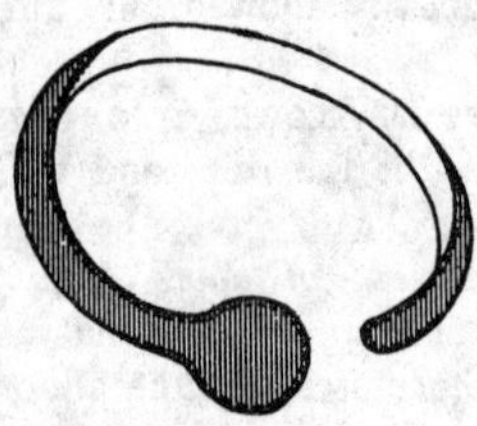

Fig. 28. *A TRUSS is made of spring steel well padded and covered on the inner body side with soft chamois leather. The widened end covers the hernia and holds it firmly in position.*

TRUSS. Only a hernia which is completely reducible can be controlled with a truss. It must be able to retain a hernia in all positions of the body and in the presence of ordinary stresses such as coughing, sneezing and laughing. The real test of a truss is its ability to retain the hernia while the patient sits on the edge of a chair with the trunk bent fully forward, and the legs widely separated. If in this position the hernia is retained during coughing, the truss is likely to prove efficient. The object of a truss is to prevent the hernia from ever coming down. It must therefore be applied before the patient rises in the morning, and it should not be removed before he lies down at night.

Umbilical Hernia

Hernia of the navel is not uncommon in infants, and it often appears when the child is a few weeks old. Two matters are important in the management of the condition. Firstly, all causes of abnormal abdominal distension should be discovered and removed, and secondly, crying should be reduced to a minimum. Pressure should be applied over the protuberance by means of a small flat pad. A penny wrapped in cloth is very suitable for the purpose. It must be firmly fixed over the site of the hernia by strapping and kept in position continuously for three to six months, though the strapping may be renewed every week or two. If this does not result in cure, or if the condition recurs, an operation should be undertaken after the child has reached the age of two years. Most hernias of this type disappear spontaneously, however, within the first year of life.

Diaphragmatic Hernia
(*Hiatus Hernia*)

In diaphragmatic hernia there is protrusion of the abdominal contents through the diaphragm into the thorax. The reverse never occurs. The opening through which the esophagus passes is the most vulnerable part of the diaphragm, and it is through this opening that most hernias of the diaphragm occur.

This condition is fairly common and may simulate almost any upper abdominal disorder. The contents are usually composed of the upper part of the stomach.

Symptoms. The chief symptom is burning pain after food, and particularly on lying down, which may prevent the patient from sleeping or may actually waken him from sleep. It is due to the acid of the gastric juice rising into the esophagus and irritating the mucous membrane in its lower third. In severe cases it may be associated with actual ulceration and bleeding.

Persistent vomiting in young infants is sometimes due to this disorder; it can be confirmed by X-ray diagnosis.

Heartburn is a common symptom during the later months of pregnancy, and is due to herniation of the stomach resulting from increased pressure caused by the enlarged uterus. The symptom usually disappears after delivery.

Treatment. This consists in raising the head of the bed on wooden blocks nine inches high, the patient being propped up with pillows during the night. Antacids should be given, combined at night with atropine or with one of the synthetic antispasmodics.

INTESTINAL AND OTHER PARASITES

Amoebiasis

Amoebiasis in man is caused by the parasite *Entamoeba histolytica.* It is not a worm but a small mobile single-celled organism which digests red blood cells (see Fig. 1). When this infestation is confined to the bowel it is called AMOEBIC DYSENTERY. (Bacillary dysentery is described in Fevers and Infectious Diseases, p. 270.) The parasite tends to form abscesses elsewhere, especially in the liver, and the disease is then named after the organ which is infected, e.g. HEPATIC AMOEBIASIS.

See also Amoebic Abscess of the Liver, p. 378.

This infestation has appeared in most parts of the world with outbreaks in Great Britain and the U.S.A. not being uncommon. It is most prevalent, however, in China and India.

Amoebiasis has a great tendency to spread through families because of poor sanitation and unclean habits of members of the family. The cysts (and entamoebae) appear in the stools of the infested person and are transmitted by flies, rats, or by direct contact with the food of the next victim.

The parasites form small cysts and ulcers in the cecum and wall of the large bowel and rectum. Some of the parasites may be carried to the liver where they produce abscesses and symptoms of hepatitis.

Symptoms. Amoebiasis is a chronic disease. The incubation period is from one week to three months. Diarrhea is usually the most obvious symptom and is mostly of the intermittent variety. The stools are copious and there is blood intermingled with the feces. The smell is very offensive. Fever is very uncommon unless the liver is involved, but there is marked loss of weight. Vomiting rarely occurs, but there is often tenderness of the abdomen over the course of the large bowel. The complications are those of perforation of the bowel wall, hemorrhage, and exhaustion.

Diagnosis is made by examining the stools for cysts and for the motile amoebae. The appearance of the bowel wall can be examined by means of a sigmoidoscope (a tube with a light and with a magnifying lens, used to inspect the bowel via the anus). The blood shows a mild leucocytosis.

Treatment. 1. Metronidazole has greatly simplified in recent years the treatment of amoebic dysentery; 800 milligrams daily for 5 days will give a satisfactory clearance in acute attacks.

2. To protect the liver from invasion, the acute attack can, alternatively, be treated for about fourteen days with a combination of tetracycline, diloxanide furoate, and chloroquine.

3. In severe attacks, especially in children and debilitated patients, the patient should be confined to bed and kept under the doctor's close care. Several treatments are available.

(a) Metronidazole 800 milligrams should be given three times a day for five days combined with tetracycline and diloxanide furoate as in treatment 2.

(b) Emetine hydrochloride 65 milligrams daily by intramuscular injection for about five days until the dysentery clears, together with tetracycline and diloxanide furoate.

(c) Dehydroemetine 1.5 milligrams per kilogram of body weight by intramuscular injection for five to ten days combined with tetracycline and diloxanide furoate.

For hepatic amoebiasis, 400 milligrams of metronidazole three times a day for five days should clear the condition.

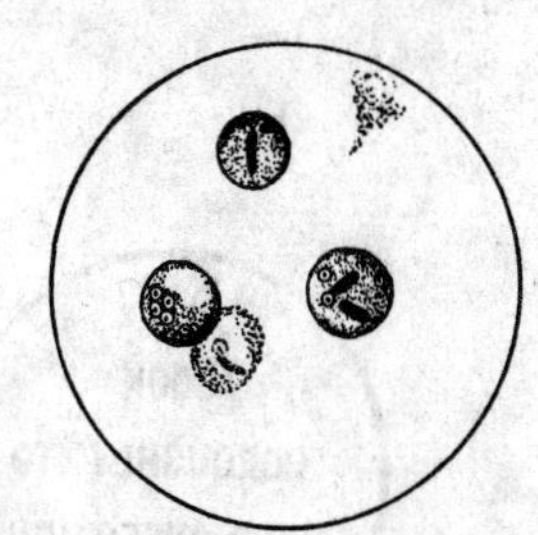

Fig. 1. *CYSTS OF ENTAMOEBA. As the cystic forms of the organism mature the single nucleus divides to form two and then four nuclei. The four-nuclei forms can survive in the bowel for about two days, but do not split (or hatch) until ingested by a new host.*

An alternative combined treatment with emetine hydrochloride for 10 days, chloroquine for 28 days, and diloxanide furoate for 10 days is also very effective.

General Management. In the acute condition, the patient needs kindly and careful nursing for he is usually much undernourished. If emetine has been given, its toxic side-effects on the heart muscle will be much reduced if the patient remains strictly resting in bed. Once the diarrhea is controlled he can be given a good mixed diet rich in any of the meat, fish, and dairy proteins. Vitamin content (see pp. 68-71) of the foods should be high. Fluids should be taken freely.

Patients in bed should be given a bath daily or take one when ambulant.

Prevention. This is relatively simple and merely entails the washing of one's hands after toilet usage and before meals. All vegetables should be cooked and drinking water boiled. Proper methods of sanitation should be installed. Wire mesh on windows and doors, fly sprays and rat killers will exclude the vectors. Finally, carriers of the disease (but who show no obvious signs of it) should be treated thoroughly and kept from occupations which take them where food is prepared.

WORM INFESTATIONS

Worm infestations are very common in tropical and subtropical countries and create much misery. They have been a cause of suffering from ancient times as evidenced by the discovery of calcified eggs of *Schistosoma* in Egyptian mummies. Medical papyri around 1000 B.C. record the symptoms of blood in the urine due to worms and they noted the existence of tapeworms.

Certain worms gain admittance to their victim directly while others require a vector, e.g. the filarial parasite is transmitted to man by the bite of a mosquito.

The life-span of the different kinds of worms which may infest man vary greatly. In patients who have been inadequately treated, tapeworms have been known to survive for twenty years. In threadworms, the life cycle is two weeks.

General Diagnosis

Some worms or their eggs are easily seen in the feces as are those of roundworms and beef tapeworms. Others require a more meticulous search, using a microscope to inspect samples of blood, feces, urine, skin, or muscle.

Certain tests may be made of a person's blood or his skin to detect the presence of worms in the tissues. One example is the Casoni test in which a small amount of substance is injected into the patient's skin and his response to the injections will show whether or not he has a hydatid infestation.

Ancylostomiasis

(Hookworm Infestation)

Hookworm is common in tropical and subtropical countries.

The eggs pass out in the feces of an infested person and, after a period of development in the soil, the larvae penetrate the human skin, from whence they migrate via the veins to the alimentary canal, especially

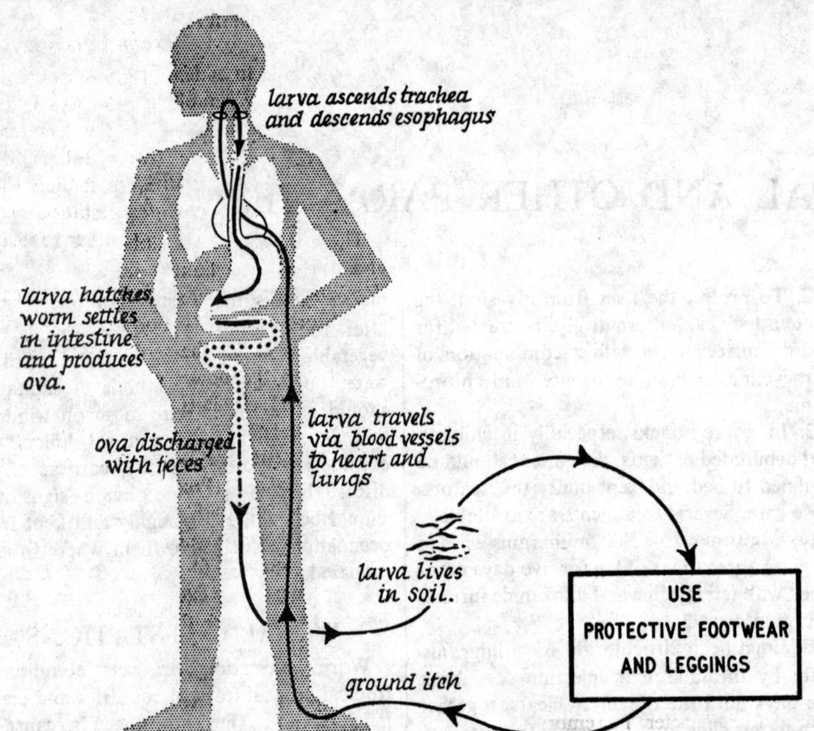

Fig. 2. *LIFE CYCLE OF THE HOOKWORM. After the eggs of the hookworm are expelled from the host's body in the feces, they undergo a period of development in the soil (usually in the top inch). They are able to remain in this larval stage for up to two years, and enter the human host by piercing the skin (usually of the feet), often causing 'ground itch' sores. In about seven days, the larvae make their way via the blood vessels to the heart and lungs, then to the trachea and downwards to the intestines. There they mature, mate and the eggs are laid. Adult hookworms are about ½ inch in length.*

the small intestine, and there they adhere to wall and extract blood (see Fig. 5).

Symptoms. The predominant symptoms are lethargy and weakness due to a severe anemia. This anemia leads to slow or retarded development in children. Abdominal pain and attacks of fever are not uncommon.

Treatment. Tetrachloroethylene is the drug of choice. The adult dose is 4 milliliters and it is given with a saline purgative, such as sodium sulphate. The dose for a child is 0.2 milliliters for each year of life. Two or more courses of treatment are required. It is important to remember that tetrachloroethylene deteriorates in a hot climate and so it must be stored in a cool dark place.

Bephenium hydroxynaphthoate has also been used with success against the hookworm. The dose is 5 grams of granules for all ages; purgation is not needed. No food should be eaten for two hours after a dose.

The anemia is corrected by the administration of iron-containing preparations, e.g. ferrous sulphate or ferrous gluconate tablets, and by eating a well-balanced diet.

Ascariasis

(*Roundworm Infestation*)

Ascaris lumbricoides is found in most parts of the world. It is a pale yellow worm up to 25 to 35 cm. in length. Infestation occurs as a result of eating contaminated food, the contamination usually being due to handling foodstuffs with unwashed hands. The eggs are swallowed and they hatch out in the duodenum and the embryos find their way to the lungs.

Symptoms. Vague digestive symptoms of nausea and malaise with occasional abdominal pain is usual. Sometimes a child will develop a cough and bronchopneumonia with the production of blood-stained sputum. The adult worm lives in the small intestine and remains there often without producing any symptoms.

Treatment. Piperazine is most effective. Piperazine citrate syrup is given to adults in a dose of 24 milliliters which contains 3 grams of piperazine citrate. For a child under 45 pounds of body weight a suitable dose is 16 milliliters.

This is given as a single dose at night, purgation being unnecessary.

Piperazine adipate tablets (0.3 gram) may be used and the doasge employed is 100 milligrams per 2.2 pounds of body weight to a maximum of 4 grams for children, and 4 grams for adults. This medication, is taken as a single dose with food. It may then be followed next morning by a saline laxative.

Prevention. In endemic areas one must not eat uncooked vegetables, and the hands must be thoroughly washed before eating.

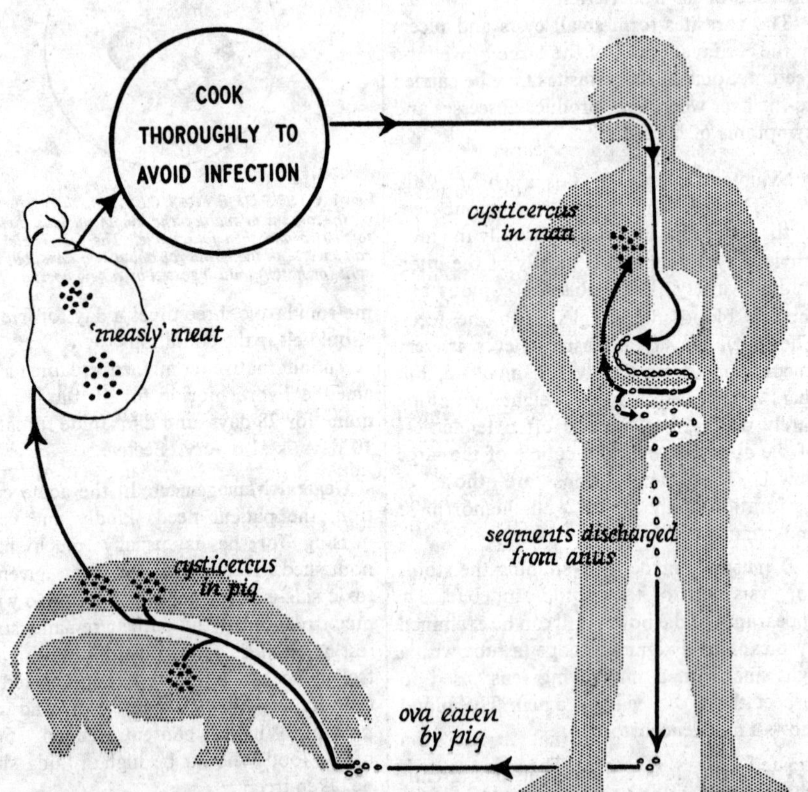

Fig. 3. *LIFE CYCLE OF PORK TAPEWORM. The adult worm inhabits the upper part of the small intestine, and when the egg segments (see text) are mature, they pass out in the feces, and are consumed by pigs (occasionally sheep or dogs) rooting around in the soil. The larvae (cysticerci) migrate to and live in the pig's muscle. If this infected pork is eaten by man, the larvae develop into tapeworms.*

Cestodiasis

(Tapeworm Infestation)

The tapeworm is a ribbon-shaped worm and inhabits the human intestinal tract. It does not have an alimentary tract of its own but absorbs its host's food from its surface. One end is called the scolex by which it is attached to the bowel wall. The remainder is composed of short segments jointed together, the last segments being full of eggs. These segments are known as proglottids.

(PORK TAPEWORM). This worm varies in length up to 12 feet. Its scolex or head consists of suckers and two rows of hooklets anterior to the suckers. Persons become infested by eating undercooked pork in which there are living tapeworm larvæ (see Fig. 3).

(BEEF TAPEWORM). This is larger and may be several feet in length. The scolex is the size of a pin head and has four suckers. Persons become infested by eating undercooked infected beef.

Symptoms. In the acute phase the symptoms are fever, diarrhea and colic, but these may vary, and there may be loss of weight and increased appetite. In the chronic phase there may be anemia and the appearance of gravid proglottids (egg segments) in the feces and underclothing.

Treatment. The most effective drug treatment is either niclosamide 2 grams or dichlorophen 6 grams given on each of two successive days. Tablets are crushed or chewed before swallowing. If no gravid segments are passed three months later, the patient is cured.

During, or for a few days after treatment, the hands of all in contact with the patient must be kept scrupulously clean.

METHOD. For 48 hours an adult patient is given fluids only. Saline laxatives are administered night and morning. About 1.0 gram of quinacrine is given often premedicated with a sedative to reduce vomiting.

The patient should remain in bed during the whole day of treatment.

Prevention. Thorough cooking of meat, especially pork, is essential. Where pork tapeworm is endemic, pork should not be eaten unless it comes from certified clean slaughter houses. Raw vegetables in tropical countries should be avoided. Scrupulous cleanliness is most necessary when dealing with patients who are infested. Medical aid should be obtained immediately tapeworm is suspected.

Cysticercosis

This is a complication that occurs in untreated cases of tapeworm. The eggs penetrate the tissues, and cysts occur in the muscles, under the skin, and sometimes even in the brain. Surgical treatment may be necessary in these cases.

Hyatid Cysts

These are caused by the *Echinococcus granulosus*, the tapeworm that infests dogs, sheep, and cattle. It affects man mostly through the dog. This tapeworm forms cysts which grow to a large size particularly in the liver and lungs, although the kidneys, stomach, brain and bones may be affected too, causing pressure symptoms.

Diagnosis. A Casoni test, given by subcutaneous injection of hydatid fluid from a sheep, is reliable in 85 per cent of cases in diagnosing the disease. On no account should the needle be inserted into the cyst itself.

The cysts may be removed surgically, but if so they must be removed whole.

Dracontiasis

(Guinea Worm Infestation)

This disease is due to infestation with the parasite *Dracunculus medinensis* and is found in parts of India and Africa. The embryo worm is about 0·5 mm. in length and the adult female 30 to 100 cm. in length and 1·5 mm. in diameter. The embryo spends part of its life cycle in a fresh-water flea of the cyclops family and, since the water fleas inhabit open wells, they are often swallowed in the drinking water.

Symptoms. The worm matures in man's intestine and travels to the lower extremities. After a time a small ulceration appears and the patient complains of a burning sensation and the desire to immerse the foot in water. If a drop of water is placed on the ulcer a whitish secretion appears and this contains a great number of guinea worm embryos.

Skin rashes, vomiting, malaise, diarrhea, asthma, giddiness, and fainting may occur. These are probably due to the poisons produced by the worm. If the worm becomes damaged while lying in the leg the surrounding tissues may become very inflamed and cause damage to the muscles, joints, and tendons.

Treatment. Niridazole, 25 milligrams per 2.2 pounds body weight given twice daily for seven to ten days, destroys the worms by making degenerative changes in them. The extruding worm can then be wound around a thin clean stick during a period of several days. Pain is relieved and the ulcers heal rapidly.

Prevention. Drinking water needs to be protected from pollution by infected people. The cyclops can be killed easily by heating the water a few degrees above the temperature in which they live. Certain species of fish which eat cyclops may be introduced into infested wells.

For immediate use, water can be cleared of cyclops by the simple expedient of straining it through calico.

Enterobiasis

(Threadworm or Pinworm Infestation)

This is due to intestinal infestation with a small white worm, *Oxyuris vermicularis*, from 2 to 13 millimeters in length. The female lays her eggs around the anal opening and her movements cause the intense itching which often occurs at night. The infestation occurs by eating raw vegetables, or other foodstuffs handled by infected persons whose unwashed hands or finger nails retain the eggs; or they may be passed by hand from child to child if hands are not well washed after using the toilet (see Fig. 4).

Symptoms. The symptoms in the child are digestive disturbances, irritability, mucus or slime in the stools, sleeplessness, and often grinding of the teeth.

Diagnosis is made by rubbing a small piece of cellophane, on a glass rod, over the anal orifice and then examining it under a microscope for the eggs. One may see the threadworms themselves as fine pieces of cotton thread if one looks at the child's anus in the evening.

Treatment. A viprynium tablet (50 milligrams) for an adult and viprynium suspension for a child (a 5-ml spoonful) to be followed seven days later by another dose of a tablet or suspension will get rid of the worms. Piperazine, as for ascariasis, p. 386, is also effective.

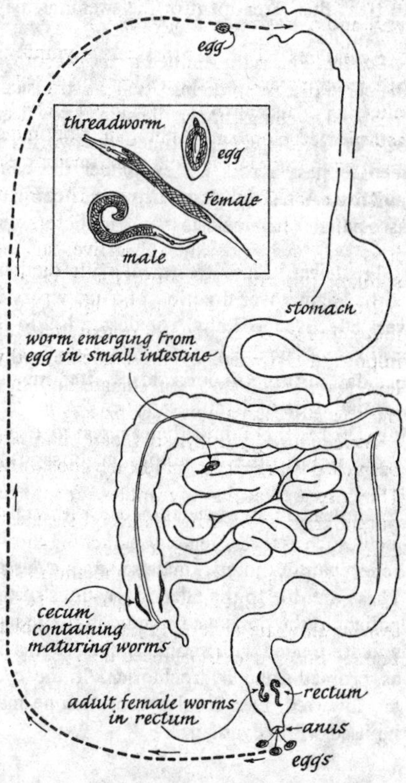

Fig. 4. *LIFE CYCLE OF THE THREADWORM. The microscopic eggs are swallowed, hatch in the small intestine, and mature to adult worms in the cecum. When the female is ready to lay eggs she migrates close to the anal opening and deposits her eggs outside, usually at night. The eggs are commonly transferred from the anus to the mouth on unwashed fingers.*

Viprynium colors the stools red and, if spilled, stains linen red.

Prevention. Hands should be washed frequently and well, especially before eating.

Bedroom dust which may contain eggs should be kept to a minimum by frequent use of a vacuum cleaner on the bed, bedding, and floors.

If there is more than one child in the household it is advisable to treat the whole family to prevent cross-infection.

Filariasis

This disease is predominantly found in Africa and three of the filarial species of worms are of interest to man.

Onchocerca volvulus. This is transmitted by a species of Simulium (biting gnat) and causes intense itching and thickening of the skin. Small lumps appear all over the body and may sometimes cause blindness. Lumps containing adult worms require surgical removal.

Wuchereria bancrofti. This filaria causes a disease known as elephantiasis. Certain mosquitos are responsible for its spread. Gross swellings of the legs and external genitalia occur due to blockage of the lymphatics by the filariae. Bacterial infection often follows and antibiotics may be required to treat this. Treatment of the swellings may be surgical.

Loa loa. This is transmitted by the mangrove fly. The disease presents itself as transient localized swellings under the skin, known as *calabar swellings.* Sometimes the worm is seen to pass across the eye under the conjunctiva. A painful dermatitis with itching is associated with loaiasis.

Treatment. Mass treatment with diethylcarbamazine over a period of three weeks is very effective medically. The dosage is 2 to 12 milligrams per 2.2 pounds body weight per day in three divided doses after meals. A small dose of 1 milligram per 2.2 pounds is given for three days then increased every 2 days until the 12-milligram dosage is reached.

Unpleasant side-effects occur with treatment, such as fever, generalized itching, headache, painful joints, malaise, and nausea. These are due to the allergic reactions of the patient to the destroyed filariae in his tissues and are treated with antihistamine drugs such as promethazine hydrochloride. If the eyes are involved, then local hydrocortisone may be used with advantage.

Prevention. In endemic areas precaution is the only method of prevention. Mosquito nets must be used and gauze fixed to doors and windows. Spraying or dusting frequently with dicophane (DDT) is very effective in destroying insect vectors.

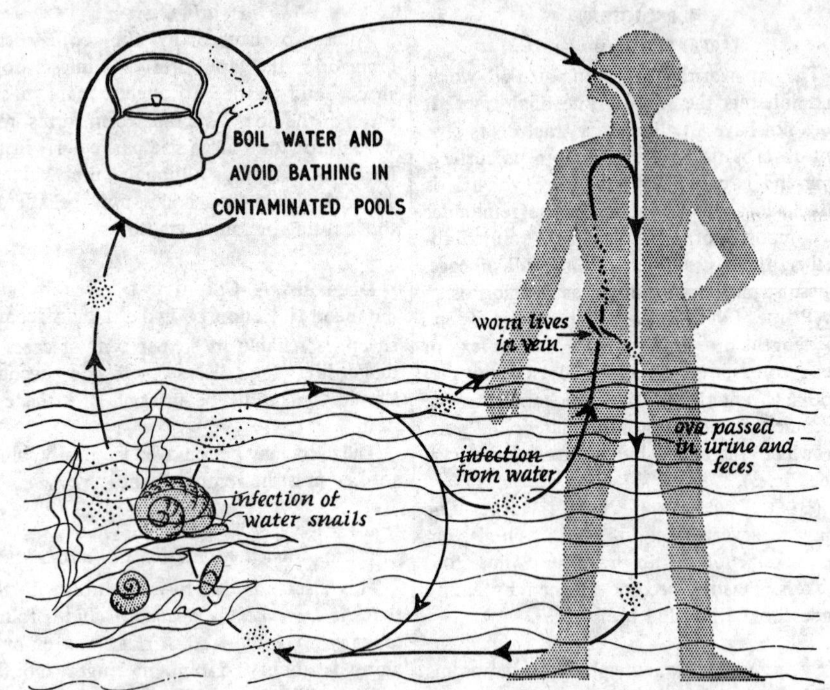

Fig. 5. *SCHISTOSOME LIFE CYCLE. The white male schistosomes are folded lengthwise around the slightly longer females (about ½ inch long) and they live in veins. The eggs bore through the host's body tissues to be excreted in the urine or feces. In soil water or canals the miracidia hatch out and bore into water snails (especially* Bulinus) *where, after a few months, they develop into* cercariae *which leave the snails to find a human host (via drinking water or during bathing). In about six weeks they have changed to adult mature schistosomes.*

Schistosomiasis

(Bilharzia)

Schistosomiasis is the cause of a great deal of suffering, especially in Africa and Egypt. Today it vies with malaria as a major scourge of mankind. Bilharz found in 1851 the organism responsible for the disease. Later it was found that this schistosome (Fig. 5) inhabited a fresh-water snail during part of its life cycle. The building of new waterways and dams has encouraged the spread of the snails (and the schistosomes) despite the finding of a chemical to destroy them.

So heavily infested can an irrigation area become, that even dewdrops in rice fields have been found full of the larval forms.

Symptoms. Some weeks after the larvae of the schistosome have pierced their way through the skin, symptoms of fever, abdominal pain, cough, skin rash and diarrhea develop, accompanied by swelling of the spleen and liver. After months or years, cystitis occurs with passage of blood in the urine. Anemia is very common.

Treatment. The well-tried elaborate treatment using sodium antimony tartrate is still employed and is effective despite its uncomfortable side-effects but it has largely given place to that using tablets of niridazole; dosage is 25 milligrams per 2.2 pounds body weight daily for seven days).

Two new drugs are now being used—hycanthone in South America and metriphonate in East Africa.

The cystitis leads to stones in the bladder, cancer, ulceration, and fistulae which will require surgical treatment.

Prevention. Bathing and washing in irrigation ditches or pools, in areas where the disease is prevalent, should be avoided. Ordinary clothes do not give protection. Rubber thigh boots and gloves are essential to persons who work in infested waters.

Drinking water should be filtered, sterilized by boiling, or stored out of contact with snails for two to three days. Chlorine concentrations used to kill ordinary bacteria do not kill the larvae. Public Health measures may be taken by spraying the land to kill the snails.

Strongyloidiasis

Infestation by *Strongyloides stercoralis* occurs in tropical countries. It causes severe bouts of diarrhea and often skin manifestations of a long-standing nature.

Treatment is thiabendazole 25 milligrams per 2.2 pounds body weight twice a day for two days.

Prevention. As for ancylostomiasis.

Trichiniasis

This disease is due to an infestation with *Trichinella spiralis* which comes from rats via the pig. After infested pork has been eaten, the embryos migrate to the muscles (see Fig. 6) of the body causing inflammation and rheumatic-like pains. In severe cases, symptoms of gastric disturbances occur and may resemble ptomaine poisoning. Mild cases recover in about two weeks but severe cases are much more prolonged.

Treatment. Tetrachloroethylene followed by vigorous purgation (as for Ancylostomiasis p. 386).

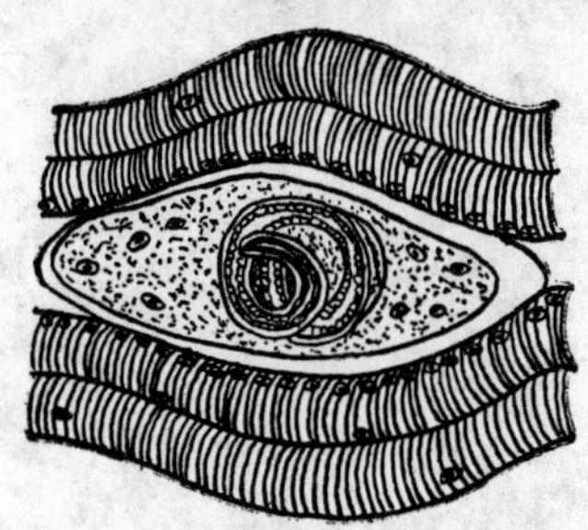

Fig. 6. *CYST STAGE OF TRICHINELLA. The embryos, produced by the female worm living in the pig's intestines, migrate to muscle tissue where they develop a protective coat, becoming cysts. Infested inadequately cooked pork, eaten by man, releases the cysts and he becomes infested.*

Prevention. The first step is to prevent infested rats from passing on the parasite to pigs. This is done by eradicating the rats with poison, and by fencing the pigs carefully. All rubbish needs to be burned and garbage stored in rat-proof containers to prevent the rats breeding. Secondly, a high standard of inspection must be maintained at the slaughter houses to prevent bad pork being sold to the consumer; and finally great care must be taken to cook pork thoroughly and so kill any possible worms.

DISEASES OF METABOLISM

The cells that make up the human body are constantly using foodstuffs, oxygen, and water to provide energy for them to carry out their vital functions. The same cells are also getting rid of breakdown products such as carbon dioxide and urea, and these have to be eliminated. The whole process of cell life, using foodstuffs and making waste products, is known as *metabolism* and any upset in the fine balance of breakdown and building causes a constitutional upset. (For fuller details concerning metabolism, see Physiology, p. 247:)

The diseases that are discussed here are examples of such an upset in the delicate balance of metabolism.

Gout

The causes and origin of gout are not clear, but the disease is often hereditary and runs in families which are said to be of a gouty stock. Exposure to cold, worry and fatigue also predispose to attacks of gout. Uric acid accumulates in the blood in the form of urates which are deposited in and around the joints, causing attacks of acute arthritis with severe pain. Rheumatism usually attacks the large joints (except in rheumatoid arthritis), but gout generally attacks the smaller joints of the fingers and toes, especially the big toe. The disease may be acute or chronic, and is most common in men in middle life; it is especially likely to occur in those who indulge habitually in rich foods and alcohol. Alcohol, particularly beer and red wines, is recognized **as predisposing to gout, and constant indulgence in rich foods is likely to precipitate an attack in persons of a gouty constitution.**

There is truth in the humorous description of the pains of gout and rheumatism: 'Place your joint in a vice; turn the screw till you can bear it no longer; that gives you an idea of rheumatism; now give the instrument one more turn, and you have gout.' Although gout is commoner among well-to-do persons, it is also seen in the less prosperous classes or in persons who do not habitually subsist on a rich diet.

Symptoms. An acute attack of gout generally begins in the night. Its unsuspecting victim is first awakened by an intensely burning or wrenching pain in the ball of the great toe or some other small joint, which becomes swollen and red and very tender. This pain, with accompanying fever, continues for

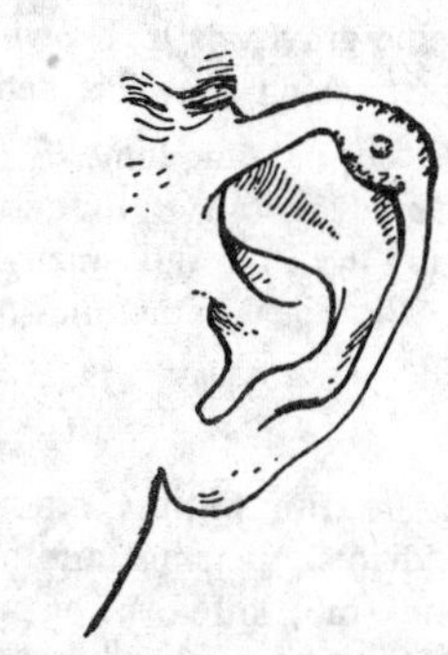

Fig. 1. TOPHUS ON THE EAR. This deposit of urates in the cartilage beneath the skin indicates that the patient has gout. Deposits in the cartilage of joints can be the cause of severe pain.

twenty-four hours; there is then a remission, when the sufferer may get some sleep. Similar attacks occur during several succeeding days and nights, until the disease subsides.

Recurrences follow the first series of attacks, usually at intervals of months or years.

Recovery from the first attack may be complete, the skin peeling off from the red and swollen joint and leaving it quite flexible; but after several attacks the joint becomes stiff and often deformed due to the deposit of concretions in ligaments and joint cartilages.

Gout is a disease which is by no means entirely confined to the joints. It affects the system generally, and is occasionally shown by general symptoms long before the local symptoms are produced by one of the attacks. Irritability of temper, depression, dyspepsia, and various disturbances of the body are often premonitory signs. The swelling about the joints is often increased by white deposits called *tophi* formed under the skin and in the cartilage of the ear. These may break through the skin, and be discharged. The swelling and redness of the back of the hand in gout may closely resemble an abscess. Chronic gout is often associated with arteriosclerosis, nephritis, and dyspepsia.

Treatment

Acute Attack. In an acute attack the patient is best confined to bed.

The most effective drug for relief is colchicine, but its exact mode of action is not known. It is prescribed in the form of tablets of the alkaloid colchicine, the dosage being 0·5 mg taken every two hours until the pain is relieved. During an attack joint symptoms may subside after 4 or 5 doses have been taken. The onset of nausea, vomiting, or diarrhea is a signal to stop the tablets.

Phenylbutazone is preferred by some patients. Pain is relieved in eight to twelve hours and treatment only lasts three to four days. Indomethacin is suitable, too, for some 80 per cent of cases of acute gout.

Heat should be applied to the inflamed joint by means of a kaolin poultice, and the pressure of the bedclothes may be avoided by means of a 'cradle.' Fluids should be taken freely, 4 to 5 pints of water being drunk daily.

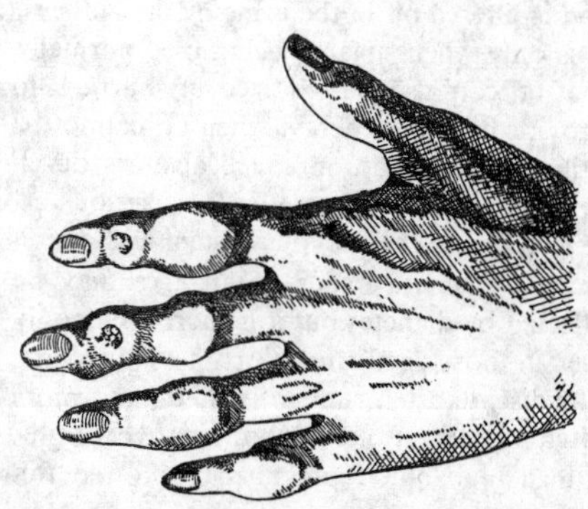

Fig. 2. GOUTY FINGERS. Chalky deposits in the joints produce smooth swellings known as tophi. They sometimes ulcerate, as shown on the first and second fingers of the hand.

Diet. The diet should be selected from the following foods: white fish, poultry, sugar, jam, fruit, bread, cereals, root and green vegetables, and eggs, while a moderate portion of red meat may be allowed each day. Peas, lentils, cocoa, meat extracts, liver, kidney, fish roe, tripe and sweetbreads should be avoided, and alcohol should not be taken.

Between Attacks, plenty of fluid should be taken and the following articles excluded permanently from the diet: fish roe, sweetbreads, whitebait, sprats, sardines, heart, venison, herring, mussels, liver, goose, kidney, bloaters. A moderate helping of meat, red or white, should be allowed during one meal of the day, and an average portion of fish or chicken at night. Strawberries, spinach and rhubarb are best prohibited, but otherwise plenty of green vegetables and fruit should be taken. Cereals, milk, cheese, eggs, jams, sugar and honey need not be restricted.

A little whisky, preferably diluted with water, may be allowed, but beer is best avoided.

It is advisable to take allopurinol regularly for the prevention of acute attacks. The drug acts by inhibiting the enzyme responsible for the formation of uric acid.

If the patient is overweight, it is important that the weight should be reduced. Exercise in moderation is of value, but over-exertion may precipitate an acute attack. Clothing should be warm, and there should be no undue exposure to cold and damp. Sufferers from chronic gout derive great benefit from an annual visit to a spa, where general treatment takes the form of vapor, hot air and immersion baths. Local treatment to the joints, in the form of mud and heat packs, wax baths, etc., does much to reduce pain and stiffness.

Diabetes Mellitus

Diabetes mellitus is a disease in which starch foods and sugar cannot be used normally in the body, so that sugar is passed in the urine; the disorder is due to lack of insulin which is produced by the pancreas, but the cause of this deficiency is not known. Much of the energy of the body is produced from sugar, but this can only be burned up when there is sufficient insulin. When this is deficient the sugar accumulates in the blood and is filtered off in the urine by the kidneys. It is only when sugar is being used normally that fat can also be oxidized or 'burned' to provide heat and energy; when fat cannot be utilized, the condition called acidosis develops, and when this is present to a serious extent it affects the nervous system and causes *diabetic coma.* Persons of all ages may be affected by diabetes but it is more commonly seen in those aged from thirty to sixty years. The disease often runs in families, and more often occurs in men who are overweight, with a high blood pressure, and often follows mental strain and anxiety.

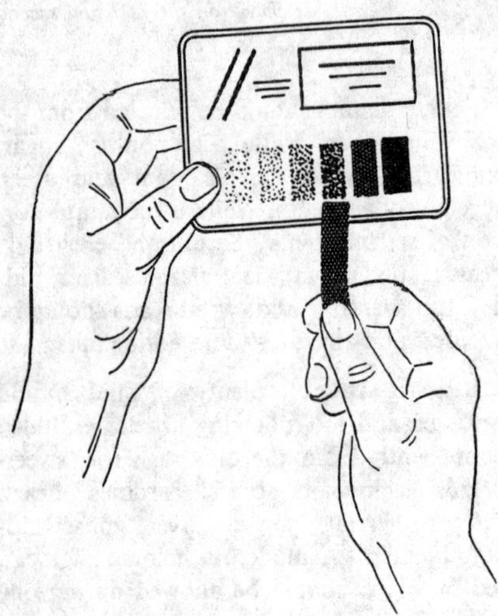

Fig. 3. *A TAPE COLOR-TEST FOR SUGAR IN URINE. The piece of prepared impregnated tape is dipped in the urine specimen, dried for a minute, and its color compared with that on a color range to find the proportion of sugar in the urine.*

Symptoms. The onset is generally gradual, the patient suffering from thirst, greatly increased appetite, constipation and weakness; there is also often great loss of weight. The thirst is generally relieved by drinking fluids copiously, so that a large quantity of urine is passed; there is often irritation or pruritus around the urethra, and women may develop gross irritation and inflammation around the vagina. Constipation is common and in severe cases the tongue is dry and red. Sexual feeling may be lost and the circulation is often poor. Rarely diabetes mellitus develops suddenly, and the patient may become comatose and die before the true condition is diagnosed.

THE URINE. The urine is often increased to five or seven pints a day; it is pale in color but the specific gravity is high owing to the sugar present, which may be detected by testing by the patient himself (see also Urinary Diseases, p. 405). In acidosis the urine contains acetone and smells of new-mown hay. Albumin is sometimes present in addition.

Complications. BOILS AND CARBUNCLES are common in diabetic persons, and are apt to be recurrent, the latter being especially dangerous. Irritation of the skin around the vulva and rectum is often complained of.

In old people GANGRENE of the toes sometimes occurs, which may spread and become very severe, so that amputation of the limb is necessary.

TUBERCULOSIS is an occasional complication, especially in severe cases of diabetes.

HIGH BLOOD PRESSURE, hardening of the arteries, and thrombosis (or clotting) of the blood in the vessels of the brain or heart are liable to develop.

EYE CHANGES, such as cataract and inflammation of the retina, are also common, causing impairment of vision or loss of sight.

NEURITIS, with tingling, pain and sometimes numbness is often complained of.

COMA is the most serious complication, but since treatment with insulin has been introduced it is now less often seen than formerly. It is sometimes heralded by pain in the abdomen, loss of appetite and constipation, and then drowsiness increases until deep coma may be reached, unless treatment is given. The pulse is fast and feeble, and there may be deep sighing, or 'air-hunger.'

Treatment. Diabetics fall into two main categories: those below middle age with severe symptoms, and those at the middle age who are obese but have milder symptoms. This differentiation is important when considering treatment.

The general health of the patient must be given every care. Any form of infection, such as boils, pyorrhea, etc., must be promptly dealt with, as sepsis affects the sugar tolerance, and the resistance to infection is generally poor.

Before the use of insulin, which was introduced by Banting in 1922, diabetes was treated by reducing the starch and sugar in the diet until the urine became and remained sugar-free, the fats also being restricted to avoid acidosis.

INSULIN is the preparation used by diabetic patients, to enable them to take a varied and adequate diet. The dose of insulin required has to be estimated for each individual case. There are several types available at the present time, including *protamine insulin,* which has a delayed action, beginning about 4 hours after injection and lasting up to 12 hours, also globin insulin. *Protamine zinc insulin* has a still further delayed action, beginning to act 8 to 12 hours after injection and continuing for 14 to 16 hours or longer. Now on the market is another form of insulin which differs from the first two in that it is not combined with a protein. This is the *Lente insulin* of which there are three types, the semi-lente, the lente and the ultra-lente. The difference in the speed of absorption is used by doctors to 'cover' patients for the full twenty-four-hour period. Ordinary soluble insulin is required in diabetic coma when treatment must be prompt.

Insulin is usually administered by the patient himself by means of a hypodermic syringe and sterile needle, following instructions given by a doctor. The dosage often requires to be increased when the patient is suffering from any form of infection such as influenza, boils, etc. It must be clearly understood that insulin does not cure diabetes, and that continued treatment under medical supervision is likely to be necessary during the patient's lifetime, although it may be possible to reduce the dosage of insulin, or occasionally to suspend its administration.

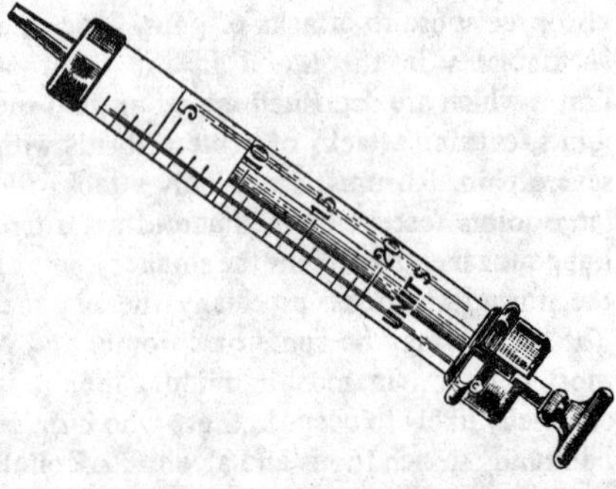

Fig. 4. *INSULIN SYRINGE (to hold 20 units). A fine stainless steel needle is fitted in to the nozzle of the small syringe when the injection is to be made.*

DIET AND INSULIN. As a general rule the following food quantities are allowed per day:

	Grams
Carbohydrate (starch and sugar) . .	100 to 250 (average 150 grams)
Protein	60 to 90
Fats	60 to 100

1 gram of carbohydrate food supplies 4 calories, 1 gram of protein supplies 4 calories, while 1 gram of fat supplies 9 calories. The above amounts thus yield 1,200 to 2,200 calories per day. A man weighing 140 lbs. requires a diet supplying about 2,100 calories a day, with an increase up to 20 per cent if he performs active muscular work. An elderly diabetic woman who leads a

sedentary life requires about 1,700 calories per day. An approximate figure for other weights is obtained by multiplying the body weight in pounds by 11.3. Insulin is given according to the needs of the patient, the dose being adjusted to each individual case.

In cases of mild diabetes, the patient's urine may usually be rendered free of sugar by restriction of diet only, on a low diet providing about 1,500 calories a day. The diet (including extra carbohydrate food) is then increased gradually to meet the patient's normal requirements, and by following a routine diet he may be able to do without insulin. In other cases insulin will be needed to allow a diet sufficient to maintain his weight. In severe and emaciated cases insulin is prescribed at once to avoid the danger of coma developing. Diabetic children nearly always require insulin, while adult diabetics require extra dosage when they are suffering from any infection, from diabetic gangrene, or before surgical operations.

Pregnant Cases. Successful pregnancy is now more common in diabetic women since insulin has become available, but diabetics tend to be less fertile than normal. During pregnancy the diabetic must take special care as her insulin requirement can fluctuate rapidly. She must be delivered in a hospital, preferably one used to dealing with diabetic problems.

The expense of insulin, and the inconvenience of continual administration by hypodermic injection, make it desirable to dispense with it when it is not essential.

Hypodermic Injection. When pain follows a hypodermic injection the needle has probably not been inserted sufficiently deeply beneath the skin. The usual sites of injection are on the outer side of the thighs or in the abdominal wall, but the sites should be continually varied. Ordinary soluble insulin is usually given about half an hour before a meal.

Oral Treatment. Treatment of diabetics by tablets of non-insulin drugs, such as tolbutamide, is now possible but it should only be done under strict medical supervision and usually only suits the older diabetic with mild symptoms.

Sugar in the Blood. The sugar in the blood must be kept within certain limits, or symptoms arising from a lack of sugar quickly develop. These are at first clammy sweating, tremor, anxiety, hunger, coldness and pallor, and sometimes double vision, followed by disorderly behavior, or by fainting or collapse with loss of consciousness, which may be prolonged into coma. In children lassitude and sleepiness are usually seen when the blood sugar is low. These symptoms are likely to occur about one or two hours after insulin has been given, unless the sugar or carbohydrate intake is sufficient. The patient should, therefore, always have sugar or barley sugar ready to take with a drink of water if the above warning symptoms develop; if he remains conscious he will be able to take them by mouth, but if he collapses glucose solution may be given by a doctor by means of a nasal tube, or by injection into a vein.

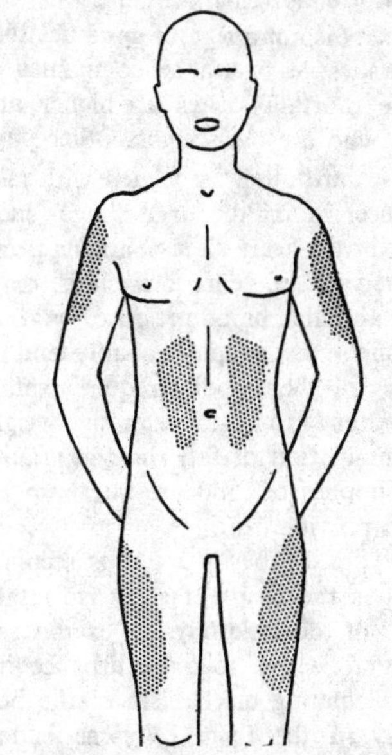

Fig. 5. *INJECTION SITES. The shaded portions indicate the areas suitable for insulin injections. The site chosen should be varied frequently.*

To decide whether a patient is suffering from diabetic coma due to want of insulin, or to lack of sugar in the blood, the urine should be tested; if the urine is free from sugar, glucose is required; if it contains sugar the bladder should be emptied by means of a catheter, and a second sample collected and retested. If this later specimen also contains sugar, soluble insulin and glucose are given.

The following table shows the difference, between diabetic coma and shortage of sugar in the blood:

	Diabetic Coma	*Shortage of Sugar in the Blood*
Onset	Slow	Often sudden
Skin	Flushed; dry	Pallid, sweating
Tongue	Dry	Moist
Breath	Smells of acetone	No characteristic smell
Breathing	Deep sighing	Shallow breaths
Pulse	Fast and weak	Normal or full
Abdominal pain	Often present. Sometimes vomiting	A sense of constriction may be felt

Diet in Diabetes Mellitus

The question of a correct and balanced diet often presents some difficulty in diabetes. All the items of food must be weighed accurately.

Insulin should be given if the urine still contains sugar after a diabetic patient has taken Diet V for 3 days, or has reached Diet III. The correct dose of insulin requires to be estimated by a doctor, after the blood sugar has been tested.

The diabetic patient should understand about the disease and the reasons for his diet. He should also be able to test his urine by using Clinitest tablets or by Benedict's test (see Urinary Diseases, p. 407).

Many pancreatic preparations and herbal remedies are advertised for diabetes, to be taken by mouth, but they are without value. Laxatives, however, are required, and a thorough daily evacuation is essential. General tonics to improve the health may also be taken.

The outlook and treatment depend on the type of diabetes and the behavior of the patient. Diabetics should always be under medical care and, provided they follow instructions, most can live a full and healthy life.

LADDER DIET SCHEME

DIET		I	II	III	IV	V	VI	VII	VIII	IX
	Tea, coffee, lemonade and meat extract as required. Vinegar, saccharine									
Eggs... ...		1	1	1	1	1	1	1	1	1
Butter ...	ounces	1	1	1	1	1	1	1	1	1½
Vegetables (cooked) (uncooked)	Vegetables such as asparagus, cabbage, cauliflower, celery, cucumber, French beans, lettuce, mustard and cress, rhubarb, radishes, sea-kale, spinach, water-cress, Brussels sprouts, may be eaten as required. Other vegetables are selected according to caloric requirements.									
Meat ...	ounces	6	6	6	6	6	6	6	6	6
Bacon ...	,,	—	—	—	—	—	1	1	1	1
Potatoes ...	,,	—	—	—	—	—	3	3	3	7
Milk ...	,,	12	12	12	12	12	12	12	12	20
Apple ...	,,	—	—	—	—	4	4	4	4	4
Orange ...	,,	—	—	—	—	4	4	4	4	4
Banana ...	,,	—	—	—	—	—	—	2	2	2
Bread ...	,,	1	2	3	4	4	4	5	6	6½
Jam ...	,,	—	—	—	—	—	—	—	—	½
Carbohydrate	grams	30	45	60	75	95	110	135	160	200
Protein ...	,,	62	64	66	69	69	73	75	85	86
Fat	,,	74	74	75	75	75	86	86	110	110
CALORIES ...	,,	1,060	1,130	1,200	1,270	1,352	1,528	1,639	1,890	2,055

Diabetes Insipidus

This is a rare chronic disease, in which the patient passes large quantities of pale dilute urine which is free from sugar and albumin. In some cases there is no discoverable cause, and the condition may apparently be a hereditary disorder which usually affects men, through several generations. It is due to an inability in the kidneys to secrete concentrated urine.

In a second type of case diabetes insipidus is due to some disease of the pituitary gland in the brain, such as a tumor or other organic brain disease. Injury is also an occasional factor. The symptoms are characteristic, with abnormal thirst, a copious flow of urine, and constipation. The patient is generally thin, and the skin tends to be dry, but the general health may be quite good.

In cases in which there is no discoverable disease the patient may live for many years. In the second group when there is some brain disease the duration of life depends on the extent and severity of the changes in the brain.

Treatment. Injection of pituitary extract effectively controls the excessive output of urine, but may need to be administered twice daily. Occasionally other pituitary compounds with a longer effect may be used and they only require one injection a day. However, this is only substitution treatment and is not a cure. A snuff of pituitary powder is sometimes of use when injection is contra-indicated.

The fluids taken by mouth should be gradually reduced in amount but *not after* the quantity of urine ceases to become less. A salt-free diet, with a low protein content, is sometimes advised, dairy foods, fish, vegetables and cereals being permitted.

See also Diseases of the Endocrine Glands, p. 403.

Obesity

Excessive obesity is due to abnormal deposits of fat in the body. The condition is a symptom rather than a specific disorder, and may be due to various causes. Obesity is especially common in Eastern races, especially in women, and often runs in families. It may be due to excessive intake of food, especially starches and fats, combined with inactivity, or there may rarely be endocrine glandular disturbance, the mechanisms of which are still not fully understood.

The fat accumulates in all the areas usually containing fat, such as the tissues beneath the skin and the omentum within the abdomen, and the heart may become fatty and diseased. The obese patient generally complains of sweating, shortness of breath, sleepiness, and perhaps pains round the heart. There may be anemia, or a plethoric condition with high blood pressure. In the latter type of case the patient is liable to develop bronchitis, or apoplexy, while in both groups heart failure and respiratory diseases are common sequels.

Recently it has been more generally realized that obesity is not a sign of good health, and the statistics of insurance companies show that the mortality rates are higher among persons who are overweight. Other physical disabilities are often associated with general corpulence, in middle or old age, such as osteo-arthritis, heart disease, angina pectoris, flat foot, varicose veins, bronchitis, diabetes mellitus and high blood pressure.

Although most people probably tend to eat in excess of their bodily requirements, not everyone tends to put on excessive weight by the accumulation of fat, since generally the excess supplies of food are burnt up in the body to provide heat.

Two types of obesity are thus recognized: the first is the result of excessive intake of food, or of too little physical exercise, while the second is due to a disturbance in the weight-regulating mechanism of the body—generally in the form of some endocrine disorder. Many cases are probably due to a combination of the above factors.

Treatment. This consists in a *gradual* reduction in obesity, with restrictions in the diet, and graduated exercises and increased activity, within the limits of the heart's capacity. The patient should be under medical observation. The diet should provide for a gradual and general decrease in the total quantity of food taken; the sugar, starchy and fatty types of foodstuffs especially should be reduced by degrees. Small meals should be taken at short intervals, to reduce the appetite, and fluids should not be drunk with meals. About two pints of fluids may be drunk daily; this amount is necessary for adequate elimination of the impurities and waste products of the body. In general a diet providing up to about 1,200 calories is advised, though up to 1,500 calories may be required for a working man. Diets providing less than 1,000 calories cannot generally be adhered to, unless the patient is kept in bed, since they lead to weakness and an unduly rapid reduction in weight.

Cereals (rice, tapioca, oatmeal, macaroni, breakfast cereals, etc.), cream, thick soups, rich sauces, rich or fatty meats and fish, such as pork, bacon, duck, goose, mackerel, sardines, salmon and herring, are to be avoided, and butter, margarine and fried foods must be used sparingly. Sweet wines, beer, ale, alcohol, carbonated drinks,

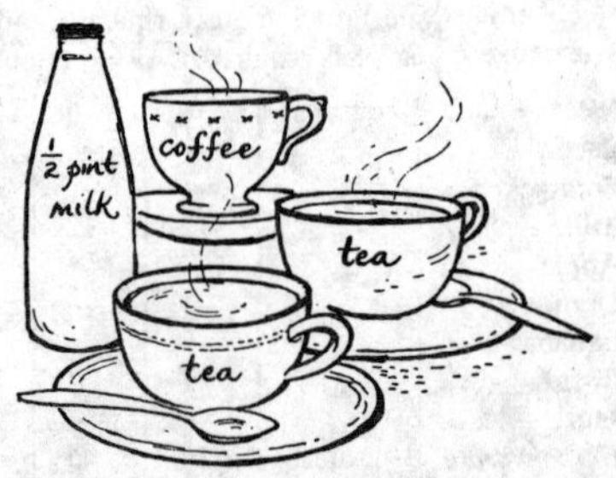

Fig. 6. *TWO PINTS OF LIQUID DAILY. With the restricted diet for reducing weight, about two pints of liquid should be taken each day for health's sake, but this amount should not be exceeded.*

sugar, jam, cakes, pastry, sweets, potatoes, nuts, dried fruits, or fruits in syrup, should be avoided.

Steamed fish, such as cod, whiting, haddock and flounder, lean meat, green vegetables, clear soups, cheese, eggs, and fruit, may be taken freely. Bread, 2 to 4 ounces a day, butter ½ ounce, milk up to 8 ounces, are allowed. Meat extracts, gelatin, egg-white, tea, and weak coffee without much sugar, may be taken.

In most cases the diet should provide *at least* 1,200 calories a day, and the loss of weight should not be more than 8 to 12 pounds a month. The patient should be weighed every week. Excessive activity must be avoided during the period of dieting.

THYROID EXTRACT, which may assist in reducing obesity, must only be given under the supervision of a doctor, since its administration, to be effective, must be carefully controlled, and it may cause ill-health if taken over too long a period or in too large amounts. The usual dose is given as tablets of 30 to 60 milligrams of the thyroid extract daily.

It takes at least a month for a daily dose of thyroid to give its full effect. Occasionally it causes tremor, nervousness or diarrhea in persons with intolerance. Many obese persons with fatty hearts may develop palpitation and a fast pulse if given thyroid, and serious damage to the heart may result from such treatment. In all cases the pulse rate should be the main guide to the use of thyroid for the reduction of weight.

DEXEDRINE is a drug used in the modern treatment of obesity since it acts by depressing the appetite and the distressing desire for food. It also helps to overcome the lassitude and depression which are often complained of by people living on a restricted diet. It is prescribed in 5-milligram doses to be taken before breakfast and before the midday meal. It should not be taken later in the day since it tends to cause insomnia. Some people are intolerant to dexedrine, even in small doses, since it gives rise to palpitation and tremor.

The use of common salt may be curtailed, and salty foods should be avoided.

A very obese woman should not attempt to reduce her weight to the ideal standard quoted for her height.

The loss of weight is usually most rapid in the first few days of taking a restricted diet. After this period the weight usually falls more slowly.

Cases of long-standing obesity often benefit from dietary treatment, but there is often a tendency to regain weight if the treatment is discontinued. A modified, though less strict, diet should usually be maintained.

Diet for Obesity: To Reduce Weight

1. **To provide 1,000 calories**

Carbohydrate: 100 grams.
Protein: 60 grams (daily average).
Fat: 40 grams (daily average).
Saccharine should be used for sweetening.

Note: Bread and butter should be weighed, and milk carefully measured. Milk: ½ pint skim milk. Butter: ¾ ounce. *No* sugar. Water: 2 pints per day.

BREAKFAST

1 orange, or ½ grapefruit (without sugar).
Bread: 1 ouce (1 thin slice).
Butter, from daily allowance.
1 egg, *or* 1 ounce of lean cold ham or tongue.
Tea or coffee, with milk from daily allowance.

DINNER

Clear soup.
Lean meat, chicken, rabbit, tripe or white fish: 2 to 3 ounces.
Vegetables: select from greens, green salad, cauliflower, kale, French beans, asparagus, cucumber, leeks, celery, mushrooms or tomatoes.
Apple, pears, stewed fruit or rhubarb sweetened with saccharine.

MID AFTERNOON SNACK

Fresh salad or tomato.
Bread: 1 ounce.
Butter, from daily allowance.
Tea, with milk from daily allowance.

SUPPER

Bread, 1 ounce.
1 egg, *or* ¾ ounce cheese. or medium helping of white fish, lean meat, chicken, or lean ham or tongue.
Butter, from daily allowance.
Coffee, with milk from daily allowance.
1 orange or apple.

2. **To provide 1,100 calories.** To increase the above diet to provide 1,100 calories, use whole milk instead of skim milk.

3. **To provide 1,200 calories.** Add ½ ounce of butter.

4. **To provide 1,500 calories.** Add another ¾ ounce butter, ¾ ounce of cheese or 1 egg, and ¾ ounce of milk.

General Rules

For constipation take extra green vegetables, or All-Bran at breakfast instead of bread.

In cases of hear: disease, very little fluid should be taken with meals. Vegetables should be sieved, and taken at midday. Supper should be taken early.

The patient should be weighed weekly while taking this diet, and the average loss of weight should be from two to three pounds a week. If the weight loss is more rapid the diet should be slightly increased. If it is less rapid this may be due to a not very strict observance of the diet scheme.

Chocolates, sweets, or sweetened drinks between meals should *not* be taken.

When the weight has been sufficiently reduced there is often a tendency for obesity to return unless a somewhat modified type of the normal dietary is adopted. The greater the original degree of excessive weight, the greater is usually the response to treatment, and the relaxation of the strict low-calorie diet must be made with care.

Other Inborn Errors of Metabolism

Of recent years, more and more has been discovered about some of the rarer disorders which are due to inborn defects of the chemical processes carried on by the enzymes in the tissue cells. The enzymes are all under genetic control and the defects are therefore likely to be passed on hereditarily.

Phenylketonuria

This inborn error of metabolism is due to the lack of a digestive enzyme in the child, which prevents the proper digestion of a certain protein in food—the amino-acid called phenylalanine. Because the alanine is not modified to the body's needs, infants and children with this defect suffer from severe mental retardation.

Symptoms. Since brain growth is severely impaired, the children have a very low intelligence quotient (I.Q.), usually under fifty. They are mostly fair-haired. A specific sign of the disorder is the presence of certain substances in the urine which will turn green when tested with ferric chloride.

Treatment. The child must be given a diet containing no phenylalanine.

If the child is partly grown when the condition is diagnosed, the chances of improvement on a special diet are reduced the older and more abnormally developed he has become. Early diagnosis is most important. Fortunately the condition is very rare.

The Porphyrias

Persons with these disorders excrete abnormal metabolic substances—porphyrins—in their urine, which is often wine-red in color.

In the acute intermittent form, the defect may be latent until it is precipitated by the patient taking a barbiturate or a sulphonamide drug. Nervous symptoms often develop, the patient becoming delirious and confused. Abdominal pain may be severe and blood pressure raised.

In the cutaneous form, the patient develops swelling of and blisters on the skin of the face and hands after exposure to bright light. After healing, the skin is scarred and pigmented.

Treatment. Good nursing is essential. Barbiturates and sulphonamides must never be taken. If the patient shows sensitivity to bright light, he must reduce exposure as much as possible. There is no known specific remedy.

Hereditary Spherocytosis

This blood disorder is due to a hereditary defect of the red blood cells which, instead of being disc-shaped, are more or less round in shape. There is a related abnormality of metabolism of phosphates by these red blood cells.

Removal of the spleen relieves the anemia but the defective cells remain unchanged.

HEIGHTS AND AVERAGE WEIGHTS OF WOMEN

(Weights taken in stocking feet and with indoor clothing)

HEIGHT			AGE 20		AGE 25		AGE 30		AGE 50	
ft	in	cm	lb	kg	lb	kg	lb	kg	lb	kg
5	0	152·5	114	51·7	117	53·1	120	54·4	133	60·3
5	1	155	116	52·6	120	54·4	123	55·8	135	61·2
5	2	157·5	120	54·4	122	55·3	125	56·7	138	62·6
5	3	160	123	55·8	124	56·2	128	58·1	142	64·4
5	4	162·5	126	57·2	128	58·1	132	59·9	146	66·2
5	5	165	128	58·1	132	59·9	136	61·7	150	68·0
5	6	167·5	132	59·9	136	61·7	140	63·5	154	69·9
5	7	170	136	61·7	140	63·5	144	65·3	159	72·1
5	8	172·5	140	63·5	144	65·3	148	67·1	164	74·4
5	9	175·5	144	65·3	148	67·1	152	68·9	168	76·2
5	10	178	147	66·7	151	68·5	155	70·3	173	78·5
5	11	180·5	153	69·4	155	70·3	158	71·7	177	80·3
6	0	183	157	71·2	159	72·1	162	73·5	180	81·6

HEIGHTS AND AVERAGE WEIGHTS OF MEN

(Weights taken in stocking feet and with indoor clothing)

HEIGHT			AGE 20		AGE 25		AGE 30		AGE 50	
ft	in	cm	lb	kg	lb	kg	lb	kg	lb	kg
5	0	152·5	116	52·6	122	55·3	125	56·7	134	60·8
5	1	155	119	54·0	124	56·2	127	57·6	136	61·7
5	2	157·5	121	54·9	127	57·6	131	59·4	139	63·0
5	3	160	124	56·2	130	59·0	134	60·8	142	64·4
5	4	162·5	128	58·1	134	60·8	137	62·1	145	65·8
5	5	165	132	59·9	138	62·6	141	64·0	149	67·6
5	6	167·5	136	61·7	142	64·4	145	65·8	154	69·9
5	7	170	140	63·5	146	66·2	149	67·6	158	71·7
5	8	172·5	144	65·3	150	68·0	153	69·4	163	73·9
5	9	175·5	148	67·1	155	70·3	158	71·7	168	76·2
5	10	178	152	68·9	159	72·1	163	73·9	173	78·5
5	11	180·5	156	70·8	164	74·4	168	76·2	178	80·7
6	0	183	161	73·0	169	76·7	174	78·9	184	83·5
6	1	185·5	166	75·3	174	78·9	179	81·2	189	85·7
6	2	188	171	77·6	179	81·2	185	83·9	195	88·5

DEFICIENCY DISEASES

Vitamins are essential food factors which occur in various foods in small quantities and which are required to maintain normal growth and health; the properties of some of them are now fairly clearly understood.

From a medical point of view the most important are the fat-soluble group, vitamins A and D, and the water-soluble group including the B complex and vitamin C. If a lack of any of these vitamins or accessory food factors occurs in the diet of human beings, certain so-called deficiency diseases develop.

Effects of Deficiency. Lack of vitamin A induces night-blindness, retarded growth and increased liability to infections.

Vitamin B_1 prevents the disease known as beri-beri, a condition common in India where the people feed mainly on polished rice, and also protects against nutritional neuritis. Pellagra, a disease occurring in countries such as the southern states of the United States, Egypt, Italy, and the Balkan countries, where milled maize is a main article of diet, is due to the lack of nicotinic acid in the complex vitamin B. This complex vitamin also contains riboflavine which may protect against certain skin diseases in human beings.

Vitamin B_{12}, or cyanocobalamin, protects against pernicious and nutritional anemias.

Vitamin C, or ascorbic acid, is the factor in our diet which prevents scurvy and possibly certain bleeding disorders.

Vitamin D is the protective factor against rickets in infants, and the associated conditions of infantile nutritional tetany, celiac rickets, and osteomalacia, a deficiency disease common in women in India.

Sterility and repeated abortions in women may be due to lack of vitamin E, but definite evidence regarding the action of this factor has not yet been obtained.

Vitamins are found in fresh vegetables and protein-rich foods. For details see section on Food and Nutrition, p. 68; see also Physiology, p. 247.

The Vitamin Content of Foodstuffs

The chief foodstuffs of mankind can be grouped according to their nature into the following categories: (1) seeds, (2) tubers, (3) roots, (4) meat, (5) fish, (6) eggs, (7) leaves, (8) fruit, (9) milk and milk products, and fats.

A diet consisting of seeds, tubers, roots and meat may be deficient in fat-soluble vitamin A and in calcium; the inclusion of leaves (green vegetables) and of milk in the diet corrects these deficiencies.

The process which food undergoes in preparation may impair its vitamin content; thus flour may be deprived of much of its water-soluble vitamin B complex in milling. Lard may lose in the process of manufacture any fat-soluble vitamin A which it may possess, and margarine made from vegetable oils, lard and 'hardened' fats may also be deficient in fat-soluble A and D vitamins.

The antiscorbutic vitamin C is readily destroyed by drying; exposure to temperatures of 80° to 100° C for one hour destroys 90 per cent of the vitamin C content of vegetables, and the destruction is still more rapid if the vegetables are boiled with an alkali such as soda. Water-soluble vitamin B_1 withstands drying, but is gradually destroyed at 120° C. Fat-soluble vitamin A is destroyed by heating to a temperature of 100° C for one or two hours in the presence of the oxygen in the air.

In the making of bread, the addition of yeast is probably sufficient to correct the loss of the water-soluble vitamin B_1 incurred in milling.

There would seem to be greater risk of a diet being deficient in fat-soluble A than in water-soluble vitamin B complex, since vitamin A is not so widely distributed among food materials as the vitamin B complex. By suitable selection and variety it may be feasible to construct an adequate diet consisting of seeds, roots, tubers and meat, i.e. the staple material of most diets, which may contain all that is necessary for normal nutrition; but the possibility cannot be ignored that a diet constructed from these important foodstuffs, while being adequate in regard to energy production, may be deficient in certain respects, notably in fat-soluble A and D vitamins. The addition of milk, and leaves (green vegetables) and cod-liver oil to such a diet would appear to be sufficient to raise it into the plane of safety, and for this reason milk and green vegetables have been termed 'protective foods.'

In adult life the need for the essential vitamin constituents is probably less than during the period of growth, so that a diet which is satisfactory during this period is almost certain to be adequate for adult life, assuming that a sufficient energy supply is assured.

Value of Varied Diet

In order that a diet should include all the essentials for nutrition it should be as varied as possible. All the evidence indicates the undesirability of limiting a diet to a few varieties of food. A satisfactory diet would include milk and green vegetables, together with the most readily obtainable foods from the class of seeds (flour, oatmeal, bread, etc.), the legumes (peas, beans and lentils), potatoes and roots (carrots, parsnips, etc.), sugar and fat of all kinds, as well as fish, meat and meat by-products. Many of the more expensive and luxurious foods are superior only in regard to esthetic qualities.

The palatability and digestibility of food are largely dependent upon good cooking, and the nutritive value of much food is impaired by lack of care in this respect.

People who are most likely to suffer from a deficiency disease are (1) those who cannot afford to buy the expensive foods regularly (including millions in underdeveloped countries); (2) faddy persons, grown-ups and children, whose food intake is not well mixed in kind; (3) children whose parents do not trouble to provide a balanced range of the foods for healthy growth; (4) those with disorders of the digestive tract which prevent proper absorption of foods; and (5) tired lonely old people subsisting on tea and flour foods.

All pharmacists stock a range of tablets and syrups containing one or a mixture of the vitamins for supplementing a deficiency.

Scurvy

Scurvy is one of the group of deficiency diseases, and is a nutritional disorder caused by the lack of ascorbic acid (vitamin C) in the diet. Vitamin C is present in the citrus fruits (oranges, lemons), tomatoes, rutabagas, cabbage, spinach, and potatoes, and to a lesser extent in other vegetables and fruits, meat and milk. Even in the Middle Ages it was known that fresh fruits and vegetables prevented and cured scurvy, which was especially prevalent among sailors who, during their long sea voyages, were often deprived of fresh fruit and vegetables and as a result developed scurvy.

Symptoms. The disease is generally slow in onset and may take about four to eight months to develop in a person living on a diet poor in vitamin C. It causes swelling and sponginess of the gums, general debility, dizziness, languor and apathy, anemia, ulceration of the mouth, and a tendency to hemorrhages, so that comparatively minor injuries may cause severe bruising. In severe cases the gums bleed easily and the teeth may fall out. Pain is often felt in the calves of the legs, and later there may be

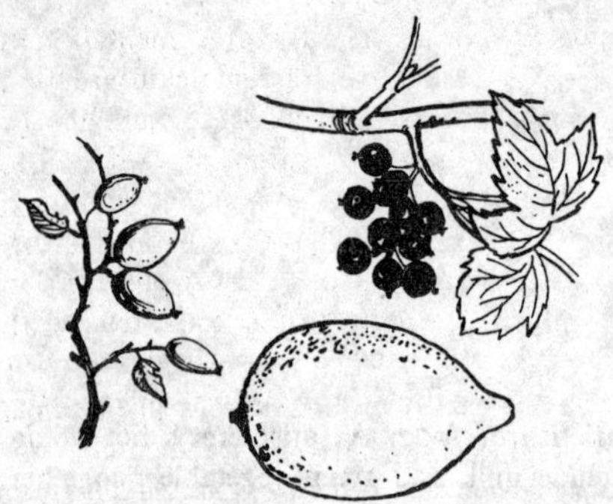

Fig. 1. *RICH SOURCES OF VITAMIN C. Blackcurrants and lemon. The fresher the fruit, the greater the content of vitamin C.*

swelling of the ankles. The patient looks ill and haggard, and suffers from breathlessness and palpitations due to the anemia. Nose bleeding, bleeding from the mouth, and intestinal hemorrhages may occur. Dyspepsia and constipation are common, although diarrhea sometimes develops.

Complications. Gangrene of the lungs is a late complication which may prove fatal, and bronchitis may also supervene.

The diagnosis is usually easily made, and the outlook is favorable except in grave cases. Recovery, however, is often slow and arthritis, or scars from skin ulceration, may persist.

Treatment. Scurvy may be prevented by a diet providing from 25 to 50 milligrams of vitamin C per day. When symptoms of scurvy have developed additional supplies of vitamin C must be given, so that 1,000 milligrams are supplied daily for a few days and then at least 100 milligrams are required daily until the patient has completely recovered. Iron tonics should also be given, and other vitamin preparations may be needed if the diet has lacked them.

The gums should be treated with weak disinfectant such as dilute hydrogen peroxide.

Sub-scurvy

A condition known as sub-scurvy is now recognized in which the symptoms remain latent, but wounds heal slowly and there is a tendency to bruising or small hemorrhages. A liberal supply of foods containing vitamin C should be taken.

Infantile Scurvy

Scurvy is particularly liable to develop in young children, especially between the eighth and twelfth months after birth. It is often associated with rickets, and is most commonly seen in babies fed on condensed milk or prepared milk foods. The baby is pale but not necessarily thin, and the symptoms of scurvy may develop suddenly. The child screams when picked up, and is fretful and anemic, often refusing food. The limbs especially are tender, and there may be swellings near the knee, formed by bleeding close to the bones. The gums are less seriously affected than in adult persons. Occasionally fractures or hemorrhages into the joints occur, or blood may be noted in the urine.

The condition may be mistaken for rheumatism which, however, is very rare in children under two years of age.

Preventive Treatment. Infantile scurvy is preventable by care in providing the proper diet both before and after weaning. An infant fed on breast or cow's milk is unlikely to develop scurvy, but bottle-fed babies who are fed on dried milk products should also be given daily orange juice, blackcurrant juice, or some other source of vitamin C. If a child ceases to gain weight, or loses weight for no very apparent reason during the first year, and becomes peevish and refuses his food, the possibility of early scurvy must be considered.

Active Treatment. This consists in plentiful supplies of vitamin C in tablet form, 50 to 100 milligrams being given daily. Orange juice and tomato juice should be introduced into the diet, and fresh boiled milk is preferable to canned products. The limbs should be wrapped in cotton, and the child should be very carefully handled and may be carried on a pillow for support.

Rickets

Rickets is a deficiency disease in children but, owing to improved schemes of infant welfare and to improved maternal care of infants, it is much less common than early in the century, when it was prevalent in large towns and poor overcrowded areas. The disease is described under Diseases of the Bones and Spine, p. 539. It especially affects the growth of bones and causes a tendency to anemia and catarrh. It generally develops between one and two years of age, especially in bottle-fed infants, and is due to deficiency of vitamin D and excess of carbohydrate (starch) foods in the diet, combined with lack of fat, sunshine and fresh air. Normally the skin can manufacture vitamin D by the action of the ultraviolet rays in sunlight, so that rickets is most likely to develop in children who live in densely built-up areas with high buildings and a smoky atmosphere. The bones are imperfectly developed and typical changes occur.

Symptoms. The child is fretful and restless, and often perspires on the head at night; he is often unusually plump, but flabby and anemic. The teeth are cut late and the bones become deformed. The skull becomes square and like a hot-cross bun, with protuberance of the forehead and soft areas in the bones. The ribs and wrists may show small swellings on the bones, and the chest is 'pigeon-breasted.' The legs are bowed outwards below the knees, the thighs being bent forwards and outwards, and greenstick fractures are not uncommon. Slight attacks of fever may be noted. The muscles are very flabby and soft, and there may be kyphosis (curvature) of the spine, with a distended 'pot-belly.' Diarrhea with pale stools, bronchitis, and convulsions are other common symptoms.

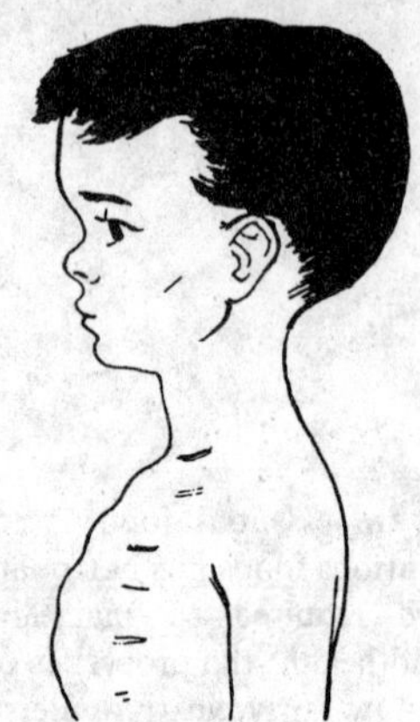

Fig. 2. *RICKETS. When there is a long-established lack of vitamin D in the infant's and small child's diet, the bones develop imperfectly: the child has a squarish skull, protuberant forehead, pigeon chest with 'beaded' ribs, and bowed leg bones.*

Treatment. Rickets is a serious disease even in its minor forms, and predisposes to other infantile disorders such as broncho-pneumonia and diarrhea. It is therefore very important to recognize the earliest symptoms, and to correct the diet and general management so that bony deformities and other defects are prevented. Breast feeding for the first six or seven months, when the mother is adequately fed, is the best means of prevention, although rickets may be produced by keeping a child too long on the breast.

After weaning, the diet must provide sufficient animal fat, and must not contain too much starch. Fresh air and sunlight are important; and good quality cod-liver oil, starting with two drops per day, increasing by one drop every other day, to ½ to 3 teaspoonfuls should be given daily to children from one month old to five years.

When rickets has developed the quantity of cows' milk should be increased to 1½ pints a day during the second year, and yolk of egg and cod-liver oil given also. Iron may be beneficial if anemia is marked. Sun baths or ultraviolet light, with tepid showers and massage, are sometimes given.

Splints may be required to correct the bowing of the legs.

Beri-Beri

(Multiple Neuritis)

Beri-beri is a disorder due to deficiency in thiamine (aneurine or vitamin B_1), and it generally occurs in tropical countries where the staple article of diet is rice which has been dehusked (polished).

Polished rice and white wheat flour are deprived of their protein, phosphorus, fat and vitamin B_1 content, and the products made from white flour, such as breakfast cereals and macaroni, are thus also lacking in B_1.

Symptoms. The symptoms are those of multiple neuritis (a polyneuropathy), but different forms of the disease are seen. A patient suffering from beri-beri gradually develops nausea, vomiting, diarrhea, with palpitation and breathlessness, and later patchy numbness of the legs. The limbs feel heavy and the calf muscles are tender. The patient becomes weak and edematous, and swelling of the legs may appear. The heart muscle is affected, causing dilatation and fatty degeneration.

In dry beri-beri, or nutritional neuropathy, the patient is very thin. Degeneration of the motor nerves results in wasting of muscles until the patient becomes bedridden. Chronic alcoholics and pregnant underfed women show similar symptoms.

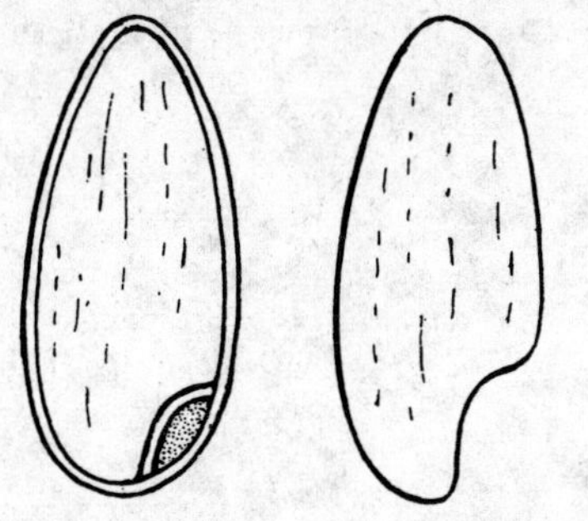

Fig. 3. *RICE GRAINS. The whole grain on the left still retains its embryo which contains protein, fat, vitamin B_1, and other food supplements for the nourishment of the young rice seedling. The grain on the right has been put through a polishing mill and lost its nutritious embryo and its outer bran coat.*

Treatment. Beri-beri may be prevented by adequate supplies of the whole vitamin B complex. When symptoms have developed, 10 milligrams of thiamine hydrochloride should be taken daily, or larger doses may be required to be given by injection when the heart is affected.

The diet should contain oatmeal, eggs, haricot beans, lentils, liver, meat, and ham. Milk and butter should also be plentifully supplied. Rest in bed, with splinting of the limbs, and later massage and electrical treatment, are required in severe cases.

Pellagra

Pellagra is a chronic disease which generally affects persons for whom maize is a staple article of diet, and is due to protein and also to nicotinic acid deficiency.

Symptoms. Pellagra is insidious, gradually giving rise to poor appetite, loss of weight, dyspepsia, nausea or vomiting, constipation or diarrhea, insomnia, headache, palpitation, vertigo, irritability and mental confusion; later the characteristic skin eruption develops on areas exposed to sunlight or friction, with inflammation of the mouth, diarrhea, and mental symptoms, although each patient may not show all these signs. The symptoms often become more severe in the spring. If the disease is untreated, death may occur from heart failure, exhaustion, or some secondary disease such as pneumonia. The patient becomes very melancholic, and suicide is not uncommon, He finally may become demented.

Treatment. In the early stages treatment gives good results. When marked mental symptoms have developed the outlook is less favorable. Vitamin B complex, with liver, kidneys, eggs, milk and cheese should be given. The diet should be rich in protein, with a reduction in carbohydrates and fats; it must be easily digestible. Yeast and green vegetables should also be taken plentifully. The skin should be protected from sunlight, and soothing ointments applied.

DISEASES OF THE ENDOCRINE GLANDS

The endocrine glands, or ductless glands, each produce one or more secretions that are absorbed directly into the bloodstream. Their work in the body is of very great importance, since they control many of the activities that are connected with growth, digestion, fertility and pregnancy, the nervous system, the general energy of the body, menstruation and lactation, the quality of the skin and the maintenance of the normal bodily functions, and normal mental activity and well-being. The proper working of each gland is dependent on that of its partners, so that if one becomes diseased or disordered the others are likely to be affected. See also Physiology, p. 260.

This important group of glands includes the pituitary gland in the brain, the thyroid and parathyroids in the neck, the adrenal or suprarenal glands above the kidneys, the sex glands (the testes and the ovaries), and the pancreatic islets of Langerhans. The secretions produced by each of these glands may be more or less than the normal amount generally formed at any particular period of life, and if this variation is marked or continues for a long time there will be some alteration in the individual's health, appearance, or activities.

The pituitary gland regulates the activities of the other endocrine glands, and normally controls growth.

THE THYROID GLAND

The thyroid gland is responsible to a great extent for the general energy of the body and brain, and is concerned in normal activity, metabolism, growth and development. It needs iodine for its formation. In some areas where iodine is lacking in the drinking water, the thyroid gland becomes permanently enlarged in its efforts to make thyroxine, giving rise to the familiar type of goiter. The thyroid gland sometimes becomes slightly enlarged at puberty and during pregnancy. Any chronic enlargement of the thyroid may be called a *goiter*, but there are different kinds. Tumors such as cysts, innocent solid growths, or malignant growths may also occur in the thyroid gland.

Hyperthyroidism
(Thyrotoxicosis)

In Grave's disease, or exophthalmic goiter, the thyroid gland becomes overactive and produces too much thyroxine and this has various effects in the body. The pulse becomes too fast, causing palpitations, the patient is excessively nervous, and there is tremor, especially in the hands. The digestion may be disordered. Sweating occurs readily, the eyeballs often protrude (exophthalmos), and, if untreated, marked wasting, loss of weight and heart weakness or heart failure, with auricular fibrillation follow. There may be difficulty in swallowing, owing to pressure by the gland.

Cause. The exact cause is not understood, but sometimes thyrotoxicosis develops after an emotional disturbance, influenza, or some septic condition, and it is more common in women, especially those under forty years. Menstruation is generally affected. Hyperthyroidism may also be caused by a tumor of the thyroid gland, known as a toxic adenoma.

Treatment. There are now various successful methods of treatment of hyperthyroidism. In severe cases the patient should be kept resting in bed for a period of three weeks or more. The diet must be generous, light and nutritious, with plenty of milk, eggs and cream, but no alcohol, and very weak tea or coffee. All worry and excitement must be avoided since even slight shocks may cause serious relapse. Phenobarbital is often prescribed to allay mental excitability.

ANTITHYROID DRUGS. Methyl and propyl thiouracils and carbimazole (in tablet form) interfere with the formation of thyroid hormone. They are used in children, during pregnancy, and in young women with moderate thyrotoxicosis without large goiters.

RADIOACTIVE IODINE (^{131}I). This isotope produces marked depression of the overactive thyroid gland. It is used in the patient who is over forty-five years of age, in cases which have (rarely) recurred after operation, and in those in which operation would be risky, such as in marked heart failure.

SURGERY. Operation is indicated in the thirty to forty age group (especially in men) and when the antithyroid drugs have failed or caused ill effects. Under the age of thirty it is used if the goiter is large or the symptoms are severe. When an operation is performed, about three-quarters of the gland is removed, and the results are generally strikingly successful. The patient puts on weight and general health returns. When there is any possibility of malignant disease, an operation is usually undertaken, and cases of adenoma of the thyroid should generally be treated surgically.

Before the operation the patient is given a course of antithyroid drugs, followed by iodine in the form of potassium iodide for 10 to 14 days. The iodine makes the gland firmer and less vascular, and so reduces the risk of bleeding at the operation.

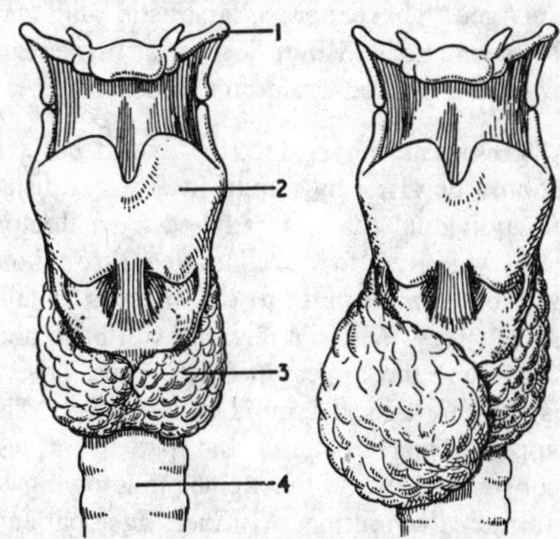

Fig. 1. *THYROID GLAND Normal gland* (left) *surrounding trachea below the larynx:* 1. *Hyoid bone.* 2. *Larynx.* 3. *Thyroid Gland.* 4. *Trachea. Enlarged goitrous gland* (right)—*the growth may affect one side only or both.*

Hypothyroidism

Cretinism. Children born with a lack of thyroid activity develop into cretins if the condition is not recognized early and treatment given. The typical cretin as a rule shows definite signs at about six months; he is a dwarf, backward in mental and physical development, with a flabby body, protruding abdomen, and short limbs. The skin is rough and dry and the hair coarse and scanty, while the tongue often protrudes. If tablets of thyroid extract are given early, that is between the third and sixth months of infancy, growth and brain development may become normal; otherwise the child becomes stunted and an imbecile, with an intelligence quotient below 70 per cent.

Treatment. Thyroid extract should be given in fairly large doses to produce normal growth, but must of course be ordered by, and progress supervised by, a physician. The initial doses should be small, and are increased gradually. In later childhood, thyroxine tablets are substituted for the thyroid extract. Treatment must be continued throughout life, in spite of apparent cure. Growth and bone development may be assessed by X-ray photographs taken at regular intervals.

Thyroid administration started after the age of about twelve years is generally useless and may make the child irritable and unmanageable, instead of being a placid imbecile.

Myxedema. In adult persons lack of thyroid secretion causes symptoms opposite to those in hyperthyroidism. Women are generally liable to be affected between thirty and fifty years, when the gland shrinks and becomes inactive; the patient gradually puts on weight, becomes slow in her movements and speech, mentally dull, and suffers from poor memory. The skin is dry, with puffiness below the eyes, the nails are brittle, and the hair often falls out. The pulse is slow, and the blood pressure is low; angina pectoris is not uncommon, and the heart may be enlarged. The patient is apathetic and may be melancholic. Minor degrees of myxedema with less marked symptoms also occur.

Treatment. Thyroxine (or thyroid extract) should be given by mouth in doses adjusted to individual cases, as advised by a doctor, and will need to be continued throughout life, but the response to treatment is usually satisfactory. Within a few weeks of beginning treatment the appearance improves, speech is clearer, and the mind more active. The appetite increases and the patient is less constipated, while the weight falls owing to an increased output of urine. Most patients keep well and free from symptoms on a maintenance dose of thyroxine which is judged by the patient's response to this drug. Treatment should be started by giving small doses, especially if the patient is elderly and the heart is affected. Excessive loss of weight, nervousness, or a fast pulse, indicate that the dose of thyroid given is too large.

Juvenile Myxedema. Juvenile myxedema should be distinguished from cretinism, since the former condition is not present at birth but develops after a variable period of normal growth. The outlook is better than in cretinism.

A dosage of 0.15 to 0.3 milligrams of thyroxine per day will usually be sufficient for maintenance treatment, but smaller doses should be given at the beginning. Treatment must be continued through life.

THE PARATHYROID GLANDS

These small bodies lie in the neck behind the thyroid gland and they are concerned in the use of calcium and inorganic phosphorus in the body, these substances being needed for the growth of bones and for the nervous system.

Tetany

When there is a very low calcium level in the blood a condition known as tetany develops, with cramps and spasm of the hands and feet. This condition is sometimes seen in cases of persistent vomiting of acid gastric juice causing alkalosis, as may occur in pyloric stenosis. Tetany may also occur in poorly nourished babies, as in rickets, in which cases calcium and vitamin D (calciferol) should be given and a more suitable diet provided. Deficiency of parathyroid secretion may occur after surgical removal of a goiter in which case the above treatment is given. Dihydrotachysterol may be used instead of calciferol. See also p. 517.

Hyperparathyroidism

Excessive parathyroid secretion is due to an adenoma, carcinoma, or hypertrophy of the glands. The symptoms include weakness, loss of appetite, and bone pain. Anemia and recurring kidney stones are common.

The treatment is surgical.

THE ADRENAL GLANDS

The adrenal, or suprarenal, glands are situated just above the kidneys. The inner part of the gland, the medulla, secretes adrenaline, which raises the blood pressure, dilates the pupils, makes the skin cold as in 'goose-flesh,' and increases the sugar in the blood. Adrenaline is produced rapidly in states of fear or alarm, so that the changes mentioned above occur almost instantaneously.

The outer part of the gland, the cortex, secretes three groups of hormones.

1. Hydrocortisone which affects carbohydrate and protein metabolism.
2. Aldosterone which regulates salt and water and potassium excretion.
3. An androgenic steroid which is a type of sex hormone.

Addison's Disease

This disease is due to deficiency of the adrenal hormones caused by tuberculosis or by atrophy of the adrenal glands. It is a rare disease, somewhat commoner in men than in women.

Symptoms. The exhaustion of the adrenals causes gradual but slowly increasing weakness, loss of weight and wasting, loss of appetite, indigestion, nausea or vomiting, and the development of brown patches, or 'bronzing,' of the neck, face, arms and hands, legs and other parts of the body, which are characteristic of Addison's disease. The blood pressure is very low and the patient feels exhausted and tends to collapse at the least exertion. In the later stages there is difficulty in writing and in speech, the pulse is weak and the patient is severely emaciated and exhausted; if untreated, the disease leads to death from extreme general debility.

Treatment requires complete rest, avoidance of cold, and prevention of excitement or worry, with a diet containing easily digested food. Soups, broths, and meat extracts should be withheld.

The most recent drug treatment consists of the administration by mouth of fludrocortisone and cortisone daily. This has largely replaced injections or pellets of DOCA (an artificially prepared adrenal substance) inserted beneath the skin.

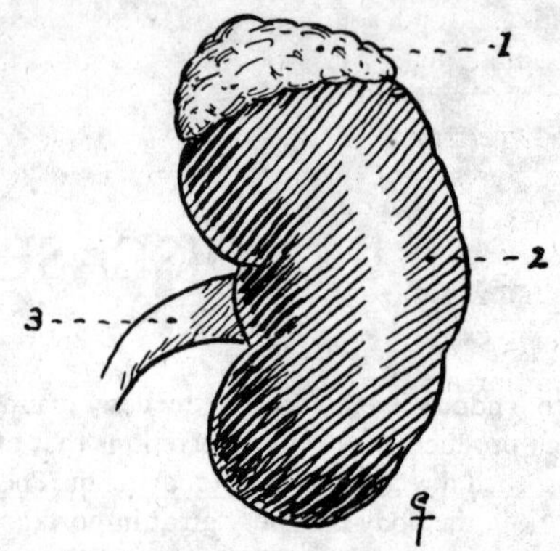

Fig. 2. *THE ADRENAL GLAND.* 1. *Adrenal gland.* 2. *Kidney.* 3. *Ureter. Although the adrenal gland lies so closely on the upper surface of the kidney, the two organs are completely unrelated in function.*

The patient must lead a quiet life and not expect to undertake much activity; there must be plenty of rest, and freedom from anxiety or responsibility. Investigation of possible tuberculous disease should be made and treatment instituted if necessary.

Crises, or sudden increase of symptoms, especially of weakness or collapse, with vomiting and extremely low blood pressure, sometimes occur. A crisis should be treated in hospital with glucose-saline transfusions and intravenous hydrocortisone supplemented by intramuscular injections of DOCA.

Patients with Addison's disease should not be given morphine or general anesthetics whenever these can be avoided, since they are liable to provoke a crisis.

The Adreno-Genital Syndrome

An excessive secretion of the androgenic steroids (due to hypertrophy or tumor in the adrenal gland) will alter the sexual characteristics. The effects produced depend on the age at which this occurs and on the sex. In embryonic life, female pseudohermaphroditism occurs. In children there is precocious sexual and physical development (infant Hercules). In young adults virilism or feminization occur.

Virilism. Virilism, or the development of masculine characteristics, is seen in young women or girls at puberty. The woman does not menstruate normally and hair develops on the face and other areas where hair normally occurs in males. Adiposity also often occurs, and the voice becomes deep. The womb may be small and under-developed, while the clitoris may be enlarged, resembling a small penis. The breasts are often small, although this may be masked by the fat deposits. Brown coloration round the eyes may be seen, as in Addison's disease. The patient may be homosexual, or may suffer from some mental disorder or psychosis, but in other cases the mental outlook and disposition may be typically 'feminine,' although the patient is generally sterile.

Treatment. The case must be carefully investigated and, if a tumor of the adrenal glands is found, it must be removed surgically; malignant tumors, however, tend to recur.

In hypertrophy, intramuscular injections of large doses of cortisone may be used to suppress the overactive gland.

Electrolysis is a useful method of treatment for removal of facial hair.

Feminization. When adrenal overactivity or an adrenal tumor occurs in a male, the opposite condition develops and is known as feminization, but this is uncommon and is generally due to a malignant tumor, which often proves fatal.

Cushing's Syndrome

Increased secretion of all three cortical hormones (see p. 402) gives rise to this rare condition. The features vary according to the predominant hormone secreted. The clinical picture includes obesity with a 'moon' face and 'buffalo' hump on the back, purple streaks on the buttocks and thighs, weakness and wasting, and maybe virilism.

The cause is either a hypertrophy of, or a tumor in, the adrenal glands.

Treatment. The treatment is either surgical removal of both adrenals with consequent life-long cortisone substitution therapy, or injections of cortisone may be given to suppress the overactivity.

THE PITUITARY GLAND

This gland lies within the brain and possesses a front and a hind lobe, either of which may become diseased. The front lobe is associated with the various processes of growth, so that disease or disorder of this lobe may give rise to variations in development and

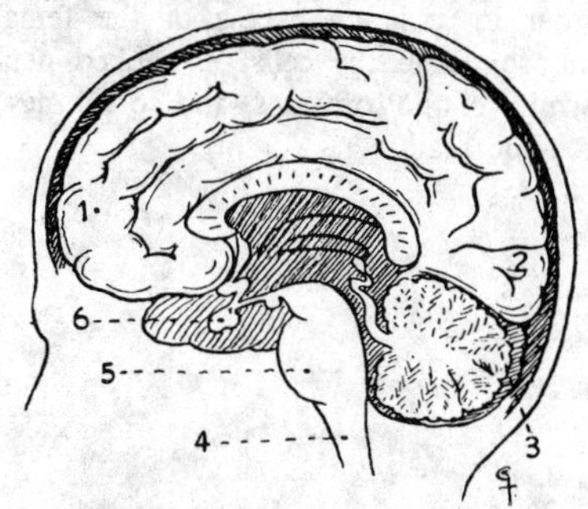

Fig. 3. *PITUITARY GLAND. Section of the brain showing the position of the pituitary gland:* 1. *Frontal lobe.* 2. *Occipital lobe.* 3. *Cerebellum.* 4. *Medulla Oblongata.* 5. *Pons Varolii.* 6. *Pituitary gland.*

physical appearance. It also regulates the activity of the other ductless glands, including the sex glands, the thyroid, and the adrenals, and is thus of great importance in the maintenance of health and well-being. The hind, or posterior, lobe of the pituitary secretes two hormones, one of which regulates the excretion of water, and the other governs contractions of the pregnant womb.

In young people overactivity of the front lobe of the pituitary causes extremely rapid and excessive growth, or gigantism, while in adults similar overactivity produces acromegaly.

Gigantism

In gigantism there is very rapid overgrowth of the bones causing unusual height of the individual. This occurs during childhood, before growth has ceased. If the overactivity continues, acromegaly also develops. There is no actual dividing line between tall persons and giants, and tallness is probably a racial or familial characteristic.

The treatment of gigantism is the same as for acromegaly (see below).

Acromegaly

Acromegaly develops in middle life before the age of forty years. It may progress rapidly, being fatal within three or four years, but usually it is more gradual. In the early stage there may be increased sexual and mental capacity, but soon lassitude, physical and sexual weakness, poor memory and incapacity for concentration are noticed. The face and head become larger, especially the lower jaw, and the hands and feet increase in size, so that the patient has to wear larger hats, gloves and shoes. The lips become very thick and the tongue is large, so that speaking may be difficult. The nose is broad, and the ears big. The hands are wide and 'spade-like' with sausage-shaped fingers, and both hands and feet sweat considerably. The back becomes bent and the head is thrust forward, like a gorilla; muscular pains and neuritis are often complained of, and sugar may be passed in the urine. When acromegaly is due to a tumor of the pituitary gland, the pressure within the brain may cause blindness.

Occasionally surgical removal of the pituitary gland is carried out; in other cases radiotherapy is given.

Dwarfism

In pituitary dwarfism there is a failure of growth with abnormal shortness of stature, due to insufficient production of the growth hormone in the front lobe of the pituitary gland. There may also be other abnormalities and sexual development may be incomplete (infantilism). Dwarfism is also seen in other conditions such as achondroplasia (see Diseases of Bones and Spine, p. 537) cretinism (p. 401), and other less common disorders.

The child ceases to grow at an early age.

Treatment. This includes administration of androgens by mouth, by injection or by pellet implantation, both to male and female patients.

Simmond's Disease

(*Hypopituitarism*)

In this disease there is a deficient secretion of all the front lobe hormones. It may result from tumor or infection, but the commonest cause is thrombosis of the gland following a hemorrhage after childbirth. Lactation fails, there is no menstruation, and the axillary and pubic hair is lost. All hormone production in the body may be affected.

Treatment consists of administration of cortisone by mouth, and testosterone preparations and thyroid if necessary.

Diabetes Insipidus

Diabetes insipidus is a rare chronic disease in which excessive quantities of pale urine are passed persistently, and there is abnormal thirst. The urine does not contain sugar as in diabetes mellitus. The disease generally occurs in young or middle-aged people, and the patient is often thin, the muscles appearing to be wasted, with a dry skin and general coldness of the body. Appetite is fairly normal. From fifteen to twenty pints of urine may be passed in a day; it is of low specific gravity, being very dilute. The disease continues over a long period, and the general health may remain fairly good.

Causes include tumors of the hind lobe of the pituitary gland or of the hypothalamus in the brain, or operations affecting this region, chronic encephalitis, syphilis, injuries to the head with fracture of the base of the skull, and cerebrovascular accidents with hemiplegia and acute delirium. Occasionally a hereditary or familial form is seen.

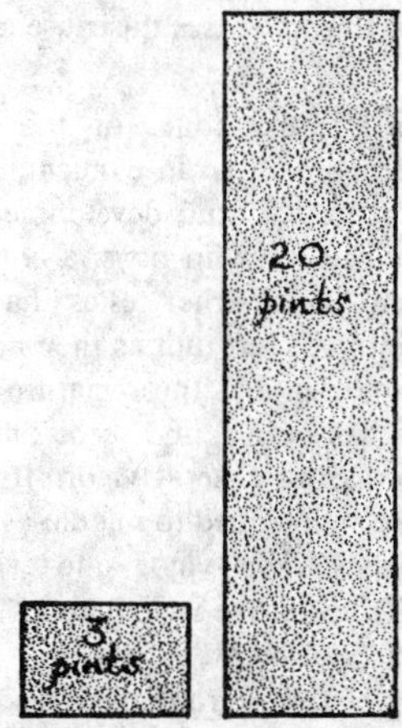

Fig. 4. *DAILY URINE EXCRETION. The normal person excretes about* 3 *pints of urine daily and in diabetes insipidus about* 20 *pints.*

The condition must be diagnosed from chronic nephritis, diabetes mellitus, hysterical thirst, and overactivity of the parathyroid glands. The outlook depends upon the underlying cause. See also p. 394 .

Treatment. Vasopressin is given, in the form of pitressin tannate in oil, by injection at intervals of one to three days or more; the dose is reduced until the water balance is established and the thirst and urine output are controlled. The use of salt should be restricted.

Powdered posterior pituitary is also used in the form of a nasal spray when injections are not available. In cases of syphilitic origin, vigorous anti-syphilitic treatment is essential. See Venereal Diseases, p. 290.

THE SEX GLANDS
(*Gonads*)

The Testes

The activity of the testes, or male glands, is controlled by the pituitary gland in the brain. The two main functions of the testes are to produce the spermatozoa for reproduction, and to form a hormone known as testosterone.

Male Hypogonadism or testicular deficiency. The signs of such deficiency depend on whether the condition develops before or after puberty. In the former case a condition of *eunuchoidism* may occur, with excessive growth of the limbs, a high-pitched voice and lack of secondary male characteristics such as hair on the face and body. If the deficiency does not develop until after puberty the person will be of normal height but there will be some obesity, softness of the skin and hair, reduced sexual function and often small sexual organs.

The cause of hypogonadism may be deficiency in the pituitary, or destruction or damage of the testes. The latter may be due to injury, tuberculosis, syphilis, gonorrhea, and mumps. In some cases the cause may not be found.

Treatment. Testosterone, or the related fluoxymesterone, is used in eunuchoidism to assist natural growth and development, and for undescended testes in boys, a congenital condition in which the testes have not descended into the scrotum as they normally do in a full-term-infant. In premature senility testosterone has been found to be of limited value in increasing general vigor. It is also sometimes recommended to middle-aged men who are losing their vigor and who feel depressed. Testosterone is sometimes used in advanced cases of breast cancer.

Any form of testosterone medication must be supervised by a doctor.

The Ovaries

The ovaries, like the testes, are regulated in their activities by the pituitary gland. During the active fertile life of women, while the eggs are being developed for fertilization, the ovaries form certain hormones known as *estrogens.* These hormones stimulate the growth of the lining of the womb. During the second half of the menstrual cycle, *progesterone* is produced; it has a complex action not only on the cycle but also on the pregnant womb.

In actual practice no pituitary extract preparations are available to stimulate inactive ovaries in cases of sterility, since they are very unstable and are also difficult to prepare. A hormone obtained from the blood of pregnant mares has, however, been used for ovarian stimulation in cases of sterility due to ovarian inactivity. The results of this form of therapy have proved very disappointing.

Estrogen is used in a number of conditions, but synthetic compounds such as stilbestrol, hexestrol, dienestrol and ethinylestradiol, which have estrogenic activity, are used in practice. Their use may be indicated in the following conditions.

1. Metropathia hemorrhagica.
2. Menorrhagia: excessive menstruation.
3. Amenorrhea: no menstruation.
4. Dysmenorrhea: painful periods.
5. Inhibition of lactation.
6. Menopausal symptoms.
7. Early arthritis in the menopause.
8. Pruritis vulva in senile vaginitis.

For full details of these conditions and their treatment, see section on Diseases of Women.

Intersex Anomalies

Pseudo-hermaphroditism. In this condition of 'false hermaphroditism' only one type of sex organ is present but the external genital parts are of a mixed type or resemble those of the opposite sex. In a boy the scrotal folds may remain separate and enclose a cavity similar to a vaginal passage, or the penis may be incomplete or underdeveloped. The boy is probably brought up as a girl until puberty, but when he fails to menstruate, or masculine hair development occurs, the internal sex organs are found to be abnormal and the testes are discovered to be in the abdomen. The boy is often eunuchoid in type.

The female pseudo-hermaphrodite has ovaries, but is masculine in type, with external genital structures similar to those of a male.

Pseudo-hermaphroditism may be either genetically determined (more commonly in the male), or due to excess secretion of androgen from the adrenal glands in the female (see under Virilism, p. 402). If the condition is seen in early childhood, the correct sex should be determined by skin biopsy so that the child may be brought up appropriately.

If advice is sought in adult life, treatment must be in accordance with the patient's inclinations. Plastic surgery now offers a means of correcting the sexual abnormalities.

Hermaphroditism. In true hermaphrodites both male and female sex glands or elements are present in the same individual, but such cases are very rare.

Klinefelter Syndrome. This is a form of gonad disorder characterized by excretion of normal male with some female hormones, failure to produce sperms, and sometimes enlarged breasts. Most individuals are males. The disorder is due to faults in the chromosomes, those particles in the cell nucleus which carry the 'pattern' of each person.

Turner's Syndrome. In this chromosomal disorder there is an excess of the female chromosomes in the cells, a webbed neck, deformity of the forearms, and sometimes a heart abnormality.

DISEASES OF THE URINARY SYSTEM

The urinary organs consist of the kidneys, the ureters, the bladder, and the urethra (the water passage); a fuller description of these organs can be found on pp. 251 to 253. The kidneys filter off the waste products from the blood in the form of urine, which passes down the ureters to the bladder; this holds the urine until it is voided through the urethra.

Fig. 51, p. 227, shows the external view of the left kidney. The kidneys lie in the loins at the back of the abdominal wall, being supported by the surrounding fat, the other organs in the abdomen, and the connecting

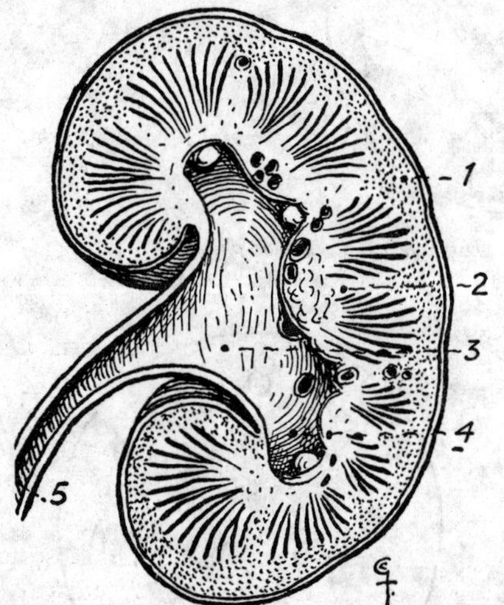

Fig. 1. *SECTION THROUGH THE LEFT KIDNEY.* **1.** *Cortex, or outer zone.* **2.** *Medulla, or inner zone.* **3.** *Pelvis of ureter.* **4.** *Calyx.* **5.** *Ureter.*

blood vessels. Each kidney consists of three kinds of tissues—the secreting tubules which begin the outer zone or cortex and then pass through the inner zone or medulla, the supporting framework, and the blood vessels with tufts of tiny capillary vessels (glomeruli) projecting into the outer ends of the tubules.

One of the most important functions of the kidneys is to keep the blood stable in composition. They filter off water, and any excess of salts or other substances not required by the body; toxins, drugs, and the products of wear and tear are separated from the blood and pass out from the body in the urine. If the kidneys are damaged or diseased they may fail to filter urea (one of the waste products in the blood), and if this accumulates in the system it produces serious symptoms (uremia). The normal average quantity of urine produced in twenty-four hours by an adult is up to 1.8 liters, but this may vary from about 900 milliliters to 1.8 liters.

Diseases of the urinary organs may be investigated in various ways, as follows:

1. By the examination of the urine, using various tests.
2. By the chemical examination of the blood.
3. By the direct surgical inspection of the bladder by means of a cystoscope, Fig. 10.
4. By X-ray examination of the kidneys, ureters and bladder, including pyelography.

EXAMINATION OF THE URINE

Characteristics of Urine. Healthy urine is usually a light amber color and transparent. It has different degrees of density (or concentration), its specific gravity varying from 1·010 to 1·025. It has an aromatic or ammoniacal smell, and a bitter disagreeable taste.

Urine which is passed a little time after drinking much water is pale, and has a low specific gravity, varying from 1·002 to 1·009; urine which is passed soon after the digestion of a full meal has a specific gravity from 1·020 to 1·030. Urine which is secreted before eating or drinking in the morning has a specific gravity of from 1·015 to 1·025. For some routine tests, a mixed specimen of urine collected over a period of twenty-four hours is used.

Methods of Examination of Urine

Acidity and Alkalinity. Urine is usually acid, but may be alkaline first thing in the morning.

A piece of blue litmus paper is first dipped in the urine; if this is acid, the color of the paper will be changed to pink. Should the blue color remain unchanged, then use a piece of yellow turmeric or pink litmus paper; if the urine is alkaline, the turmeric paper will become brown, and the pink litmus paper will turn to blue. If the color in both cases remains unaltered, the urine is neutral, that is, neither acid nor alkaline.

Odor. Alkaline urine often smells of ammonia. In diabetes mellitus the sugar in the urine gives it a sweetish smell, like apples or new-mown hay. Acetone in the urine gives the smell of peardrops.

Cloudiness or turbidity may be due to:

URATES; these are cleared by warming or filtering the urine.

CALCIUM OR MAGNESIUM PHOSPHATES; these are cleared by a few drops of strong acetic acid, or by filtering.

BACTERIA OR PUS CELLS are not cleared by the above methods.

MUCUS, ALBUMIN, AND OXALATE OF LIME also make the urine turbid.

Color Changes. Concentrated or 'strong' urine is generally of a deeper color than dilute urine, but in diabetes mellitus, when the urine contains a considerable quantity of sugar, it may still be pale.

Certain characteristic color changes in the urine are found to occur, and should be noted.

BRIGHT YELLOW URINE is found after taking santonin in the treatment of roundworms, or mepacrine in the treatment of malaria.

PINK OR RED URINE may be due to blood, or to drugs such as senna or rhubarb, or may occur after eating sweets colored with eosin coloring. Fresh blood appears bright red, while old blood makes the urine appear 'smoky.'

BLACK OR BROWN URINE may contain bile, or it may be seen in cases of poisoning with carbolic acid or lysol, or in some cases of cancer.

BLUE OR GREEN URINE may be passed after drugs containing dyes such as methylene blue have been taken.

Quantity. In adults, about 1 to 1.5 liters of urine is generally passed in twenty-four hours. If much extra fluid is drunk, or in cases of diabetes mellitus or chronic nephritis, much more may be passed; but if the fluids in the diet are reduced, or after heavy sweating, and in acute nephritis and fevers, the urine output may be small. Urine may cease to be formed ('suppression' or anuria) in severe acute nephritis, in cases of kidney stone and in other severe conditions.

Retention of urine in the bladder may be due to some obstruction, such as an enlarged prostate gland, or stricture of the urethra.

Urinary Deposits. When normal urine is left to stand for a time, a woolly deposit of mucus tends to settle at the bottom. In alkaline urine a heavier deposit of phosphates is often seen, while in acid urine the urate salts are pale pink.

Blood appears as a brownish or red deposit, whereas pus is creamy.

Specific Gravity. This is easily tested by means of the urinometer (Fig. 2). This instrument is also called a hydrometer; it is usually made of glass and has a graduated scale by which the density of liquids may be read. When placed in distilled water, it will sink to a certain level; since all bodies immersed in fluid displace a volume of the liquid corresponding to their own mass, it follows that in a fluid denser than water the instrument will not sink so deep as in water, because less fluid is displaced. The space above the large bulb of the urinometer is marked off into degrees which denote the different densities of urine samples.

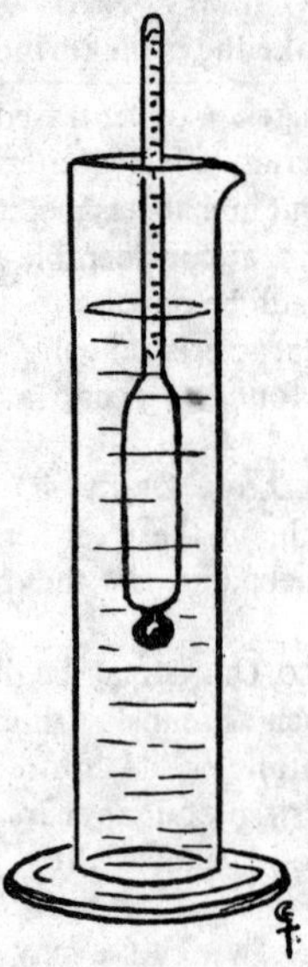

Fig. 2. *THE URINOMETER for testing the density of the urine.*

When this instrument is immersed in urine and has come to rest, the number on the graduated scale which is shown at the surface of the liquid represents the ratio of the specific gravity of the fluid compared with that of water, which equals 1·000. If, for example, the surface of the liquid corresponds with 1·009 on the scale, the specific gravity of the urine will be 1·009; if the fluid level on the scale is shown at 1·025, the specific gravity will be 1·025.

By noting the specific gravity of the urine, the physician may often gain important information, since it indicates how much soluble or solid matter it contains.

Chemical Deposits. The main abnormal substances which may be found in urine by chemical tests are albumin, sugar, ketone bodies, blood, pus, and bile.

Albumin in the urine generally indicates that there is some disturbance in the kidney function, although there may not necessarily be any actual disease.

The commonest causes of albuminuria are:

Acute fevers;

Congestion of the kidneys as in heart failure, or irritation from some poison;

Kidney diseases such as nephritis;

Tuberculosis;

Cancer of the kidneys;

Eclampsia, a condition which sometimes occurs in pregnancy;

Inflammation of the pelvis of the kidney (pyelitis), or of the bladder (cystitis);

CRYSTALLINE DEPOSITS IN URINE AS SEEN UNDER A MICROSCOPE

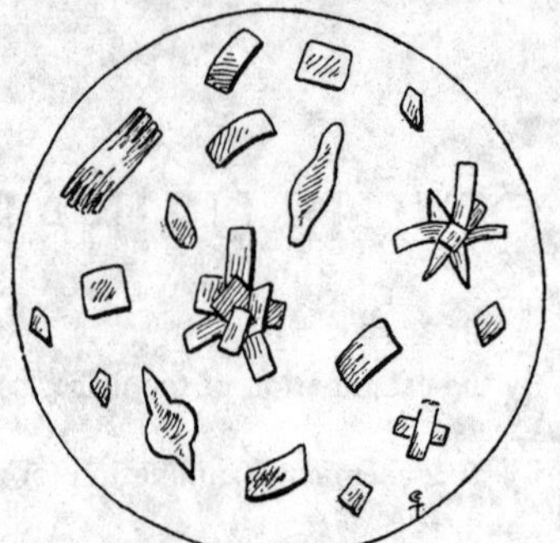

Fig. 3. *URINE CRYSTALS. Uric acid*

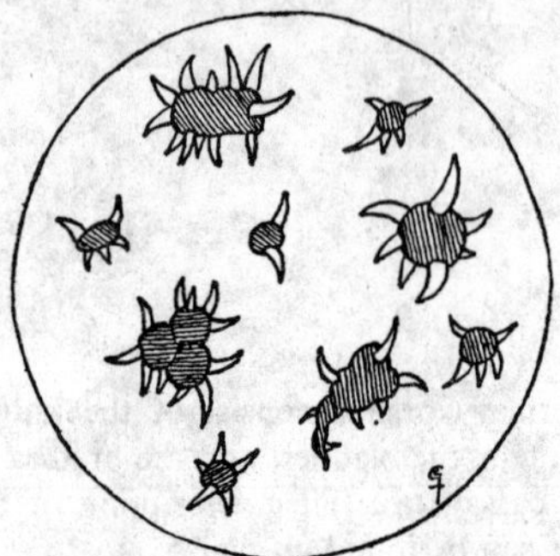

Fig. 4. *URINE CRYSTALS. Ammonium urate*

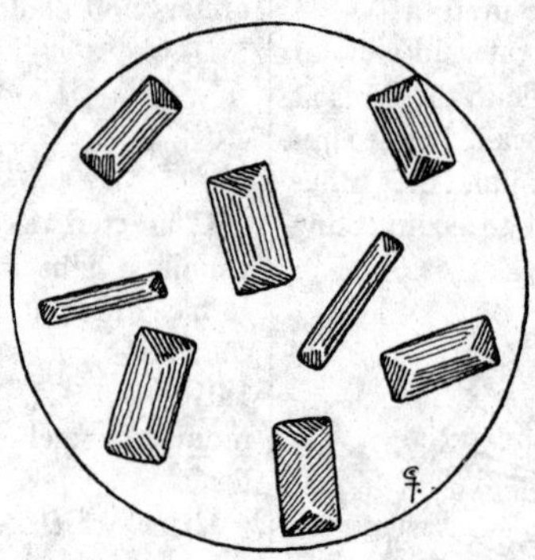

Fig. 5. *URINE CRYSTALS. Ammonium phosphate and magnesium phosphate*

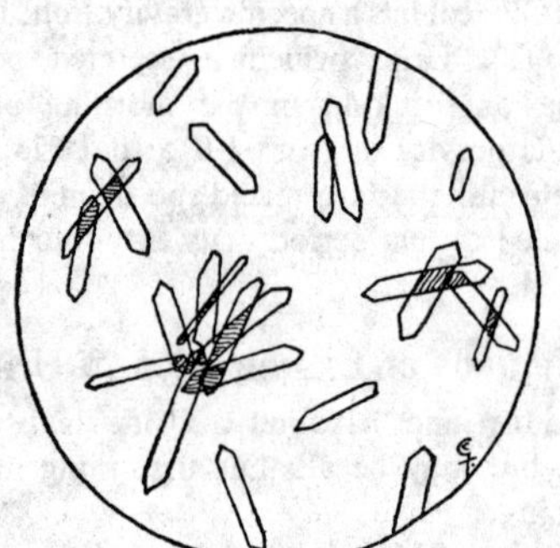

Fig. 6. *URINE CRYSTALS. Stellar phosphates*

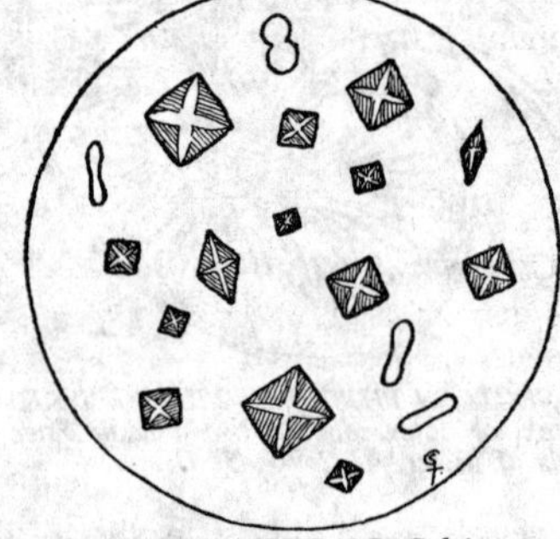

Fig. 7. *URINE CRYSTALS. Calcium oxalate*

Orthostatic or postural albuminuria which is sometimes seen in young men during adolescence. In this condition albumin is absent in the morning after a night's rest, and is not due to disease of the kidneys.

Tests for Abnormal Constituents of Urine

Albumin in the urine may be tested for in various ways, the most usual methods being the boiling test and the sulpho-salicylic acid test.

THE BOILING TEST. If the urine is cloudy it should be filtered. A test-tube is then filled two-thirds full of the filtered urine; the tube is held over a Bunsen gas burner or spirit lamp until the upper part of the urine boils. The mouth of the tube should be held away from the person to prevent the hot urine causing injury if it boils over. If no cloudy layer appears in the upper boiled part, albumin is not present in the urine. If a cloudy haze appears, a few drops of dilute acetic acid should be added; if the cloud remains it indicates that albumin is present, but, if it dissolves, the deposit was due to phosphates. The greater the quantity of albumin in the urine, the denser will be the cloud formed on boiling.

SULPHOSALICYLIC ACID TEST. This test does not require heat. Cloudy urine should be filtered: 5 milliliters of urine is then placed in a test-tube and 6 drops of 20 per cent sulphosalicylic acid added. The formation of cloudiness indicates albumin.

Albumin is sometimes estimated quantitatively by *Esbach's method*, a simple way of finding the amount in the urine; this test is used in cases of acute nephritis, as an aid in estimating the progress of a patient.

Sugar in the urine is found in diabetes mellitus, and occasionally in some other

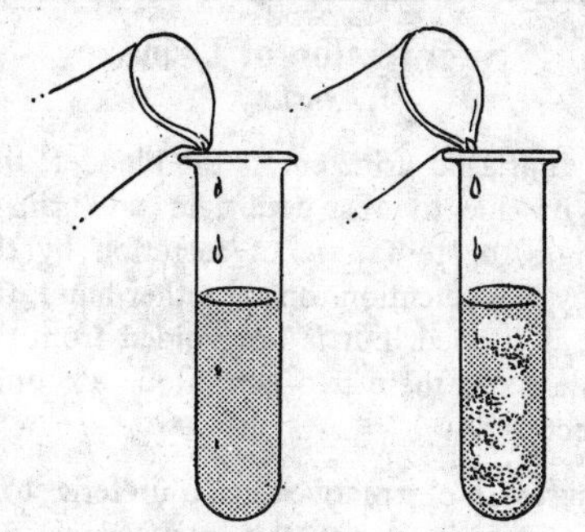

Fig. 8. *TEST FOR PROTEIN (albumin) IN URINE. The sulphsalicylic acid test. Normal urine* (left) *remains clear; albumin in the urine produces cloudiness* (right).

conditions; the presence of sugar in the urine is called glycosuria, and may be discovered by various easy tests.

1. FEHLING'S TEST. A small quantity of Fehling's solution is boiled in a test-tube, and is then added to an equal quantity of boiling urine in another tube; if an orange or red cloud or precipitate appears, it indicates the possible presence of sugar. If, however, the patient has recently taken aspirin or any salicylic acid drug, or if there is much uric acid present, these may also give a positive result as above, and the urine should be retested later, or another test should be used.

2. BENEDICT'S TEST. This is a rather more delicate test for showing small traces of sugar in the urine. Five milliliters of Benedict's solution is added to eight drops of urine in a test-tube, and the mixture is boiled for about two minutes. In the absence of sugar the solution remains blue, while a small amount of sugar causes a green color to appear within fifteen minutes, and a larger quantity produces a red or yellow color.

3. CLINITEST TABLETS. These tablets contain copper sulphate reagent and are very easy to use as no heating is required. They are especially useful for diabetics who are able to check their own urine when necessary.

Blood is found in the urine (hematuria) in any condition in which bleeding occurs in the kidneys, ureters, bladder or urethra. It may follow an injury, or it may be due to a stone, growth, or some form of inflammation such as tuberculosis, or other infection—a common type being pyelitis due to *Escherichia coli* infection from the intestines. Acute nephritis is another cause of hematuria. Tumors, either innocent or malignant, and various general diseases such as blood diseases, fevers, malaria, or certain poisons or drugs may also cause blood to appear in the urine.

BENZIDINE TEST. Blood in the urine may be detected by putting a little benzidine (to cover a knife point) into a test-tube and adding 2 to 3 milliliters of glacial acetic acid. This should be well shaken and an equal volume of hydrogen peroxide (10 volumes) added. Urine is then added drop by drop. If blood is present, the solution becomes deep blue or greenish blue.

Pus occurs in the urine in various infections of the urinary organs when pus is formed, such as in abscess of the kidney, pyelitis (infection of the kidney pelvis), cystitis (or inflammation of the bladder), and urethritis (or inflammation of the urethra). Pus is generally detected by miscroscopical examination by a doctor.

Bile may be present in the urine in jaundice, and causes a dark greenish-brown color.

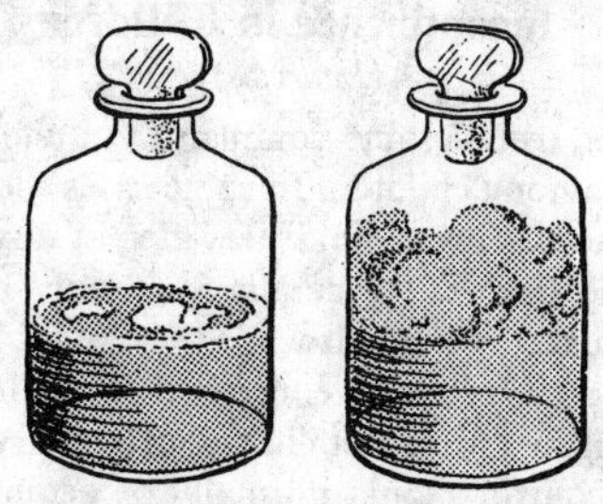

Fig. 9. *TEST FOR BILE IN URINE.* (left) *Scanty white froth is produced when urine in the bottle is shaken.* (right) *Copious yellow froth is produced if bile is present.*

TESTS. A simple way of detecting bile is to shake the urine in a stoppered bottle. If bile is present a large amount of yellow froth is

Other abnormal constituents of urine are generally found by chemical or microscopical examination. They include hemoglobin from the blood cells, bacteria, casts, drugs and crystalline drug deposits.

Recently, chemical examination of the urine has been simplified by the production of strips of paper with the reagent sealed in the end. The strip is dipped into the urine specimen and any color change noted. Sugar and albumin can be tested for in this way.

Kidney Efficiency Tests

Certain tests are used to discover the efficiency of the kidneys when the action of these organs is thought to be impaired.

BLOOD UREA TEST. The amount of urea in the blood may be estimated in a small sample of blood drawn off from a vein.

The UREA CONCENTRATION TEST demonstrates the capacity of the kidneys to filter off a dose of 15 grams of urea taken in water, within periods of one hour, two hours, and three hours. In normal cases at least 2 per cent of urea is present in one sample of the urine. In cases where less than 1·5 per cent is present, the outlook is serious.

Other more complicated kidney efficiency tests may sometimes be necessary.

EXAMINATION OF THE BLADDER

Cystoscopy

By this means of examination many diseases of the urinary organs may be investigated. The cystoscope is an instrument designed for inspecting the interior of the bladder, and is used by surgeons. It is introduced through the urethra and has an illuminated light bulb, so that the walls of the bladder and the ureteric openings are plainly seen. It

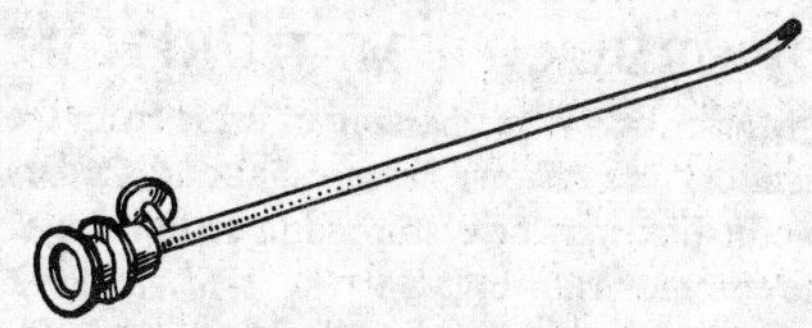

Fig. 10. *A CYSTOSCOPE. This viewing instrument is used for inspecting the interior of the bladder.*

is thus possible to see if blood or pus is passed down the ureter from either kidney, and the urine from either ureter can be collected separately for examination.

EXAMINATION OF THE KIDNEYS

Pyelography

Pyelography is an investigation which is carried out to obtain information as to the condition and function of the kidney, its pelvis and the ureters on each side.

A substance which is opaque to X-rays, is given by intravenous injection. X-ray photographs of the kidneys are then taken at intervals, and these show opaque shadows which reveal abnormalities of the shape, size, or position of the urinary organs.

Food and drink are not taken for twelve hours before the injection is given.

DIAGRAMS SHOWING X-RAY APPEARANCES OF KIDNEYS, NORMAL AND DISEASED

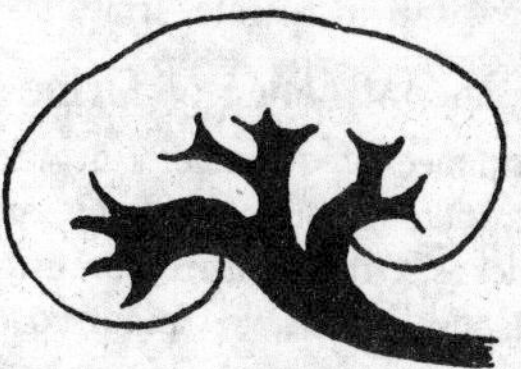

Fig. 11. *Diagram showing X-ray appearance of a normal kidney as seen in pyelograms.*

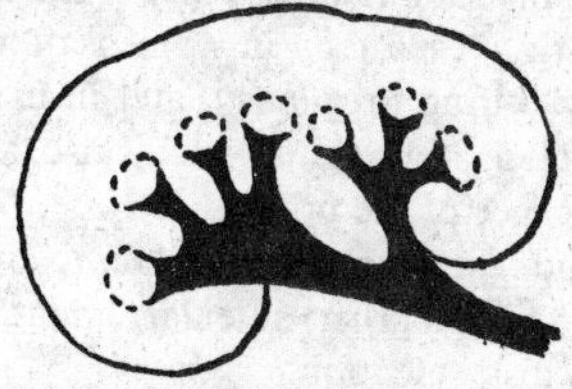

Fig. 12. *Normal kidney, with calyces and ureters filled with opaque fluid.*

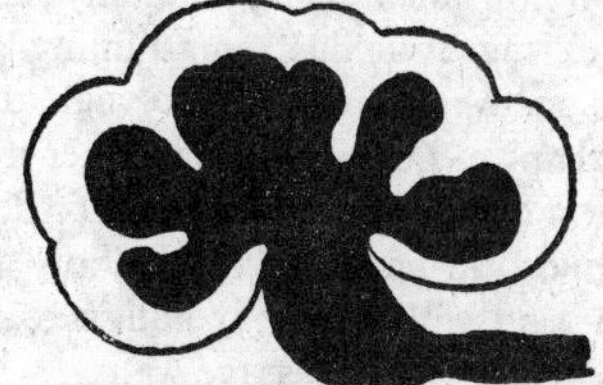

Fig. 13. *Enlarged kidney with advanced hydronephrosis showing greatly distended pelvis and calyces, and compression of kidney tissues.*

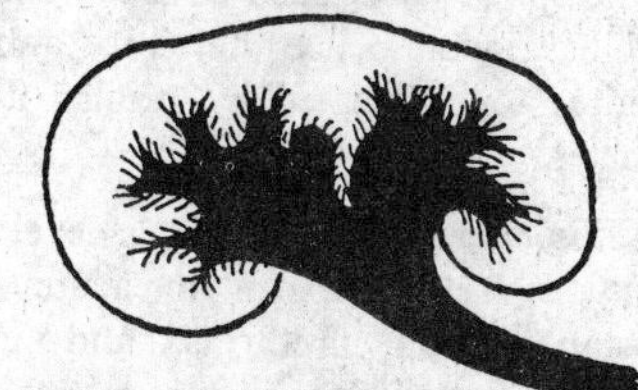

Fig. 14. *Kidney damaged by tuberculosis.*

DISORDERS OF MICTURITION

Micturition is the passing of urine from the bladder. In various diseases and disorders micturition may be disturbed in certain ways, the commonest being:

1. INCONTINENCE, or leakage and involuntary passing of urine. This may occur in brain disorders, unconsciousness, or as a result of laxness of the urethral muscles, particularly in women.
2. RETENTION, or inability to pass urine from the bladder. This may be sudden or acute in onset; or the retention may be chronic, with dribbling away of urine due to overflow.
3. FREQUENCY OF MICTURITION is very common. It may be due to nervousness, or to drinking large quantities of fluids, and is a common symptom of diabetes and chronic nephritis (Bright's disease). Local disorders of the bladder such as stone, inflammation, urethral inflammation, or pressure upon the bladder by tumors or by the womb in pregnancy, also cause frequency, which can be very troublesome and distressing.
4. PAINFUL OR DIFFICULT MICTURITION (dysuria) is a symptom of disorders such as inflammation of the bladder or urethra, stricture, enlargement of the prostate gland, or certain nervous diseases.
5. In ANURIA, no urine enters the bladder, either as a result of obstruction, or because the kidneys fail to secrete urine.

Incontinence of Urine

Incontinence of urine may occur in brain disorders such as epilepsy, idiocy, or disseminated sclerosis, or in other conditions when consciousness is lost, in spinal cord disease or injuries, or as a result of weakness of the urethral muscle in old age or in severe illnesses. Any state causing laxity of the urethral muscle ring, especially in women after childbirth or during pregnancy, and in cancer of the bladder and vaginal walls, also leads to incontinence of the urine.

Incontinence may also be due to overflow of urine, as in prostatic enlargement, where there is also retention.

Mechanical Incontinence. This is fairly common in women, being especially liable to occur during coughing or straining, when there is some relaxation of the vaginal walls and perhaps of the urethral sphincter muscle. This form of incontinence is likely to develop after child-bearing or difficult labor, and is usually dealt with by an operation to repair the stretching of the passage walls.

Nervous Incontinence. In certain diseases of the spinal cord, such as tabes dorsalis in syphilis, incontinence develops and often requires to be treated by regular use of a catheter.

Spasmodic Incontinence. This develops as a result of severe spasm in acute cystitis, prostatitis, and urethritis, and may be alleviated by sedatives such as morphine, and by treatment of the causative condition.

General Treatment of Incontinence

Care must be taken to prevent soreness of the back or legs; the bed linen and clothes must be changed as often as necessary, and the skin of the parts affected should be carefully dried, gently massaged with alcohol, and then powdered.

Incontinence in Children

(Enuresis)

This troublesome complaint is quite common among children. In some cases the child has no ability to hold its water at any time of the day, but generally it is only passed involuntarily at night while the child is asleep in bed. In adult life enuresis is less common, except in old or debilitated persons. Voluntary control should normally be acquired in children by the age of four years, and in some cases incontinence after this age is due to lack of careful training.

Causes. In the majority of cases no organic cause can be found. Various factors such as an insecure home background and other psychological states, bad training and heredity are thought to play a part in these cases. In 10 per cent of cases there is some actual urinary tract disease, and occasionally enuresis may be the only sign of other organic disease such as petit mal epilepsy. Incontinence is common in mentally deficient children.

Treatment. Any organic disorder must be recognized and attended to, and the urine should be carefully examined for albumin, pus, and sugar.

It is important that parents should do everything in their power to cure the habit early. The bedclothes should not be too heavy, and the child should not be allowed to get overtired before bedtime. Care should be taken to see that the child urinates before going to bed. The skin should be washed all over every day with cool or cold water, and vigorously rubbed with a coarse towel.

All sources of irritation should be removed. Highly-strung children require plenty of sleep, and late hours should not be allowed. A child who is incontinent should not be scolded severely, but should be encouraged and praised when control is achieved. The parents should not discuss the condition in front of the child, or show undue concern. The urine should always be tested by a doctor, since incontinence in young girls is sometimes due to pyelitis with infected urine.

The treatment advised by the doctor may be one of many. A rigorous bladder training régime may be instituted, or various tablets such as ephedrine, amphetamine, belladonna, or propantheline (Pro-banthine) may be prescribed. Or the use of an electrical 'buzzer,' waking the child as soon as he has passed urine, may be advised (see p.126).

Suppression of Urine

(Anuria)

In anuria no urine enters the bladder; this may be due to obstruction in the urinary passages, or to failure of secretion by the kidneys. In retention, on the other hand, the urine is formed, but is not voided from the bladder, and these two conditions are quite distinct.

Causes. In obstructive cases a ureteric stone is a common cause; this may block one ureter, and anuria follows if the other kidney is diseased. A growth in the bladder may also compress both ureters, causing obstruction to the passage of urine through these tubes.

In cases where there is no obstruction to the urine, acute nephritis, acute fevers (in which the suppression is usually temporary and seldom fatal), operations or injuries to the urinary system, cholera, or poisoning due to lead, turpentine or phosphorus, may be responsible. Another cause of anuria is the development of a 'lower nephron nephrosis' following burns, abortion, heat stroke, or an incompatible blood transfusion.

Symptoms. There may be no symptoms for several days in obstructive cases of anuria; then nausea usually develops, with thirst and constipation, and perhaps vomiting. The temperature is low, the pupils of the eyes are small, and soon drowsiness follows, with wandering of the mind, incoherent talk, twitching, hiccup, stupor and perhaps eventually death from heart failure. These symptoms are caused by the retention of urea which acts as a poison to the nervous system. Before death the perspiration has a strong smell of urine.

In non-obstructive cases the symptoms are typically those of uremia.

Treatment. The treatment must necessarily vary with the cause. The patient must be in hospital where accurately calculated fluids may be given intravenously and the acid-base balance corrected if necessary. Ureteral catheterization or nephrostomy may be performed in obstructive cases. The artificial kidney apparatus (p. 411) may be used to remove waste products from the body.

The pulse must be carefully watched for signs of impending collapse.

In ureteric obstruction exploratory operation on the kidney or ureter may be necessary after the anuric crisis has been treated by the above measures.

Retention of Urine

This condition is most common in men, and various causes may be responsible. There may be obstruction to the passage of urine by an enlarged prostate gland, or an abscess of the prostate. Urethral stricture, or inflammation, or a stone, growth, or foreign body in the urethra may be present. In the bladder there may be a stone, or a large blood clot obstructing the outlet; and certain diseases of the spinal cord, or poisons such as arsenic, mercury or lead may give rise to retention. Occasionally spasmodic retention develops after surgical operations in the pelvic region, or in cases of hysteria. Typhoid fever may very often be accompanied by retention of the urine. Pelvic tumors, and a retroverted pregnant uterus, are other cause.

Acute retention is usually complete and sudden in onset, while chronic retention is more often incomplete, and is a common symptom of enlargement of the prostate. The distended bladder can be felt in the lower part of the abdomen, and there is frequency of micturition but the bladder fails to empty completely.

Treatment. In acute retention after operations or childbirth, certain measures may be taken to help the patient to pass urine in the normal manner. The sound of water running from a faucet is sometimes sufficient to start micturition, while hot wet cloths over the bladder change of position (as from lying to sitting, or the 'knee-chest' position), hot drinks, or hot baths may prove helpful. If these methods are not successful, the doctor or nurse will be required to pass a soft rubber tube or catheter (p. 566), to allow the bladder to be emptied. Strict asepsis is essential and no force must be used.

Retention with overflow should never be allowed to develop, since it can be prevented by suitable measures for draining the bladder by a trained nurse or doctor; when it occurs, infection of the urine, with consequent inflammation of the bladder, often follows. Another danger is damage to the kidneys themselves due to 'back pressure.'

The bladder may have to be drained by a surgical operation when the above methods fail. In chronic cases the bladder should not be emptied at once, the urine always being allowed to pass very gradually.

Blood in the Urine
(*Hematuria*)

Blood passed in the urine may come from the kidneys, the ureters, the bladder, or the urethra, and is a symptom associated with many different types of disease.

Symptoms. The passage of the blood may be preceded by pain in the region of the bladder or kidneys, and is often accompanied by faintness. If pain is felt at the end of the penis, the bleeding probably arises within the bladder, while renal colic suggests kidney or ureteric disease. Bleeding from the bladder is generally seen in the urine passed at the end of micturition, while urethral bleeding is shown in the urine voided in the first part of the act.

It is sometimes difficult to decide whether the red discoloration of the urine is really due to blood as certain drugs may give rise to a red urine, e.g. senna and sulphonal. In such cases microscopic examination will demonstrate the red blood cells (corpuscles), if these are present (see Fig. 15).

In blackwater fever the urine is dark in color, owing to the presence of hemoglobin from the red blood cells.

When the bleeding is profuse a stone or growth may be present. If the color is bright red the blood probably comes from the bladder or lower part of the urinary tract.

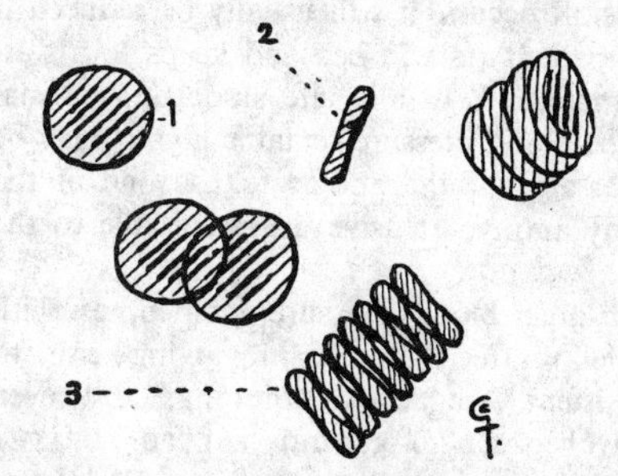

Fig. 15. *THE ERYTHROCYTES, OR RED BLOOD CELLS. 1. Red cell, front view. 2. Red cell, side view* (*biconcave*). *3. Red cells in 'rouleaux.*

Causes. These may be general affections such as BLOOD DISORDERS, leukemia, purpura, scurvy, specific fevers, malaria, and heart failure; or the hematuria may be due to KIDNEY DISORDERS such as:

Acute glomerulonephritis, or less commonly chronic glomerulonephritis;
Stone in the kidney;
Hydronephrosis;
Injuries;
New growths;
Polycystic kidneys;
Pyelonephritis.

Less commonly the following are responsible:

Infarction, as in endocarditis or mitral stenosis:
Early tuberculosis of the kidney.

Certain POISONS, e.g. carbolic acid, turpentine; or sulphonamide drugs which tend to make crystals in the kidney.

Certain AFFECTIONS OF THE URINARY PASSAGES may lead to blood in the urine. They include:

Stone in the ureter;
Bladder affections, such as growths, stone, tuberculosis, or cystitis (acute);
Prostatic tumors;
Stone in, or gonorrhea of, the urethra;
Injuries.

ESSENTIAL HEMATURIA is a condition where there is no discoverable cause, and it is seldom dangerous.

In older persons a stone or growth is a likely cause of hematuria, while in young people tuberculosis may be responsible. Painless hematuria occurs in growths and tuberculosis of the kidney.

Treatment. This must of course vary according to the nature of the case, and the immediate cause producing it.

In cases where the diagnosis is not obvious, the cause of the hematuria must be carefully investigated by a surgeon. This investigation will probably include cystoscopy, pyelography, and X-ray examinations.

In cases of injury, tuberculosis, stone, or growths of the urinary tract, the treatment may require a surgical operation.

DISEASES OF THE KIDNEYS

Nephritis

Nephritis, or Bright's disease, is the name which in the past has been given to several types of kidney disease, and it has been used to include cases of actual inflammation of the kidneys, as well as those in which degeneration or destruction of the kidney tissue or of its blood vessels has taken place.

Nephritis may be grouped into the following types:

Acute glomerulonephritis;
Subacute glomerulonephritis.

The effects of the disease depend on which portions are most affected; in most cases the kidney as a whole is generally damaged so that each part suffers to some extent.

Type 1: Acute Glomerulonephritis

This consists in acute inflammation of the kidneys, especially of the glomeruli (see p. 252). The disease generally develops in seven to twenty-one days after some streptococcal infection, especially of the throat; this may have been quite slight and have escaped notice at the time.

Causes. Acute nephritis is often a sequel to infectious fevers, especially scarlet fever, or tonsillitis, and may also follow exposure to cold and damp. The infecting micro-organism is usually found to be a strain of *Group A Streptococcus* which has an affinity for kidney tissue.

Onset. The disease generally starts suddenly, with pains in the back, headache, sickness and constipation. The patient is feverish, with a fast pulse, and there is a very typical white swelling, or edema, of the eyelids and face. There may also be some dropsy of the legs and/or abdomen and chest, and the blood pressure may be raised.

The kidneys are red and swollen, and the tubules become blocked. Only a small amount of strong (concentrated) urine is passed, that is about half a pint in 24 hours, but there may be complete suppression in very severe cases. When urine is passed, it is seen to be red or 'smoky,' owing to the presence of blood, and it contains a large amount of albumin.

The diagnosis is generally apparent from the appearance of the patient, and from the evidence afforded by the urine tests.

Course. Most young patients with acute glomerulonephritis recover after two to three weeks. In adults, however, there is usually much greater damage to the glomeruli and a higher degree of blood pressure. Recovery depends on the extent of the damage and as this is often progressive the patients may survive only for weeks though sometimes for a few years.

Complications. Damage to the glomeruli usually results in renal failure of varying degree, often leading to uremia. (p. 411). The increased blood pressure may cause brain disturbances with headache, convulsions, paralysis, or loss of sight. In cases with dropsy there may be heart failure and breathlessness; pleurisy and inflammation of the heart sac (or pericardium) sometimes occur.

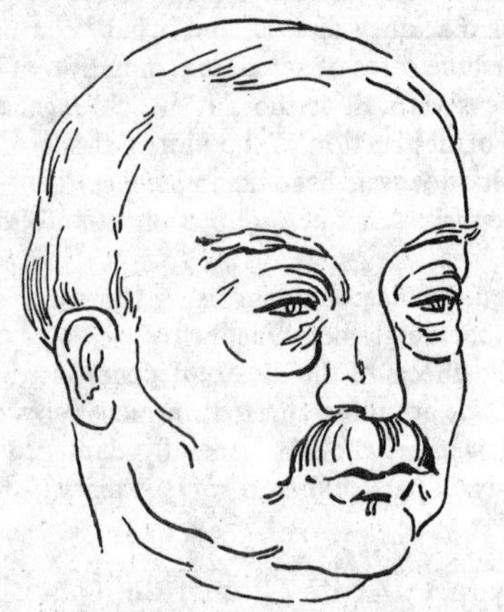

Fig. 16. *NEPHRITIS. A typical sign of this disease is puffiness around the eyes due to edema.*

Treatment. It is very important from the earliest stage to rest the kidneys as far as possible. The patient must rest in bed and be kept warm until the urine is free from albumin, the blood pressure is normal, and complete recovery has taken place. The period of rest in bed varies from two to four weeks to several months depending on the severity of the disease.

Woolen blankets should be used in place of sheets, and all risks of chill should be avoided, especially during washing. If there is much dropsy the patient's position should be changed frequently to prevent waterlogging or severe edema of the back parts.

DIET. Protein foods such as meat, cheese, and eggs, and meat extracts should not be given because they increase the work of the kidneys. Salt should not be added to food or used in cooking. Only moderate quantities of fluids should be given, since otherwise the dropsy is increased.

In mild to moderate cases the following dietary points should be observed.

FLUID should be restricted to 1 liter (1¾ pints) per day, plus about ¾ pint of milk.

FOOD of high carbohydrate content, e.g. bread, biscuits, cereal, sugar, can be given as the patient wishes. Unsalted butter, cream, and fruit are also suitable.

In cases with vomiting and anorexia (no wish for food) 1 pint of 30 per cent glucose in water (flavored with fruit juice) and 1 pint of milk per day, is given alternately in small two-hourly feedings. Fluids may have to be given rectally. In two to three days most patients will be able to take solid foods.

After about a month eggs are allowed, and finally fish, poultry or lamb may be given in small quantities if the patient's progress is satisfactory. At this stage tests of the kidney function may be made (see p. 407).

DRUGS. A full course of intramuscular penicillin is given to clear up any residual streptococcal infection.

Treatment of Complications. Where HYPERTENSION occurs, it will usually be reduced if the patient rests in bed and keeps to a salt-restricted diet to alleviate associated edema. If the blood pressure remains high it may be necessary for the doctor to use one of the many antihypertensive drugs suitable to the case.

If high blood pressure (sometimes with uremia) affects the brain, giving rise to persistent headaches, vomiting, and even convulsions, the general ENCEPHALOPATHY may be treated with the prompt administration of an injection of pentolinium 0·5 to 1 milligram. More doses may be needed and the patient must rest quietly in bed sedated with barbiturates. Recovery is usual.

DROPSY. Dropsy must be prevented as far as possible. Salt should be withheld, potassium chloride being used instead.

When there is much fluid in the chest or abdomen, it may be drawn off by a doctor by mechanical means (*paracentesis*). See Medical and Technical Procedures, p. 568.

HEART FAILURE. In cases where heart failure sets in, complete rest is essential. Digitalis is generally ordered by the doctor.

A patient with glomerulonephritis should always be under a doctor's care and observation, and careful nursing with a strict regard to the diet is essential.

Convalescence. After recovery takes place the patient must be especially careful to avoid damp or chills. A restricted diet is generally unnecessary.

Type 2: Subacute Glomerulonephritis

In this disease, certain cells of the glomeruli, different from those in type 1, are deranged. The condition is known as minimal lesion glomerulonephritis. In a similar disease in older patients, yet other cells become thick and twisted. This is known as membranous glomerulonephritis.

Either disease produces similar characteristics which constitute the *nephrotic syndrome*. There is massive loss of protein (largely albumin) in the urine and generalized edema.

Causes. It may follow acute glomerulonephritis in children but in other age groups it may also develop after systemic diseases such as diabetes mellitus, lupus erythematosus, polyarteritis, multiple myeloma, or congestive heart failure.

Symptoms. The chief symptoms are considerable swelling or puffiness round the eyes, especially in the morning, with dropsy of the feet, the legs, and other parts; there are also headache, normal or reduced volume of urine, poor appetite and increasing weakness.

Course. The onset is gradual, and the acute stage may subside with an interval of normal health before the chronic stage of the disease develops.

Complications such as pneumonia or pericarditis may develop. The outlook is always serious, and infective conditions are always liable to develop. Life may be prolonged for some years if care is taken, and there may be long periods when dropsy is absent.

Treatment. Bed rest is necessary when the dropsy is severe. A fairly liberal diet is permitted. Salt is withheld, even in butter; a minimum is used in cooking.

A high-protein diet is given, 125 grams a day of protein being allowed if the patient can take it; this amounts to 8 ounces of meat, 1 egg, and 1 pint of milk. Milk should only be given in measured amounts, owing to its salt content.

DRUGS. Small injections of diuretics, may be used to diminish dropsy, but they are of limited value and must be used carefully. The fluid may also be removed from the body by 'tapping' (*paracentesis*) by a doctor.

Cortisone or corticotrophin (ACTH) may be tried when other measures fail, and may cause relief of symptoms. It cannot, however, cure the disease. Supplementary vitamins and iron tonics should be given.

After-care. When dropsy is absent the patient may perform his ordinary occupations, but must be very careful to avoid chills.

Renal Failure

An acute decrease in the functioning of the kidneys may have many causes.

1. Conditions which reduce the quantity of blood circulating through the kidney tissues. These include high fluid loss from vomiting, hemorrhage, burns, or shock; heart failure; serious infections; and crush injuries to limbs.

2. Those in which infection or poisons have damaged the functional kidney tissues, such as in acute glomerulonephritis, pyelonephritis, carbon tetrachloride or ethylene glycol poisoning.

3. Obstruction in the urinary tract. This may be due to stone in the ureters, carcinoma, accumulated pus, uric acid crystals, or fibrosis.

Symptoms. The early symptoms are insidious, and include pallor, difficulty in mental concentration, irritability and sleeplessness, with perhaps bilious attacks and loss of appetite. Dropsy is slight or absent.

Course. Neglect of the condition leads to chronic renal failure with extension of the disease to both kidneys and irreversible destruction of the nephrons. Blood pressure rises to high levels with breathlessness, giddiness, palpitations, and even convulsions. Headaches, generalized weakness, digestive disturbances, and disorders of vision are common. Anemia develops. Bone pain arises from calcium imbalance. Edema increases and congestive heart failure with uremia may prove fatal.

Treatment. The first essential is to find the precipitating disorder and give specific treatment. This is particularly important in acute failure so that it will not progress to the dangerous chronic state. Antibiotics will be used against infections.

The second essential is to take every measure to prevent the development of uremia.

It is advisable that patients are treated in hospital, in special units, particularly chronic cases. Constant urine testing, adjustment of water lost and taken in, balance of sodium to potassium, and a low protein diet to remedy nitrogen retention require skilled care.

Dialysis with an artificial kidney may be required in severe cases.

Uremia

Uremia occurs when the kidneys are unable to carry out their normal work of ridding the body of waste products and poisons, so that these accumulate in the bloodstream. The most important of the substances retained is a substance called urea.

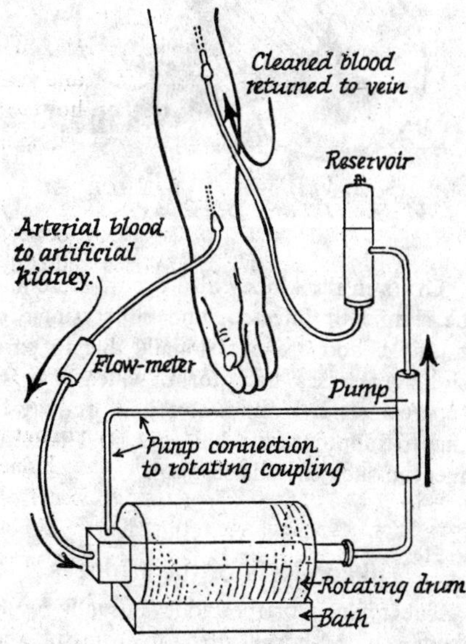

Fig. 17. *ARTIFICIAL KIDNEY. A diagram illustrating the principle on which a small artificial kidney operates. Arterial blood flows from the patient into the purifying bath and the cleaned blood is returned into a vein. The cleansing of the blood is done on the principle of osmosis.*

Symptoms. When a considerable amount of urea circulates in the blood it causes typical symptoms of uremia, such as headache, nausea, shortness of breath, hiccup, vomiting, cramps, and in serious cases delirium, mental disturbances, insanity, twitchings, convulsions, blindness, and unconsciousness.

Uremia is seen in severe cases of nephritis, and in anuria, suppression of urine, tuberculous disease of the kidneys, hydronephrosis, stone, and other gross diseases of the kidney substance.

Treatment. This must be directed to the cause and to the uremia itself. It includes a careful adjustment of the fluid and electrolyte balance with administration of calcium if tetany develops, sedation, blood transfusion, and digitalization when necessary. Urea itself may be removed by (a) use of the artificial kidney, (b) exsanguination transfusion, and (c) continuous gastro-intestinal lavage.

The outlook is serious, especially when the kidney disease is chronic. Death may follow in a few hours in acute uremia, with profound coma, or the condition may become chronic.

Pyelitis and Pyelonephritis

Inflammation of the kidney pelvis (pyelitis) is due to infection by bacteria but as the condition is usually short-lived it is often neglected and is probably the starting point for an extension of the infection into the deeper tissues of the kidney which is known as pyelonephritis.

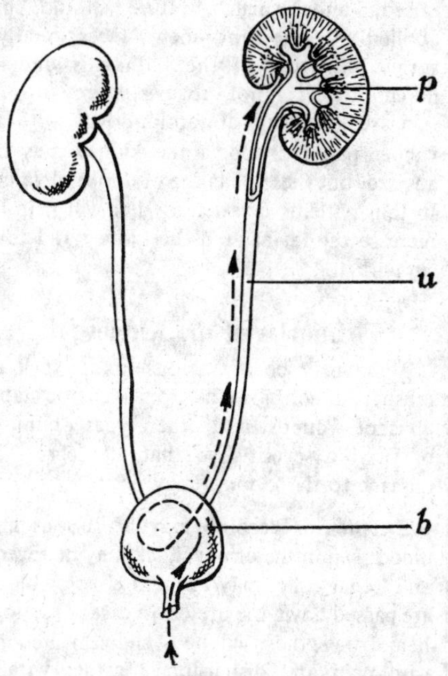

Fig. 18. *PYELITIS. Infection in the bladder (b) often extends upwards through the ureter (u) to the kidney pelvis (p) causing pyelitis.*

The condition may arise, via the blood stream, from existing infection in colitis, cystitis, tuberculosis, influenza, or fevers, or from congestion due to pregnancy, tumors, or stone whereby bacterial infection of the bladder ascends the ureter. The usual infecting bacteria are *Escherichia coli*, commonly found in the intestines, and *Staphylococcus aureus*.

Symptoms are variable. The disease may develop as an acute fever, or as a more chronic disorder with an insidious onset and malaise. In most cases there are usually backache and pain, with cloudy urine and frequency of micturition. In the acute state there is a fairly high temperature, with chills, prostration, headache, lumbar pain, and sweating. In old people the bladder inflammation tends to be aggravated by prostatic enlargement in men, and by vaginal prolapse in women. The presence of pus and bacteria in the urine should be confirmed by tests and microscopical examination by a doctor. A mid-stream urine specimen should be utilised; a catheter may reinfect the patient.

In *chronic pyelonephritis*, symptoms are again very variable. Some patients have no symptoms and only when examined for some associated hypertension or complication is the condition revealed. Others have lumbar backache, pus in the urine, and pain on micturition while a third group shows weight loss, general malaise, and ill health. There is usually a reduction in output of urine and such renal failure requires investigating with cystoscopy and retrograde pyelography.

Treatment in acute or semi-acute cases consists of rest in bed, with investigation of any underlying condition or general systemic disorder and its specific treatment.

When there is much dull pain in the loins or abdomen, hot bottles or an electrically heated pad may be applied to the back, and aspirin may be prescribed. The high temperature may be brought down by careful warm sponging.

Fluids such as fruit juices, barley water, and weak tea, all given with plenty of glucose, and also milk, amounting in all to up to four to five pints a day, should be given while the fever persists.

As soon as the fever has cleared, the patient is quite able to take a mixed diet with cereals, fish, eggs, meat, vegetables, and fruit.

For the infection itself, the choice of an antibiotic, e.g. ampicillin or cycloserine, will depend upon the micro-organism found in a culture of the urine. Drug therapy is continued until the urine remains sterile after treatment has stopped. The urine should be cultured four days after the end of treatment and again about four weeks later. If the culture indicates infection, though the patient shows no outward symptoms, longterm follow-up may be required in order to prevent chronic irreversible disease.

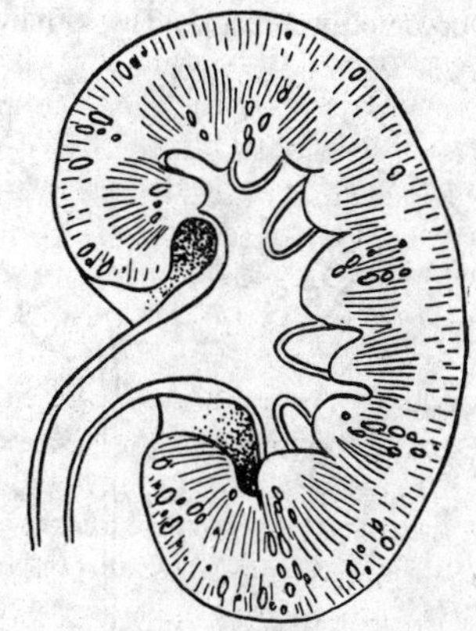

Fig. 19. *ABSCESSES IN KIDNEY. Section showing sites of numerous small abscesses throughout the substance of the kidney in pyelonephritis.*

When the temperature runs a normal course, the patient can be allowed to get up for a short time each day but must be very careful to avoid a chill. Exertion must be limited until convalescence is well advanced. Regulation of the bowel action is very important in any attack of pyelonephritis.

Treatment in chronic cases may be surgical to remove a stone or a diseased kidney. In recurrent cases antibiotics may be helpful. Treatment is less successful than in the acute form of the disease.

Prevention. Frequent cleansing of the ano-genital area, especially by both partners in sexual intercourse, will prevent many cases of infection leading to chronic pyelonephritis, which in turn is the usual cause of later renal failure.

Perinephric Abscess

In this condition, an infection elsewhere (boils on the skin, infection in nearby organs), usually due to *Staphylococcus aureus*, has reached the kidney via the blood stream. Abscesses form in the cortex of the kidney.

Although the onset of the condition is gradual it leads to high fever and to edematous swelling in the lumbar region. The urine is often clear and on examination no infecting organisms are found but if the abscess(es) ruptures into the renal pelvis the urine contains pus in which the organisms can be identified.

Treatment. With clear urine, the doctor can only prescribe antibiotics blindly; with pus-laden urine the most suitable drug can be selected. Occasionally, surgical drainage is necessary.

Floating Kidney
(*Movable Kidney*)

In some people the kidney is more freely movable than normal, usually when there is a general dropping (or visceroptosis) of the abdominal organs due to weakness of the muscular abdominal walls. The condition is more often seen in women who complain of aching in the loins, with nausea, vomiting and constipation. The kidney on the right side is more commonly affected. The kidneys have usually some degree of movement during the act of breathing, and this mobility may be greatly increased so that the whole organ can be pushed freely about inside the abdomen. The condition may be discovered by accident in the first place, when the patient is perhaps being examined by a doctor for some other reason. One-third of all cases of floating kidney have no symptoms, in which case no treatment is necessary.

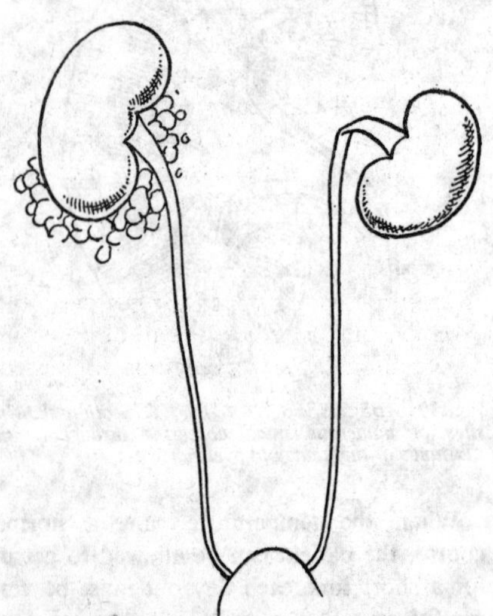

Fig 20. *FLOATING KIDNEY. The healthy kidney is well fixed into the surrounding fat and tissues. The other kidney is poorly attached and may float freely within the abdomen, the movement often causing kinking of its ureter.*

Occasionally, sudden attacks of severe pain occur, and blood may be passed in the urine; in such attacks the kidney may become twisted, or the ureter kinked, and such attacks are apt to be recurrent.

Treatment. Operation is seldom necessary. The foot of the bed should be slightly raised, and warm bottles should be applied to the abdomen. Occasionally, surgical fixation of the kidney is undertaken but it is not always successful. A specially designed abdominal belt with a rubber pad to support the kidney may be advised, but these belts are of doubtful value. In thin patients a fattening diet will help to increase the fat around the kidney and thus support it.

Injuries of the Kidneys

These may be of various kinds, such as crushes, direct blows as from kicks or stabs, gunshot wounds, and other types of injury of varying severity, so that all degrees of damage to the kidneys may occur.

Symptoms. Bleeding may be serious and blood seen in the urine; shock may be severe, and 'renal colic' may occur if clots of blood are passed down the ureter. In cases of serious hemorrhage there will be swelling in the loin, with pain and distension, together with a rapid pulse, thirst, pallor, and distress.

Treatment. The patient must be kept recumbent and treatment should be carried out in hospital. The doctor may give morphine or some other sedative, and a blood transfusion may be required. Surgical treatment may be necessary to control the hemorrhage, the operation being either a repair of the kidney or removal of the kidney if damage is extensive.

Tumors of the Kidneys

These are rare, and may be either benign or malignant. Benigh tumors include fibrous, lipomatous (fatty), and nevoid growths. Malignant growths may be primary or secondary and consist of various types, but fortunately none is very common.

Benign Types. An adenoma or papilloma may develop; the latter usually grows in the renal pelvis, and may later become malignant. These growths give rise to obstruction, pain, blood in the urine, and sometimes hydronephrosis, or stone. Occasionally seedling growths arise in the ureter or bladder.

Malignant Growths. Cancer and sarcoma are malignant tumors which are sometimes seen, the latter occurring in children under five years, and being rapid in growth.

Symptoms. Blood in the urine is a common symptom except in sarcoma of children; the bleeding is painless and irregular, but renal colic may be felt if the blood forms clots in the ureter.

Pain is felt when the growth extends outside the capsule of the kidney; at first there is a dull aching in the loins, but later the pain becomes more widespread.

In children a swelling may be felt, but is less easily detected in adults. Pressure by the growth on the spermatic vein may cause a varicocele, which aids the diagnosis. Cystoscopy and X-ray examination must be carried out in suspected cases, and removal of the kidney may be undertaken if secondary growths have not developed. Radiotherapy may be advised as well.

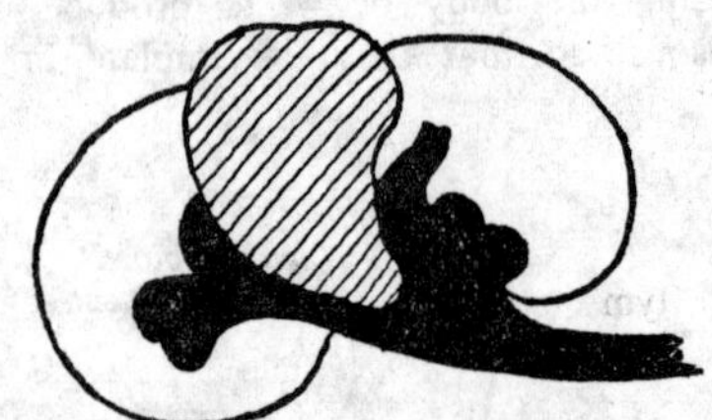

Fig. 21. *KIDNEY WITH A TUMOR PARTLY FILLING THE PELVIS.*

Cysts in the kidney also occur; these may be simple or infected, and either single or multiple, and are occasionally due to parasites. Abscesses may form, which may be tuberculosis or pyemic in origin, or may be due to suppuration within a cyst. The treatment in such cases is surgical.

Tuberculosis of the Kidneys

Tuberculosis of the kidneys usually results from a blood-borne infection from tuberculosis elsewhere in the body, and less commonly occurs by lymphatic spread. The disease is more common in women than in men.

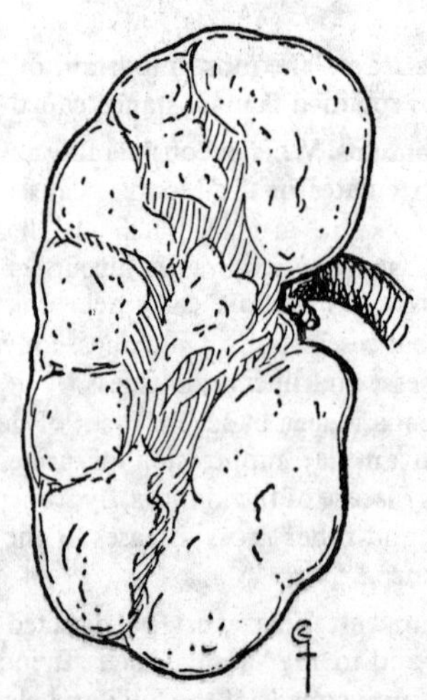

Fig. 22. *TUBERCULOSIS IN KIDNEY. Section showing large areas containing pus.*

Symptoms. The blood-borne type generally affects one kidney at first, and gives rise to general debility, pain in the affected region, frequency, and perhaps turbidity of the urine owing to pus and blood in small amounts. Later there may be blood in the urine, and infection may descend into the bladder. Fever may be only slight, but loss of weight occurs in active cases. Renal colic may be felt when tuberculous material enters the ureter from the diseased kidney.

Where the disease is spread by the lymphatic system, the outlook is less favorable, since the infection probably involves both sides; the kidney symptoms tend to be masked by the cystitis until the kidney disease is advanced.

Treatment consists of confirmation by cystoscopy and X-ray investigation, with microscopical examination of the urine. In blood-borne infection, surgical removal of the kidney is usually carried out if the kidney on the opposite side is not affected. Intensive medical treatment, preferably in a sanatorium, is given for three to six months before the operation.

In lymphatic spread the general health must be carefully guarded, and the usual hygienic or sanatorium treatment of tuberculosis provided. Streptomycin, sodium PAS (para-aminosalicylicacid) and isoniazid are the drugs used.

Hydronephrosis

This is the dilatation of the kidney pelvis (see Fig. 1, p. 405) with a collection of nonpurulent fluid resulting from obstruction to the downward passage of urine. The condition may be congenital, with a twisted or deformed ureter, or it may be caused by a stone or tumor, or by tuberculosis, or the kidney blood vessels may be in the wrong position. In many cases, however, no apparent cause can be found. The kidney tissue becomes

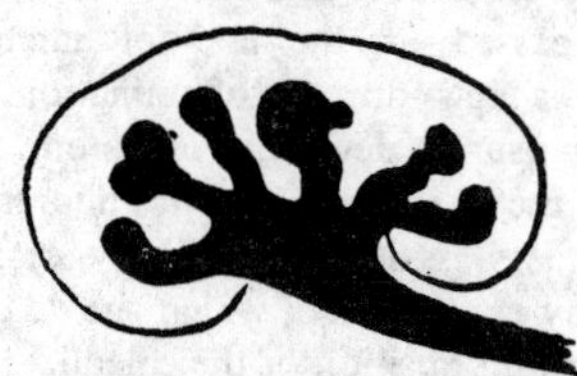

Fig. 23. KIDNEY IN EARLY HYDRONEPHROSIS. An X-ray diagram showing the dilated pelvis and calyces.

shrunken (atrophied) from back pressure and distension, and the ureter may also be distended, depending on the site of the obstruction; the other kidney may become enlarged to carry on the increased work. The condition may be intermittent, with the periodic passage of the urine, and the sac then refills. The pelvis of the kidney becomes enormously distended, and finally the whole kidney becomes a sac of fluid. A tumor may be felt in the abdomen, but in the earlier stages is often absent. The condition is twice as common in women as in men and most cases occur under the age of 30. The diagnosis is made by the position of the tumor, which is freely movable, and by X-ray examination or pyelography.

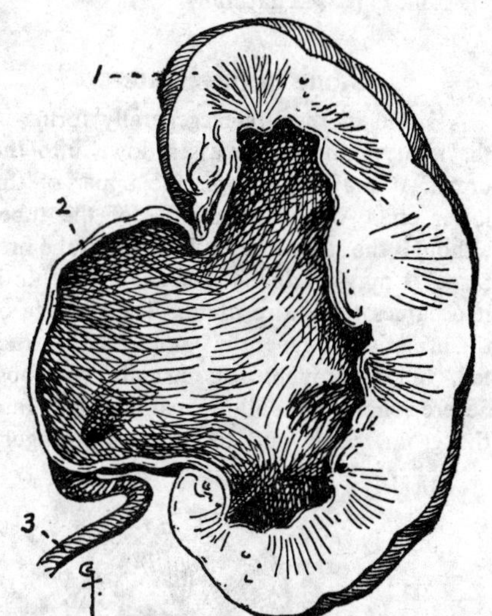

Fig. 24. HYDRONEPHROSIS. Section through enlarged kidney showing hydronephrosis due to injury. There are adhesions round the entrance of the ureter blocking the passage of the urine. 1. Kidney tissue. 2. Dilated pelvis of kidney. 3. Ureter.

Symptoms. These correspond to those of a tumor, together with the particular cause of the hydronephrosis. They may be entirely absent, but usually there is a dull aching in the loin, with pain passing down into the groin. Gastro-intestinal symptoms may be a prominent feature. Blood often appears in the urine and, if both kidneys are affected, uremia develops. Micturition may be frequent, or the urine may be diminished in amount.

Treatment is always surgical. When infection occurs in a hydronephrosis, prompt antibiotic treatment is required to clear the infecting organisms.

DISEASES OF THE ADRENAL GLANDS

Addison's Disease

The adrenal glands are small and are situated above the kidneys (Fig. 51, p. 227) but, since they are made of completely different tissue, they are not affected by kidney diseases.

They are subject to a comparatively rare disease, which is usually tuberculous in origin, called Addison's disease. For a general description and treatment see p. 402.

Tumors of the Adrenal Glands

Tumors or overgrowth of the cortex of the adrenal glands may be associated with unusual sexual disturbances. In children there is remarkable sexual precocity. In boys great adiposity occurs, the 'infant Hercules' type being produced; but in women a masculine distribution of hair, a deep voice and a change of personality develop, so that the woman resembles a man in outward appearance. (See also Virilism, p. 402.) The overgrowth of the glands may be shown by X-ray examination, and the tumor may be removable by surgical operation.

In tumors of the medulla or central part of the gland, there are sudden attacks of high blood pressure, with severe headache, cramps, colicky pains, pallor, breathlessness and sweating. These tumors may also be treated surgically in a few cases, but tend to invade the inferior vena cava (or great vein of the abdomen) before they are diagnosed.

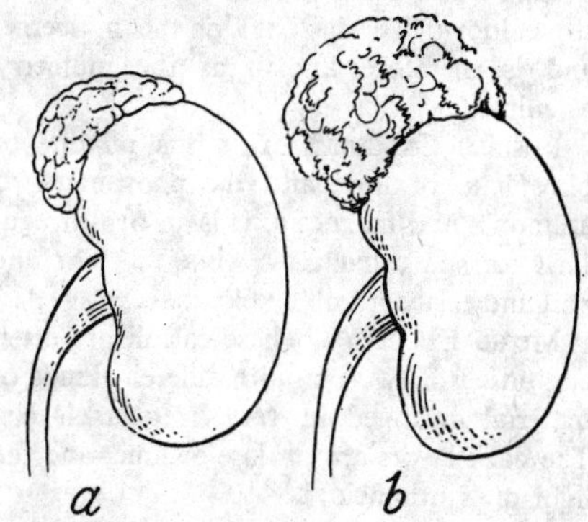

Fig. 25. ADRENAL GLAND TUMOR. a. Normal gland situated above the kidney. b. A tumor of the adrenal which is usually due to overgrowth of the cortex (outer portion).

STONE
(*Calculus*)

The causes of the formation of stone in the urinary tract are imperfectly understood. Diet is thought to have some effect, but probably the most important contributing factor is chronic infection of the tract which disturbs the function of the kidney and its associated organs.

Kidney Stone

Kidney stones are usually found on one side only, although the other kidney may be similarly involved later. Persons who lead quiet sedentary lives, especially men, are more likely to be afflicted.

Kidney stones also occur in hyperparathyroidism and in certain bone diseases.

Stones are composed of various chemical substances or crystals of one type or of mixed composition. Urinary crystals are illustrated in Figs. 3 to 7, p. 406. The commonest stones in adults contain calcium.

URIC ACID CALCULUS. A common stone in children is the uric acid calculus; it is generally smooth or slightly nodular on the surface, and varies in color from a pale yellowish-fawn to a reddish-brown. When cut through the center the layers will be found to be fairly regular, but of quite different thickness.

URATE OF AMMONIA CALCULUS. These

stones are generally small in size, smooth or slightly irregular upon the surface, and are of a very pale slate or clay color. When they are heated before a blowpipe, they gradually disappear.

PHOSPHATE OF LIME CALCULUS. This has a smooth polished surface, and shows regular layers which separate easily when the calculus is cut; it has a pale fawn or stone color. Dilute nitric or hydrochloric acid will dissolve the stone without effervescence.

OXALATE OF LIME CALCULUS. This is often found uncombined with other material, but more commonly its nucleus consists of uric acid or urate of lime. It usually has a brown, dark-olive, or dirty-purple color, with an irregular and somewhat rough surface; the stone looks like the fruit of the mulberry, and is therefore known as the mulberry calculus.

FUSIBLE CALCULUS. This is a mixture of phosphate of lime and the phosphates of ammonia and magnesia. It is an oval irregularly formed calculus, is white in color and soft and easily crumbled like chalk.

MIXED CALCULUS. These calculi are often composed of two or more different kinds of material arranged in very irregular layers. The dark layers are oxalate of lime, and the light ones uric acid.

Symptoms. Kidney stones may cause no particular symptoms, especially when they are large and are lodged in the pelvis of the kidney. Smaller stones may give rise to pain in the loin, especially when the patient lies down. If the stone passes into the ureter, there is intense pain called *renal colic*, which is very sudden in onset and shoots down to the groin or testis and is made worse by any movement. The patient may vomit, and micturition is painful; scanty blood-stained urine is passed, or the urine may be loaded with crystals. The stone may pass right down into the bladder, or it may lodge in the ureter and obstruct the flow of urine, causing hydronephrosis (p. 413). To confirm the diagnosis, the stone may be detected by X-rays, and cystoscopy shows blood coming from one ureter.

Treatment. The pain can be relieved by rest, with morphine and atropine given by a doctor. Surgical treatment is generally necessary after the acute pain has subsided. The kidney may need to be removed if bleeding continues, or if stones are quickly reformed.

Anuria due to Stone

This condition is generally seen in middle-aged men, as a result of obstruction of the ureter by a small stone which usually lodges at the upper end of the tube. If the other kidney is diseased or absent, or if there are stones on both sides, anuria follows. The condition may develop suddenly, with renal colic, or it may be insidious and painless; the affected kidney is swollen and tender. An interval of a week or more may follow with complete cessation of the passage of urine, or there may be occasional micturition. If the condition remains untreated, uremia then develops, with nausea, headache, and finally delirium or coma.

Surgical treatment may be required unless the stone is passed naturally.

Stone in the Ureter

A stone in the ureter generally forms in the kidney, and then passes down into the ureter. It may lodge near the upper or the lower ends, or in the middle of the tube; although the stone is usually small in the first place, it may gradually increase in size until it occupies the entire ureter. The passage of the urine is not generally completely obstructed, but hydronephrosis usually develops. Severe colicky pain follows, passing down into the groin, penis and testis, with strangury (slow, painful micturition). Small amounts of blood-stained urine are passed before the stone finally descends into the bladder.

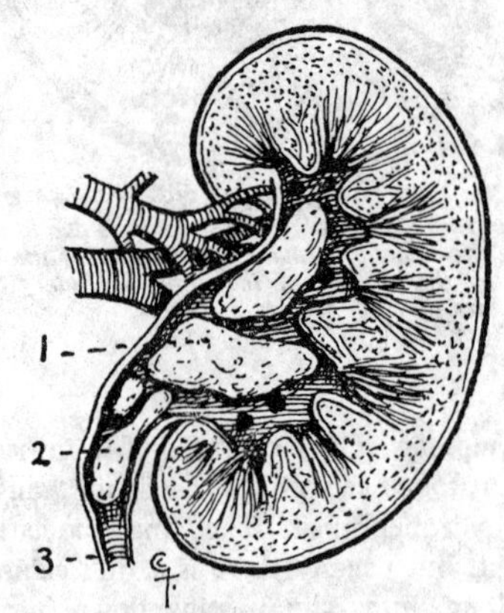

Fig. 26. *STONES BLOCKING URETER OPENING. Stones* (1 *and* 2) *are formed in the kidney pelvis and if they pass into the ureter* (3) *they cause acute pain.*

Several weeks may elapse while the stone moves down the ureter, and surgical treatment may be delayed during this time if the other kidney is healthy. If the stone becomes firmly impacted (as shown by X-ray examination), surgical treatment may be required.

Stone in the Bladder

Causes. Stones of the bladder are generally formed in the kidney and, descending through the ureters into the bladder, are prevented from passing out through the water-passage or urethra. Remaining in the bladder, they soon become encrusted and enlarged. These stones are commoner in men and children than in women, and may be solitary or numerous. There is often a history of previous attacks of renal colic.

The center part or nucleus of the stone is often composed of oxalate or uric acid, while the main body consists of layers of calcium oxalate, phosphates, uric acid, etc. When infection occurs, with decomposition, soft phosphates are deposited as a crust round the stone. A mixed phosphate type of stone is particularly likely to form in cases of obstruction to the passage of urine by an enlarged prostate gland. Phosphate stones tend to grow rapidly, while oxalate stones are slower in their rate of growth. Both forms are often round or oval in shape.

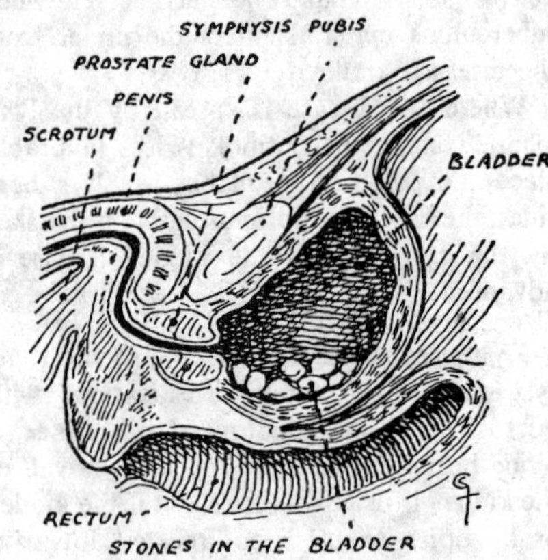

Fig. 27. *STONES IN THE BLADDER. The stones are formed in the kidney, pass via the ureter into the bladder. They lodge at the bottom of the bladder and sometimes block the urinary exit to the urethra.*

Symptoms. When a stone in the bladder reaches a certain size—especially if it is rough—it causes pain, with frequency of passing water; these are the earliest symptoms, and a dull aching pain is felt at the end of the penis, although in some cases pain is trivial or absent. The desire to pass water is frequent, and there is a sense of weight in the perineum. Sometimes the stream of urine is suddenly stopped, and retention occurs, owing to the stone falling against the orifice of the urethra. In children there is often incontinence, and pain causes screaming. As the bladder becomes nearly emptied it embraces the stone, and the pain is increased; jolting in a vehicle also causes great pain. Mucus is passed in the urine, and sometimes small amounts of blood and albumen, the blood being passed at the end of micturition, usually a few drops. Inflammation of the bladder usually develops. The stone may be felt by rectal examination in children, or in other cases is demonstrated by cystoscopy or X-ray examination, which shows the size, number and position of the calculi.

Treatment of Bladder Stone is a choice between certain operations: lithotrity (litholopaxy), or suprapubic cystotomy. SUPRAPUBIC LITHOTOMY consists in making an incision into the bladder above the pubic bone (cystotomy) and taking out the stone or stones whole.

LITHOLOPAXY consists in crushing the stone *in situ* by means of the lithotrite, and syphoning out the debris.

General Treatment for Stone. Treatment is usually surgical, but stones tend to recur after operation and certain medical measures and attention to diet may lessen the tendency

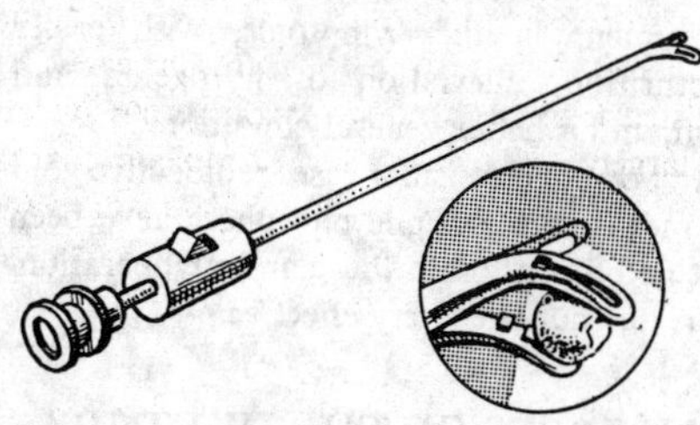

Fig. 28. *A LITHOTRITE. After the insertion of the lithotrite into the bladder, the stones are picked up by the head of the instrument and crushed to pieces. The debris is then syphoned out.*

to recurrence by reducing the crystalline deposits in the urine. Renal colic, suppression of urine and infection may also be amenable to medical methods of treatment. Any patient who appears to be likely to redevelop a stone should take large amounts of fluid by mouth: natural mineral waters, water and barley water, or lemon drinks, etc. are suitable, and up to 5 pints a day is advised. Where considerable quantities of urates or oxalates occur in the urine, potassium citrate is prescribed in doses of 1 to 2 grams three times a day, this to be continued for some months.

If there are signs of colic or irritation, 1 to 2 milliliters of tincture of belladonna, three or four times a day for two or three days, are prescribed by a doctor. When there is a tendency to form phosphatic stones, the urine is kept slightly acid with sodium acid phosphate (600 milligrams in water every four hours.)

Protein foods such as meat and eggs are reduced, but fruit and vegetables are allowed in plenty; kidney, liver, sweetbreads, beef and coffee should be avoided.

DISEASES OF THE BLADDER

Injuries of the Bladder

The bladder may be ruptured, or torn, as a result of falls, blows or kicks, etc., when the bladder is full, and the pelvis is often fractured at the same time. Surgical treatment must be given immediately.

Foreign Bodies in the Bladder

These are sometimes introduced through the urethra by children or lunatics; hairpins, or other small objects may be pushed up and, if they are left in the bladder, are likely to cause cystitis. They can usually be identified by X-ray examination, and should be removed by a surgeon.

Inflammation of the Bladder

(*Acute Cystitis*)

Causes. This condition is commoner in women than in men, and is due to bacterial infection. Virulent bacteria may invade the bladder without other predisposing causes, but cystitis is usually favored by some obstruction to the proper emptying of the bladder. The disease may be acute or chronic; acute cases generally clear up with appropriate treatment.

Cystitis may also be produced by taking drugs or poisons such as ethylene glycol and turpentine; by foreign bodies being forced into the bladder, or by the use of catheters; by stone; by retained infected urine; by external injuries; by growths; by gonorrhea or tuberculosis; and by chill. Infection also extends into the bladder in pyelonephritis, and sometimes in urethritis.

Symptoms. In acute cases burning and throbbing pain is felt in the region of the bladder, especially on micturition. The pain extends to the perineum, and in some cases to the testes and thighs, and is much increased by pressure while the perineum feels sore to the touch. Pain is much less pronounced in chronic cases, but the urine is foul and contains much pus. The desire to pass urine is incessant, but the effort to do so may be ineffectual, leading to incontinence; occasionally urine is retained, causing distension of the bladder with great distress; this form of retention is usually seen in cases of prostatic enlargement.

Mucus, blood and pus from the inflamed bladder are present in the urine. Nausea, vomiting and fever may occur, but the temperature is usually normal unless the infection spreads upwards to the kidneys.

Treatment. The patient should be kept in bed, and the diet should be non-irritating and non-stimulating, with plenty of bland fluids.

If the urine is retained, it may be drawn off with a catheter, to prevent distension. (See Retention of Urine, p. 408.)

Warmth should be applied upon the lower part of the abdomen; frequent warm sitz or hip baths also give relief, and should be used once a day or oftener. The bowels should be opened with Epsom salts.

Drinks must be taken very freely, as long as there is no acute distension, and barley water or other bland fluids are allowed. If the urine is acid, alkalis are useful in allaying pain and with water every three or four hours; when the urine is alkaline, sodium acid phosphate is prescribed.

Suppositories of belladonna or opium and belladonna to be inserted into the rectum may be ordered by a doctor to allay the frequent micturition and pain, and to relax the spasm of the neck of the bladder. Antibiotics are usually prescribed by the doctor if the infecting organism has been identified in analysis of the urine.

Chronic Inflammation of the Bladder

(*Chronic Cystitis*)

This is more common than the acute form of the disease. It often arises from the same causes which produce acute inflammation of the bladder, and may follow this disease, being an especially common affection among old people; or the condition may be of gradual onset from the beginning.

Symptoms. Slight darting pains are felt, with a feeling of heat in the region of the bladder, and there is a sense of weight and tenderness in the perineum; a frequent desire to pass water is present, with occasional spasmodic action of the bladder. The urine is loaded with albumin and sometimes pus is present. When the urine has stood for a time, mucus settles at the bottom of the vessel, leaving the fluid clear above. Large quantities of urine are sometimes passed.

Frequently there are disturbances of the appetite and digestive functions as well as thirst; white or brown fur upon the tongue may be noted, with a harsh dry skin, and general debility, especially in the back and loins. Sometimes there is slight fever.

Treatment. Chronic or recurrent cases of cystitis should be investigated to exclude any underlying condition, such as stone, tuberculosis, or cancer.

Confinement to bed in the early stage, and a light diet with cereals and vegetables are recommended. Potassium citrate should be given in water every three or four hours to lessen acidity of the urine.

To relieve pain and strangury, belladonna and opium may be ordered by a doctor, or a morphine suppository, 15 milligrams, may be used per rectum.

Antibiotic treatment is also often ordered by the physician.

Tumors of the Bladder

Papilloma

The only benign tumor of the bladder which is commonly met with is a papilloma; this may be a very small growth, or it may occupy the entire bladder, being spread over the walls in multiple growths which 'seed' themselves. Although these tumors are usually described as being benign, they often become malignant.

Symptoms. Painless and recurring hematuria, which starts suddenly and lasts for a few hours or days, is the common characteristic symptom, and there may be long intervals between the attacks. Occasionally, the passage of urine is obstructed if a piece of the growth enters the urethra. When a surgeon examines the bladder with a cystoscope he sees a soft pale pink branching growth, semi-translucent, and with finger-like projections.

Surgical treatment is required either to remove the growth or destroy it by electrocoagulation. As papillomas tend to recur, periodic cystoscopic examinations are advisable after the operation.

In some cases part of the bladder wall is excised, or the entire bladder is occasionally removed, the ureters being transplanted into the descending colon.

Cancer

The symptoms of cancer of the bladder are somewhat similar to those of papilloma, but there is more likely to be frequency in passing the urine as well as hematuria, and cystitis often develops early. Pain is often felt in the sciatic nerve. When the condition is confirmed by cystoscopy, surgical treatment or radiotherapy, or both, give good results if the condition is diagnosed early.

DISEASES OF THE PROSTATE GLAND

The commonest of prostatic diseases are gonorrheal inflammation, stone in the gland, malignant growths, and a generalized benign enlargement which often occurs in late middle life. Malignant growths are usually seen in men between forty and fifty-five years of age, but are moderately uncommon.

Prostatic Enlargement

The common type of an enlarged prostate gland occurring in elderly men, usually over fifty years of age, gives rise to difficulty and delay with straining in passing the urine, and also frequency of micturition. In most cases the gland is considerably enlarged and causes the bladder to become pouched.

Symptoms. These may remain slight for years, but slowly tend to become more severe and gradually affect the general health, giving rise to headache, retention of urine, sexual irritation, rise in blood pressure, and finally, in severe cases, uremia. The same symptoms may develop when the prostate is not much enlarged, but is hard and fibrous.

When cystitis (inflammation of the bladder) develops, urgency of micturition is sometimes accompanied by slight incontinence of urine.

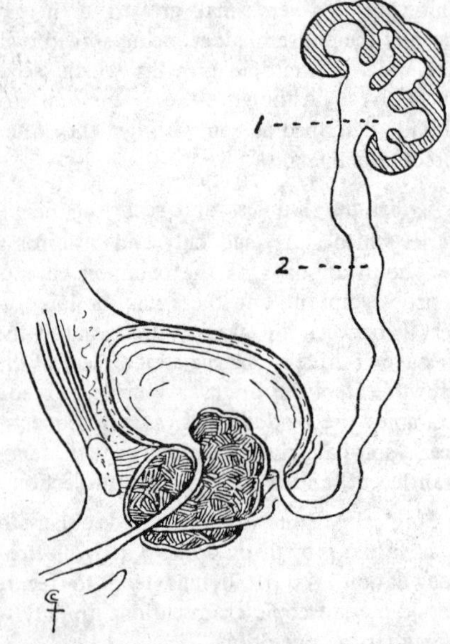

Fig. 29. *SIMPLE ENLARGEMENT OF THE PROSTATE GLAND causing the bladder to become pouched: this in turn prevents a free flow of urine via the ureter and urethra. Hydronephrosis usually results.* 1. *'Water-logged' kidney pelvis.* 2. *Dilated ureter.*

The stream is passed, feebly at first, with a gradual increase of force, and then final dribbling; or there may be an interruption of several minutes before the bladder can be emptied. Cold and alcohol, or delay in regular micturition make the passage of the urine more difficult, and may cause retention.

In many cases at least three ounces of urine are retained in the bladder, and later this residual urine may increase up to ten ounces, so that the bladder is constantly semi-distended. In acute retention, extreme distress and pain are present until a catheter is passed to draw off the urine. Hematuria is often noticed, but this symptom may be absent, and sexual irritation sometimes occurs. The condition is diagnosed by examination, made by a surgeon inserting a finger in the rectum and feeling the enlarged prostate gland, and by cystoscopy.

Retention of urine, infection, stone, stricture, and kidney failure are complications which are liable to develop in long-standing cases.

Treatment depends on the age and condition of the patient, and on the state of the gland itself. Surgical removal is recommended in many cases, the alternatives being frequent catheterization, or a permanent supra-pubic drainage of the bladder. Testosterone, a male hormone, is also used to relieve the symptoms of prostatic enlargement, but it does not actually cure the condition.

General measures, which may be taken to avoid the necessity of an operation in mild cases of enlargement, are avoidance of alcohol, prevention of chills, plenty of rest, a plain diet and regular attention to the bowels.

Tumors of the Prostate Gland

Cancer of the prostate may develop in a case of simple enlargement, and is most often seen in men about fifty years of age. In malignant cases the gland may be fairly small, but usually it is bulky and hard, with nodules; in other cases soft tumors are found.

The growth may rapidly invade the bladder, the rectum, lymphatic glands, and pelvis; or the primary growth may remain small while secondary growths are formed in the bones of the body. As the gland enlarges, the symptoms similar to those found in simple enlargement develop; pain is sometimes felt early. Hematuria is uncommon, but pus is present in the urine when the bladder ulcerates, and constipation is often noted.

Rectal examination reveals an irregular and hard nodular tumor, which may be adherent to the rectum.

Treatment. Surgical treatment is usually unsatisfactory unless the condition is seen early enough, and palliative treatment is usually resorted to.

The use of stibestrol, an ovarian hormone preparation, together with bilateral orchidectomy (removal of both testes) has given good results in the treatment of cases of cancer of the prostate, causing the growth to be arrested. There is generally striking improvement in the symptoms, with easier micturition, alleviation of headaches and pain, and a better general condition.

In hormone-resistant cases radioactive gold or radioactive chromic phosphate have been injected directly into the gland at operation. This has not been very effective.

DISEASES OF THE URETHRA

Urethral Stone

A stone may become impacted in the urethra, causing sudden blockage, pain, strangury, and retention of urine. A smaller stone may cause partial obstruction, with discharge, pus in the urine and frequency of micturition. These stones can generally be removed by a surgeon, either by a crushing procedure (p. 414), or by opening the urethra.

Stricture

The urethra may be narrowed congenitally from birth or, more commonly, as a result of inflammation or injury; the condition is generally seen in men over twenty years of age.

Inflammatory stricture develops after urethritis, ninety per cent of such cases being due to gonorrhea; the condition is often made worse by the use of strong antiseptics, indulgence in alcohol, and phimosis. The passage of water becomes difficult in some cases, the jet being sprayed or twisted, but in others a chronic discharge may be the main symptom. Pain and frequency, with pains in the lower part of the back, often follow.

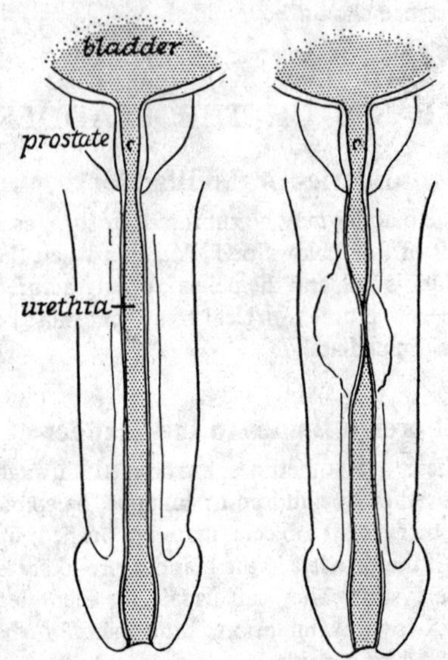

Fig. 30. *STRICTURE. A normal urethral passage from bladder to tip of penis, and a urethra narrowed by abscesses causing stricture, with consequent difficulty and pain in passing water.*

Acute retention of urine may develop after chill or alcoholic excess; in the former case cystitis will then be an added complication, the infection tending to ascend to the kidneys. Urethral abscess, infection of the prostate, stone, fistula, or cancer may also follow.

Treatment consists in either dilatation by a surgeon or, if this fails, an operation may be undertaken.

Urethritis

Inflammation of the urethra is frequently due to gonorrhea, but may also be due to *Escherichia coli* infection (as in cystitis) or other bacteria. See Cystitis, p. 415.

Treatment is similar to that used in cystitis, with potassium citrate, 1 to 2 grams, taken 4-hourly in water, and free administration of bland foods and fluids. Penicillin or other suitable antibiotic is also prescribed by the physician. (See also Treatment of Gonorrhea, in Venereal Diseases, p. 291.)

Urethral Caruncle

A urethral caruncle is a small tumor, often about the size of a pea or a bean, which is fairly common, generally occurring in elderly women. It is bright red and firm, bleeding fairly easily, and tender when touched. This small swelling is seen protruding from the opening of the urethra, and often gives rise to frequency and pain in passing urine.

Treatment. Pain can be reduced by taking an alkaline mixture such as mixture of potassium citrate, and the caruncle may easily be removed by a surgeon. A caruncle sometimes recurs after incomplete removal of the part inside the urethral passage.

DISEASES OF THE PENIS

Phimosis

Phimosis, or the inability to draw the foreskin from the glans or end of the penis, is usually an acquired condition. Even if the foreskin is adherent at birth, it usually frees itself within a few years. Circumcision should be carried out if the foreskin is very long or tight after the age of three years; or if the opening of the water passage is very small, causing difficulty in micturition at any age; or if the foreskin is firmly adherent to the glans. Removal of the foreskin by circumcision should leave sufficient of the foreskin to cover part of the glans, or tip of the penis. There is some evidence to suggest that carcinoma of the penis does not occur in patients who have been circumcised before the age of five years.

In Paraphimosis the foreskin is slipped back tightly over the glans and cannot be returned, so that considerable swelling of the glans follows. It may occur as an accident after coitus, or as a result of gonorrhea. The foreskin must be replaced as soon as possible. This may be possible if the glans can be carefully compressed; but if there is much swelling, iced compresses may be needed to reduce the swelling before the foreskin can be drawn forward. A surgeon's assistance may be needed to divide the foreskin, and circumcision should be performed after all the swelling has subsided.

Priapism

This consists in a painful erection of the penis, without sexual desire. Injury, alcoholism, excessive coitus, or leukemia are occasional causes. The penis becomes tender and micturition may be difficult. Sedatives such as potassium bromide (1 to 4 grams) may be tried, but if the erection continues, minor surgical treatment may give relief.

DISORDERS OF THE TESTES

Non-descent of the Testes

(*Cryptorchidism*)

Occasionally it is found in newborn infants that one or both testes are not descended down into the scrotum where they should

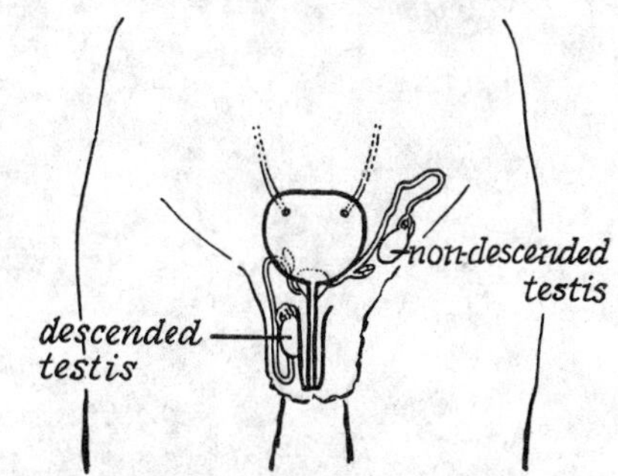

Fig. 31. *DESCENDED AND NON-DESCENDED TESTES. One testis has descended normally into the scrotum, the other has not passed through the canal and may require surgical attention.*

normally be present. The condition is often overlooked, but in some cases the condition may be wrongly suspected, since in boys the testis is easily withdrawn into the canal above. If, however, there is actual non-descent, a doctor's advice should be sought, since it may later give rise to twisting (torsion) of the spermatic cord.

Treatment. Doses of fluoxymesterone by mouth are given at about the age of ten or eleven to stimulate the descent of the testis; in some patients smaller maintenance doses may be needed. If this does not prove successful, surgical treatment is usually carried out at the age of eleven.

Orchitis

(*Inflammation of the Testes*)

This may be acute or chronic, and may follow infection of the bladder or prostate,

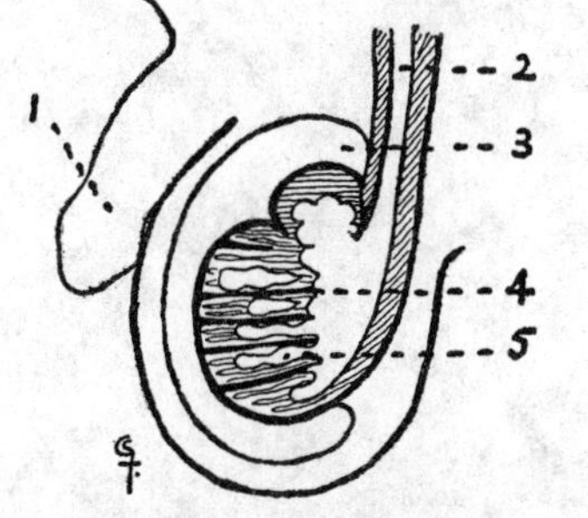

Fig. 32. *GONORRHEAL INFECTION OF THE TESTIS (with small hydrocele). 1. Penis. 2. Vas deferens. 3. Small hydrocele. 4. Fibrous partitions. 5. Spread of infection along the tubules.*

or the condition may develop after typhoid fever, gout, syphilis, mumps, or injury to the testis. Young adults generally suffer from this complaint. The testes are hard, tender and painful, with redness of the scrotal skin.

Treatment consists in attention to the underlying cause such as cystitis or gonorrhea. The testes should be supported in a suspensory bandage; or the patient may be kept in bed, with the testes resting on a

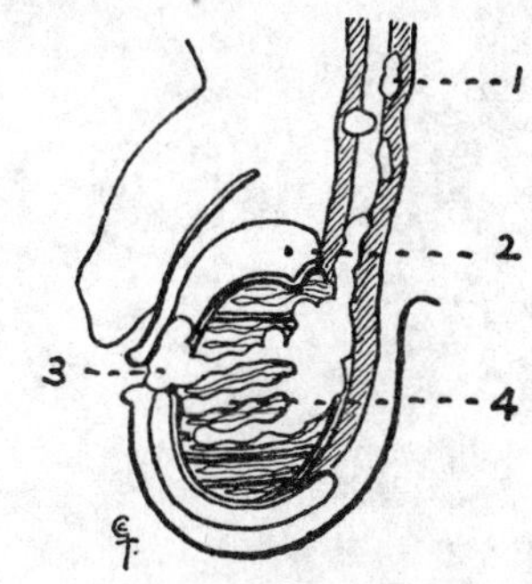

Fig. 33. *TUBERCULOUS INFECTION OF THE TESTIS. 1. Nodules. 2. Secondary hydrocele. 3. Tuberculous sinus. 4. Tuberculous infection spreading along the fibrous partitions.*

pillow. Warm compresses are usually soothing. Antibiotics are used where indicated. In mumps orchitis, prednisone may give some relief. If pus forms, surgical drainage is necessary. Occasionally the affected testis later becomes wasted and ceases to function in older persons.

Hydrocele

A hydrocele is a collection of fluid, other than blood or pus, in the scrotum (or sac containing the testes).

A PRIMARY hydrocele may be either acute or chronic; the acute type is uncommon, but may be due to rheumatism or some other infection. Chronic hydrocele is more common, and the cause of this condition is unknown. Elderly men are most often affected, but sometimes children or young men develop this form of swelling in the scrotum. There is no pain, but the weight causes discomfort, and the swelling may interfere with the passage of urine. The tumor is somewhat the shape of a pear, and is translucent to light. It may rupture, in which case there will be a sharp pain, and an alteration in the feel of the swelling which becomes softened; or inflammation may follow, occasionally with the production of pus.

A HEMATOCELE is a similar type of swelling which contains blood; this may be produced by the bursting of a blood vessel, during the tapping of a hydrocele, from twisting of the testis, or as the result of a malignant growth.

A SECONDARY hydrocele follows injuries or inflammation of the testis, or it may be due to tuberculosis or a tumor. If pus forms, it must be drained off as from an abscess.

Treatment. The treatment of the common or primary hydrocele containing clear fluid may consist in palliative measures, regular tapping being done to remove the fluid. An irritant fluid is sometimes injected into the sac to cause it to shrink down. Other patients will prefer removal of the sac by an operation.

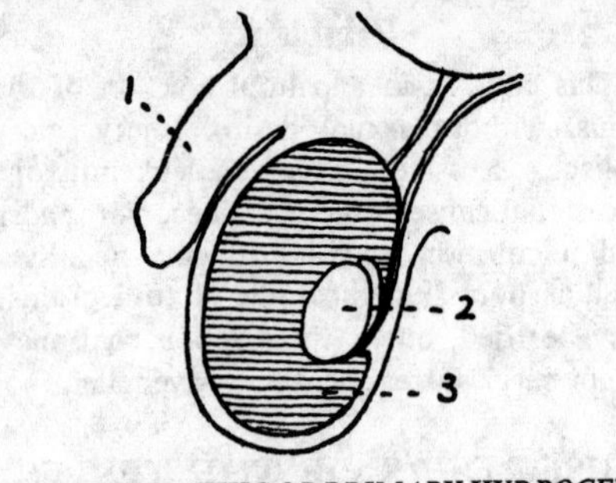

Fig. 34. *IDIOPATHIC OR PRIMARY HYDROCELE.* 1. *Penis.* 2. *Testis in scrotum.* 3. *Hydrocele.*

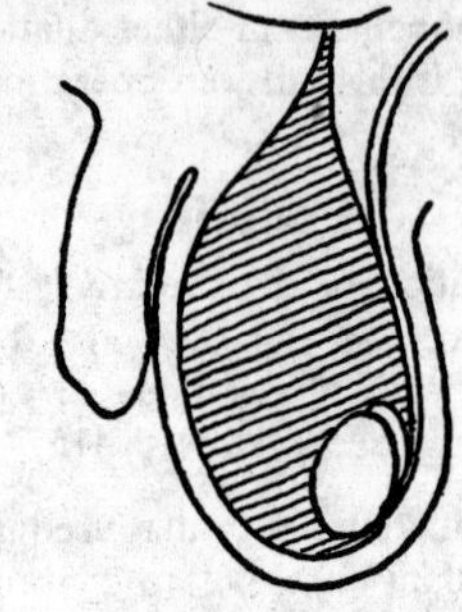

Fig. 35. *INFANTILE HYDROCELE*

DISEASES OF THE NERVOUS SYSTEM

(See also Anatomy of Brain and Nerves, pp. 230-32, and Physiology, pp. 256-59.)

Symptoms of Disease of the Nervous System

Any patient who is suffering from some disease of the brain or spinal cord will generally complain of one or more of the following symptoms.

1. **Paralysis,** or loss of muscular power. This, together with loss of sensation, is the most important symptom in diseases of the nervous system. The patient may complain merely of weakness of a limb or some other part of the body, or of complete inability to move it. A paralysis which affects one side of the body, such as that which may follow a stroke, is known as a hemiplegia. If it affects both legs without involving the face (as after an injury to the spinal cord) it is known as a paraplegia, and when affecting all four limbs it is a quadriplegia. Paralysis is often followed by wasting of the affected muscles, and by contraction or shortening, as in poliomyelitis.

2. **Anesthesia,** or loss of sensation. This may involve loss of the sense of touch, pain, temperature or vibration.

3. **Paresthesia** may occur at the edge of an anesthetic area. This consists of tingling and a 'pins and needles' sensation.

4. **Pain** along the course of a nerve or its branches. This is known as neuralgia.

5. **Convulsions,** or fits (epilepsy). Fits are due to irritation of the brain. They may be localized to one part of the body, or generalized over the whole body, in which case they are usually attended by loss of consciousness.

6. **Involuntary Movements** (tremors). These may be rhythmical and regular, as in paralysis agitans, with its 'pill rolling' movements of the hands, or they may be irregular, as in chorea, in which the movements are quick and apparently purposeless, occurring in any part of the body.

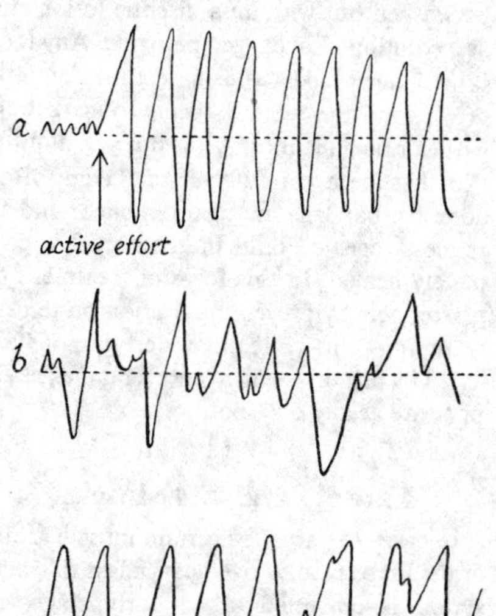

Fig. 1. *TREMORS. Tracings indicating patterns made by various types of tremor. a. After active effort. b. Due to athetosis. c. Senile tremor.*

Reflex Action in Diseases of the Nervous System

Reflex action is an immediate muscular response to a stimulus applied to certain parts of the body. Thus, when the white of the eye is touched, almost immediately there is an involuntary closing of the eye to protect it from injury. Similarly, when the legs are crossed one over the other so that the uppermost limb is allowed to dangle loosely at the knee joint, a sudden tap on the ligament below the knee-cap results in a prompt contraction of the muscles of the front of the thigh, which causes the leg to be extended forwards with a jerk. This reflex is known as the knee-jerk. The ankle-jerk is a similar kind of reflex which may be elicited by tapping on the broad tendon at the back of the ankle. Different diseases of the nervous system give different responses to the tapping stimulus which is applied to the tendon. In some diseases the jerks are absent, e.g. locomotor ataxia; in others, they are exaggerated, as in paralysis following a stroke.

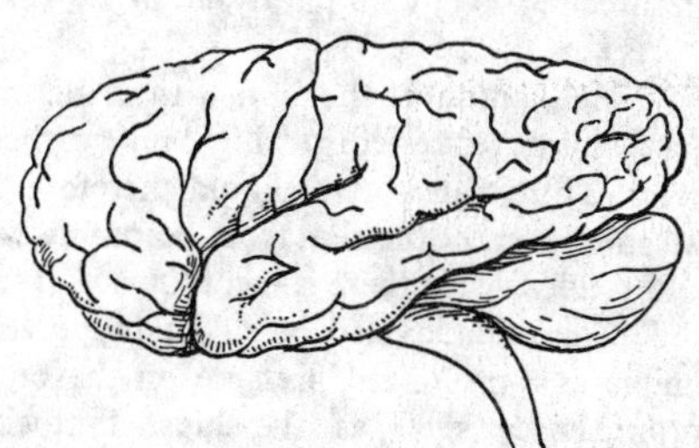

Fig. 2. *BRAIN OF A MENTALLY DEFECTIVE CHILD showing small convolutions, especially in the occipital (rear) region, with unusual conformation.*

The act of passing water is a complex process, which in normal health is largely under the voluntary control of the brain, the stimulus to the act being the distension of the bladder with urine. The voluntary control of the bladder, however, may be lost in some nervous diseases which interrupt the higher control. In such cases sudden micturition may occur, since the patient cannot control the urgent desire to pass urine. This is another example of reflex action in nervous disease. At the onset of severe acute nervous diseases, retention of urine may occur, which later gives way to incontinence with dribbling.

Special Investigations in Diseases of the Nervous System

Lumbar Puncture

Many diseases of the nervous system are investigated by examining a specimen of the cerebrospinal fluid which is secreted in the cavities of the brain and percolates all over the brain surface and the spinal cord in the space existing between them and the inner wall of the skull and vertebral column. It is withdrawn by tapping the lower part of the spinal canal by means of a special hollow needle. The cerebrospinal fluid is normally a clear colorless fluid, but in conditions of disease it may contain abnormal constituents such as pus (as in meningitis), or blood, or it may undergo alteration in its chemical contents (salt, sugar, albumin, etc.) Examination of the cerebrospinal fluid is particularly valuable in cases of meningitis and syphilis of the nervous system. See also Medical and Technical Procedures, p. 568.

Electroencephalogram

Electrical recordings of the brain's activity are taken and they may assist localization of the disease in the cerebral hemispheres of the brain.

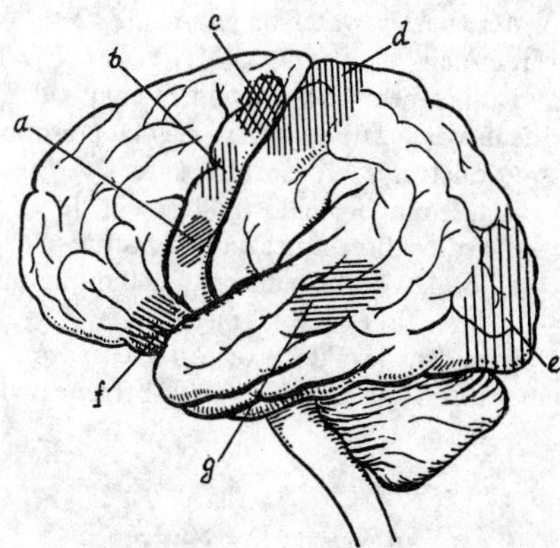

Fig. 3. *BRAIN CENTERS. Localization of the cortical centers. The marked areas are the centers controlling the following functions. a. Voluntary movements of face and tongue. b. Voluntary movements of arm. c. Voluntary movements of leg. d. Sensation. e. Sight. f. Speech. g. Hearing.*

Special X-ray Examination

As well as the ordinary X-ray photography of the skull, sometimes radio-opaque substances may be introduced into the cerebrospinal fluid to show up disease in the various parts of the nervous system.

GENERAL MEASURES IN TREATMENT

For many disorders of the nervous system there is no known specific treatment, and proper management calls for a great deal of thought and nursing attention. Such conditions are difficult to relieve, and much patience will often be required. In certain conditions, e.g. disseminated sclerosis, improvement often occurs, or the symptoms may remain stationary for many years, and in many of these diseases the patient often adjusts himself to the future with surprising equanimity.

In acute diseases of the nervous system such as meningitis, apoplexy, or injuries to the head or spine, the patient is usually helpless, semi-conscious or actually comatose, and frequently paralyzed. He should be in bed in a quiet well-ventilated room which may with advantage be darkened. Paralyzed and comatose patients should be nursed on foam rubber mattresses. It is important to remember the danger of placing hot water bottles against the skin of any patient who is paralyzed or unconscious. The head should be kept low, with not more than one pillow. Headache may often be relieved by applying cold to the head by means of compresses or an ice bag. If the patient is unconscious, breathing should be carefully watched and skilled care is required to keep a clear airway.

Feeding may be a matter of some difficulty. No attempt should be made to feed an unconscious patient by the mouth. When consciousness returns, small amounts of liquids may be given at frequent intervals, care being taken that no food enters the air passages. During the acute stages it should be restricted to fluids (milk, beef tea, soups, etc.), while thirst may be relieved by giving water, barley water or lemonade. (See also Treatment of Coma, p.442.)

Restlessness and excitement may call for the use of sedatives, which may be prescribed by a doctor. Useful sedatives are:

- potassium bromide in doses of 1 to 1·2 grams three times daily for adults;
- chloral hydrate in doses of 600 milligrams three times daily for adults;
- paraldehyde in doses of 1 to 2 teaspoonsful: this is the safest, and can be repeated if necessary.

Care of the Bowels

At the outset the bowels may be freely opened by a good purge (100 to 250 milligrams of calomel for an adult, followed in 4 to 6 hours by two teaspoonsful of Epsom or Glauber's salts). Frequently care must be taken to avoid distension of the rectum with feces, and the best method of regulating the bowels is by an enema of soap and water every other day. In addition, mineral oil may be taken regularly, as it helps to prevent the formation of hard masses in the bowel. Cascara or senna may be given if necessary twice weekly.

Care of the Bladder

Paralysis of the bladder is a common complication of acute diseases of the nervous system, resulting in retention of urine and distension of the bladder. The chief danger of retention of urine is infection of the bladder, which is almost certain to occur, especially if the bladder is allowed to become distended. It is thus particularly important to catheterize at least once every 8 hours. Catheterization must only be done with strict aseptic precautions (sterilization of the catheter by boiling, meticulous cleaning of the hands with soap and water, etc.). It should be noted that dangerous distension of the bladder may pass unnoticed especially during the first twenty-four hours of an acute disease or injury involving the nervous system. When infection has actually developed it may be necessary to give the patient an antibiotic particularly suited for clearing urinary infections, e.g. cephaloridine and cycloserine.

Care of the Skin: Bedsores

Prevention. Particular attention should be paid to the care of the skin, as bedsores are very liable to develop unless the following points are attended to.

1. Hot water bottles must never be placed in direct contact with paralyzed or sensitive parts.

2. The soiling of the skin with urine and feces is a potent predisposing cause of bedsores. The greatest care should therefore be taken to prevent the skin from becoming wet and sodden when there is incontinence.

3. Care should also be taken to prevent undue and prolonged pressure on the bony prominences such as the hips, buttocks, sacrum (lower part of the back) and heels. An air ring for the sacrum may be necessary. Pressure on the heel may be diminished by resting the lower part of the leg on a shallow pillow so that some of its weight is borne by the back of the calf. The heels should be carefully watched for the development of blisters which may develop into bedsores; rest the heels on pads of lamb's wool. The bedclothes should be kept off the legs by using a leg or foot cradle (see Figs. 5 and 6 in Home Nursing, p.46).

All pressure on the skin of the back should be relieved by turning the patient on to his side every four hours. Opportunity is then taken to keep the skin clean by washing it with soap and water, drying it carefully, and then rubbing it with methylated alcohol or toilet water. Finally the skin is sprinkled with a dusting-powder containing equal parts of zinc oxide and starch. These measures harden the skin. If the skin tends to be dry, the following ointment may be rubbed in, in order to soften the skin around the anus or in skin folds.

Zinc Ointment	8 parts
Castor Oil	4 parts
Compound Benzoin Tincture	1 part

For some patients a thinly smeared film of a silicone ointment is a more suitable protective against bedsores.

After the skin has been attended to, the patient's bedclothes and drawsheet must be carefully smoothed out before he is returned to his former position.

4. All movements which cause rubbing of the skin must be avoided. The patient should therefore never be pulled across the bed, but always lifted or turned into a new position.

Treatment of Bedsores. If, in spite of the above precautions, parts of the skin show signs of rubbing or chafing, a large Band Aid should be applied to the threatened area of skin, and left in position for four or five days.

If actual bedsores develop, the method of strapping with adhesive bandage gives better results than other forms of treatment, besides relieving the nurse of innumerable dressings. It does not, however, diminish the need for preventing any avoidable pressure on the sore. It is carried out as follows: strips of wide adhesive bandage are applied unstretched across the area of the bedsore, so that the discharges of pus are completely prevented from escaping from the wound. The strapping is left in position for four or five days, being removed earlier if the discharge begins to escape from the sore. When the strapping is removed, the wound should be washed out with an antiseptic lotion such as a solution of hydrogen peroxide. Any loose skin is removed at the same time, and the skin round the wound cleaned and rubbed with surgical alcohol. After the surrounding skin has been carefully dried, layers of the adhesive bandage are again applied, and the process repeated until the bedsore has completely healed. In this form of treatment the plaster acts by preventing friction on the surrounding skin, while the underlying pus acts as a cushion which prevents excessive pressure at any one spot.

Care of Paralyzed Muscles

In cases of paralysis, certain muscle groups of the limbs tend to overact. Unless this overaction is corrected at an early stage, the affected muscles will become contracted, thus causing a permanent deformity of the limb, with fixation of the arrested joint in an undesirable position. The shoulder joint becomes stiff, the elbow and knee are fixed at an angle, and the wrist and ankle become stiff in the positions known as 'dropped wrist' and 'dropped foot.' The prevention of faulty positions of the joints is therefore of the greatest importance. For patients in bed, careful adjustment of the limbs between supporting pillows or sandbags may be all that is required in the earlier stages, but often splints are needed to prevent deformities. They should be made of the lightest materials —molded plastics, aluminum or leather, and interfere as little as possible with the voluntary movements of the joints.

A useful type of splint for a slightly mobile person is that in which springs are used, the springs being just strong enough to control the resting position yet with enough 'give' to provide movement of the weak muscles. Enfeebled muscles in other cases may be spring-assisted by walking calipers with toe-raising springs.

Movements. From the earliest stages it is of the greatest importance that passive movements (or, if possible, assisted active movements) of the joints should be performed daily with the help of a physiotherapist or attendant, in order to prevent contractions of muscles, with resultant adhesions and stiffness of the joints. Pain which is referred to a paralyzed limb is often due to lack of movement of the joints and can be prevented by frequent passive movements of the limbs. The shoulder joint is especially liable to be affected in this way. All the usual range of movements of the affected limbs should be covered by the physiotherapist or nurse who is responsible for assisting the patient. See also Physiotherapy, p. 177.

Exercises. As soon as voluntary movements are possible, the patient should be encouraged to perform them daily through the fullest range of which he is capable. The next step is the relearning of movements by a careful system of graduated exercises which at first should be as simple as possible.

If the patient is confined to bed, he should lie flat on his back with the bedclothes removed and his head raised on pillows so that he can use his eyes to control the movements. For exercising the legs, three or four small sandbags or pillows should be arranged along the foot of the bed, the exercise consisting of lifting up one leg and moving it slowly and steadily from one sandbag to another, so that the heel is placed accurately in the center of each bag.

A paralyzed person should be got on to his legs and encouraged to try to walk as early as the returning power in the muscles allows the attempt to be made. When he is able to get out of bed, walking exercises may first be practiced by means of a wheel chair, and as soon as he is able to walk without actual support, he may practice walking along a straight line drawn along a non-slippery floor. He should be instructed to walk along the line with the right foot just to the right, and the left foot just to the left of it. When good progress has been made, he may practice walking heel to toe along the center line. Later exercises should consist in placing the feet in a series of footprints marked along the floor, walking sideways, and standing on one leg.

For the arms and hands, five-finger exercises may be practiced, followed by building with small bricks. A box of checkers also provides material for a useful exercise, the patient being instructed to pile one on top of the other as many of the pieces as he can. This exercise requires both accuracy and steadiness of movement.

Occupational Treatment. In all cases of nervous disease in which prolonged convalescence or permanent disability is anticipated, occupational treatment is of the greatest value to the patient for obtaining exercise and stimulating mental interest, and thus maintaining his morale. For this purpose knitting, typewriting practice, basket weaving, rug-making, leather work, etc. may all be of the greatest use. (See also Occupational Therapy, p. 181.)

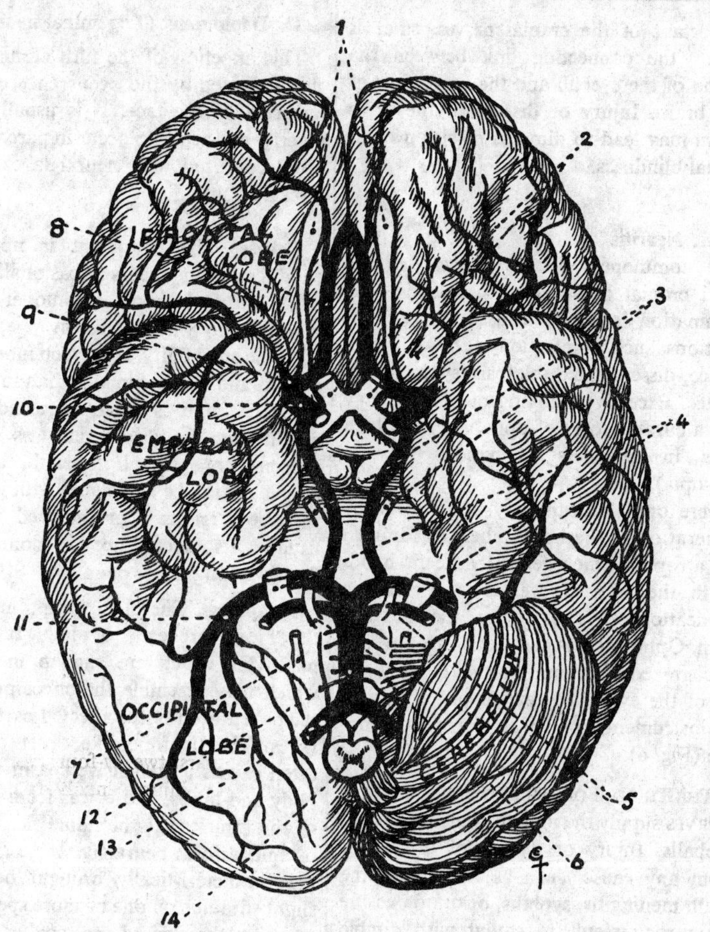

Fig. 5. *BASE OF THE BRAIN, SHOWING CRANIAL NERVES AND ARTERIES.* 1. *Olfactory nerve (of smell).* 2. *Optic nerve (of sight).* 3. *Oculomotor nerve (to move muscles of eyeballs).* 4. *Trigeminal nerve to face.* 5. *Abducens nerve of eyeball.* 6. *Glossopharyngeal nerve.* 7. *Auditory nerve (of hearing).* 8. *Anterior cerebral artery.* 9. *Middle cerebral artery.* 10. *Internal carotid artery.* 11. *Posterior cerebral artery.* 12. *Basilar cerebral artery.* 13. *Vertebral artery.* 14. *Beginning of spinal cord.*

DISEASES OF THE NERVES

Affections of the Cranial Nerves

There are twelve pairs of cranial nerves but only those which are commonly involved in disease processes will be referred to here.

THE SECOND CRANIAL NERVE (optic nerve, or nerve of sight). This is the most

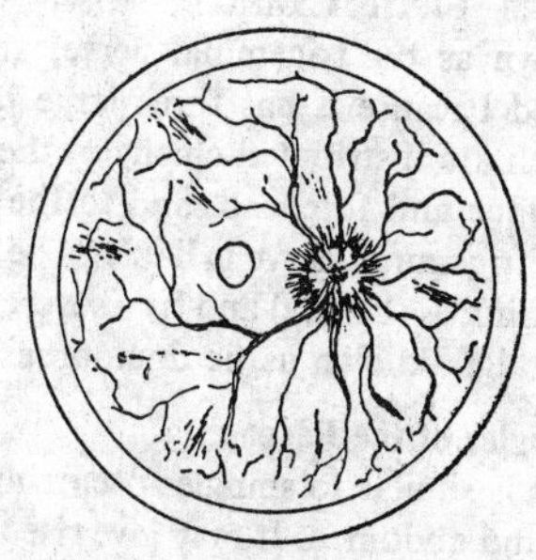

Fig. 4. *OPTIC NEURITIS. The nerve of the eye spreads out over the retina that lines the eyeball. In optic neuritis the retina is grayish and the point of emergence (disc) of the nerve is blurred and swollen; the veins are dilated and tortuous.*

important of the cranial nerves, since it forms the connecting link between the retina of the eyeball and the nerve cells of the brain. Injury or disease of the optic nerve may lead to dimness of vision or to actual blindness.

Optic Neuritis

The commonest disease process of the second cranial nerve is optic neuritis. The inflammation may be caused by various conditions, such as infection in the sinuses of the face, disseminated sclerosis, syphilis, and diabetes. Excessive smoking of tobacco may cause a curable form of optic neuritis which results in mistiness of vision (tobacco amblyopia).

Severe optic neuritis may be followed by degeneration of the nerve fibers, leading to optic atrophy, which generally means blindness in the affected eye. It is a common complication of syphilis of the nervous system. Optic neuritis and optic atrophy can be recognized by examining the retina at the back of the eyeball by means of an illuminated instrument known as the ophthalmoscope (Fig. 6).

THE THIRD, FOURTH AND SIXTH CRANIAL NERVES supply the muscles which move the eyeballs. Injury or disease of the nerves from any cause, such as fracture of the skull, meningitis, syphilis, or tumor of the brain may result in squint with double vision, or unequal pupils, or drooping of the upper eyelid.

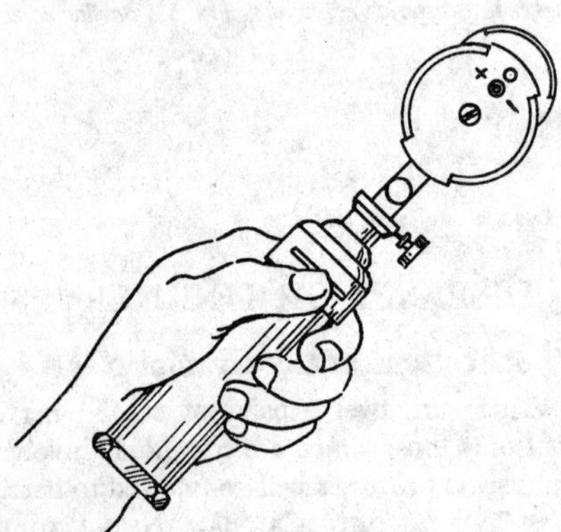

Fig. 6. *AN OPHTHALMOSCOPE for examining the retina lining the eyeball.*

THE FIFTH CRANIAL NERVE. This is known as the trigeminal nerve, and is so called because it has three large branches which are distributed chiefly to the skin of the face and forehead, and to the tongue. The trigeminal nerve is liable to be affected by shingles (herpes) and by a severe form of neuralgia known as tic douloureux.

Shingles of the Face

This is similar to shingles occurring on the chest and abdomen. It may give rise to severe scarring, and to ulceration of the front of the eye. It is accompanied by severe pain which may persist for months. (See also Herpes Zoster, p. 427).

Tic Douloureux (Trigeminal neuralgia)

This affection of the fifth cranial nerve is characterized by the occurrence of pain on one side of the face. It is usually of great severity and tends to occur in paroxysms. It is often confused with neuralgia caused by a diseased tooth.

Causes. The complaint is not seen in childhood, but occurs occasionally in early adult life. It becomes commoner and often more severe with increasing age, especially after the age of fifty. It is much more common in cold and damp climates than in warm and dry ones, and is often preceded by some debilitating influence such as overwork, influenza or general ill-health. In younger people it may be associated with infection of the nasal sinuses or infected teeth, but usually its occurrence is commonest in highly strung, tense people.

Symptoms. The chief symptom is pain in the face, forehead, or jaw. It occurs in paroxyms which are sudden in onset and which may resemble the effect produced by the penetration of the affected part by red hot wires. The lightning-like onset of the pain often causes a convulsive spasm of the face, body and limbs, and it was from this feature of the attack that the name tic douloureux, or epileptiform neuralgia, arose. The attacks are characteristically brought on by some slight stimulus on one or more specific trigger areas on the skin of the face, as may occur while shaving or putting on make-up. The paroxysms are at first short, but gradually they become more frequent and severe, and of longer duration. The paroxysmal pains are usually followed by more lasting dull continuous pain of a boring character.

Treatment. The older the patient, the more intractable as a rule is the pain. The complaint needs to be carefully distinguished from dental neuralgia, or face-ache due to defective teeth, and in all cases the teeth should be carefully examined, and any infected teeth removed.

The patient should be careful to avoid draughts on the face, and the general health should be improved by means of diet, hygiene and tonics. Vitamin B is occasionally beneficial and may be given as tablets, or by injection.

In some cases the spasm may be relieved by inhaling 15 to 20 drops of trichoroethylene from a piece of gauze. The patient should be lying down when this is done, and the inhalation should not be repeated more than five times in the twenty-four hours.

For the pain itself, aspirin will provide temporary benefit.

The irritating sensations take about two years to ease off.

For very severe and persistent cases, the treatment is surgical. Injection of the nerve with alcohol may be tried, and relief will often be obtained for months, or even up to five years. Usually, however, the pain recurs, and subsequent injections are apt to be less effective. Permanent ease may be obtained by removal of one root of the nerve itself by an operation. This operation requires great skill on the part of the surgeon, but the results are usually very satisfactory, and it is often performed even on patients over eighty years of age. A permanent result of the operation is numbness of one side of the face.

THE SEVENTH CRANIAL NERVE (facial nerve). The seventh nerve controls the movements of all the muscles of expression on the corresponding side of the face.

Bell's Palsy

A paralysis of the facial nerve is more common than that of any other nerve in the body, usually occurring as an isolated nerve paralysis, and generally without any obvious cause. It leads to the condition known as facial palsy, or Bell's palsy.

Cause. It occurs in both sexes equally and at all ages, though it is commonest in early adult life. It comes on rapidly, generally after exposure to wet or cold, or to drafts on the side of the face. An exactly similar type of facial paralysis may occur in cases of acute inflammation of the middle ear, or after operations on the mastoid.

Symptoms. The onset is usually sudden, and the paralysis is generally complete from the first. If it is incomplete, the lower part of the face is more affected than the upper. The first symptom is that the patient feels one side of his face to be stiff when he attempts to move it. The paralyzed side of the face shows a striking contrast with the normal side. It is smooth and free from wrinkles, and devoid of any form of expression, so that the patient cannot laugh or weep or frown or express any feeling or emotion, while the features of the normal side are in full play. The eye cannot be closed because of the drooping of the lower eyelid, and the mouth cannot be moved on the affected side so as to expose the teeth. Speaking becomes difficult, and fluids may escape from the mouth on drinking, and saliva dribbles away.

Course. The duration of the paralysis varies within wide limits. Quite slight cases may recover in ten to fourteen days. Others remain unaltered for many weeks or months, but recovery usually occurs finally, and as a rule within two years. The recovery always appears first in the upper part of the face.

Treatment. For immediate relief of stiffness apply heat to the region of the ear by means of warm compresses.

The administration of corticosteroids will reduce the inflammation in the affected nerve and also prevent damage due to pressure in the nerve canal.

Attention should be paid to the eyes and mouth. The eye on the paralyzed side should be protected by a loosely applied eye shade, and should be bathed with weak boric acid lotion (600 milligrams in 30 milliliters of warm water) night and morning.

The Eighth Cranial Nerve (auditory nerve). The eighth nerve is the nerve of hearing and balance, and diseases of this nerve may give rise to deafness, to noises in the head (tinnitus) or to dizziness (vertigo). In cases of deafness it is of course important first to exclude local causes in the ear, such as wax in the ear passage or perforation of the ear drum.

Noises in the Head (Tinnitus)

Causes. Persistently recurring noises in the head which are referred to the ears may be produced by wax in the ear passage, perforation of the ear drum with disease of the middle ear, or by any condition of congestion or inflammation in the region of the inner ear. They may be associated also with anemia and with high blood pressure, or may occur after taking certain drugs such as quinine and salicylates.

Symptoms. To begin with, the sounds are faint and occur only at intervals, usually at night when everything is silent. Later they become louder and more persistent. The sounds may vary from a low rumble like distant traffic to loud hissing, rushing or bell-like noises. They are commonly compared by the patient to the hissing of a steam engine or to the noise of revolving machinery. The hearing often remains normal for many years, but there may be some deafness on one or both sides.

Treatment. Some cases of tinnitus may be corrected simply by the removal of wax from the ear, but as a rule the noises persist in spite of all treatment.

Phenobarbital, 30 to 60 milligrams, may lessen the symptoms while the general health should receive attention, tonics and vitamins being prescribed if necessary.

Dizziness (Vertigo)

In this affection stationary objects have the appearance of moving round the patient. It is often accompanied by vomiting.

Causes. It is a common symptom of disturbances and diseases of the internal ear.

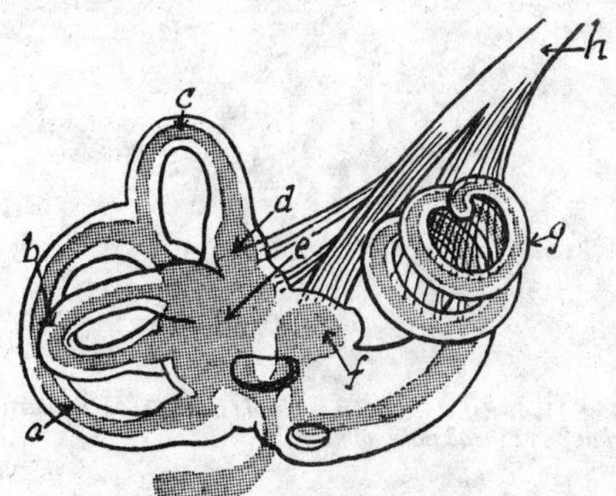

Fig. 7. *INNER EAR. Diagram of the labyrinth of inner ear, showing three semi-circular canals* (a, b, *and* c). *A special organ, the ampulla* (d) (*see also Fig.* 8) *lies at the end of each canal where they run into the common vestibule, the utricle* (e). *With the saccule* (f) *and the spiral cochlea* (g) *these organs of the inner ear all act as organs of balance. The hearing nerve* (h) *runs from the inner ear to the brain.*

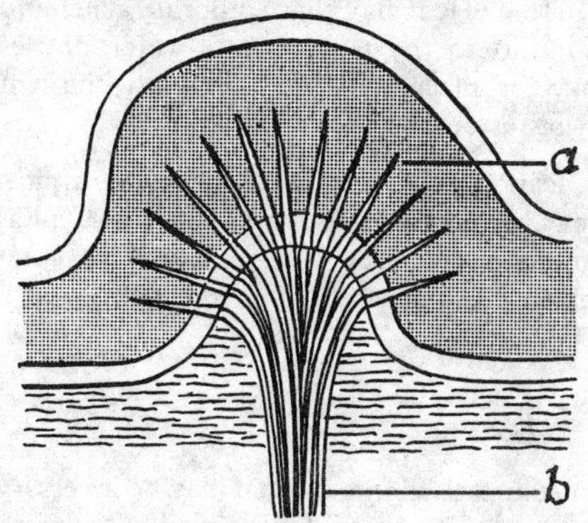

Fig. 8. *AMPULLA. Section through the ampulla* (*compare Fig.* 7) *to show the sensory hairs* (a) *supporting minute particles of chalk which move when the head is moved and help to maintain the balance of the body:* (b) *is the auditory nerve.*

It occurs also in a variety of other conditions such as swinging and seasickness, which are associated with unnatural disturbance of the organ of balance in the internal ear, and with disturbances of the cerebellum (or lower part of the brain). It may occur also in various general conditions, such as the administration of anesthetics, excess of alcohol or tobacco, fevers, irregularities of the blood supply to the brain as in anemia and fainting, in hardening of the arteries with high blood pressure (when it may be a symptom of impending apoplexy), and in migraine and epilepsy.

Treatment. This consists mainly in relieving the cause. Alcohol and late meals should be avoided, and a light diet prescribed. If vertigo occurs frequently, cyclizine tablets (50 mg) may be taken three times daily to prevent attacks.

Menière's Disease

This is due to distension of the fluid in the inner ear so that the sense of balance is disturbed. At irregular intervals the patient has sudden attacks of severe dizziness associated with noises in the head and deafness. With each attack the tinnitus and deafness increases. The attacks may be so intense that the patient often falls to the ground as if he had been shot. He may actually lose consciousness for a few moments, and generally vomits. Recovery may occur within a few minutes to twenty-four hours. Slight persistent vertigo may, however, remain between the attacks.

The attack is distinguished from an epileptic fit by the absence of convulsions. The illness is dangerous for those whose occupation exposes them to the risk of injury in case of a fall, e.g. bricklayers, or for car drivers.

Treatment. Phenobarbital is prescribed in doses of 15 to 30 milligrams thrice daily. It needs to be taken regularly to help reduce the frequency of the paroxysms. The diet should be low in salt. As an alternative to table salt, potassium chloride may be taken. The doctor may prescribe a diuretic.

Neuritis

This is a form of fibrositis of the nerves of the body due to inflammation of the connective tissues which surround the nerve fibers and bind them into nerve trunks. It is often associated with fibrositis in other parts of the body.

The sciatic nerve of the leg is by far the commonest seat of the disease, producing the condition known as sciatica. Next in frequency come the main nerves of the arm, resulting in brachialgia (below), the nerves of the neck and back of the scalp, and the nerves of the chest wall, in the so-called intercostal neuralgia.

Causes. Neuritis often arises without any obvious cause, but it may result directly from exposure to cold (especially after a cold wind has been playing on a particular part) or from injury such as muscular strain, especially sudden strain, such as in lifting heavy weights. It is often associated with sepsis, such as infected teeth or infection in the nasal sinuses, and with anemia, arthritis, gout, or diabetes. In all cases of neuritis the urine should therefore be examined for sugar.

Symptoms. The symptoms are the same whatever nerve is affected, and consist of:

1. pain in the area of distribution of the nerve, often increased by pressure or movement;
2. tenderness of the affected nerve to pressure;
3. tingling, numbness and muscular cramps; and
4. wasting of the muscles of the area.

Neuritis of the Arm (Brachialgia)

This is a common complaint, especially in women who are weak and anemic, and in those who are suffering from prolonged physical strain. The pain is at first intermittent, but soon becomes continuous and spreads down the whole arm. Tingling and numbness in the hand are the rule.

Neuritis of the Leg (Sciatica)

This is the commonest form of neuritis. It is not met with in childhood, but it begins to be common soon after puberty, and it occurs most frequently in early middle life.

Causes. The most common cause is displacement of the gristle-like discs between the spinal bones with pressure on the spinal nerve roots affecting the whole leg. It is sometimes associated with arthritis of the hip joint, and may occasionally be due to pressure on the sciatic nerve by growths in the lower part of the abdomen or pelvis. It is often seen in patients who are suffering from diabetes, and in every case of sciatic pain the urine should be tested for sugar.

Symptoms. As a rule the symptoms begin gradually with pain in the buttock and back of the thigh, later spreading downwards to the calf and foot. At first the pain is noticed only when the leg is moved, but it gradually

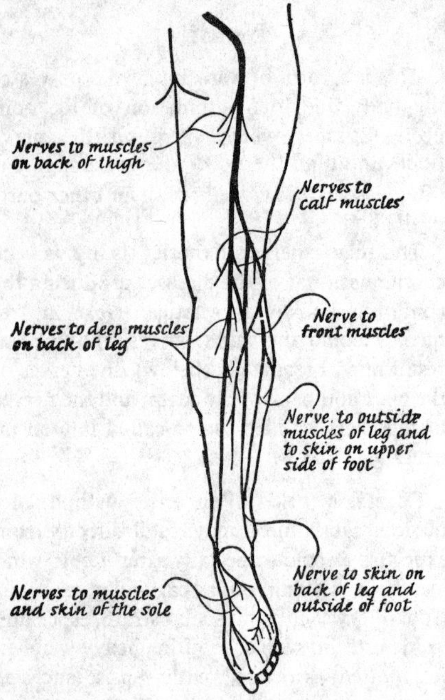

Fig. 9. *THE GREATER SCIATIC NERVE. Pain traveling along the length of the nerve and its branches can be highly disabling to the whole leg.*

becomes more severe and continuous, and is usually worse at night. Cramp in the leg is common, with tingling and numbness of the skin. In walking, the patient limps with the knee and hip joints slightly bent, and is often unable to straighten the knee completely. The nerve, which passes down the back of the thigh, is usually extremely tender to pressure.

Most cases of sciatica take several weeks to clear up, but it is a remarkable fact that severe sciatica rarely occurs twice in the same leg. In slight cases, however, subsequent attacks may occur.

General Treatment of Neuritis

All patients who are suffering from any form of neuritis should be given a generous diet, with extra milk, butter, cream and cod-liver oil. Diet is particularly important in anemic and debilitated patients. Attention should also be given to the provision of sufficient sleep, healthy exercise and, as far as possible, freedom from anxieties and mental strain.

REST. The first essential is to secure rest for the affected part, and to avoid anything which excites or increases the pain.

When the arm is mildly affected, it may be sufficient to support it in a sling. In more severe cases, the patient should rest in bed. He may need intermittent traction of the neck which will require the services of a physiotherapist. Between treatments, the neck may need to be immobilized with a plastic or light metal collar.

When the nerves of the leg are affected, as in sciatica, the patient must lie on a firm mattress (preferably a hair type) under which fracture boards are placed. Only one pillow should be given. The patient may not sit up because it is important to keep the spine horizontal, so patient care is more arduous for home nursing.

HEAT. Heat may give temporary relief and comfort to the patient. Hot-water bottles may be placed around the sciatic patient lying in bed.

DRUGS. For the relief of pain, aspirin may be required in doses of 600 to 900 milligrams every four hours. It may be combined with phenacetin and codeine:

Aspirin	600 mg
Phenacetin	600 mg
Codeine	30 mg

SURGERY. In rare cases, it may be necessary to remove the protruding portion of the disc.

Polyneuropathy

(Multiple Neuritis)

Polyneuropathy is not a disease entity but a condition to be found in a number of illnesses. Many nerves are involved at the same time, the affection usually being symmetrical on both sides of the body and the symptoms worse at the ends of the limbs. The older term 'multiple neuritis' is not quite accurate since inflammation does not always occur.

Polyneuropathy is seen in chronic states of poisoning by alcohol or by lead, arsenic, mercury, and other heavy metals and by some insecticides; it is then known as *toxic neuropathy*. It also occurs in nutritional deficiency, diabetes mellitus, myelomatosis, vitamin-deficient diseases such as beri-beri and pellagra, after severe influenza, and in cancer of the bronchus.

In some cases the prolonged taking of mineral oil may in course of time lead to the loss of absorption of B vitamins and so cause a polyneuropathy due to vitamin deficiency.

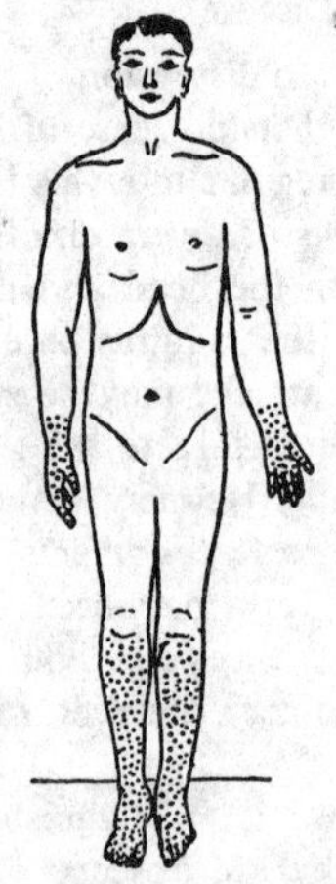

Fig. 10. *PERIPHERAL NEURITIS. 'Glove and Stocking' type of loss of sensation to touch and to painful stimuli such as pin-pricks.*

Symptoms. 1. Disturbances of sensation. These are often the first evidence of the disease, and usually consist of numbness and tingling in the hands and feet, which are generally severe and persistent, especially in alcoholic cases, and may be accompanied by loss of sensation in the hands and feet. Painful cramps may occur in the calf muscles of the legs, and are usually worse at night. The skin may become thin and glossy, and the nails furrowed and brittle.

2. Disturbances of muscular power, varying from slight weakness of the muscles to complete paralysis of the affected part. The muscular weakness may lead to dropping of the wrist and dropping of the foot, and muscular wasting may follow.

Treatment. The first step lies in the discovery and removal of the cause. In toxic neuropathies the patient must be removed from further contamination.

Rest in bed is essential in all but the mildest cases, and may be necessary for several weeks. The limbs should be wrapped in raw cotton, and the legs protected by leg or foot cradles from the pressure of the bedclothes.

A very important point in the treatment is the prevention first of bedsores (see p. 420) and secondly of contractions and deformities of the paralyzed muscles (see pp. 420-21). Care must be taken to counteract the positions of wrist-drop and foot-drop, as well as the tendency to bending (flexion) of the knee joints. In cases in which there is paralysis at the ankle joint, the feet should be prevented from dropping below a right angle either by the use of sandbags, or by placing a padded board across the bed, against which the feet may rest. During the acute stage when the muscles are still painful and tender, physiotherapy must be avoided, but it may be useful in the later stages.

Many forms of multiple neuritis should be treated with vitamin B, both by mouth and by injection.

See also General Treatment of Neuritis, above.

Alcoholic Neuritis

In this form of polyneuropathy the tenderness of the legs may be so extreme that they need to be wrapped up in raw cotton and protected by a cradle from even the lightest touch of the bedclothes. In addition to the local symptoms of neuritis, there are as a rule the general symptoms of chronic alcoholism, such as irritability, agitation, gross failure of the memory, and sometimes hallucinations.

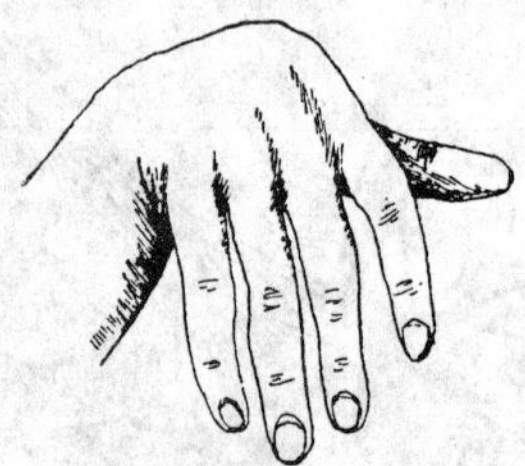

Fig. 11. *WRIST DROP in multiple neuritis, particularly that due to lead poisoning.*

Feeding often requires special attention, and small nutritious meals of milk, eggs, soup, purées of fish and chicken, etc., should be given every two hours. Vitamin B given by injection often has a particularly good effect on the patient.

Lead Neuritis

(See also Lead Colic, p.370)

This form of neuropathy is associated with chronic lead poisoning, as in plumbers and painters. It affects the nerves which supply the muscles, and it is rare to find any disturbances of sensation. As a rule only the arms are affected, resulting in a typical wrist-drop. It may take months for the arm to recover completely.

Treatment. For the wrist-drop, a light metal 'cock-up' splint should be worn, and treatment by physiotherapy must also be carried out.

Diabetic Neuritis

This often appears in the form of severe neuralgic pain in the distribution of one of the larger nerves. It is commonest in the legs, where it may be mistaken for sciatica. The muscles of the legs are often tender, and perforating ulcers may be present in the feet. It is usually seen in elderly patients who are also suffering from hardening of the arteries. The essential part of the treatment is that of the diabetes itself.

MENINGITIS

This is an inflammation of the membranes, of which there are three, which cover the outer surface of the brain and spinal cord. The inflammation is caused by the entry of micro-organisms, particularly the meningococcus. Other bacteria sometimes cause meningitis—pneumococcus, streptococcus, staphylococcus, tuberculosis organisms, and influenza organisms, the most dangerous being the pneumococcus.

Menigococcal infections (p. 267) are notifiable. The incubation period is three to seven days.

The micro-organisms enter the nasal passages, get into the blood stream, and thence to the meninges.

In a rigid cavity like the skull there is very little room for the accommodation of the products of inflammation, which therefore give rise to pressure on the surface of the brain and to irritation of its surface.

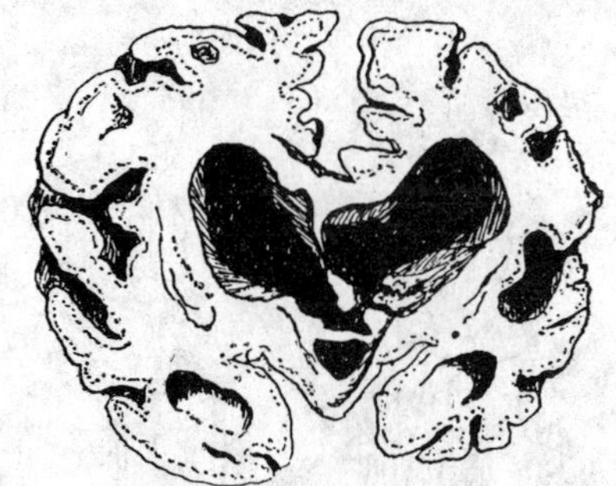

Fig. 12. *SYPHILITIC MENINGITIS. Section of a child's brain showing wasting and softening of brain tissue; the ventricles are dilated and cavities have formed.*

In all cases of suspected meningitis, lumbar puncture should be performed by a doctor. This means the withdrawal of cerebrospinal fluid from the lower end of the spine through a long hollow needle. In meningitis the fluid is infected with bacteria and contains an excess of white blood corpuscles in the form of pus.

Meningitis is always a dangerous disease, but recovery may be expected even in the tuberculous form if suitable treatment is started at an early stage.

Acute Meningitis

This is usually due to extension of infection to the meninges from adjacent structures. Thus, it arises commonly from chronic infection of the middle ear, infection of the scalp, fractured skull, and bullet wounds of the head.

At the time of injury the patient may merely feel upset, but deeper trouble may be taking place inside the skull. For this reason all injuries to the head, even though they may appear to be trivial, should be carefully watched. In all cases where meningitis is suspected the ear drum should be examined.

Symptoms. As in all forms of acute meningitis, there is headache, vomiting and drowsiness, accompanied by high fever with chills (attacks of shivering as the temperature rises). Later there is restlessness with delirium, and a painful stiff neck so that the head is drawn backwards.

Treatment. A darkened room is necessary, because the patient is intolerant of light. The high fever creates great thirst so plenty of fluids, sometimes given intravenously, are essential.

Penicillin is usually administered by injection; sulphonamides have proved useful adjuncts.

Complications in peripheral nerves arise in about five per cent of cases but most clear up.

The patient may get up on the twenty-first day of the illness and needs a month or more to recover strength.

Tuberculous Meningitis

This is most frequently met with in the second and third years of life, but may affect young adults or older people. The infection is carried to the pia mater by means of the bloodstream from some already existing focus of tuberculous infection, such as tuberculous glands in the chest.

Symptoms. The onset is usually gradual, with signs of vague and slight illness for several weeks before any definite symptoms appear. The child is noticed to be out of sorts and peevish, and neglects his amusements and play. There is headache and loss of appetite, so that he gradually loses his healthy look and grows paler and thinner. Vomiting is frequent at an early stage of the disease, and usually there is a distinct dislike of light. At a later stage stiffness occurs at the back of the neck, so that the head is pulled backwards on the shoulders—a characteristic sign of irritation of the membranes of the brain. Convulsions are common, and squint may develop.

Spinal lumbar puncture assists the diagnosis.

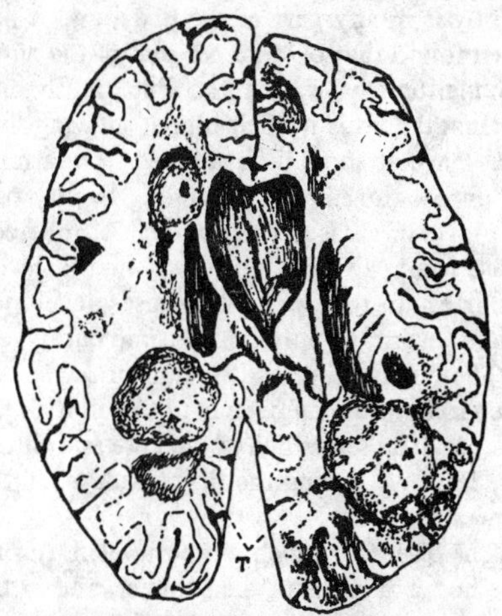

Fig. 13. *TUBERCULOUS MENINGITIS. Section of brain showing large tuberculous masses (T) lying in the brain substance, with areas of softening.*

Treatment. It is vitally important for diagnosis to be made as early as possible. Untreated cases are invariably fatal within a few weeks from the onset.

With modern treatment the outlook depends upon when this is started; up to 95 per cent of patients may recover when only meningeal signs are present, and there is no disturbance of consciousness. The patient must be in hospital, and is given streptomycin, PAS, and isoniazid. Treatment must be continued until all signs have disappeared, and may continue for six months or longer. Attention must be given to proper nutrition throughout.

VIRUS DISEASES OF THE NERVOUS SYSTEM

There are certain viruses which are particularly liable to attack the nervous system, leading to damage or destruction of the nerve cells which are involved. The virus usually gains an entry into the system through the pharynx (at the back of the nose and throat).

Poliomyelitis

The old name 'infantile paralysis' is no longer acceptable because poliomyelitis is by no means a disease only of infancy.

Cause. Poliomyelitis is caused by infection of the nervous system by a virus which gains entry through the nasopharynx and breeds in the intestinal mucous lining. It is expelled in the feces. The bloodstream carries the disease to the nervous system. There the virus attacks the cells lying in the gray matter of the brain and spinal cord, and in a case of very severe infection certain of these nerve cells may be entirely destroyed. This affection of the nerve cells leads to the characteristic symptom of the disease, namely muscular paralysis.

A striking feature of the disease is its occurrence in young people, in adolescence and early adult life, but it is rare after middle age. During an epidemic the virus may attack many persons without giving rise to actual paralysis in any part of the body, and it has been found that over 50 per cent of the adult population have the specific antibodies against the virus in their blood, showing that they have at some time suffered from a mild or unrecognized attack. Among twenty-two contacts of a case of poliomyelitis, fourteen were found to have the virus in the feces. Fourteen of the twenty-two cases developed slight fever, but only one became paralyzed.

The disease is spread by human carriers of the virus, who may or may not be ill with the disease. The secretions of the nose and throat are infective during the first ten days of the illness.

The disease is much more prevalent during the hotter months of the summer, and in the European climate it reaches its maximum frequency in August and September. The incubation period is very variable, between six and twenty-one days. The disease is notifiable to the public health authorities. Epidemic outbreaks may occur.

Symptoms. Poliomyelitis begins suddenly with fever lasting one to five days; the temperature may rise to 40° C (104° F). The patient is usually flushed and drowsy, but may be very irritable, and vomiting and convulsions may occur. There is headache, with pain in the neck and back, and tenderness of the limbs. The symptoms at this stage are similar to those seen in many other acute infectious diseases, though special significance should be attached to severe pains in the limbs and tenderness of the muscles.

THE STAGE OF PARALYSIS. In one to five days the characteristic signs of paralysis appear in one or more groups of muscles. In older children and adults the paralysis is usually present within twenty-four hours of the onset. It develops rapidly and appears to have its maximum limit of distribution from the moment it appears. It is, in fact, usually much more widespread at the onset than it is destined to be permanently. At first all four limbs may appear to be completely helpless, but after some days a rapid recovery occurs from much of the paralysis, and only one limb may be finally affected.

The reduction of the initial paralysis begins to appear after the end of the first week, and any muscle which is going to recover its power will have done so before the end of the first month. The muscles which are permanently paralyzed become wasted, and in course of time they tend to become contracted or shortened. This shortening may lead to considerable deformity of the part unless it is prevented by suitable treatment.

The paralysis may affect any of the muscles of the body, but those of the leg are the most commonly involved. When a child's limb is paralyzed there is usually some slowing up of growth, and the limb may remain stunted. The trunk muscles may also be affected, giving rise to deformity of the spine.

There is little or no loss of sensation, but there may be severe local pains in the limbs, back and neck, which may persist for many weeks. Second attacks rarely occur.

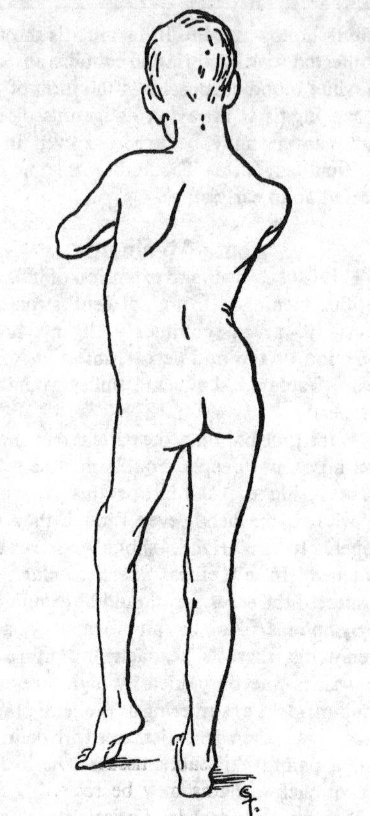

Fig. 14. *DEFORMITY AFTER POLIOMYELITIS. In this child there is deformity of the spine and wasting of the left leg, with club foot.*

Prevention. Children in contact with a case must be kept away from school and other crowded gatherings for three weeks, and should be under medical supervision, the temperature being taken morning and evening. It is not advisable to close boarding schools when an outbreak has occurred, but all contacts of a case should have their temperatures taken, and be carefully watched for the three weeks. Discharges from the nose and throat must be carefully collected on tissues and promptly burnt, and the urine and stools should be disinfected.

Adult contacts may continue their occupation provided it does not entail mixing with children. They should, however, avoid social activities for three weeks from the date of the last contact, and should carefully avoid playing with children, or kissing them.

During an epidemic active exercise should be avoided as fatigue greatly increases the risk of severe paralysis. As much time as possible should be spent in the open air, and children should not sleep together in the same bed. Crowded gatherings and swimming pools must be avoided. A gargle of salt and water (one level teaspoonful to the pint of water), or potassium permanganate (1 in 5,000 solution) may be used three times daily with advantage

During an outbreak of poliomyelitis no operation should be performed for removal of tonsils or adenoids in any child who may have been exposed to infection. All operations of this nature should be postponed until the epidemic has subsided.

A person who has recovered from the disease should as far as possible avoid contact with children for three months after the date of apparent recovery.

VACCINES. The advent of Salk and injection vaccines made from killed viruses and also the Sabin oral vaccines of living viruses has revolutionized control of the spread of poliomyelitis. Widespread use of these preventive vaccines in children has greatly lowered the risk of contracting infection, and those who have been infected seem to have a less severe form of the illness.

Treatment after Infection

A patient suspected of suffering from poliomyelitis *must* be isolated for at least three weeks from the onset of the first feverish symptoms. He should be kept at rest for several days with a diet suitable for fevers. Feeding utensils must be disinfected and kept separately. Any discharges from the nose and throat must be disinfected by soaking handkerchiefs in 1 in 20 carbolic lotion, or lysol, or by using and subsequently burning small pieces of linen or tissue. Urine and feces should likewise be disinfected.

Tepid sponging should be used if the temperature is high, and sedatives for restlessness. Special note should be taken of pain in the back or limbs and, if it occurs, a doctor should be sent for without delay. Particular attention should be paid to the urine, since retention of urine may occur during the first two weeks in paralyzed cases. Aspirin, 150 to 600 milligrams, every four hours is useful for relieving pain and fever.

Treatment of Paralysed Muscles

WARMTH. It is essential that the paralyzed limbs should be kept warm by wrapping in hot dry raw cotton and by the use of extra hot water bottles. When the legs are affected, long woolen stockings should be worn, and particular attention must be paid to keeping

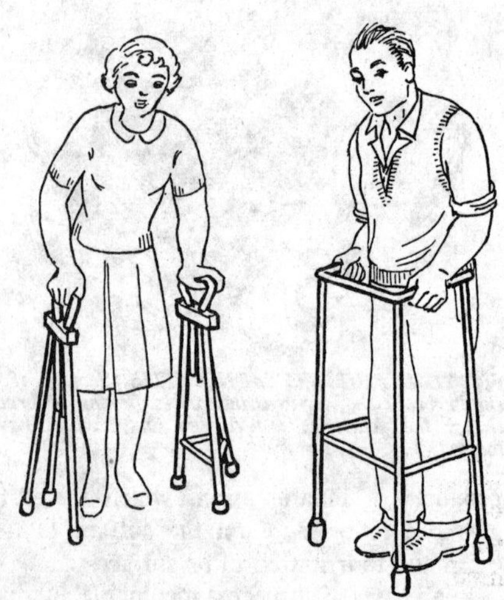

Fig. 15. *WALKING AIDS are used for the retraining of poliomyelitis patients. They vary in type according to the disability of the individual patient.*

the limbs warm at night, since limbs which are continually cold will take much longer to recover. A cradle should be used to ease the pressure of the bedclothes.

PREVENTION OF CONTRACTIONS AND DEFORMITIES (see also p. 421). The position of the paralyzed limbs should be such as to secure complete relaxation of the paralyzed muscles, and appropriate positions can be maintained by the use of pillows, sandbags and splints. If splints are necessary, the lightest possible molded splints, which are almost weightless, should be used.

Massage should not be given until all tenderness of the affected muscles has disappeared, but after a few weeks have elapsed massage and passive movements should be regularly used in order to restore the tone of the paralyzed muscles, and re-educational exercises are begun as soon as there is sufficient power to perform them. In the re-education of the legs for walking, walking aids of various kinds are necessary. Contractions and deformities which hinder the action of a limb may later require surgical treatment.

In cases in which the respiratory muscles are involved, an artificial respiration apparatus known as the 'iron lung' may be necessary.

Encephalitis Lethargica

This must be distinguished from the African disease of sleeping sickness (trypanosomiasis) which is caused by the bite of the tsetse fly (see p.280).

Encephalitis lethargica is an acute feverish disease, occurring in epidemics, which is due to infection of the brain and spinal cord by a virus, which appears to enter the body by way of the mouth and nasal passages. The incidence of this serious disease has diminished in recent years. The incubation period is uncertain, but it may vary from one day to as long as three weeks.

Symptoms. The disease usually begins gradually as an apparent attack of influenza, with headache, giddiness and fever (100° to 103° F) which lasts for about a week. This is followed in many cases by an increasing drowsiness or lethargy which often becomes very deep and may last for three weeks or longer, but which may persist for months.

MENTAL SYMPTOMS. Mental changes of all kinds are a common and important sequel to encephalitis lethargica. There is considerable deterioration in the mental capacity of the patient, who becomes incapable of any sustained work. At the same time there is a change of character, usually in the direction of a depressed and neurasthenic state which may border on the melancholic type of insanity.

PHYSICAL SYMPTOMS. The most important change is the gradual development of the condition known as Parkinsonism. There is weakness, rigidity and slowness of movements so that the face becomes mask-like, the neck stiff and the limbs rigid. These symptoms are generally accompanied by a tremor consisting of rhythmic involuntary movements.

Treatment. The patient should be promptly isolated and children who have been in contact with a case should be excluded from school and placed in quarantine for a period of three weeks from the last date of contact. The noses and throats of contacts may be sprayed with a 1 in 5,000 solution of potassium permanganate in normal saline (one level teaspoonful of salt to the pint of warm water) night and morning.

FOR THE DEVELOPED DISEASE, there is no actual cure. During the acute stage, the patient should be in bed for at least four weeks, and should only be wakened for meals. At least four pints of glucose lemonade should be given daily. Special feeding utensils should be provided, and all personal linen must be carefully disinfected. The patient should use a spray of potassium permanganate, as above, for the nose and throat. Discharges from the mouth, nose and eyes must be carefully collected on disposable tissues, and burnt. Headache and pains may be relieved by an ice-bag and by the administration of aspirin (600 milligrams) and codeine (15 milligrams) every six hours.

CONVALESCENCE is usually slow and tedious, and the patient should be in the open air as much as possible. After a varying period of apparent recovery, the distressing sequels of mental changes and Parkinsonian rigidity (already mentioned) may appear, leading to chronic invalidism. For severe mental disturbance the patient may require treatment in a mental hospital or, if a child, in a special school. For the rigidity, massage may be of value. (See also treatment of paralysis agitans, p. 433.)

Herpes Zoster
(Shingles)

The name of shingles is derived from the Latin word *Cingulum*, which means a girdle. It refers to the distribution of the rash in a girdle-like eruption round one half of the chest. This distribution corresponds with the area of skin supplied by the branches of one or more of the main spinal nerves as they follow the course of the corresponding ribs from the backbone forwards to the breastbone.

Shingles is an acute infection of the roots of one or more spinal nerves by a virus, which leads to great pain and the appearance of a crop of vesicles in the affected area of skin. The virus is related to that of chickenpox. The majority of cases occur in the spring and early summer. Second attacks are very rare.

Symptoms. The onset is often accompanied by fever which may last for two to four days. From the first there is pain in the area of skin supplied by the affected nerve, which means that the pain appears before the rash.

The eruption appears on the third or fourth day of the illness, and consists of small vesicles filled with clear fluid. From the fifth to the tenth day the vesicles dry up and shrink until scabs are formed, which finally drop off, leaving as a rule a considerable amount of scarring which is usually permanent. The pain in the affected area of skin may be intense, and in frail and elderly persons it may persist for months or even years after the eruption has disappeared, in the form of a most intractable neuralgia.

In older persons the disease may also affect the fifth nerve of the brain, giving rise to shingles on one side of the face and forehead. The condition is characterized by intense pain and is often followed by a particularly intractable form of neuralgia, while subsequent scarring is often severe. In some cases there is ulceration of the front of the eyeball, which may be followed by scarring and marked impairment of vision. Shingles may also appear in other areas such as the thigh and upper arm.

Treatment. The vesicles should be kept dry and free from infection. For this purpose a dusting-powder of equal parts of starch and zinc oxide may be used; or starch, 60 grams, zinc oxide, 30 grams, and powdered camphor, 1 - 2 grams. The area of the eruption should then be covered with a warm pad of dry raw cotton.

Pain may be relieved by aspirin, but the neuralgia which often follows in elderly and feeble persons may persist for years, and it may be very difficult to relieve. Some patients benefit from tetracyclines (usually Aureomycin) given at the time of onset of the herpes in that this mitigates its severity and may prevent the post-herpetic pain.

Rabies
(Hydrophobia)

Hydrophobia means literally 'fear of water.' The bite of a mad dog or mad wolf, or any other animal affected by rabies, is one of the most dangerous of all poisoned wounds. Since the virus of the disease is located in the salivary glands and central nervous system of the infected animal, the disease is transmitted to man by the bite of the animal, the virus being carried in the saliva. From the wound in the skin the virus is carried to the nervous system of the victim, where it produces degenerative changes in the nerve cells of parts of the brain and spinal cord.

The interval between the bite and the appearance of the disease (i.e. the incubation period) varies as a rule from one to two months, but may be as short as eleven days or as long as a year. The incubation period seems to be related to the distance of the bite from the brain, for infected bites of the face may cause symptoms much more rapidly than those of the arms which, in turn, have a shorter incubation time than bites of the legs. It should be noted that the wound may be completely healed long before the symptoms of the disease appear.

Symptoms. The onset of the disease after the long incubation period is usually sudden, and begins with headache, loss of appetite, sleeplessness, fever and a rapid pulse. It is followed in twenty-four to forty-eight hours by great excitement and irritability. After a day or two, difficulty in swallowing appears, together with fear of water which consists of a sudden spasmodic contraction of the muscles of the mouth and throat. A typical attack may be brought on by offering the patient some water to drink. As the glass approaches the mouth, the head is drawn back with a series of spasmodic jerks accompanied by gasping respirations. Any water which may reach the mouth is immediately rejected, together with frothy saliva which collects in the throat. The attacks are characterized by the most intense fury or the most abject terror. These spasms of hydrophobia may also be brought on even by the sight or mention of water, or by the sound of liquid shaken in a vessel. In the intervals between attacks the patient rests quietly in bed with a clear mind. Death may occur during a paroxysm, or the patient may gradually sink into coma. Once the symptoms have appeared, death always occurs after four or five days.

Treatment. This is entirely preventive. Once symptoms have appeared, treatment is useless, although palliative treatment of the painful spasms should be given.

In countries where the disease is prevalent, dogs showing signs of becoming morose and irritable should be handled with great care, since these are often the first signs of rabies. The fingers should never be put into the mouth of the dog. If a person has been bitten by a dog, the suspected dog should not be killed, but should be chained up, muzzled, and kept under observation for ten days. If the animal is alive at the end of this time, it is proof that the bitten person has not been infected with rabies. This is because an infected dog never survives for longer than six days from the onset of its symptoms, while its saliva is never infected for more than four days before the symptoms appear. Persons who have merely been licked on the unbroken skin are not in danger.

LOCAL TREATMENT OF BITES. In locales where the disease is prevalent, dog bites should be promptly treated. The sooner the treatment is undertaken the better is the outlook for the patient. If seen within thirty minutes, bleeding should be encouraged by applying a tourniquet just sufficiently light to compress the veins of the part without obstructing the artery, and the bite should be bathed with a solution of potassium permanganate. Subsequently, each tooth mark should be treated with pure carbolic acid, and the wound should not be stitched for at least three days.

ANTI-RABIC VACCINATION. Patients who have been bitten by a suspected animal should be promptly treated by the injection of serum prepared from the spinal cord of a sheep or rabbit which has been infected with rabies. This is followed by daily injections of rabies vaccine given subcutaneously on each side of the abdomen. During the course the patient is instructed to undertake no vigorous exercise, and to abstain from alcohol. These injections reduce the mortality of an otherwise fatal disease to less than 1 per cent. In suspected cases, especially in bites of the head, face and neck, treatment should be given immediately, and discontinued if the dog survives. Should the dog die or be killed, its body should be sent for examination to a skilled pathologist for signs of the virus in the brain. This may help in deciding the treatment for the patient.

SYPHILIS OF THE NERVOUS SYSTEM

Syphilis is one of the most common diseases of the nervous system, and also one which responds most readily to treatment if begun in time. The disease may involve any part of the nervous system, including the brain, the spinal cord and their blood vessels and their meningeal coverings. The various forms of damage which may be caused by syphilitic infection are so great that almost any disease of the nervous system may be imitated.

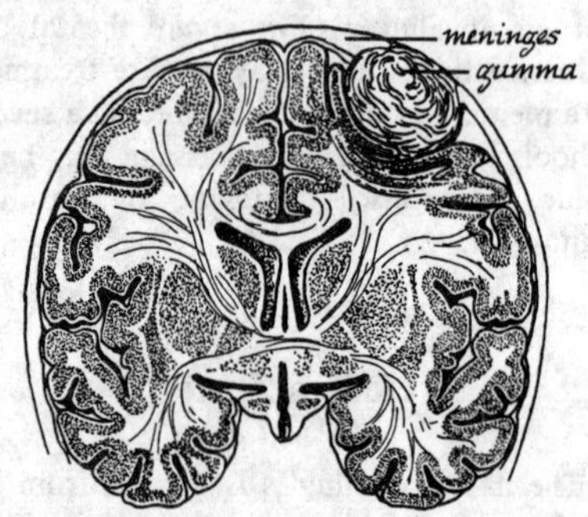

Fig. 16. *A GUMMA OF THE BRAIN. The syphilitic gumma deforms the convolutions of the brain, and is adherent to the meningeal membrane on the outer surface.*

In untreated cases of syphilis, the nervous system may be affected very early, often with only very slight symptoms, such as headache or pains in the limbs. Usually, however, the infection becomes more strikingly evident only in the later, or tertiary, stage of the disease. In general, the symptoms appear in one of three main forms.

1. SYPHILITIC MENINGITIS, chiefly involving the blood vessels and meningeal coverings at the base of the brain, will develop in 15 per cent of patients.
2. TABES DORSALIS (locomotor ataxia), chiefly involving the spinal cord, will develop in 5 per cent.
3. GENERAL PARALYSIS OF THE INSANE (G.P.I.), chiefly involving the brain itself, will develop in 5 per cent.

Any of these forms may be associated with a syphilitic aneurysm of the aorta.

Whenever syphilitic disease of the nervous system is suspected, a lumbar puncture should be performed by a doctor, and a specimen of the cerebrospinal fluid withdrawn for examination. In these cases it is generally found to be altered in quality and to react positively to a Wassermann test.

The most effective treatment of syphilis of the nervous system is preventive, and this consists of adequate treatment of the early or primary disease. All cases should be under strict medical supervision. (See also Venereal Diseases, p. 290.)

Syphilitic Meningitis

The syphilitic infection is concentrated chiefly in the blood vessels of the brain and in the meningeal coverings, especially those at the base of the brain.

Symptoms. Since any part of the brain may be affected, a great variety of symptoms is possible. Headache is a common early symptom. It is often severe and persistent, and is usually worse at night. All mental and physical effort becomes exhausting, the memory is poor, the character alters, and epileptiform fits may occur. The pupils of the eyes are generally unequal or irregular, and drooping of the eyelids and squint are common, from paralysis of cranial nerves.

Treatment. This is as for primary syphilis (p. 290). Penicillin is the treatment of choice. Courses should be repeated every four months for two years. At the end of two years examinations of the blood and cerebrospinal fluid should be made.

Tabes Dorsalis

This is always caused by previous infection with syphilis which may have taken place from two to twenty years before the first symptoms of tabes appear. It usually begins between the ages of 30 and 45, and is ten times more common in men than in women.

Marriage should not be undertaken by any person suffering from tabes, except possibly in very special cases where both parties are fully aware of the nature of the disease and of its possible consequences.

Symptoms. These are mainly concerned with sensation. The earliest and most important symptoms are pains, usually in the legs, of sudden onset and short duration. These pains usually recur very rapidly in one place for a few seconds (e.g. in the bony prominences round the knees). They have been compared with the timing of a machine gun which is firing short bursts, with intervals between each burst. These pains have been given the name of 'lightning pains.' They

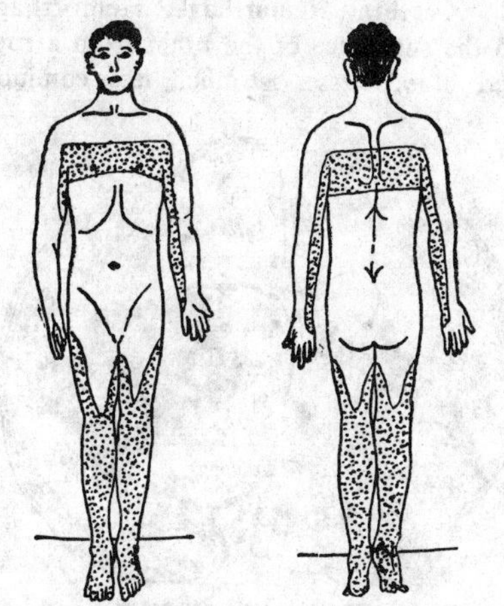

Fig. 17. *TABES DORSALIS. Dotted areas show the extent of loss of sensation to painful stimuli. The analgesia is usually both superficial and deep.*

vary with the weather, and are often put down to rheumatism.

At a later stage, loss of sensation appears in certain areas of the skin, so that a band of numbness appears to stretch round the chest, extending also along the inner borders of the arms. The feet also are affected, causing the sensation of walking on air or raw cotton, while areas of numbness appear also on the nose and round the anus. Gradually the loss of sensation spreads downwards from the chest, upwards from the feet, and outwards from the nose and anus in concentric circles, so that ultimately the sensation all over the body is diminished or completely lost.

At the same time the muscles gradually lose their tone and become flabby, so that the limbs develop an abnormal range of movement. Later the most characteristic feature of tabes appears, incoördination, or loss of control over the muscles, so that they do not move in harmony with each other. This leads to difficulty in keeping the balance, so that the patient reels from side to side (ataxia) as if drunk. In walking he picks the feet well off the ground, and stamps them down unnecessarily hard. It becomes necessary for him to have the support of one or two walking sticks, and finally walking becomes impossible. The same unsteadiness affects the arms, so that the patient becomes unable to feed himself.

In a few cases, a peculiar condition of the joints may occur, called Charcot's joints. The knee, hip, shoulder, elbow and ankle joints may gradually become swollen with fluid, and then completely disorganized, so that the range of movement becomes greatly increased, making dislocation especially liable to occur. Although these joints show all the changes of severe arthritis, they remain completely painless at all stages.

It is a characteristic sign in tabes that the ankle jerks and knee jerks are lost at a fairly early stage. A swaying symptom is noticed if the patient tries to stand with the heels together and the eyes closed. He is unaffected if the eyes are open, but sways violently and may fall if they are closed.

The pupils in tabes are usually irregular in outline, and in many cases the sight begins to fail and may end in complete blindness, from atrophy of the nerve of sight. Deafness is common.

Disorders of the bladder occur frequently. At first there is difficulty in passing water, but later this gives way to incontinence or dribbling of urine, which is especially troublesome at night. Sexual desire and power are lost early in the course of the disease. Occasionally attacks of severe abdominal pain come on suddenly with repeated vomiting (gastric crises). They may last for three to seven days, and may be mistaken for acute intestinal obstruction.

Course. The disease may last as long as twenty to thirty years. It runs a variable course, usually slowly and steadily downhill, the patient eventually becoming bedridden and possibly blind. Even in arrested cases lightning pains in the legs may persist for years and constantly torment the patient. Most persons are rather susceptible to other diseases, particularly cystitis.

Treatment

A complete cure cannot be looked for. Any treatment which is found to be effective must be continued throughout the patient's life, but with diminishing intensity as the years go by.

Anti-syphilitic Treatment. Patients with tabes have rarely had a proper course of anti-syphilitic treatment. The treatment of the syphilitic infection will inevitably extend over two or three years, but in most cases it is followed by a considerable relief of symptoms. Courses of arsenic and bismuth are given by injection four times a year and, in the intervals, potassium iodide may be taken by mouth, but penicillin in proper courses remains the most valuable agent. The progress of the patient is assessed by examination of the cerebrospinal fluid every six months, and treatment should continue at least until the blood and cerebrospinal fluid give a negative Wassermann reaction.

General Treatment. A generous diet should be provided in order to prevent any rapid loss of weight, which is commonly seen in tabes. Cod-liver oil and malt should be taken, with vitamin B (or yeast). The patient should be very moderate in the use of alcohol and tobacco. He should be examined for any kind of chronic infection, since this often aggravates the symptoms. Septic teeth and infection of the bladder are especially common, and should be appropriately treated. Unsuitable occupations may have to be changed. Thus, it is unsafe for a person with tabes to drive a vehicle or to work on a railway.

Over-exertion is harmful, and the physical and mental activities of the patient may have to be modified to prevent fatigue. He should not be confined to bed, however, until it becomes essential owing to weakness and lack of muscular control.

Treatment of Symptoms. Ataxia, or staggering gait. The success of any form of treatment will depend largely on the degree to which the self-confidence of the patient can be restored. By persevering with treatment, complete recovery of the capacity to walk is possible except in the most advanced cases.

A person with tabes should not be confined to bed unless it is absolutely necessary. If he is in bed, however, regular simple exercises will help to restore the weak muscles. As soon as possible he should be encouraged to get up, to stand and to try to walk. Walking exercises are of great value (see p. 421). He should be encouraged to step forward with confidence, and to look, not at his feet, but at some object in front of him.

Lightning Pains in the Legs. Pains may be relieved by tablets each containing:

Aspirin	300 mg
Phenacetin	300 mg
Codeine	30 mg

These may be taken if necessary every four hours. Attacks of pain are often brought on by wet weather so that, if possible, the patient should live in a dry and sunny climate.

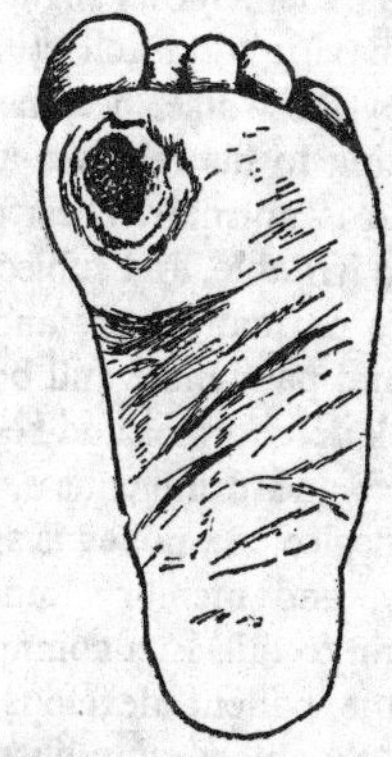

Fig. 18. *PERFORATING ULCER on the sole of the foot in tabes dorsalis.*

Disorders of the Feet. Patients should be warned of the dangers of cutting corns or callouses, since ulcers may form which rapidly lead to a painless destruction of the bones of the feet. When present an ulcer should be treated by the careful removal of any thickened horny material, followed by dressings of zinc oxide and iodoform or other suitable paste and a pad to relieve any pressure on the affected part.

Retention of Urine. The patient should get into the habit of emptying the bladder at regular intervals, not longer than three hours, and he should empty it completely before retiring to bed at night and again in the morning on waking. These precautions are necessary in order to avoid the risk of retention of urine, which may occur if the bladder has not been emptied for many hours.

For Incontinence, drugs to improve the tone of the muscles of the bladder may be prescribed but, when the incontinence is uncontrollable, a suitable apparatus may have to be worn by the patient in order to collect the urine.

CONSTIPATION. In many cases the normal urge to empty the rectum is not felt and, unless regular efforts are made to empty the bowel, severe retention of feces may occur. Enemas or glycerin suppositories should be given as required.

Fever Treatment. In cases where the above methods of treatment have failed, treatment in a fever-heat cabinet is occasionally employed.

General Paralysis of the Insane

(*Dementia Paralytica*)

Like tabes dorsalis, G.P.I. is due to degenerative changes in the nervous system caused by the spirochete of syphilis. The main changes occur in those areas of the brain where the higher intellectual functions are performed. The onset of the disease is insidious, and is commonest ten to twenty years after the original infection with syphilis.

Symptoms. In the course of the disease two quite definite groups of symptoms occur.

MENTAL SYMPTOMS. At the beginning of the illness the patient shows slight changes in character, behavior and intellectual capacity which, as they get worse, become more and more distressing to his relatives and friends. The man who is normally cheerful becomes depressed and irritable, and subject to violent rages. If he is normally quiet and unassuming, he becomes passionate and boastful. His moral outlook deteriorates and he indulges in sexual excesses and drunkenness. Work and business are neglected, money is spent rashly and unwisely, and memory and power of judgment begin to fail. In a common form of the disease the patient develops expansive delusions of the most grandiose character (megalomania), imagining himself to be a great personage of extraordinary ability, or the possessor of untold wealth. It is characteristic of the disease, however, that the patient will always readily reveal his delusions.

The speech becomes slurred, and syllables are omitted from words in speaking and writing. Instead of British he may say Brrsh, and instead of South Africa he may say Safric.' The handwriting shows a tremor and whole words are left out. As time goes by, memory fails completely and the delusions are forgotten.

PHYSICAL SYMPTOMS. The limbs become weakened, resulting finally in almost complete paralysis, with incontinence of the bladder and bowels. Once established, the disease runs a steadily progressive course so that the patient becomes unable to move from his bed, where he lies paralyzed and speechless, and unable to control the evacuations of the bladder and the bowels. If untreated he finally dies, usually in less than three years from the time the disease was first recognized

General Treatment. Rest is of the greatest importance for the mind of the person who is suffering from G.P.I., and a quiet and well-ordered life at home is best. It must always be remembered, however, that the patient is usually unable to look after himself, so that he will probably need a skilled attendant. He must be forbidden to take any alcohol, and must be guarded against physical fatigue. Particular care must be taken to prevent injury to himself or others as a result of his delusions. In the later stages great care in nursing is essential since there is a great likelihood of bedsores and cysitis (see p. 420). A diaper frequently changed may be necessary for incontinence. If adequate nursing is impossible at home, the patient may need to be certified at an early stage of the disease.

A full course of antisyphilitic treatment with penicillin, arsenic, and bismuth must be given and may be repeated every four months for two years. (See also Venereal Diseases, p. 290.)

Fever Treatment. Although malaria therapy for G.P.I. has yielded to penicillin, fever-heat treatment is used for patients who do not respond to the antibiotic, if they are otherwise physically fit. It should not be given to those who are over the age of fifty or sixty unless they are exceptionally robust. It is quite unsuitable for patients who are bedridden.

There is often no improvement in the mental state until some weeks or months have elapsed after the fever treatment, the best results being usually seen about six months later. In general the grandiose type shows greater improvement than the depressed type of case. It is an advantage for the patient to spend several months of his convalescence in a mental home, or resting quietly somewhere in the country, so that he is not affected by the strain of ordinary life.

DISEASES OF THE BRAIN

Apoplexy

(*Cerebral Stroke*)

By the term apoplexy, or stroke, is meant a sudden local disturbance in the circulation of the brain, without preceding injury. There are three distinct ways in which this catastrophe can occur, all of which cause similar symptoms, although they may differ in degree.

Causes

1. **Cerebral Thrombosis.** Clotting of blood in the blood vessels of the brain is by far the commonest cause of a stroke in persons who are over the age of sixty-five, with degenerated arteries of the brain. It is particularly likely to occur when a blood pressure which is habitually high is temporarily lowered so that the blood is circulating less vigorously than usual. The clot of blood blocks an artery, thus cutting off the blood supply to the corresponding region of the brain. This results in softening of the brain, and the affected part loses its function.

2. **Cerebral Hemorrhage.** Hemorrhage into the substance of the brain from a ruptured blood vessel is much less common than thrombosis but, like thrombosis, it occurs in cases of high blood pressure. It results from weakness of the walls of the arteries of the brain, which may be a direct consequence of a previous thrombosis. Bright's disease, alcoholism and previous syphilitic infection may also lead to weakness of the vessel walls.

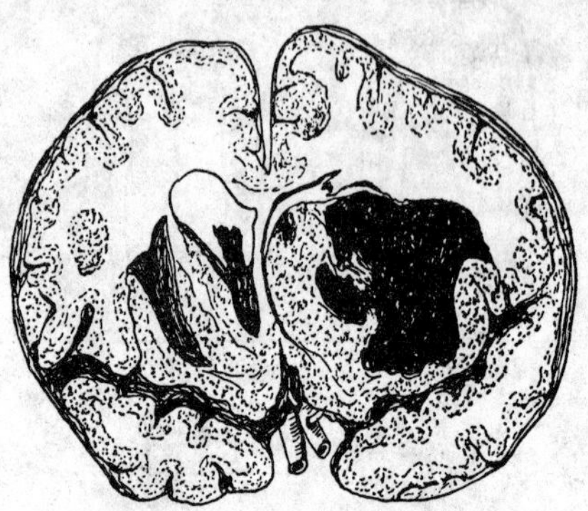

Fig. 19. *CEREBRAL HEMORRHAGE. A large recent hemorrhage is shown on the right side of the brain, and an old healed patch of hemorrhage on the left side.*

Such weakened blood vessels are liable to rupture when there is any sudden increase in a blood pressure which is already raised. Such an increase may result from some sudden activity or strain such as coughing, sneezing, straining at stool, or lifting heavy weights. It may also occur from over-exposure to the sun or to severe cold, or to the bad air of overcrowded rooms. Not uncommonly it follows an emotional disturbance such as shock or anger, which produces a sudden rise of blood pressure. Such hemorrhage is most commonly seen in men over the age of fifty.

3. **Cerebral Embolism.** Obstruction of a blood vessel of the brain occurs when an embolus, or clot of blood, is brought from a distant part. When a clot of blood in the auricles of the heart becomes loose (as in

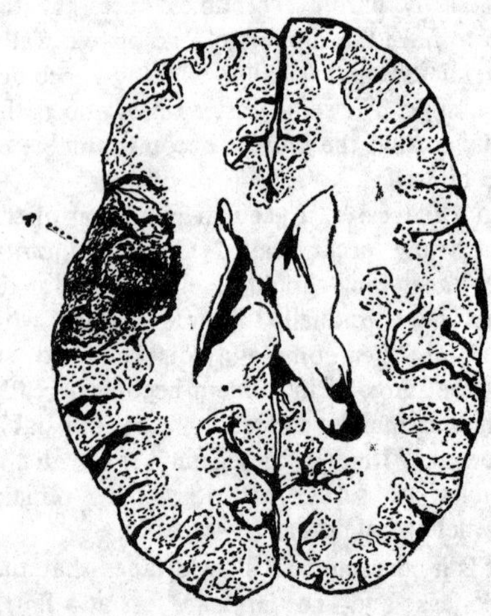

Fig. 20. EMBOLUS OF THE BRAIN, with thrombosis leading to hemiplegia in the case of a child with congenital heart disease. The clot had traveled from the heart through the blood vessels and lodged in the brain causing thrombosis (T) and softening of the brain.

cases of mitral stenosis) it may be dislodged and carried by the bloodstream until it reaches an artery too small to allow it to pass. The artery is then blocked up, as in thrombosis, and the blood supply to the part is cut off. When this takes place in an artery of the brain the same serious results follow as in thrombosis. Embolism is a not uncommon cause of a stroke in young persons between fifteen and thirty years of age with heart disease.

Symptoms. The actual onset of the stroke may be gradual or rapid, according to the cause. In cerebral thrombosis the onset is often gradual, and the patient may notice certain premonitory symptoms such as headache, dizziness, temporary weakness in one or both limbs of one side, tingling, double vision, faltering speech and inability to remember words. These symptoms may pass away, or they may become intensified during the following twenty-four hours, reaching a maximum with the appearance of the actual stroke. Cerebral thrombosis may produce extensive paralysis, without any great shock or actual loss of consciousness. The patient frequently survives.

In hemorrhage the onset is always rapid. The patient sinks to the ground and soon loses consciousness, rapidly becoming comatose, with marked congestion of the face and neck. Unlike thrombosis, cerebral hemorrhage is usually fatal within a few hours or a few days from its onset. This is one of the important distinctions between apoplexy due to thrombosis and that due to hemorrhage.

In cerebral embolism the onset of the stroke is always instantaneous, instead of being gradual as in thrombosis.

Paralysis due to Apoplexy

(Hemiplegia)

The commonest result of an apoplexy, whether it is due to thrombosis, hemorrhage, or embolism, is paralysis of one side of the body. When an entire half of the body is affected (namely the face, arm and leg) it is called *hemiplegia*. In some cases of apoplexy due to embolism, however, only a single limb may be affected (*monoplegia*). When the damage is on the right side of the brain, the paralysis appears on the left side of the body, while damage to the left side of the brain produces paralysis on the right side of the body. When the right side of the body is paralyzed, speech is often lost. When the face is involved in paralysis, the mouth is drawn to one side, the lower lip on the paralyzed side hanging down so that saliva dribbles away (see also Bell's Palsy, p. 422).

In cases of apoplexy which survive (usually those due to cerebral thrombosis), a considerable degree of recovery may occur after a few weeks or months, since the actual damage to the brain is often less than the original stroke suggests. The leg usually shows the earliest and most extensive recovery. All degrees of recovery are possible,

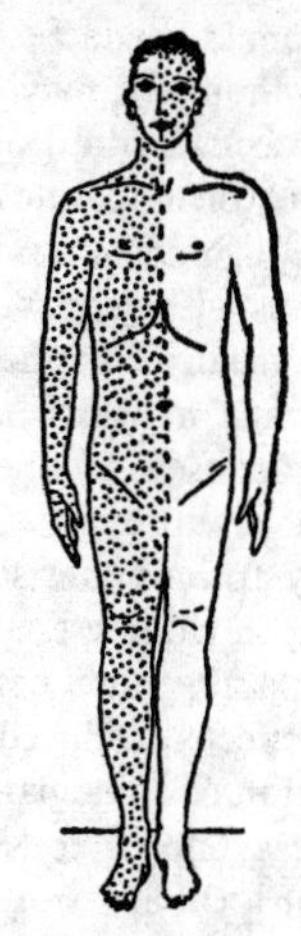

Fig. 21. *HEMIPLEGIA. Effect of a blood clot in the left side of the cerebellum. The dotted areas show the regions where there is loss of sensibility to pain and to different temperatures.*

and many patients survive for years without any recurrence. Some will recover almost completely, while others may be left with imperfect speech, a dragging leg, or an arm hanging useless at the side.

Treatment

Prevention. When a condition of hardening of the arteries with high blood pressure is known to be present, the only thing which can prevent the danger of a stroke is moderation in all things (see Treatment of High Blood Pressure, p. 306).

A light diet should be taken, largely vegetable; meat fat and alcohol must be avoided. Constipation should be corrected, sexual intercourse limited, and direct exposure to the sun avoided in summer.

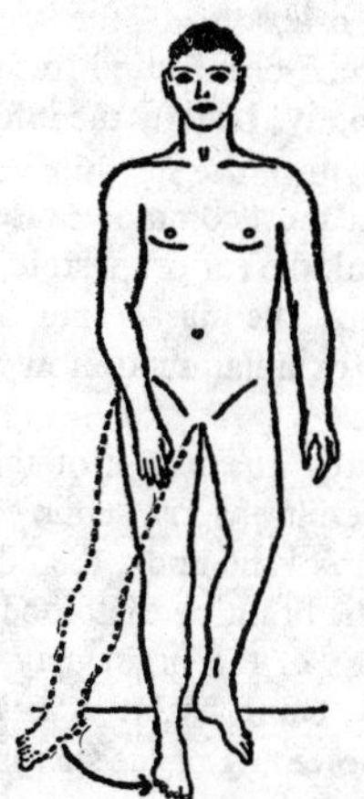

Fig. 22. *MODE OF WALKING IN HEMIPLEGIA. The affected leg is stiff and extended, and is swung round at each step to prevent the toe dragging on the ground.*

First Aid for Stroke. At the onset of a stroke the clothes should be loosened, particularly the collar and tie. If the patient is unconscious, the head and shoulders should be turned on one side so that the tongue does not fall back and cause difficulty in breathing. No attempt should be made to feed an unconscious patient by mouth, but if consciousness returns, small amounts of liquids containing glucose may be given at frequent intervals, care being taken that no food finds its way into the air passages. (See also Treatment of Coma, p. 442.)

Paralysis. In cases which survive the first few days, passive movements should be used daily for all the joints of the paralyzed side, to prevent the stiffening of the limbs. The prevention of deformities and contractures in the paralyzed limbs is of the greatest importance. A hemiplegic patient should be got on to his legs and encouraged to walk as soon as the returning power in the muscles allows the attempt to be made. For the care of the bladder and bowels, the prevention of bedsores, and care of paralyzed muscles, see pp. 420 to 421.

Hydrocephalus

(Water in the Brain)

Hydrocephalus is a distension of the cavities inside the brain by an accumulation of fluid within them. This distension is associated with considerable enlargement of the skull.

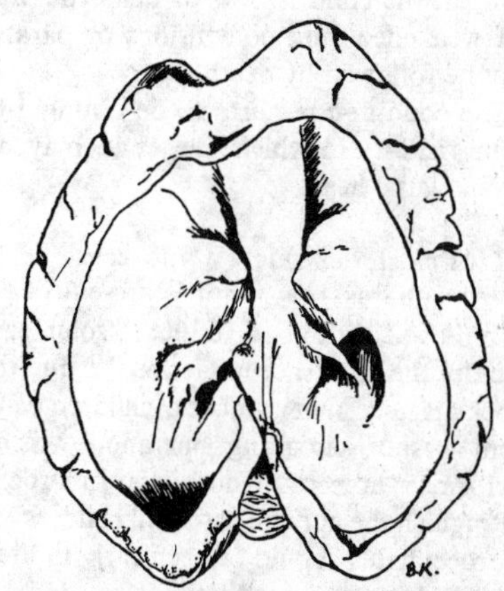

Fig. 23. *BRAIN SECTION IN CONGENITAL HYDROCEPHALUS showing the great dilatation of the ventricles.*

Causes. The disease is chiefly one of infancy and childhood. It may be congenital, when it is present from birth, and is often associated with other abnormalities such as hare-lip, cleft palate, or spina bifida. In other cases it arises after birth, usually following meningitis, though it may occasionally be due to a tumor of the brain.

Symptoms. The most striking feature is the enlargement of the head caused by the pressure on the soft skull bones from within. The skull may reach an enormous size, the forehead being particularly prominent and rounded, and projecting forward. The face is triangular, and contrasts markedly with the size of the forehead, which appears to overhang the eyes, displacing them downward and giving them a sunken effect. The hair is scanty and the general nutrition of the child is poor.

The enlargement of the skull is often associated with persistent headache, vomiting, convulsions and retardation.

The final outlook depends on the cause and the rate of progress of the disease. In mild

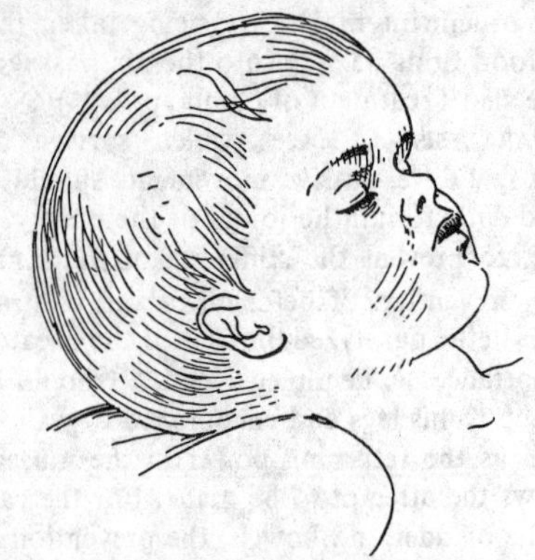

Fig. 24. CHILD WITH HYDROCEPHALUS showing huge head and bulging forehead. When the child is awake the eyes are usually staring.

cases it may be arrested, and the patient may live to adult age with a fairly normal mentality. In cases where the brain is much affected, or when epileptic convulsions are frequent, little or no improvement can be hoped for. The senses gradually become blunted, the child is deaf or blind, the intellect weakened, and convulsions or paralysis may be followed by death.

The condition requires to be distinguished from rickets, in which the child may also have a large head.

Treatment depends on the cause of the hydrocephalus. If a tumor is present, it may be removed with good results in some cases. Should the fluid accumulation be due to a blockage, a certain number of children benefit from a short-circuiting operation which is performed at certain hospitals. In order to distinguish the curable cases, all children with hydrocephalus should be seen early in life by an expert in these conditions.

Tumors of the Brain

The brain is one of the commonest sites of new growths in the body, and in young persons tumors affect the brain more frequently than any other part of the body.

The tumor may be a primary tumor of the brain substance, or it may be secondary to some primary growth elsewhere in the body. Sometimes a brain tumor is due to cysts resulting from infection by the tapeworm.

A tumor of the brain differs in two important respects from tumors occurring in other parts of the body. First, it is growing in contact with very delicate tissues which are easily destroyed. Secondly, it is growing inside a bony cavity which allows little or no room for expansion. The consequences of even small tumors are therefore very serious even in the early stages.

Symptoms. A tumor of the brain may exist for a long time without any definite symptoms, and when these do appear they may be of great variety, depending first on the size and secondly on the situation of the tumor. Symptoms thus fall into two groups.

1. The general effects of increased pressure within the skull. As a rule, the first and most constant symptom is headache. This is rarely strictly located, though it may be referred to the nape of the neck. It is a deep, steady, dull type of headache, of moderate intensity, and aggravated by coughing or straining at stool. It rarely interferes with sleep. Vomiting occurs later, and is usually of the type called 'cerebral vomiting,' in which the sickness is not preceded by nausea. Dimness of vision is common from compression of the optic nerves. Other symptoms consist of slowing of the pulse rate, with giddiness, mental lethargy and drowsiness, and general convulsions.

2. The local effects produced by the irritation or destruction of some particular part of the brain. These effects consist usually of localized fits, or local areas of paralysis.

In all cases of suspected tumor of the brain, the blood should be tested for the Wassermann reaction, and if this is found to be positive, the patient should be treated as for syphilis.

Treatment. Where possible, the treatment is surgical, but when removal of the growth is impossible, an operation known as 'decompression' may be performed. In this operation, a portion of the skull is removed to relieve the pressure inside the skull, and to prevent such serious complications as blindness, mental derangement, and intolerable headache.

For the headache, aspirin, phenacetin and codeine may be required. For convulsions, full maintenance doses of phenobarbital are prescribed. (See Treatment of Epilepsy, pp. 437-38.)

Abscess of the Brain

Causes. An abscess of the brain is always due to a spread of infection from some other part of the body. Usually the infection has its point of origin in the neighboring tissues of the brain, the most common cause being infection in the middle ear or mastoid, while septic conditions of the nasal sinuses, carbuncle of the neck or inflammation in the scalp are other causes.

Occasionally an abscess of the brain may occur as a result of some septic condition in a distant organ of the body, the infection being carried to the brain by the bloodstream.

An abscess of the brain may vary in size, occasionally being as large as a hen's egg. It causes a softening of the surrounding brain tissue.

Symptoms. In most cases the symptoms are slight, and are apt to be masked by the symptoms are very like those of a tumor of of the middle ear or mastoid, empyema of the lung, etc.). At a later stage, an increase of pressure develops inside the skull, so that the symptoms are very like those of a tumour of the brain. Headache is rarely absent and may be severe, and vomiting is almost constant. Dimness of vision, drowsiness and slowing of the pulse may follow. These symptoms are accompanied by fever which helps to distinguish the condition from a brain tumor.

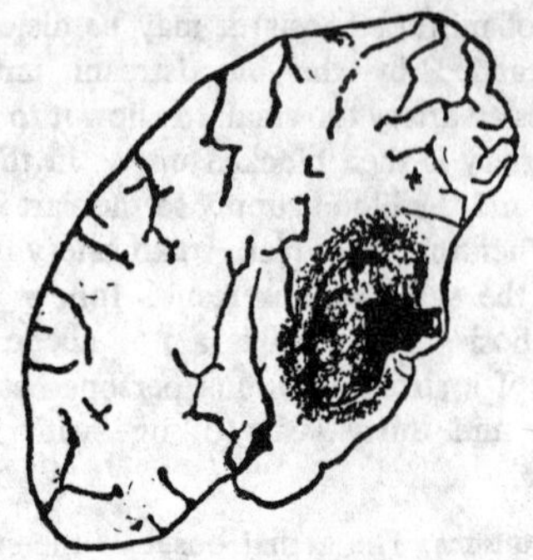

Fig. 25. CHRONIC ABSCESS OF BRAIN. Longitudinal section showing abscess and destruction of surrounding brain tissue.

Usually the abscess enlarges and, unless an operation is performed, death occurs—usually from rupture of the abscess which leads to general meningitis.

Treatment. Whenever the condition is suspected, the ears should be examined. Any infection of the ear, nasal sinuses, or scalp must be vigorously treated until it is cured. The only treatment for a developed abscess is surgical, and consists of drainage with possible later removal of the abscess capsule.

Disseminated Sclerosis
(*Multiple Sclerosis*)

This, together with apoplexy, syphilis of the nervous system, and tumor of the brain, is one of the commonest organic diseases of the nervous system.

Cause. The cause is quite unknown, but there is evidence to suggest that it is due to an infection resulting in the appearance of small patches of inflammation scattered irregularly throughout the brain and spinal cord. Later on these patches are replaced by small scars, which destroy the part of the nervous system involved. The disease most frequently begins between the ages of sixteen and thirty.

Symptoms. Since the patches of scarring may occur in any part of the brain or spinal cord, it is evident that the symptoms may be extremely variable. The onset is insidious.

The symptom for which most patients first seek medical advice is weakness in the legs. This begins with a feeling of stiffness, or heaviness in one or both legs, which gradually increases, so that after a period which varies between a few weeks and several years, it leads to complete paralysis of the legs.

In the arms there is often a feeling of uselessness and loss of power, and in some cases the arms are affected before the legs. The arms show a characteristic shaking or tremor which may be noticed first in finer movements such as threading a needle or writing. In the advanced stages of the disease this tremor may be so marked as to prevent any useful movements of the arms so that the patient becomes unable to do anything for himself. Other early symptoms are numbness and tingling, or 'pins and needles,' in the hands and feet.

Highly characteristic of the disease are attacks of double vision, and any young person who complains of this symptom should be carefully examined by a doctor. In nearly every case, there is sooner or later an actual diminution of vision from inflammation of the optic nerve. Deafness, giddiness and noises in the head are common.

Although some patients with disseminated sclerosis are morose and depressed, the majority of them are surprisingly cheerful, in spite of considerable physical handicaps.

Course of the Disease. In a large number of cases the course of the disease is interrupted by remissions, or periods of apparent recovery, the improvement sometimes lasting for months or years. During these remissions the signs of the disease are apparently capable of lying dormant in the body. After an interval, however, they rewaken and produce a fresh crop of inflammatory patches in the nervous system, with a corresponding renewal of the symptoms. Any kind of feverish illness, injury, or surgical operation, or any condition of physical exhaustion is likely to aggravate the disease, with an increase of symptoms.

The later in life that disseminated sclerosis makes its first appearance, the milder is its course, and patients may sometimes reach old age without any very great disablement. Generally, the patient becomes weaker and weaker until the failure of muscular power eventually confines him to bed.

Treatment. Up to the present there is no treatment which exerts any constant or appreciable influence on the course of the disease. New methods of treatment are reported every year, but there is no proof that any are of value. In any case it is very difficult to assess the use of any form of treatment since the characteristic periods of improvement are a very striking feature of the disease.

While no specific treatment is available, it is advisable that the patient with disseminated sclerosis should lead an ordered life with the minimum of fatigue. Any intercurrent illnesses should be treated vigorously for they have a deleterious effect on the malady.

Nursing. In the early stages of the disease a patient should not be kept in bed more than is absolutely necessary. He should take a reasonable amount of exercise each day, but it is very important that he should avoid becoming overtired. Gentle massage and passive movements three or four times daily are of value in overcoming the stiffness of the limbs, while walking exercises may also be practised.

For constipation, a simple enema given every other day, or a glycerin suppository may sometimes be employed.

In the later stages careful nursing is required to deal with incontinence of urine and to prevent bedsores (see p. 420; also Home Nursing, p. 47).

Marriage. The question of marriage has often to be considered, since the first symptoms of the disease commonly appear in the twenties. While there is no appreciable risk of the disease being transmitted to the next generation, the fact that the disease is likely to cause serious paralysis in the future may be sufficient justification to advise against marriage.

Pregnancy itself has no effect on disseminated sclerosis although some patients have an exacerbation after delivery. Certainly if the patient with this condition becomes pregnant there is no indication to interfere with the pregnancy.

Paralysis Agitans
(Parkinson's Disease)

This disease was first described in 1817 by James Parkinson, who gave it the name of shaking palsy. It is due to a degenerative process affecting certain parts of the brain, the cause of which is unknown. It appears to be aggravated by excessive worry and mental strain, but is not due to the excessive use of tobacco or alcohol. Paralysis agitans affects elderly persons, usually between the ages of sixty and seventy, and occurs in men twice as often as in women.

Symptoms. The disease is characterized by two particular signs:

1. rigidity or stiffness of the muscles;
2. rhythmic tremors, or shaking of the limbs.

RIGIDITY. The onset is always very gradual, and nearly always the first symptom to appear is rigidity of the muscles. At first the stiffness is more pronounced on one side than on the other, but later it spreads over the whole body, and affects the muscles of the face, neck and trunk to a greater degree than those of the limbs. The face tends to become fixed, staring and mask-like, without expression, and with emotional changes reduced to a minimum. The patient smiles little or not at all, and the mouth is often slightly open, a distressing result of which is the constant dribbling away of saliva. The voice loses its inflexions and becomes monotonous.

Rigidity of the limbs causes a peculiar shuffling gait with short steps so that the patient appears to be hurrying forward. When standing up, the head is depressed on the chest, the shoulders are bowed, and the knees and elbows slightly bent. In walking he does not swing the arms, and because of the stiffness, all movements of the body are difficult and slow. The patient may find it almost impossible to turn over in bed because of increasing stiffness. It is often noticed, however, that if he is angry or frightened he can move rapidly. There is often a dull aching pain in the muscles of the trunk and limbs.

TREMOR. This is present in most cases, and usually begins in the hand and forearm. The arm seems to be constantly shaking, while the thumb is rolled upon the fingers in movements resembling those used in making pills. Later the tremor extends to the whole arm and to the leg on the same side, and finally to other parts of the body, so that it becomes impossible for the patient to write or read.

Mentally the patient may be entirely normal, though mental depression may develop as the symptoms get worse. High blood pressure is uncommon in the subjects of paralysis agitans, and the bladder and rectum are not affected by the disease.

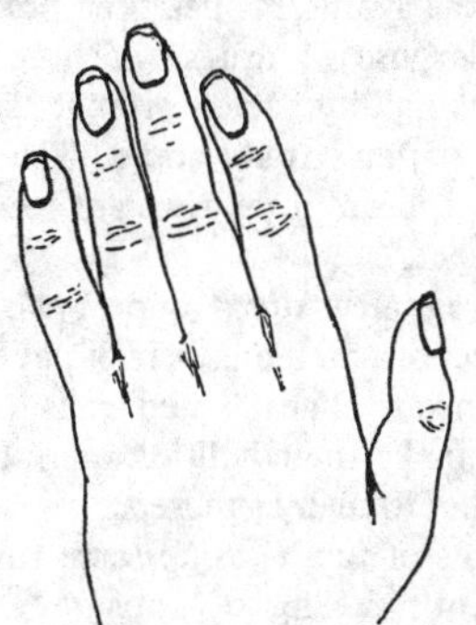

Fig. 26. *OUTWARD DEVIATION OF THE FINGERS in a case of paralysis agitans. Such deviation does not occur in the Parkinsonism which follows encephalitis lethargica.*

Course. The course is generally slowly but steadily downhill. In older patients the disease may remain stationary for years, and on the whole paralysis agitans has remarkably little tendency to shorten life, the average duration of the complaint being as long as ten to fifteen years, unless some intercurrent disease develops. For many years the patient may be able to get about reasonably well and live a useful life, but sooner or later the disease advances to a disabling state.

Treatment. For the condition of Parkinsonism which may be due either to paralysis agitans or to encephalitis lethargica (see p.427) no treatment is known which either prevents the condition from developing or arrests its progress.

An important point in the management of paralysis agitans, however, is to keep the patient up and about as long as possible, as a certain amount of movement prevents the disease from reaching a disabling stage. The patient must therefore be encouraged to continue his work, and to take plenty of exercise, and any kind of occupation which is within his capacity should be followed. Mental exercise is quite as important as physical, and the mistake is often made of advising people who suffer from this complaint to retire and give up their work or business interests.

Massage may be given to the limbs although it is not of great value, and electrical treatment is useless. When the rigidity of the muscles is advanced it may cause considerable pain in the affected limbs, which is partly due to the fixation of the joints in one position. Pain may be relieved by daily passive movements of the joints which should be carried out by a nurse or attendant when the patient is not able to perform them for himself.

Changes of position also give considerable relief to patients who are confined to bed in the advanced stages of the complaint. In such cases, great care must be taken with the skin, since the stiffness of the trunk causes a great likelihood of bedsores (see p. 420).

Constipation is common and should be treated with laxatives.

DRUGS. Although no treatment is known which will cure the disease, a considerable relief of the symptoms has been obtained by the regular use of drugs which reduce the muscular rigidity, and prevent salivation which is often troublesome. The tremor, however, appears to be resistant to all forms of treatment.

Each year new drugs appear which have some effect on small numbers of patients with Parkinsonism. These medicines do not cure but make the condition more bearable, giving relief to many sufferers.

Vitamins of the B group serve to increase the patient's feeling of strength and well-being. Sedatives used alone have the effect of increasing the stiffness and feeling of weakness.

SURGERY. In very severe cases of disability a brain operation may be undertaken by a skilled surgeon for patients under fifty years of age.

Chorea

(Sydenham's Chorea)

This affection of the nervous system is probably due to rheumatic infection of the brain. Females are affected at least twice as often as males, and the disorder is commonest between the ages of five and fifteen. Chorea occurs particularly among nervous, high strung and anemic children, in whom it is apt to appear after emotional shocks. After the age of twenty it is uncommon, except occasionally in pregnancy, when it may appear during the first three months.

Symptoms. The onset is usually gradual, the child becoming slightly more nervous and clumsy in her movements. She is anemic and has a poor appetite, and gets tired very easily. The disease is characterized by irregular, involuntary and purposeless movements and by muscular weakness.

MOVEMENTS IN CHOREA. Gradually there appear slight involuntary movements of the face and fingers, which become more marked as time goes on, spreading to the limbs. At first the child may simply appear to be making faces, which is liable to be mistaken for insolence. Later the face becomes twisted into all kinds of grimaces, the tongue being put out and rapidly snatched back like that of a serpent, or like a Jack-in-the-box, the jaws snapping together after it like a trap. The child can no longer keep still, and becomes liable to drop things from sudden involuntary movements of the arms when picking them up. When she tries to carry food to her mouth, her hand goes part of the way and is suddenly jerked back. The legs are perpetually moving so that walking becomes irregular and clumsy, the feet incessantly shuffling on the floor as if they wanted to dance (hence the popular name, St. Vitus' dance).

The movements of chorea are usually more evident on one side of the body than the other. They are increased when the child is being watched, or when she is self-conscious, but disappear during sleep. The limbs gradually become weaker and the child tires easily, and in severe forms there is much sleeplessness. As a rule there is a good deal of psychological disturbance, which betrays itself in the form of restlessness, agitation and facile laughter or tears.

Complications. Other manifestations of rheumatism may occur during the course of an attack, or they may become evident only after an interval of several months or years. Thus tonsillitis is fairly common, and 'growing pains' or rheumatic pains in the joints may cause considerable distress. Chorea, like any other form of rheumatism, may cause damage to any part of the heart, so that a murmur may appear at the mitral valve after the chorea has apparently been cured.

Course. The disease usually tends to clear up spontaneously after a period varying from six weeks in a mild attack to six months or more in a severe one. The sooner the patient is brought under careful treatment, however, the more likely is its course to be shortened. The ultimate outlook for recovery is nearly always good, but in one-third of all cases there is a recurrence of the disease, usually after an interval of one to three years from the first attack. The greater the number of attacks, the more likely is the heart to be affected.

Treatment

REST. By far the most important item of treatment is rest in bed, which should continue until all movements have disappeared for at least a month, and the pulse is normal and regular. If the heart is affected, a longer period of rest up to several months may be necessary. Mental rest is as important as physical, and the child should be isolated in order to avoid excitement. In severe cases no visitors should be allowed.

The room should be light, quiet and airy. When the movements are really violent a nurse should be in constant attendance, and the child should be prevented from falling out of bed by securing the bedclothes firmly beneath the mattress. If a cot is used, the bars should be protected by pillows bandaged in position, so that the child cannot bruise herself. It may be necessary to protect the limbs from injury by padding them with large pieces of cotton, which should be firmly bandaged on.

DIET. Since children with chorea are usually undernourished, thin and anemic, they should be given a nutritious diet, with extra milk, cream, eggs and fresh fruit. Cod-liver oil and malt should also be given.

It is important that the child should not be allowed to use feeding vessels or utensils made of glass or china, in order to prevent the risk of pieces being bitten off and swallowed. Plastic feeding cups or a spoon should be used instead.

DRUGS. Aspirin helps to combat the rheumatic infection causing the disease. This is given in doses of 600 milligrams three times daily after meals for a child between the ages of six and fourteen years, and should be continued until convalescence is complete.

In severe cases, one of the phenothiazine tranquilizing drugs, e.g. chlorpromazine, is now found to be the most effective of sedatives for chorea. Chloral hydrate is still sometimes used for calming affected children.

For sleeplessness, the best remedy is a larger dose of aspirin given at night.

During convalescence, tonics are helpful, and anemia must be treated by iron tonics.

Convalescence. When active signs of the disease have disappeared, the child should be encouraged to use her limbs, and simple exercises, with games such as dominoes or checkers, are valuable for re-educating the control of the hands. Sewing and knitting can also be practiced. Later, exercises given under supervision, and simple forms of drill are useful. Any recurrence of involuntary movements, however, must be the signal for an immediate return to bed.

After an attack of chorea the child should not be allowed to do much mental work for several months. She should be given a long holiday in healthy surroundings, and this should be repeated for some years at intervals of not more than six months.

Huntington's Chorea

This is a rare malady of the middle-aged occurring as an inherited disease.

Symptoms. Jerky purposeless movements of the face and limbs occur and, gradually, a mental deterioration develops resulting in maniacal outbursts. The disease runs a downhill course and recovery is unknown.

Treatment. No specific treatment is known but heavy sedation keeps the patient tranquil.

DISEASES OF THE SPINAL CORD

The spinal cord is a continuation of the brain from which it extends through the center of the vertebral column, or backbone. In order that a person may feel what takes place in any part of the limbs or trunk, and in order that the will, acting through the brain, may have the power to move any of these parts, it is necessary for the nerve fibers which connect the part in question with the brain to be continuous and unbroken. These fibers are collected together in the form of compact bundles in the substance of the spinal cord.

Compression of the Spinal Cord

When any part of the spinal cord is subjected to pressure, whether it be the sudden pressure produced by crushing of the cord after an injury to the back, or the gradually increasing pressure of a tumor of the spine, all the nerve fibers below the level of the injury or pressure will be damaged and destroyed. Whether this destruction will be sudden or gradual depends on the cause. The result of such pressure is that all the parts of the body which receive their nerves from below the point of injury in the cord become both paralyzed and numb, that is they lose both their power of movement and their sense of feeling.

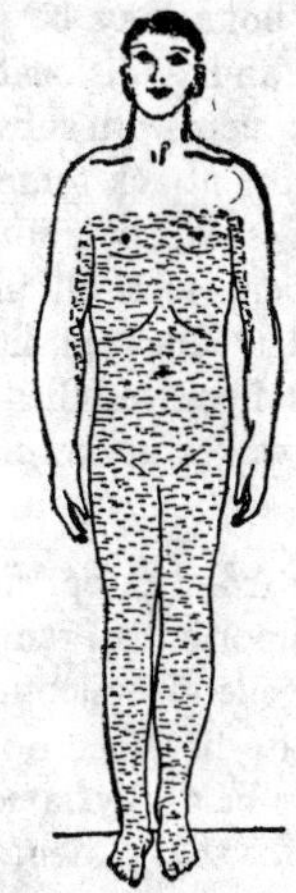

Fig. 27. *FRACTURE-DISLOCATION OF SPINE IN THE NECK produces loss of sensitivity to touch, pain, heat, and cold in the areas indicated by shading.*

If the lower part of the spinal cord is affected, both the legs will become paralized and numb, a condition known as paraplegia. If the middle part of the spinal cord is affected (as in the lower chest or back) not only the legs, but also the lower part of the trunk, together with the bowels and other organs, will lose their powers of movement and feeling. When the compression is in the upper part of the cord, in the neck, the arms as well as the legs and trunk will be paralyzed. If the compression is sufficiently rapid (as in broken neck, etc.) the breathing and circulation also will stop, and death is the immediate consequence. Disease or injury in the upper part of the spinal cord is therefore considerably more dangerous than in the lower parts of the cord.

Rapid Compression. The commonest causes of quick compression are fracture or dislocation of the spine, which occurs most often after a fall from a height on to the feet or buttocks, or after a blow on the back. Such an injury produces complete paralysis of the parts below the level of the injury, together with total loss of sensation. These changes are permanent. Bedsores often develop with great rapidity, and the bladder is very likely to become infected.

Gradual Compression of the spinal cord is commonly due to tuberculous disease of the spine (Pott's disease), which occurs most often in children. Other causes are tumors of the spinal cord and its membranes, which may be secondary to cancer elsewhere in the body.

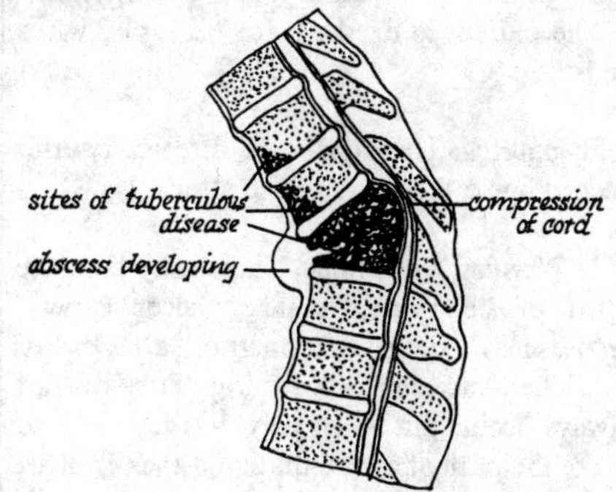

Fig. 28. *POTT'S DISEASE (tuberculosis of the spine) in the lower part of the spine, showing two diseased and collapsed vertebrae which have fused together, the intervening disc having been destroyed by the disease. Note the angulation of the spine and consequent compression of the spinal cord.*

Symptoms. An important early symptom is pain in the part of the body which is at the level of the disease. It is greatly aggravated by movement. As the pressure increases, the parts below the level of the disease show gradually increasing loss of power, with weakness of the knees and legs. At a certain stage the compression quite suddenly causes paralysis of the legs (paraplegia) from which there can be no recovery. Inability to control the bladder and rectum leads to retention of urine, and constipation, and later to incontinence—the urine and feces being passed involuntarily.

Treatment. It is important that the pressure on the spinal cord should be relieved by surgical operation as soon as possible. For nursing treatment, see pp. 420 to 421.

Subacute Combined Degeneration

Cause. This is a degeneration of certain fibers of the spinal cord which is always preceded by an anemia caused by a specific lack of vitamin B_{12}. The actual cause of the disease is unknown, but probably there is a common cause which is responsible both for the nervous disease and for the anemia. It is commonest from the age of forty onwards, increasing in frequency up to the age of sixty, and it affects both sexes equally.

Symptoms. The disease begins with tingling and numbness in the tips of the fingers and toes, which gradually spread up the limbs. Creeping sensations, burning pain and coldness are also common. Later, fatigue appears on exertion, with weakness of the leg muscles and dragging of the feet, leading to unsteadiness in walking. The muscles of the calf become tender on pressure, and there is general wasting of the muscles. Finally the disease may incapacitate the patient completely, with loss of bladder and rectum control.

As in pernicious anemia, the tongue is always clean, and the skin is usually lemon-colored. Other symptoms of anemia are commonly present—breathlessness, headache, and swelling of the ankles.

Treatment. The disease can be arrested if properly treated. If treatment is neglected, however, the disease progresses, leading to irreparable damage to the spinal cord, with resulting paralysis of the legs. Whatever the degree of anemia present, intensive treatment, generally with vitamin B_{12} (hydroxocobalamin) both by mouth and by injection, is essential, and the patient should be under proper medical supervision. It requires larger doses and for a longer period than ordinary uncomplicated pernicious anemia, and doses must be continued indefinitely in order to prevent any relapse.

Decayed teeth must be attended to, and every care taken to prevent the development of bedsores and cystitis which occur very readily in this disease (see p. 420).

Remedial exercises under the supervision of a physiotherapist are often needed to retrain the patient to walk properly.

Progressive Muscular Atrophy

This is due to a degeneration of certain nerve cells and fibers of the spinal cord, and is characterized by a gradually increasing weakness of the skeletal muscles. The same type of weakness is found, in an acute form, in poliomyelitis. Usually no cause can be found, though it is occasionally associated with preceding syphilitic infection. It begins between the ages of thirty and forty-five.

Symptoms. The onset of the disease is usually very gradual, and its course is often interrupted by long periods when it is stationary. The most characteristic feature is weakness and wasting of the muscles, which may begin in any group of muscles, especially those of the hand and arm, either around the shoulder joint or in the hand. Paralysis and wasting of the small muscles of the hand leads to various deformities, such as 'claw hand,' and 'flat hand,' or **'monkey's hand'** from wasting of the muscles of the ball of the thumb. Loss of power accompanies the wasting which usually begins in one limb and spreads symmetrically to the other. The muscles of the back may be affected, with increasing difficulty in holding the head up. The disease progresses very slowly, and may last for many years before causing death.

Treatment. The disease appears to be uninfluenced by any form of treatment. If syphilis is found to be present it must be treated. Every effort should be made to improve the general health, and septic teeth, etc. should be dealt with. Massage may be given. Patients with progressive muscular atrophy should not be confined to bed until the paralysis becomes so advanced as to make it necessary.

EPILEPSY

Causes. An epileptic attack is characterized by abnormal and uncontrolled discharges of energy from the cells of the brain. Since such attacks may be due to a number of causes, it would be more correct to use the term 'the epilepsies.' Each form of epilepsy has its own variant of fit.

The conditions which may precipitate an epileptic fit are:

1. A genetic predisposition (idiopathic epilepsy). Fits in children are more likely to be due to such a cause. It is often possible to trace a hereditary or familial tendency to the disorder, and other nervous affections such as migraine, hysteria or asthma are often found in the same family. The direct transmission of epilepsy from parent to child, however, is somewhat exceptional and probably does not occur in more than 30 per cent of all cases. Repeated attacks of infantile convulsions may often indicate a predisposition to epilepsy in later life;

2. A structural lesion of the brain caused by the pressure of a cerebral tumor or abscess; epilepsy from this cause is not likely to occur until after the age of 25;

3. Vascular disease of the brain blood vessels in older persons;

4. Severe hypoglycemia in diabetics, and states of poisoning due to chronic kidney disease, etc. or to drug poisons such as cocaine or absinthe;

5. Infections reaching the brain, e.g. meningitis and syphilis;

6. Injury to the brain from any cause, such as a fractured skull, gunshot wounds, etc. The fits may first appear at any time after the injury and in some cases they do not occur until several years have elapsed;

7. Infestation by tapeworms or other parasites. The cyst stage of the pork tapeworm sometimes reaches the brain and its disintegration some years later produces intense irritation causing epilepsy and personality changes.

Periodicity of Fits. While some patients may have fits at any time, the majority show a tendency for the attacks to occur at certain times and not at others. A well-recognized form is the epilepsy of sleep (nocturnal epilepsy). Another common type is the attack which occurs when the patient gets up in the morning. In many young women the attacks are related to the monthly periods, occurring as a rule just before or just after menstruation. Finally it is not uncommon for a patient to have a series of attacks occurring together in the course of a single day. Such groups of attacks are often repeated at regular intervals of seven, fourteen or twenty-eight days. Occasionally there is an interval of several months between the attacks.

The fits are not as a rule aggravated by pregnancy, nor is the pregnancy itself unfavorably affected. It is unusual for an epileptic attack to occur when the attention of the patient is fixed as, for example, when he is at work.

Symptoms. These fall into three categories according to the stage of the attack.

1. **Warning Symptoms.** These may take the form of headache, lethargy, sleeplessness, restlessness, unusual appetite, attacks of giddiness, sneezing or yawning. They do not always occur, but when they do they seem to make the patient aware that an attack is near.

2. **The Aura.** This is really the first part of the actual epileptic fit. It may assume many different forms, but is generally constant for the same individual.

(a) Disturbances of sensation, such as tingling in one hand, or unusual sensations in the limbs.

(b) Disturbances of the special senses of sight, smell or taste.

(c) Disturbances of muscular movement such as localized twitchings in certain groups of muscles.

(d) Psychic disturbances.

3. **The Epileptic Attack.** There are three main types of epileptic attack.

(a) Minor Epilepsy (Petit Mal). This is a mild form of epilepsy, with only a slight loss of consciousness lasting a few seconds. The patient may only sway slightly, with a vacant expression, and be unable to describe what has happened, or he may suddenly fall without warning, so that the head reaches the ground first and the forehead becomes bruised. He regains consciousness immediately and picks himself up. In this type of epilepsy the forehead may show many scars caused by repeated falls. Such attacks are commonly seen in patients who also suffer from grand mal, but they may occur quite independently.

(b) Epilepsy with Convulsions (Grand Mal). This type of seizure is usually preceded by an aura. If standing, the patient suddenly feels giddy and falls to the ground, often with a peculiar noise—the 'epileptic cry' produced by a spasm of the larynx during inspiration. In the first part of the attack, the muscles of the whole body are in continuous rigid contraction, with the hands and jaws clenched, while a temporary stoppage of the breathing causes blueness of the face and enlargement of the neck veins. During this stage the tongue is often forced out of the mouth and bitten by the sudden closing of the jaw. This first phase of contraction (tonic stage) lasts for about half a minute, and then begins to break into a series of jerky shock-like movements which affect the whole body almost simultaneously. The movements increase rapidly in extent, and then diminish both in frequency and size, becoming less regular and occurring at longer intervals, until after about two or three minutes the muscles give a final jerk and then become perfectly limp. During the convulsive stage the movements of respiration return, and frothy saliva may appear at the mouth. It is often bloodstained from injury of the teeth or tongue. Some patients always bite the tongue, and others only occasionally. It is always bitten on the same side and at some distance from the tip. During an attack it is a common feature for urine to be passed involuntarily, and occasionally the bowel may be evacuated as well. In some patients the spasms of the muscles may be so powerful that a bone may be broken or a joint dislocated, and a dislocation so produced will always recur with subsequent fits.

At the end of the attack there is complete loss of consciousness which gradually returns. Usually the patient feels ill and mentally confused, and has a severe headache. He often vomits, and then sleeps heavily for some hours. When he wakes up he may feel quite well.

Danger to Life from an epileptic attack is not great. It is important to remember, however, that in a general epileptic convulsion the patient usually lies face downward, so that he may easily be asphyxiated by his own pillow. Moreover, the patient may vomit while he is still unconscious, so that there is some danger of choking from inhaling vomited material.

Fire, water, and machinery provide the main dangers to the epileptic.

(c) Focal Fits (Jacksonian Epilepsy). These fits are caused by the irritation of the white cortex of the brain, and occur usually as a result either of injury or of organic disease of the brain. Such localized irritation causes the fits to start in the same group of muscles on each occasion, but usually does not lead to loss of consciousness.

The common points of onset of such a fit are the corner of the mouth, the thumb or index finger, and the great toe. The convulsive movements may remain localized to these situations, or they may spread widely so as to involve a whole limb or even half the body. In some cases there are disorders of behavior, particularly automatism, so that this form is often termed *psychomotor epilepsy.*

Course of Epilepsy. Many patients with epilepsy keep their intellectual capacity unimpaired. If the attacks are infrequent or confined only to the sleeping hours or to the menstrual periods, the ultimate outlook is good, and the attacks may cease spontaneously. In many cases of convulsive attacks in infancy and early childhood, the attacks tend to disappear after the age of five to six. Moreover, the earlier that treatment is started, the more likely is it to bring about a cure.

One of the most curious features of epilepsy is the tendency for the patient to be unaware of the attack, and to pass into a condition known as 'post-epileptic automatism' in which he behaves in a strange manner, sometimes assuming a second personality with habits which are quite different from those of his ordinary life (i.e. the Jekyll and Hyde type of personality).

In some patients who are subject to frequently repeated attacks of epilepsy, mental deterioration is apt to occur. This is one of the most serious features of the disease, since once established it is likely to be progressive, so that the ultimate outlook is bad. Mental deterioration first shows itself in defects of memory which may be followed by failure in concentration and attention, and every degree of mental impairment up to complete dementia may occur. Some of these patients with chronic epileptic insanity are subject to impulsive attacks of a vicious kind, and constitute a dangerous type of case.

Status Epilepticus. This is a dangerous but fortunately uncommon condition, in which one severe convulsion follows another at short intervals without any return of consciousness during the intervals. It may develop suddenly in any kind of epilepsy, but as a rule only in patients who have been subject to major attacks of grand mal. It may be brought on by excitement or overexertion, but usually it occurs when medicines such as phenobarbital, which have been taken regularly for a considerable time to keep the fits in check, are suddenly stopped. During an attack, the temperature and pulse rate rise and marked exhaustion follows. Death may occur rapidly, or after the lapse of a few days.

Treatment of Epilepsy

Since it is quite common for a doctor to visit an epileptic patient on many occasions without ever seeing a fit, it will usually be necessary for him to rely on descriptions of the attacks by any witnesses who happen to have seen them in progress. *No opportunity should therefore be lost, by relatives or members of the patient's household, of seeing the patient in a fit if this is possible, and of observing the type and distribution of the convulsive movements, and of the duration of unconsciousness.* The course of the fit is of great importance in the recognition of epilepsy, and particular attention should be paid to the following points. 1. The aura; 2. The epileptic cry; 3. The 'tonic' stage of rigid muscular contraction; 4. The 'clonic' stage of convulsive spasms; 5. The stage of coma, passing into sleep; 6. Biting of the tongue, with frothy blood-stained sputum, and involuntary passing of urine.

Treatment of the Epileptic Attack. The main points in the treatment of the attack are to protect the patient from being injured by the violence of the convulsion, and to avoid unusual accidents. He should be moved into a safe position where he cannot be injured by water, fire, moving vehicles, etc., and placed flat on the floor, or on a bed or couch. To prevent the tongue from being bitten, the teeth should be separated at the side of the mouth by some object such as a tightly rolled handkerchief, a strong cork, a piece of rubber tubing, or a soft wooden wedge such as the handle of a hairbrush. Dentures should if possible be removed. The head should be slightly raised, and the collar and any tightly fitting clothing should be loosened. The patient should be carefully watched for possible choking from food remaining in the throat after vomiting.

It is important to remember that in an epileptic attack the patient often lies face downwards so that he may easily be asphyxiated by his own pillow. A patient who is subject to nocturnal attacks in bed should therefore not be allowed to sleep alone, and when the attack occurs, care must be taken to see that he does not turn on to his face.

On no account should the patient be disturbed immediately after an attack, and he should be allowed to sleep without being roused. He must, however, be kept under careful observation until any post-epileptic confusion has passed off.

Treatment of Status Epilepticus. This condition calls for prompt and vigorous treatment, since it may easily cause death. The patient must be placed in bed at once. The convulsion may usually be controlled by giving relaxant drugs under proper medical supervision, but the fits tend to recur as soon as the drugs are stopped. The doctor will inject sedatives to stop the fits.

As soon as the convulsions have been arrested, *it is of the greatest importance that the lower bowel should be thoroughly emptied.* Often the rectum will be found to be loaded with hard fecal matter, and it will then be necessary to inject 60 to 90 milliliters of warm olive oil or mineral oil into the rectum, and follow it up with an ordinary soap enema after two hours. If the patient is sufficiently conscious he may be given, in addition, 30 milliliters of castor oil by mouth.

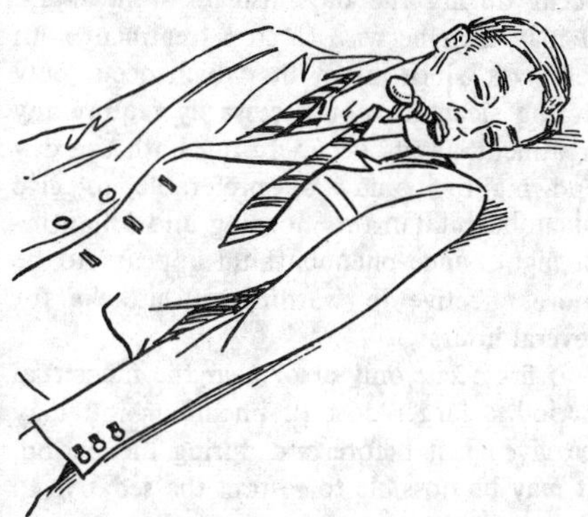

Fig. 29. *EPILEPTIC FIT. When the patient is in the convulsive stage, insert a rolled handkerchief or spoon between the teeth to one side to prevent the tongue being bitten. Loosen the collar.*

The evacuation of a loaded bowel is often all that is necessary to stop the fits, but, if they persist, they can usually be controlled by giving paraldehyde by the rectum.

At this stage the unconscious patient must be transferred to hospital for skilled care.

If home treatment is continued and the temperature rises above 39·4° C (103° F) the patient should be continuously sponged with tepid water. If the fever persists, the patient may be immersed in a tepid bath, and this will sometimes have a dramatic effect.

When the convulsions and the fever have been controlled, and the bowels well moved, the only food should consist of 120 grams of glucose in 300 milliliters of water, in order to control the acidosis in the system. It is essential for the patient to have complete rest in bed for several days.

General Management of Patient's Life

The chance of improving a patient who is subject to epilepsy is much greater if the patient can live as normal and satisfying a life as possible. Thus, children and adolescents should attend school, since mental exercise does no harm. They should have regular physical exercise and long hours of sleep. Adults should follow their regular employment, provided they are working in suitable surroundings. On the other hand, improvement is much less likely to occur if education is stopped, all forms of pleasures and sports forbidden, and the patient condemned to a gloomy narrow life because he has a few fits.

It is, however, always advisable to avoid any circumstance which might precipitate an attack or endanger life. It is impossible to guard against all risks, but it is a good thing for the patient to know that he is unlikely to have a fit during mental concentration, e.g. while crossing a busy street, or while faced with a situation requiring careful and intensive thought. On the other hand, emotional disturbances and excitements should be avoided, and the neurotic and over-conscientious type of child should not be allowed to take part in competitive tasks or games. He should always go to bed early. For the less nervous type of patient ordinary games can nearly always be allowed.

WATER, FIRE AND MACHINERY are the main dangers for the epileptic. Bathing is apt to precipitate an attack, and he may be drowned in a few inches of water while swimming or boating. He should only take a bath if there is someone at hand who knows the risks. He may fall into a fire while having a fit, and should be warned against this danger. He must not be allowed to work near machinery, fire or water, or on a ladder.

An epileptic patient should be forbidden, of course, to drive a car or ride a motor cycle.

THE DIET should be liberal and nutritious but free from condiments, and the patient should not go too long without food. If he is exposed to such risk he should carry sweets or chocolate to bridge the gap. Alcohol must be absolutely forbidden, and abnormal quantities of fluid should not be drunk at any one time.

CONSTIPATION. It is particularly important that constipation should be avoided, since obstinate constipation, with the retention of masses of hard dry feces in the rectum, is commonly associated with status epilepticus. Thus, a free daily evacuation of the bowels must be secured, a precaution doubly necessary in patients who suffer from repeated convulsions, and in cases of mental deterioration.

MARRIAGE. Since not more than 30 per cent of all epileptics inherit the disease directly from one or other parent, it is hardly justifiable for an epileptic who is otherwise normal to be advised against marriage, provided that he does not suffer from the disease in a severe form. Speaking generally, marriage itself rarely has any adverse effect on the patient who suffers from epilepsy in its milder forms, and there is no special danger in pregnancy. Patients with severe epilepsy, however, should in general be advised against marriage.

MANAGEMENT OF PATIENTS WITH SEVERE ATTACKS. Children and adolescents who suffer from severe and frequently repeated attacks are best educated at home. Since these children always tend to become self-centered and egotistical, it is important that the child should not become obsessed with his complaint, and as little attention as possible should be paid to the actual fits.

INSTITUTIONAL TREATMENT. In cases where no adequate care can be provided at home, and especially if the patient is of low-grade mentality, and if the disease interferes with a normal education, treatment in an institution for epileptics is advisable, where the regular work and interest help to relieve the burden of the complaint. Plans are being made to lessen the need for institutions, however, by having epileptic clinics in general hospitals where, in residential units, the patients can be watched in everyday conditions.

If well-marked dementia is established, it may be necessary for the patient to be certified as insane, and admitted to a mental hospital.

Medicinal Treatment

Apart from the points already mentioned, the treatment of epilepsy is almost entirely by means of sedative drugs, which in most cases are able to reduce considerably the number of fits. It is generally impossible to treat any but the mildest cases without the regular use of some sedative drug.

There are two main types of drug in use for epilepsy, the barbiturates and the anticonvulsants, which are given in regular dosage. Their effectiveness depends on continuous treatment.

PHENOBARBITAL is a very powerful drug, and must be used with care. It can only be obtained with a doctor's prescription. The usual dose for epilepsy is 60 or 100 milligrams night and morning, and a total daily dose of 200 milligrams should rarely be exceeded. It is usually taken as a tablet.

There are, however, minor drawbacks to treatment with phenobarbital, and some patients show the effects of sensitivity even with quite small doses. It may give rise to rashes, chiefly on the arms, but other signs are giddiness, unsteadiness in walking, nausea and mental dullness. On the other hand, a tolerance to the drug may be acquired fairly rapidly, so that the effective dose may have to be increased.

ANTICONVULSANTS are specific in preventing attacks; one of the safest is Dilantin®, 100 milligrams twice or three times a day, which is usually given in conjunction with phenobarbital.

VARIATIONS IN DOSAGE. Epileptic fits often tend to occur at certain times of the day or night, or at certain times in the month, and when this is the case the sedative should be given so that it anticipates the occurrence of the fit and exerts the maximum effect with the minimum dose.

If the attacks take place at a certain time during the day, a larger dose of the sedative should be taken an hour or two before the attack is expected. Thus, when the attacks occur on rising in the morning, the patient should take a cup of tea and a biscuit in bed, with the appropriate dose of phenobarbital or other drug. He should then remain in bed for half an hour before rising. A second dose may be given if necessary in the afternoon. If the fits occur only during the night, a single dose of phenobarbital at night may be very effective. In cases of nocturnal epilepsy, however, a sedative taken before going to sleep may cause some of the fits to occur during the day instead of at night. It may then be wise to stop treatment with sedatives, since minor fits which occur only during sleep do not necessarily require any treatment. If fits occur during both the day and night, it may be preferable to give phenobarbital in the morning and Dilantin® at night, since phenobarbital appears to be more effective in warding off attacks for several hours.

If fits occur only at or near the menstrual period, a larger dose of phenobarbital may be given just before and during the period. It may be possible to restrict the sedative to the week before and the week after the beginning of each period. Operations to stop menstruation are of no value in diminishing the fits.

In any feverish illness in which the temperature is raised above 37·8° C (100°F), the dose of sedative may be reduced, since it is rare for attacks to occur at such a time. Moreover, a severe feverish illness may be followed by freedom from attacks for as long as six months.

CHOICE OF DRUG. While some patients do well on phenobarbital alone, and others need a combination of drugs, the best course can only be decided after trials. In general, phenobarbital is very suitable for younger patients and for mild petit mal.

Other useful drugs are ethosuximide for petit mal; methoin; primidone often used in conjunction with phenobarbital for grand mal.

Many anticonvulsants have undesirable effects and have to be administered with great and constant care.

Duration of Treatment. The most important point in the administration of sedatives is that it should be continuous and prolonged and, once the effective dose of the drug is chosen, it will have to be continued regularly for a period of many years. *It is very important to remember that intermittent treatment is extremely bad and if the treatment is suddenly stopped the very serious condition of status epilepticus may quickly follow. Even if a single dose is omitted, a fit will usually occur.* When the fits are under satisfactory control, the treatment must be continued steadily for at least two or even three years after the last attack. After there have been no attacks for six months or longer, the dose may be cautiously and gradually reduced, but the medicine must be continued for at least two years after the attack, and in severe cases a diminishing dose is required for a third year.

HEADACHES

Migraine

(*Sick Headache*)

Migraine is one of the most common complaints of civilized people. It takes the form of recurring intense headaches accompanied by nausea or vomiting, which usually develop on waking in the morning.

Causes

PREDISPOSING CAUSES. The attacks may begin in childhood, but more often they begin at puberty, and then persist until middle age, disappearing in women at the change of life. They are very uncommon in old age. Heredity plays a considerable part and several subjects of migraine or of epilepsy and asthma may be found in the same family. The subjects of migraine often suffer from travel sickness, but are otherwise generally quite healthy, and are usually of an active and intelligent mentality.

PRECIPITATING CAUSES. An attack is commonly precipitated in susceptible persons by worry, emotional disturbance, mental or physical fatigue, or indiscretions of diet. Migraine headaches are therefore common during weekends, immediately after holidays, and just before menstruation. For school teachers, they are apt to occur in the early autumn, and for business people during rush seasons. Patients with migraine often have fixed days of the week when their headaches occur. Eyestrain, disease of the nose, or infected teeth may be associated conditions which may bring on an attack.

Symptoms. The essential symptom is headache, which may be so intense as to make the patient extremely ill for the time being. The attack may come on at any time of day or night, although it generally occurs on waking in the morning. On raising the head from the pillow, the patient has a feeling of giddiness with nausea and confusion of vision, which closely resembles the beginning of an attack of seasickness. Vomiting often occurs at once, but is sometimes delayed for several hours. The association of vomiting with the headache often causes migraine to be referred to as a bilious attack, especially in childhood.

The headache follows shortly after these early symptoms. It usually begins on one side as a sharp boring pain, at a spot which is constant for each individual patient, in the temple, forehead or eyeball. From this localized spot it gradually spreads. The headache may be confined to one side, or to the front or the back of the head, or it may be felt all over the head. As it increases, the face becomes pale, the patient being prostrated and irritable and unable to take any food. The pain is aggravated by noise and movement of any sort, so that he only wishes to be left in absolute quiet.

In some cases there are characteristic disturbances of vision, in the form of zig-zag figures, colored lights, or flashes in front of the eyes. Occasionally there may even be temporary blindness.

After several hours the patient falls into a heavy sleep for the rest of the day and following night, and generally awakes next morning rather weak but otherwise well. Sometimes the attacks may last for several days, and have been known to persist for as long as three weeks. After an attack the patient usually experiences a feeling of well-being and buoyancy, and a striking feature of migraine is the complete freedom from headache between prostrating attacks.

Treatment

Treatment of the Acute Attack. Any person who has an attack of migraine should lie down and keep warm in a semi-darkened room, preferably in bed, and should not be disturbed, in order that he may sleep at the earliest possible moment. A cool evaporating lotion, such as Eau-de-Cologne or cold water, may be applied to the head. The patient may get some relief by having a hot bath, and glucose in water or lemonade should be taken whenever the vomiting does not prevent it. In some patients, a teaspoonful of Epsom salts or a Seidlitz powder may be successful in shortening an attack. Many subjects of migraine derive great benefit from a headache powder, which should always be carried and used at the first appearance of the sick headache. The following prescription may be used:

Aspirin	225 mg
Phenacetin	150 mg
Caffeine	30 mg

Proprietary preparations of unknown composition should be avoided unless prescribed by a physician.

A distinct advance in treatment is provided by ergotamine tartrate. It is most effective by injection in doses of 1/4 to 1/2 milligram, and repeated after one hour if necessary. In mild cases one tablet of ergotamine tartrate, containing 1 milligram, taken by mouth may give relief. The same amount may be repeated one or two hours later if necessary. This drug should not be used during pregnancy, and should only be given under the supervision of a doctor. Ergotamine tartrate does not relieve any type of headache other than migraine.

When the attacks last for more than twenty-four hours, it is very important for the patient to sleep, for which purpose sedatives may be prescribed. He must also be persuaded to take a sufficient amount of nourishment, and glucose should always be at hand.

Prevention of Attacks. Between attacks of migraine an effort should be made to improve the general health and nutrition. Any obvious mental strain or anxiety should if possible be corrected, and the patient should avoid becoming overtired. Sometimes the number of attacks may be diminished by taking a rest in the middle of the day, or by avoiding evening work or amusements and by going to bed earlier. In the case of frequent and severe attacks, a long holiday will often bring about a lasting improvement. While fresh air and regular exercise are beneficial, excessive physical exertion should be avoided.

A good diet is essential, although articles of food which appear to precipitate attacks should not be taken, and overeating must be avoided. In all cases, particular attention should be given to a satisfactory daily movement of the bowels. Eyestrain should be corrected, and eyeglasses prescribed if necessary, and any infection of the nose or teeth should be appropriately dealt with. The blood may require to be tested for evidence of anemia, which if present should be treated.

In children and adolescents when acidosis may be the exciting cause, glucose should be given in doses of 2 teaspoonsful per 2 tablespoonsful of barley water, lemonade, etc., three times daily.

Other Forms of Headache

Headache is an extremely common complaint, and is found most often among civilized people.

Causes. Although headache is often due to trivial causes, it should not be neglected. Apart from migraine (see above), which is one of the commonest of all head complaints, the most usual causes of headaches are the following.

1. ANXIETY AND EMOTIONAL TENSION, which may lead to tightening of the muscles at the back of the head and neck, with resultant pain. In hysteria the headache may be felt as a weight on top of the head. Such nervous headaches are often associated with insomnia, and a person who complains of long periods of loss of sleep because of headache is usually anxious or depressed.

2. RHEUMATISM. In cases of fibrositis of the scalp (rheumatic headache) painful nodules can often be felt at the back of the head.

3. FEVERS. In childhood, a headache is usually more serious than in adults as it may indicate the approach of an infectious illness. In tropical countries it is an invariable symptom of the onset of an attack of malaria. Headache is also common in adults with low-grade fever, as in tuberculosis.

4. POISONING OF THE SYSTEM. Headache may result from poisoning by chemical agents such as alcohol or carbon monoxide (as from exposure to a leaking gas pipe, fumes of a car exhaust, etc.).

5. DISORDERS OF THE EYES, usually due to errors of refraction, especially far-sightedness. Such headaches are caused by overtaxing certain groups of muscles or by fixing the eyes too long on one objective point, as in prolonged study or reading, especially with a bad light. The headache is usually dull, being situated mostly in the forehead and over the eyes, and is often accompanied by nausea. It usually begins toward the end of the day.

Another common cause of headache of this kind is astigmatism or the inability to see equally well horizontal and vertical lines. It is often so insidious in onset as to escape attention. The eyes should be tested without delay by an ophthalmic surgeon.

Glaucoma, a serious eye disease accompanied by headache above the affected eye, is characterized by defects in color vision and by the appearance of colored rings about lights.

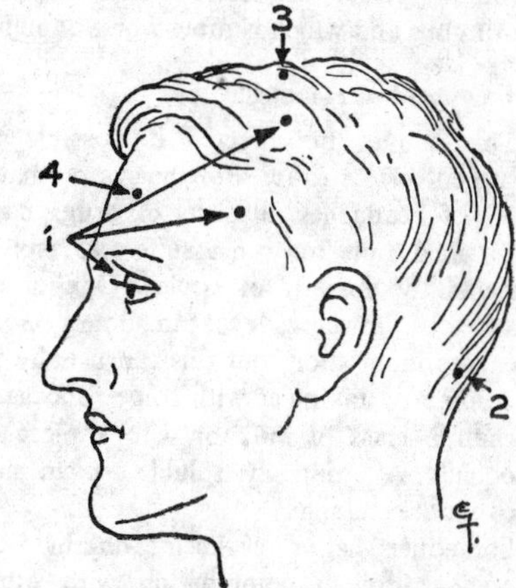

Fig. 30. *LOCALIZATION OF HEADACHE in various disorders.* 1. *Headache at onset of migraine (worse in early morning) and in cases of raised blood pressure.* 2. *Occipital headache due to anxiety and nervous tension, or to rheumatic fibrositis of the scalp.* 3. *Headache due to hysteria is felt as a weight on top of the head.* 4. *Headache in eyestrain or other eye disorders, or in frontal sinusitis.*

6. DISEASE OF THE THROAT AND NOSE, from infection of the teeth, tonsils, or nasal sinuses. Headaches which are associated with nasal disease are usually more common during the winter months, when colds and sore

throats are most prevalent. In infection of the nasal sinuses, the headache usually begins in the morning, persisting during the waking hours of the day, and often ending towards the evening. It is increased by shaking the head and by coughing. It may persist in this intermittent form for weeks or months. When the frontal sinuses are infected, the headache may be localized to the forehead.

7. Diseases of the Circulation. Headaches associated with high blood pressure usually begin, like migraine, in the early hours of the morning, so that the patient awakens with the pain which increases steadily until breakfast but is often relieved on taking food. It may be prevented by taking a mouthful of food and some fluid immediately on waking.

A more persistent type of headache in cases of high blood pressure begins later in the day, steadily growing worse under the pressure of work and exertion, and increased by the stagnant air of crowded rooms, to become totally disabling by the late afternoon or evening. It is accompanied by a sense of fullness and throbbing over the temples, and by dizziness and a mist before the eyes. Lying down after lunch before the pain has developed may enable the patient to do without medicines and to resume activities which he has had to give up.

Headaches are commonly associated with chronic nephritis and with anemia.

8. Organic Disease of the Brain. The least common type of headache is that which is due to actual organic disease of the brain such as meningitis, tumor of the brain, etc. Patients who have been infected with syphilis, however, commonly suffer from a chronic type of headache which may be continuous and which is often worse at night.

Treatment of Headache

This should be directed if possible to treatment of the cause. For the symptomatic relief of headaches all sorts of drugs have been tried but, for most sufferers, aspirin remains the remedy of choice. One of its drawbacks, however, is that in some persons it causes indigestion, but this can usually be overcome by taking it with some food such as half a glass of milk or with a piece of chocolate. Alternatively, soluble aspirin may prove more suitable.

Sometimes better results are obtained by giving aspirin in combination with other drugs such as caffeine or codeine, or:

Aspirin	250 mg
Phenacetin	250 mg
Codeine Phosphate ..	8 mg

Paracetamol, either alone or in combination with other drugs, suits some patients better. For tension headache chlordiazepoxide or meprobamate may be prescribed in addition.

Patent cures for headache should not be used unless they have been approved by a doctor.

DISORDERS OF SLEEP

Insomnia

The number of hours of sleep which a person requires depends largely on his age. The young child needs between ten and fourteen hours, and the average adult seven or eight. The habit of sleep, however, is very variable in different individuals, and what is a normal amount of sleep for some may be quite inadequate for others. It should also be remembered that people generally sleep more than they think they do, and that the serious evils which are commonly supposed to result from loss of sleep are generally much exaggerated.

Causes. A careful inquiry should always be made in order to discover the cause of insomnia. It may be due to some obvious external cause, but in many cases a searching physical examination will be needed, and sometimes an exploration of the mental and emotional condition of the patient as well.

1. External Causes. Insomnia may be due to disturbances from certain irritating external conditions such as the discomfort of unaccustomed noises or light, a badly ventilated room, an uncomfortable bed, with too heavy or too light bedclothes, or excessive heat or cold. The disturbing effect of cold feet in bed is often insufficiently recognized, and the bedclothes should be properly tucked in at the bottom of the bed.

2. Physical Causes

(a) *Pain.* Insomnia may be due to some obvious cause such as discomfort or pain from injury or disease.

(b) *Dietetic Faults.* A common cause is some error of the diet, such as the excessive consumption of tea, coffee or alcohol in the evening, often accompanied by too much smoking. A heavy meal in the evening, leading to flatulent distension, will often be followed by a sleepless night. On the other hand, insomnia may be caused in some persons by insufficient food. Chronic constipation is another common cause.

(c) *Fatigue.* Sleepless nights may be caused by excessive physical and mental fatigue such as may follow working late at night right up to going to bed.

(d) *Disorders of Circulation.* Defective circulation through the brain, as in chronic heart disease, often associated with high blood pressure, or defective circulation through the muscles, leading to muscular cramps. These conditions are especially seen in elderly patients with hardening of the arteries.

(e) *Fever.*

3. Mental and Emotional Unrest, due to anxiety or worry, or to emotional states of grief or fear. Such patients often aggravate their condition by worrying about the possible consequences of their insomnia, fearing that it may end in some mental disorder.

Treatment

Removal of Cause. The cause must be found and removed if this is possible.

1. Removal of external disturbances: change lights, new mattress, adjust the bedclothes, hot-water bottle or electric blanket, etc.

2. Treatment of existing physical disease or symptoms.

In persons who are fatigued from overwork, a holiday may be the best treatment, but high altitudes are usually best avoided.

3. In cases of psychological unrest, every effort should be made to discover the cause of the worry or anxiety, and the necessary adjustments made. The patient should be reassured that loss of sleep will not cause any permanent ill health, either physical or mental, and it should also be pointed out that as people get older they can do with very much less sleep than in their younger days. For cases of insomnia due to emotional causes some form of sedative is nearly always required, at least for a time.

General Measures for Prevention. Daily exercise in the fresh air is advisable, but fatigue should be avoided. Some people benefit by a quiet walk, lasting from fifteen to twenty minutes, shortly before retiring. Others prefer relaxation, or some amusement or light occupation which is neither exciting nor over-fatiguing.

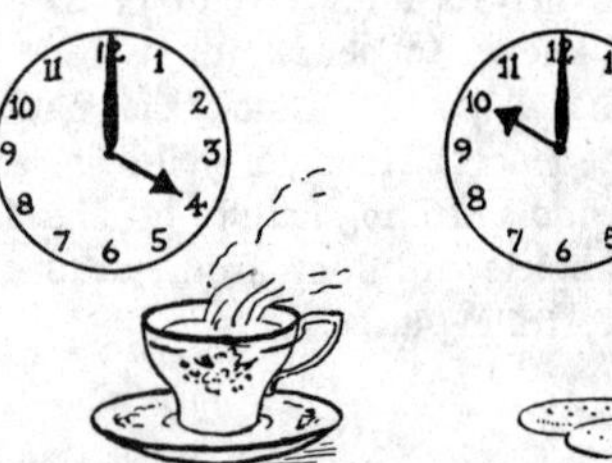
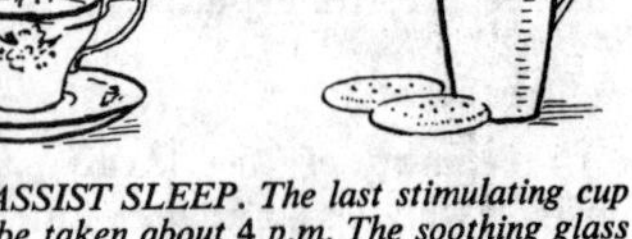

Fig. 31. *TO ASSIST SLEEP. The last stimulating cup of tea should be taken about* 4 *p.m. The soothing glass of hot milk with crackers at* 10 *p.m.*

Stimulants such as tea or coffee should not be taken within five hours of going to bed, and over-indulgence in alcohol and tobacco must be avoided. No copious drinks should be taken to cause the patient to wake up during the night to urinate.

If the insomnia results from taking insufficient food, however, a glass of hot milk or Ovaltine with a biscuit or a slice of bread and butter at bedtime may be sufficient to ensure a good sleep. Flatulent distension may be relieved by taking half a tumblerful of hot water containing a pinch of bicarbonate of soda about twenty minutes before bedtime, or chewing one or two compound magnesium trisilicate tablets.

The patient should train himself to relax physically as soon as he retires, and a hot bath taken at night is often a great help. He should preferably sleep alone in a well-ventilated quiet bedroom. The custom of reading in bed for ten or fifteen minutes is often useful and effective to induce sleep. The reading matter, however, should not be too stimulating, and should not be connected with business matters, and the bedside light should be within easy reach. In obstinate cases of insomnia, the patient may benefit from massage, which should be given after he has retired to bed.

Medicines for Sleeplessness

The above mentioned measures will often be sufficient, but if the insomnia persists, and especially in anxiety or worry, it may be necessary for the doctor to order some form of hypnotic. It should be explained, however, that taking a hypnotic does not mean that the patient will become addicted to it and unable to give it up.

Whatever hypnotic is used, it is important that a sufficiently large dose should be taken at the outset to make certain of a good sleep. This dose is then taken for a period of say, two weeks, so that the habit of sleep can be regained. The dose may then be reduced and subsequently taken every second or third night, and as soon as it is feasible it should be stopped entirely. After several good nights' rest, it is a good plan to let the patient have a single dose of the medicine at his bedside, to take later if he wakes. Large quantities, however, should never be allowed at the bedside.

The following types of sedatives are in common use.

1. **Alcohol.** In cases of mild insomnia, especially in elderly patients who are accustomed to taking a little alcohol, a small quantity of whisky, or a glass of beer taken with the evening meal, may make all the difference between a good and a bad night. Alcohol should not be used, however, by young persons, or by anyone affected with anxiety or a nervous temperament.

2. **Chloral Hydrate.** This is a very useful sedative for children which acts quickly as a rule, giving prolonged and quiet sleep. It should be given in solution in a dose of 0.6 to 1.2 grams. It is particularly valuable for occasional use, and for cases of insomnia of recent origin. For severe cases with restlessness, the dose may be repeated every two hours until sleep occurs.

3. **Paraldehyde.** Taken in doses of 5 to 10 milliliters (1 to 2 5-ml spoonsful). Owing to its strong flavor, it is best taken diluted with water, or flavored with tincture of orange. It acts quickly and has no dangerous effects on the heart or lungs, and produces no depressing effect the following morning. For these reasons it is particularly suitable for old people. Unfortunately it has the drawback of giving the breath an unpleasant odor the following day.

4. **The Barbiturates.** These are perhaps the most widely used sedatives at present. They are especially useful in insomnia arising from mental anxieties, depression, or nervous restlessness. They act best when absorbed quickly from an empty stomach, and no food should be taken for an hour before the tablets are due, since food delays their absorption. Generally they produce sound sleep without subsequent depression. They do not give rise to addiction.

They must always be prescribed by a doctor, and should never be taken except under strict medical supervision. They should not be prescribed in large quantities, and the patient should never be allowed to have the bottle at his bedside. Caution should be used if they are required for a long period, especially in cases of chronic disease of the heart, lungs or kidneys.

(a) *Phenobarbital*, often taken in doses of 30 to 60 milligrams at night. It is useful for patients who fall asleep easily, but who waken early in the morning, and is given for the insomnia associated with high blood pressure.

(b) *Pentobarbital* is a similar type of barbiturate, the effect of which wears off in three to six hours. Doses of 100 to 200 milligrams are used for those who have difficulty in getting to sleep.

(c) *Butobarbital* in doses of 100 to 200 milligrams acts quickly and is useful in milder cases of insomnia.

(d) *Cyclobarbital* in doses of 100 to 400 milligrams is taken with a warm drink shortly before retiring; it is a convenient barbiturate, inducing sleep quickly so that an hour or so later natural sleep continues; the patient wakes more refreshed than after using phenobarital, for example.

(e) *Amylobarbital* in a dose of 100 to 200 milligrams half an hour before bed-time gives a quick result in inducing sleep.

Several proprietary preparations exist of combinations of these barbiturates and are useful at the doctor's discretion for patients with irregular insomnia.

Insomnia in Children

Sufficient rest and sleep are essential for every growing child. The newly born infant should wake up only for feedings. A child of three months requires eighteen hours' sleep out of twenty-four, and a child of six months, sixteen hours. At the age of one year, the child should sleep fourteen hours a day. After this age the amount of sleep should gradually be reduced to about twelve hours by the time the child reaches the age of five years.

Causes. As with adults, sleeplessness may be due to external disturbances such as noisy surroundings, or it may be dependent on physical or mental causes. In young infants, cold, hunger, thirst, indigestion and teething are perhaps the commonest causes. In older children insomnia is often associated with rheumatism, constipation, irritation of the skin, earache, or dental troubles. The neurotic child is often a bad sleeper.

Treatment. A warm bath at night is usually of some help in insomnia. Children are often sent to bed hungry, being allowed nothing after supper for fear of digestive disturbances during the night. A warm drink such as milk, may help in producing sleep. Glucose or barley sugar should also be given and is of great value. Older children may be given a light supper.

In nervous children, much patience may be needed before a good habit of sleep is acquired. Over-fatigue and excitement in the evening must be avoided. If the child is afraid of the dark, he may be allowed to sleep with a night light or shaded lamp, and it should be explained that his fears are really without foundation. If necessary, a small dose of chloral hydrate may be given an hour before bedtime over a short period. If pain is present, children's aspirin may be given, the dosage depending on the age of the child.

Nightmares

Causes. Nightmares are apt to affect children of a nervous and imaginative disposition between the ages of three and eight, and it is uncommon for them to persist beyond the tenth year. They may appear for the first time after some emotional disturbance. They may be brought on by indigestion from a heavy meal taken late in the evening, and are not uncommon in children with enlarged tonsils and adenoids. They are often accompanied by bed-wetting.

Symptoms. Nightmares generally occur during the first three hours of sleep, and it is rare for them to recur during the same night. The child is in a state of dreaming, and suddenly sits up with a scream, in a condition of great emotional excitement. Although he may not be fully awake for some time, he slowly becomes aware of his surroundings, and finally sinks back exhausted into sleep. The same experience may be repeated for several nights in succession.

Treatment. Children who are nervous and subject to nightmares should be shielded from terrifying suggestions and ideas, and should not be told alarming stories, or watch exciting scenes on television before bedtime. They must be protected from overpressure of work, and evening excitements should be avoided. A child who has been having nightmares should be sympathetically told during the day that he has only been having a nasty dream, and that there was really nothing to be frightened of.

An improvement can often be brought about by restricting the starchy foods in the diet, and a doctor's advice should be sought before using sedatives.

Children who are afraid of the dark may be allowed to sleep with a shaded lamp or night light, but the presence of shadows on the wall may actually be the starting point of nightmares in imaginative children.

Sleep-walking

Sleep-walking (somnambulism) is an uncommon condition which rarely occurs before the age of eight. It may appear in normal children, but is usually found in association with some slight illness.

Symptoms. While still asleep, the patient gets out of bed and, usually without dressing, walks about the house or even out into the street, finally coming back to bed again. He usually avoids obstacles and may carry out various complicated actions. The following day he has no recollection of the event.

Treatment. A patient who is discovered in the act of sleep-walking should not be roughly awakened, but should be gently led back to bed. In the case of recurrent sleep-walking in a child, the habit may be prevented by tying him down lightly in bed. He should wear a belt which is made to fasten at the back. Attached to the belt is a ring through which a bandage may be passed and tied underneath the bed. A net placed over the bed will be an additional safeguard. In rooms where there is a danger of falling from a window or landing, some further precaution should be taken, such as the insertion of bars or a railing which should prevent an accident of this kind.

COMA AND CONCUSSION

Coma

By coma is meant a state of unconsciousness much deeper than ordinary sleep, from which the patient cannot be roused. The breathing is usually noisy.

Causes. There are many different causes, but among the commonest are:

INJURY TO THE SKULL, causing concussion or compression of the brain, or to some other part of the body causing hemorrhage or severe shock.

APOPLECTIC STROKE (cerebral thrombosis or hemorrhage).

ILLNESS OF LONG DURATION, of which the coma may be a symptom, e.g. diabetes, Bright's disease, epilepsy, or duodenal ulcer with internal hemorrhage.

ALCOHOLISM. This is a common cause.

POISONING, either by accident, or with suicidal intention. Among the likely poisons are opium or morphine, bromides, chloral, sleeping tablets of various sorts (especially the barbiturates), and carbolic acid. Poisoning by coal gas is another fairly common cause.

SUNSTROKE, especially in tropical climates.

Examination of Patient. In order to arrive at a decision as to what has caused a patient to become comatose, it is necessary to make the following examinations.

1. *Examine for signs of injury*, especially of the scalp or skull. Examine the ears for escape of blood. Any signs of injury should be reported to a doctor.

2. *Examine for signs of paralysis.* Lift each limb in turn and compare the two sides. A paralyzed limb may be recognized, even though the patient is unconscious from a stroke, by the 'dead' or limp manner in which it falls after being lifted up, compared with the unaffected limbs. In cases of apoplexy the face is often congested.

3. *Smell the breath for alcohol*, and always remember that though the patient may have been drinking, it is possible that he may be injured as well.

OTHER INVESTIGATIONS. If the cause of the coma is not obvious, further examinations and inquiries are therefore necessary:

4. Smell the air for escaping gas.

5. Search the room for bottles or boxes containing poisons, tablets, etc. and for hypodermic syringes.

6. Inquire if possible about any previous attacks of the same sort, and about previous illnesses or symptoms suggesting diseases such as diabetes, Bright's disease, epilepsy, high blood pressure, alcoholic excesses, drug-taking habits or suicidal tendencies.

7. A specimen of urine should be obtained if possible, and examined for sugar (as in diabetes) and albumin (as in Bright's disease). It may be necessary for a nurse or doctor to pass a catheter for this purpose.

Treatment. When a person is found in a state of unconsciousness or coma, he should be turned half over on his side, in order to prevent the tongue from falling back and causing difficulty in breathing, and also to prevent the secretions of the nose from being inhaled into the lungs. Since a comatose person is unable to swallow, no attempt should be made to feed him by mouth, and food may have to be given in some artificial way, as for example by means of a tube passed through the nose into the stomach. If and when the patient becomes conscious again, small liquid feedings containing glucose, in the proportion of 1 tablespoonful to the pint, may be given at frequent intervals, the greatest care being taken that no foo finds its way into the windpipe.

A patient who is unconscious is likely to suffer from retention of urine, which may easily pass unnoticed, and it may be necessary to pass a catheter at eight-hourly intervals. The bowels may require to be emptied by means of an enema.

See also treatment of the various causes of coma (concussion, apoplexy, poisoning, diabetes, etc.).

Concussion

Concussion is a condition of widespread paralysis of the functions of the brain, which comes on immediately after a blow on the head. Such an injury may cause a momentary squeezing of the brain with resultant slight damage to its substance. Concussion is sometimes associated with more serious conditions such as a fractured skull, or hemorrhage on to the surface of the brain.

Symptoms. At the onset the patient is unconscious and in a state of shock. In mild cases without complications the concussion lasts as a rule for only a short time, and recovery occurs within twenty-four hours. In more severe cases, however, headache may persist for some time.

Treatment. In cases of concussion due to injury to the skull or brain, the greatest care must be taken to deal thoroughly with any injury to the scalp, since it may lead to infection inside the skull. Even the smallest scalp wounds must not be neglected. Care must be taken to search for other injuries which may be present and which might be overlooked.

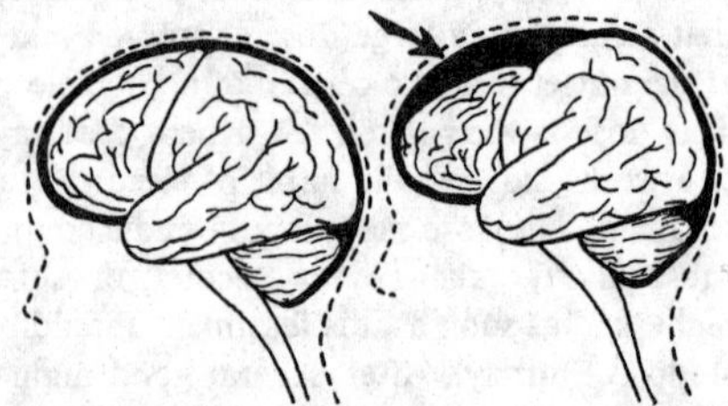

Fig. 32. *CONCUSSION. A blow on the forehead temporarily squeezes the brain tissues together and damages them.*

If, instead of being followed by a return of consciousness, the coma becomes deeper, some complication is probably developing which may require urgent surgical treatment.

In uncomplicated cases, however, after the first stage of shock has passed off, the patient should gradually become more conscious, passing through a stage of restlessness and confusion which indicates a step towards recovery.

The most important point in the early treatment of cases of head injury is rest in bed in quiet surroundings. With the reappearance of consciousness, a small soft pillow may be allowed, and a laxative should be given as soon as the patient can swallow. If the patient has not voided urine for some hours, it may be necessary to pass a catheter.

Rest in bed must be maintained until the acute symptoms such as headache and giddiness have passed off. Whatever the severity of the injury, it is important that the patient should be surrounded by an atmosphere of confidence concerning his quick recovery. If the injury has only been slight, and the patient is free from symptoms, he may be allowed to read and get up for a short time, within a week of the accident. If the headache is persistent, however, he may have to remain in bed for two or three weeks. It is often possible for the patient to return to work within a few weeks, and even in cases of severe injury, he should seldom stay away from work for a longer period than three months from the date of the injury.

After-effects of Concussion. Slight symptoms often persist for many months, but rarely cause any disability unless the patient develops a neurosis. Headache, giddiness, loss of powers of mental concentration, nervousness, irritability and sleeplessness are symptoms which commonly follow severe concussion, and they are often associated with a state of anxiety neurosis.

In such cases, the patient should be removed if possible to a hospital or nursing home and surrounded by a cheerful atmosphere of confidence and optimism regarding his recovery. He should rest in bed without making any mental effort such as reading, and may be given a mild sedative such as phenobarbital, 60 milligrams, at night. Often he will be most comfortable with his head well raised. Following a period of rest in bed, graduated exercises are of great value.

MISCELLANEOUS DISORDERS OF FUNCTION

Fainting

(Syncope)

Causes. Fainting is caused by a temporary lessening of the blood supply to the brain. It is likely to occur after long standing in in a hot stuffy atmosphere with poor ventilation. It is sometimes brought on by sudden surprises and emotions, and by the sight of blood. While it is by no means necessarily associated with serious disease, it may occur in general debility or weakness, and is often associated with anemia, internal hemorrhage, abdominal colic, fever, epilepsy (petit mal), etc. It is not, however, a typical symptom of a diseased heart.

Symptoms. A fainting attack may be preceded by a feeling of 'swimminess' in the head, sickness, and coldness of the hands and feet. Everything appears to grow dark, and the patient falls down, becoming more or less unconscious of what is going on around him. The face is pale and the pulse at the wrist is small and feeble.

Treatment. The patient should be placed on his back with his head low, and the collar loosened, in order to allow the blood to flow to the brain as quickly and as freely as possible. He must be surrounded by a good supply of fresh air. Cold water may be sprinkled on the face and smelling salts held to the nose. As soon as the patient is able to swallow, half a teaspoonful of aromatic spirits of ammonia in water or a teaspoonful of brandy may be given.

Any person who is subject to fainting attacks should be medically examined to see if there is any underlying cause for the attacks, and this, if present, should be treated. He should not wear tight clothes, and should avoid going into crowded rooms where the ventilation is inadequate.

Cramp

Cramp is a painful muscular contraction which cannot be relaxed at will. It is a common symptom and it may be due to various distinct causes.

Simple Cramp

Many normal people suffer occasionally from a sudden, violent and painful contraction in a group of muscles which appear to be drawn up into knots. It usually occurs in the calf of the leg, but it may also affect the muscles of the abdomen. It may come on while the muscles are at rest, occurring most often at night, usually as a result of overfatigue and indigestion during the day.

Treatment. It is usually necessary to remain still for as long as the attack is on. The part should be kept warm and massaged, if possible, with warm water. When the attack occurs in the leg, a handkerchief tied around the leg above the affected muscle may quickly bring relief. Nocturnal cramp may be very troublesome to deal with. A light meal only should be taken in the evening, and the tendency to cramp may sometimes be lessened by raising the foot of the bed.

Cramp Due to Swimming

This often occurs during swimming in cold water, due to overstraining a group of muscles with a temporary insufficiency of the blood supply to the muscles in question.

Heat Cramp

This is apt to occur in persons who perform muscular exercises when exposed to high temperatures, e.g. soldiers marching in hot climates, stokers on board ship, and furnace-workers. See Disorders due to Physical Agents p. 561.

Occupational Cramp

It occurs in persons who are called upon to carry out precisely co-ordinated movements in rapid succession for long periods, e.g. telegraph operators and tailors.

Cramp Due to Underlying Disease

Rheumatism may be the cause of painful muscular cramps, especially in children ('growing pains'), while cramp may also occur in the disease known as tetany which is associated with a deficiency of calcium in the blood (see Diseases of Young Children, p. 517).

A special form of cramp, due to narrowing of the arteries of the legs, with insufficient blood supply to the muscles on exertion, is known as intermittent claudication (see p. 303).

Nocturnal 'Jumps'

Some persons complain that as they are falling asleep, they are suddenly awakened by a spasmodic jumping of both legs. This may be due to a momentary anemia of the brain, and may sometimes be prevented by sleeping with the head as low as possible or by raising the foot of the bed.

The Tics

(Habit Spasms)

A tic is a constantly repeated movement or group of movements, consisting of sudden rapid involuntary twitches, always of the same nature and in the same region. A great variety of such habit spasms may occur. The usual regions affected are the face, neck and arm.

Simple tic is a common disorder of late childhood, most cases occurring between the ages of five and ten years. It often appears without obvious cause in quite healthy children who are usually highly strung and intelligent.

Causes. A tic may be regarded as a psychoneurosis, or expression of unrest in a person with a highly sensitive and possibly unstable nervous system. In such a person a tic may be brought on by any form of mental strain or by an illness, or by such conditions as eyestrain, enlarged adenoids and infected tonsils, diseased teeth, constipation, or worms.

Signs and Symptoms. The usual site of the spasm is the head or neck. A common example of a tic is the continuous blinking of an eye. The blinking may originally have been necessary to remove a speck of dust from the eye, but its persistence after the cause has been removed is abnormal, and occurs in persons of a nervous disposition. Raising and lowering the eyebrows, tossing the chin in the air, side to side movements of the mouth, sudden movements of the tongue and shrugging the shoulders are other types of tic which are commonly met with. The movements are increased by excitement and observation, and they stop during sleep. When the child reaches adult life, the condition generally disappears.

It is important to distinguish a tic from Sydenham's chorea (p. 434), the main point of difference being that in a tic the same movement is performed repeatedly.

Treatment. Recovery from a tic will usually occur within two or three months in young people, but in elderly patients in whom the symptom has existed for a long time, it may be very difficult to eradicate.

Any source of mental or emotional worry should be discovered and if possible removed. A quiet life with sufficient rest and plenty of time for sleep is equally important. In children it is unwise to draw attention to the movements or to make remarks about them, since any factor which tends to increase the self-consciousness of the child causes the tic to become uncontrollable. Children should be encouraged to control the movements and when the tick affects the limbs, much valuable re-education in control can be achieved by means of games, and by such manual occupations as carpentry, sewing, knitting, etc.

Any defects of the general health should be attended to, and a generous diet provided, together with extra milk and cod-liver oil.

Spasmodic Torticollis, or wry-neck, is usually a tic of psychological origin, and is exceedingly resistant to treatment.

Stammering and Stuttering

Stammering is a defect of speech leading to a sudden check in the utterance of words. It is due to spasm of the muscles of the lips, tongue or vocal cords. Stuttering is a rapid repetition of the initial syllables or consonants of words, and occurs most commonly with the 'explosive consonants' such as P, B, T, D, G, K. The stammerer never stammers in the speech of thought, or when talking aloud to himself, or when singing.

Cause. Stammering is not due to any changes in the nervous system or organs of articulation. It first appears as a rule about the fifth or sixth year, when reading and writing are being acquired. Boys are affected four times as often as girls. It is caused by shyness and self-consciousness, and is most likely to appear at some definite epoch of childhood or adolescence, such as going to school, or puberty. It may appear after a sudden fright, or in conditions of debility such as measles or diphtheria. It often follows the attempt to make a left-handed child use his right hand, which disturbs the speech center in the brain.

Treatment. When stammering occurs in a left-handed child who has been made to use the right hand, a return to left-handedness often leads to considerable improvement. Most children who stammer tend in any case to improve spontaneously with the passage of time. Recovery is always hastened, however, by systematic treatment, and in the course of time perseverance will almost always bring success. It is hardly necessary to say that persons with a stammer must be sympathetically treated, the most important factor in treatment being the development of confidence and self-reliance. Impatience and irritability are fatal to progress.

In many cases it will be found that faulty respiration is present, in which case the capacity of the lungs should be increased by regular breathing exercises (p. 196). The patient should then speak, read or recite in a large room slowly and deliberately, using a loud and full voice, and during speech the chest must always be kept well filled with air. When he comes to a word on which he tends to stammer, he should direct his attention more to the vocalization of the subsequent vowel sound than to the articulation of the initial consonant, e.g. in the word BAT, his energies should be concentrated on the final syllable AT, at the same time raising his voice, as if to make it carry further. For many patients singing exercises and gymnastics are very useful.

Lessons should be short rather than long, but in all cases reading exercises must be carried out daily. The best results are to be obtained by an experienced teacher, but whether this is possible or not, the patient should practice at home alone in a large room. Speaking through a megaphone, or in time with a metronome, are also useful devices. There is often a good deal of difficulty at first in persuading the stammerer to carry out the principles of his teaching in his daily life. (See also Speech Therapy, p.189.)

Hiccup

(Hiccough)

Causes. Hiccup is due to a sudden spasmodic contraction of the diaphragm, the muscular partition which separates the contents of the chest from those of the abdomen. It may be due to various causes.

1. Gastric causes. In most cases hiccup is a temporary condition associated with some form of dyspepsia. Thus, it may occur from sudden overfilling of the stomach with food or drink, and from irritation of the stomach with highly spiced foods, pepper, pickles, condiments, etc. It may occur as a symptom of gastritis (especially alcoholic gastritis), enteritis, etc. In children it may be associated with teething and with worms.

2. Nervous causes. In hysterical subjects it may result from fright, shock, or other sudden emotion.

3. From irritation of the diaphragm, as in diaphragmatic pleurisy, and in acute abdominal disease such as peritonitis.

4. As a terminal symptom of chronic disease. Persistent hiccup, which exhausts the patient, may be a terminal symptom of chronic nephritis with uremia, or cirrhosis of the liver, or of serious disease of the bowel, such as intestinal obstruction.

Treatment. Simple hiccup may often be relieved by holding the breath for as long as possible, or by pressure on the chest. One of the most effective remedies is heavy pressure on the collar bones. It may sometimes be stopped by inducing an attack of sneezing, or by vomiting. Ammonia, smelling salts, ether, or spirits of chloroform may be inhaled with beneficial effect.

In cases which are due to gastric disturbances, a teaspoonful of sodium bicarbonate in a tumbler of water may be effective by relieving flatulence, and the same effect may be produced by carminatives such as half a teaspoonful of aromatic spirits of ammonia in water, or two tablespoonsful of peppermint water. In severe cases it may be necessary for the stomach to be washed out through a stomach tube with a solution of one teaspoonful of sodium bicarbonate to the pint of water, as hot as can be comfortably borne.

Myasthenia Gravis

In this disease the muscles tend to become abnormally fatigued, so that they become incapable of sustained activity. In the earlier stages a short period of rest is sufficient to restore the affected muscles to their normal condition, but finally they fail to recover even after prolonged rest, and they remain permanently paralyzed. The disease affects particularly those muscles which are in constant use, especially those which are responsible for the movements of the eyes, eyelids, face, lower jaw and neck. It is equally common in women and men.

Causes. The biochemical changes essential for transmission of impulses from nerve to muscle fail to function properly and the muscle cannot respond.

It is thought by some research workers that the thymus gland produces a substance which prevents the transference of these cholinergic impulses from nerve to muscle and in many patients the thymus gland is enlarged and a small tumor may be present.

Symptoms. The onset is usually insidious, the commonest early symptoms being dropping of the upper eyelids and double vision. Affection of the muscles of the jaw makes it increasingly difficult for the patient to masticate his food without frequently stopping, and in severe cases the mouth hangs open. Speaking becomes difficult as the muscles of the lips and tongue become affected. The muscles of the neck become very easily fatigued so that the head tends to fall forwards or backwards, and in the later stages the patient may not be able to raise his head from the pillow.

Treatment. The failure of transmission of impulses at the myoneural junction can be corrected by drugs known as anticholinesterases. Too large doses can reverse the pattern, so dosage has to be very carefully assessed.

Pyridostigmine bromide is the drug most frequently used, one or two tablets (60 milligrams each) being taken every three to six hours to suit the patient's needs. Neostigmine bromide is also used but its effects do not last so long.

Injections of neostigmine are often effective but should be reserved for special occasions when the patient particularly wishes to be relieved of symptoms for several hours.

Referred Pain

Referred or displaced pain is not a disorder of the nervous system, but is due to the patient being aware of pain in a part of the body other than that which is infected or injured but which is served by the same nerve carrying the pain sensations. In certain cases it may even be felt along another branch of the main nerve trunk.

This disparity may misdirect attention to a part of the body where there is no disorder while the sick area may be overlooked. It is therefore a very important factor in diagnosis. The following are some of the commoner instances of referred pain.

Abdominal Pain which is obviously not due to a disorder of the bowels may be referred from the chest (as in pneumonia or pleurisy), or from the spine (as in tuberculosis, or arthritis of the spine, or growths on the spinal cord).

NEURITIS OF THE ARM OR FINGERS may be due to the pressure of a cervical rib.

EARACHE may be due to tonsillitis, pharyngeal growths, herpes, or influenza where the ear is not directly involved.

GIRDLE PAINS, apart from spinal disease, commonly occur in pelvic cancer, in pellagra, and in the tabes dorsalis of syphilis.

SCALP TENDERNESS may arise from diabetes mellitus, headache, rheumatism, or malaria.

NEURALGIA may have its source in eye disorders such as astigmatism, iritis, or glaucoma, or in inflammation of the tongue, or in decayed teeth.

PAIN IN THE LEFT SHOULDER may be referred pain from some form of heart disease, while pain in the right shoulder may have its source in gall-bladder affections.

See Fig. 23 in Diseases of the Digestive System, p. 380.

PSYCHIATRIC DISORDERS

The human mind can be studied in two ways. An investigator can ask a person for an account of his inner experiences or he can observe the behavior and reactions of the person in various situations. The scientific study of information obtained by either method constitutes 'psychology.'

Everyday experience suggests that either method will show that people differ widely. In fact, wide differences are normal; that is, wide limits have to be set to include the majority of people. But what is regarded in everyday life as 'normal,' however, is liable to be much narrower since it is usually a matter of convention and often merely a reflection of prejudice, varying from generation to generation and from community to community.

In general, psychiatric illness exists when these conventional bounds of normality of inner experience or of behavior are exceeded, and when definite inconvenience is thereby caused, or seems likely to be caused, to either the person concerned or to those around him. For example, inner experiences such as fear before a possible car smash, or apprehension before a dental appointment, are common and accepted as normal. Fear and apprehension without a conventionally acceptable cause or with a cause too trifling for the intensity of feeling, may prompt the sufferer to seek medical advice. Again, to be suspicious of strange men is at times a wise precaution for females. To be suspicious of all men all the time is excessive but the inconvenience may be balanced by the pleasure of feeling such a center of attraction. However, if public accusations follow that all the men around her have designs on her virtue, then the neighbors of such a lady are likely to press her to seek medical advice.

The study and treatment of all such personally or socially inconvenient forms of experience or behavior is termed 'psychiatry.'

DEVELOPMENT AND FUNCTIONING OF THE MIND

Learning in the Earliest Weeks

It is characteristic of human beings that, in the developing phase of their lives, they are constantly doing different things to satisfy their curiosity. This is seen very early in life and is certainly present from soon after birth. Combined with it is a very great ability to store past experience. Memories which give a framework of reference to new experience are gradually accumulated and this at the same time provides an increasing store of past actions from which can be chosen those which are appropriate to present needs.

An action which provides some benefit tends to be repeated and retained whereas one which results in nothing beneficial or even in something unpleasant tends to be dropped. Benefit here means either the production of a sensation apparently pleasurable in itself, or the relief of an apparently unpleasant sensation. From fairly soon after birth, a kind of transmitted pleasure from the parents becomes an additional source of benefit, and their transmitted disapproval a source of unpleasantness.

Development of Skills

The ability to put the hand into the mouth is acquired because some of the random movements of the arms result in a hand arriving there. The pleasure of sucking encourages this action and it becomes progressively more easily and certainly carried out. Somewhat later, when the co-ordinated activity of the diaphragm, larynx, tongue and mouth is being tried out, various noises of many kinds are produced. Sooner or later 'Da' or 'Pa' occurs when the father is present. If he is American his evident pleasure encourages the infant to repeat 'Da' rather than 'Pa.' If he is French, however, 'Pa' is encouraged. Ultimately 'Dada' or 'Papa,' according to nationality, is achieved, and later still, by ever greater refinement of the process, recognizable English or French is spoken.

Development of Social Sense

It would appear, therefore, that pleasure or its opposite have a completely predominant influence on the infant's activities, with the complication that some forms of pleasure or discomfort arise from within himself and others derive from his parents. Sooner or later these sources diverge. Initially they coincide; the infant feels hungry, cries and his mother gladly feeds him; her pleasure is transmitted to him, increasing his enjoyment.

Later, however, some compromise takes place between his desire to eat whenever he is awake and his mother's desire for a rather more regular schedule. Generally, the mother has her way and modification of his 'natural' desire occurs in response to parental influence. The external source of pleasure or displeasure has prevailed over the internal one. Weaning results in an even greater curb on the infant's 'natural' tendencies. Totally different and unfamiliar foodstuffs are presented and gradually replace the familiar milk. In the security of his mother's communicated pleasure when the infant eats them, they become in the end a source of enjoyment in themselves.

Rudimentary 'Right' and 'Wrong.' It seems likely that this kind of parentally-induced change of behavior represents the rudimentary beginning of conceptions of 'right' and 'wrong.' Until very much later in life, 'right' is what pleases the parents and 'wrong' what displeases them.

This becomes even more apparent in the great modification of spontaneous behavior that occurs with regard to bladder and bowels. Initially, a full bladder or bowel is immediately relieved. Sometimes, however, generally in the second year of life, parental pleasure begins to show when the child is dry or clean and displeasure when wet or dirty. Sooner or later these parental reactions become a sufficient inducement for the unfamiliarity of a full bladder or bowel to be tolerated for longer and longer periods and for their evacuation into a strange pot instead of the familiar diaper to be performed. 'Good' and 'bad' are terms that are more positively applied now; partly because speech has developed to some extent and these actual words may be used, and partly because many parents are excessively emotionally concerned about the speed or slowness with which their children acquire toilet training. Control of these functions is considered 'good,' and lack of control 'bad.'

Development of Emotional Expression

Simultaneously, other types of behavior tend to become associated with parental approval or disapproval, and they, too, are classified as 'good' or 'bad.' This applies to the extreme of behavior which is aroused by apparent frustration of some desire.

Rage and Anger. At first, when displeased, the infant reacts instantly but the reaction is unco-ordinated; he strenuously roars, waves his arms and kicks. Later, as more purposeful activities are acquired, these are also enlisted to express his rage. The acquisition of teeth is of importance for the expression of rage or aggression; they are a more effective means of grappling with the world than the naked mouth; they can inflict pain; they can apparently destroy by chewing and swallowing. In adult life, teeth are ground with rage, under extreme provocation. Other activities such as co-ordinated hitting or kicking are recruited and they too become subject to parental sanctions.

As activities acquire the coloring of right or wrong, they can be used if necessary to express aggression by flouting the parental training. Thus, anger can be expressed by spitting out food instead of swallowing it dutifully, by wetting or by evacuating the bowels in the wrong place or at the wrong time, or by not wetting or not evacuating or by being willfully independent or by being irritatingly more childish or infantile than is habitual.

The genital regions generally become included in the right-wrong system. Their stimulation appears to give the infant pleasure and if he or she succeeds in finding a way of doing this on his or her own, by rocking or rubbing or handling, parental alarm may be aroused by this infantile masturbation, and the activity rapidly acquires a strong toning of 'wrong.'

Prohibitions vs Tolerance. There is a wide variation in the intensity with which all these activities are felt to be 'good' or 'bad.' Some children learn more quickly or readily, some parents teach more ardently, and the strength of the children's impulses vary. Extremes of prohibitions rather than of tolerance are likely to produce biases in development which may play a part in the production of neurotic reactions later in life. This may be because in general a parent who is over-enthusiastic in prohibiting and controlling is an anxious parent, and the communication of his or her anxiety is more dominant than the training.

The Growth of Sexual Awareness

At some time, roughly between four and six years of age, socially determined differences in emotional attitudes according to the sex of a child become established. A boy is 'Mommy's little boy' on the one hand, while at the same time he is encouraged to feel himself similar to and as one with his father. A girl is 'Daddy's little girl,' while being encouraged to feel similar to and as one with her mother.

Intense rivalries with the parent of the same sex may develop and the death or destruction of this rival may, in imagination, be thought of as leading to exclusive possession of the parent of the opposite sex. If this rivalry is unusually intense, then feelings of guilt may be aroused; the more so if aggressive feelings have come to be regarded as excessively bad.

These feelings may become associated with the anatomical differences between the sexes, which have become apparent to the child from observation of his parents or brothers and sisters. The boy may fear the loss of his penis, which would turn him into a girl, in punishment for wishing to supplant his father; and the girl may fear that she has already been punished and has lost an imaginary male organ. These early feelings and fears may be reawakened in later life in relationship to the opposite sex and then play an important part in producing neurotic illness.

The presence of brothers or sisters, younger or older, provides another source of rivalry and possible guilt feelings from their imagined elimination. The reawakening of such feelings later in life may contribute to neuroses in connection with one's equals or with one's children, when they are felt to be rivals in some way.

The Pattern is Set. By the age of about five or six years the broad pattern of right and wrong as acquired from the parents has become part of the child's personality. His basic emotional activities—those connected with the gratification or frustration of pleasure, with the excretory habits, with the aggressive impulse and with the male or female role will have been established. Formal education and widening social contacts in subsequent years merely modify or intensify and make more complex the patterns derived from the primary family group.

AN ACCOUNT OF MENTAL FUNCTIONING

How Emotions Influence Actions

It is customary to assume that human beings are reasonable and that they act logically, forming sound judgments of situations and persons. But in actual fact, equally 'reasonable' people often sincerely disagree about what happens before their eyes—a fact made use of by lawyers in courts. Two apparently 'reasonable' people often find themselves unable to convince each other of their own 'reasonable' and 'obvious' points of view.

Sometimes it is easy to recognize that behavior is affected by what is felt emotionally. Even so, it is not always admitted that strong emotions of pity, anger, fear or love can affect judgment very greatly. Indeed, it is conventionally assumed that these emotions are firmly under rational or conscious control. Equally, it is pleasant to think that when anger or contempt is felt, these feelings are justified by the circumstances. Such a view of emotional life is not only seriously incomplete; it is quite misleading.

Duality of Feelings. At times anger is felt towards people for whom it may be asserted there is only love. Sometimes feelings of irritability arise which are not to be accounted for by the circumstances in which they occur. A sudden outburst of temper may show that feelings are not always in control. 'I didn't mean to do it' or 'I didn't mean to say it' may be the excuse, but nevertheless it happened.

The concept of the rational man, in full control of his feelings, conscious of all his motives, and able to bring reason to bear in the face of all his difficulties, is comforting rather than true. But if we acknowledge that a great deal of mental functioning is neither rational nor conscious, we can gain a clearer understanding of human behavior.

Identification and Conscience

In the process of growing up each person learns to live with both the civilized demands of society and the primitive drives and feelings which give form to early behavior. The difficulty in coming to terms with these very different demands is reflected in mental functioning.

Some impulses, such as greed, destructiveness and certain sexual drives, are often unacceptable to society. But for the young child 'society' is the family—parents or guardian, brothers or sister. Behavior is strongly influenced by this early society. Often attitudes and actions will seem to be modeled on very close relatives, especially when they are loved and admired and there is a wish to follow their code of conduct. This process, which takes place largely unconsciously, is called 'identification.' But identification does not only occur with the pleasing or good aspects of our relatives but also with their forbidding aspects as well; those aspects which can instill fear, punish, or threaten with retribution.

Consciously, this process of identification can be felt as 'conscience,' as if there is something inside which tells whether what is done is 'right' or 'wrong,' 'good' or 'bad.'

Repression and Reaction Formation

Where greed, destructiveness and sexual drives are felt to be unacceptable either to society or to 'conscience' they can sometimes be controlled by conscious effort. At other times, however, the existence of such impulses is not even consciously admitted, especially if they are particularly strong or potentially frightening. In such cases it is said that these impulses are 'repressed.'

The value of repression is that it permits conformity to the needs and demands of society, as well as inner standards, while preserving a feeling of safety from impulses, emotions or wishes which might otherwise be disturbing or dangerous. But sometimes, when forbidden feelings are exceptionally strong, a person may go to the opposite extreme to avoid expressing them. For example, he may react to someone whom he hates by being excessively polite and by showing him a deference which goes far beyond ordinary social politeness. This process, in which one conspicuously adopts an attitude which is the very reverse of the unconscious one, is called 'reaction formation.'

Projection and Displacement

There is a form of behavior in which people disguise, for example, their own destructive impulses by a noisy opposition to some special form of cruelty yet all the while wishing to see the practitioner of that cruelty himself savagely punished. This tendency to attack in others feelings or attitudes which one fears to find in oneself is called projection, and is one of the commonest forms of preserving an internal sense of comfort. It is always easier to see 'badness,' destructiveness or rapacity in others than it is to see these tendencies in oneself.

Often, of course, these projected feelings arise only within oneself and may be worlds away from the real feelings or attitudes of the person who is attacked.

Displacement. Sometimes, one feels endangered by a person one dare not attack. In such a case one may turn from the object of hatred to someone else to whom it is safer to show such feelings. This is often a conscious process, as it is when the unjust strictures of the boss are suffered without protest and it is later 'taken out' on the office boy. But a similar process can occur when one does not wish to recognize the true source of displeasure. The henpecked husband who does not recognize his anger with his wife may well kick the cat instead. In such an instance his choice of animal may not be entirely a matter of chance!

Regression and Denial

When a person has to meet situations of danger and difficulty he often longs to return to an earlier period of life which was free from such dangers. In a painful adolescence a youth may behave as a little boy who has no adolescent anxieties to face. Sometimes, when one has a cold or when things are not going as well as they might at work, the solicitude of an indulgent wife or mother may be welcomed. A hot-water bottle can be taken to bed and 'mothering,' as it were, allowed. This return in behavior to an earlier stage of development is called 'regression' and it is often an unconscious mechanism. It is seen at its most striking in some forms of psychiatric illness.

Denial. Another way of dealing with unpleasant reality is simply to deny its existence. The custom of having an elaborate reception after a funeral helps to deny the painful nature of the occasion. 'Denial' is particularly easy to observe in children. In children's games a boy may pretend to be a great warrior and conqueror, and so deny the essential weaknesses of childhood and the feelings of insecurity that go with them. Equally, wild animals in the form of toys may become pets, so that their frightening aspects are denied. And a little girl with a doll may behave as if that doll were her child, and so deny her inability to be grown-up and have a baby like her mother.

Defense Mechanisms. All these mechanisms of defense against unpleasant or frightening feelings will be met again, both in the succeeding section and in the section on the types of psychiatric illness. All the mechanisms of defense have not been discussed; those which are less easy to see in 'normal' people and easier to detect in ill patients have been reserved for later discussion.

Ambivalence

It will be clear from this brief account of mental functioning that every individual is trying to deal with opposing forces. This conflict of opposites is seen when contradictory impulses—such as love and hate—coexist. The tendency to hurt as well as to love and preserve may often be recognized in any human relationship. This coexistence of conflicting tendencies is technically known as 'ambivalence,' and, while it is universal, it is seen at its most intense in certain psychiatric illnesses.

ABNORMAL MENTAL FUNCTIONING

The mechanisms just described serve, quite literally, to preserve peace of mind. Sometimes, of course, they fail to prevent unpleasant tensions, which are then experienced as anxiety. But anxiety can be avoided by the operation of these mechanisms—identification, repression, projection, etc.—to a degree uncommon in the normal person.

Lost Memory. For example, a very painful period of one's life may sometimes be blotted from memory by wholesale 'repression.' A young woman, painfully crossed in love, may lose her memory not only for the event but for the whole period of her life concerned with it. In such a case her last recollections may be of a time of life when she felt happy and secure, and she may have no knowledge of her subsequent career.

Excessive Guilt. In 'identification,' the threatening or punishing aspects of the person with whom we identify may seem so strong that we feel as if we ourselves are 'bad' inside. This kind of excessive guilt, a feeling of great wickedness, is seen at its most extreme in some forms of depression and may be a feature in the sort of suicide which occurs when a person feels he doesn't deserve to live any longer. But here again the real accusation of 'badness' is against the person with whom we identify, though it cannot be allowed to be felt as such. Something of an opposite nature occurs in 'projection.'

Delusions and Hallucinations. In 'projection' our own badness is attributed to someone else, not to ourselves. Such badness is often aggressive feelings or forbidden sexual ones.

In some forms of psychiatric illness, projection can be so marked that the patient feels persecuted by the wickedness and malevolence of his supposed enemy. It can take the form of a delusion, that is, a false belief which is not open to reason and which cannot be accounted for by the prevailing social or cultural conditions. Sometimes projection takes the form of an hallucination. An hallucination is a perception of something which is not really there; a vision, a voice, a touch, a smell or an internal sensation. If, for example, a patient is feeling that he is a very wicked or a bad person, he may hear a voice telling him this, so that his wickedness appears to originate from without.

Other mechanisms are easily recognized in different forms of psychiatric illness and will be discussed in the appropriate sections.

THE CAUSES OF PSYCHIATRIC ILLNESS

Illness is generally the result of a number of different factors operating together rather than of a single cause. For example, an illness such as pneumonia may be regarded as an infection of the lungs by bacteria, but mere contact with such organisms does not necessarily lead to pneumonia. A person's inherited susceptibility to chest infection, his own acquired resistance to the bacteria and his general state of bodily health may all influence the result. In addition, his body's reaction to the infection may modify the severity of the illness.

Similarly, the causes of a psychiatric illness may include an immediate precipitating cause, emotional or physical, an inherited liability to emotional disorder, and the susceptibility which a person may develop in his own lifetime. The nature of the illness will depend on all these factors and also on the individual personality.

Inherited Influences

These are transmitted through certain structures in the germ cells of the mother and father. They are independent of the parents' influence on the developing child. The inherited characteristics may be tendencies to develop particular illnesses or a general greater-than-average liability to emotional disorder. In very few conditions is the inherited factor the chief cause, and types of psychiatric illness in which all blood-relatives are affected are very rare. Unaffected persons from an affected family, however, may sometimes transmit the tendency to their children.

The majority of psychiatric illnesses occur without any pronounced inherited contribution and most children born of psychiatrically ill parents do not inherit the condition.

Influence of Personality and Psychological Development

Everyone knows that members of any given family may have similar personalities and temperaments, and that in some families there is a common tendency to be 'high strung.' This can be partly accounted for by truly inherited traits, as above. But perhaps even more important is the influence which members of the family have on each other's development. The effects on developing personality of family relationships and, later, of wider social contacts, have been described.

Varying Responses. Different people respond to the same situation in different ways. They show tendencies to react quickly or slowly, aggressively or submissively, in a hostile or friendly manner, suspiciously or trustingly according to their inherited qualities and the ways in which they have learned from their experience. Most people will respond at different times in each of these and many other ways. Often the personality and the way it has developed will decide the nature of the response as much as the person or incident arousing it. Often a person's responses will be consistent in that he will react similarly to a particular type of situation as it recurs. For example, he may show particular respect or particular rebelliousness in the face of authority. He may show undue aggressiveness or undue submissiveness when he feels uncertain of himself.

Recurring Difficulties. Everyone meets situations which for him are peculiarly difficult to deal with. Often he will not be fully aware of the nature of the difficulty and, in that case, the difficulty will tend to recur with unpleasant emotional accompaniments, the source of which is unrecognized. If this experience is severe or prolonged or leads to difficulty in managing his life, he will be said to be suffering from an emotional disorder. He will be aware of repeated and apparently unfounded feelings of anxiety, fear, guilt or depression. Such difficulties may begin in early life, and persist unrecognized and unsolved only to be encountered once more in later years when the individual concerned is under stress.

Immediate Emotional Causes

It is widely recognized in medicine that emotional stress may lead to illnesses, physical or emotional. Overwork and disturbed sleep are often blamed, probably too often. Prolonged and severe worries, shocks, bereavements and disappointments often contribute, as may debilitating physical illnesses.

As described above, certain persons are likely to face the same difficulties in a given set of circumstances over and over again. When these circumstances arise they stir up the unpleasant emotions associated with them. In consequence they may be dealt with unrealistically or unconstructively with the result that the original difficulty may be prolonged and intensified. This then is a type of 'cause' arising in the environment which operates more because of the individual's personal difficulty in his emotional life than because of any difficulties inherent in the situation. Since no situation difficult in itself is apparent, it may seem to the person concerned, or to the observer, that there is no reason for the emotional discomfort experienced. His reactions to the situation may thus appear inexplicable and irrational.

Physical Factors

Psychiatric disturbances occur as an occasional accompaniment to physical illness. Delirium following high fever or poisoning is a well-known example. It is usually a short-lived disturbance and clears up when the physical condition improves. Physical illnesses which affect the brain, such as injury or encephalitis (inflammation of the brain as a result of infection), are particularly prone to disturb its function. In most cases there is no permanent damage and recovery takes place.

Injury, Old Age, Tumors. Sometimes damage to the brain occurs as a result of various diseases or injury, and may lead to long-lasting or permanent psychiatric abnormality. In old age the brain, in common with other parts of the body, wears out and the structure of the nervous tissue deteriorates. Failing memory, diminished power of thought and, later, confusion about places and people and time usually ensue gradually. When severe this deterioration is referred to as dementia. Similar mental deterioration may occur as a result of other sorts of brain damage, e.g. that due to diseases of the blood vessels, to tumors, or occasionally following serious head injuries. A rare group of illnesses occurs where dementia takes place early—they are therefore called presenile dementias. In some of these disorders heredity plays an important part.

Chemical Disorders. Disorders of function of the chemical and hormonal processes of the body may result in psychiatric disorder. Certain rare types of psychiatric illness have been shown to be due to such chemical abnormality and it is likely that other illnesses, whose cause is at present unknown, are due in part to comparable disorders (see p. 458).

THE TYPES OF PSYCHIATRIC ILLNESS

THE PSYCHONEUROSES

Anxiety and the Anxiety State

On pp. 448-49 some forms of psychological defences were described. These serve to prevent various mental conflicts from resulting in the unpleasant state of tension technically termed 'anxiety.'

'Anxiety' covers all degrees of fear from mild apprehension to uncontrolled panic. Its sources are, frequently, unconscious. Paradoxically, this is still true even in the so-called phobias, which will be discussed below under the heading of Anxiety Hysteria.

Causes. Most people have experienced anxiety in some degree, though not everyone is equally prone to it. It is not known for certain why this is so. Genetic factors may have a bearing, and it seems fairly well-established that certain events in childhood play a significant part. It is possible that these two factors are complementary. Whatever its more distant origins, anxiety is often precipitated by some form of current stress. In some cases, the stress will be self-evident, as in loss of one's home through fire or flood, serious physical illness, financial catastrophe, difficulties in marriage, threatened or actual loss of employment and indeed in all circumstances where the individual feels threatened or insecure. In other cases the stress will be less obvious, and the significance of unconscious factors altogether greater.

Clinical Features. Anxiety may be acute (may begin suddenly) or chronic (prolonged). It may also start gradually. Often it is very short-lived, though it can and does recur. It may produce certain secondary effects, although these are not pronounced in the milder forms. Restlessness is an example, and varies considerably. The same is true of impaired concentration and disturbed sleep.

Physical changes, when they occur, are temporary and reversible. Thus, the pulse-rate may rise and is sometimes experienced as palpitations. The blood pressure may increase. Occasionally, there is a tendency to diarrhea or to the frequent passing of urine. Other bodily changes are often present, but clinically they are not of any great importance.

Treatment. Short-lived anxiety, unless severe, rarely calls for treatment. But long-standing anxiety often brings a patient to his doctor. The doctor may prescribe a sedative or a tranquilizer, or may discuss with the patient whatever difficulties may seem to underlie the condition. Sometimes he may refer the patient to a specialist for more detailed psychotherapy.

Simple uncomplicated anxiety of any considerable duration, however, is not often seen by the psychiatrist. It is almost always complicated by further symptoms, usually of an hysterical or obsessional kind (see below).

Hysteria

There are two main clinical kinds of hysteria: anxiety hysteria, in which the patient develops phobias; and conversion hysteria, in which the patient develops bodily symptoms. In addition, there are certain striking disturbances of consciousness which are more difficult to classify. They are described under the heading of 'dissociation hysteria.'

Anxiety Hysteria

In this condition the anxiety relates to an external situation, object or person. But unlike the anxiety present in the face of a very real danger, the fear in anxiety hysteria seems irrational. Thus there may be fear of open spaces, streets, elevators, subways, water, spiders, or children, to name only a few examples. Such irrational fears are termed 'phobias.'

The apparently irrational nature of these fears springs from the fact that the sources of the anxiety remain unconscious, while the fear is displaced from the original object or objects on to a relatively harmless substitute. But the choice of object or situation is itself significant since it represents, in a symbolic form, the original dangerous object or person.

Causes. A man afraid of a crowded subway train may be unable to face his fear of a tangled domestic situation from which he can see no escape. A modest girl of strict upbringing may be unable to allow herself to recognize the temptations which strangers represent for her, and thus be confined to her home by an apparently irrational fear of streets. These are simplified examples; as a rule, the determinants of the phobia are rather more complicated.

A dangerous *internal* impulse is sometimes symbolized by a phobia. A man who is afraid of knives may, in this way, be expressing his alarm at his own destructive feelings.

But whatever the phobia symbolically represents, its success as a defence rests in the opportunity it gives the patient to avoid the apparently threatening situation and so maintain some peace of mind. But the price the patient pays may be heavy. For while a patient with a fear of subway trains may manage perfectly well as long as he travels by bus, a patient with a severe street phobia may be seriously incapacitated.

Conversion Hysteria

Just as in anxiety hysteria inadmissible unconscious factors are symbolized by a phobia, so, in conversion hysteria, they are symbolized by bodily symptoms. The anxiety is now said to be 'converted,' that is, its sources are represented by the bodily change. Usually, this form of hysteria is a more successful defense against anxiety than the phobia; indeed, in some cases of conversion obvious anxiety may be entirely absent.

Clinical Features. The forms which conversion may take are as limitless as the varieties of phobia. Very striking disabilities such as blindness, deafness or paralysis are less common than they were fifty years ago, but they still occur from time to time. On the other hand, hysterical loss of voice, muscle weakness, pains of all kinds, headaches and disturbances of sensation such as numbness still occur with the greatest frequency. An inevitable result of this is that some patients are referred to general hospitals for specialist medical and surgical advice, where investigations fail to reveal a physical basis for the disorder.

It used to be thought that hysteria of this kind occurred almost entirely in women. This idea originated from the notion of the ancient Greeks that the symptoms of hysteria were due to a wandering of the womb or 'hysteros.' Today it is recognized that hysteria is common in men.

Symbolic Paralysis. A hypothetical example may help to demonstrate some of the symbolism to be found in conversion hysteria.

An attractive young woman whose mother had recently died had to cope unaided with a tyrannical and bedridden father. Her sense of duty allows her no protest in spite of an intense longing for a young man whom she often meets during the course of her daily shopping. One morning she wakes to find both legs paralyzed. The unconscious conflict between desire and hostility has been converted into a bodily symptom which has three immediate results. First, she can no longer meet the young man she admires. Secondly, she can no longer care for her father since she is now unable to climb the stairs. Thirdly, her sexual conflict is symbolized by the paralysis.

This case is oversimplified, but it may serve to illustrate not only the process of symbolization but also the gain from the illness which results from the production of symptoms. This so-called 'secondary gain' explains why conversion hysteria is not always easy to cure.

Dissociation Hysteria

This group of conditions is closely allied to conversion hysteria. The main difference is that, in dissociation, the disturbance is one of consciousness while in conversion the disturbance is bodily.

To this category belong certain 'dream states,' somnabulism or sleep-walking, massive loss of memory, wandering from one town to another with no recollection (fugues) of the journey, and the very rare cases of 'multiple personality.' In these remarkable, rare cases a man may live part of his life in an apparently ordered way, without any knowledge on his part that he lives the rest of his life in an entirely different way, perhaps in a different place and under a different name. In fiction the best-known example is Stevenson's 'Dr. Jekyll and Mr. Hyde,' but there are a number of startling though authentic cases on record.

In all forms of dissociation a whole area of the patient's mental life which he does not wish to recognize is excluded from consciousness.

The Hysterical Personality

A large number of people, who cannot necessarily be regarded as psychiatrically ill and who may never develop hysterical symptoms, show certain personality traits which together constitute what is known as the 'hysterical personality.'

These people are often said to be emotionally shallow, able to form impulsive and fickle relationships but rarely ones of a lasting or deeply felt kind. They are often sexually capricious or frigid. They are said to be fond of the limelight and tend to dramatize their actions and relationships. Where these traits are sufficiently pronounced to interfere seriously with the patient's life, treatment may be called for.

The Obsessional Neurosis

Unlike hysteria, the major disturbance in obsessional neurosis is of thought, word or deed, so that the patient feels compelled repeatedly to think certain thoughts or perform certain actions. In each case the symptom is determined by unconscious factors, and often seems perverse, alien or absurd to the conscious mind.

The obsessional symptom is characteristically recurrent, occurs against the patient's conscious wishes, and cannot be dismissed by an act of will. These features distinguish the obsession from all other forms of pre-occupation.

Obsessional Thoughts. There are countless varieties of obsessional thoughts. There may be disturbing ruminations of killing a loved one, or of spreading infection or poisoning people. Such thoughts occasion a great deal of guilt. Elaborate defenses may be involved in a constant fight to prevent any such thought from being translated into action. But sometimes the thoughts concerned seem trivial or even meaningless. In such cases the trivial thoughts may sometimes occupy the patient more and more until, occasionally, more important thoughts are virtually excluded. In some cases the thoughts take the form of unwanted philosophical speculations, such as 'Why am I?' or 'What is God?' Sometimes thoughts appear in flagrant contradiction of the patient's conscious attitudes. A religious man, for example, may feel plagued by blasphemous ideas, and a woman who prides herself on her purity may find herself preoccupied with obscene thoughts.

Sometimes the thoughts refer to recent actions. The patient may find himself constantly wondering whether or not he has turned off a gas tap, locked a door or switched off a light, even when he knows perfectly well that he has done so. In other cases the thought of doing some definite and purposeful act may be followed immediately by the thought of doing its opposite. Such a condition may be characterized by extreme indecision.

Obsessional Speech. Some people are obsessed by words rather than by thoughts. A man may find himself compelled to mutter an obscene, trivial or frightening word, and then feel very embarrassed in case he has been overheard. More rarely, he may shout. As with all obsessions, a conscious fight against these activities results in anxiety which may be very considerable.

Compulsive Actions. When we consider compulsive actions, we find them equally varied. The patient may feel compelled to remember every single event of the day and to record it in a diary, even when he feels the task overwhelmingly beyond him and stays up half the night in a vain endeavor to complete his notes. Or he may find himself compelled to write on lavatory walls, to his continued astonishment, guilt and disapproval. Sometimes he has to touch a series of objects, often in a carefully organized manner and order. Such activities may become so involved and elaborate that his life is seriously dislocated by them.

Although such compulsive actions may remain isolated they are often built up into complicated rituals. A woman may have to dress in a certain order, have everything 'just so,' and may take several hours to get the seam of her nylons straight.

Guilt is a striking feature of obsessional neurosis. It explains the constant need to eliminate objectionable thoughts, to check and recheck whether or not one has done any damage. Ambivalence—in this case the coexistence of destructive and reparative tendencies—is more pronounced in this disturbance than in any other neurosis.

Many of the defenses described on pp. 448-49 are employed by the obsessional subject to allay his anxiety. A return is often made to earlier levels of development when magical devices, such as crossing one's fingers, touching wood, walking round ladders and stepping between cracks on the pavement, were used for supposed self-protection (as in young children). Another defense is displacement. In obsessional neuroses, the fight against unconscious forces takes the most devious routes.

The Obsessional Personality

As with the hysterical personality, the obsessional personality shows a number of traits which are shared by many people who cannot be considered psychiatrically ill, unless these traits are so pronounced that everyday life is seriously interfered with.

They can be considered 'careful' or 'mean' according to taste and according to the general regard in which they are held. They are punctual and set great store by time. They are sticklers for exact usage of words, custom and social order. They demand a great deal of themselves and set high standards for others. They tend to take strict moral attitudes to the point of being puritanical. They are active, hard-working and scrupulous. They are often excessively neat and clean. They are the natural enemies of dirt, carelessness and disorder. But faced with a choice between two similar attitudes, or courses of action, they may become utterly indecisive and uncontrollably anxious. Such a situation will, of course, call for treatment.

Mixed Neuroses

Often the conditions described under the headings of 'hysteria' and 'obsessional neurosis,' as well as those conditions predominantly characterized by anxiety, are not present in pure form but show features of different types of neurosis. Anxiety with some conversion symptoms, and phobias occurring in obsessional states are common examples of 'mixed' neuroses.

Neurotic Depression

It is doubtful if the term 'neurotic depression' can be regarded as a diagnosis in its own right. Depression, a subjective feeling of sadness and misery, occurs in its milder forms in normal people but in the neuroses the depression may be of considerable duration and intensity.

Depression can occur in any of the neuroses so far described. It is closely related to feelings of guilt, though the guilt is by no means always conscious. It is often present in hysteria. If often colors an otherwise obsessional picture. When depression is the leading symptom in the neurosis, some doctors prefer to diagnose 'neurotic depressive reaction.'

Feelings of depression are often precipitated by an external event which may be striking, as in bereavement, or relatively trivial. But it is important to recognize that what determines the quality of the depression is not the magnitude of the external stress, but its unconscious significance for the patient. Indeed, consciously, the precipitating event may be entirely overlooked.

Associated with the depression there may be impaired concentration, loss of appetite, varying feelings of hopelessness, variable degrees of self-reproach, anger and irritability. But, with the possible exception of self-reproach, these features are not specific, and may occur in any form of neurosis even when little depression is evident.

Other Neurotic Illnesses

Other conditions are sometimes referred to as if they were separate neuroses.

Depersonalization. In this condition the patient complains that he does not feel real, that his body feels as if it is not his, that he feels a puppet or automaton, or that he feels as if he is acting in a play. In our view this condition is almost always part of another neurosis or psychosis, and constitutes a special defense against unpleasant or disturbing feelings.

Hypochondria. Some doctors also describe 'hypochondriasis,' in which there is fairly persistent preoccupation with bodily health or ill health, as a separate entity. We believe that the condition is usually part of another illness such as hysteria or the obsessional neuroses. It is also very common in depression and other psychoses.

The Sexual Perversions

Human sexual behavior varies so widely that it is not always easy to say what is normal and what is perverse. Indeed, the concept of sexual 'normality' is often a social one. Male homosexuality, for example, was entirely accepted in the Greek City State but is not tolerated in most Western countries today. On the other hand, female homosexuality, which can hardly be regarded as less 'perverse,' rarely arouses so much condemnation, at any rate where the law is concerned.

It is difficult to give a satisfactory psychological definition of sexual perversion. In general, however, the perverse sexual act tends either to exclude or replace male-female or heterosexual genital intercourse, or to relegate it to a subordinate role. Thus the exhibitionist or the peeping Tom gets sexual satisfaction without indulgence in intercourse; the homosexual may never have sexual relations with women or, if he does, he will find relations less satisfying than those with men; and the fetishist finds the excitement he gets from the article of clothing concerned of primary importance, even when intercourse takes place.

Homosexuality in either sex may be active or passive and both forms may be practiced at different times by the same person. The partners may be of any age. Some male homosexuals (probably a fairly small percentage) show a preference for children. Some homosexual attachments are very constant and the partners may live together, sometimes in great affection. Other homosexuals are promiscuous.

Fetishism. In fetishism the subject, invariably a male, is excited by some particular article of female clothing such as a stocking, a piece of underwear or a shoe. Not all fetishists require a partner to wear these items to get sexual satisfaction, but when they do the article itself is sexually more important than the person who wears it.

Exhibitionism. The man or woman concerned gets satisfaction from exposing the body, while in 'voyeurism' the voyeur gets his sexual enjoyment from spying on couples making love.

Sadism and Masochism. In sadism the sadist derives sexual pleasure from inflicting pain, while in masochism the reverse is the case.

These are the commonest perversions met with in clinical practice, though only a small proportion of perverts seek treatment.

Causes. The factors producing a perversion in a given individual are difficult to elucidate. In some adolescents perversions are merely forms of sexual experiment and have no special significance. In some homosexuals genetic factors seem to be important, especially in men with pronounced feminine physical characteristics and, equally, women of masculine build and appearance. But psychological factors can rarely be excluded.

In the earlier section on psychological development it was explained that the growing child passes through important stages where his relationship with parents, brothers and sisters make him aware of the fundamental sex differences. It was also explained that, during these stages, attitudes of passivity or assertion, and feelings about masculinity and femininity are encountered and dealt with. Failure to negotiate these stages satisfactorily has important consequences in later sexual development. In perversions, such early difficulties have been pronounced. In addition, problems at these stages are reinforced by pathological attitudes developed even earlier in childhood.

Treatment. The majority of people with perversions never come to treatment. The fact that the symptom is in itself pleasurable tends to weaken the incentive to seek help. If, in addition, the pervert has a fairly stable and well-adjusted private life he may only wish to be left in peace.

LEGAL ASPECT. If his activity causes him anxiety or guilt, however, he may seek medical advice. It may then be possible to relieve his anxiety even when the perversion itself cannot be uprooted. But sometimes the pervert seeks help not because he wishes to change but because he has fallen foul of the law or feels afraid that he may do so. Again, he may have been referred by a court of law, or treatment may have been a condition of probation. In these cases the outlook is poor unless the patient has some other inner incentive to get well.

Various factors affect the outlook where treatment is concerned. For example, the homosexual who has never had any heterosexual (male-female) relationships is, in general, more difficult to help than one who has.

PSYCHOTHERAPY offers the best, if not the only, hope of resolving the mental conflicts behind the perversion, though its use is limited. Sometimes, especially in fetishism, a form of 'deconditioning' has been used. In some male perversions, where the urge to practice the perversion is particularly strong, synthetic hormones have been used to damp down the sexual drives.

Alcoholism and Drug Addiction

Development of Addiction. Because alcohol and various drugs temporarily reduce anxiety, dull the intensity of depression or of feelings of inadequacy, and in some circumstances produce a positive feeling of well-being, persons with almost any psychiatric condition may seek comfort from them. Once a habit has been established dependency on alcohol or drug is likely to follow, and the consequences of this dependency may completely overshadow the original psychiatric condition. In general, increasing quantities are required. This leads to an increased financial burden. It may lead to incapacity at work and the loss of the job. Disruption of social relationships or of marriage may ensue, with ultimate decline to the status of a 'down-and-out.'

Secondary consequences of alcohol or drug taking may follow—confusional states, malnutrition and peripheral neuritis. Indulgence in the alcohol or the drug may be continuous or intermittent. People vary in the ease with which they become dependent on alcohol or a drug. This may be hereditarily determined or caused by their personality development.

Withdrawal Symptoms. As well as this dependency, some drugs, such as morphine and heroin and probably alcohol, produce withdrawal symptoms. These are bodily reactions consisting of cramps, aches, nausea, vomiting and even collapse, with intense anguish at times. They occur when the patient suddenly stops taking the drug. Clearly such symptoms are likely to be the more intense when dependence has been very marked.

Treatment. In general, in-patient hospital treatment is required in the first instance for alcoholism and drug addiction. The outlook is often rather poor, because although almost any psychiatric condition can be the starting point, the commonest underlying disorder is a psychopathic personality (see 457). Also, by the time a patient comes under treatment, very often considerable and irreparable havoc has been played with his former way of life and former relationships. These consequences may cause relapses into further alcoholism or drug-taking.

General Treatment of Neuroses

About three-quarters of all cases of neurosis are likely to recover within a period of less than two to three years, whatever treatment is given. In fact, many people who suffer from a neurosis never seek medical advice and put up with the discomfort and inconvenience. Whether someone does ask for treatment or not depends mainly on how much his every-day life, or that of his relatives, is disturbed by the symptoms.

With this high natural recovery rate, the efficacy of various treatments, whether psychological or by drugs, is hard to assess accurately. Certainly it appears that symptoms can often be speedily reduced in severity and possibly the natural duration of the illness shortened. This may, of course, be due to the effect of suggestion. Almost any system or regime or drug, in which the patient firmly believes, will produce at least temporary benefit.

The more intensive forms of psychological treatment, such as psychotherapy (described more fully in the section on treatment, 458), may effect an alteration in personality so that the patient is less liable to further breakdown, although this is by no means certain. On the other hand, however doubtful the curative effect may be of any treatment so far devised, it cannot be denied that the partnership in therapy of someone (the doctor, psychiatrist, or other therapist) who is trying at least to accept, understand and help, makes more tolerable the inexplicable difficulties, the mental discomfort or anguish and the discouragement to the point of despair, which may be the daily companions of a patient.

Main Forms of Treatment. In general terms, treatment of neurosis may be (1) by psychological methods which are intended to reassure, to provide helpful practical advice or to promote self-understanding, or (2) by drugs, which are intended to allay anxiety and tension, or else (3) by both. Treatment by prolonged drug-induced sleep (prolonged narcosis) or with daily doses of insulin (modified insulin therapy) to increase appetite and weight, are decreasingly used. Occasionally, when all other methods have failed, brain operations such as prefrontal leucotomy, intended to diminish inner tensions, may be advised.

DEPRESSIVE ILLNESS AND MANIA

DEPRESSION in its psychiatric sense means a mood of dejection accompanied by a tendency to be unduly self-critical. The majority of normal people have such moods from time to time, and it is only when they are unduly intense or long-lasting that they are regarded as abnormal. Many patients with psychoneurosis have such feelings. When depression overshadows all other symptoms and is accompanied by intense and usually unfounded self-blame, then the condition is termed a depressive illness.

Various types are recognized, such as 'reactive depression,' 'melancholia,' 'involutional depression,' according to the secondary features of the clinical picture.

MANIA. The term 'mania' is applied to a state of mind which is, in many ways, the opposite of depression. It refers to elation of mood, when the subject feels unusually cheerful, and is overactive and overtalkative. When the condition is mild, it is termed 'hypomania.' Those persons who show mania or hypomania at some times and depression at others are termed manic-depressive. The duration of each contrasting spell is rarely less than a week and often may last for months. The mercurial type of person who one moment is ostensibly in the depths of gloom and five minutes later on top of the world is not a manic-depressive subject.

Causes. A tendency to develop depressive illness or mania often seems to run in families and some genetic influence in its causation is likely. This predisposition can be very marked in certain families.

Severe depression and mania may be accompanied by changes in the regulation of the physiological and biochemical processes of the body; it is likely that faulty functioning of these regulatory mechanisms contributes to the development of these illnesses.

CYCLES. Depression and mania may occur in regular cycles. Often, however, an attack of depressive illness or mania follows some triggering-off situation. Commonly this is some bereavement, loss or failure (for which the patient blames himself), but sometimes the circumstances may appear to others to be trivial or unimportant. The loss may be actual, threatened, or present only in fantasy. In some instances the patient has feelings for and against the person he feels he is losing, so that unconscious destructive feelings towards that person occasion the severe guilt which is such a prominent feature of the illness. In mania, similar feelings are involved but are dealt with by denial; hence the unbearable guilt and the misery it occasions are not directly experienced. Physical factors may directly contribute to depressive illness, in particular infections and debilitating illness, such as influenza.

Depressive illnesses are more common after the age of forty than in previous years. Middle-age is often a particularly difficult period of life, when new adjustments have to be made. In women, the physical changes associated with the menopause and in men the decline in physical vigor entail readjustments of bodily function. Such changes may present an emotional threat. The growing-up and dispersing of the family, the death of parents and the comparison of early ambitions with a life-time's achievements often occur about this time. While physical and psychological adjustments are made in most cases without great upset, a minority of people develop depressions apparently as a result of these changes.

Clinical Features of Depression

Depressive illnesses may range in severity from a slight exaggeration of normal depression of mood to stupor with a complete absence of response to anything in the surroundings. The very severe forms of depression do not necessarily have a worse outlook, as regards effective treatment, than the milder ones.

PESSIMISM. The onset may be gradual or sudden. The most prominent feature is the feeling of sadness and pessimism. The patient feels that he is a failure, that he has let people down, and is a burden to his family, that there is no good in him and that he has not the capacity to carry on. He tends to blame himself for all sorts of misfortunes, real and imaginary. In severe cases, extreme feelings of guilt and hopelessness lead to suicidal ideas and sometimes to attempts at suicide. The patient may have delusions that he has committed great and unforgivable sins, or even that he is responsible for all the evil in the world. In addition he may think that retribution is imminent and that he and his family are about to be destroyed. With such ideas the patient may believe that others are aware of his badness, that they talk about him or plan to have him arrested and punished. In this respect the delusions may resemble those of a paranoid illness.

In other subjects the pessimistic beliefs may take the form of preoccupations with supposed ill-health and sometimes with an unshakeable belief that he has some incurable disease.

LOSS OF APPETITE AND WEIGHT are usually present and sleep is usually disturbed; characteristically, the patient wakes early and lies awake brooding on his worries. There is a general loss of interest, and sexual desire diminishes. The ability to concentrate is reduced; in severe cases, intellectual powers may appear impaired. The patient's appearance reflects his depressed mood. There is little play of expression and all activities and speech are slow and the voice monotonous.

Agitated Depression. This is a variety of depressive illness where the mood changes, and the preoccupation and delusions described above are accompanied by great anxiety and restlessness. Weeping and wringing of hands accompany the recounting of guilt and expectations of tragedy. This form of depression is common in later years and is sometimes referred to as 'involutional depression.'

Prognosis and Treatment. Depressive illnesses carry a good prognosis, in that they almost always clear up completely in time, even without treatment. Untreated, however, depression may last for many months or years and while it lasts there may be risk of self-injury or of deterioration of physical health because of the patient's neglect of his bodily needs.

With treatment, recovery is often prompt and dramatic. The principal treatments available are electroplexy, antidepressant drugs and psychotherapy, and it is almost always possible to cut short an attack of depression with one or other of these treatments. In many cases treatment may be given without the patient's entering hospital, but in severe cases admission is necessary in order that the patient may be adequately supervised and cared for. In addition to these main treatments, various drugs may be used to relieve some of the symptoms; sedatives to help sleep, and sometimes stimulants to help overcome the lack of energy.

Clinical Features of Mania. Just as some people experience periods of depression at times, so they also have periods of increased cheerfulness and energy. In mania there is an exaggeration of these features to an extent which inconveniences and incapacitates the subject.

In mild cases the patient is restless and overactive, and he has an increased feeling of self-importance and a tendency to flit from topic to topic in conversation. Although he is often in an elated and over-expansive mood, he is easily antagonized, thinking that others are obstructing his wonderful ideas and activities. He may be interfering and he may launch over-ambitious schemes involving him in financial and other troubles.

In severer cases the restlessness is so extreme and continuous as to lead to serious exhaustion. The patient is often in a mood of wild elation, which turns easily into extreme anger and possibly violence. New thoughts follow so rapidly on old ones that coherence is lost. Grandiose delusions are often present. The patient may believe himself to be some famous person or even the savior of the world and may act accordingly. Rarely, hallucinations of vision and hearing may occur.

Prognosis. Recovery usually takes place in time without treatment, but an attack may last for months. Recurrences are common.

Treatment. In mild cases the patient can be treated as an out-patient and given one of the tranquilizer group of drugs. Supervision may be necessary to avoid the personal neglect or the consequences of the excessive and ill-judged activities.

Severer cases require hospital treatment and this may be urgent when exhaustion or disturbed behavior exists. Tranquilizers and sometimes electroplexy are usually given.

Recently, medication with lithium (an element resembling sodium) has been thought to be effective in some cases, in both the treatment of attacks of mania and in the prevention of further attacks.

SCHIZOPHRENIA

Schizophrenia (pronounced 'skittsofreen-ya') is a group of illnesses characterized by varying degrees of social withdrawal, together with certain disorders of thinking and feeling. Further, most patients show evidence of delusions or hallucinations, and behavior is often strange and disturbed. In many instances these features are so striking that hospital treatment is likely to be given in the early stages.

While a schizophrenic illness is often very serious and results in a protracted stay in hospital, it must be emphasized that an increasing proportion of patients suffering from the severe forms of the illness recover or improve, and that, in many mild cases, the outlook is good.

Causes. There are probably many different illnesses included in the group, so that the causes vary with the individual case.

HEREDITY. Sometimes hereditary features seem important, in that there is a history of one or more relatives (parent or grandparent, sister or brother, aunt or uncle) who have also suffered from schizophrenia. This inheritance may predispose to the physical abnormalities which are observed in some cases. Abnormalities reported include certain trends of bodily build and certain glandular and chemical disorders.

Environmental. A predisposition to schizophrenia is not necessarily inherited. Childhood experiences often play a part in the patient's susceptibility. These experiences include deprivation of maternal love and care, possibly through bereavement, enforced separation, or emotional disorder on the part of the mother of such a nature that she finds adequate mothering difficult or impossible. These and other disturbances in early childhood may cause the child to grow up shy, solitary and lacking in confidence.

Only a small proportion of such predisposed people, who meet particularly unfavorable circumstances in adolescence or early adult life, develop schizophrenia. Adversities encountered in the process of loosening parental ties, falling in love, starting new careers or meeting unfamiliar social situations often immediately precede the start of the illness.

Clinical Features. All persons with schizophrenia show some degree of loss of contact with the real world so that fantasy may be preferred to reality. This is often the first abnormality, especially in the younger patient. There may be a progressive loss of interest in the people and events around him, ranging from mild apathy to an apparently total loss of awareness. In other cases there is a narrowing of interests around a group of preoccupations which eventually become the sole topic of thought and which the imagination elaborates into a set of delusions. What begins as a daydream in which the dreamer sees himself in the romantic role of a secret service agent may develop into a hardened conviction that he is hounded by international forces who join in league against him. In such a case all his everyday failures, disappointments and frustrations may be laid at the door of the conspirators.

At the same time the ability to think becomes affected in a characteristic way. The logical sequence of thought is broken. To begin with this shows itself in an artificial and stilted manner of speech. Later, successive sentences may be unrelated, answers to questions quite beside the point, and sentences cut short in the middle with a total inability to carry on. Sometimes a continuous repetition of a word or phrase takes the place of ordered thinking. Meaningless words may be invented or existing words telescoped together so that a single word carries a number of different meanings.

Disturbed Emotion. The emotion shown by the patient is inappropriate to the circumstances or to what he is saying. He may show little emotion where emotion is called for, and may show feelings which seem quite out of place. Thus he may be unmoved by catastrophe and greatly distressed by trivialities. He may laugh while recounting his imagined persecutions.

Strange and Irrational Beliefs frequently develop. The most commonplace event may be regarded as something of the greatest personal significance. There is a tendency to develop false beliefs of self-importance and of persecution. The patient may think himself to be the Messiah, or the subject of malicious conspiracies which he may attribute to Communists, Fascists, Freemasons, Jews, Catholics, or any other easily identified group. A chance occurrence or an innocent remark overheard in the street may be interpreted to fit these beliefs.

In many cases the patient hears imaginary voices which give further expression to these ideas. Thus he may hear people plotting his downfall, threatening and accusing him. Sometimes he experiences strange and unpleasant sensations in his body which appear to him to be the result of radio waves or some sort of magical device operating from a distance and trying to destroy him.

The above account applies generally or at least in part to most cases. Great variation in severity and type occurs, but it is customary to distinguish four main types of the illness. These divisions are by no means hard and fast.

Schizophrenia Simplex
(*Simple Schizophrenia*)

The onset is often in the late 'teens and is gradual. Performance at school or work falls off. Indifference and self-neglect increase. Jobs of progressively lower grade succeed each other. Interest in, and feeling for relatives, friends and social activities decrease. Good fortune or adversity means nothing. The patient may drift into petty crime or prostitution. The outlook for full recovery is poor though the patient may adjust himself to a lower level of achievement.

Hebephrenic Schizophrenia
(*Hebephrenia*)

This condition often begins gradually in the late 'teens or the twenties. A tendency to pointless joking, witless mischief, unpredictability and fatuousness develops. Increasingly, new and strange words are used and the talk becomes more and more nonsensical. Interest in other people diminishes. Hallucinations of hearing are common, and may take the form of instructions to commit the various mischievous and unpredictable acts that are performed. The outlook for complete recovery is bad.

Catatonic Schizophrenia
(*Catatonia: Katatonia*)

The onset of this type of schizophrenia is usually more abrupt, and often occurs in the early twenties. Episodes of illness may alternate with long periods of complete remission, or exacerbations may occur without full recovery between them. There may be one, two or more acute episodes without any subsequent attack. The episodes may be either stupor or excitement. In stupor the patient may be quite unresponsive, say nothing, answer no questions and maintain any posture in which he is placed for quite a long period. He may refuse all food and drink and pay no heed to his bladder or bowels. He may appear to be in an intense state of terror or ecstasy. Subsequently he may recall that he experienced vivid hallucinations of sight or sound.

If, however, the patient is in a state of catatonic excitement (as opposed to stupor) intense abrupt activity occurs. Speech may refer to strange feelings or experiences, or even be quite incomprehensible. There are outbursts of violence against the self or others.

In spite of these severe disturbances the outlook for complete recovery is better than it is in any other form of schizophrenia. Even so, a fairly large proportion of patients do not recover completely.

Paranoid Schizophrenia

Onset is usually in the late twenties or in the thirties. The subject develops various delusions which may have only the loosest connection with each other or which, on the other hand, may be built up into the most logical system. All kinds of ideas of persecution may be expressed, together with delusions which indicate an inflated self-importance.

Generally, some degree of emotional flattening is present, but frequently sufficient emotion and drive remains to take action against the supposed persecution.

The outlook is not very good for complete recovery, but in many cases the patients manage to live outside hospital without too much social friction. They may, however, make life difficult for their relatives.

Paraphrenia. A term applied to a similar condition when it begins in middle age.

Paranoia. A rare condition when little change other than a highly developed and complex system of delusions is present. This may persist unrecognized for years and may never require hospital treatment.

General Treatment of Schizophrenia

This will vary with the individual case. In patients whose illness is mild, out-patient treatment may suffice and often consists of medication with tranquilizing drugs, and regular interviews in which advice and guidance are given to the patient, his family and relatives. Working and living conditions will often need adjustment.

In the severer cases, admission to hospital is necessary. In addition to the measures described, courses of electroplexy or of insulin shock therapy may be given. Active measures to minimize deterioration of social habits are very important, especially in the artificial setting of a psychiatric hospital.

On discharge from hospital a period of after-care supervision is necessary to help the patient to take his place once more in normal society.

ORGANIC ILLNESS

Psychiatric disorders may arise when the structure of the brain is physically altered or when its chemical composition is changed. Structural changes may be produced by head injuries, by deterioration in old age, by degeneration of the blood vessels or by certain degenerative conditions whose cause is yet unknown. Chemical substances such as alcohol, drugs, or coal gas, abnormal in quality or quantity, may come from outside the body, or others may come from within the body when they are produced, for example, by severe kidney disease or during infections. Sometimes there may not be enough of a normal substance, such as in vitamin deficiencies or when the oxygen supply is inadequate because of disease of the heart or lungs.

Although these chemically produced changes are generally reversible, permanent damage to the brain may result if they persist for a long time.

The so-called organic disorders thus produced all cause some degree of impairment of intellectual powers or of consciousness, as well as various other psychiatric abnormalities. They fall into three groups: the acute, of sudden onset and brief duration; the chronic, of gradual onset and long duration; and the subacute, intermediate between the first two.

Acute Disorders causing Confusion and Delirium

In these acute conditions there is an impairment of consciousness termed confusion, in which decreased awareness of one's surroundings, difficulty of comprehension, and bewilderment occur. A common form is delirium where the confusion is accompanied by restlessness, hallucinations and often by fear. It may be caused by infections of the brain or its delicate coverings, by high fever, by poisoning, by certain vitamin deficiencies, by heart failure, or by injury. Delirium tremens is one form of the condition and is caused by alcoholism.

Clinical Features. The confusion usually fluctuates in severity, commonly being worse at night and, when it is severe, the patient may not recognize his relatives or his surroundings. He may be disturbed by visions of a frightening nature and he may believe that awful catastrophes are happening. He is usually very restless and may attempt to escape from the frightening things which he sees.

Prognosis and Treatment. The condition as a rule lasts for a few days and clears up with the underlying cause, which should of course receive appropriate treatment. In addition the patient may be treated with sedatives, and care is needed to ensure that he receives adequate nourishment and that he does not injure himself as a result of his restlessness. It is often found helpful to keep his room well lit at night, since he may be less troubled by visions if he can see clearly the objects around him.

Subacute Disorders causing Korsakov's Syndrome

This is most often a consequence of severe vitamin B deficiency, of alcoholism, or of head injury, though it may be caused by any of the conditions which can result in delirium. The onset is gradual and may follow delirium. The patient may appear superficially normal and often rather cheerful, but he has, however, impairment of memory and fills in the gaps in memory with fictitious accounts. He often does not know where he is, or the time of day, or the date (disorientation).

Some recovery takes place over a period of weeks or months as the damaged nerve cells recover; in many cases, however, the damage is permanent, and the intellectual powers are not recovered. The condition is treated by large doses of vitamin B.

Chronic Disorders causing Dementia

In these conditions there is a progressive loss of intellectual powers as a result of deterioration of the cells of the brain. This loss of mental abilities is termed dementia, and often occurs in senility. In other cases it may be due to brain damage in diseases of the blood vessels, to inflammation of the brain in syphilis or encephalitis, to brain tumor and other diseases of the brain, as well as to serious brain injury. There is also a rare group of illnesses, the presenile dementias (Pick's disease and Alzheimer's disease) and Huntingdon's chorea, where dementia takes place in early or middle years as a result of degeneration of the tissues of various parts of the brain.

Psychiatric Changes in Old Age and Senility. Sooner or later in old age, a degree of impairment of intellectual powers and of mental energy and flexibility is inevitable, but great variation exists and everyone has known old people who retained their faculties, abilities and interests into very advanced years. While degeneration of brain tissues leads to dementia, other factors appear to play an important mitigating role in the degree of disability. The subject's personality, his breadth of interests, his ability to retain activity and interests within any limitations which physical changes may impose on him, may greatly offset the effects of the decline in functioning brain tissue which takes place in senility. In addition, common everyday care contributes to well-being—an adequate and varied diet and reasonable precautions over bodily health are at least as rewarding in old age as in the younger years.

Intellectual power reaches a peak in the late 'teens and probably begins to fall off very gradually in the late thirties. This, however, may be more than compensated for by increasing experience and increasing emotional maturity—benefits which continue into old age. Old age is, however, usually accompanied by a constriction of interests, an inability to accept and deal with new ideas and experience, while some degree of memory difficulty is usual and normal. Only if these difficulties become severe is the condition described as dementia.

Senile Dementia

In the early stages, this condition is chiefly manifested by difficulties with memory and with comprehension. As this becomes more severe the patient begins to forget where he has put things, begins to forget recent happenings and to be more preoccupied with earlier memories which are better retained. These difficulties may be accompanied by irritability and petulance and sometimes by suspicions that people are hiding things from him, or maltreating him. Speech difficulties often occur, such as a difficulty in finding the right word at times, even though the word is a simple and common one. In more severe disorders of speech the subject cannot construct intelligible sentences. Later, he begins to fail to recognize people and becomes disorientated for time and place. Personal habits may deteriorate. Delusions and hallucinations may accompany this dementia.

There is no curative treatment for senile dementia because the damaged tissues cannot be replaced. Help may be given by medication to reduce irritability or restlessness. Sometimes because of his failure to take proper care of himself, the patient lives on a most inadequate diet and suffers from vitamin deficiency; appropriate measures may then result in a degree of improvement. In later stages the patient may require care in a nursing home or hospital.

Arteriosclerotic Dementia

This condition of intellectual impairment results from diseases of the arteries of the brain. Arterial diseases are common conditions. In some kinds the arteries of the brain become narrowed, thus restricting the blood supply and damaging the brain tissues. The condition resembles senile dementia generally, but commonly occurs earlier in life, in the sixties. The subject is often keenly aware of loss of intellectual power, and depression and agitation are common. Attacks of headache and dizziness or confusion may occur, and minor or major strokes as a result of artery disease may accompany the illness.

In mild cases, the patient may continue with his work and ordinary life, but an ordered routine with reduction of physical exertion and responsibility are necessary. A good diet is essential. In severe cases of arteriosclerotic dementia, hospital care is required.

Presenile Dementia

While dementia before the age of senility occurs in arteriosclerotic dementia, and sometimes in brain tumors and other conditions, the term 'presenile dementia' is usually reserved for two particular and rare diseases, Pick's disease and Alzheimer's disease where deterioration of the brain tissue takes place from causes as yet unknown. These are two very similar forms of progressive dementia which occur in the late forties and fifties and which advance more rapidly than senile dementia. In Alzheimer's disease the dementia is frequently accompanied by marked difficulty in speech and writing, by paralysis and by epileptic fits. Pick's disease is commoner in certain families than in the general population.

Huntington's Chorea

This is a rare inherited disease occurring in certain families, where progressive dementia commencing between thirty and fifty years of age is accompanied by involuntary and uncontrollable writhing movements of the face, limbs and trunk. No effective treatment is known.

Psychiatric Illness Caused by Syphilis

If untreated, advanced syphilis frequently affects the nervous system, resulting in both neurological and psychiatric illness. The psychiatric condition is one of progressive dementia and of delusions and it may also be accompanied by various paralyses.

Symptoms. Psychiatric symptoms usually first appear some years after the original untreated infection. Often the first noticeable feature is a deterioration in personal habits and the early decrease in intellectual power and memory may not be noticed. Delusions frequently develop early in the illness and this may be the first noticeable abnormality. The patient may believe that he is a very famous and rich person, and his claims are often in marked contrast to his dilapidated appearance and inactivity. Eventually dementia becomes severe, with the loss of almost all intellectual activity.

Treatment. Syphilis is effectively treated by penicillin and this should be given soon after the original infection. It is still often effective in arresting the disease in the later stages, but much improvement is then unlikely because of the damage already done to the brain tissues.

Psychiatric Changes with Cerebral Tumors

Irritability and depression are fairly common accompaniments of cerebral tumors. In addition they may cause confusion, delirium, or dementia.

PSYCHOPATHY
(Psychopathic Personality)

There are some people who are consistently unsuccessful in providing and obtaining love and friendship, whose worldly achievements do not satisfy them and who disrupt their social group, sometimes by criminal activities, yet who do not suffer from psychosis, neurosis or mental subnormality. They are termed psychopaths. This difficulty in living in reasonable harmony with other people often appears in childhood, is most marked in adult life and may decrease in middle age. Because it seems enduring and deeply engraved, it is often described as an attribute of personality, hence the term 'psychopathic personality.'

Causes. The causes are uncertain. Heredity may play a part but the influence of early adverse circumstances seems more striking. Emotional instability on the part of the parents with rejection of the child, sometimes due to their own psychiatric illness or psychopathy, or else adverse environmental circumstances, such as poverty or illegitimacy, often appear to have been present. On the other hand a psychopath appears sometimes to have had, as far as is known, the best of homes. Sometimes behavior indistinguishable from psychopathy may follow head injury with brain damage. In fact a high proportion of adult psychopaths actually show electrical abnormality of their brains when tested by the electroencephalogram; often the abnormality is similar to the records obtained from young children, as if the psychopath's brain had not matured in some way.

Clinical Features. Generally there is a history going back to schooldays of poor social adaptation, as shown by bad work record, lack of sustained effort and frequent dishonesty or untruthfulness. Some may have become alcoholics, established criminals, drug addicts or sexual perverts. Others may come to attention because of their tendencies to tell the most fantastic lies for no other reason than apparently to gain attention and a temporary feeling of importance. More careful scrutiny will reveal that the subject has fairly consistently been unable to foresee the consequences of his actions, has been unable to postpone satisfaction of his desires or expression of his impulses, has been unable to consider other people's needs or rights, and has been apparently unable to establish a normal emotional relationship with anyone. There may have been a tendency to explode on very slight provocation into violence, sometimes directed at other people, sometimes at the self. Such people often readily express regret for their past misdeeds, promise repentance and may have considerable plausibility and charm of manner in doing so. Neither the repentance nor the charm is likely to last very long if their suggestions and desires are not acceded to.

A psychopath in general does not seem to appreciate other people or persons in their own right; he seems to regard them merely as pawns to be manipulated. When a 'pawn' shows signs of having a will of his own the psychopath may seem quite genuinely surprised.

Treatment. The majority of psychopaths probably never come under medical care. Those who break the law may become habitual criminals and may end up in preventive detention. Others who are not criminally antisocial, may be repeatedly in and out of psychiatric hospitals, following episodes when too much trouble has accumulated for them or for their relatives to tolerate. The majority continue throughout life, making trouble for themselves and other people, sometimes occupying positions of considerable responsibility in many walks of life.

The treatment of these psychopaths, other than custodial, is unsatisfactory. Various endeavors have been made to provide specialized surroundings in which they can learn to increase their impaired abilities of social functioning, but the results so far are not very encouraging.

MENTAL SUBNORMALITY
(Mental Deficiency)

Some individuals lack the ability to develop their general mental powers to a level which is high enough to allow them to deal with the everyday hazards, difficulties and requirements of life. They are unintelligent to a greater or less extent, their emotional reactions are childish and simple, and their abilities to persist in a task or an idea or to exercise foresight is reduced.

Such persons can be divided into two main categories.

Group 1. The larger group consists of subjects who just happen to be unlucky in their genetic inheritance. Just as a few people have a physical stature which is very small without any actual disease causing this, so some people's intellectual stature is small. This happens quite by chance, and there is no way likely to be found of avoiding it. It is as if, in a sweepstake, as well as there being a few tickets which win prizes, there were others which carry a forfeit.

It is true that the parents of such children often tend to be somewhat below the average level of intelligence, but for as many children as they produce who are less intelligent, there are likely to be a similar number who are brighter than their parents. Suggestions of sterilization or so-called eugenic measures would therefore not affect appreciably the incidence of this type of mental subnormality.

Group 2. The second group consists of a number of rarer conditions, generally associated with a definite disease process which is usually inherited in some way. The forms of subnormality produced tend to be severer than in the first group. The inheritance may be of two kinds. First, it may be 'dominant,' that is to say, a parent is affected with the same condition. Secondly, and more commonly, it may be 'recessive,' that is to say both parents are normal, but happen to be carrying the same hereditary predisposition which when combined in reproduction produces the subnormality in the offspring. The recessive form of inheritance is more common because, in general, affliction by these conditions usually reduces a person's fertility and certainly reduces the chance of finding a mate.

A small number of cases in this group arise from non-inheritable conditions (a) due to maternal infections affecting the unborn child, such as German measles during early pregnancy, (b) to damage during birth, or (c) to childhood infections such as meningitis.

Clinical Features of Group 1. The majority of cases do not show any striking physical abnormality, although minor peculiarities are not uncommon. These minor differences may include marked facial asymmetry, being undersized or poorly proportioned, or awkwardness in posture and gait.

SEVERE CASES. Broadly speaking, the more severe the degree of mental subnormality, the earlier in life it is apparent. In infancy, for example, the child seems inert and takes little interest in his surroundings. He may be difficult to feed. Later on, there is a tendency to be late in reaching all his milestones of development such as lifting up his head, sitting up, teething, walking, getting control over his bladder and bowels, and learning to play. It is worth emphasizing that it is the overall backwardness that is important; many perfectly normal children may be late in reaching one or two of these attainments.

Once the child has gone to school, lesser degrees of backwardness will become apparent. Compared with other children of his age, he cannot do as well, learn as quickly, or adapt as easily to the circumstances of school life.

MILD CASES. The mildest degrees of all may not be detected until adolescence or early adult life. After an indifferent performance at school, difficulty in learning a job or in settling down to one, or persistent delinquency often of an inept and stupid kind, may lead to the correct diagnosis.

Clinical Features of Group 2. A number of relatively uncommon conditions with characteristic physical abnormalities compose this group.

Mongolism is associated with abnormalities of the chromosome number in all the tissue cells. Generally born late in the mother's life, these children have a rounded skull, a flattened face with obliquely set eyes, a large fissured tongue, a fresh complexion and short hands with very short little fingers. The degree of subnormality may be mild or severe. Their disposition is generally placid and friendly. Death in childhood is quite common.

Hydrocephaly. The child has an abnormally large head either at birth or starting in the first few years of life, sometimes after an infection. There is an excess of fluid formation inside the skull and atrophy of the brain. Early death is common. The degree of deficiency is often severe.
(See also p.431.)

Microcephaly. In this disorder the child has an unusually small head and brain. The scalp may show deep furrows, as if it were of normal size on the too-small skull.

Phenylketonuria. Children with phenylketonuria have an inherited inability to metabolize the amino-acid phenylalanine and consequently development of the brain is severely impaired. They are always fair-haired and are generally severely subnormal.
(See also p.395.)

Other rarer conditions include epiloia, amaurotic family idiocy, gargoylism, and toxoplasmosis, associated with subnormality and various physical peculiarities.
(For toxoplasmosis, see p. 280.)

Treatment. Most of the severer cases (mainly group 2) require institutional care. Some of the less severe cases (mainly group 1) may also need such care, particularly if behavioral disturbances such as emotional instability or delinquency have occurred. For the subnormal to develop their limited capabilities to the fullest extent possible, skilled training and handling is required. They are unlikely to receive this other than in an institution, or a special school. When they are grown up, special sheltered conditions of employment are likely to be required for the higher grades to maintain stability and use what abilities they have.

PSYCHOSOMATIC ILLNESS

This term is applied to conditions in which emotional stress appears to precipitate or perpetuate illness with actual physical changes in the organs concerned. Examples are asthma, migraine, peptic ulcer, mucous colitis, ulcerative colitis, some skin diseases, and fibrositis or muscular rheumatism. Emotional factors can play a part in tuberculosis, rheumatoid arthritis, high blood pressure, thyrotoxicosis, some menstrual disorders, infertility and probably many other conditions.

The organs involved in these disorders are probably affected through the autonomic nervous system (see Anatomy, p. 230). This is not under voluntary control but is profoundly influenced by emotions. It regulates blood flow (through skin, muscles and internal organs), the contractions and relaxations of involuntary muscle (e.g. in stomach, intestines, bladder, lungs and bronchial tree), the secretion of glands (e.g. sweat, digestive, thyroid, adrenal), and, in part, the cyclical changes of menstruation. Thus, for example, fear produces sweating, embarrassment often causes blushing, and disgust produces vomiting.

Causes. It is thought that unresolved (and so enduring) states of emotional conflict in a predisposed person may affect the autonomic nervous system so as to disturb the proper working of an organ. A particular organ may be vulnerable because it has been diseased before, or because it has some symbolic significance in terms of the emotional conflict or else because of an inherited susceptibility.

Asthma illustrates these three points. Sometimes emotionally precipitated attacks only begin after a lung infection such as bronchitis. In other cases, it may affect physically normal lungs because an attack symbolically represents a repressed desire to cry or weep. Lastly, asthma often runs in families in a way suggesting its inheritability.

General Treatment. The physical changes in the organs concerned generally require the appropriate physical treatment; peptic ulcer for instance, needs rest, medicine and special diet. To speed recovery and so reduce the likelihood of relapse, it is often desirable to reduce or remove the emotional stress which, if unrelieved, may cause the physical treatments to fail. Simple removal from or avoidance of the stressful situation can be sufficient. Otherwise, psychotherapy of some sort may be indicated.

Immediate anxiety and tension can be reduced by sedatives or tranquilizers and the vicious circle broken whereby anxiety leads to disease which leads to further anxiety about the disease.

THE TREATMENT OF PSYCHIATRIC ILLNESS

PSYCHOLOGICAL TREATMENT

General Measures or Simple Psychotherapy

Any contact between doctor and patient has psychological aspects. A simple act, such as writing a prescription, has a psychological meaning. This depends on the setting in which the act occurs, the way it is carried out and the respective psychological attitudes, conscious and unconscious, of patient and doctor towards each other. To one patient the prescription may convey only kindness and consideration. To another it may be seen as a gesture which silences him, which stops him talking about his troubles and, by implication, tells him to take them elsewhere.

Reassurance and Suggestion. Often the doctor deliberately tries to influence the patient's symptoms by psychological methods. He may try by persuasion, reassurance and encouragement. He may offer advice on the patient's management of everyday affairs. Sometimes he tries suggestion. This means that the doctor uses his authority and influence with the patient to convince him he is getting better or that a particular course of action will be helpful.

Abreaction. General discussion of the patient's difficulties may also help by allowing him to 'get things off his chest' and unburden himself to someone he can feel is an interested observer, yet who is more impartial than his family and friends. Sometimes the release of pent-up emotion during such discussion leads, at least, to temporary relief. This process is called 'abreaction.'

Such methods can be termed 'simple psychotherapy,' to distinguish them from the 'dynamic' treatments described below. It should be added that this distinction has nothing to do with efficacy.

Dynamic Psychotherapy

Dynamic psychotherapy or interpretative psychotherapy covers those methods of treatment where an attempt is made to use the doctor-patient relationship to increase the patient's knowledge of himself. This means that some of his unconscious motivations are brought into consciousness. The basic assumption is that, if this is done, the patient's more pathological defenses, from which his symptoms result, become unnecessary.

The first form of dynamic psychotherapy was psycho-analysis. It will be discussed at some length, to help in understanding the modified and shorter techniques.

Psycho-analysis

A basic assumption in psycho-analysis is that there is a reason for all mental events, however haphazard they appear.

Free Association. In ordinary social conversation many ideas which occur to the speaker are not expressed, because they may be irrelevant, out of place, or in bad taste. But in psycho-analysis the patient is asked to tell the doctor everything that occurs to him —thoughts, feelings, fantasies, sensations—as he experiences them during the session and without any reservations whatsoever. This is known as 'free association' and is the basic rule for the patient. The doctor's role is that of an interpreter. This means that he listens carefully to all that the patient tells him and, as occasion fits and the pattern of mental events becomes clear, interprets to the patient the emotional significance of what he says. The process is gradual, but this does not mean that there is any attempt to avoid painful or anxious feelings. These, like any others, must sooner or later be faced.

In its pure form, this treatment avoids any direct use of methods of influencing the patient. This means that the measures described as 'simple psychotherapy' are never deliberately practiced. Thus it is held, for example, that the best form of reassurance is a correct interpretation, since it shows the patient clearly that the doctor is in touch with his feelings.

Regression. Treatment is aided by a very remarkable fact. The situation fosters regression (see p. 449) and in this way the patient's childhood, in a sense, is again accessible to observation, as more childish ways of thinking or feeling replace adult ones, and the patient behaves, often in spite of himself, as if the doctor were an important figure in his childhood, such as a parent. Surprisingly, this occurs irrespective of the age, sex or appearance of the doctor.

Transference. This displacement of feelings from a parent or other important person to the doctor is known as 'transference.' Because it may have all the violent qualities of love and hate felt towards the original figure, the doctor-patient relationship can become the central and most important object of study. Consequently, one aim of the doctor is the interpretation of events occurring in the transference. From this he can try to show the relationship of these events to others in the patient's life, whether past or present.

Character Change. If treatment is successful there is usually some degree of character change, so that aspects of the patient's behavior which increased his difficulties are modified. This cannot happen quickly. Few analysts would expect substantial changes in less than eighteen months or two years, even when the patient attends for an hour five times a week.

Doctor and Patient. In orthodox psycho-analysis, the patient lies on a couch while the doctor sits out of sight, because it is thought that both patient and doctor are thereby more relaxed, the patient better able to concentrate on 'free association' with less distraction, and the doctor freer to devote his attention to the patient's productions and their meaning. Patients, of course, often try to discover whether the doctor approves or disapproves of what they are saying, and they may fancy that it is easier to do so when they can watch the doctor's facial expression. Perhaps we should add that during this treatment, and in all forms of dynamic psychotherapy, the doctor is careful not to express moral criticism, since this would be an attempt to influence the patient's behavior without trying to understand it. It would also seriously interfere with the patient's ability to follow the basic rule of free association.

As far as we can see at present, analysis is more likely to be useful in the neuroses than in the psychoses, though attempts are sometimes made to treat the latter. It is not usually indicated in people much older than forty or who are unintelligent. But the most serious disadvantages of psycho-analysis lie in its great length and in its expense.

Shorter Forms of Psycho-analysis

Because of the length of time and expense involved, psychiatrists have sought short cuts in interpretative psychotherapy. In these shorter techniques it is not always possible or desirable to avoid reassurance or advice. But almost without exception all forms of dynamic psychotherapy use the concept of transference in their work with the patient.

Sessions vary in length and frequency, but are usually from half to one hour once or twice a week. Most doctors agree that the longer the interval between sessions, the more difficult the task. If intervals are too long it becomes particularly hard to interpret the transference material correctly.

Modification of Pressing Conflicts. Before treatment itself starts, a careful history of the patient is taken and the likelihood of psychotherapy being helpful is assessed. Many doctors find it convenient to set themselves a particular goal in treatment. This need not be an ambitious one. It may be concerned with the modification of the patient's more pressing conflicts by interpretation of his more prominent defenses. It is unrealistic to set these goals too high. In general, less urgent conflicts will be ignored in short-term treatment.

In shorter methods of psychotherapy it may be necessary to direct the patient's attention to particular periods or aspects of his life, even when his free association is not leading in that direction. This may have to be done by questioning. But the emphasis will still be on interpretation of what the patient communicates to the doctor and especially of the transference relationship.

Face-to-Face Interview. In many forms of dynamic psychotherapy the couch is discarded in favor of a face-to-face interview. There are many practical reasons for this. One is that the use of a couch occasions much anxiety in itself, partly because it produces a greater degree of regression (see above, p. 449). Many psychiatrists prefer not to invite this state of affairs when they have less time than the analyst to deal with this situation. However, the face-to-face technique can be exacting for both parties and, while the doctor must be natural in his manner, he must try not to convey, unintentionally, attitudes detrimental to the patient's free expression.

No Rigid Rules. The kinds of dynamic psychotherapy vary greatly in detail as do the conditions in which they are practiced. However, certain basic conditions seem necessary. The patient's time must be respected; for example, it seems important for him to know in advance the times and duration of his sessions. Consistency in appointments is desirable. Free expression must never be discouraged. But when this has been said, it must be emphasized that there are no rigid rules in dynamic psychotherapy. Techniques need to be adaptable and imaginative. They call for great skill, which is why not every psychiatrist would care to use them.

Finally, more than anyone else, the psychiatric patient is inclined to feel that no one has time for him or is willing to help him. To feel that he can be respected as well as tolerated is in itself a corrective emotional experience.

Dynamic Group Psychotherapy

Before the Second World War some attempts had been made to treat small numbers of patients collectively in groups. An increasing emphasis on psychiatric treatment stimulated by the war revived interest in these methods.

Free Discussion. In dynamic group psychotherapy the patients, usually six to eight in number, sit in a circle together with the doctor. The length of the session varies. The 'free association' of individual therapy is replaced by 'free discussion'—there is no set subject and the doctor does not direct the discussion. As in individual treatment, his role is essentially that of interpreter. Here again he tries to avoid those methods of influencing patients described on p. 458 as 'simple psychotherapy.'

Open vs Closed Groups. Groups are of two kinds: open and closed. In an open group patients may join and leave at different times during the course of the group. As each patient goes he is replaced by someone else, so that the composition of the group changes. In a closed group, on the other hand, all patients start and finish their treatment at the same time.

An open group can be rather unsettling for patients who need long-term treatment. A closed group is better for such people. Patients who seem able to benefit from two or three months' treatment are, on the other hand, perhaps best treated in an open group. An open group can also be useful for an initial period of observation and assessment. If found suitable, a patient can then be transferred to a closed group. A closed group may continue for anything from six months to a year, sometimes much longer. In the case of out-patients the group meets once or twice a week, but in a few in-patient centers five sessions a week are offered.

The Interpretation. The doctor may interpret the behavior of the group as a whole, or he may interpret that of a given individual. Most doctors prefer to interpret principally group behavior in the early stages, to help the group to work together as a coherent unit. But individual interpretations are important and will certainly be made as the group progresses. There are, of course, no rigid rules and the technique needs to be adapted to the situation prevailing in the group at the time.

As in individual therapy, special importance is placed on the interpretation of transference. Here again, the aim of treatment is to examine a current situation in an attempt to bring to light unconscious factors in the illness.

While patients with many different kinds of psychiatric illnesses can be helped in groups, there are indications that some patients with long-standing personality disorders can benefit more from group therapy than from individual treatment.

Other Forms of Group Therapy

There are other kinds of group therapy where no attempt is made to conduct the treatment on dynamic lines. Mutual discussion of personal problems is the usual basis of a supportive group. Some doctors conduct groups where the emphasis is on explanation rather than interpretation. Some combine these methods and also include active counselling. Some hospitals use larger groups in which patient and staff—including nursing staff—meet to discuss everyday problems of running the hospital. In groups such as this the patients often receive other forms of treatment as well.

Drug-assisted Techniques

In these methods, psychotherapy is used together with some form of stimulant, sedative or anesthetic.

The patient lies on a couch and the doctor sits at his side. Most drugs are given by injection into a vein, usually in the forearm. In the case of an anesthetic such as ether, the patient's face is covered with a mask on to which the ether is dropped.

For Abreaction. One use of this method is to facilitate abreaction (see p. 459). If it is felt that the illness is largely concerned with a single disturbing episode (as in some wartime cases of battle neurosis), the patient may relive the disturbing scene, thus 'abreacting' or giving vent to his pent-up emotions of fear, rage or grief. It is hoped that, if this is repeated a number of times, the individual can be brought to face his disturbing past more easily. The drugs which are often used for this purpose are those of the sedative group, and ether. In each case, the aim is to give just enough of the drug to make the patient drowsy and a little 'drunk.' He can then usually be persuaded to relive the scene concerned without too much difficulty.

For Narcoanalysis. The sedative group of drugs is also used to facilitate exploration of those events in the patient's past which may have a special significance for the present neurosis. This is sometimes called 'narcoanalysis.' Here the aim is to make the patient relaxed, so that he can survey his past without too much anxiety.

For Amnesia. An intravenous sedative can also be used for patients with a massive hysterical loss of memory. It is often possible, in this way, to re-establish the events of the period covered by the amnesia.

For Reticent Patients. When a patient finds it difficult to talk about himself and his difficulties a stimulant can be used. Methylamphetamine injected into a vein often makes a reticent person feel talkative.

Hallucinogens. A further group of drugs, the hallucinogens such as L.S.D. (lysergic acid diethylamide), mescalin, and psilocybin, have recently been used to enable a patient vividly to relive his childhood. Their usefulness is at present uncertain.

'Truth Drugs.' These methods are sometimes described in newspapers as treatment with the 'truth drug.' While their aim is indeed to help a patient tell the truth if this is repugnant or embarrassing to him, no drug yet discovered can *make* him do so if he does not wish to.

Hypnosis

Hypnosis is used as an abreactive technique or for exploration, with the same aim as the administration of sedative drugs. Commonly, it is used to reinforce suggestion.

The technique varies: most hypnotists develop their own. One method is to ask the patient to relax, preferably on a couch. The hypnotist then stands in front of him and holds a small bright object in such a position that a very slight strain is imposed on the patient's eyes. The room is darkened a little. The hypnotist then repeatedly assures the patient that he can't keep awake, feels drowsy, is very relaxed, and so on. Once the patient is hypnotized, the hypnotist 'suggests' that the patient's disability will grow less or disappear and that he will not remember it in the waking state. Many sessions of treatment may be required.

The procedure is so frequently followed by relapse and so liable to produce an abnormal dependence on the hypnotist that many authorities consider it of little use in psychiatric illness.

Pavlovian and Learning Theory Methods

Conditioned Reflex. Pavlovian methods of treatment are based on Pavlov's discovery of the conditioned reflex and the branch of biology deriving from this. Pavlov demonstrated that an organism can be trained to respond automatically to a given stimulus and to repeat this response in an identical way on subsequent occasions. For example, whereas the mouth normally waters in response to food, an animal can be trained to salivate at the sound of a bell.

Attempts to apply findings of Pavlovian physiology to the treatment of certain psychiatric disorders have been made in recent years in Great Britain, Russia and the United States of America.

'Learning theory' makes use of Pavlovian ideas together with knowledge gained from watching young animals and young children and studying their processes of learning. Neurotic symptoms are regarded not as part of a disease process but as habits developed on the lines of conditioned reflexes.

Treatment aims, broadly speaking, at conditioning the patient to respond in new and more satisfactory ways, and at deconditioning him from undesirable responses. Many methods of treatment have been devised, of which the following are only examples.

Buzzer for Enuresis. One device which has been developed is designed to help nocturnal enuresis (bed-wetting). When the sleeping patient begins to pass urine an electric circuit is completed and a loud bell or buzzer, placed at the bedside, rings. This wakes the patient who can then complete urination in the toilet. This procedure is repeated nightly for several weeks. The patient then begins to associate a full bladder with the bell-ringing and with awakening. The hope is that, even when the device is withdrawn, the full bladder will now cause the patient to awaken and use the toilet.

Cat Phobia. A method of treating phobias has also been devised and recently applied in the case of a patient who was terrified of cats and everything connected with them. She was first shown furry materials and later encouraged to touch them. Eventually she was able to hold and even stroke the material. She was soon prepared to tolerate photographs of cats. and later to stroke small kittens. In due course she was able to encounter cats without fear. Other phobias have been treated in a similar way.

Writer's Cramp is one example of a hysterical condition which has been treated by related methods. In this case small, repeated electric shocks are passed which make maintenance of the 'cramp' difficult. Eventually the patient may learn to use a pen without the intervention of the machine.

Aversion Therapy. A form of treatment known as 'aversion therapy' has been used to treat alcoholics. The patient is given injections of a drug which causes vomiting; apomorphine and emetine are examples. He is given alcohol to drink just before the drug can be expected to work. Again, the hope is that in due course he will come to associate the drinking of alcohol so strongly with vomiting that such drinks will revolt him. The procedure may have to be repeated separately for beer, gin, whisky and so on.

Finally methods have also been evolved whereby some sexual perversions, notably fetishism, can be treated. These rely on training the patient to become actively averse to the article of clothing concerned instead of becoming excited by it. But it must, of course, be emphasized that none of these methods, even when successful, does anything to resolve the mental conflicts underlying the symptoms.

Occupational Therapy

This term is used to cover a wide range of activities in which patients participate, under the guidance of trained staff, as part of the treatment of medical, surgical and psychiatric illness. At its simplest it provides a series of handicrafts to occupy and divert patients who are bed-bound or otherwise incapacitated. More active and complex programs are used for rehabilitation and retraining. Individual requirements of psychiatric patients differ greatly, but most in-patients and day patients need a full occupational regime at some stage in their treatment.

Graded Tasks. A patient recovering from a severe illness may be given a series of tasks which can be stimulating or soothing. These may be graded from simple to more complex tasks as the patient's condition improves, to give increasing exercise in concentration and the regaining of self-confidence. He or she may begin with undemanding work such as basket-making, proceed to handicrafts requiring more skill and later take up activities akin to his or her own work. Many occupational therapy departments can provide facilities for housecraft, woodwork, metal work and typing and clerical work. At this stage it is particularly encouraging for the patient if the work is of immediate use to the other patients or to the hospital.

Social Aspects. Patients in hospital for a considerable period tend to lose touch with social activities and with everyday responsibilities. This may impede return to full health. One aim of a psychiatric hospital is to provide for its less incapacitated patients the facilities for a full regime of work, social activity and physical exercise. It is usually helpful for the patient to feel that he retains responsibility for himself, and some hospitals encourage patients to arrange the details of their work and leisure, and to organize work projects and social activities such as dances and discussion groups.

The idea of the hospital as a small community of people representing both the family and civic group is an important one. Most psychiatric illnesses are characterized to some extent by an impairment of ability to live happily in reasonable harmony with relatives and society. Through the various activities described and particularly during the course of psychotherapy, the patient may be helped to improve his relationships with people, to function in a way both satisfying to himself and to the community, to accept the needs of the group when they conflict with his own, and to contribute to the group. His day-to-day experiences in the hospital community may be discussed in psychotherapy sessions and may give him a wider understanding of himself and his difficulties.

Acting a Role. Some additional occupational activities have special aims. In play-readings and psycho-drama, patients may gain understanding of personal problems by acting roles allotted to them. For example, a young girl playing the role of a mother may come to understand more clearly her own mother's interests and difficulties. Art therapy provides the satisfaction of self-expression and the patient may, in depicting his own experience and emotions, gain greater self-awareness. (For fuller details of the work of an Occupational Therapy Department, see section on Occupational Therapy, p. 181.)

PHYSICAL TREATMENTS

Treatment by Drugs

The various drugs used in the treatment of psychiatric illness fall into four main categories: sedatives, stimulants, tranquilizers and antidepressants. They are all used empirically, that is, while they are known to have particular effects, the way in which they act is unknown or only partially known.

Of recent years many new drugs have been discovered and developed, notably the tranquilizers and the antidepressants. Some of them have greatly improved the management of many disorders and, in some illnesses, have appreciably altered the outlook. With other drugs, however, the initial optimistic claims have not been confirmed by medical experience. The greatest care is necessary in the close study of a new drug to establish its usefulness.

Sedatives. These are drugs which reduce the activity of the brain and the rest of the central nervous system. In small doses they reduce restlessness, feelings of anxiety and tension. In larger doses they induce sleep. In very large doses their effect is powerful enough to abolish breathing. Until the discovery of the tranquilizers they were the only medicines available for the control of anxiety, restlessness and excitement.

They have certain disadvantages. They cause sleepiness, and sometimes depression in all but the smallest doses. There is a tendency for the system to become accustomed to them and larger doses may be required or addiction may develop.

This group includes many drugs having very similar effects, but which differ chiefly in the speed and duration with which they are effective. Medium and long-acting ones are used in relatively small doses for their calming effect. Medium and short-acting ones are used in larger doses to induce sleep in cases of insomnia or in sleep treatment.

Sedatives are usually taken by mouth, but they may be given by injection when a more marked and powerful effect results. The more commonly used sedatives are:

Barbiturates:
- Phenobarbital
- Amylobarbital
- Pentobarbital
- Hexobarbital

Paraldehyde
Chloral Hydrate

Tranquilizers. Tranquilizers have a calming effect in certain conditions and cause less drowsiness than the sedatives. They can therefore be used in larger doses, leaving the patient alert. They also have the advantage of not depressing respiration even in very large doses and they are to this extent safer than the sedatives. Tolerance and addiction are also much less likely to develop. Some tranquilizers have a number of side-effects, including dryness of the mouth, fall in blood pressure and stiffness of the muscles.

Tranquilizers are frequently used in the treatment of anxiety or restlessness accompanying any psychiatric condition. The older tranquilizers are used chiefly in schizophrenia, mania and in organic states, being relatively ineffective in the psychoneuroses. Newer tranquilizers, such as chlordiazepoxide and thiopropazate are more effective in these latter conditions.

In schizophrenia, these drugs may be strikingly effective in reducing disturbed behavior, hallucinations, delusions and thought disorder.

The better known tranquilizers are:

Chlorpromazine
Promazine
Meprobamate
Trifluoperazine

Antidepressants. Their name is self-descriptive. Unlike the stimulants they have no effect on people who are not depressed. They may be used in cases where a mood of depression exists, whether in depressive illnesses or in neuroses with depression. They are frequently used for patients who would previously have been given electrical treatment.

Their side-effects include dryness of the mouth and fall in blood pressure. It is customary for these drugs to be taken in tablet form:

Imipramine
Phenelzine
Tranylcypromine
Amitriptyline

Stimulants. These drugs, especially the amphetamines, produce increased wakefulness, postpone the need for sleep and may increase the flow of mental activity. They do not, however, markedly improve a mood of severe depression. They may produce or increase anxiety. Amphetamines are sometimes given as an aid to slimming, because they tend to diminish appetite. In large doses, usually over a period of weeks or months, acute toxic confusional psychoses may be produced.

Patients with unstable personalities may become addicted to stimulants.

Amphetamines are often prescribed combined with a small dose of sodium amytal in the same tablet. This counteracts the tendency for anxiety to be produced. The more commonly used stimulant drugs are:

Caffeine
Amphetamine Sulphate
Dexamphetamine Sulphate
Methylamphetamine
  Hydrochloride
Phenmetrazine Hydrochloride

Electroplexy
(*Electroconvulsive Therapy*)

The development of electroplexy arose out of the observation that spontaneous convulsions appeared to have a favorable effect on various sorts of mental illness. The supposed rarity of epilepsy in schizophrenia led to the conclusion that these two conditions were opposed to each other.

In 1936 the first attempts were made to treat schizophrenia with drug-induced convulsions. In 1938 the production of a convulsion using an electric shock was developed and this is the method commonly used now.

In modern techniques the treatment is usually administered under light anesthesia, such as may be used for dental extractions, and the muscular convulsion is reduced by a muscle-relaxant drug. The patient may sometimes be given this treatment as an outpatient. He receives an injection containing the anesthetic and the muscle relaxant, then an electric current of appropriate strength and duration is passed between two electrodes placed on his temples. The procedure takes a few minutes and the patient may be able to walk about after a short period of rest.

Electroplexy is usually given two or three times a week, though in certain circumstances it may be given more frequently. Improvement usually begins after three or four treatments but a course of six to eight is usually necessary.

Electroplexy is used in the treatment of depressive illness, of mania and in schizophrenia. It is most effective in depressive illnesses, 80 per cent of cases making a complete and prompt recovery.

Insulin Coma Therapy

Insulin is a substance, produced in the pancreas, which controls the storage of sugar in the body. It is given by injection in the treatment of diabetes and in psychiatric treatments. One of its effects is to reduce the amount of sugar in the bloodstream and, in large doses, the reduction of blood sugar has the effect of producing coma.

Chance observations that a coma so produced had beneficial effects in cases of schizophrenia led to the use of insulin coma as a treatment for schizophrenia. The subsequent discovery of the tranquilizer drugs and of their efficacy in such illnesses, has reduced the need for insulin coma treatment, but it is still used for some patients.

Producing the Coma. Injections of increasing dosage are given on successive days until a coma is produced. Thereafter a coma is produced each day with the appropriate dosage until between 25 and 30 comas have been produced. Each coma is allowed to continue for half to one and a half hours, and is then interrupted by giving the patient sugar either by injection or by stomach tube.

Since great care is needed in order that the treatment may be given with the minimum of risk, insulin coma therapy is only given in special units under the supervision of specially trained staff. The best results are obtained in early acute cases of the disorder. There is usually a progressive improvement in schizophrenic symptoms and a steady gain in weight during the course of treatment.

Modified Insulin Treatment. Before the discovery of insulin coma treatment for schizophrenia, small doses of insulin given over a short period of time were known to have a sedative effect, to reduce tension, and to increase appetite and weight. Modified insulin therapy is therefore used in cases of psychoneurosis or mild depression where there is considerable tension and, in particular, if there has been weight loss. The treatment usually results in a general improvement in bodily health and in a feeling of well-being.

Prolonged Narcosis
(*Sleep Treatment*)

During attacks of severe anxiety or depression occurring in the course of a psychiatric illness, a period of continuous sleep is sometimes thought desirable. This can be induced by giving large doses of sedatives, or combinations of sedatives and tranquilizers, to achieve deep sleep for most of the day and night and heavy drowsiness for the remainder. The treatment may last for one or two weeks. It is necessary for the patient to be under close supervision in hospital.

Prolonged narcosis is usually given where the illness is reactive to extremely traumatic or painful circumstances which have become too much for the patient to cope with. It may tide him over the period of acute reaction. When this has been relieved, the patient is able to continue with other forms of treatment.

Brain Surgery in Psychiatry

Prefrontal Leucotomy (lobotomy) is the most commonly used of operations for the relief of psychiatric illness. Certain nerve fibers from the frontal lobes of the brain are cut, in order to reduce severe anxiety, tension, depression, or the excessive excitability and activity that occurs in some disorders.

Various brain functions such as sensation or movement have been located in different parts of the brain. The conscious experience of emotion depends to a certain extent on the cortex (the outer shell of gray matter covering the brain) of the frontal lobes, and a certain collection of gray matter at the center of the brain. Severing of the communicating fibers between these centers results in the reduction of the degree of emotional intensity experienced, without interfering with other functions. The reduction of feeling, however, may result in some degree of apathy, of loss of tact, and of diminution of energy. Several variations of the operation have been devised in order to minimize these undesirable effects, while retaining the maximum benefits.

Indications for Surgery. Leucotomy is aimed at the reduction of undesirable emotions and drives, rather than at the cause of any particular illness. In the most favorable cases, however, complete recovery is achieved. Surgical treatment is usually only used in severe and protracted illnesses which have not responded to drugs or psychotherapy, or which relapse frequently after electroplexy. The cases of schizophrenia which respond best are those in which there is overactivity, in which there is marked depression, in which the patient is greatly disturbed by hallucinations, or in cases characterized by recurrent attacks of the illness with normal periods intervening. Tranquilizing drugs are particularly effective in these forms of the illness and have greatly reduced the number of cases requiring surgery. Prefrontal leucotomy is often extremely effective in cases of severe depressive illnesses which originally respond to electroplexy, but which relapse repeatedly despite electrical treatment.

In severe psychoneuroses, much suffering and incapacity may result from continuing symptoms, and brain surgery may afford great relief. It is most often used in chronic states of anxiety or tension, and in cases of obsessional neurosis. The operation is not indicated in cases of psychopathic personality, in many cases of drug addiction, and in mania.

A period of convalescence, rehabilitation and retraining is required after leucotomy.

Other Forms of Brain Surgery in psychiatry include the removal of parts of the frontal lobe cortex or of parts of the central gray matter. Ultrasonic waves or proton beams have been used to give an effect similar to surgical leucotomy.

PSYCHIATRIC TREATMENT IN THE HOSPITAL

General Practice and Out-patient Psychiatric Clinics

The majority of emotional disorders are treated by the patient's family doctor. In most cases his long knowledge of the patient and his thorough acquaintance with the family and background place him in an ideal position to understand the precise nature of the difficulties which the patient is undergoing and to provide guidance and short-term psychotherapy.

Where the general practitioner wishes to have specialist advice, he may refer the patient to a psychiatrist in the out-patient department of a general hospital or to a clinic attached to a psychiatric hospital. Here the patient is interviewed and examined by the psychiatrist and, in most instances, his relatives are interviewed by a psychiatric social worker, and any necessary investigations performed.

The patient's family doctor may then be advised on the further management of the case, or the patient may continue to attend the out-patient department for treatment, or he may be admitted to hospital. Most forms of treatment can be provided in out-patient departments in suitable cases, but here as elsewhere there is usually insufficient staff to provide detailed psychotherapy without a long wait.

In-Patient Treatment

This may be given in one of the large psychiatric hospitals, in a general hospital or in one of a number of special psychiatric units. In any case, admission is almost always completely informal and on exactly the same basis as admission to general medical or surgical wards.

The large **Psychiatric Hospitals** are the erstwhile mental hospitals. They have all the usual facilities for treatment and sometimes have attached to them units for special treatments such as neurosis units. It is true that their large size is in some ways a disadvantage and that the buildings are frequently old-fashioned but, as a rule, no restrictions are placed on patients apart from the immediate demands of treatment.

Other Psychiatric Units are generally of four kinds.

1. General psychiatric hospitals of small size and recently built: they provide in more advantageous circumstances the same facilities as the large psychiatric hospitals.
2. Units for special types of care, e.g. for children, for adolescents, or for cases of personality disorder.
3. Units where more adequate time can be devoted to psychotherapy.
4. Day Hospitals, where patients are treated during the daytime and return to their homes at night. Many cases which are treated as in-patients are suited to this sort of management which has the special advantage of avoiding long separation from the family.

These special units are few as yet and form only a very small proportion of psychiatric hospital facilities.

Community Care

Treatment of some types of psychiatric illness is often a long business entailing a long stay in hospital. In addition, popular and administrative prejudice isolates the psychiatric hospital, frequently placing it a long way from population centers. This creates great difficulty for the convalescent patient who is ready to take his place in his family, in the community and at work.

PSYCHIATRIC DISORDER AND THE FAMILY

People get on together by adapting to each other's habits, emotions and personalities. Of course, no relationship is completely smooth, and irritation and conflicts arise. These negative aspects are as much part of the friendship as the obvious affection and regard. The relatives and friends deal with their differences partly by modifying aspects of their behavior which might otherwise be disagreeable, partly by accepting each other's idiosyncrasies and partly by learning to have their disagreements while retaining mutual respect and affection. A family, therefore, or a group of friends becomes a distinctive group with its own varied patterns of behavior and interactions.

Other Members Involved. As is only to be expected, it is frequently found that when one member of the family has an emotional disorder other members are involved, or the difficulties arise out of their interaction. For this reason the relatives of a patient are often invited to attend when he seeks treatment. They may add to the information which the patient gives and make his problems more comprehensible. They may be given advice or be offered help on their own account. This is particularly likely with the parents of children and adolescents who attend psychiatric clinics. Husband and wife frequently attend together to discuss their problems.

Family Reactions to Psychiatric Illness

When a member of a family becomes ill, a new stress is placed on the relationship.

Self-blame. The relatives are naturally anxious about the patient's illness, but in addition they often feel guilty or have guilt of which they are unconscious. Usually there is no realistic cause for self-blame, which may arise out of the ambivalence towards the sick relative. The guilt may result in various responses.

Frequently relatives are over-solicitous and over-attentive, feeling an urgent need to perform services though these may have little bearing on the actual difficulties, or finding solutions to the sick person's difficulties though this may be far beyond the scope of their abilities. This attitude commonly shows by repeated, forceful and sometimes unreasonable demands on the patient's medical advisers. In many instances the self-blame is projected on to the doctors who may be blamed for not doing enough to help.

Unrealistic Assurances. The sick person often makes many demands on his family. They may be pressed for repeated reassurance and their own anxiety may lead them to give unrealistic reassurances and promises, which the patient may then resent as much as a complete lack of sympathy. The repeated demands may arouse hostility in the family who may feel that more is being asked of them than they can give and this may in turn increase their guilt feelings.

Understanding but not Anxiety. In general, the family can best help by being aware of these pressures, and by offering understanding and sympathy while at the same time not increasing the patient's fears by a great show of anxiety. They should accept the patient's need to regress, but recognize at the right time the patient's need to deal in realistic terms with his life. They should also be willing to make any necessary modification of their own behavior as it bears on the origins of the patient's disorder.

Relatives' Attitude to Phobias and Obsessions

As has been described these symptoms are in themselves irrational, though the underlying anxiety is very real. The patient is only too well aware that his feelings or actions are irrational, so that admonitions or encouragements to 'be sensible' are unhelpful and may put extra strain on the patient. The relatives should accept the presence of these symptoms, and acknowledge the anxiety which accompanies them.

Relatives' Attitudes to Delusions and Hallucinations

These false beliefs and perceptions are usually quite real to the person who suffers from them. They frequently represent feelings which are of great importance to the patient and which are arising out of his illness. To contradict or deny them is therefore unavailing and will be seen by the patient as an act of hostility or lack of sympathy. At the same time, it is usually possible with tact to avoid appearing to share these false ideas in case they are reinforced.

DISORDERS AND DISEASES OF THE SKIN

The skin is the pliant membrane which covers the external surface of the body; it varies in thickness in different regions. The interior passages, like the exterior surface, are likewise covered by tissue called mucous membrane. At the various openings of the body the outer and the inner membranes are united, forming a continuous covering structure. For anatomy of skin, see p.235.

A disease of the skin may spread to the mucous membrane, and a disease of the mucous membrane may affect the skin. This is seen in herpes, or the breaking-out around the lips after colds.

Structure of the Skin. The skin is a complex structure, but here may conveniently be described as consisting of two main layers; these become separated from each other when a blister is formed. The thin portion which is raised up by the fluid of a blister is called the epidermis; the lower layer is the sensitive skin, the dermis, or the true skin. The epidermis is horny and insensible, and serves as a sheath to protect the more sensitive true skin beneath. The dermis is well supplied with nerve endings which enable one to appreciate heat and cold, pain, pressure, the texture and shape of things, and so on. The hair roots lie in the dermis—the hair and nails being specialized forms of skin.

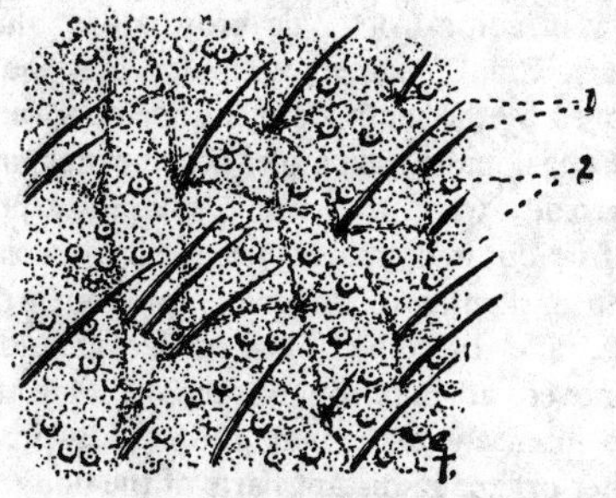

Fig. 1. *THE BACK OF THE HAND. The texture of the skin on the back of the hand is rather different from that of the palm. It has more hair follicles and smaller pores.* 1. *Hairs.* 2. *Pores.*

Both these layers may be involved in different skin diseases, either separately or concurrently.

Functions of the Skin. The four main functions are regulation of the body temperature, protection of the underlying structures, the capacity to feel sensation through the nerve endings (see above), and to act as a lesser excretory organ through the pores.

In regulating the body temperature, healthy skin has the capacity of narrowing down the skin blood vessels and closing the pores to conserve heat on a cold day, and reversing the process in hot weather.

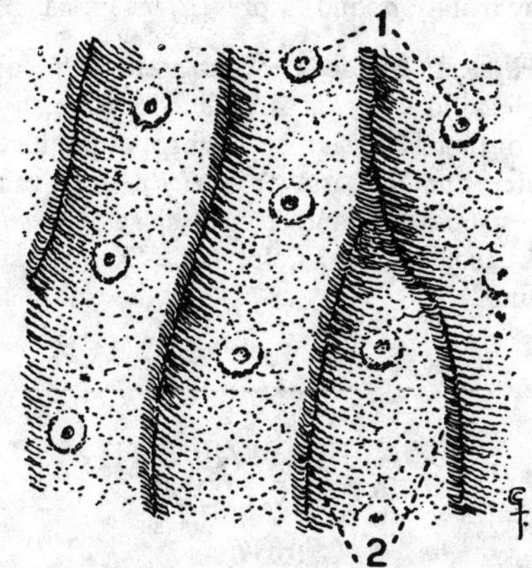

Fig. 2. *THE PALM OF THE HAND. The permanent creases of the skin are shown clearly in this highly magnified section and the large pores of the sweat ducts lie between the creases.* 1. *Pores.* 2. *Creases.*

One or more of these functions may be disturbed in skin diseases.

Causes of Skin Diseases

The causes of skin diseases are very numerous, since the skin may be injured by many factors which do not affect the inner organs and tissues. There may be predisposing or exciting factors, and immediate causes.

Predisposing Conditions include climate, race, age, sex, occupation, diet, constitution and temperament.

Immediate Causes are: (1) hereditary defects, or maldevelopments; (2) physical causes such as friction, heat and cold, irradiation, or pressure; (3) chemical agencies, such as acids, alkalis, drugs, tars, dyes, vegetable and plant irritants, and proteins; (4) parasites, mainly bacteria, fungi and viruses; (5) circulatory disorders; (6) nervous disorders; (7) disorders of the glands and their hormones; (8) systemic diseases.

An understanding of the causes is necessary to arrive at a correct diagnosis, and to do this the sequence of the disturbing symptoms must also be followed. The eruption must be examined as to color, size and shape, distribution, character of surface, nature of lesion (pustule, vesicle, weal, etc.), duration of symptoms, and occupation of patient; and finally, it must not be forgotten that two separate diseases may exist together.

Signs and Symptoms of Skin Diseases

Associated with most skin complaints are a wide range of lesions or eruptions and a more limited number of symptoms.

Symptoms. The chief of these are itching, tingling, burning, pricking, increased and decreased sensitivity, crawling sensations, and pain; itching is the commonest symptom, and may be intermittent or continuous, while pain is less usual.

Lesions include primary or secondary manifestations; the primary may be in the form of macules or spots, papules or pimples, nodules, tumors, weals, vesicles or small blisters, and bullae or large blisters. The secondary effects may appear as scales, fissures, excoriation, crusts, ulcers, and rarely malignancy.

Various terms are used to describe the conditions seen in different skin diseases, and it may help the reader if these are briefly explained here.

A **macule** is a small flat patch or spot of discoloration, not raised above the surface of the skin. A larger lesion of this type is called a **plaque**, whereas large reddened areas are referred to as **erythema**.

A **papule** is a raised solid pimple, not larger than a pea.

A **tubercle** or **nodule** is a similar raised eruption of larger size.

A **vesicle** is a small raised spot containing fluid; a **bulla** or blister is larger than a vesicle.

A **pustule** is a small raised lesion containing pus; a **furuncle** or boil is a large pustule.

A **scale** is a dead flake of the epidermis or outer horny skin.

Crusts and **scabs** consist of skin cells, fibrin, dried serum, white blood cells and sometimes pus cells.

A **weal** is a transitory raised lesion of the skin, with edema in the part concerned.

Scars are formed by fibrous tissue, and may be red in recent cases, or white in long-standing cases.

An **excoriation** is an abrasion of the epidermis.

A **fissure** is a crack of variable depth.

An **ulcer** is a local lesion with loss of skin tissue.

General Treatment in Skin Diseases

The practical measures to be considered include general hygienic measures, diet, investigation for presence of septic foci in the body, medicines and external applications, and physical treatment.

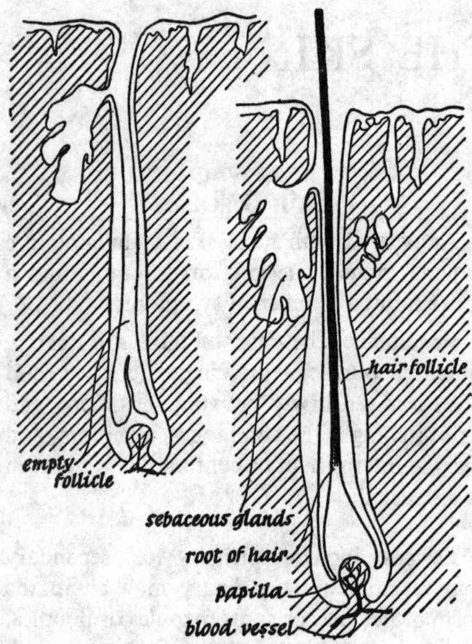

Fig. 3. *HAIR. Each hair on the skin grows from a separate follicle which lies deep in the true dermis. Each hair root is fed by blood capillaries and lubricated by oily secretion from the sebaceous glands.*

General Hygiene. In acute or extensive skin eruptions the patient is best in bed, which provides rest, and makes the application of remedies easier. The bowels should be kept regular.

Hard water is often irritating to the skin, but artificial water-softeners, such as bath salts, are often unsuitable. Soap should be avoided in irritative conditions such as eczema or dermatitis.

Diet must be suitable, nourishing and well balanced, with avoidance of items known to disagree, as for example, shell fish in cases of urticaria, or alcohol in acne or rosacea.

Baths. Prolonged immersion baths are sometimes used for the treatment of dermatitis. Continuous irrigation may be used for extensive burns; it greatly reduces pain and prevents infection of large areas.

Applications may be dry or moist, and may or may not contain medicaments.

POWDERS are used as drying and astringent agents. They are also soothing and absorbent.

LOTIONS are useful for large areas; they may be astringent, antiseptic, sedative, etc.

PLASTERS are used spread on cloth (cotton or linen) for close contact and prolonged application.

OINTMENTS and PASTES are two of the commonest skin applications. Vaseline, lanolin, olive oil, etc., form common bases for incorporating medicaments.

CREAMS are soft ointments, which are easy to spread.

POULTICES are used to allay inflammation, and to reduce pain and congestion in septic conditions. They may be made of starch, linseed, kaolin, simple bread, or lint fomentations, and may contain medicaments such as ichthammol or boric acid.

Drugs are selected according to individual requirements, and idiosyncrasies must be recognized. Sedatives are often required to allay irritation, and to prevent insomnia.

Physical Methods of treatment include application of *cold*, as carbon dioxide snow for birthmarks; *heat*, in the form of poultices, cautery and diathermy; *electricity*, in galvanic baths, ionization and electrolysis; and *irradiation*, such as ultraviolet light, X-rays, and radium.

CONGENITAL SKIN AFFECTIONS

Ichthyosis

Ichthyosis is a harsh dry condition of the skin, usually appearing in the newborn infant or in early life; scales, warty growths and fissures may be associated. There are various degrees of severity, minor cases being called 'xeroderma.' The disease may not interfere with the general health, but in rare cases the child may live only a few days. Ichthyosis generally becomes worse in cold weather, and the skin tends to be easily injured or excoriated; the condition becomes worse up to puberty, then becoming stationary. Eczema may supervene in adult life and the skin is particularly susceptible to irritation by external agents.

Treatment. Since many patients show signs of malnutrition, a good mixed diet is helpful. Thyroid extract has been tried with only moderate success. Large doses of vitamin A may be helpful.

Emollient ointments or creams are often required. Avoidance should be made of any irritating cheap soap or clothes, and starch or bran baths are valuable for removing accretions of scales and sweat. A superfatted soap should be used. Warm clothing is essential in cold weather.

Albinism

Albinism denotes a hereditary lack of pigment in the skin, hair and eyes; 'albinos' are characteristic in appearance, and have white skin, pink irises, and very fair hair. They are generally rather delicate, suffer from a dislike of light, and readily develop sunburn. No treatment is effective, but protection of the eyes by tinted glasses is advisable. The general health requires care.

Nevi and Moles

Birthmarks are common on the face, but may occur in any region and are often associated with other defects such as hare-lip or webbing of the fingers. Those containing blood vessels are known as 'port-wine stains' and 'strawberry marks,' and are of a reddish or purple color. The former type often disappear within a few months of birth; if they do not, they may be treated by electrolysis or diathermy by a doctor, or by cautery or application of carbon dioxide snow.

The 'strawberry marks' are generally found on the face and scalp, and tend to increase in size for a few months after birth; they may then disappear about the fifth year. A less common type increase rapidly in size in adult life. If they cause disfigurement on the face or scalp they may be removed surgically, or be treated with carbon dioxide snow, or by the injection of sclerosing solutions.

Spider nevi are very small marks, bright red in color, with small blood vessels radiating outwards. They are not very disfiguring but sometimes bleed easily, and, since they do not often disappear spontaneously, they may be obliterated by cautery, electrolysis, or carbon dioxide snow.

Pigmented Moles and hairy moles vary from very small patches to large areas; pigmented moles are very common and most people have several small scattered moles in different parts of the body. Giant moles are much less common, but often cover a large part of the trunk or body. Pigmented moles vary in color from pale brown to a bluish-black. Small pigmented moles may be removed by the methods mentioned above.

Occasionally such moles become malignant, especially when they are constantly exposed to friction; malignancy is generally associated with darkening of the color, rapid growth in size, and bleeding. Such moles should be removed at once by a surgeon since they are intensely malignant and rapidly invade other organs in distant parts of the body.

Sebaceous Cysts
(*Wens*)

Wens are cysts occurring in the sebaceous

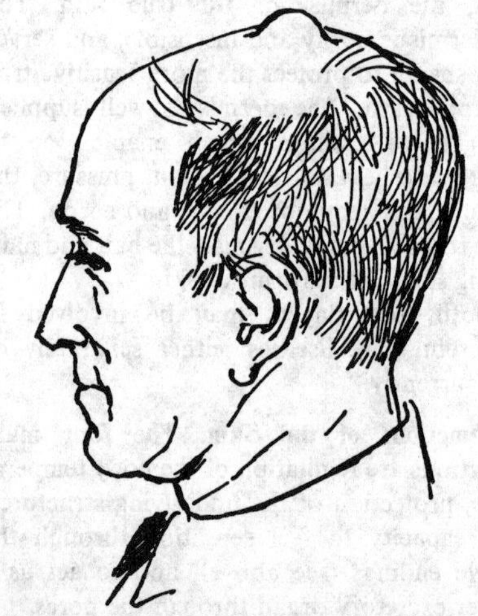

Fig. 4. *A WEN. This is a cyst occurring chiefly on the scalp. It is very easily removed by a local operation.*

glands, being especially common on the scalp, neck, scrotum and vulva in young adults. They often measure about an inch across, and are yellowish or white in color, from the fatty cheesy material they contain.

Treatment consists in removal of the entire cyst with its sac wall. Occasionally such cysts become inflammed and suppurate, in which case they must be treated as a boil until the infection subsides.

DISEASES DUE TO PHYSICAL CAUSES

Corns and Callosities

CALLOSITIES are thickenings of the horny layer of the skin occurring, as a result of irritation, on the soles, palms, and other parts. A corn may form in a callosity, but often develops independently.

A CORN is a small localized deep-seated horny formation, commonly found on the toes and soles of the feet, the apex of the corn pressing down upon the corium of the skin. It is a popular belief that the development of corns is confined exclusively to the foot. It is true that these growths are most frequently seen on the feet, but they often occur between the fingers or on the hands of persons who are engaged in manual labor.

Hard Corns

The hard corn is the most common variety and originates through pressure and friction. This first produces irritation of the cutaneous nerves, causing an increased blood supply to the part, and congestion takes place immediately beneath. The corn itself is composed of the horny layer of the outer skin, which becomes much thickened and, owing to the external pressure, projects inwards in the form of a cone. This causes pain as a result of pressure on small nerves in the deep layer of the skin.

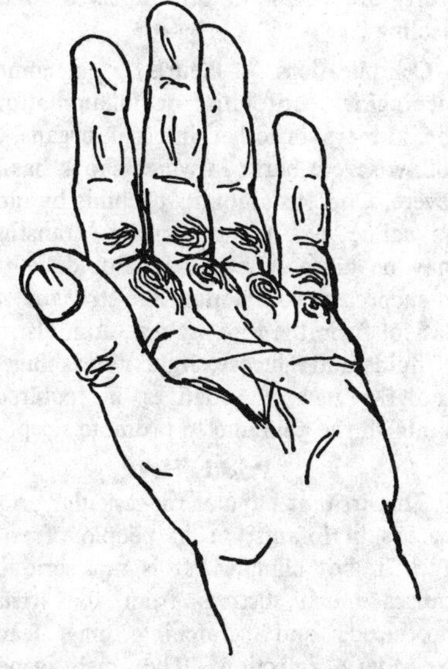

Fig. 5. *CORNS ON THE HAND are due to pressure or friction.*

Causes. Hard corns are commonly caused by intermittent pressure or friction of ill-fitting shoes; the shoes may be too tight, thereby causing pressure, or they may be too loose, causing friction. Corns may also be caused by some roughness in the finish of the shoe, or by the sole of the shoe being too thin.

Stockings are important factors in producing corns; knots or poor workmanship in darning are often responsible for these minor troubles. A stocking that is too short presses the toes together, at the same time causing flexion, with the result that the toes are pressed against the upper of the shoe, causing direct pressure. A similar stocking is often responsible for the first stages of bunion.

Treatment. Preventive methods should be adopted in the first case. A simple corn may be frequently shaved off at intervals of a few days, using a suitable instrument such as one of the numerous types of safety corn razors, taking care not to draw blood, or infection may follow. As a precautionary measure before cutting the corn, the corn razor should be immersed for a few minutes in an antiseptic such as methylated alcohol, and the area surrounding the corn painted with weak solution of iodine, again using iodine after the operation. Pumice-stone is also useful for rubbing down large calloused places on the sole of the foot.

To prevent pressure from the shoe, a circular adhesive felt shield may be applied *around* the corn. For the sole of the foot thin zinc oxide felt or chamois leather plaster afford relief on account of their resiliency. In no case should felt or a piece of plaster be cut to the exact size of the corn, since this will merely cause the pressure to be increased by the shoe.

Patent remedies and strong acids are often injurious and, when used, frequently injure the normal tissues, causing inflammation or possibly suppuration, before affecting the compact structure of a corn. X-rays have been used for relief of pain in corns, and to arrest their growth.

Note: People requiring the services of a chiropodist should be careful to go to a properly qualified practitioner.

Soft Corns

These develop between the toes, and are associated with ringworm of the clefts between the toes. A soft corn has a white sodden appearance, with the consistency of rubber. The symptoms vary with the degree of pressure brought to bear upon the toes. Sometimes there is a sensation as if there were a foreign body between the toes, and as the growth develops, the pain becomes worse. Others give similar pain to that caused by a hard corn—shooting pain, throbbing, or a scalding sensation. The sweat glands continue to function but the parts, being pressed together, do not allow the perspiration to evaporate.

Treatment. Scrupulous cleanliness and correct footwear should be observed. Bathing the feet night and morning with spirit will assist in drying up the skin between the toes, especially where excessive moisture is general. Applications of weak solution of iodine twice daily for one or two weeks will often clear up the condition. Pledgets of raw cotton placed in between the toes tend to relieve pressure, and small plain felt pads are resilient and protective.

Chapped and Cracked Skin

Cracked skin may occur as a result of constant softening from moisture (as with housewives' hands), or in dry conditions of the skin with loss of elasticity, as occurs in chapping. Grease or cold cream should be used to soften the skin, and water, soap and alkali should be avoided, especially when the condition is the result of constant immersion in water and washing preparations.

Effects of Cold

Frostbite

The first effect of cold applied to the body is to contract the small blood vessels of the skin; the circulation is delayed in the vessels near the surface, and the fingers, toes, ears, nose, etc., become waxen and white. The capillary or hair-like vessels then dilate while the arterioles remain contracted, and the skin is red. If severe cold be continued sufficiently long, the capillaries are paralyzed, the circulation ceases in the surface tissues, and there is clotting in the small blood vessels.

With intense cold the tissues are frozen, heat ceases to be evolved and, on thawing, necrosis (death) of the parts follows. Parts affected in this way are said to be frostbitten; the fingers, toes, nose and ears are most often affected, since a large surface area is exposed. The part becomes white, hard and numb. On thawing it becomes purple, swollen and painful, and may be blistered or ulcerated and sloughing. Free circulation of oxygenated blood is essential to the continuance of sensation and consciousness; hence, when the circulation is seriously impeded by cold, the body becomes numb, and languor and torpor follow. Drowsiness supervenes, followed by sleep, from which there may be no waking.

Treatment. In restoring frostbitten parts or persons benumbed with cold, warmth must only be applied very gradually and cautiously, *after* the circulation has returned. On no account bring the affected part near a fire or a hot-water bottle, or use massage. To restore a frozen limb or part, wrap it in dry sterile dressings and thick raw cotton; keep it absolutely at rest. Give the patient warm blankets and hot drinks, but *no* alcohol. Do not take the patient into a warm room until the circulation is restored in the affected parts.

After thawing and when sensation has returned, the parts should be warmed very gradually, but direct heat must *not* be applied. Blisters should not be opened. (See p. 309.)

If a person be reduced by cold to insensibility and if signs of life appear, wrap him in warm blankets and put a drop of brandy on the tongue; finally give tea, or coffee, or hot milk and glucose when the patient can swallow. Oxygen is sometimes beneficial at high altitudes.

Chilblains

These are local areas of congestion caused by exposure to cold or damp in persons of feeble circulation, and affect the ears, fingers, toes, and heels, with irritating or painful inflammatory swelling of a red, purple, or bluish color. The skin may be red in patches, and the part is swollen, with itching, tingling, pain, and stiffness or lameness. There may be blisters, around which the skin is blue or purple, or there may be ulceration and sloughing. Young girls and women are mainly affected. Anemia and tuberculosis are sometimes associated conditions.

Treatment. To prevent chilblains, promote a better circulation by exercise, tonics, and good food, particularly dairy foods. Wear woolen gloves and warm stockings in winter.

When the chilblains have developed, painting with weak solution of iodine, or with ichthammol, or rubbing with an ointment containing menthol or iodine are useful. If there is ulceration, use zinc cream and cover loosely with a bandage. Tablets containing nicotinamide and acetomenaphthone are given for the prevention and treatment of chilblains. (See also p. 309.)

Acrocyanosis

Plump adolescent girls sometimes develop a chronic dusky reddening and some swelling of the limbs, feet and hands. It is painless, apart from slight tenderness and occasional tingling. The treatment should be on the same lines as that for chilblains.

Raynaud's Disease

This is a symmetrical pallid and bloodless spasmodic affection of the hands and feet, and occasionally the nose or ears, caused by cold, and ranging from discomfort to gangrene of the parts. It is commonest in women, and the extremities appear cold, insensitive and stiff, the middle fingers of the hands being the most commonly affected parts. An attack may last from a few moments to some hours or days and as the numbness subsides, tingling and burning occur. In rare cases ulceration subsequently develops. See also Vasomotor Disorders, p. 309.

Treatment requires fresh air and exercise, nutritious food and warm clothes, with tonics and cod-liver oil. At the onset of an attack, friction and warmth with liniments are beneficial, and galvanic baths may be useful for reducing the spasm. Occasionally, operations on the sympathetic nerves to the hands are helpful in suitable cases.

Effects of Heat

Burns and Scalds

A burn is the effect of flame or heated solids, electrical currents, lightning, or friction, acting upon living tissues. Other types of burns are caused by strong corrosives, or by irradiation from X-rays or radium. The effects are inflammation, and sometimes destruction of the skin or structures below.

A scald is an injury produced by applying hot water or other fluids or hot gases or moist heat to the skin or mucosa. The natural temperature of the human body is about 37° C (98·4° F), that of boiling water is 100° C (212° F). Bringing the skin in contact with a fluid heated so far above it produces redness and pain. If nothing is done instantly to prevent injury, the outer skin becomes raised from the skin in the form of a blister filled with fluid. The degree of danger from a burn or scald depends upon the extent of the injured surface, and also upon the depth of the injury. An extensive scald or burn may prove fatal in a few hours.

Shock. The symptoms of shock and collapse in a burn of any considerable extent are often very severe, and may be fatal. The pulse becomes feeble and rapid, the temperature subnormal, and the skin cold and clammy. Injuries from burns are especially dangerous upon the head, neck, chest and abdomen. Children and old or debilitated persons run the greatest risk of severe shock after burns and scalds. Shock is increased by the loss of fluid from the body in severe burns, and must be counteracted by administration of fluids to the patient. The internal organs may also be affected.

In one to two days the stage of reaction follows, with improvement in the pulse, rise of temperature due to toxemia in severe cases, and vomiting or convulsions may develop in children. (See also p. 558.)

There are various degrees of burns, and the treatment varies accordingly.

First Degree Burns. Despite reddening and tenderness, there is no real destruction of the tissues. A non-greasy mild antiseptic cream or a paste of sodium bicarbonate may be applied, and the burn lightly bandaged.

Second Degree Burns cause superficial injury to the skin, with blistering. These blisters should be bathed with an antiseptic solution; if very large they may be punctured with a sterilized needle or other instrument to allow drainage. The burn may be dressed with pieces of vaseline-impregnated gauze which may also contain an antibiotic.

Third and Fourth Degree Burns. When the burn causes partial or total destruction of the skin, the patient must be treated for shock with warmth and sedatives. Morphine is often required to be given by a doctor. Later the clothes are gently removed by soaking, if necessary, in saline or sodium bicarbonate

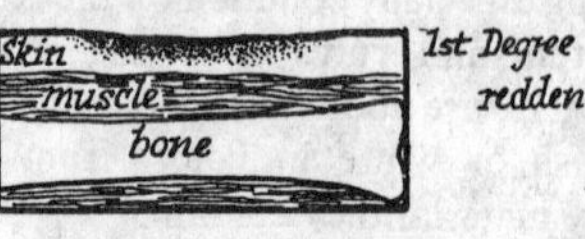

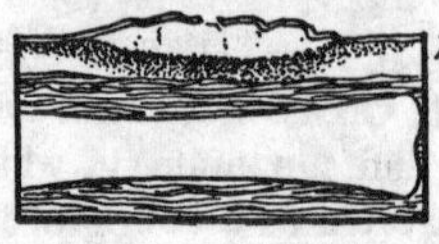

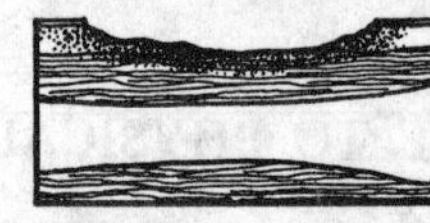

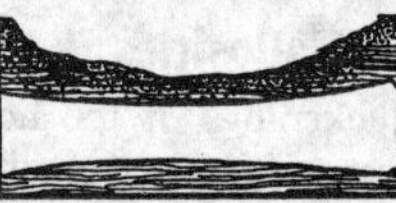

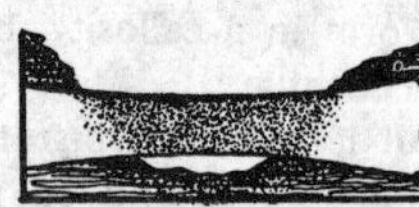

Fig. 6. *BURNS are assessed according to the degree or intensity of the damage done to the part or limb. Usually six degrees of burn injury are recognized: see text.*

solution. The burnt area must be cleansed and, because the procedure is so painful, anesthesia is often required.

In Fifth Degree Burns the muscles below the skin are burned, while in **Sixth Degree Burns** the whole limb or part is charred.

The choice of dressing depends on the facilities available. In extensive burns (except of the face, hands, feet and chest), the treatment of choice is exposure to the air under sterile conditions. This means that the patient must be in hospital and preferably under the care of a special burns unit. In burns of the face, sterile gauze dressings with an antibiotic cream may be applied. If the eyes are involved they should be bathed frequently with boric acid solution.

If burns become septic, the appropriate measures must always be applied. Skin grafts are useful in certain cases to assist healing (see p. 560).

Complications. Pleurisy, pneumonia, meningitis, peritonitis, or inflammation of the kidneys or other internal organs, may follow severe burns in which shock has been severe. Copious amounts of fluids by mouth, or saline per rectum or by transfusion, may be given. Great care should be taken in such cases to maintain the strength of the patient from the first, by rest, administration of fluids and glucose, light nourishing diet, and the use of sedatives if required to diminish the pain and to promote sleep.

Prickly Heat

This irritant papular or vesicular eruption occurs in infants, or in people of varying ages in hot climates. It is not serious but causes much distress from the irritation produced, and scratching may lead to secondary infection. The rash generally affects the trunk, neck, arms, and thighs, or the exposed parts. (See also p. 561.)

Treatment should be directed to avoidance of direct sunlight or unnecessary heat, to strict cleanliness, light dry cotton clothing next to the skin, and a light diet without alcohol, meat, or coffee; water should be drunk plentifully, and the bowels should be kept regular. Calamine lotion may be applied to soothe the affected area.

Sunburn

Sunburn is a form of heat rash familiar to most people, and is produced by excessive stimulation from the ultraviolet rays in the sunlight. A protective reaction occurs which results in pigmentation of the skin, but prior to the deposition of the pigment there may be much redness and blistering, as in an ordinary burn.

When redness occurs the parts should be covered with calamine or a non-greasy cream; exposure to the direct sunlight should be avoided for long periods, until the skin is inured. (See also p. 561.)

It is particularly important to avoid sunburn in young babies and children, in whom the skin is very sensitive. A young baby should not be exposed to bright sun. The sunlight is less intense at 5 p.m., which is a suitable time to allow exposure in babies in hot weather. The eyes should always be directed away from the sun, and the nape of the neck should be protected.

Freckles and other Pigmentations

Freckles are circumscribed patches of pigment found mainly on the face, neck, arms, hands or legs; they tend to be increased by sunlight, but generally give no trouble. When considered unsightly they can sometimes be bleached by hydrogen peroxide (10-volume strength) after light scraping by a doctor.

Chloasma, a brownish pigmentation of the face, especially the forehead and neck, is often seen in pregnancy, and may also develop during the menopause. Pigmented patches may also develop in old scar tissue, such as burns, or on the legs as a result of constant exposure to the heat of a fire (erythema abigne).

Irradiation dermatitis occurs after exposure of the skin to strong sunlight, X-rays, or radium. Severe sunburn is treated as indicated above, and may be prevented by the use of brown grease paint before exposure, which should only be undertaken for short periods until the protective reaction of pigmentation has developed.

DERMATITIS DUE TO CHEMICAL AGENTS

Dermatitis, or inflammation of the skin, is shown by redness, swelling, heat and pain, or irritation. Chemical substances which give rise to dermatitis may affect the skin directly by contact from outside, or as a result of the chemical being carried around in the blood. Individuals vary considerably in their susceptibilities to irritants, and in the intensity of the reaction. In some cases 'sensitization' occurs after repeated exposure to certain substances.

Vegetable and Animal Irritants

Vegetable irritants which are prone to affect human beings are nettles, some primula plants, mayweed, tulips, chrysanthemums, tomato plants, orchids, daffodils and other bulb plants, poison-ivy, lacquer preparations, various woods, especially teak, satinwood and ebony, and other less common plants. The volatile oils obtained from plant sources such as mustard oil, turpentine and arnica are well known for their irritant properties.

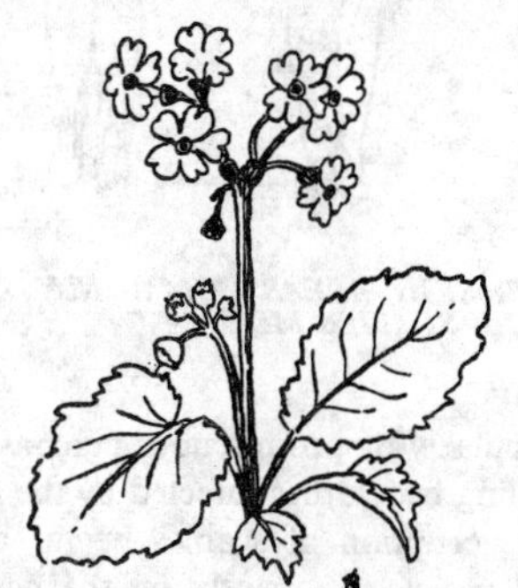

Fig. 7. *A PLANT CAUSING DERMATITIS: Primula obconica.*

Animal irritants which give rise to dermatitis of varying degree may be divided into two groups: those due to an actual secretion, e.g. jellyfish stings, bites of red-brown ants, and those of an allergic nature such as the hairs of wooly caterpillars, and the fur of animals.

Treatment consists in avoidance of the irritant substance, and in the application of lead or calamine lotions, or zinc cream to allay irritation. Antihistamine creams or ointments (see p. 482) are useful in allergic cases.

For the treatment of jellyfish stings see p.36 .

Mineral Irritants

Mineral irritants cause a large number of the cases known as industrial or occupational dermatitis. The hands and arms are commonly affected since they are the parts most exposed to direct contact; the face or any other part, however, may be involved. In some cases it may be the cleansing agents used that cause an eruption.

Mineral irritants may be gritty substances, causing mechanical irritation, cleansing agents which soften and crack the skin (soda, ammonia, etc.), or irritating substances such as petroleum or turpentine derivatives, strong irritants, such as chromic acid, tar, aniline dyes, acids and alkalis, oils and greases, metals, plastics, rubber substances, paints and varnishes, and so forth.

Drugs may also cause eruptions when used externally; arnica, belladonna, carbolic acid, formalin, iodine, mercury, picric acid, sulphur, and turpentine are common examples.

The dermatitis produced may be of all grades of severity from reddening or vesicles to weeping dermatitis with crusts, scaling, or suppurating conditions with ulceration. In rare cases, cancer of the skin may develop after prolonged contact with tar, soot, or other strong irritants.

CERTAIN FORMS OF OCCUPATIONAL DERMATITIS are now recognized, the main being:

- Analysts and chemists: from chemicals.
- Bakers and grocers: from flour and sugar.
- Barbers and hairdressers: from soap and some hair dyes.
- Bronze workers: from arsenic.
- Builders: from lime and dust.
- Carpenters and French polishers: from dust, turpentine, resin, and oils.
- Chromium platers: chrome ulcers.
- Compositors: from benzene and bichromate.
- Dyers and painters: from various dyes and pigments.
- Farmers and gardeners: from agricultural sprays and pesticides: from fruits, plants, soil, etc.
- Furriers: from dyes.
- Metal workers: oil acne from oil.
- Mill-hands and cotton-winders: from cotton and potash of alum.
- Munition workers: from T.N.T., nitroglycerine, and other explosives.
- Miners: from coal and soot.
- Surgeons, dentists, and nurses: from certain drugs, disinfectants, soap, etc.
- Tar-workers: from contact with tar.
- Housewives: from detergents, strong soaps, and frequent immersion of the hands in water.

Treatment resolves itself into removal or avoidance of the irritant substances, or protection against them by suitable clothing. It is often necessary to change the occupation.

Soothing applications, such as zinc ointment, calamine lotion or ointment, should be applied to the affected areas, and attention should be paid to the general health. In some cases greasy preparations are not suitable in the early stages, but when the acute symptoms subside, oily applications may be used. In chronic cases zinc paste is protective. X-ray treatment is useful in some resistant cases, but must be used with great caution.

Diaper Rash

This is common in young babies, affecting the buttocks, thighs, genital organs and groins. Such a rash may be due to faults in washing the diapers, such as insufficient rinsing, or the use of harsh detergents. Commonly, diapers are washed in too strong a solution of one of the modern detergents and, following this, inadequate rinsing leaves granules of the detergent on the diapers. Infrequent changing of diapers, diarrhea, and thrush are other causes of eruptions in these areas, and rashes may be avoided by scrupulous attention to hygiene and cleanliness.

Treatment. When a rash develops, zinc and castor oil cream is a protective preparation which is suitable for application. Before the cream is used the parts must be gently and carefully dried after bathing. A few applications of picric acid lotion, 1 per cent, will often clear up sore buttocks which are resistant to other forms of treatment.

To prevent a rash, soak the diapers, after washing, in benzalkonium chloride solution, following the directions on the label; allow to dry without rinsing to retain the protective film.

Attention must be paid to thrush or digestive disturbances when these are present.

Eruptions due to Drugs

Taken Internally

Certain drugs taken internally tend to produce eruptions in some persons who seem to be especially susceptible or to possess an idiosyncrasy to particular substances.

The ASPIRIN group, the IODIDES and the BROMIDES are common examples, the former giving an urticarial or scarlatiniform rash, while the two latter may produce an erthematous or papular acne eruption.

ARSENIC sometimes causes eczema or urticaria or, if taken over a long period, produces brown pigmentation.

QUININE and BELLADONNA and sometimes SULPHONAL give scarlatiniform rashes. GOLD salts cause purpuric rashes in some patients.

SANTONIN, the IODIDES and QUININE occasionally give rise to urticaria, while the SERUMS that are used for inoculation purposes are a very common cause of a generalized giant urticaria, called a *serum rash.*

SULPHONAMIDES, (p. 595), PENICILLIN and other antibiotics (p.598) may produce various types of eruptions.

Treatment is usually simple; the drug should be discontinued, and the patient rested and given a laxative, with plenty of fluids and demulcent drinks. Calamine lotion may be used to allay urticarial irritation.

SKIN PARASITES

Scabies

(*Itch*)

Scabies is a contagious disease due to infestation by the mite called the *Acarus scabiei*, which has its habitat in the human skin. The female, after fertilization, burrows into the skin, while the smaller male soon dies. In the burrow the female lays her eggs at the rate of about 2 or 3 a day, which in their turn grow into adult mites and infest new areas. The adult is a small organism with legs and suckers, which is just visible to the naked eye as a pearly white speck. The disease is usually contracted from a bed-fellow,

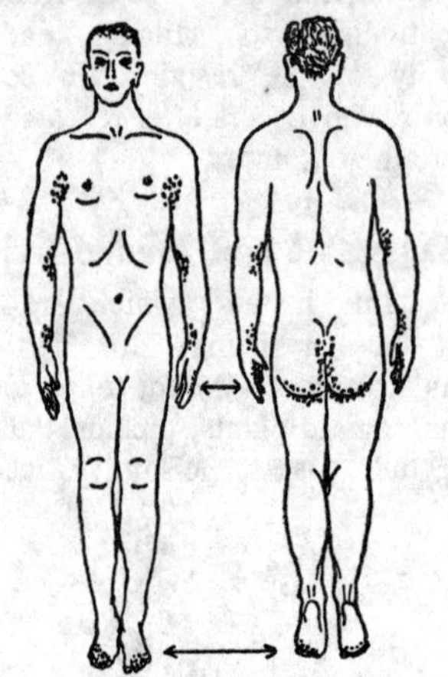

Fig. 8. *SKIN AREAS COMMONLY AFFECTED BY THE SCABIES MITE.*

particularly by promiscuous persons, or from handling bedclothes infected by the acarus.

The eruption of scabies begins as a very small vesicle, frequently on the hands, feet, wrists and ankles, armpits, abdomen, breast and penis, which is followed by a small burrow reaching up to half an inch in length and causing great irritation, although this may not develop for about a month after infection. The irritation is generally severest at night. Scratching produces secondary excoriations and pustules.

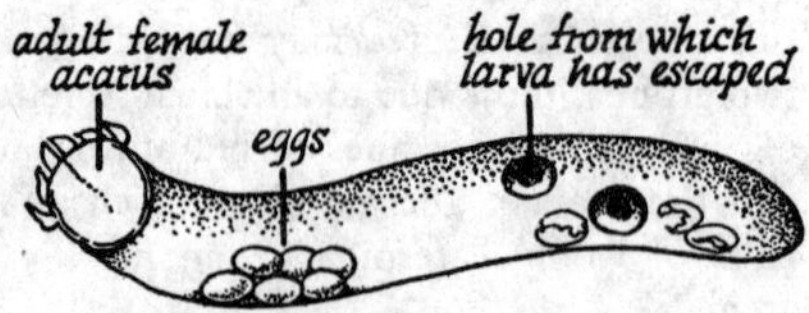

Fig. 9. *THE BURROW OF A SCABIES PARASITE IN THE HUMAN SKIN*

Treatment. The best treatment is to discard all clothing for disinfection, to apply gamma benzene hexachloride (0.5% cream base) to cover the whole body, and allow to dry. Repeat twice, with 12-hour intervals. Twelve hours later, patients should have a bath, put on clean underwear, and change their sheets.

The itching generally ceases, and in most cases the disease is arrested, but occasionally some further treatment is required. To allay irritation, a zinc cream or an oily calamine lotion may be used on the skin. Severely infected patients must be kept in bed.

Lice

Pediculosis is a contagious animal parasitic affection, characterized by the presence of pediculi on the skin or hair of the body. They are small six-legged creatures without wings and are about 3 millimeters ($\frac{1}{8}$ inch) long. There are three varieties named according to the site they infest. They all cause great discomfort and itching, since they obtain their food by biting the skin and sucking out the blood.

The Head Louse (*Pediculus capitis*) is found on the scalp, and has a long oval greyish body with six legs furnished with nails; it has an oval head with two prominent eyes and two horns.

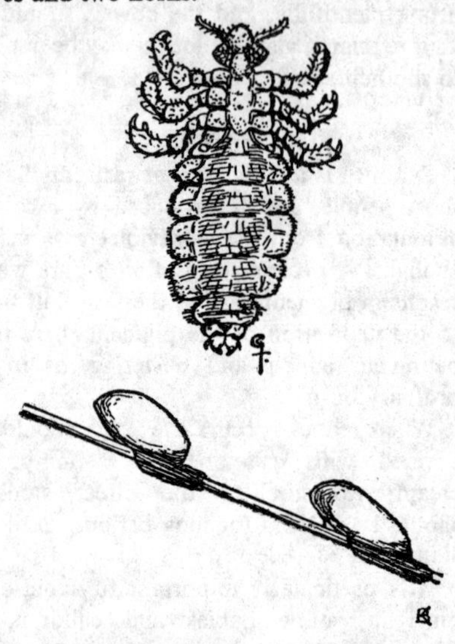

Fig. 10. *HEAD LOUSE. The adult female, and the nits (eggs) 'glued' to a hair.*

NITS are the eggs or ova. They are small whitish bodies which adhere to the hairs and look like small pieces of dandruff. One or two are deposited on a hair, and hatch out in from six to sixteen days.

The lice are most numerous on the sides and back of the head, and occur for the most part in school children brought up in unhygienic surroundings and are thence communicated to others. Lice cause extreme itching and scratching, so that often the irritation is unbearable and the sticky serum of the blood mats together the hair, forming crusts, or impetigo develops. Sleep is often interfered with and ill-health results. The lymphatic glands of the neck may become swollen or form abscesses from the scalp infection.

The Body Louse (*Pediculus corporis*) is generally found on the underclothing. It is somewhat larger than the head louse, and deposits its eggs in the seams of the clothing, remaining on the body only long enough to gain sustenance. The young are hatched in five or six days. The louse reproduces again in eighteen days.

The bite of the parasite is visible as a small red spot which produces extreme itching, and subsequent scratching results in long lines of excoriation. The chief locations for this parasite are the shoulders, back, chest, abdomen, buttocks and thighs. The middle-aged and elderly are more apt to be attacked than the young. Uncleanliness is again a prime factor in its occurrence. Typhus and other diseases are transmitted by the body louse where such infections are prevalent.

The Crab Louse (*Pediculus pubis*) is a smaller, shorter, stouter parasite than the two preceding types, and particularly attacks the pubes, but is also found in the armpits and over the eyelashes and beard of the male.

They may be seen clinging closely to the skin with remarkable tenacity. The nits are attached to the pubic hair or the hair of other regions.

Crab lice occur on adults and produce the same lesions as the other varieties. This infestation is often the result of promiscuous sexual intercourse. In cases of pruritus ani and pruritus vulvae, these regions should be carefully examined for lice.

Treatment. The main object in the treatment of these filthy diseases is the destruction of the parasite. The lesions they produce disappear with the disappearance of the lice, although some pigmentation of the skin may remain. The most effective drug for exterminating lice is DDT but its international danger is well known so other remedies, chiefly gamma benzene hexachloride (GBH) are often used. It need hardly be said that strict cleanliness of person is a *sine qua non*.

In the case of the head louse the simplest treatment for young children is to use a GBH shampoo. The hair may be cut to get rid of the nits more easily. Hats must also be cleansed.

To get rid of body lice treatment must also be directed to the clothing, which needs to be changed often and baked, or treated with GBH or 5 per cent DDT powder. This process is to be repeated until no more parasites are found.

After a hot bath, cresol solution, 2 per cent, or xylol, 25 per cent, in equal parts of lanolin and vaseline, is also effective. The body hair should be shaved off.

The itching of the body is best allayed by carbolic acid lotion, one teaspoonful to a pint of water. DDT, 10 per cent, in water, is used for de-infesting clothes.

The crab louse may be destroyed by using a 25 per cent benzyl benzoate application, or a 5 per cent DDT dusting-powder. It must be persisted in till no more 'crabs' are found and no itching is noticed.

Prevention. Infestation with lice is now preventable by the use of dusting-powder or cream containing either GBH or DDT which may be applied to the body or clothes and will destroy the lice and prevent their breeding on the body.

Bed Bugs

Bed bugs are flat brown insects about 5 millimeters (¼ inch) long, with an objectionable smell. They live in the crevices of woodwork and walls, and can live for many months without food.

The best preventives against these bugs are corrosive sublimate and pyrethrum powder. Purchase a small bottle of corrosive sublimate tablets (**poison**), usually sold at the druggists for surgical purposes, and dissolve one in a quart of water. This solution is to be used freely around the cracks of the bed, after it has been taken apart, and also around any wooden furniture of the room as well as the woodwork. The pyrethrum powder is then to be used freely. This process is to be repeated several times, since it is difficult to eradicate the bugs. Fumigation and DDT preparations are also used.

The bites themselves are best relieved by carbolic lotions, vinegar and water, ammonia and water, etc. (see also the preparations recommended for flea bites).

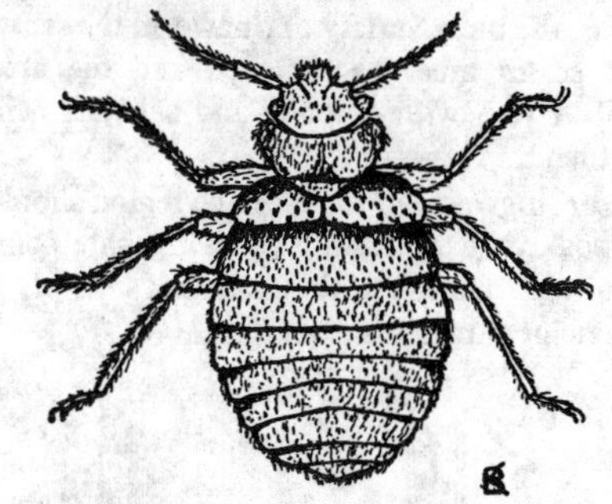

Fig. 11. *BED BUG, FEMALE. These grayish-brown insects are about a quarter of an inch long and can live for many months without food.*

Fleas

Some persons are much more susceptible to flea bites than others. Flea bites are visible as small red spots with a darker central spot. Animal fleas sometimes infest human beings, and rat fleas are carriers of bubonic plague infection.

Flea bites may be prevented by the use of oil of pennyroyal or by DDT. After bites have occurred, irritation is reduced by applications of weak carbolic acid lotion, or an ointment containing 2 per cent of carbolic acid, 2 per cent menthol, and 12 per cent coal tar solution. DDT is efficacious in the destruction of fleas, and may be sprinkled in the clothing, but see under Louse Treatment.

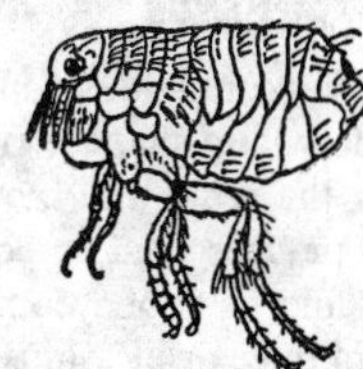

Fig. 12. *HUMAN FLEA, FEMALE. This flea is brown, but sometimes human beings may become temporarily infested with animal fleas, some black, some grayish-brown, according to the species of animal host.*

Harvest Bugs, Wasps, Horse Flies, etc.

Harvest Bugs (Chiggers). Harvest bugs may attack the legs or other exposed parts, their bites causing severe irritation. They may be warded off by DDT (see Louse Treatment, above) and the bugs may be removed from the skin by applying benzyl benzoate application or.

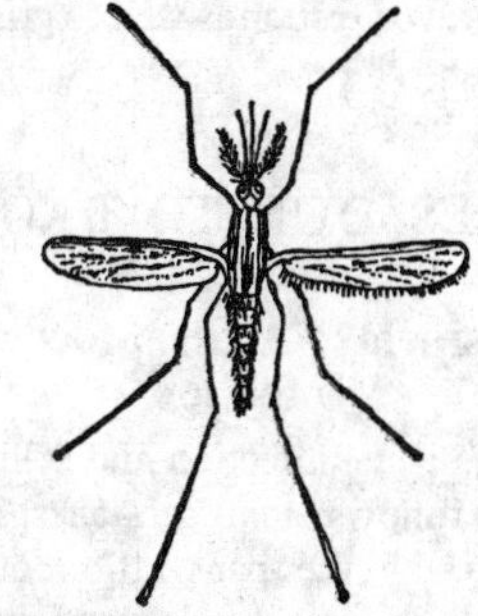

Fig. 13. *MOSQUITO* (Anopheles). *This mosquito carries the micro-organisms of malaria in its stomach and injects them into the human being when it pricks the skin.*

Bees, Wasps and Hornets. The stings of these insects may give rise to considerable pain, and occasionally they may cause severe symptoms if they involve a blood vessel or occur on the tongue or mouth. Bee stings should be removed, and ammonia, or sodium carbonate or bicarbonate solution dabbed gently on. For wasp stings, lemon juice or vinegar alleviate the pain. For the bites of small **gnats** and **midges,** weak carbolic lotion relieves the irritation, or bites may often be prevented by using oil of lemon or 40% dimethyl phthalate cream on the skin.

Use an antihistamine cream for severe reactions to bee stings or get medical attention.

Horse Flies and Mosquitoes. Treat as for midge; bathe with sodium bicarbonate lotion (a teaspoonful in half a pint of water); apply crotamiton lotion.

DISEASES DUE TO FUNGI

Thrush

Thrush is a fairly common affection occurring in the mouth in bottle-fed infants. White patches are seen on the tongue and lining membrane of the mouth, and the child will probably have sore buttocks. Scrupulous attention should be paid to cleanliness of bottles and nipples, these being boiled after each feeding and kept immersed in cold boiled water between feedings. The patches in the mouth should *not* be cleaned after the child has had a feeding.

Thrush infection sometimes occurs in adults, especially in the genital areas, causing a form of intertrigo. It may also cause peeling and oozing between or beneath the toes, or give rise to white leathery patches between the fingers.

These eruptions may be treated by local application of nystatin ointment or crystal violet (gentian violet) solution, while nystatin tablets may be given by mouth. For infants, nystatin suspension may be applied to the inside of the mouth three times daily.

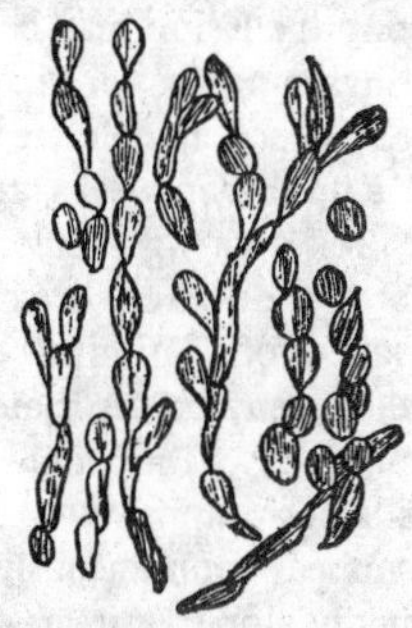

Fig. 14. *THRUSH. This fungus, which often affects the mucous membrane of the mouth especially in bottle-fed infants, grows in short chains of cells.*

Occasionally thrush round the nails is seen in housewives or cooks, the areas being swollen, red and tender; the condition tends to be chronic unless the hands are kept dry. A 2 per cent solution of crystal violet (gentian violet), or a 1 in 1,000 solution of proflavine should be applied, and sometimes X-ray treatment is used in very chronic cases.

Dandruff

(Seborrhea Sicca)

Dandruff is a mildly infectious disease of the sebaceous glands of the scalp, characterized by the copious production of horny white or yellow scales. The secretion may be so thick as to mat together the hair, or so dry as to fall off the head in a shower when the hair is combed. It is a common cause of early baldness, especially of the temples and crown, and causes irritation of the scalp; seborrheic dermatitis may develop on other parts of the body. There is often reddening of the forehead along the margin of the hair. The heads of babies may be infected soon after birth by scales of dandruff from the mother's hair.

Treatment. Should the amount of scales be considerable, especially if there are crusts as in the case of small children, the best procedure consists in oiling the scalp overnight with olive oil, and washing off the oil in the morning with soft soap and water. The scalp needs a shampoo two or three times a week with selenium sulphide solution. For excessive oiliness, a 10 per cent solution of sodium sulphacetamide is excellent. A more chronic case may require resorcinol lotion or ointment.

Ringworm

(Tinea)

The different forms of ringworm are due to various fungi which may attack the scalp, body, skin or nails. The varieties more commonly seen are:

TINEA CIRCINATA, in the body.

TINEA TONSURANS (capitis) in the scalp.

TINEA BARBAE, in the beard region.

A rarer form called TINEA CRURIS or DHOBI ITCH occurs in the groins and thighs, while TINEA PEDIS is well known as athlete's foot, and the nails may be affected by TINEA UNGIUM.

On the body the lesion may be papular, in pink scaly rings, nodules, or plaques. On the scalp it usually occurs in children; the incubation period is up to two weeks, and the patch begins as a pink area with scales around the hairs which are dry and broken and can easily be pulled out. It must be borne in mind that there may be associated eruptions such as seborrhea or impetigo which may mask the ringworm appearance. The disease tends to disappear spontaneously at puberty, but occasionally alopecia areata follows.

Treatment of ringworm of the scalp necessitates isolation, and segregation of the patient's towels and toilet articles. The hair should be cut close over the affected area. All older treatments have been superseded by griseofulvin, an antibiotic derived from strains of *Penicillium*, which is given by mouth as tablets for three to six weeks. As the new hair grows in, it is then resistant to the fungus.

For the body variety of ringworm the crusts and scales must be removed and the area rubbed well with sulphur and salicylic acid ointment.

For ringworm of the toes, the region should be soaked in potassium permanganate solution and painted with Castellani's paint; a fungicide powder is then dusted on.

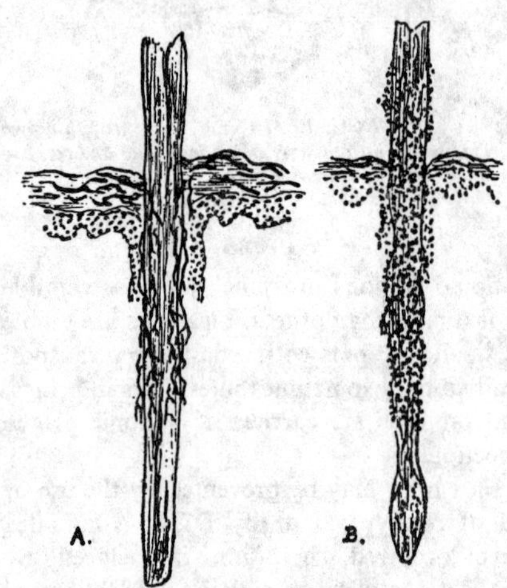

Fig. 15. *HUMAN HAIR INFECTED BY RINGWORM. A. First stage, with fungus at the mouth of the hair follicle and spreading downwards by a loose meshwork. B. Later stage of infection, with the fungus forming a sheath around the hair; some threads of the fungus and spores lie within the bulb of the hair.*

Favus

Favus is also a contagious fungus disease producing yellow cup-shaped crusts which first appear on the scalp and may spread to the body. The patches tend to coalesce, and form a mass like a honeycomb; an unpleasant odor of mice or of a musty nature is characteristic. The hair is very dull, but does not break as easily as in ringworm. Bald areas, however, are produced in time and the disease often proves very intractable. The treatment is again to prevent contagion, while an ointment containing mercury, salicylic acid, and resorcinol in lanolin is used, the crusts being removed with olive oil, and a soap and spirit shampoo given. Like ringworm, favus responds well to griseofulvin.

DISEASES DUE TO BACTERIA

Erysipelas: A Streptococcal Infection

This is an acute infection and is highly contagious. It follows small scratches, abrasions or wounds, by the penetration of streptococcal bacteria into the deeper layers of the skin, Infection is favored by debilitated states, dirt and alcoholism, and the outbreaks are most common in the spring.

The eruption most often occurs on the face, after an incubation period of about two to five days, and is preceded by malaise, headache, fever, dry tongue, chills, and vomiting. The infected area is of a bright red color with a hot shiny surface, and usually starts with a single patch with definite raised edges and irregular outline, which spreads rapidly with small vesicles at the edge. There is much swelling and if the disease affects the face the patient may be almost unrecognizable, while the disease may spread into the mouth. On the limbs red streaks of lymphangitis may be visible.

The rash lasts about a week and then abates, unless the infection extends into underlying structures, causing complications such as meningitis, pleurisy, pneumonia or pyemia, in which general exhaustion may end fatally. The disease is especially fatal in infants and old people.

Treatment requires isolation with rest in bed. The case should be treated by a physician. A light or fluid diet is required.

Given immediately the disease is diagnosed, sulphonamides rapidly control the infection so that skin treatment is seldom needed. For recurrent attacks, for babies, and for elderly patients penicillin is often preferred. Glycerin and ichthammol lotion, or simple hot compresses, may be used to relieve the pain and edema.

See also Fevers and Infectious Diseases, p. 270.

Impetigo: A Mixed Infection

Impetigo contagiosa is an infective inflammation of the skin, often staphyloccal in origin, with vesicles which suppurate and when they break yield a serous or honey-like exudate which forms characteristic yellow crusts. The infection enters through an excoriation or scratch, and generally affects children, especially in the region of the mouth or scalp. It is often secondarily affected by streptococci, spreads rapidly, and is very contagious.

Treatment consists in careful bathing off of the crusts and removal of any hair. An application of 1 per cent crystal violet (gentian violet) in 25 per cent alcohol is effective. A better application is an antibiotic cream put on freely after removal of the crusts; the skin should be clear in about a week.

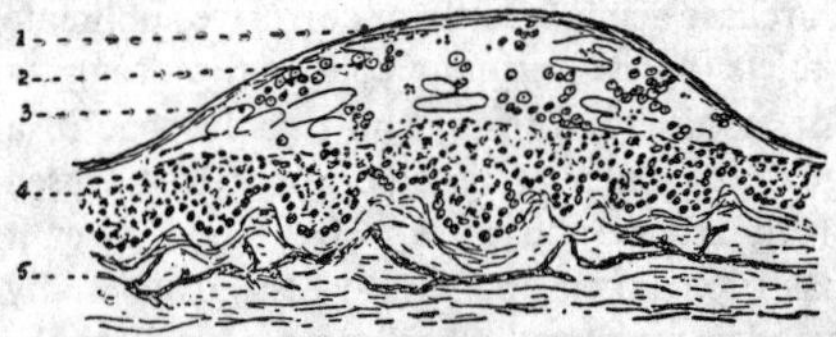

Fig. 16. *A SKIN VESICLE IN IMPETIGO. 1. Surface of vesicle. 2. White blood cells and microbes (streptococci). 3. Dried serum. 4. Swollen epidermis. 5. Dilated capillary blood vessels, and inflammed tissues.*

In extensive eruptions, warm starch compresses may be used to assist separation of the scabs, the skin being then swabbed with spirit. The patient's towels, brushes, and clothes should be segregated, and school children should be kept from school. Gloves may be required to be worn to prevent scratching.

IMPETIGO OF BOCKHART is a milder form than that described above, and is papular rather than vesicular, occurring in connection with hair roots in hairy areas. The treatment is the same as that already described, with tonics for the general health.

Sycosis: A Staphyloccal Infection

(*Barber's Itch*)

Sycosis is a pustular eruption with crusts, which somewhat resembles impetigo contagiosa. The crusts occur in the hair follicles of the beard region; it is often very intractable and is highly contagious. As the pustules dry and heal new foci appear, so that the infection spreads, and the hairs gradually drop out of their infected follicles. Sometimes secondary infection with boils, eczema, or impetigo develops, while the condition occasionally affects the scalp, eyelids, armpits, or pubes.

Treatment is similar to that used for impetigo but is often protracted, since the infection is deeper and is less easily destroyed. The hairs should be pulled out with forceps, and any deep pustules may be opened. It is generally advisable to discontinue shaving, since this may cause reinfection of abrasions; in any case the shaving brush should be kept disinfected. Alternatively the hair of the affected area may be clipped short.

Antibiotic creams may be ordered by a doctor. When the skin is much inflamed poultices of 1 in 4,000 mercury perchloride solution may be used before more active treatment is started.

Pemphigus Neonatorum: A Staphylococcal Infection

Pemphigus neonatorum is a staphylococcal infection affecting newborn babies, and has no connection with ordinary pemphigus. It is generally transmitted from the mother, but is becoming increasingly rare. There are two types, a benign, and a 'malignant' or septicemic form. Large vesicles or blisters appear at, or shortly after, birth and these spread and coalesce, on any part of the body except the soles and palms. The vesicles break and leave raw areas, or crusts may be formed. The outlook used to be serious and some cases end fatally.

Apply 1 per cent aqueous crystal violet (gentian violet) solution after the vesicles have been opened. Any septic foci, such as the umbilical stump, must be dressed with antiseptics. The child should be isolated from other infants, and careful precautions taken against spreading the disease. Intensive courses of antibiotics are given.

Boils

(*Furuncles*)

A boil is a localized infection of the skin, arising in a hair follicle or sebaceous gland. It usually proceeds to abscess formation. At first a tender nodule or hardness is felt just under the skin, which soon begins to look red. A painful tumor now begins to show, of a dusky red or purple color, which increases to the size of a pea, a hazel-nut or a walnut. Some time between the fourth and eighth day it becomes pointed and white at the top, when the skin breaks and lets out a little pus mixed with blood, and exposes a core. In two or three more days this core comes away, leaving a cup-like cavity which gradually fills up, and the boil then gradually heals in two or three weeks.

Boils are liable to occur in parts exposed to friction, such as the neck and buttocks. Very often crops of boils occur over a period of some weeks or months. In the passage of the ear, boils are exceedingly painful, while on the nose or upper lip a boil may cause infection of a vein leading to the brain and may prove fatal.

A 'blind boil' is slow in pointing, and may persist for some weeks.

There are various causes of boils, but they are commonly associated with debilitated conditions, dirt, or irritation of the skin by friction. Diabetes mellitus is often associated with recurrent attacks of boils and carbuncles.

Treatment. General cleanliness by use of antiseptic soaps is indicated, coal-tar soap or carbolic soap being suitable. Any sources of irritation, such as frayed collars, should be avoided when boils occur on the neck.

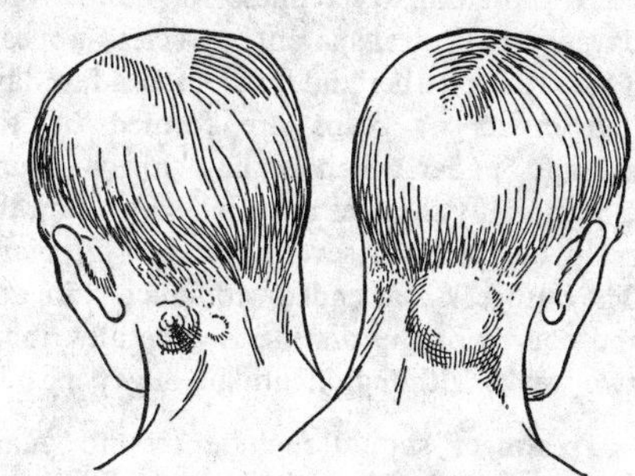

Fig. 17. *A BOIL AND A CARBUNCLE. In a boil the infection usually arises in a hair follicle causing the formation of a small abscess. A carbuncle resembles a compound boil with the inflammation spreading from one follicle to another; a carbuncle may be about two inches in diameter.*

Locally, apply glycerin and ichthammol (10 per cent) on a bandage until the boil points, and then incise gently to allow drainage. Regions such as the axilla should be shaved and not compressed, since the surrounding hair follicles tend to become infected. A paint of 1 per cent solution of crystal violet or brilliant green should be used daily (these solutions dye the skin). After the boil has opened, apply small dressings of glycerin and magnesium sulphate paste, or use glycerin.

Paint the surroundings of the boil with iodine, which will prevent a crop of pustules appearing round the boil. General tonic treatment, with an iron mixture, is usually required.

Antibiotics may be given if the boil is in a dangerous situation, as on the upper lip, or if there are signs of general spread.

An open-air holiday is often beneficial, and the diet should contain plenty of green vegetables and fruit, with restriction of sugar.

Carbuncles

A carbuncle is somewhat like a boil, only much larger and more painful. Instead of one hair follicle being inflamed, as in the case of a boil, a carbuncle is a confluent mass of boils in several follicles. The surface is flatter than that of a boil, the inflammation is more severe and the constitutional symptoms are more acute. Like boils, a carbuncle develops most often upon the nape of the neck, the shoulders, the back, the buttocks or the thighs. The diameter may be two or three inches, and the surface is dusky red and painful for about seven to ten days until the center softens and perforates, often at several points. Pus is discharged, and a large slough eventually separates. The central cavity heals slowly, leaving a large scar.

Carbuncles most often occur in men over middle age, and diabetes mellitus, alcoholism and albuminuria are often predisposing causes. They cause much pain, great suffering, and sometimes prove fatal, especially in old or debilitated people. Upon the head or neck they are more dangerous than in other situations.

Treatment. During the formation of the carbuncle apply kaolin or magnesium sulphate compresses. The skin around the carbuncle may be painted with 1 per cent brilliant green solution. A surgeon may excise the carbuncle, or scrape out the cavity under a general anesthetic. In other cases make two incisions in the form of a cross, when the core is formed. Antibiotics are also usually given.

Ultraviolet light therapy may be beneficial. The general health requires great care, with rest, fresh air, and a nourishing diet.

Lupus Erythematosus

Lupus erythematosus is also a disease of the skin, generally affecting the face and causing redness, scaliness, and sometimes much scarring later on. This form of lupus may be associated with tuberculosis in other parts of the body, or with some other infection, or with Raynaud's disease. Bright light or sunshine appears to aggravate the disease. Some cases clear up spontaneously, while others persist for some years. Occasionally the disease is widespread and such cases may end fatally.

Patients with the acute disease are usually admitted to hospital where cortisone has proved most effective in treatment.

Leprosy

Leprosy is a general disease with extensive skin manifestations; it is caused by the *Mycobacterium leprae,* but the mode of invasion remains obscure. The disease may be contracted by contagion from leprous sores or discharges from the mouth or nose of a leper. It is associated with dirt and squalor.

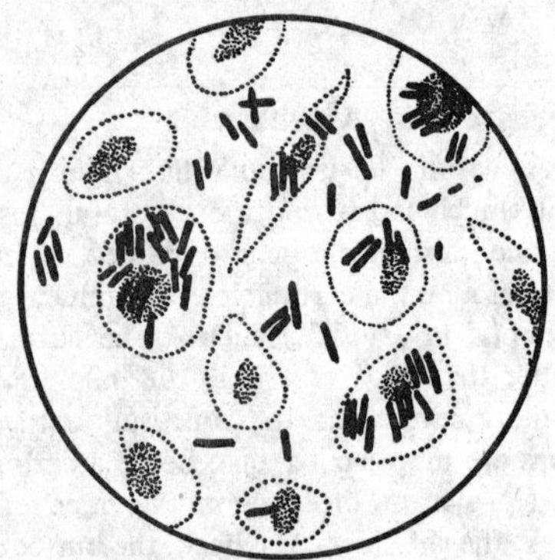

Fig. 18. *LEPROSY BACILLI. Small rod-shaped organisms are shown lying in bundles among scar-tissue cells.*

The incubation period may be several years; after a long interval there may be vague malaise, drowsiness, pains and pricking sensations. In the lepromatous nodular skin affection, fever occurs in bouts and there are nodules in the skin and mucous membranes. In tuberculoid leprosy an erythematous rash appears with patches on the arms, hands, feet, and face; later these may become numb, lose sensation, and form ulcers. The eyes are generally involved also, and in the last stages the toes, fingers and indeed the whole limb may undergo dry gangrene and drop off. The disease is very chronic.

Treatment. Sulphone drugs, dapsone and solapsone, have revolutionized the treatment of leprosy. Although treatment may have to be continued for up to five years, a number of cures have been effected. Treatment always requires the care of a physician. See also Fevers and Infectious Diseases, p. 271.

DISEASES DUE TO VIRUSES

Herpes Simplex

Herpes simplex, that is herpes of the lips, face, buttocks, and genital organs, is a common eruption which is mildly infectious and often occurs in association with a cold, pneumonia, malaria or other illness, but may follow pregnancies, menstruation, the use of certain drugs, or exposure to sunlight. The small blebs which develop dry up into yellow crusts and generally heal within about ten days. Recurrences, however, are common.

Treatment. The patch should be kept clean and dry by swabbing with dilute Milton or spirit of camphor, and dusted with zinc oxide or calamine powder. Hydroderm ointment (containing hydrocortisone) has proved useful in clearing herpes of the lips.

Shingles
(*Herpes Zoster*)

This disease occasionally occurs in epidemics, and generally affects older adults; it often follows debilitating conditions such as influenza, spinal injury, or tuberculosis, and is an inflammatory and painful affection of the nerves to the skin, bearing close relationship to chickenpox. One attack confers immunity for life.

Course and Symptoms. The onset is acute, with slight fever and neuralgia of the part, which generally only affects one side where, after a preliminary redness for about three days, small transparent vesicles appear. These run together and break after a few days and crusts or scabs are formed by the exudate, under which healing slowly occurs. Occasionally the eyes are affected, and on the scalp or forehead severe scars may remain. The outbreak is attended with much pain, and the course of the disease is generally about two weeks, although neuralgia may persist.

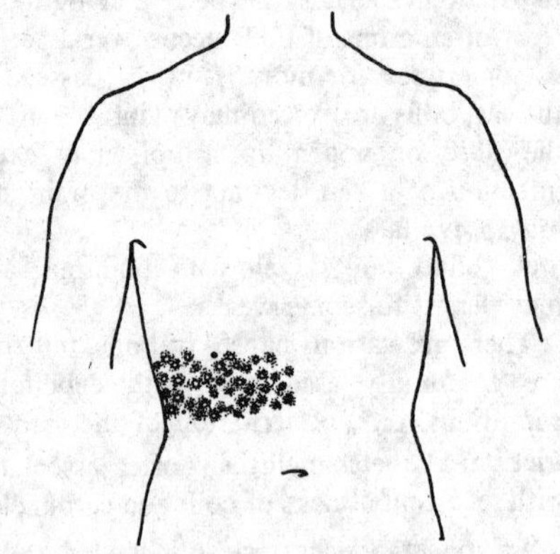

Fig. 19. *SHINGLES* (Herpes zoster). *Zoster means 'girdle.' At the waist the one-sided rash follows the course of an affected spinal nerve.*

Treatment should include rest to guard against prostration, with a light nutritious diet. Sedatives such as aspirin or phenacetin may be given, especially at night to procure sleep.

The vesicles themselves should be dusted with starch and boric acid powder; when situated on the chest or limbs, menthol collodion paint often gives relief. If they become infected compresses must be used, and ruptured vesicles should be dressed with calamine lotion or zinc cream.

Warts
(*Verruca Vulgaris*)

Warts are due to a contagious virus infection of the skin, and various forms are commonly found. RAISED WARTS are commonly met with on the hands. FLAT WARTS occur chiefly on the hands and faces of children, in great numbers, the plane juvenile wart being sometimes an early stage of the raised, flat-topped wart. PLANTAR WARTS occur on the ball of the foot or heel, being similar to the common wart on the hand and sometimes mistaken for corns; other elongated or filiform forms of warts are sometimes seen.

CONDYLOMATA are flat venereal warts which occur on the genitals, often in large numbers. Some may be contracted in conjunction with syphilis.

Common raised warts may be single or multiple, and may be irregularly distributed or grouped, sometimes in a cluster around a larger central one. They are situated most frequently on the backs of the hands and fingers, and more rarely on the face, scalp, and arms. In size, they vary from a pin's head to a pea or larger, and may coalesce to form irregular masses. They first appear as small grayish-yellow or pinkish translucent papules, practically the color of the normal skin; after a time they become raised up to about a quarter of an inch and flat-topped, the surface being grayish or blackish from dirt, and rough from the presence of small horny points. Plantar warts are commonly seen in school children, and often make walking painful.

Warts of all types are outgrowths of the dermis, covered with an overgrown epidermis which is more granular and rougher than the normal skin; they are sometimes pigmented, and bleed easily. Warts are slightly infectious, and are often auto-inoculated.

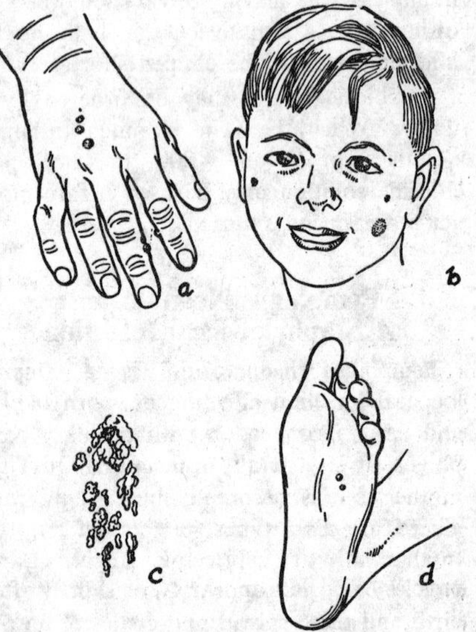

Fig. 20. *WARTS OF VARIOUS KINDS.* a. *Raised warts.* b. *Flat warts, usually on children.* c. *Condylomata, or venereal warts, usually on the genitals.* d. *Plantar warts, usually on the soles of the feet.*

Treatment. Silver nitrate and nitric acid are useful caustics which can be used for repeated application at intervals with good results; the outer dead layer is scraped away before a fresh application is made. Another method is to take a piece of diachylon plaster, cut a hole in the center the size of the wart and stick the plaster over, leaving the wart projecting through; then touch it daily with 2 to 4 per cent salicylic acid ointment.

Warts of the feet are often a more serious trouble, owing to their position and, unless warts in general speedily respond to treatment, a medical man should be consulted. Small plantar warts can be treated by formalin foot soaks each night for six to eight weeks, the foot staying in the solution for twenty minutes each time.

Warts may also be destroyed by diathermy, carbon dioxide snow, X-ray or cautery .

Prevention. For children and young persons, footwear should be worn in gymnasiums; those with warts should not use swimming baths. Feet should be kept dry and rubber soled shoes avoided.

DISEASES DUE TO NERVOUS DISORDERS

Pruritus

There are several varieties of this common complaint, which signifies 'itching,' and it is symptomatic rather than a separate disease. It may be localized in one part as in pruritus vulvae or pruritus ani; or it may be generalized as in the senile form, or in jaundice, or accompanying other skin affections such as eczema, urticaria, and parasitic infections like ringworm and scabies. Either form may be followed by secondary infection from uncontrollable scratching during the severe spasms.

The essential form met in the anal or vulval regions may not be associated with an antecedent lesion, but is singularly distressing; the irritation is usually intermittent, and may be so severe as to lead to exhaustion. In the anal and genital area, worms, cystitis, diabetes mellitus, piles, anal fissure, seborrhœa, pregnancy, rectal or vaginal discharge, or pelvic tumors may be responsible for setting off the irritation.

Of the diffuse type, there are many causes, such as gout, nephritis, alimentary disorders or parasites, senility with dryness of the skin, external conditions of temperature, chemical substances, dust, or irritation from clothing, while neurotic or highly strung persons are often susceptible.

In some cases the condition appears to be psychological in origin.

Senile Pruritus is frequently associated with a slight atrophy of the skin which can be restored to condition again by lubrication with grease and creams, plentiful vitamins in the diet, and regular attention to elimination by kidneys and bowel.

Treatment consists of recognition and, if possible, removal of the cause, and attention to the general health, particularly in regard to constipation, worms, pyorrhea, anemia, and any liver, kidney or diabetic disorders.

The diet should be light and unstimulating, and include plenty of bland fluids. Alkaline baths are recommended, and scrupulous attention must be paid to cleanliness. Starch and bran baths (see also p. 377) are also soothing.

Sedatives by mouth are helpful in many cases, especially promethazine given with amylobarbitone.

TOXIC RASHES

These generally consist in diffuse reddening of the skin, and may be caused by foods, sera, drugs (p. 470), or infective bacteria Such rashes usually cause irritation, and there may be general malaise and slight fever. A generalized rash sometimes occurs in rheumatic fever in children.

Erythema Nodosum

Erythema nodosum is another form of eruption, the origin of which is uncertain, but which may sometimes be due to latent tuberculosis or some other bacterial infection. This disease usually occurs in young persons up to twenty-five years of age, especially girls and women, and causes fever, malaise, and joint pains, with hard tender red swellings from one to three inches long on the legs and forearms. After a few days the patches resemble bruises, and there may be a succession of crops of these swellings. The course usually lasts for two or three weeks, the patches then disappearing, without scars.

Treatment consists in aspirin 300 to 600 milligrams thrice daily, rest in bed, and compresses for the limbs. Sulphonamides and poultices for the limbs. Sulphonamides and antibiotics may be ordered by a doctor, and have been effective in some cases in cutting short the disease.

Afterwards special care should be paid to the general health to guard against tuberculous disease, which often shows itself within a year after erythema nodosum.

Urticaria

(Nettlerash)

This is a vasomotor disturbance with damage of the walls of the capillary blood vessels by toxins.

Causes. It is often associated with ingestion of certain articles of food such as fish, shellfish, or drugs. In some cases the reaction belongs to the group of 'allergic' phenomena of which asthma and hay fever are other examples. The term 'allergy' denotes particular susceptibility in certain individuals to various protein substances. Emotion, too, may precipitate an attack. (See p.481).

Less commonly urticaria is caused by insect bites, nettle stings, or the stings of jellyfish, or by drugs (aspirin or quinine), serum injections, penicillin, cold or heat, or some source of infection.

Symptoms. The eruption may be ushered in with slight fever, and raised blotchy areas or weals suddenly appear, generally in white patches on an erythematous background, and somewhat resembling a nettle sting. Sometimes very slight injury or pressure on the skin, such as a small scratch, will produce such an effect. Where the condition is due to food 'allergens' the weals may appear and disappear in various parts of the body with great rapidity. They are accompanied by intense irritation which the patient tries to relieve with scratching, and may produce severe excoriation or eczema. A 'giant' form, called angioneurotic edema, is met, which is accompanied by much swelling.

Most cases are acute and the attack lasts for a few hours or for some days.

Treatment. The cause or exciting irritant should, whenever possible, be discovered and avoided, possibly for life.

Saline laxatives may help to cut the attack short, and calamine lotion should be applied externally to relieve the itching. Local antihistamine ointments (see p.482) combined with antihistamines by mouth or by injection are rapidly effective in this condition.

In recurrent or chronic cases skin tests of various proteins, or diet tests, should be carried out, and desensitization by inoculation may be attempted.

In some cases, giant urticaria of the tongue, mouth or larynx may cause suffocation by sudden swelling and obstruction of the air passages, and no time should be lost in sending for medical aid, when an injection of adrenaline by a doctor may give prompt relief.

Purpura

In purpura there are scattered small areas or large patches of bleeding in the skin, which do not fade on pressure, and this condition may be caused by various agencies; it is a symptom rather than a disease. Rheumatism or other fevers are often responsible; septicemia, tuberculosis, blood diseases, nephritis, endocarditis, heart disease, cancer, senility, scurvy, drugs, typhus, smallpox, cerebrospinal meningitis, and local diseases such as varicose veins, jaundice and numerous other general disorders also give rise to purpuric rashes, which should always be investigated by a doctor.

Causes. Although the skin is affected secondarily, the basic causes are usually disorders of the blood, the blood vessels or the blood-forming organs.

ECZEMA

Eczema is an inflammatory acute or chronic non-contagious skin disease characterized at first by redness, little pimples, vesicles or pustules, and attended by more or less burning and itching. This process terminates either in the formation of crusts as the result of dried sticky serum, or else in infected patches, or eventually in the formation of fine scales. At this stage the condition often relapses, and the weeping state recurs. Certain forms of eczema are allergic in character, that is the individual possesses some special sensitivity to certain irritants.

The source of irritation may be outside the body (clothes, dust, dirt, etc.), or may be some foodstuff, or septic focus in the body, or some cause in the skin itself. Nervous exhaustion or emotional disturbances may cause attacks of eczema.

Eczema may begin in early infancy and continue during life, or may occur in infancy and then disappear, or in other cases it may appear for the first time in adult persons or in old age. In most cases eczema is caused by some form of irritation which does not affect most normal persons, that is to say there is some particular predisposition in the patient with eczema. Other members of the family may suffer from asthma or hay fever.

These attacks may, after various relapses, subside with complete healing of the skin, but in many cases the skin becomes scaly, thickened, pigmented and harsh; the irritation continues and constant rubbing makes the eczema persist. Other cases of eczema remain dry and scaly from the beginning, and there is no oozing of serum; these cases tend to be chronic. When the surface becomes infected in moist eczema, impetigo may develop.

Eczema may develop in a few small patches, or may be spread over most of the body. In nearly all cases the itching and burning are made worse by washing with soap and water, and by fatigue or heat.

INFANTILE ECZEMA is common in babies under two years, and is often caused by eggs, tomatoes, milk, oatmeal, fish, oranges, or cod-liver oil. Woolen clothing and soap may also give rise to eczema in susceptible babies. Overfeeding, with indigestion and constipation, may be a common cause. In many cases there is a family history of eczema, and the condition often begins during the winter months. Infantile eczema is usually worse at nights and commonly affects the face, scalp, forearms, legs and trunk.

Many babies with infantile eczema show sensitivity to any foodstuffs, and these cases are often rather resistant to treatment.

In infants eczema often disappears after teething is completed.

EXFOLIATIVE DERMATITIS. A severe chronic type in older persons is known as exfoliative dermatitis, with prolific production of scales which causes extremely severe irritation. The disease often persists for years.

Eczema may be confused with many other skin disorders, and should only be diagnosed when other possible conditions have been excluded.

Treatment. With so many clinical varieties of eczema, there is no simplicity of treatment.

GENERAL MEASURES. The first essential step is to try to trace any cause of the eruption; if this can be discovered it must be avoided, or in some cases desensitization may be attempted. The skin must also be protected from irritation and scratching, to encourage healing. Emotional or psychological causes should also be looked for in chronic or recurrent cases.

In severe cases the patient should rest in bed, and the diet be kept light and nutritious.

LOCAL TREATMENT is of great importance. Water and soap are generally injurious to eczematous areas, and should be avoided. Crusts may be removed with olive oil, or starch poultices; lead lotion is very soothing. The more chronic cases may be treated with zinc ointment or a cortisone ointment.

Infants should be restrained from scratching by light cardboard splints tied to the arms.

PSORIASIS

Psoriasis is a common non-infectious disease characterized by patchy areas often situated on the elbows, knees, palms, soles, and scalp; these areas are pink and covered with dry silvery scales which are not easily removed. The nails also may be affected. The cause is unknown, but in some cases the condition is hereditary; psoriasis usually develops between five to fifteen years, or later, and may be favored by ill-health. Slight scratches or mental strain may cause recurrent attacks. At the onset there are numerous small papules which become larger and run together as the scales appear. The scales vary from a thin layer to a thick mass. Sometimes the patches are circular or disc-like. Tonsilitis may precede a generalized attack, and in some severe cases arthritis also develops. There is generally no itching or other disturbance; the patches may disappear, but others usually follow. The eruption is often chronic or recurrent.

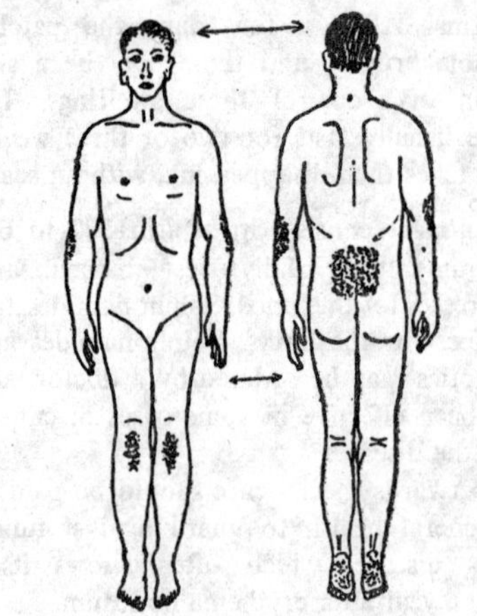

Fig. 21. *SKIN AREAS COMMONLY AFFECTED BY PSORIASIS*

Treatment must be directed to general health measures and great care must be taken to avoid irritating or damaging the skin.

LOCAL APPLICATIONS in the form of zinc cream or calamine lotion may be used in acute eruptions.

Diet should be nutritious, and alcohol should not be taken. Chronic cases, if the rash is extensive, may, when the scales have been washed off, be treated with an ointment containing:

Ammoniated mercury	..600 mg
Coal tar solution	.. 3·5 ml
Soft paraffin ..	to 30 grams

X-ray treatment and ultraviolet light are often used with success in localized psoriasis.

When all other treatments fail, cortisone may be successful.

For the scalp use oil of cade (12%), camphor (4%), and yellow mercuric oxide (4%) in emulsifying ointment. The hair should be washed twice a week with ordinary shampoo.

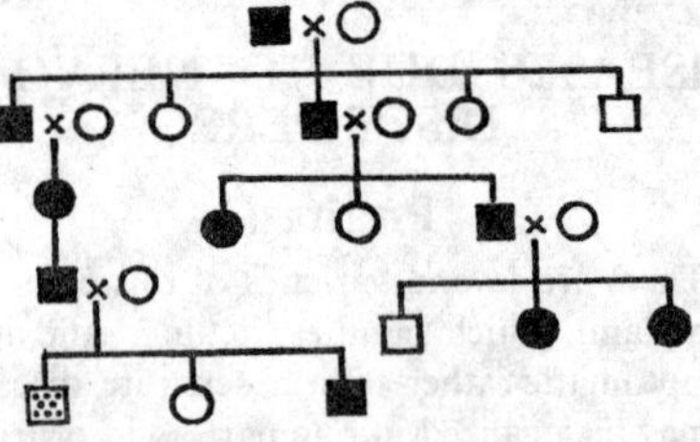

Fig. 22. *DIAGRAM SHOWING A FAMILY CHART OF FOUR GENERATIONS WITH INHERITANCE OF PSORIASIS. Black: a severe case. Dotted: a mild case. Squares=Males. Circles=Females.*

Pityriasis Rubra

Pityriasis rubra is a form of dermatitis which occurs in adults, and gives rise to a branny condition in which fine scales are shed from the skin surface. It usually first appears on the backs of the hands and sides of the neck. The onset is either acute or chronic, and there may be slight fever; the area affected assumes a bright red tint and this spreads until a wide surface is hot to the touch. Later desquamation follows with much exfoliation of scales; there is not much complaint of irritation. The course is often long, up to two months, but the disorder is seldom recurrent. The exact cause is not known, but it may be due to a vitamin A deficiency.

Treatment includes attention to cleanliness and soothing lotions in the early stage. Salicylic acid ointment may be given to assist desquamation in the later stages, although in some patients ointments are not well tolerated. Weak potassium permanganate baths may also be used daily.

A high vitamin-A diet (butter, milk, carrots, eggs, etc.) and vitamin A medication should be taken.

DISORDERS AND DISEASES OF THE HAIR AND NAILS

The hair is an outgrowth of the skin, and may be affected by various disorders. It may also be deficient, or may appear in abnormal places as on hairy moles. Premature baldness may occur, or the hair may become gray unusually early; occasionally one strand only turns white or gray, and this is often due to shock or severe nervous strain.

Alopecia Areata

Alopecia areata is the name given to irregular patchy baldness seen in persons of either sex, chiefly between five and forty-five

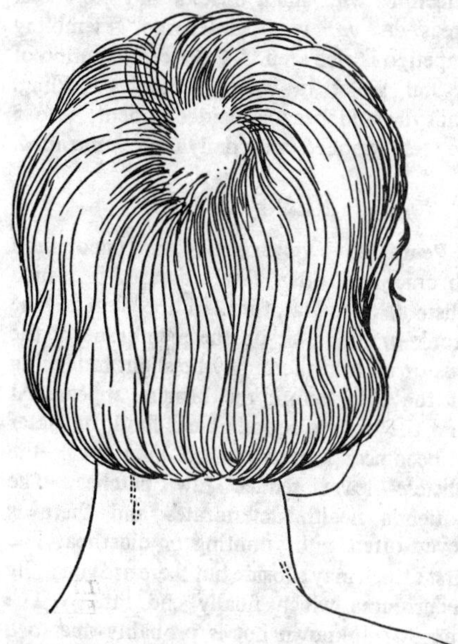

Fig. 23. ***ALOPECIA AREATA. A mild case of irregular patchy baldness on the head of a young woman.***

years, and of which the exact cause is undetermined. It is often ascribed to debility, endocrine or nervous disorders, but there may be an infective organism, as epidemics are described as occurring. Often these patches correspond to the area of skin supplied by one nerve affected by peripheral neuritis.

The patient generally requires rest, and the general health should be attended to; dandruff should receive appropriate treatment. Ultraviolet light treatment is recommended as giving good results. The patches may be painted daily with a weak iodine solution. The condition usually subsides after a few months, but sometimes recurs, or may progress to total baldness.

Baldness
(Alopecia)

Baldness or scanty hair on the front of the head may be due to old age, hereditary tendency to early baldness, seborrhea, or dandruff.

General baldness or loss of hair all over the scalp may follow debilitating conditions, glandular disorders, various skin diseases, e.g. scleroderma, or X-ray treatment.

Scattered patches of baldness in any part of the scalp may be caused by alopecia areata, ringworm, favus, scars, or habitual maltreatment of the scalp.

Preventive Treatment. A good head of hair exists when a proper supply of good blood nourishes the hair roots in a clean healthy scalp. Therefore it is necessary to maintain general good health and to keep the head clean and absolutely free from dandruff. If a hat or any tight head covering compresses the blood vessels of the scalp, the blood cannot reach the hair roots and they become impoverished and fall out.

Prevent dandruff by washing the head once a week with warm water and pure superfatted or castile soap, or a good quality shampoo, rub dry with a rough towel, then massage the scalp with vaseline if the scalp is dry, or with a touch of almond oil if it tends to greasiness. Hats should be loose and soft.

The only common forms of baldness which usually benefit from treatment are loss of hair due to dandruff, ringworm, and alopecia areata, and the baldness associated with thyroid deficiency.

Canities
(White Hair)

Whitening of the hair during old age generally begins on the temples and front of the scalp. This process may begin at about the age of thirty in some individuals, or occasionally the hair 'turns white overnight' as a result of shock or emotion. In other cases the hair becomes gray or white as a result of severe illness, or prolonged mental strain.

Treatment seldom leads to a return of normal color, but iron tonics, vitamins and care of the general health may delay the progress of whitening.

Hirsutes
(Excessive Growth of Hair)

Excessive growth of hair is generally only complained of by women when it occurs on the face or legs; in most cases the woman is normally healthy, but in a few cases the overgrowth of hair in such regions may be due to an adrenal gland disorder, as in virilism (see p. 402).

Treatment. In ordinary cases electrolysis (see p. 166) or diathermy are safe forms of curative treatment, or the hairs may be removed by forceps, shaving, or depilatories; the last-named are apt to cause soreness which may be relieved by emollient creams such as zinc cream. Pumice stone may also be used to rub off the hairs on such parts as the legs. Sometimes it is sufficient to bleach the hairs with hydrogen peroxide so that they are less conspicuous.

Ingrown Toe-nail

A so-called in-grown toe-nail is not due to actual ingrowth of the nail itself, but to overgrowth or inflammation of the soft parts at the side of the nail, which become raised over the edge of the nail; this condition is generally seen in the big toe. An in-grown toe-nail is generally due to pressure from the boot or shoe, and as a result the toe may become infected. The toe should be kept scrupulously clean; in early cases the overgrowth of the soft parts may be checked by

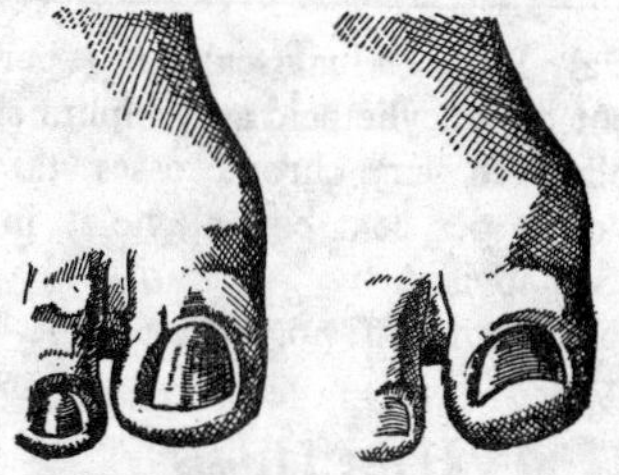

Fig. 24. *IN-GROWN TOE-NAIL is caused by overgrowth at the sides of the big toe (left). When the nail is cut back in the center, and thinned, the pressure on the sides is released.*

the use of a piece of thin metal foil inserted under the nail edge, and wide shoes must be worn. Sometimes, however, it is necessary to have a part of the nail removed by a surgeon, and the soft overgrowth is pared away. Sterile dressings must then be applied, and the toe carefully protected from infection or friction until the nail has regrown.

DISEASES OF THE SEBACEOUS AND SWEAT GLANDS

In order to keep the skin supple and healthy, an oily secretion is produced by certain glands in the dermis (see Fig. 3 on p. 466), called the sebaceous glands. The sebum secretion passes up to the surface of the skin by means of a short duct; the sebaceous glands are more abundant in some parts of the body than in others, notably in the face and scalp region. The proper function of these glands depends on general health and cleanliness, or their ducts are liable to become blocked with the sebum secretion and debris from the skin.

Seborrhea Oleosa

Seborrhea oleosa is characterized by an unusual degree of greasiness in the skin, with large sebaceous glands; it mainly affects the face, scalp, and trunk. The condition may develop about puberty and only last a few years. A seborrheic skin is often the site of some other skin disease such as acne, eczema or impetigo. Permanent seborrhea oleosa is often a congenital condition.

Treatment. The diet should be plain, wholesome, without excess of starchy foods, and sodium bicarbonate taken by mouth may be beneficial. Sulphur soap or sulphur lotion are also advised for local use, and the hair should be shampooed regularly.

Seborrheic Dermatitis

In seborrheic dermatitis the skin is red and moist, with 'weeping' areas, generally affecting the scalp, face and neck; it may be very chronic and resistant to treatment.

Treatment. When the scalp is badly affected the hair should be clipped short, and the crusts should be soaked off with starch and boric acid poultices. Applications of lead lotion on lint will reduce the 'weeping,' and calamine lotion or zinc cream may then be used. X-ray treatment is often very beneficial. For residual scales a 1 per cent ointment of salicylic acid and sulphur should be applied. In very chronic cases, tar ointments or 1 per cent crystal violet in zinc cream are advised.

See also Dandruff, pp. 472 and 477.

Hyperidrosis

Hyperidrosis, or excessive sweating, is a disorder of the heat-regulating mechanism in the hypothalamus of the brain. The disorder is brought about in some conditions such as tuberculosis of the lungs causing night sweats, or exfoliative eczema with its sudden drenching sweats. Excessive sweating of the hands and feet is sometimes seen in adolescents (and others in the family may be affected). If the feet are affected the odor may be very unpleasant, since the skin is constantly wet and sodden.

In other instances there is too little sweating, this is called *anidrosis*, but is less common. Sometimes the perspiration has some peculiar smell; this is called *bromidrosis*.

Treatment. Excessive sweating of adolescence can generally be corrected by cold or warm baths, tonics, and proper clothing. Talcum and boric powder may be applied locally. For the feet use a weak formalin lotion or a foot-bath containing potassium permanganate 1 in 5,000, then a powder containing:

Aluminium chloride ..	3 per cent
Salicylic acid	3 per cent
Powdered alum	10 per cent
Purified talc	84 per cent

X-ray treatment may be considered in serious cases.

Acne

Acne is a chronic infective condition of the ducts of the sebaceous glands, and is attributed to the organism called the acne bacillus. Staphylococci are also found in some pustules. It is very common in occurrence.

The underlying disorder, however, is an overactivity of the endocrine glands, most probably of certain secretions of the sex glands. These secretions in turn cause an overactivity of the sebaceous glands of the skin resulting in the formation of comedones (small, lumpy swellings often with black heads), especially on the face, and sometimes the chest, which tend to become secondarily infected with staphylococci so that pustules are formed. Acne is often present at about puberty and in young adults, and is rather more common in men than in women, in whom it may be of a severe and disfiguring type. It may be also associated with some digestive disturbances, with dyspepsia and constipation, while some drugs may cause an acne rash.

Treatment necessitates scrupulous cleansing of the skin with hot water and sulphur soap once daily, preferably at night, gently massaging in the lather. This is then removed and the face dabbed dry. A lotion containing zinc sulphate and sulphurated potash is then applied, and washed off in the morning. Repeat daily for one or two weeks.

The second part of treatment is to remove the surface skin by a sulphur paste applied at night and removed with olive oil in the morning. This is done for two nights, and a soothing paste applied on the third; the process is repeated two or three times. The blackheads are removed. X-ray therapy is then given over six weeks. Ultraviolet light is helpful in many cases especially in acne of the back.

Outdoor exercise and exposure to wind and rain can do much to improve the condition.

The diet should not be too rich, lard foods and condiments being restricted. Sugar should be taken very sparingly, bread in moderation, and fried foods, chocolates, ice-cream, etc. eliminated. Large doses of vitamin A are helpful in chronic cases.

It is important to keep the scalp washed regularly, particularly if dandruff is present, because contamination of the comedones may lead to the development of pustules. Pustular comedomes may be relieved by lancing or by an antibiotic.

Rosacea

Rosacea is a chronic congestive condition of the 'flush area' of the face, especially of the nose, and is caused by dyspepsia, chronic gastritis, and emotional upsets. It generally occurs about the age of thirty or after, and is slightly commoner in women especially at the menopause. Cold winds and sinus infections may aggravate the condition.

The face is flushed, the blood vessels are dilated, and the skin is greasy. Occasionally the nose becomes much enlarged (rhinophyma), or the eyes may be affected. There may be a papular rash in severe cases, causing disfigurement. Dandruff and seborrhea of the scalp are often also present.

Treatment. The diet should be plain, with limitation of starchy and rich foods, no strong tea or alcohol, and plenty of green vegetables. No fluids should be drunk during meals. Sodium bicarbonate, with water after meals three times a day, is helpful. Vitamin B may be taken daily. The patient should avoid sitting in front of a hot fire. Physical exercise in the open air is often helpful in improving the blood flow.

The face should be cleaned with 2 per cent boric acid in surgical alcohol, or gently washed with soap and cool water. Rhinophyma is best treated by plastic surgery or by the electrical cautery.

Intertrigo

Intertrigo is a condition affecting the skin of the armpits, the folds of the abdomen and genital regions, and the lower part of the breasts. It is generally seen in obese persons who sweat profusely, and may be a form of thrush, or due to a streptococcal infection. The area is smooth, moist, and red, with a white sodden edge. The parts should be frequently washed with soap and water, and zinc oxide and talcum powder should be applied to keep the skin as dry as possible.

Intertrigo is sometimes caused by fungus infection, with small blisters and red moist areas. A variety of intertrigo resembling impetigo is also seen. A 2 per cent solution of crystal violet in water promotes healing. Salicylic and benzoic acid ointment, 1 to 5 per cent, applied twice daily is recommended.

PEMPHIGUS

Pemphigus vulgaris is an uncommon chronic and often fatal disease, in which blisters, or bullae, form in the skin of the trunk or limbs, or on the membrane of the lips or mouth; there may be slight reddening of the skin before the blisters appear. At first the blisters contain clear fluid, but later it becomes purulent; when they break the blisters leave tender raw patches. The patient's health deteriorates and there is fever, often with vomiting or diarrhea. The first attack may subside but there are generally recurrences which finally end fatally. The cause is unknown but is probably due to a virus infection which may become secondarily infected.

The disease usually occurs in persons over forty years of age. In children the outlook is better. Pemphigus vulgaris is often confused with another uncommon form of dermatitis known as dermatitis herpetiformis.

Treatment consists of rest in bed, with a nourishing diet and daily warm baths. Blood or saline transfusion, or iron medication may be beneficial. Local antibiotic ointments are helpful. Cortisone has improved the outlook for these patients for it suppresses the symptoms, checks complications, and allows other therapy to take effect.

TUMORS OF THE SKIN

Cysts and other Innocent Tumors

Innocent tumors of the skin include:

(1) DERMOID CYSTS, which contain hair, etc., and occur on the face, neck, and genital regions;

(2) MILIA, which are very small white swellings on the face;

(3) LIPOMATA or fatty tumors, which may be large or small and may develop in any part of the body;

(4) KELOIDS or hard plaques forming in old scars;

(5) XANTHOMATA or yellow plaques, generally found on the face, especially the eyelids, or limbs; this type is sometimes seen in diabetic patients.

Other innocent growths such as warts, moles, and sebaceous cysts have already been described.

Treatment of the above types is surgical removal.

Malignant Growths

Malignant growths are unfortunately moderately common.

RODENT ULCERS or locally malignant ulcers, occur on the face in middle or old age.

EPITHELIOMATA. Cancerous ulcers known as epitheliomata are more malignant and are sometimes caused by chronic irritation from sun, tar, various oils, lupus, X-ray burns or injuries.

Rodent ulcers and epitheliomata must be distinguished from syphilitic ulcers, lupus, and ulcerative conditions.

PAGET'S DISEASE OF THE NIPPLE is a local form of cancer which starts as a hard red plaque which may be scaly like psoriasis. An internal breast cancer is often also present. (See Diseases of Women, p. 488.)

Treatment for all these malignant conditions must be instituted as soon as possible, and includes wide surgical excision, with radium treatment or X-ray irradiation. Plastic surgery may improve the cosmetic results.

DISEASES DUE TO CIRCULATORY DISORDERS

Varicose Disorders

Varicose ulcers and varicose eczema are due to deficient circulation in the legs, with dilatation and twisting of the veins, incompetence of the valves, and resultant susceptibility of the skin to injury. The skin becomes discolored, purplish and scaly, causing dermatitis or eczema. When the skin breaks it does not heal readily and a painful chronic ulcer often develops, generally on the lower part of the leg or foot.

Treatment. Rest and elevation of the leg are required, with mild antiseptic dressings to prevent infection, a common sequel. In some cases healing is promoted by injection of clotting agents into the veins of the part; this must of course be carried out by a doctor, but is contra-indicated when there is thrombosis of the deep veins.

Elastoplast or varicosan bandages are often used to exert compression; they are applied spirally from the foot to the knee. A pad of sponge rubber is sometimes also used between two layers of the bandage. If the leg is very swollen the bandage will require to be changed frequently. In diabetes mellitus and some other diseases such as arterial disease or severe varicose eczema, Elastoplast bandages should not be used.

See also Diseases of the Heart and Blood Vessels, p. 304.

Bedsores

Bedsores are caused by continued pressure with obstruction to the circulation in debilitated parts, so that the sites most commonly affected are the buttocks, spine and heels. The area is at first red and sore and then the skin may break to form an ulcer, which is painful and slow to heal.

Treatment should be preventive when possible, with daily massage with surgical spirit, cleanliness and good nursing, but if ulceration occurs the pressure must be relieved, and antiseptic dressings applied. Silicone barrier creams often allow the ulcer to heal under the best conditions. A nourishing diet is essential. (See also p. 420.)

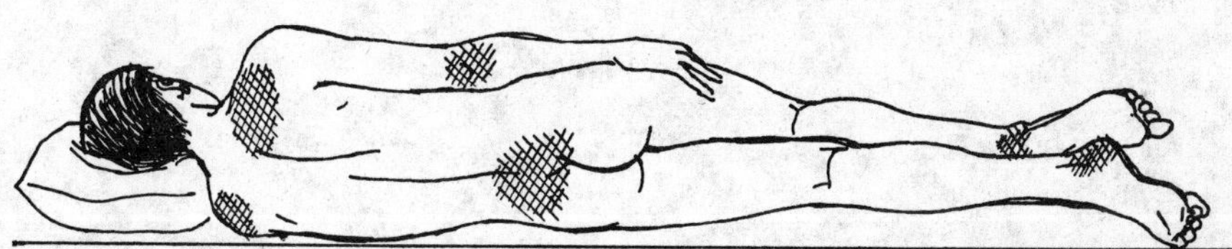

Fig. 25. *BEDSORES occur in the areas upon which the bedridden patient is likely to rub or press most heavily*

ALLERGY

Allergy is a hostile reaction, appearing in susceptible sensitized persons, to a foreign substance or agent which is irritating and disturbing to the body tissues, especially the skin and mucous membranes. The substance which is foreign to the body is known as the *allergen*. The word 'allergy' is derived from the Greek, and means 'altered reactivity.' As research progresses so the explanation of how and why an allergic manifestation is produced becomes clearer and more complete, if complex.

A susceptible person on first contact with the allergen shows no outward signs of allergy but his tissues become sensitized—in most instances by forming *antibodies*. At the next contact with the foreign agent, be it pollen, eggs, or an emotional disturbance, an allergic reaction results.

The basic terminal mechanism involved is the same in all cases of allergy whether the result is hay fever, vomiting, or nettle rash.

Pathology

The tissues involved in the production of an allergic reaction are the skin and various membranes (lining tissues).

In hay fever the mucous membrane of the nose is affected, in asthma the mucous membrane of the small air passages (bronchioles) leading to the lungs, in intestinal allergy the mucous membrane of the gut, and in nettlerash (urticaria) the skin.

The Basic Mechanism. The allergic stimulus causes dilatation of the small blood vessels (capillaries) in the affected part, and these capillaries become more porous. The effect of this is that an excessive amount of blood flows into the capillaries, and as they are now more porous the fluid part of the blood seeps into the surrounding tissues and causes swelling. The capillaries then contract tightly. It is this resultant swelling that is responsible for most allergic symptoms.

Role of Histamine. What initiates these events? Research has shown that the dilatation of the capillaries is the result of the liberation of a substance called *histamine* (or one closely allied to it). Histamine is present in every tissue of the body in an inert state. It is released as a response to various influences such as infection, injury and allergic stimuli. In the former two conditions the release of histamine is usually moderate and of a defensive nature. In allergy its output is excessive and the results injurious.

Other influences which are thought to play

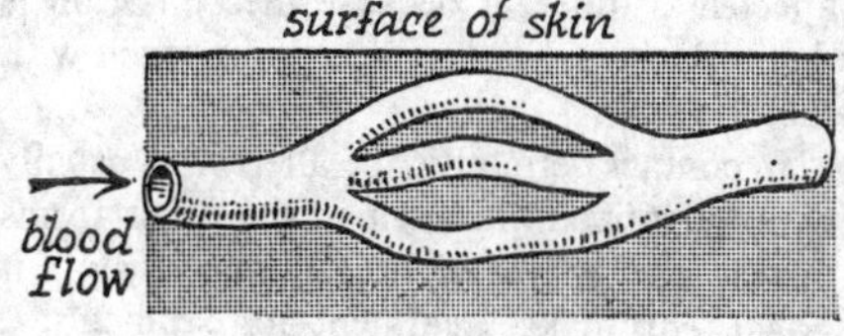

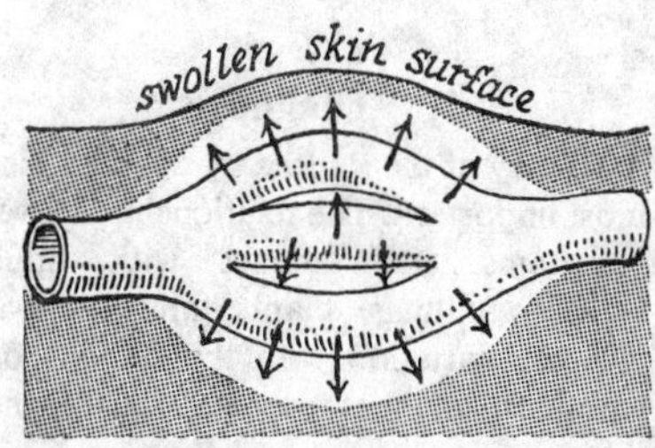

Fig. 1. *SKIN REACTION IN ALLERGY.* (Top) *Normal blood flows through the fine capillaries near the skin surface.* (Below) *Blood carrying abnormal allergens causes the fine skin of the capillaries to dilate and become porous. The blood serum or fluid seeps through into the surrounding tissues which become water-logged and cause blistery swellings on the surface.*

a part include the vegetative (autonomic) nervous system and the endocrine glands, especially the pituitary and the adrenals.

Causes of Allergy

Possible allergens may be divided into four main groups:

1. protein substances;
2. non-protein substances;
3. physical agents;
4. emotional factors.

Protein Substances. A vast number of substances come into this group. Some of the better known are:

dust, cat hair, wool, feathers, pollens; eggs, shellfish, pork, some fruits (e.g. strawberries, tomatoes, plums), insect bites; sulphonamides, antibiotics, bacteria, fungi.

The initial mechanism with the majority of protein allergens is as follows.

At the first contact with the allergen no physical effects of allergy are experienced but the tissues are stimulated to produce defensive substances known as allergic antibodies. The person is now sensitized. When next he meets cat hair, or eats shellfish, or takes a sulphonamide drug the allergen particles combine with the allergic antibodies which are on the cell surfaces. This combination injures the cell, histamine is released, swelling occurs, and allergic symptoms result.

Put symbolically, the mechanism is:

Allergen + Antibody *leads to* Allergic Reaction.

Non-protein Substances. Into this group come the simpler drugs, oils, metals, chemicals and such agents as primula plant juice and adhesive plaster. A wide variety of drugs, among them aspirin, morphine, the barbiturates, gold salts and quinine, can cause any of the allergic reactions.

Some of these substances are said to unite with the blood protein forming a protein linkage which then stimulates the production of allergic antibodies. With other substances, antibodies have not been demonstrated and it is believed that the cell is directly injured by the particular allergen, thereby causing histamine release and subsequent allergic signs and symptoms.

Physical Agents. Allergic reactions to heat, cold, sunlight, mechanical irritation, and burns can all occur. These agents are usually harmless, but some persons appear to have unusually sensitive tissue cells which release histamine excessively when they are exposed to one or more of these agents.

Emotional Factors. Some people who are allergic to physical substances are especially susceptible to psychogenic influences. For example, a woman whose asthma was caused by roses developed an attack whenever she came into contact with artificial ones (see also Asthma, p. 344).

Acute or chronic emotional conflict in a person whose personality is 'unstable' may be the sole cause of some cases of allergy. The vegetative (autonomic) nervous system is directly stimulated by such conflict. As the parasympathetic component of this system is affected, and this system triggers off the dilatation of small blood vessels and increases their permeability (thereby causing swelling), it can be seen how over-stimulation of these nerve pathways can cause allergic symptoms.

Heredity. There is a family history of allergy in 50 to 75 per cent of persons showing allergic reactions. The chances of a child showing some type of allergy are greater if both parents are 'allergic' types. Where one parent is allergic, one half of the offspring are likely to develop allergy, where both are allergic, nearly three-quarters.

It is the tendency to allergy that is inherited and not the specific illness or sensitivity: thus the parent may have asthma and the offspring eczema, or the parent may be allergic to house dust, the offspring to strawberries.

Allergic Symptoms and Manifestations

The commonest sites of allergy are:

the nose: causing hay fever, etc.
the chest: causing asthma, etc.
the intestines: causing intestinal allergy
the skin: causing urticaria, etc.

An allergic subject may show one or more, or all, of these forms. Furthermore, most allergens are capable of producing symptoms at any of these sites. In the following brief descriptions we shall see how the basic end-result of allergy, i.e. swelling of mucous membrane and skin, results in the various symptoms of the allergic diseases.

Nasal Allergy

SEASONAL HAY FEVER is the commonest form. The swollen mucous membrane lining the nose is responsible for the symptoms of sneezing, itching in the nose, stuffiness and excessive running. The sneezing, which is often violent and distressing, is an attempt to get rid of the swelling which is being treated as a foreign body. (A more detailed description is given on p. 483.)

Chest Allergy

ASTHMA is the result of an allergic reaction in the small chest tubes, the bronchioles. The swollen mucous lining gives rise to difficulty in breathing, which produces the typical wheezing as air passes in and out of the affected tubes. The coughing (like the sneezing in hay fever) is an attempt to get rid of the swelling (see also Chest Diseases, p. 344).

Gastro-intestinal Allergy

The commonest type of intestinal allergy takes the form of nausea, vomiting and diarrhea, following the eating of food to which the subject is allergic. There may be an associated urticaria of the skin.

Skin Allergy

In URTICARIA (nettlerash) the superficial skin is involved, and the swelling is seen as raised white areas surrounded by large irregular areas of redness. The redness is due to the rush of blood into the dilated blood vessels under the skin. Itching is an annoying characteristic of nettlerash and is due to the stimulation of local nerve endings by the increased pressure of the swelling.

In ANGIONEUROTIC EDEMA the deeper parts of the skin are swollen. The joints, and the lining of the lips and larynx, may also be involved. The swellings may be enormous and may involve the eyelids (shutting the eyes), the lips, the face or any other part of the body.

If the larynx becomes swollen then breathing may become obstructed and emergency tracheostomy (making a hole in the windpipe) will then be necessary.

ECZEMA is a skin condition which usually appears in infancy but may affect any age group. The characteristic lesion is blistering which breaks and oozes. Itching is intense. Later, crusting and perhaps secondary infection occur. The most commonly affected areas are the folds of the skin, e.g. behind the knees, and on the face.

Infantile eczema usually spontaneously disappears by the age of four or five. Fortunately no scarring or disfiguration results.

In CONTACT DERMATITIS the lesion is similar to that seen in eczema but the area affected is different because the condition is due to some substance directly in touch with the skin.

In contact dermatitis the allergen is usually easily identified although in the other forms of skin allergy it is often impossible to pin it down. This makes treatment more difficult.

Diagnosis

History of the Patient. A detailed history is most important. The relationship between the symptoms and contact with household articles, animals, plants, and the patient's job, the variation with the seasons or with emotional changes must be carefully inquired into.

When such a history suggests an allergic basis for a person's condition, then various tests can be done to confirm or identify the allergen.

The Skin Test. The skin test depends on the allergen and antibody reaction. A small amount of extract of the possible offender is inoculated intradermally (into the skin) by the scratch or prick method. A positive reaction is shown by redness and swelling at the site of contact within ten to twenty minutes. Pollens, dust, animal hair, and face powder are a few examples of the agents which can be tested in this way.

The results must be interpreted with care as a number of normal people give positive reactions but never show any symptoms of allergy.

The Patch Test. The patch test is used in testing the offending agent in contact dermatitis. In this condition the skin test is usually negative. A minute amount of the possible allergen is applied to a lightly abraded portion of the skin and left in contact for forty-eight hours. A positive reaction is shown by a patch of dermatitis developing over the test area.

Treatment

Prevention. If the specific allergen (or allergens) has been identified, then it is possible in many cases to avoid it either completely or partly by taking certain precautions.

In gastro-intestinal allergy, the offending food must be eliminated from the diet. Air conditioning and flue filters may cut down house dust. People who are sensitive to a drug, penicillin for example, should be told of this fact and it should be recorded on their medical record card. A wise precaution, in case of an accident, is for the patient to carry a card which states that he is penicillin-sensitive.

If a bacterial allergy is present, then any suspected focus of infection should be removed, e.g. infected teeth or tonsils.

Psychotherapy may help where an emotional basis to the allergy is suspected.

DESENITIZATION. Where the cause cannot be eliminated from the person's environment then desensitization may be advised. Hay fever due to pollen allergy may be treated in this way. The course consists of a series of injections with pollen extract (or other allergen), starting with very small doses and increasing them at regular intervals, usually weekly. In the case of hay fever the course usually has to be repeated each year.

Drug Treatment

ADRENALINE. As the action of this drug is to constrict the small blood vessels, it is therefore logical to use it for treating the allergic state.

Adrenaline is given by injection in acute allergic conditions such as severe asthma or progressive angioneurotic edema. It can also be inhaled from a nebulizer, the adrenaline acting directly on the swollen bronchial lining.

ANTIHISTAMINE DRUGS. This group of drugs acts by blocking the action of histamine, and in this way can prevent the development of many allergic symptoms. They are a valuable form of treatment for hay fever, urticaria and some cases of allergic asthma, especially in children. Antihistamines, however, are not effective in some forms of allergy. Furthermore, apart from their antihistaminic action, they have a depressive action on the central nervous system. Thus side-effects can occur, such as drowsiness, dizziness and blurring of vision. They also potentiate the action of the barbiturate drugs and of alcohol.

As new antihistamines are developed it is hoped to cut down these side-effects, but the perfect antihistamine has not yet been produced.

Antihistamines can be given by injection, but are most commonly taken in tablet form. Examples include promethazine hydrochloride, diphenhydramine.

Antihistamine eye- and ear-drops, may relieve running nose and eyes in hay fever.

Corticosteroids. The steroids are the most effective medicaments in allergy therapy, but they must be used with caution and only in severe cases because of their side-effects (see Cortisone and Corticosteroids, in Pharmacy section, p. 591). One of their actions is to reduce the permeability of the small blood vessels, and they thus prevent or reduce the typical allergic swellings.

The cortisone group of medicaments, e.g. prednisone and prednisolone, are used in tablet form, as injections, nose- and eye-drops, creams, lotions, or snuff.

SOME COMMON ALLERGENS AND HOW TO LIVE WITH THEM

Allergen	*Usual Symptoms*	*How to Avoid Reaction*
Detergents	Red or blistery rash on hands	Use soap. Wear cotton-lined rubber gloves. Use weaker solutions of the detergent.
House Dust	Sneezing. Running nose (i.e. allergic rhinitis) Asthma	House free of dust traps such as drapes, curtains, books. Avoid housework: if impossible, wear mask and use suitable vacuum sweeper. Flue filters: air conditioning
Feathers	As for house dust	Replace feather pillows with foam rubber. Avoid feather quilts
Eggs	Nausea. Vomiting	Do not eat them
Lipstick	Rash around lips which may spread on to face	Use special 'non-allergic' lipstick
Nickel	Irritating rash where suspenders, etc., touch the skin	Wear rubber-ended suspenders, etc.
Shellfish	Vomiting and / or skin rash	Do not eat them
Wool	Eczematous type of rash at sites of contact	Wear loose-fitting cotton, linen, or nylon garments

HAY FEVER

This complaint makes the summer months a miserable time for many sufferers. It is due to pollen allergy, the commonest 'culprit' being grass pollen (the pollinating season May to July). Tree and weed pollen allergy is less common. A person may be sensitive to one, two, or all three. The commonest age of onset is the second and third decade.

Symptoms. The symptoms come on abruptly at the start of the season and gradually subside as the season ends. The severity of the symptoms depends on the degree of the person's sensitivity and on the weather which influences the amount of pollen in the air. A high wind, for instance, will bring a larger amount of pollen.

The mucous membrane of the nose is always affected in this condition but the eyes, the soft palate, the throat, and sometimes the Eustachian tubes may also be involved.

The main symptoms are a running, clogged and itchy nose, sneezing and, commonly, watering red eyes. When the other sites are affected then itching of the ears, palate and throat, loss of taste and smell, and dullness of hearing may result.

Treatment. The sufferer should avoid heavy pollinating areas such as the open country. Windows of a car, train and house should be kept shut when possible.

Preseasonal courses of desenitizing injections help a certain proportion of people. Antihistamine drugs and eye- or nose-drops are useful during the attacks. Some sufferers claim that a nasal filter is of help.

See also p. 334.

AUTOIMMUNITY

This is a little understood subject at present. The body knows 'self' and 'not self.' When foreign tissue is grafted or introduced into the body, it reacts by producing antibodies, within a week or so, to destroy the 'intruder.' Unlike trees, which can bear two kinds of fruits, man generally rejects another person's tissues (with a couple of exceptions, corneal grafting and blood transfusion). This is the reason why the successful transplantation of a kidney, or any other organ, is so difficult. The actual surgical procedure is relatively simple compared with the problem of overcoming the natural rejection tendency of the body.

Minimizing the Resistance. Until more is known the antibody production (prior to transplantation) is minimized, first by choosing a donor with similar 'tissue make-up,' e.g. identical twin or close relative, and secondly by depressing the systems producing the antibodies by giving the patient radiation or antimetabolic drugs. This means that the natural resistance to infection is virtually abolished. Antibiotics, special sterile wards and sterile food are some of the precautions which must be taken.

A few successful kidney transplants have been achieved with the above measures.

New Research. Autoimmunity is thought to be the body reaction to some of its own proteins, as if they did not belong to it. Many research workers think that this may be the basis of those strange diseases for which no other explanation has been found, e.g. Hashimoto's disease of the thyroid. Much work must be done before the picture becomes clear.

FUNCTIONAL CHANGES AND DISEASES OF WOMEN

There are certain diseases which are specific to one sex and which cannot occur in the opposite sex. This demarcation may be due to one of two factors. The first is a genetical one, determined by the genes in the inherited chromosomes. Thus no woman can have true hemophilia, although she can hand it on to her male children. The second factor is an anatomical one for, although most organs of the body occur in men and women, a few of them only occur in one sex. These are the organs concerned with reproduction. Thus only men can get a cancer of the prostate for the woman has no such organ in her body. Alternatively, a man has no uterus or ovaries and he has only rudimentary breasts so he cannot suffer from gynecological disorders.

It is with the diseases and conditions of the special reproductive organs of the woman that this section concerns itself. Some women, who would willingly go to their doctor with a painful hand or a broken nose, are too shy or embarrassed to approach him in connection with something associated with the breast or vagina. Naturally, a certain reticence exists in everyone in connection with discussing their private and intimate life and thoughts. It should be remembered, however, that diseases like cancer are no respecters of such thoughts. While people need not tell the whole world of their troubles, their doctor is a privileged person to whom they may confide. He or she may then be able to help them diagnose an illness, and treat and cure the condition. Only by co-operating with the doctor can such a happy result occur. Delay in going to see a doctor because of shyness or embarrassment may result in a disease only being seen at a stage too late for simple treatment.

In order to understand a little of the illnesses that affect a woman's special organs, something of their structure and working should be known.

THE SEXUAL ORGANS

These are the reproductive organs in the pelvis (Fig. 1) and the breasts.

In the pelvis the uterus and ovaries are suspended between the bladder in front and the rectum behind (Fig. 2). The uterus is connected with the outside by a tube, the vagina, which opens on the surface of the body between the legs at the vulva (Fig. 3). Just in front of the opening of the vagina is the end of the urinary tube (the urethra) and just behind is the rectum and its opening, the anus.

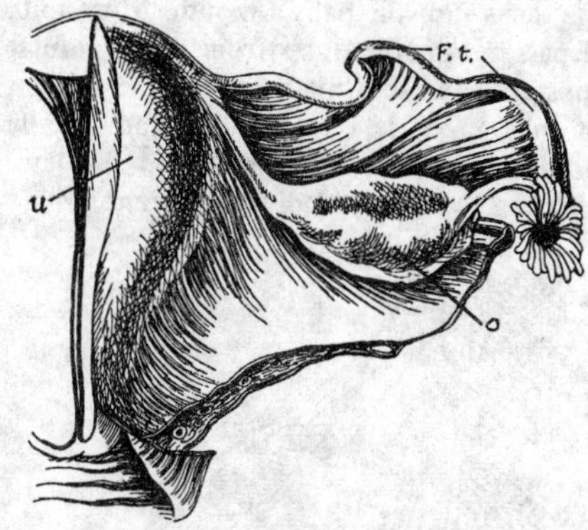

Fig. 1. *OVARY AND FALLOPIAN TUBE. Opened uterus (u), seen from the back, showing ovary (o) and a Fallopian tube (F.t.) with fimbrial fronds.*

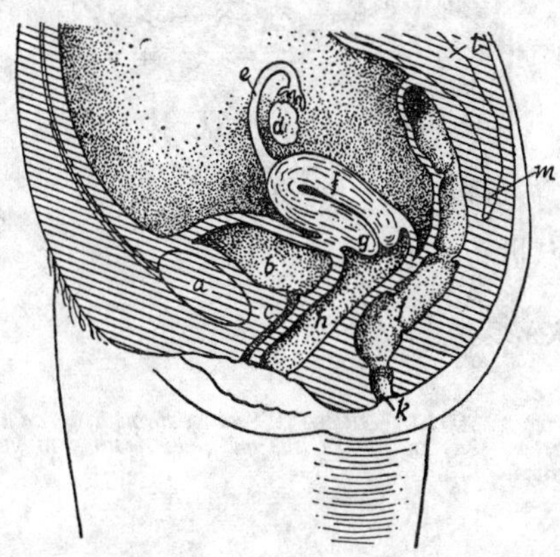

Fig. 2. *ORGANS IN THE PELVIS (side view). a. Pubic bone. b. Bladder. c. Urethra. d. Ovary. e. Fallopian tube. f. Uterus. g. Cervix, or neck of uterus. h. Vagina. j. Rectum. k. Anus. l. Sacrum. m. Coccyx.*

Vagina. The vagina is a flattened tube passing about three inches into the body. At its upper end is that part of the uterus that protrudes downwards, the cervix or neck of the womb. This tube has much elastic tissue in its walls for it has to expand to become the birth canal when a baby is being born.

Labia. On either side of the opening of the vagina are two fleshy lips, the labia. Just inside these is a shelf of skin called the hymen. In young girls this is intact (Fig. 4) but after intercourse has occurred, or after internal sanitation has been worn, the shelf becomes stretched and no longer closes over the vaginal entrance.

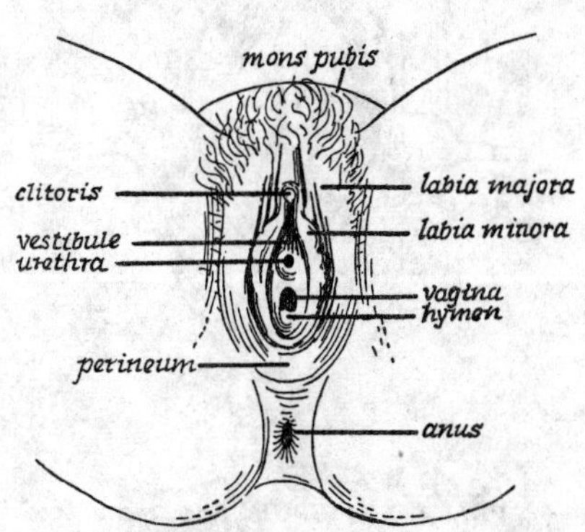

Fig. 3. *EXTERNAL GENITALIA OF A NORMAL WOMAN*

Uterus. The uterus is suspended in the pelvis. It is about the size of a pear, being three inches long and two inches wide at its upper end. Its lower part, or neck, protrudes into the vagina and, through the channel in this neck, sperms can pass up after intercourse, to reach and fertilize the ovum. Fig. 5 shows the uterus opened and one can see the thick muscular wall and the hollow cavity. This cavity is lined by a vascular layer rich in blood vessels—the endometrium. Every month, if pregnancy does not occur, this thick lining is cast off. At the same time there is some bleeding, and it is the passage of this blood, with the uterine lining in little pieces, that constitutes the regular menstrual period.

Fallopian Tubes. From either side of the uterine cavity a tube passes out to the side of the pelvis. This is the Fallopian tube (Fig. 1); it is made of muscle surrounding a very thin cavity. The opening down this tube is a little smaller than the lead in a thin pencil and it is along this tube that the sperm must swim to meet the ovary. The meeting usually occurs in the outer part of the Fallopian tube and the resulting fertilized egg then travels back along the tube to the uterus where it settles and grows into a baby. It can be seen that the Fallopian tube is very thin and easily damaged. At the outer end, the tube is wider and around its opening are a lot of fine fronds. These are just like the tentacles of a sea anemone and they are there to help waft the egg from the ovary to the opening of the Fallopian tube at the start of its journey after its release from the ovary.

Ovary. Near the mouth of each Fallopian tube is an ovary. This is the source of all the eggs and of many of the sex hormones that keep the woman feminine. The ovary (Fig. 1) is a rounded solid piece of tissue about two inches in diameter. It is gray in

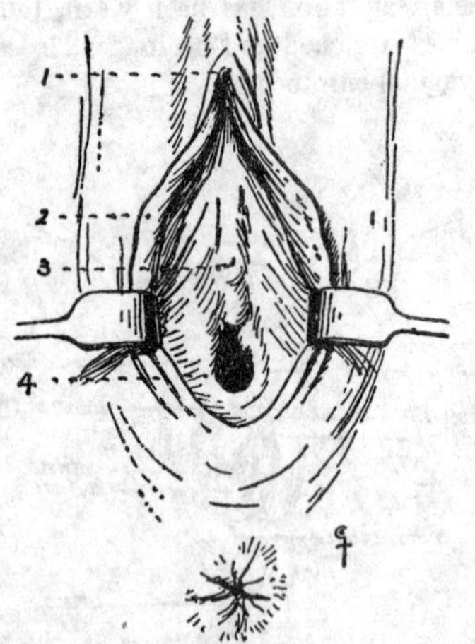

Fig. 4. *VULVA OF A VIRGIN, after separation of the labia.* 1. *Clitoris.* 2. *Inner labia.* 3. *Opening of the urethra.* 4. *Hymen covering vaginal opening.*

color and covered with a capsule through which an egg pushes its way every month. Usually only one egg is passed out each month but occasionally two may come. The egg passes to the mouth of the Fallopian tube, aided by the fimbrial fronds, and down the tube. If it meets sperm, fertilization occurs and the egg passes on as described above. If no intercourse has occurred, the egg dies after about three days in the tube and is absorbed by the tube lining.

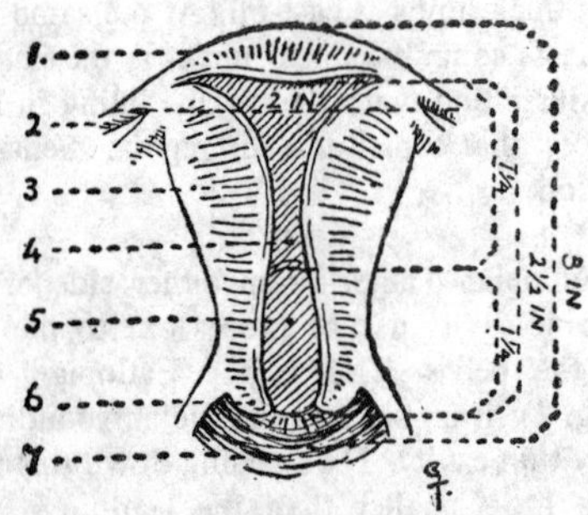

Fig. 5. *PARTS OF THE UTERUS.* 1. *Fundus, or base of womb.* 2. *Beginning of Fallopian tubes.* 3. *Body, or muscular wall, of womb.* 4. *Cavity of womb.* 5. *Canal of cervix, or neck of womb.* 6. *Cervix.* 7. *Vagina.*

Breasts. In addition to the sexual organs in the pelvis the breasts are also a source of diseases specific to women. The function of the breasts is to provide milk for the newborn infant and so they enlarge and are active in and after pregnancy. For the rest of the woman's life they are inactive.

Each breast is a rounded eminence on the chest at the apex of which is a protuberance, the nipple. Inside the breast are a series of ducts which connect the milk-making glandular tissue to the nipple (Fig. 6). When the breast is actively making milk, the infant sucks at the nipple and milk is drawn from the ducts into the baby's mouth. More milk is passed into the ducts from the glandular substance and so the baby is fed. The amount of milk made is very variable and usually production settles down to about the level required to feed the individual infant.

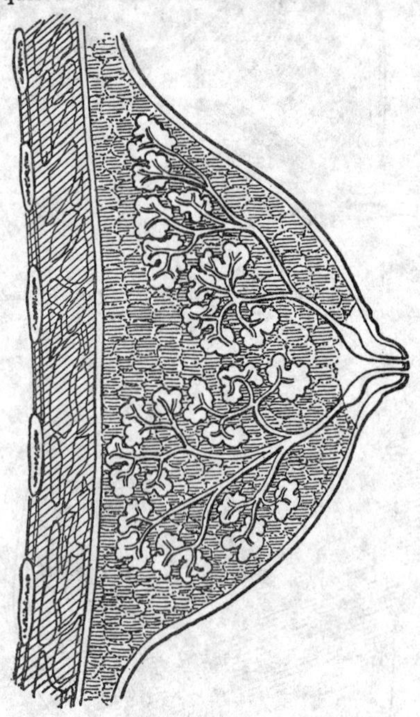

Fig. 6. *ADULT BREAST. Section through an adult breast showing gland tissue and ducts leading to the nipple.*

Apart from pregnancy and lactation, the female breast is inactive except for a small function of mild sexual stimulation before and during intercourse.

MENSTRUATION

Every month, during reproductive life, most women pass an egg from their ovaries. This ovulation starts at puberty (about 13 or 14 years of age) and ends at the menopause (about 45 to 50 years of age). The egg production is under the control of hormones (see p. 260) made by the pituitary gland in the base of the skull. Correct balance of these hormones causes ripening of an egg and its shedding towards the Fallopian tube. If the egg is fertilized, it settles in the uterus and the uterine lining provides a suitable bed for the fertilized egg to settle on. Hence no shedding of the uterine lining occurs and there are no monthly periods in pregnancy. This absence of periods is how many women are made aware that they are pregnant.

Loss of Uterine Lining. In most months, the egg in the tube is not fertilized. Then the egg dies and is absorbed. Since there is then no more use for the uterine lining the hormones controlling the uterus cause the uterine lining to be separated and passed with some blood a few days after the death of the egg. This is a menstrual period. When all the lining has gone, four or five days later, bleeding stops and preparations begin for reception of the next ovum. The accompanying diagram (Fig. 7) helps to explain the cyclical nature of the menstrual loss. It will be seen that it is entirely dependent on the egg and its fate.

Variation in Cycles. The timing and amount of menstrual loss vary considerably from one woman to another and also vary in any given woman with her age, health, and in relation to any pregnancies. Most women lose for four or five days, the loss occurring every 26 to 28 days. However, perfectly normal women may have a 21-day or a 35-day cycle and the loss may be scanty and confined to one or two days only. There is nothing wrong with such women; this is merely individual variation. Similarly, some lose heavily at the period, having to use six to eight changes of protection on each day of the period. Again this is within the normal range of loss, for just as there is no exact timing of the cycle so the 'normal' loss is variable.

Puberty. The starting of periods in puberty is accompanied by an activity of the organs of reproduction. The girl goes from child to woman, her breasts enlarging and hair appearing on the body. The internal sexual organs, too, grow rapidly, the ovaries and uterus increasing in size. The first few menstrual periods may not be accompanied by the production of an egg but the cyclical hormone changes go on and monthly bleeding may occur.

This is a time of emotional and mental stress for many girls. It is wise for parents to maintain a close liaison and friendship with a young girl at this time in her life. She should be warned in advance of the onset of menstruation with a simple explanation of its cause and nature. Further, a mother should explain about the preceding vague aches and headache that may accompany menstruation. The whole tone of the discussion should, however, emphasize the normality of the event. Possibly the parent may feel that this is an opportunity to take the matter further and discuss sex generally but this is very much an individual point and is best left to the mother's discretion. How-

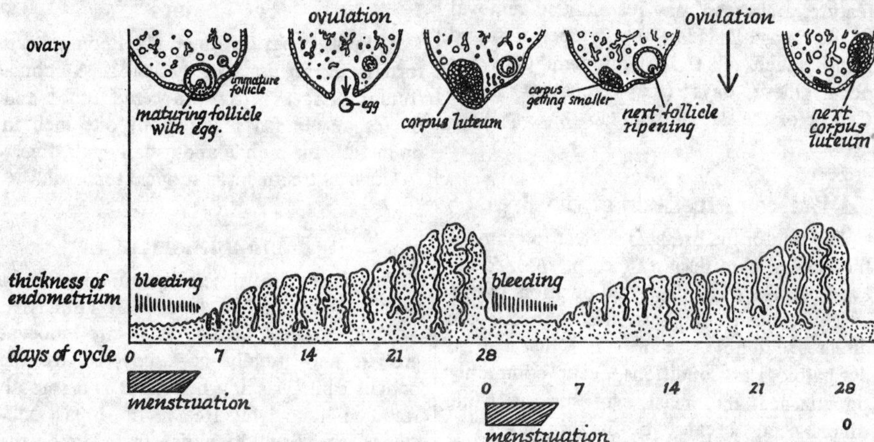

Fig. 7. *ENDOMETRIUM IN MENSTRUAL CYCLE. A diagram of two consecutive menstrual cycles to show how the stages in egg production (top of diagram) are related to the thickness of the endometrium which lines the womb.*

ever, the young girl should be prepared carefully for the onset of menstruation by intelligent anticipation and frank discussion.

Menopause. Most women continue menstruating every 28 days (with the exception of pregnancy and lactation) through all their middle years until the mid-forties. Like the other statistics of menstruation this is a variable age and, while most women reach the menopause at about 45 to 47, many normal women stop within seven years on either side of this time. Thus a woman could expect to stop menstruating in her forties but no one can prophesy exactly when. A guide is sometimes given in that those who start their periods later in life (16, 17, 18) may well finish a little earlier (40 to 45). The menopause may be accompanied by a few months of uncomfortable symptoms. Although these are not serious, they are often worrying and very uncomfortable. Hence, although the cessation of periods is in itself a normal event, the menopause may be a time of great stress for many women. (See also p. 144.)

DISEASES OF THE BREAST

Although the female breast is an inactive organ except in pregnancy and lactation, a little secretion can occur from its ducts and may collect at the nipple. This makes small crusts and these should be removed gently in the bath by soaking in warm water.

Brassières. The breasts should be supported well by a comfortably fitting brassière. Fashion and vanity demand women to give an external appearance of breasts of certain size and shape. While those with a small bust probably do themselves no harm by exaggerating their breast size, women with large fleshy breasts may do damage by trying to cram such organs into tight constricting garments. As well as being uncomfortable, the breast tissue may be bruised and movement of the chest is restricted.

At the time of puberty, when a girl's breasts are increasing in size, a carefully selected brassière is essential and many manufacturers are aware of the problems of this time of life. A mother should advise her daughter carefully about the choice of support. Similarly, in pregnancy and during lactation, the breast is bigger and heavier. A better support is then required and the nursing brassiere (Fig. 3, p. 94) is well designed for such a purpose.

Abnormalities of Function

Very rarely a baby may be born without one or both breasts. Occasionally also, extra breast tissue may be present above and below the normally sited breast (Fig. 8).

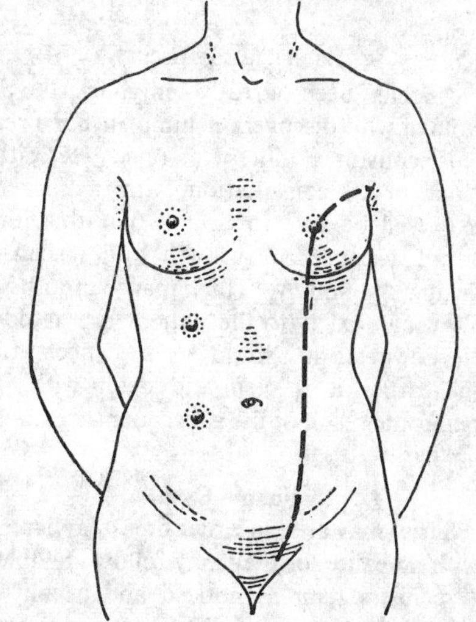

Fig. 8. *ACCESSORY BREASTS. The broken line indicates the positions in which additional breasts can occur in some women. The 'breasts' are usually only nipples.*

This tissue may be stimulated, in later life, to make milk and, in the rare event of there being an accessory nipple also, the milk may be secreted to some degree by such an orifice.

At birth some children have slight enlargement of the breasts and may even secrete a little milk. This is due to the powerful hormones circulating in the mother's blood which have passed through the placenta and into the baby, thus stimulating the infant's breast tissue. Within a few days of birth, with no more hormones acting, the breasts subside and secretion stops. The old midwives trick of 'breaking the breast cords' is to be greatly condemned. It can do no good and may well damage immature breast tissue.

Cracked Nipples

Soreness and cracks of the nipples may occur during breast feeding. They may be avoided by proper prenatal care of the breasts. In the last months of the pregnancy, a little clear fluid is often secreted by the breast as it is preparing for its task of milk-making. The nipple should be kept clean by daily washing with warm water and soap. A little lanolin ointment may be rubbed in and, if the nipple itself is flat or retracted, gentle massage and pulling out is recommended (see also pp. 94 and 100.).

DURING BREAST FEEDING, allow the child about five minutes only to each side at first, to allow the nipple skin to accustom itself to the rather vigorous massage of the baby's gums. Should any cracks occur, care must be taken to prevent their becoming inflamed and leading to infection of the breast. The infant should be fed only from the healthy breast for a few days while the affected breast is emptied by hand or with a gentle milk pump. Local anesthetic ointments are helpful to relieve pain. Warm bathing and careful drying of the affected nipple is soothing and may hasten healing. On restarting feeding, a nipple shield should be used for about two or three days.

Inflammation of the Breast

This nearly always follows a crack in the nipple or blockage of the milk ducts during breast feeding. Germs get into the warm milk and multiply rapidly leading to inflammation of the tissue with, if neglected, abscess formation. Infection rarely occurs in those who are not secreting milk.

Symptoms. The first symptoms are usually pain in the breast accompanied by a fever. Examination often shows a sore crack in the nipple and that quadrant of the breast behind the crack is tender and engorged. There may be redness and heat of the overlying skin and later on the area becomes very swollen and throbs. The lymph glands in the armpit may become enlarged.

Treatment. Prevention of cracked nipples (see above) is the best treatment. Once inflammation of the breast is present, local hot compresses are pain-relieving and may help healing. The breast should be seen by a doctor who may well prescribe antibiotics. If the inflammation is advanced, it may be wise to stop breast feeding and the milk can then be dried up with hormones.

Should pus be present, it must be released and this means a small incision, best performed under anesthesia. After such an abscess is opened, the arm is kept supported in a sling and the breast held up by proper dressings. The woman should stay in bed and all lactation must be stopped. When all the pus has drained away, and this often takes several days, the patient may get up and resume her tasks. During this time a nourishing diet with extra vitamins and iron is helpful.

Chronic Infection of the Breast

Real chronic breast infection is rare. Occasionally the acute form continues for months and recurs. The breast becomes perforated with abcess cavities and is most resistant to treatment. Very rarely tuberculosis can affect a breast. This nearly always comes from an internal source (bloodspread, or from a rib or lung) and usually the patient is known to be suffering from tuberculosis. Treatment is with antituberculous drugs as described on p. 353.

Mastitis

The so-called chronic mastitis of the breast is not really an inflammation but an exaggeration of normal changes occurring in the breast, induced by a mild imbalance of hormones. The breasts become knotty and lumpy while occasionally a single large cyst of one breast presents itself. The woman may feel pain in the breast and 'drawing' sensations are often noticed. In the younger woman pain may be felt but in those around the menopause the condition is usually pain-free. Occasionally a little dark discharge occurs from the nipple.

This condition is not cancer but only a proper examination by a doctor can distinguish between the two diseases. Even then, if a doubt exists in the doctor's mind it is wise to have a minor operation to remove a little piece of tissue of the breast. This tissue is then examined carefully under the microscope by a pathologist and he can give an exact diagnosis.

Any woman with a discharge from the nipple, or a lump in the breast, must see a doctor. It is useless to take the advice of an older woman, however well intended it may be.

Treatment of mastitis is by a suitable supporting garment. Often the discomfort of the affected breast is aggravated by an ill-fitting bra which grips the breast, or a portion of the breast, at its base. Any cysts may be emptied by a small needle puncture.

Should pain be a continuing and worrying feature, a surgeon may recommend removal of the breast. This is a simple operation and brings much relief. Disfigurement does not occur these days (see discussion under Cancer of the Breast, see below).

Diseases of the Skin of the Breast

The skin of the breast is subject to many of the general skin diseases (see p. 465). However, because of its protected position and its lack of exposure in Western countries, some diseases tend not to occur on it. Other general dermatological conditions occur commonly on skin near the breast, e.g. psoriasis, while others occur because of the breast's overhanging situation, e.g. eczema.

When a woman is fat, the area under the breast must be carefully washed, dried and powdered every day to prevent the collection of perspiration and the onset of such skin conditions.

Paget's Disease

This is a red, scaling, weeping eczema which affects the skin around the nipple. It is a chronic, long-standing affliction and usually occurs in women aged between 40 and 60. Excoriation of the skin occurs and weeping red patches are left. These crust over but the crusts soon separate to leave larger areas of rawness.

Treatment. There is a real danger that this condition, although not malignant in itself, may become a cancer. Hence the best treatment is removal of the breast. Any such skin ailment on the breast should not be treated by a succession of ointments from the drug store but should be seen by the woman's medical practitioner.

Lumps in the Breast

As has been already emphasized, any woman who discovers a lump in her breast must consult a doctor at once. He, either alone or in consultation with a surgeon, may well be able to decide that this lump is not a cancerous growth and it can be dealt with simply. Thus many months of gnawing anxiety to the patient are avoided. If, however, it should be a cancer, then the earlier it is seen and dealt with, the better the result of the subsequent treatment.

Simple Cysts

These may arise in either breast, apparently with no cause, or they may follow childbirth. A painless lump is noticed and usually no other symptoms occur. The best treatment is removal by a small surgical operation. This removes both the lump and the doubt that it *may* turn into a cancer later in life.

Occasionally such cysts follow a blow to the breast. In this situation internal bruising occurs and, after many months, a thick-walled cyst is formed around the fluid old blood. This, too, is best treated by removal.

Fat Tumors

As in other parts of the body, lipomata can form in the fat tissue of the breast. A lipoma (tumor of fat) is an innocent tumor and makes a rounded mass about one inch in diameter. It is mobile and usually pain-free.

The best treatment is surgical removal.

Fibro-adenomata

This is a firm, descrete, rounded tumor usually found in the breasts of unmarried women in their forties. It is an innocent growth and usually is discovered by the patient while washing herself. It is a smooth rounded lump lying free in the breast substance, not fixed to either the skin or the underlying muscle tissue. It feels mobile and often is difficult to hold under the examining fingers; hence its common name 'breast mouse.' Usually there is no involvement of the glands in the armpit.

Treatment. The best treatment is removal of the lump by surgical operation. This does not of necessity mean removing the entire breast.

Cancer of the Breast

Cancer of the breast is one of the common cancers in women. It occurs in women aged 30 to 40 and is more common in those who have not breast-fed children. Occasionally there is a family history of such a growth.

Symptoms. A hard, irregular, painless lump appears in the breast which soon is found to be fixed to deeper tissues and the skin (compare with fibro-adenomata above). A bloodstained discharge may be found from the nipple. The disorder soon spreads to the lymph glands in the armpit, the chest wall and ribs, and further afield to the liver and the bones of the spine and limbs.

SPREAD OF NEGLECTED BREAST CANCER

Early Stage	*Middle Stage*	*Late Stage*
Breast	—Lymph glands in armpit	—Arm bones
	—Chest wall	—Spine
		—Ribs
		—Liver
		—etc.

Treatment is by a combination of surgical removal of the breast, and nearby tissues, and of radiotherapy. To give these treatments the best chance of working, they should be started as early as possible in the disease. Valuable time is lost by the woman who is too shy or embarrassed to go to her doctor, and in this time the cancer is spreading further, reducing the chance of complete removal. It must be stressed that such growths are pain-free and may be quite small when first noticed. All breast lumps must be seen by a doctor as soon as they are noticed.

Many women are alive and well today, years after having had a cancer of the breast properly treated. If seen in the early stages and operated upon, the patient is out of bed in the hospital a few days after operation and often goes home two or three weeks later.

ARTIFICIAL BREASTS. Permanent disfigurement need not occur nowadays for various artificial substances can be worn to simulate the removed breast. So good are these prostheses that some women who have had a breast removed, wear such artificial breasts even with bathing costumes and can defy detection. The fear of looking asymmetrical has in the past kept women from consulting their doctors until too late for help. This fear need not exist in these days of good post-operative prostheses.

DISORDERS OF THE GENITAL ORGANS

Abnormalities in Structure

In the fetal development of the genital tract, two tubes, one from each side of the body, come together and fuse side by side (Fig. 9). If this joining up is incomplete, then instead of a single uterus in the middle of the pelvis, there will be a pair of smaller tubes, partly or completely separated (Fig. 10a and b). Should the tubes join, but the tissue of their common wall not be absorbed, then a septum or partition is left down the middle (Fig. 10c and d).

In the vagina of the embryo, a horizontal septum (thin dividing wall) is found just above the level of the hymen. This is usually absorbed while the female infant is still in the mother's womb. In rare cases absorption does not occur. The baby is born and appears normal, but when she grows up and menstruation commences, difficulties start. The lining (endometrium) of the womb is shed each month in accordance with cyclical hormonal stimulation (see p. 486). With this shedding of the lining, bleeding occurs. The blood is not lost to the outside but retained by the septum. Each monthly period adds gradually to this pool of blood and, although a small amount is absorbed, much is left in the upper vagina. This organ soon balloons out and, with each period of bleeding, pain is felt. If the process goes on long enough, and it may not be diagnosed for two or three years, the uterus itself may be stretched and the retaining septum bulged down the vagina until it appears at the entrance.

Treatment. Once diagnosed, the condition can be corrected by a small operation. This, however, must take place under anesthesia in a hospital to prevent infection. Recovery is usually rapid and, if the womb and vagina have not been overstretched for too long, the girl will have normal periods and can subsequently bear children.

Discharges from the Vagina

The normal woman makes a little moisture from the genital organs, just as she does from the salivary glands or from the sweat glands. In health this is not noticeable and causes no trouble. When, however, the moisture is excessive, offensive, or irritant, the woman's notice is drawn to it. This discharge may be clear, white, yellow, green, or blood-stained.

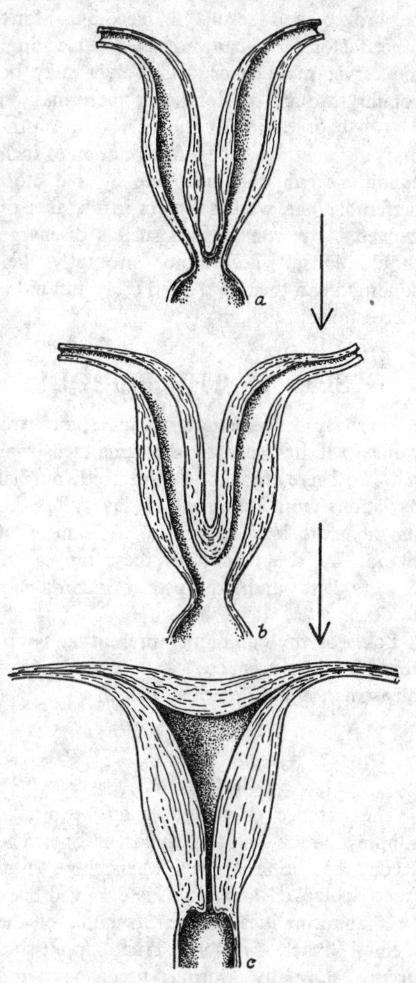

Fig. 9. *FORMATION OF A NORMAL UTERUS. a. In the developing embryo two tubes lead into the vagina. b. At a later stage the walls between the tubes begin to fuse. c. The dividing wall is absorbed to form the fundus of the womb, leaving a single cavity.*

Clear Discharge

A clear thin discharge may just be an excess of the normal production of mucus from the cervix and the vaginal wall, and is a normal variation just as some people perspire more than others do. It may, however, be the result of an increased blood supply to the pelvis as happens in pregnancy, pelvic inflammation, or over-indulgence in sexual stimulation.

White Thin Discharge

White vaginal discharge is variable—it may be thin, foamy, and white (like watered-down milk), or thick, white, and curdy. The thin discharge is due to infection by an organism, *Trichomonas vaginalis* (Fig. 11). The discharge is very irritating on the skin and causes the patient to scratch and soon make herself raw.

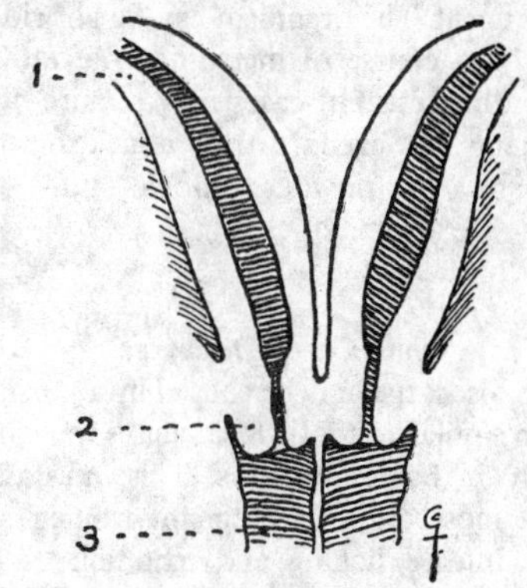

a. DOUBLE UTERUS, or uterus didelphys, with two cervices and two vaginas. 1. *Left uterus.* 2. *Cervix on left side.* 3. *Vagina on left side.*

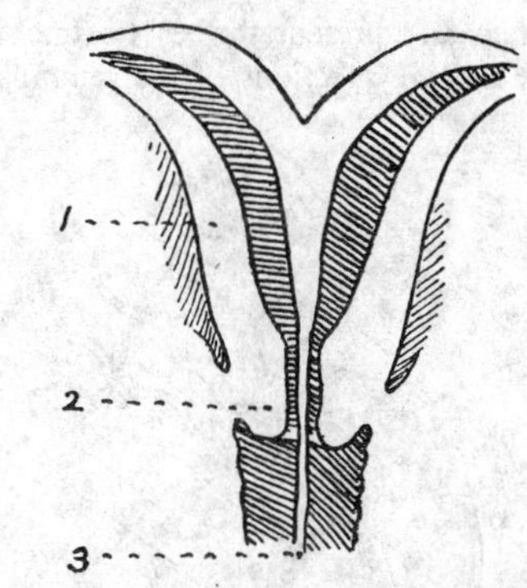

b. TWO-HORNED UTERUS, or bicornate uterus, with a partition in the cervix and vagina. 1. *Left uterine horn.* 2. *Cervix.* 3. *Partition in vagina.*

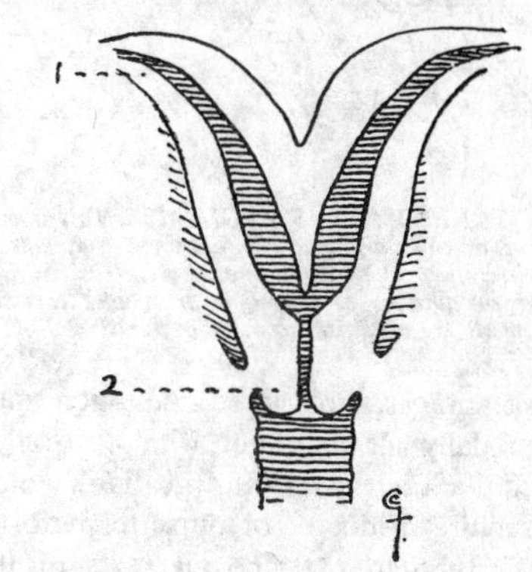

c. TWO-HORNED UTERUS, or bicornate uterus, with a single cervix. 1. *Left uterine horn.* 2. *Cervix.*

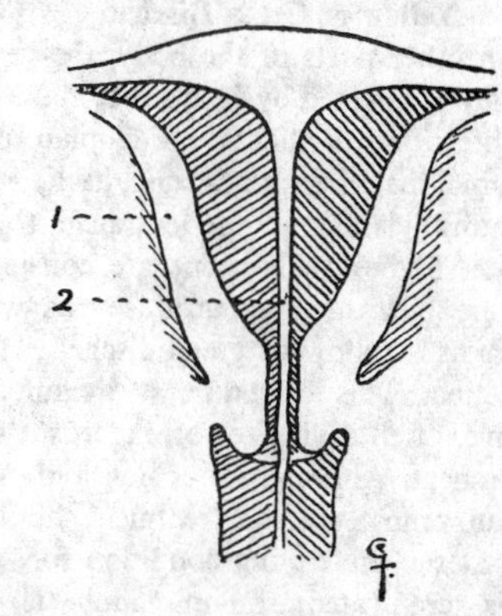

d. UTERUS WITH A SEPTUM. 1. *Uterine wall.* 2. *Septum or partition.*

Fig. 10. DIAGRAM SHOWING DIFFERENT TYPES OF UTERINE ABNORMALITIES

Treatment. The organism can be got rid of either by a course of metronidazole tablets by mouth. Resistant cases may require both treatments, or even further attack on the organisms by powders blown into the vagina. See also p. 293.

White Curdy Discharge

This discharge may be caused by a yeast infection similar to that which causes the curdy 'thrush' in babies' mouths. This infestation occurs most often in pregnant women and causes intense itching and irritation of the skin around the vulva. The area may be so scratched that secondary infection follows and this causes more redness and swelling.

Treatment. At present, the best treatment of yeast (*Candida*) infections of the genitalia is mycostatin.

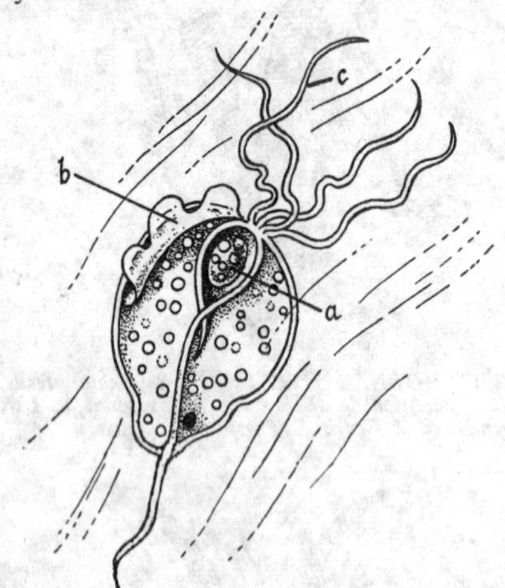

Fig. 11. *TRICHOMONAS VAGINALIS. This micro-organism (much enlarged) can infect the vagina causing a thin irritating white discharge. a. Nucleus. b. Undulating membrane. c. Flagellae, or mobile threads, which enable the organism to move in fluids.*

Resistant cases of yeast infestation may require daily cleaning out with a strongly colored dye such as crystal (gentian) violet. This requires a doctor or nurse to perform, using a tube to examine all parts of the vagina.

Yellow or Green Discharge

As in other parts of the body, the genital tract can be infected by germs that make pus. Such infection can affect the Fallopian tubes, the uterus, the cervix, the vagina itself, or the lubricating glands at the entrance to the vagina. All these conditions are considered elsewhere but any may produce pus which appears as a yellow or green discharge from the vagina. This discharge is irritant and offensive, often drying to form a crust.

Treatment. Although douching and swabbing can remove the pus, treatment should be aimed at the underlying condition for, until this is eradicated, inflammation is still present and causes further discharge later.

Blood-stained Discharge

Heavy infection in the vaginal region may cause the skin of the vagina or cervix to be broken and result in bleeding. Many other factors, too, can induce such bleeding; the cervix may be eroded, polyps may be coming through the cervix, or there may be a growth or tumor of the cervix or of the body of the uterus. The differentiation of such conditions can only be made by a doctor, preferably one who is expert in diseases of women. Any woman with such a discharge should consult her doctor promptly; her condition can then be treated early and more successfully.

UPSETS IN THE PERIODS

Since women are not machines, no two women will have exactly the same menstrual pattern. There are many and perfectly normal variations from the usual 28-day cycle with its moderate loss of four to six ounces of blood. The exact limits of these ranges are hard to define and require your doctor's help to demarcate.

Some of the commoner presenting symptoms of disturbances and disorders of menstruation are described below.

Amenorrhea

The absence of periods may be a true suppression or only an apparent one. The second condition applies when the genital tract is blocked and blood is dammed back (see Abnormalities of the Structure of the Genital Tract, p. 489). True suppression occurs normally during pregnancy and lactation. Further, no periods occur before puberty or after the menopause.

Other than these normal times, amenorrhea can occur as a primary or a secondary phenomenon. In a primary case, the woman has never seen periods, despite her being well past the age when bleedings should have started. In the second instance, periods have started normally as a young girl and then, after a variable interval, they have ceased.

Primary Amenorrhea. The first group of women are usually suffering from some endocrine disease. The ovaries are under the control of the pituitary gland in the brain, and either this or the ovary itself may be in some way deficient in its action. In consequence, ovulation does not occur and no cyclical hormone changes follow. Thus the lining of the uterus is not shed and no bleeding occurs. Sometimes this primary amenorrhea is the result of lack of development of the ovaries, that is they are either absent or very small.

Secondary Amenorrhea occurs normally in pregnancy and lactation. It may also be a symptom of disease of both ovaries or of a general bodily condition such as thyrotoxicosis or tuberculosis.

Many patients, particularly younger women, have such a cessation of the periods following a disturbance in their way of life. Girls who go away from home for the first time to university, to school, to nurse, or to join the Services may have two or three months with no periods. Emotional factors obviously are also involved in those women who greatly desire, or greatly fear, pregnancy. Such women may suppress their periods for many months, the notable example in history being Queen ('Bloody') Mary. She had a secondary amenorrhea for eighteen months and was convinced that she was pregnant.

Treatment. When such a patient consults her doctor, the exact cause and type of the amenorrhea must be determined. Blind treatment of the condition with hormones, without first making a diagnosis, is dangerous and may be useless. Full examination of the patient must be made, and often special investigations are required to sort out the cause of the condition.

Should some disease outside the genital organs be discovered, treatment is first aimed at this condition. Correction of this will often allow the periods to return to normal.

If the amenorrhea is due to emotional causes, no specific treatment is required, for as soon as the woman adjusts herself to her new environment or to the new emotional situation, periods will start again. Should, however, a glandular disorder be diagnosed, treatment with hormones may be prescribed. Amenorrhea due to such causes is difficult to treat and response is not always good. This is a matter for experts and the patient should be under the care of a physician skilled in such matters.

General Care. Diet and exercise should be well regulated. Fresh air, good food, moderate exercise, and plenty of rest are valuable adjuncts to more specific treatments.

Uterine Hemorrhage

Although the amount of blood lost at each period varies in individuals, an excessive amount soon reflects itself in the patient's general health. She becomes listless and tired, she is anemic and each menstrual period presents such a profuse loss of blood that normal social life is grossly interfered with; she cannot go shopping for fear of an excessive loss, and even her household duties become too much.

Treatment. As for Menorrhagia, p. 491.

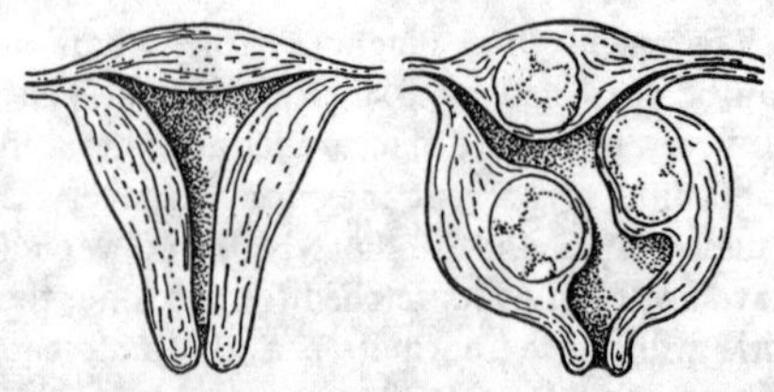

Fig. 12. *FIBROIDS IN UTERUS. In the uterus to the right, the fibroids have distorted the cavity so that it presents a much greater surface area than the normal uterus on the left. The greater the surface area, the more endometrial lining is made and shed, thus causing a heavy menstrual flow.*

Menorrhagia

This implies an extra heavy loss of blood with each period. Usually the period is too profuse while it lasts, or the period lasts a longer time than was usual for that individual patient. However, in this state the periods are still regular and no loss occurs between each period.

Menorrhagia may occur in young girls at puberty just after the onset of menstruation. Usually this is due to a lack of balance of the endocrine system. Within a few months normal balance is usually achieved and the blood-loss settles down to a reasonable amount.

Like amenorrhea, menorrhagia is a symptom rather than a disease in itself. The loss may just be heavier than usual and the body adapts itself to such a loss, or more profuse hemorrhage each month can cause an anemia and even, in rare cases, death.

Causes. The causes of this condition may be considered in two groups—general diseases, and abnormalities in the pelvis itself. The first group is a small one since debilitating diseases tend to suppress menstruation rather than increase it and, with the exception of the few instances cited, chronic disease neither causes nor aggravates excessive uterine hemorrhage. Occasionally blood diseases, e.g. thrombocytopenic purpura or a severe anemia, cause can increase in blood loss, but heart disease and high blood pressure are rarely evocative unless the patient is in heart failure. Lack of thyroid function (see myxedema, p. 402) may start with heavy periods but other endocrine diseases usually tend to suppress menstruation. Emotional upsets, nervous tension, anxiety states, unsatisfied sexual urge, marital upsets, and overwork can all cause menorrhagia, but their effects on menstruation may be delayed for six to twelve months.

Local Causes in the Pelvis. These are usually centered around the uterus itself rather than the ovaries. Should any infection lodge in the pelvis, reactive increase in blood supply to the uterus results, and this leads to heavy periods. Thus salpingitis (inflammation of the Fallopian tubes) or metritis (inflammation of the uterus) tends to cause uterine hemorrhage. The further the infection is from the body of the uterus, the less likely is menstruation to be increased. Thus chronic cervicitis or vaginitis is not often accompanied by menorrhagia. These infections often follow a pregnancy or an abortion, because inflammation occurs very readily in a uterus that has been recently pregnant.

Tumors and Fibroids: Any large pelvic tumor can cause menorrhagia simply by increasing the pelvic blood supply; an increased blood loss at each period is often the first indication that such a tumor is present. Fibroids of the uterine muscle (see p. 497) are a common cause of menorrhagia especially in women over 40 years of age. This bleeding is due partly to the increased blood supply mentioned above but also to the increase in the surface area of the uterus (Fig. 12). Also, it is possible that women who have fibroids have an increased level of estrogens (female hormone) in the blood and this may be a cause of increased bleeding.

Disorderly Uterine Hemorrhage. A large number of women who have menorrhagia, however, do not have any obvious disorders. Such patients are said to have disorderly uterine hemorrhage and their management presents a problem. Commonly such women are in the last decade of reproductive life and may have had either no children or else their pregnancies were many years earlier. It is assumed that such hemorrhages are due to an upset in the hormone balance but exactly what goes wrong is unknown.

Treatment with hormones given by mouth helps in many cases by supplementing the body's own natural hormones; by this means a regular cycle of moderate loss is restored. Recent successes have been reported from the use of aminocaproic acid for menorrhagia. The final solution is removal of the womb—hysterectomy.

Metrorrhagia

Irregular and acyclical bleeding from the uterus is termed metrorrhagia. It occurs at any time in the menstrual cycle and may vary from a continuous heavy loss of clots to a slight staining by blood. Occasionally such a loss is due to a profound disturbance of ovarian function with consequent loss of the cycle but more often it is due to a surface abnormality in the genital tract, e.g. a fibroid ulcerating through the inner lining of the uterus. This symptom demands careful assessment by a doctor expert in female diseases, for occasionally cancer may present itself in this way. A full examination is made to check the size, position and constituency of the uterus, tubes, ovaries, cervix, and vagina. If no obvious abnormalities are found, it is wiser to admit the patient to hospital for a diagnostic curettage of the uterus and a fuller examination under anesthesia.

Curettage is a scraping of the lining of the womb. It is done under general anesthesia in an operating room under full aseptic conditions. Once anesthetized, the patient is positioned and the area is carefully cleaned. A full pelvic examination is then done, for under the anesthetic the pelvic organs can be felt more easily. The cervix is then inspected using a speculum (Fig. 13) and the pouches of the vagina alongside the cervix are examined. The mouth of the cervix is then gently dilated to allow the passage of the curette. This instrument is gently drawn against the wall of the uterus and thus scrapes off a strip of the uterine lining (endometrium). By curetting the whole of

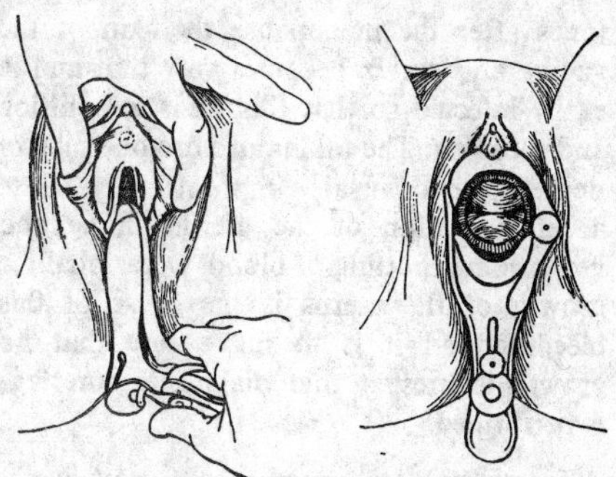

Fig. 13. *SPECULUM EXAMINATION OF THE CERVIX.* Left. *Inserting the speculum.* Right. *The cervix under view.*

the inside of the uterus, all its lining may be removed. The curettings of endometrium are then examined under a microscope after special fixing and staining. Thus this comparatively small and simple operation can give a clue to disease or dysfunction of the uterus or ovaries. It is almost completely painless and usually does not keep the patient in the hospital more than a few days.

Causes. Metrorrhagia is often caused by a simple non-cancerous condition such as a polyp of the uterus, or a fibroid. The underlying condition can be treated on its own merits. However, occasionally a cancer of the womb is found at the curettage and there is thus an opportunity for this to be treated at an early stage with much better chance of cure.

Bleeding after Intercourse

Except possibly the first time or two a woman has intercourse, bleeding should not occur on these occasions. If it does, usually there is some surface condition of the vagina or cervix which is made to bleed by the friction. Although many such conditions are not serious and can easily be treated, the symptom of post-intercourse bleeding must be taken seriously for it may herald a cancer of the cervix. Any woman with such bleeding should consult her doctor in order that a proper diagnosis may be made and treatment started. Erosions of the cervix and polyps can cause this bleeding and although they are not serious, they deserve early treatment.

Post-menopausal Bleeding

As has been mentioned previously, most women have no periods after about 45 to 47 years of age, although a few go on to the early 50's. Once the periods have finally stopped, however, any bleeding from the vagina is not normal. The amount may be nominal, a few spots or just a blood staining of a discharge, but this should not be ignored.

Causes. Many local pelvic causes can account for this type of bleeding. A caruncle (or wart) of the end of the urethra may bleed, as may a crack or fission of the skin around the entrance to the vagina. There may be an erosion of the cervix or a polyp protruding through the cervix from the uterus. Sometimes after the menopause the skin of the vagina and cervix becomes very thin and is easily infected so that this leads to splitting and bleeding. The taking of hormone pills to depress menopausal symptoms may cause a reinvigoration of the uterine lining and hence some spotting of blood. Occasionally a growth of the uterus is the cause of this bleeding and it is to make sure that no growth is present that diagnostic curettage is performed.

Treatment. Any woman with post-menopausal bleeding, no matter how little in amount nor how pain-free it is, should consult her doctor. One of the simpler causes mentioned above may be found and can be treated. If no simple cause is found, the patient should be admitted to a hospital for a diagnostic curettage (see p. 491). This can confirm whether a growth is there or not; should one be found, early treatment can be started.

Dysmenorrhea

Dysmenorrhea is a term used loosely to cover various types of painful menstruation. Up to two-thirds of women suffer some discomfort with their periods at some time or another, especially when young. Most can pass it off and carry on with their daily tasks. Some women—about one in twenty—have a severe enough pain to disable them and interfere with their work, their studies, or their social activities.

As well as those with true dysmenorrhea arising from the genital organs, any pain will appear worse at the time of menstruation. Thus the girl with the dull ache of a urinary infection will notice the ache much more at the time of her periods, but this is not a true dysmenorrhea.

Patients presenting with this symptom belong to one of two groups.

Spasmodic Dysmenorrhea. The pain comes on with the menstrual flow, is made worse by the passage of clots, and is confined to the pelvis and lower back.

Congestive Dysmenorrhea. A dull ache is felt over the whole lower abdomen for a few days before the period starts. This pain is often eased by the onset of the period and may be accompanied by vomiting which is also eased by the start of menstruation.

Dysmenorrhea is commonest in the late teens and early twenties. Usually marriage and commonly childbirth see the end of dysmenorrhea in most women, especially those who suffer from the spasmodic variety.

Emotional Causes. It must always be remembered that just as the 'pain threshold' varies from one woman to another so it may be varied in any one woman at different times. Any form of ill health will cause the woman to observe her periods more readily. During menstruation and for a few days before it, a woman may be emotionally upset and there is a tendency for a lowering of general efficiency, varying with the type of nervous make-up of the individual. Hence anything which increases nervous tension, such as unhappiness at work or marital upsets, can make the dysmenorrhea worse.

Engorged Blood Supply. An engorged or slow circulation of blood in the pelvis makes any dysmenorrhea worse, especially if it is of the congestive variety. Chronic inflammation is often first recognized because of this symptom and occasionally chronic constipation and a sedentary life may make matters worse. An unsatisfied sexual urge can lead to dysmenorrhea for the same reason—an engorged blood supply.

Treatment. The basis of good treatment rests on good diagnosis and the patient should consult her doctor. He, by means of questioning and examination, can decide which type of dysmenorrhea is being suffered and he can check for the presence of any abnormality that may be causing it. Should any abnormality be found, it is treated on its own merits, e.g. chronic infection by means of antibiotics, or endometrial disorders with hormones or operation.

It is important to remember, however, that dysmenorrhea is a self-limiting condition and always disappears in time, its going often being speeded with marriage and childbirth.

Spasmodic Dysmenorrhea. Treatment lies along the lines of improved hygienic conditions, improving the patient's exercise habits, seeing that she has a good mixed diet with plenty of roughage, adequate and regular rest including some early-to-bed nights in the week that the period is expected. A careful inquiry is made into the girl's work habits and her happiness in her job. Some women require more to occupy their minds while others are overstraining themselves. Those who are constipated should take laxatives for a few days before the expected period and have plenty of fruit and fluid in their diet at all times. Warm baths are helpful.

Congestive Dysmenorrhea is dealt with along the lines mentioned above, once any specific disease has been treated. If the uterus is displaced backwards, it may help if this is corrected (see Retroversion p. 498). Rarely, the dysmenorrhea is due to a too small opening in the cervix with a consequent damming back of the menstrual flow. This causes a colic of the uterus and may be treated by dilatation of the cervical os (opening or mouth of the cervix) under an anesthetic.

Drug Treatment. In both types of dysmenorrhea pain-relieving tablets and medicine should be taken to help the situation until the full cure is effected. Aspirin is still the best of these although codeine and phenacetin are more effective in some girls. These three are made into a variety of combinations, e.g. A.P.C. Tablets, sold over the counter at the drug store and many girls find by trial and error which combination gives them the best relief.

Operative Treatment. As well as the simple operation of dilatation of the cervix mentioned above, a very small number of girls require a bigger operation. Should the dysmenorrhea not respond to the measures suggested and the patient is still grossly incapacitated, the nerves which supply the uterus may be divided. This operation of presacral neurectomy requires the abdomen to be opened and the nerves on the back wall of the pelvis to be cut. It is a major procedure and only indicated in very severe cases.

INFERTILITY

Since pre-Christian times Man has been interested in the reproduction of his own sort. Anthropology, history and mythology can all cite examples of the great desire of men and women to prove themselves capable of having babies, and of the numerous and bizarre maneuvers they performed in the pursuit of fertility. The barren would sacrifice at the altars of Ceres and, even today, African and aboriginal tribes have complex fertility rites to aid those who do not conceive readily. In some parts of the Middle East, a man can divorce his wife should she not produce issue. This puts all the blame on the woman while we know that in about one-fifth of sterile marriages it is the man who is at fault.

It must be remembered that an embryo only grows from the fertilization of a female egg by the male sperm. As mentioned previously, the egg is produced from the woman's ovary and is shed about the middle of the menstrual cycle (see Fig. 7). This egg passes into the Fallopian tube. Sperms in the semen from the male are deposited in the vagina during intercourse. These sperms are actively mobile (Fig. 14) and many millions are present in every production of semen. Thus there is one egg and probably 100,000,000 sperms.

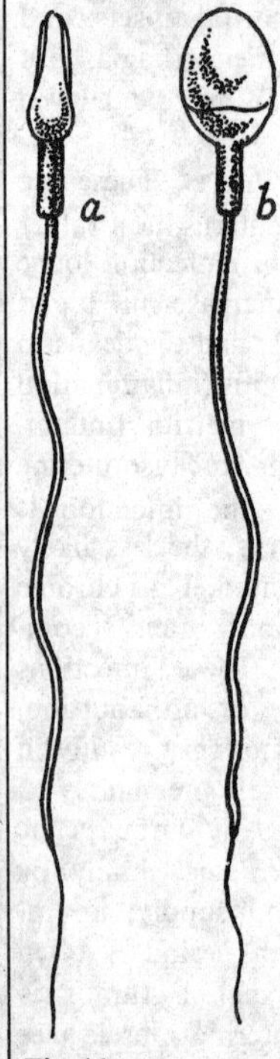

Fig. 14.
HUMAN SPERMS. a. Side view. b. Front view.

The sperm travels under the power of its actively lashing tail through the cervix and up the uterus, swimming in the thin film of fluid that covers the uterine lining. Millions of sperms die in the process but a few pass from the uterus along the Fallopian tube and eventually to the outer end. It is in this outer inch of the Fallopian tube that the sperm usually meets the egg and fuses with it. Only one sperm will fuse with an egg. Once fertilization has occurred, the egg will not allow any more sperms to penetrate.

Once shed, the egg can live for about 48 hours. Once ejaculated, the sperms may live for 48 to 72 hours. Thus it will be seen that unless intercourse occurs at the right time the living sperm and egg will not meet. For most couples there are probably only about 48 hours in each month that a pregnancy can be achieved. It is as well to bear this in mind when thinking about the whole problem of infertility.

Terminology. FERTILITY is the ability to produce offspring and INFERTILITY is the opposite. Slightly different is STERILITY. This is the inability to initiate the reproductive process. Thus sterility is absolute while infertility is relative. BARRENNESS is a loose term roughly equal to infertility. FECUNDITY is the potential capacity to produce either sperms or eggs while POTENCY is the capacity to perform the sexual act.

All these terms are loosely used to mean the same thing but it will be seen that they are all different if used precisely and correctly. A woman who has a blockage of both Fallopian tubes is quite potent (she can have intercourse) and fecund (she still makes eggs). She is sterile (reproduction cannot occur) and also infertile (she cannot produce babies). If an operation is done and the tubes are 'unblocked,' she is not now sterile (reproduction could occur) but not of necessity fertile (she still may not conceive) for although the pathway is there, egg and sperm still may not meet. A man who has lost his testicles may still be potent (many eunuchs can have intercourse) but he is infecund, infertile and sterile. It is hoped that these two examples help to clear the confusion that has arisen over the loose usage of these terms.

Statistics of Fertility. Remembering that the chances of the meeting of sperm and egg are few, it will be realized that it is hard to give a definition of infertility. If 100 healthy young married couples were to have regular intercourse without contraception the results would probably be that pregnancy would occur in 10 in the first two or three months while 80 would probably conceive within two years. Of the other 10, three would conceive in anything up to five years while seven couples would remain childless. Thus 10 per cent would be very fertile, 80 per cent fertile, 3 per cent subfertile but not sterile, and 7 per cent would be sterile. In some couples, the low fertility of one partner would be counterbalanced by high fertility of the mate. Other couples might both be so subfertile that sterility would be the result of that marriage. A small number of couples of normal fertility may remain sterile because ignorance or lack of desire has prevented proper intercourse occurring.

It is against this time background that infertility must be assessed. Most doctors who advise on these problems consider that investigation of the couple is not warranted unless two years have gone by with regular intercourse using no contraception. This is to be sure that the couple concerned are not in the group of 90 per cent of marriages who would conceive anyway. This time-limit varies with the opinions of the doctor investigating and a range of one to four years may be encountered. However, no hard and fast rules exist and each marriage must be assessed separately. Investigations would probably be justified much earlier if there were some obvious factor present which could be righted or if the couple were past the middle of reproductive life, for fertility falls off after 30 years of age in many people.

Causes of Infertility

In order to provide for fertilization each of the following three basic requirements must be fulfilled:

1. ovulation must occur;
2. active sperms must be deposited in the vagina; and
3. there should be no barrier between egg and sperms.

Factors influencing infertility can be divided into male and female groups depending on the partner. It must be remembered, however, that the problem is one of the couple rather than the individual and very few 'causes' of infertility are absolute. Hence, although a factor may be diagnosed, it is by no means certain that this is the only cause of the childless marriage.

Infertility in the Male

Lack of Penetration. Although pregnancy can and has occurred with no penetration of the male organ into the vagina, this is the exception and very rare. Usually sperms must be deposited high up in the vagina to achieve success. The male organ may not fully enter the vagina either through a fear of hurting the woman or from an ignorance of the exact site of the vaginal entrance. It has been estimated that 1 in 20 of those attending infertility clinics have never had proper intercourse because of one of these factors.

Lack of Potency. The male organ must be erect in order to enter and stay in the vagina. Some men lack this ability or, even if erection is maintained, ejaculation of semen occurs before the organ can enter the female passage. These points should be investigated by the doctor; commonly no serious illness exists but merely a mental state of fatigue or an over-exertion sexually.

Block of the Male Tubule System. Sperms are made in the testicles and pass in the collecting tubules to the vas deferens. The semen is stored in the seminal vesicles by the prostate gland and only comes from these sacs under sexual stimulation. The collecting tubules may be missing from birth while they or the necks of the seminal vesicles may further be blocked by old inflammation. In either of these situations, sperms will not get to the vagina during intercourse. If the blockage is of the tubules, then although no sperms emerge, 'seminal fluid' may still be ejaculated at intercourse for most of this fluid comes from the prostate gland and would still be made.

Treating old infections of this region and trying to cause blocked tubes to become patent again is a difficult business and is rarely attended by success.

Agenesis of Sperms. The sperms are made in their millions in the testes from the cells lining the coils of tubes inside the testicle itself. Many factors can upset this production of sperms.

The sperm-producing tissue may be absent from birth. If all the testicular tissue is not present then a eunuch results; he may have rounded female body curves and scanty facial and body hair. Sometimes only the sperm-making tissue itself is absent while the hormone-producing cells are still there. These men will be male physically.

Sometimes the testicles do not descend into the scrotum properly (see p. 129). If they stay in the abdominal cavity, it is probable that the man will be sterile. Should they partly descend then the chances of making sperms are increased but are less than those of the normal man. This condition is best treated by surgical operation in childhood (see p.417).

Testicles can be damaged in war and accident. Although in the human they seem to lie in a relatively exposed place for such fragile organs, in fact one of man's strongest responses to attack is to adopt a position where the testicles are retracted against the lower abdomen and between the thighs. Thus they are well protected in fact. However, gunshot wounds and road accidents, as well as kicks in sports such as football, can damage the testicles. If the damage is gross and much bruising occurs it is possible that no more sperms will be made but the hormones will probably continue to be produced. It is very difficult to predict in any given case, no matter how severe the damage, whether sperm production is affected or not.

Acute infections usually do not affect the testicle so much as the collecting tubes alongside it. There are, however, a few virus infections, notably mumps, which affect the testicle and may lead to permanent sterility.

If chronic infections such as syphilis or tuberculosis occur, they usually cause sterility in the patient. Their general treatment is dealt with on pp. 290 and 352.

TUMORS of the testicle usually occur in the older man who is past having children and whose wife is likely to be post-menopausal. These tumors usually cause sterility and necessitate treatment with operation and deep X-rays.

Infertility in the Female

Female infertility factors divide women into those who do not make eggs and those who make them but have a barrier to their fertilization by sperms.

Non-ovulation. In a very small number of women, the ovaries are too small or too underdeveloped to make eggs.

In most cases, such women are small with poorly developed other features of their sex. Many women, however, with apparently normal ovaries may not ovulate at certain times. For the first few years of menstruation it is not uncommon for no eggs to be shed. Later on in reproductive life any illness or time of malnutrition may cause a temporary cessation in egg production. These stoppages are probably brought about by hormonal influences. Occasionally, the hormone balance is upset because of an endocrine gland disease such as myxedema due to thyroid deficiency.

Cervical Causes. The cervix, being the entrance to the uterus, must be in good condition to allow the swarm of active sperms to pass up. Infection of the cervix, which is often accompanied by erosion, may sufficiently delay the sperms so that they die before reaching their objective.

Normally, the cervix produces a clear slimy mucus. This production is at its height in the middle of the menstrual cycle and this is just the time that ovulation occurs. Through this mucus the sperms ascend to the uterus above and, if such mucus is deficient or missing, sperm ascent is more difficult and slower.

To produce a better mucous surface, it is therefore necessary (1) to get rid of any infection of the cervix, and (2) to check on the cause of a 'dry cervix.' Many women who do not receive sexual stimulation during intercourse do not produce much mucus and it may be that a difference in technique by the husband could arouse an increased cervical outflow.

Uterine Causes. Normally the uterus is flopped forwards but a small number of women (10 per cent) have it tipped back, a position known as RETROVERSION (p. 498). This is probably a normal position for most of them but a few of this group once had an anteverted uterus (one tipped forwards) which has at some time gone back and been held there. Should some women of this last group be infertile it may be worth while correcting the retroversion so that a pregnancy may result.

PROLAPSE. A severe prolapse may interfere with fertility in that it is a bar to intercourse but, once an embryo lodges in such a uterus, it will probably stay.

FIBROIDS. In the later half of reproductive life fibroids (see p. 497) are often found in the uterine wall, and may be associated with infertility. This may be due to the fibroids distorting the uterine cavity so that the fertilized egg cannot settle, or else to the high estrogen state that often accompanies fibroids. Fibroids in the upper part of the uterus may actually press on and block the part of the Fallopian tube that passes through the uterine wall. Occasionally, fibroids are treated by myomectomy, a 'shelling-out' operation (see p. 498).

Fallopian Tube Disorders. The Fallopian tubes are very narrow (sometimes 3/100 of an inch) and may easily be blocked by spasm or by infection.

SPASM is commonest in tense women who are worried about themselves. They blame themselves for not being pregnant and are very introspective. The emotion-tension causes the nerves to the muscle of the Fallopian tube to be overactive and the tubes contract down tightly. It is of interest that such women often have spasmodic dysmenorrhea (see p. 492).

INFECTION. The other common cause of a blocked tube is old infection. After the pus stage of the infection, healing occurs by fibrosis and this fibrous tissue contracts slowly and strangles off the opening and central cavity of the tube. The original infection may be of the tube itself or of the abdomen generally. It is not uncommon for a pus-forming infection of the tubes to occur after a pregnancy, especially if that pregnancy was interfered with (see septic abortion, p. 507. Another tubal infection is tuberculosis. The general abdominal infections may be appendicitis or diverticulitis. Here pus is loose in the abdominal cavity and, as it settles in the pelvis, it causes fibrosis which kinks and blocks the tube.

Surgical Treatment. Once both tubes have been shown to be blocked (see Hysterosalpingography and Insufflation, below), it is difficult to advise on treatment. A very small number of such women may be suitable for surgical operation if the affected blocked segment is short. In such a major operation, the affected part is removed and the tube either reconstituted end-to-end or reimplanted in the uterus. Both these procedures are difficult and even after the best of surgery, fully satisfactory results cannot be promised.

At the Infertility Clinic

The brief review above of the common causes of infertility covers conditions found in about 30 per cent of couples who submit to full investigation at an infertility clinic. Of the other 70 per cent, no obvious cause of their trouble can be found.

When a couple attends the infertility center the exact investigations required depend on the doctor's assessment of the situation. The following are a few of the tests and examinations which may be used.

Health Record and Medical Examination. A carefully planned set of questions is asked to find out about the past health record of the couple and to check if there are any difficulties about their sexual relations. Perfect frankness is best at this stage. The woman's menstrual history is checked and any previous pregnancies are enquired after in detail in case there has been previous infection. Both partners have separate medical examinations to check for any obvious abnormalities of the genitals. If any abnormalities are found they are treated. If there are none, some of the following tests may be performed.

1. **Post-intercourse examination** of the woman may be performed in order to check on the semen left by her husband and its activity. If possible the test should be within twelve hours of intercourse but can be done later. Hence intercourse should be late the night before attending the clinic and the woman should not wash, bath, or douche herself afterwards. A small specimen is painlessly taken from the cervix and examined under the microscope for active sperms. If present they rule out most male causes of infertility and help to clear the cervix from being the cause of the childlessness. If no active sperms are seen, it is wise to repeat the test closer to the time of intercourse.

2. **Examination of the Semen.** If both the above tests fail to show active sperms, the husband should produce a fresh specimen for the laboratory to examine fully. There are many variations in numbers, type, and mobility of sperms and only an expert can decide on the variations available. The fertile man has millions of sperms in each teaspoonful of semen.

3. **Basal Temperature Charts.** To check if eggs are being made, the woman may be asked to keep a chart of her early morning temperature for some months. The temperature under the tongue should be taken with a clinical thermometer every morning before rising, drinking tea, and washing teeth. These temperatures are recorded, and experts can sometimes tell by the cyclical change if an egg is shed (Fig. 15) and when in the cycle this happens. They can then advise the woman about the best time for fertilization to occur.

4. **Tubal Insufflation.** A small tube is led into the uterus, and air or carbon dioxide is passed along it. The gas goes into the uterus and along the Fallopian tubes. If these are not blocked, it will pass out of the outer ends of the tubes into the abdominal cavity. This escape of gas may be noted by the drop in pressure of the gas or by listening to the bubbling through the abdominal wall with a stethoscope. This investigation may be done on the conscious patient in an out-patient department for it is rarely painful although often uncomfortable. Some doctors prefer to perform the tubal insufflation under a general anesthetic and to combine it with other tests.

5. **Hysterosalpingogram.** By passing into the uterus a fluid which is not transparent to X-rays, a 'picture' can be obtained of the cavity of the uterus and the Fallopian tubes.

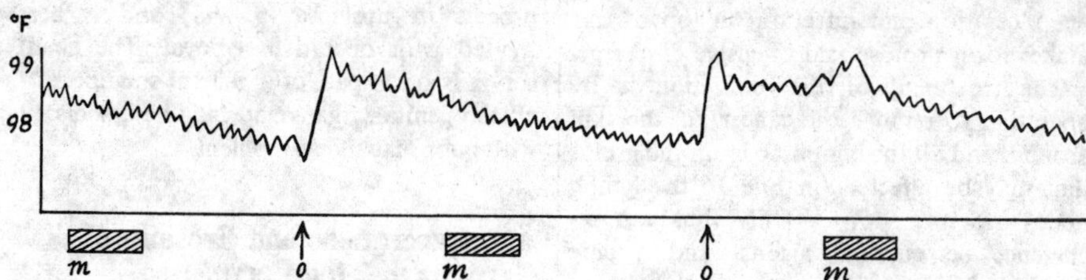

Fig. 15. *BASAL TEMPERATURE CHART showing the change of a woman's temperature during menstruation (m) and at ovulation (o) times.*

Further, if some of the material 'spills' out of the end of the tube into the abdominal cavity, this is good proof of the patency of the tubes. All these changes can be seen on the X-ray screen and can be recorded with X-ray films. If blockage occurs, the exact site is shown so that if the surgeon thinks an operation is feasible, he knows just where to cut. This investigation is usually done in the X-ray department and takes about 20 to 30 minutes. It is not usually very painful but if it is so, an anesthetic would be used.

6. **Curettage.** If the woman is admitted to hospital for a curettage, this has to be in the later half of the menstrual cycle. An anesthetic is given and a full pelvic examination is made. After dilatation (see p. 491) a few strips of the lining (endometrium) are taken and, by examination of these under a microscope, the investigator can tell if the patient is making eggs. Certain infections of the pelvis, e.g. tuberculosis, might also be detected from such curettages. This examination means only three or four days in hospital.

Infertility is an increasing problem. Forty years ago a couple accepted barrenness as inevitable, a condition about which nothing could be done. Now couples are wanting to know more about themselves, and modern treatments can sometimes help them to have a family.

DISEASES OF THE GENITAL ORGANS

DISEASES OF THE VULVA

The external genital organs consist of the labia or lips of the vagina, the clitoris and, if present, the hymen (see Fig. 3, p. 485). The area has many sebaceous and sweat glands and often a profuse growth of hair. The inner lips have no hair and no sweat glands but lots of sebaceous glands and two of these are enlarged towards the back to make the Bartholin's glands.

This area is liable to many skin diseases and these are already described in the section on Diseases of the Skin, p. 465. Further, venereal diseases can affect this region; they are dealt with on p. 289.

Malformations

Children can be born with very small lips to the vulva. Often when puberty is reached, the pubic hair is sparse and the entrance to the vagina is less well protected. Such children may have ovarian or pituitary gland deficiency.

More rarely the lips are exaggerated in size (hypertrophy). This is often just a part of the normal range of variation and is a racial characteristic. One lip (commonly the right) may be much bigger than the other. In a very few cases operations are required in adulthood if the enlarged lips are getting repeatedly inflamed or if they interfere with intercourse and child-bearing.

Some girls suffer from an excess of male-type hormone, producing the disorder known as virilism (see p. 402) and then the clitoris (Fig. 3) is enlarged. Correction of this hormone imbalance causes the clitoris to shrink to a normal size. Operations are very rarely required.

The hymen is usually a thin membrane like the frenum that anchors the tongue to the floor of the mouth. It does not completely cover the vaginal entrance but there is an opening in the middle. At intercourse this opening is usually stretched and hence a little pain may occur in the first few intercourses of the unprepared girl (see Injuries below). Occasionally the hymen is very thick, like the webs between the fingers, and requires a small operation to enlarge the vaginal entrance.

Injuries

Most injuries to the vulva occur during childbirth. To save such tears sometimes a cut or episiotomy is performed. Occasionally a fall astride a gate or manhole cover can cause much bruising and damage, while criminal assault on children may lacerate the vulva. In such cases collections of blood may form internally in the loose tissues alongside the vagina and uterus. These require operations to release the blood, and treat properly.

Sometimes too violent first intercourse tears rather than stretches the hymen. This may cause bleeding and pain. The best treatment is prevention; any virgin about to be married should consult her doctor a month or so before the marriage. He can advise her about a simple means of softening and stretching the hymen which will remove any troubles on the honeymoon. Should tears occur, however, admission to hospital and a small operation may be required.

Inflammations

The most common causes of inflammation of the vulva are from vaginal discharges especially those due to *Trichomonas vaginalis* or to *Candida* (or monilia, a yeast-like organism). (See p. 490.) Occasionally, because of the sebaceous glands and hair follicles, a crop of boils (furunculosis) can occur on the vulva. Boils occur especially in women who are run down; treatment consists of rest, local warm moist dressings, and antibiotics. The urine should be checked in case sugar is being excreted, a sign of diabetes mellitus.

The Bartholin's glands can become infected and converted to an abscess area; some swelling then occurs between the legs behind the entrance to the vagina. The area throbs and the woman feels ill and may have a rise in temperature. If left, the abscess will burst and discharge pus but it is liable to seal over before proper healing has occurred, thus causing a recurrence of the abscess. The best treatment is to open the abscess widely, the patient being under a general anesthetic, so that the area cannot close over but heals from the bottom of the abscess. Occasionally it is necessary to remove the gland a few weeks after the acute attack.

Filariasis. In Northern and Eastern Africa, the lymph glands of the groins may be infected by a parasite called *Filaria*. The infection causes a damming back of tissue fluids and elephantiasis results (see also p. 388). This usually affects the legs but can cause great swelling of the lips of the vagina. So big may these become that operation is required to remove them.

Skin Disorders in Old Age

After the menopause, the external genital area, in common with all other sexual organs, receives a diminished blood supply. This causes drying and flattening of the skin. Small cracks may occur in older women and may become infected and itch. Scratching worsens the infection and so a vicious cycle is set up.

Kraurosis. The area affected may spread to the buttocks and insides of the thighs which may be brown-stained while the relatively moister areas, which are most affected, are sodden and white. This condition is called kraurosis.

Lichenification. Occasionally the skin becomes thickened and rigid with deep cracks in it, causing great irritation. This condition is called lichenification, and must not be confused with lichen skin infection which can occur on any part of the body, including the vulva.

Both the above changes are not serious and can be treated with local drying agents and anti-itching ointments as prescribed by the doctor.

Leukoplakia. There is a further, more serious condition, that of leukoplakia. In this, white patches of skin are formed in the genital region. They itch, are scratched, and bleed. This is a progressive condition and although not a cancer itself, could turn into one in years to come. Therefore it is important that it be removed early by operation.

The differentiation between these three conditions can be very difficult despite the descriptions above because either of the first two can merge into leukoplakia. It is vitally important that such differentiation is made in order that correct treatment can be given and worse results avoided.

Caruncle

The lower end of the urinary outflow, the urethra, opens into the vulval region, just behind the clitoris (see Fig. 3). Occasionally, in older women, a wart or caruncle develops on the lowest end of the tube. This announces itself by pain or by bleeding, both occurring at the end of micturition. The swelling is the size of a pea, bright red, and bleeds easily when touched. It is best treated by cautery or removal. See also p. 417.

Tumors of the Vulva

Most warty growths of the vulva are papillomata (simple warts that are not cancerous). They are formed by local irritation of chronic inflammation. They can be treated by diathermy. Such a lipoma or fibroma is best removed by a simple operation.

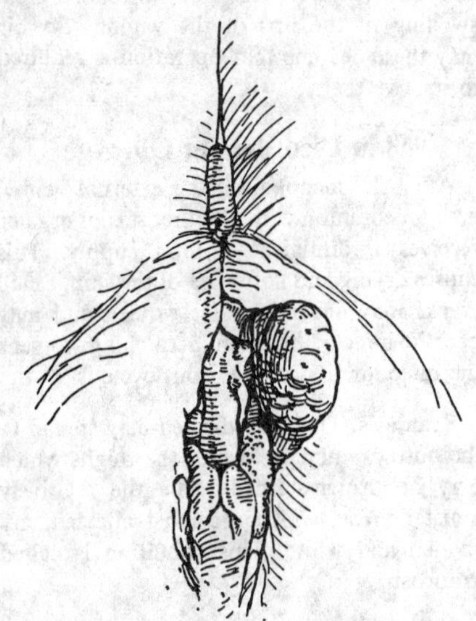

Fig. 16. *CANCER OF VULVA*

Cancer. In older women a skin cancer can occur on the vulva. It comes most commonly on the inside of the lips or around the clitoris. Often it follows leukoplakia. At first the patient has no pain but just notices a little lump (see Fig. 16). This may grow slowly and become an ulcer. A little watery matter or even blood may exude from its surface. Later on, ulceration and infection on top of this makes for a profuse and offensive discharge.

The treatment of this condition is by operation to remove the cancer, all the skin around, and all the lymph nodes in the groins that may be affected (in Fig. 16 the lymph nodes are not shown). Only thus can recurrence be guarded against and a cure sought. This is a big operation and so the earlier the growth is treated, the easier things are for patient and surgeon. All lumps in the external genital skin of post-menopausal women should be seen by a surgeon as soon as possible.

DISEASES OF THE VAGINA

Developmental abnormalities of double or imperforate vagina have already been mentioned (p. 489). Occasionally a mild degree of these will be missed until intercourse is attempted and then a small operation is required to put the defect right. Infections of the vagina are usually due to trichomonas or to monilia yeasts (p. 490), and are commonest in pregnancy.

Tumors of the Vagina

In a rare case, a small piece of embryo tissue gets cut off from the rest of its parent tissue and lodges in the front wall of the vagina. In adult life this may become filled with fluid and so a cyst is formed. It is usually about one inch in diameter and only causes mild troubles. In some cases it is bigger and presses into the vagina causing pain on intercourse. Such cysts are not serious, but if inconvenient may be removed by a small operation.

Occasionally polyps and fibroids of the vagina occur. They may be removed if causing trouble to the patient. A cancer of the vagina is rarely found; it is usually spread from another growth such as cancer of the cervix, but may be a primary solitary growth. Treatment of the secondary growth depends on the site of the primary one. The best results in the treatment of solitary growths of the vagina come from the use of radium and radiotherapy.

DISEASES OF THE CERVIX

The cervix, or neck of the uterus, (Fig. 2, p. 485) is considered separately from the main body of the organ for it suffers from diseases different from those of the uterus proper. This may well be because of its more external position, half of it being in the vagina where the secretions are different from those inside the uterus itself.

Abnormalities of Structure

The developmental abnormalities are dealt with on p. 489 but, in addition, the cervix may be very long (hypertrophy) or very small (hypoplasia). The first is usually part of a process of prolapse (p. 498) and is best treated with operative removal. The small cervix is often part of a general smallness of all the genital organs and may be associated with poor sexual development.

Lacerations and Erosions of the Cervix

When a baby is delivered, the baby's head is usually about four to four and a half inches in diameter. This has to pass through the cervix which usually dilates in labor to accommodate such a passenger. Despite the dilatation there are often small tears in the cervix after delivery (Fig. 17: compare *a* with *b* and *c*) and these tears are permanent. To a lesser extent this can happen after a miscarriage.

The resulting exposure of the delicate lining of the cervical canal to the vagina with its germs, often causes a low-grade, mild, chronic infection. This process goes on and causes much reddening of and discharge from the cervix. The condition is known as an erosion of the cervix although in actual fact no real erosion of tissue occurs, rather a heaping-up. Sometimes this process goes on inside the canal of the cervix so that the heaping-up process makes a cervical polyp protrude (Fig. 17*d*).

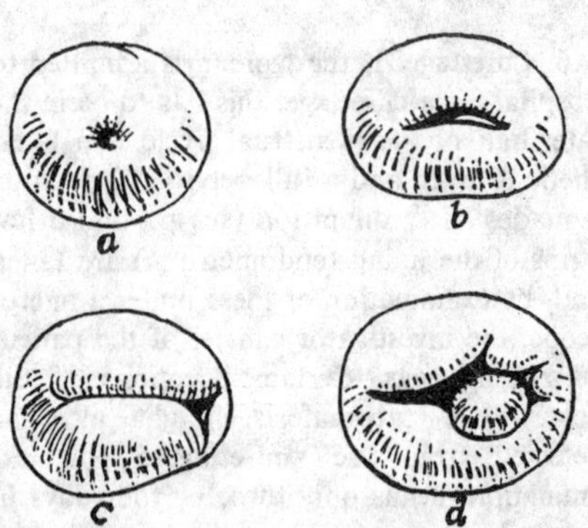

Fig. 17. *CERVIX OF UTERUS as seen by the aid of a speculum. a. Cervix of a woman who has never been pregnant. b. Cervix of a woman who has borne children. c. Cervix with a bad tear. d. A cervical polyp protruding through the opening.*

Both these conditions can give rise to bleeding from the vagina at any time, but especially after intercourse. They commonly lead to infection so that the periods are heavier and may become painful. Intercourse is often painful and conception may be difficult.

Treatment is operative. A polyp can be twisted off but this process should be accompanied by a full uterine curettage in case other polyps, which cannot be seen at the entrance to the canal, exist higher up. Cervical erosion is best treated by cautery to destroy the unhealthy tissue and to allow healthy regrowth of the lining of the cervix. Both operations necessitate an anesthetic and a short stay in hospital, but they give good results.

Cancer of the Cervix

This is the most common of all gynecological cancers and is about the fifth commonest of all malignant growths that develop in women. Since it usually occurs in fairly young women it is important that treatment starts early in order to give patients the best chance of cure.

The growth seems to develop more commonly in women aged 35 to 50 who have had children. The number of children does not seem greatly to increase the risk, but some doctors believe that the younger the mother when her first children are born, the greater the likelihood of cancer of the cervix. No one knows yet what causes this or any other cancer, but until we do, treatment must be aimed at destroying all new growths as soon as they are found. As has been affirmed above, this means that early treatment is the best treatment.

Early Cell Changes. Over the last few years, doctors have been finding that cancer of the cervix is sometimes preceded by a state of instability of the cells of the cervix. While not producing a frank cancer, the cells show rapid growth and other marked changes. If the disorder is ignored, a certain number of such women develop a true cervical cancer. These early cell changes have been called 'carcinoma in situ,' that is, cancer-like changes that are well localized and have not spread to neighboring cells.

Throughout life, the cells of the cervix are growing and the outer layers are shed. They peel away just as the outer layers of the skin flake off.

Cervical Smears. A small wooden spoon lightly rubbed across the cervix will remove a lot of cells. These *cell scrapes* can be put on a microscope slide, stained, and examined. Experts trained in this special field can sometimes find groups of cells which show 'carcinoma in situ' changes. If found, the patient should have a small operation to remove a little of the cervix tissue. This can be further examined microscopically and the diagnosis confirmed or not. Should 'in situ' changes be found in the tissue, it is possible that all the affected cells have already been removed in the small piece of tissue and experts can sometimes tell this too. If the patient has had these potential cancer cells excised, she needs no further operation although she should be seen regularly at an out-patient clinic for some time. Should however, all cells not be removed, and the patient be finished with childbearing, it may be wise to remove the uterus to prevent the onset of cancer.

Thus there is a possible means of detecting cancer of the cervix before it is at a spreading stage. The test is simple, painless, and takes ten minutes of the woman's time. Many hospitals and clinics will do this easy test freely for women who wish it in order to try to prevent cervical cancer.

Symptoms. The symptoms of cancer of the cervix should be well known. Irregular bleeding or spotting of blood is often noticed first. It may occur between the periods or even after the menopause. It may come after intercourse or after having the bowels open. This symptom demands proper investigation by a doctor and must not be ignored. If neglected, the growth may go on to cause a foul discharge. Pain is a late symptom as are bladder troubles such as increased frequency of passing urine or pain when voiding.

Examination by a doctor may show a suspicious ulcer or nodule. This should be removed under an anesthetic and examined with a microscope. If it confirms the presence of cancer, treatment should be started.

Treatment. Some growths of the cervix may respond to radiation and so treatment is given by radium pellets or by external penetrating rays beamed on to the pelvis. Other growths can be removed by operation and this means removing the cervix and uterus plus the Fallopian tubes, ovaries and lymph nodes coming from these regions. Thus potential cancer-bearing tissue is excised. Sometimes the two types of treatment, radiation and surgery, are combined one after the other to give the best chance to the patient.

If treated early, there is a good chance of full recovery but early treatment depends on early diagnosis. This in turn depends on the patient seeing her doctor as soon as any irregular bleeding occurs. Delay may allow cancer cells to spread to areas where they cannot be destroyed and this may be fatal.

DISEASES OF THE BODY OF THE UTERUS

Malformations of the uterus have been already mentioned (p. 489); they may give rise to difficulty in conceiving, to abortion, or to troubles in the delivery of a baby but usually they cause none of these. In most cases, a patient with a minor uterine abnormality is unaware of it and has no trouble with her gynecological life.

Infections

Infections are not very common and usually spread from the Fallopian tubes or up through the cervix. The most noticeable of the former is tuberculosis and it may cause congestive dysmenorrhea, painful intercourse, and sterility. Its treatment is discussed with tuberculosis of the Fallopian tubes (p. 500). Infections may ascend through the cervix especially after a delivery or miscarriage. A hundred years ago one woman in ten died as a result of such infection—puerperal fever—after childbirth. The simple measure of attendants washing their hands cut this death rate dramatically. Now, by conducting all deliveries with the strict asepsis of a surgical operation, uterine infection is rare. Most cases occur after a miscarriage, especially a criminal one where interference has taken place.

Chronic uterine infection causes the symptoms (dysmenorrhea, etc.) mentioned above, and the non-tuberculous variety is best treated with antibiotics, local heat, and shortwave therapy. It is very difficult to eradicate.

Fibroids

These non-cancerous growths are found in 1 in 10 women. They are benign rounded masses of fibrous tissue occurring in the muscle of the myometrium. They come most commonly in the mid to late thirties and no new ones are made after the menopause. Indeed, those already present at such a time usually shrink in size.

Fibroids may be single or multiple, large or small. They may come in any part of the uterine muscle and usually start as small seedlings (Fig. 18a). They enlarge, and for a while remain embedded in the uterine muscle (Fig. 18b). As they continue to grow their size or position makes them bulge either through the outer lining of the uterus (Fig. 18c) or through the endometrium (Fig. 18d). In either case they can bulge so far that they are pushed out on a stalk (Fig. 18 c and d). They are found only very occasionally in the region where the Fallopian tube enters the uterus (Fig. 18e) or in the substance of the cervix (Fig. 18f).

Symptoms. Just as the size, site, and number of fibroids in any woman is very variable, so too the symptoms she notices will vary. Commonly such symptoms occur between the ages 35 and 45 although no age is exempt. Fibroids usually make their presence known by bleeding, usually in the form of heavy or prolonged periods (see Menorrhagia p. 491). This is especially true of the fibroids shown in Fig. 18 type d. The lining of the uterus is greatly increased in size and so bleeding is heavier.

Pain is rarely a feature of fibroids unless they are outgrowing their blood supply. Occasionally this happens in pregnancy or if one twists (as might Fig. 18 type c on top of the uterus, with a thin stalk).

Sometimes fibroids grow to the size of a football and cause symptoms by pressing on other organs such as the bladder or the rectum. Sterility may be associated with fibroids (see p. 494). However, should a patient with fibroids become pregnant she will probably have no difficulties (see p. 507).

Treatment. Many fibroids are small and symptomless and require no treatment. They may be found incidentally in the course of an examination and will have caused the woman no trouble. It is probably wise for such a patient to be seen by her doctor at yearly intervals until the menopause. If the fibroids cause much bleeding or pain they are best removed.

Hysterectomy. The woman who is in her late thirties or early forties and has completed her family would probably benefit most from

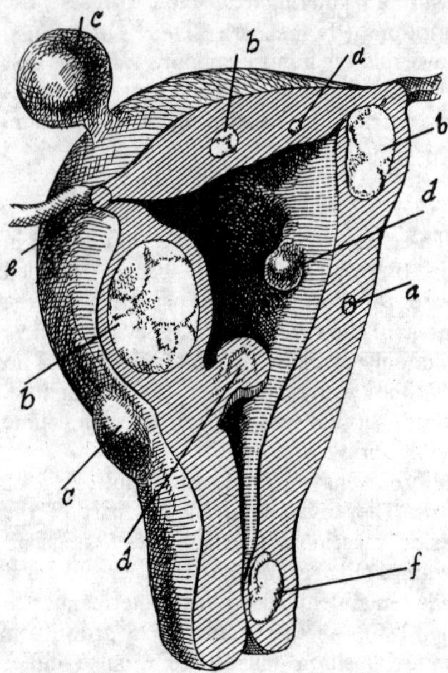

Fig. 18. *FIBROID. Section through uterus showing numerous fibroids. a. Small early fibroids embedded in the uterine wall. b. Larger fibroids in the uterine wall, distorting it. c. Fibroids bulging externally. d. Internal stalked fibroids. e. Fibroids blocking entrance to the Fallopian tube. f. Fibroid of cervix.*

a hysterectomy, or removal of the uterus. This removes the fibroids and all potential fibroid-forming tissue so that no further operations are required.

MYOMECTOMY. If the patient is younger or desires more children, then efforts should be made at operation to remove the fibroids only and to reconstitute the uterus. Such an operation (myomectomy) is difficult and can lead to troublesome bleeding. Further fibroids may grow and necessitate more operations later. However, myomectomy does leave the patient with a chance of pregnancy and this may be important to some women.

Cancer of the Uterus

Cancer in the body of the uterus is less common than in the cervix. It usually occurs in an older group of women between the ages of 50 and 60, and commonly presents after the menopause. In many cases, these women have had no children or else relatively few pregnancies which occurred early in life. There may be association between uterine cancer and obesity, diabetes, or fibroids, and often there is co-existence of these conditions.

Symptoms. The first symptom noticed by the woman is irregular bleeding. Usually this comes after the menopause but, if before, is often intermenstrual (between the periods). The bleeding may be very little in amount at first, just amounting to a spotting. It may be accompanied by a watery discharge. Pain is rare in the early stages unless the cancer has assumed a polyp-like shape and the uterus is trying to squeeze the polyp out through the cervix.

Diagnosis. Any woman with such bleeding should be examined by a doctor. He may not see or feel any gross abnormalities but the wisest course then is to send the patient to hospital for a curettage. This is the only way of finally ruling out cancer. The method described on p. 497 for checking a cancer of the cervix with cell scrapes is not so applicable for cancers of the body of the uterus and so curettage is used.

Treatment of a diagnosed cancer is either by operation to remove the uterus and all the potential cancer-bearing tissue around, or by irradiation with radium or deep external X-rays. In the past, surgical removal was used almost entirely, but a combination of both treatments is now often used. The outlook for patients so treated is better than for those with cancer of the cervix. The growth develops more slowly, is usually confined to the uterine tissues, and the women are in an older age group. However, as in any cancer, the chances of cure lessen in proportion to the length of time the growth has had to spread. Thus early diagnosis leads to good results.

Endometriosis

Other organs as well as the uterus are involved in this condition but it is discussed here for its origin lies in the uterus.

Cause. In normal women, the endometrium or uterine lining is shed each month and flows out of the cervix in the menstrual flow. In a few women, however, the endometrial tissue is found in other places. It can be deep in the uterine muscle, the ovaries, the deep lining of the abdominal wall, the rectum, bladder, or even in the arms and legs. There is much speculation as to how this tissue got to these strange sites and many doctors believe it developed there from floating cells.

Because of its origin, this endometrium is affected by the ovarian hormones each month in the same way as the lining of the uterus. The big difference is, of course, that at the end of each month, the tissue cannot break away and flow out of the body. It is trapped in deep tissues and so month after month a little more bleeding occurs and gradually a blood cyst forms. This becomes tense and painful.

Symptoms. The patient will notice this trouble in different ways depending on the site of the abnormal endometrium. If it is in the rectum or behind the uterus, there is likely to be pain before the periods, especially on opening the bowels. If it is in the abdominal wall, a tender lump is felt premenstrually. The one constant feature is the timing of the pain just premenstrually and often through the period.

Treatment is aimed at removing the pain. If the tissue is in a site from which it can easily be cut out, an operation will cure the disorder. Often, however, this is not so. Hormones can be given to stop egg production and therefore the cyclical hormone stimulation will not occur. Eventually the menopause, by stopping all egg-making, will bring the condition to a halt.

Displacements of the Uterus

The uterus is held in its place in the pelvis by a series of ligaments and muscles rather as a tent is held up by a set of guy ropes. Usually the organ is in a tipped-forward position of anteversion (Fig. 2) but it may be tipped backwards into retroversion, or in between these two it may be upright.

Causes of Displacement. With the softening and stretching of these ligaments during childbirth and their thinning with age, the uterus may not be supported as well as it might. This causes it to sag down into the vagina often taking down with it the bladder or the rectum.

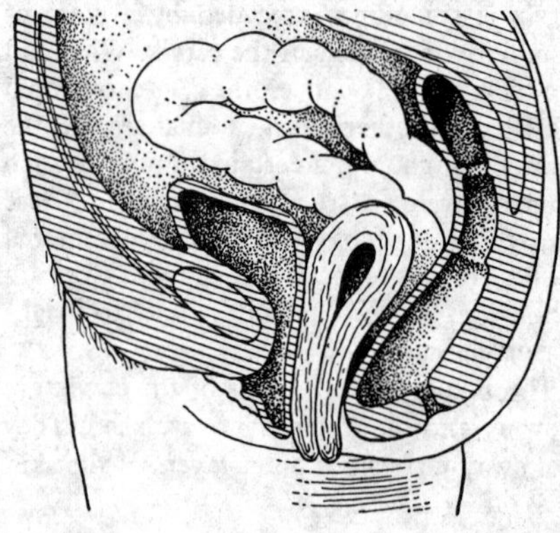

Fig. 19. *PROLAPSE OF UTERUS. Section showing a case of severe prolapse which has caused displacement of the other organs around it.*

Fig. 19 shows an extreme example of this prolapse where the cervix is outside the body and both rectum and bladder are pulled down in the back and front walls of the prolapse.

Symptoms. The sensation of 'something coming down' is often the first symptom that a patient notices. The woman may feel a lump in the vagina or just a feeling of weakness. This may be accompanied by backache. If the front wall of the vagina is involved and the bladder or urethra is pulled downwards, then the woman may well notice urinary troubles. The commonest upset is called stress incontinence of urine. This means that when the patient sneezes or strains in any way, urine escapes involuntarily. This can get so bad that mild exertion, such as carrying a shopping basket, can cause the woman to wet herself. As well as being an embarrassment, stress incontinence is soon followed by urinary infection and this causes scalding and a frequent desire to pass urine.

Should the back wall of the vagina be involved then the wall of the rectum or of the anal canal will be pulled downwards (Fig. 19). This may cause the feces to accumulate in the sac so produced and lead to difficulty in passing of feces. This in turn causes constipation.

Treatment. The best treatment of prolapse is surgical operation. In some cases, for reasons of general health, operation must be postponed, or the patient has reasons of her own for not wanting any such operation. There are devices that can be used to help control the prolapse but it should be stressed that none of these is as good as a surgical operation.

SURGICAL OPERATION. At operation, the ligaments of the uterus are buttressed up and the weakened muscles are brought together to provide a stronger, more stable support. The sacculations of bladder and rectum are corrected, and returning these organs to their usual positions often does much to correct the imperfect function. Sometimes the cervix has been elongated by its continued drooping down and this is often corrected at the same operation. Such surgery has to be performed under a general anesthetic, with a hospital stay of two to three weeks. It is wise, further, to plan a convalescence of a few weeks rather than to try to return to full work immediately.

PESSARIES. Sometimes a patient who has a prolapse is not fit to stand an operation because of a poor heart condition, raised blood pressure, or a weak chest. In addition, prolapse is sometimes found in young women who may wish to have further pregnancies. In both these situations, it would be wise not to operate but to compromise, and try to control the prolapse with pessaries. Some patients in the former group may be relieved of their symptoms provided they can retain a pessary. In the latter group, the wearing of a pessary is a temporary expedient until pregnancies have finished, when proper surgery can be performed.

'Watch Spring' and Plastic Pessaries. Most pessaries for younger patients or in inoperable cases are either of the 'watch spring' variety or made of plastic. A watch spring pessary is a flexible metal ring covered with rubber for comfort (Fig. 20). The other type is made of

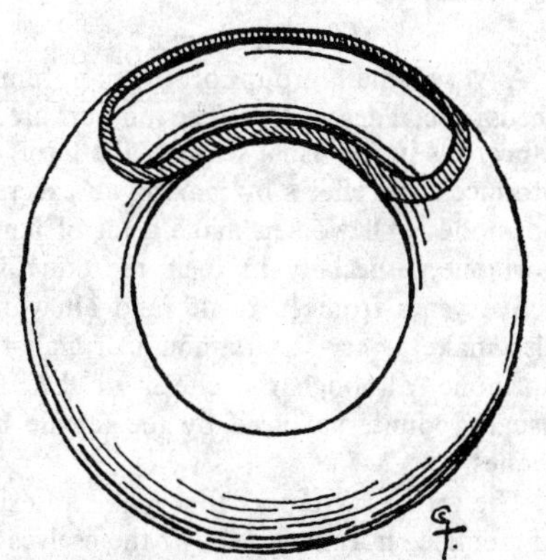

Fig. 20. *WATCH-SPRING RING PESSARY for use in prolapse of the uterus. The rubber is shown cut away to show the metal ring.*

solid plastic. Both are slightly springy and can be flattened into a long oval for inserting and removing from the vagina. When inside, however, the pessary opens out to its ring shape and, by stretching the vaginal walls, holds up the uterus.

Cup and Stem Pessary. Should the prolapse be so severe that even a ring will not hold it, a cup and stem pessary is sometimes used (Fig. 21). The upper part acts as a platform to rest the uterus while the stem is in the vagina. If necessary this is held in place with tapes.

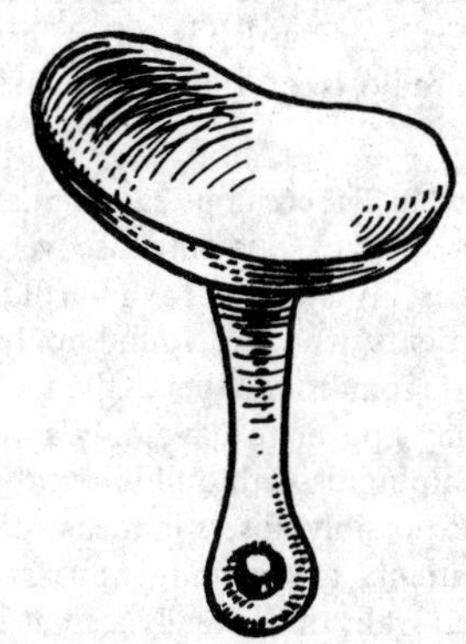

Fig. 21. *CUP AND STEM PESSARY for use in cases of prolapse of the uterus.*

Hodge Pessary. A retroverted uterus can sometimes be maneuvered forwards by a doctor while examining a patient. If he can do so, the uterus may be held in its forward or anteverted position by the use of a specially curved Hodge pessary (Fig. 22). This is kept in for six to eight weeks in an effort to cure any symptoms caused by the retroversion.

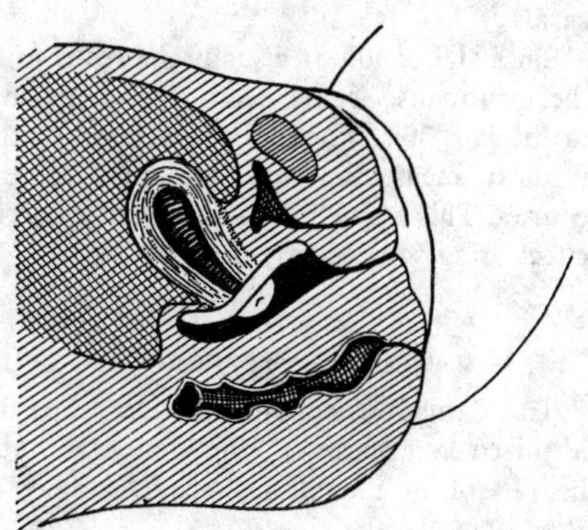

Fig. 22. *HODGE PESSARY in position around the cervix to support a prolapsed uterus.*

VAGINAL HYGIENE. Any pessary must be properly fitted by a doctor and inspected every few months. Pain should not be felt and the pessary should be comfortable and just fit snugly. A pessary worn in place for too long a time causes irritation, inflammation, and later ulceration of the vaginal walls. A persistent discharge may occur which becomes bloody later on.

It is advisable to douche regularly with salt solution (1 tablespoon of salt to a pint of water at body heat) while wearing a pessary but, if douching is impracticable, a salt bath should be taken twice a week.

Disorders of Pregnancy

The uterus, being the seat of childbearing, is liable to certain disorders particular to pregnancy. Most of these—abortion, hydatid mole, etc.—are dealt with in the section on Diseases of Pregnancy, pp. 503–9.

As the uterus of the pregnant woman stretches to accommodate the growing infant, the muscular walls 'give' a little. If previous pregnancies have occurred and there is some degree of fibrous tissue laid down in the uterine wall, this stretching process may cause discomfort. Further, the front ligaments of the uterus are put under stretch and these too are uncomfortable. A little bleeding can occur into these ligaments to give an acutely tender area in some patients.

FIBROID DEGENERATION. Should fibroids be present in a uterus which becomes pregnant, they may undergo degeneration (p. 507) and become very painful. Operation is seldom required for such conditions.

DISEASES OF THE FALLOPIAN TUBES

The anatomy of these delicate structures is described on p. 485. Developmental abnormalities of the Fallopian tubes are not rare and may be an accidental finding at an operation, or they may be discovered while investigating for infertility. Although complete absence of the tubes is uncommon, in some cases they may be small, deficient, or 'solid' so that sperms and eggs cannot pass through them.

Acute Inflammation

Causes. Acute inflammation of the Fallopian tubes is most liable to occur in women who have been recently exposed to childbirth, a miscarriage, or to a pelvic operation. The micro-organisms enter from the vagina, pass through the cervix and up the uterus to settle in the tube. Commonly, an acute abscess is found in the tube.

Course. The onset of this condition is usually rapid. The patient feels ill about a week after delivery or a miscarriage, and she may have chills or vomiting. The temperature is high, 103° to 105°F, while there is much lower abdominal pain. Examination is difficult because of the pain but the doctor may be able to feel the abscess on vaginal palpation.

Some acute infections may reach the tube by the blood stream, as happens in gonorrhea. The illness is not so sudden but when at its height it is acute. In a few cases inflammation spreads from an infected adjacent organ such as the appendix.

Treatment. The patient must be put to bed and kept on a fluid diet. Hot water bottles in the pit of the stomach bring relief. Analgesic tablets, such as aspirin, or compound codeine tablets, may be taken if tolerated. Antibiotics will be prescribed by the doctor who may take a vaginal swab for examination in order to help identify the infecting organism and check its sensitivity to the antibiotics given.

If this treatment is started before much pus has formed, response is rapid and the patient gets better in a day or so. The temperature returns to normal and the swelling of the Fallopian tubes goes down.

Should treatment be delayed, however, and pus has formed, the course of the illness is much slower and response takes many weeks. Occasionally the pus has to be released by surgical operation and this means a stay in hospital of some weeks. If the abscess bursts, a generalized peritonitis results as from a ruptured appendix. This is a very serious condition and necessitates urgent treatment.

Should the inflammation of the Fallopian tube have spread from some neighboring organ, the satisfactory treatment of that condition will resolve the tube infection.

After such acute inflammation the Fallopian tube is usually damaged. Mild degrees of infection promptly treated may not impair fertility permanently, but severe infection causes blockage of the delicate narrow tube which becomes kinked and fibrous. The power of the tube to squeeze the eggs along its cavity is thus lost, and sterility follows.

Chronic Inflammation

Recurring attacks of inflammation may occur at intervals, for infecting organisms may lurk in the recesses of the matted pelvic organs after a partly- or late-treated acute attack. These flare-ups are not so severe as acute attacks but are extremely difficult to treat and overcome.

The patient's general health is poor. She becomes tired and worn out by her symptoms and may be anemic. There is usually a discharge from the vagina due to the increased congestion or to the associated chronic inflammation that occurs in the uterus or cervix. Backache is common and so is the congestive type of dysmenorrhea. There may be deep pain on intercourse and the periods will probably be heavier than usual. A doctor examining such a woman may find thickening of the Fallopian tubes or tender areas alongside the uterus, usually present on both sides although one side is usually worse than the other. Married patients may complain of infertility.

Treatment. Management of such chronic infections is very difficult and depends on the severity of the condition and the patient's age. If symptoms are not severe and the patient is young, treatment with local heat, courses of antibiotics and analgesics can be used, and may be supplemented by short-wave diathermy heat treatment. Should symptoms be severe and the patient older, then operation must be advised. Operation involves removing the infected tubes and usually the uterus as well. Since the condition of chronic infection itself has produced sterility, then the operation of removing the tubes cannot worsen it.

Tuberculosis

Tuberculosis of the Fallopian tubes, or tuberculous salpingitis, is often associatee with tuberculosis of the urinary tract (see p.412).

Symptoms. Tuberculous salpingitis is often symptom-free and so is only discovered when a patient is investigated for infertility. Thus many patients who are found to have this condition seem to be perfectly fit women. Others may appear to have only a very mild chronic salpingitis with dull lower abdominal aches and possibly upsets in menstruation. In a few patients an opening appears on the abdominal wall; this is really a sinus draining from a tuberculous mass around the Fallopian tube.

Treatment. As detailed on p. 352, the treatment of tuberculosis rests on a sanatorium regimen, good diet, sunlight, and such drugs as streptomycin, para-aminosalicylic acid (PAS) and isoniazid (INH). These are the basic requirements for treatment of tuberculous salpingitis. Should these not control the condition, operative removal may be required but this is difficult and dangerous and requires careful pre- and post-operative care.

Since the condition usually improves after the menopause, some doctors treat patients in the late 30's, who do not respond to the medical measures, with radiation to the ovaries. This stops the making of eggs and in effect brings on an early menopause.

Ectopic Pregnancy

This dangerous condition occurs when the fertilized egg settles in the Fallopian tube instead of in the uterus. See Disorders of Pregnancy, p.508.

Tumors of the Tubes

These are very rare. Fibromata can occur and so occasionally can cancerous growths but these are usually secondary from some other site, such as the ovary.

DISEASES OF THE OVARIES

The female gonads, which produce eggs and female hormones, are rarely completely absent but occasionally they may be smaller than usual and their function depressed accordingly.

Tumors

Cysts. Many tumors are simple retention cysts, being a damming back of fluids made in the ovary. They can grow to the size of an orange. Other cysts are lined with secreting cells which cause them to grow rapidly. Such tumors can be the size of two or three footballs and fill the whole abdominal cavity. Despite their size, however, they are seldom cancerous and treatment can result in complete cure.

Solid Tumors are usually smaller. They grow more slowly and, while a number of them are simple and cause only pressure troubles, some are cancerous growths. If left untreated, these cancers spread malignant cells all over the abdomen, encouraging the collection of fluid (ascites) there.

Many women with smaller tumors are unaware of their presence and the swellings are only found on some routine examination such as that at a prenatal clinic. As the tumor grows it presses on the surrounding structures. A dull ache and tiredness are felt. Pressure on the bladder may cause increased frequency in passing urine, and pressure on the rectum may result in constipation. As the tumors grow larger, the abdominal girth increases and the abdominal wall has to stretch. Indigestion is a late symptom in these cases and loss of weight may follow a cancerous growth.

Treatment is by operation. It is often possible to tell if the growth is a cancer or not. Should the cyst or solid tumor be simple, then it can be satisfactorily removed by operation and the patient will recover with no further trouble.

If cancerous tissue is discovered, it is not always enough to remove the cancer by operation. Further treatment may be required to deal with any microscopic spread of cancerous cells. The treatment often takes the form of deep X-rays to the abdomen. A new treatment now in use, however, is of cancer-killing drugs which are used to 'mop up' any undetected cells. This treatment may last for months, being continued after the patient has gone home from hospital.

Hormonal Tumor

A very small group of ovarian tumors needs special description. The tumours are not cancerous in the usual sense of the term, but produce their effects by making an excess of hormones. All women make a lot of female hormone, especially in their reproductively active years from 15 to 45, and all women also make a very small amount of male-type hormone, although the effects of these are usually counterbalanced by the female hormones.

The group of tumors that make an excess of female hormones show themselves by causing excessive menstrual bleeding in the reproductive age and even by starting periods again in patients past the menopause.

The masculinizing tumors cause a cessation of periods and an alteration in the woman's bodily habit. Her breasts shrink, pubic hair grows, and the voice gets deeper. All these signs should alert the doctor who can perform special tests to confirm the altered hormone balance.

Treatment. The hormone upset can usually be corrected by operation, and the patient returns to her old self.

Malfunction of the Ovaries

Sometimes patients who started their womanhood normally find that their periods are stopping, that they are infertile, or that they are becoming increasingly hairy and fat. A few even notice the breasts getting smaller, or their interest in sexual matters diminishing. If special tests are performed on such women, it can be shown that they are no longer making eggs and in consequence the balance of female to male hormones in the body is altering. The exact reason for this is not known for the cause may lie in the pituitary gland, the ovary, or in any of the other endocrine (hormone-making) glands of the body (see pp. 260-61 and 404).

Treatment. After proper investigation a group of such women may be diagnosed as suffering from a condition which a small operation on the ovary can correct. The surgeon cuts a wedge from the ovary on each side. In this group the operation causes menstruation to return to normal and eggs to be produced again so that such women can conceive. The exact explanation as to how the cure works is still not known but the small amount of surgery brings good results to this group of women.

DISORDERS OF PREGNANCY

Pregnancy is a normal event which many women undergo with no more than a few minor inconveniences, carrying through to a normal labor and the production of a healthy infant. The mothers themselves are usually back to full strength in a few weeks and the whole cycle is taken in the stride of the normal healthy woman. However, this is a time when the woman is under stress and, in consequence, departures from the normal path must be watched for and corrected when they occur. It is to this end that prenatal care is conducted, although most patients pass through the prenatal clinics with nothing abnormal being found during the whole pregnancy. But it is to detect early signs of trouble that the prenatal care is given, and because of early detection simple and early corrective measures can be applied. The disorders to be corrected can be conveniently grouped into two categories, those peculiar to the pregnancy state and those which existed in the mother before the pregnancy started and which may be affected by the pregnancy.

DISORDERS PECULIAR TO PREGNANCY

Most women feel at their best in pregnancy and a great sense of well-being is often felt by young women who have been in vague ill health for some time before. However, a few minor and even fewer major disorders may affect them.

Vomiting

This is such a common disorder of pregnancy that many women regard it as a sign of normal pregnancy and accept it as such. Indeed, fifty per cent of pregnant women, especially those so for the first time, have vomiting attacks during the first few weeks of pregnancy. The nausea is usually noticed on rising from bed (morning vomiting) but often occurs in the evening. It usually starts at about six to eight weeks from the beginning of the pregnancy and is often the first indication to a woman who is irregular in her menstrual cycle that she is pregnant. The condition lasts for several weeks and usually lessens towards the end of the third or fourth month. Beyond the immediate unpleasantness of the vomiting most women are not inconvenienced for the rest of the day and are certainly not ill.

In a few women the vomiting gradually becomes more frequent and more severe, so that repeated attacks begin to interfere with their ordinary activities and their intake of food. This state will be discussed separately.

Treatment. Vomiting of pregnancy can be mitigated by a sensible regime helped by certain medicines from the doctor. It is wise to keep off highly spiced or rich foods for a few weeks at this stage of pregnancy and live on simple foods. If the vomiting is most pronounced in the morning, the patient should eat a little before getting up (a couple of crackers and a cup of tea brought to her by a sympathetic husband are a great help) If family commitments allow, breakfast should be eaten fairly soon after getting up and, during the day, frequent small snacks are better than two or three big meals.

Often the family doctor or prenatal clinic can help by giving anti-sickness tablets. Since many types of these tablets exist, the patient is best guided by her doctor as to which is preferable.

The most important thing to remember is that the vomiting always stops, usually at about the fourth month, so that wretched though it is at the time, it always settles itself.

Hyperemesis Gravidarum

This is the more serious form of vomiting in pregnancy, when the vomiting becomes intractable and weakens the woman. Occasionally a little blood may be vomited and the patient begins to lose weight and becomes sunken-eyed.

This stage of the condition is best treated in hospital when the stomach can be rested by feeding by other routes, and the patient's morale can be maintained with other treatments. The severe stage rarely lasts more than a few days and, once ended, the woman usually goes on to complete a normal and uneventful pregnancy. In a very small minority of cases the patient may lose her baby or pregnancy may have to be terminated, but this is rare.

Toxemia of Pregnancy

This is an old term which covers a wide group of more serious conditions of pregnancy which are now usually referred to as pre-eclampsia or eclampsia. It is to diagnose and treat these conditions as early as they appear that, at antenatal clinics, the patient's blood pressure is taken and her urine samples tested. Some clinics also weigh the patient at each visit as a further precaution.

Pre-eclampsia

This condition occurs mostly in those having a first baby. It is also more common in those having twins and in diabetic patients who become pregnant.

Symptoms. occur towards the end of pregnancy, commonly after the thirty-sixth week. The course of the condition is very variable, sometimes progressing rapidly but often getting only slowly worse until the birth of the infant.

The first symptom is swelling of the feet and legs. This often disappears with rest and therefore may not be present in the mornings. The condition increases slowly and may occur in the hands and face; the former make the wedding ring tight and the latter causes a puffy face. When examined, the blood pressure is often raised and later the urine contains protein which should not be present.

Treatment. Provided the onset is late in pregnancy and the progress of the condition slow, the only treatment is extra rest. At first this may be taken at home with two hours every afternoon in bed (not sitting in an armchair) in addition to the usual amount of sleep at night. This will control most patients with pre-eclampsia although sedative tablets may occasionally be used, as well. Despite these measures, a few women continue to have a raised blood pressure and swelling of hands and feet. Usually these patients should be admitted to hospital for more intensive rest treatment and further sedation.

If the pre-eclampsia continues despite these treatments and if the baby is considered to be mature enough in the uterus, then the obstetrician will consider starting labor in order to get a fit mother and child. He would begin with simple (but uncomfortable) measures such as an enema after a hot bath; if this should fail he may go on to giving drugs either intramuscularly or intravenously (by a 'drip') in order to stimulate the action of the uterus and start it contracting. If these measures should be unsuccessful he may consider starting labor by 'breaking the water,' a painless procedure.

In its most serious form eclampsia may go on to fits; this is dangerous to the mother and extremely dangerous to the infant. On the warning signs of this condition, any patient with eclampsia should be admitted immediately to a maternity unit and treated with heavy sedation in various forms.

When the danger of having fits is over, the baby must be delivered as soon as possible by the most suitable means according to the patient's stage of pregnancy; the choice usually lies between forceps delivery for those well on in labor and a caesarean section for those not yet in labor.

Preventive Treatment. Eclampsia and its associate pre-eclampsia are gradually getting less common and less dangerous; this is entirely due to better prenatal care and the early detection of abnormalities of pregnancy at clinics. For this reason alone it is essential for every pregnant woman to be seen at regular intervals at a clinic or by her family doctor in order to check her progress. By this means she can ensure the best chances for herself and her future child.

INCIDENTAL DISEASES IN PREGNANT WOMEN

A hundred years ago many children died of illnesses before reaching adulthood. Better treatment is allowing most of them to survive now, and among them are less robust young women, many of whom have children. These women cause special problems for the obstetrician and make up a great deal of his prenatal work. By careful control of the pregnancy most of these women carry through normally and bear normal children, usually by a natural delivery. In order to ensure this, constant vigilance is required throughout pregnancy and much patience is often needed on the part of the mother while undergoing treatments that appear boring and pointless to her at the time. She must remember that these very treatments have brought many women with conditions similar to her own through to a safe delivery. The incidental conditions, some serious and others trivial, will be dealt with in turn.

Heart Disease

The heart is an organ not usually affected by disease until the patient is middle-aged but a few young women in the child-bearing group have a diseased heart resulting from congenital defects or a childhood illness. Commonly the patient knows about her disability and also well knows the type of life she must lead to minimize the effects of the heart trouble. Some women, however, are unaware of any disorder and the diagnosis is only made as a result of examinations made in early pregnancy at the prenatal clinic.

Management. The management of the pregnant woman with heart disease requires skilled medical and nursing care. Delivery of the baby should take place in hospital and it may be necessary to admit the patient to hospital in the sixth, seventh and eighth month for complete rest to avoid overworking the damaged heart. Labor and delivery are usually easy and moderately quick, although the doctor may help the baby's progress at the end of labor in order to avoid the mother tiring herself.

After delivery the mother must rest for several weeks. It used to be thought that no one with heart disease should breast feed an infant as this would involve too much effort, but now, provided the patient is sensible and not distressed by the feeding, it is often allowed. However, each patient should seek expert advice on this problem.

Pulmonary Tuberculosis

The fertility rate of women suffering from tuberculosis little, if at all, below the normal and the only reason in the past for discouraging pregnancy in these cases was that the illness was too severe to allow them to marry. Now, with modern drugs and surgery, pulmonary tuberculosis is being forcefully treated as soon as diagnosis is made and usually the results of such therapy are excellent.

Any woman who has had tuberculosis in the past may become pregnant and carry through her confinement quite naturally. If her chest disease was more than two years before the delivery, it is most unlikely that either she or her baby will be affected by the old trouble.

Treatment. Women affected within two years of the pregnancy or those who are still under active treatment should take a little more care than the unaffected mother. There is no reason why, provided such care is given, events should not continue to a normal conclusion—but skilled hospital supervision is necessary. Any anti-tuberculosis treatments being given may be continued, and are not likely to affect the baby in the womb. Further, many women treated with artificial pneumothorax and thoracoplasty go through pregnancy and labor with complete success.

During the pregnancy the patient should have the best possible conditions as regards fresh air, good food and adequate rest. Extra calcium and vitamins are advisable.

After-care. The delivery is usually normal, but the patient needs special care in the lying-in period. She must have complete bed rest at this time, and breast-feeding and other intimate contact with the baby should be curtailed. This is the time when a resurgence of tuberculous infection may occur and both mother and infant must be guarded against such hazards.

This last advice, which applies only to mothers with active or recently active tuberculosis, may seem cruel but any mother will realize, with a little thought, that it is for the baby's future good health that these precautions are necessary.

Kidney Disease

Chronic Disease. Some women have chronic diseases of the kidneys and although they are a little less likely to become pregnant, modern therapy is allowing an increasing number of them to do so. Special care taken during the pregnancy and measures to prevent an increase in blood pressure will be directed from the prenatal clinic. Because of an increased risk to the baby, many women with chronic kidney disease enter hospital during the later stages of pregnancy and often it is wise to start labor off or deliver the child operatively a few weeks before term, thus ensuring a live infant.

Acute Disease. During pregnancy even the healthy woman's kidneys are put under strain and many women develop infections of the urinary tract often starting as cystitis (bladder infection) and going on to pyelitis (kidney duct infection) or pyelonephritis (kidney infection). This is most likely in the third or fourth month of pregnancy.

Symptoms. The patient starts the illness by feeling generally unwell and may have dull pain in the lowest part of the stomach, or the loin. She wants to pass urine much more frequently than usual and when she does so only a small amount comes away and this burns or stings at the outlet. Chills and shivering attacks may occur and the temperature can rise during the attacks to 103° or 104° F. The patient may vomit and will feel generally ill. In the mild case the symptoms will subside with treatment in two or three days but the severely ill patient may continue with chills and a raised temperature for several days. The sooner therapy is begun the milder will be the illness.

Treatment depends upon antibiotics, nitrofurantoin and sulphonamides, added to a high urinary output. This last depends to a large extent on the fluid intake and thus the patient can help herself by drinking large quantities of bland fluids.

It is wise to stay in bed for a few days, and a light tasty diet is good because the appetite needs stimulating. The baby is usually unaffected by this illness and frequently pregnancy continues with no ill-effects.

Infectious Diseases

Pregnant women are as likely as anyone else to become infected with infectious diseases if they come into contact with them. The common cold is a nuisance and should be treated by the usual measures of a couple of days in bed, hot drinks and aspirins. Influenza is the usual miserable disease and the patient takes the same time to get better as the non-pregnant woman. These and similar diseases usually have no effect on the growing baby in the womb, but we must consider two or three conditions that may affect the baby.

Vaccinia

Most people in this country have very wisely been vaccinated against smallpox.

For those women traveling and living in parts of the world where smallpox still occurs, it is occasionally necessary to vaccinate during the pregnancy. Most people who have been vaccinated earlier in their lives suffer no ill effects, but a small number, vaccinated for the first time, develop a mild form of smallpox (see Fevers, p. 287) known as vaccinia. This has an eruption and makes the patient unwell for a few days but it is not dangerous to the adult (and is a risk worth taking to guard against getting smallpox proper). In the early months of pregnancy it is possible for the infant to be infected in the womb and for this reason it is advisable not to vaccinate for the first time a woman in the first four months of her pregnancy.

Rubella

Rubella (German measles) is a common mild illness which affects young people, making them only slightly ill (see Fevers and Infectious Diseases, p. 283). If, however, a woman is infected in early pregnancy there is a risk that the baby may be affected so that heart, eyes, or ears may be damaged. The exact extent of this risk has been variously estimated but, if the mother has German measles during the fourth to eighth week of pregnancy, there is probably a one-in-five chance of an affected child.

It will be seen that it is hard to lay down rules about this because many women do not know at this stage that they are pregnant, having only just missed one menstrual period. Also, since most children will not be affected even if the mother is ill at the vital time, it is hard to estimate the risks in a given case.

Any woman who is infected with rubella at this stage would do well to consult her doctor or prenatal clinic where she will be given the best advice for her case.

Preventive Treatment. A good precaution is to allow young girls in their teens to catch rubella; it is only a mild disease and one attack usually gives immunity for life. In Australia they even have 'rubella camps' where girls go for two weeks in the summer to be in contact with those who have the illness. Thus about nine-tenths of them get rubella early in life and need have no fears later on.

Venereal Diseases

Syphilis and gonorrhea are both diseases which are spread by sexual intercourse and a small number of pregnant women are affected by them. Details of both these conditions are given in the section on Venereal Diseases, p. 289, and only a few points need be discussed here.

Every woman having prenatal care should tell her medical advisers if she knows she has contracted any venereal condition and should further report any discharge or sores of the vagina that may occur during the pregnancy. In addition the blood of all pregnant women should be checked in early pregnancy to see if active disease is present.

Treatment. Should syphilis or gonorrhea be found in pregnancy, energetic treatment is necessary to avoid the tragedy of the infant being affected. Proper courses of penicillin with bismuth, even if given late in pregnancy, are usually effective in protecting the baby.

Syphilis and gonorrhea lessen the chances of a woman becoming pregnant and, if she should become so, they increase the risk of miscarriage. If not properly treated, syphilis can affect the infant causing irreversible damage to the child's brain, bones, eyes and ears. If the venereal disease was contracted late in pregnancy or if the child shows any signs of syphilis (either in physical features or in the infant's blood test) then a full course of penicillin will have to be given to him.

The best prevention of syphilis and gonorrhea is to avoid the chance intercourse and thus not to come in contact with the disease in the first place; this ensures that each baby is given a fair chance of being born with a healthy body and brain.

Diabetes

With the advent of insulin in 1924, diabetics were given the chance to lead normal lives. The likelihood of a diabetic now becoming pregnant is almost as good as for any other woman and, with special care, a normal infant is produced. This is a great contrast with the situation thirty to forty years ago when diabetic patients rarely became pregnant and, if they did so, were in grave danger of losing the infants' if not their own lives.

Hospital Care. A diabetic woman who becomes pregnant should attend the prenatal clinic of a hospital that is used to dealing with such cases. The blood-sugar levels will have to be checked frequently as the urine tests may be misleading. A high carbohydrate diet (about 300 grams per day) is advisable and the insulin dosage will have to be watched carefully.

Because of the increased risk to the baby, a pregnant diabetic woman should be admitted to hospital in the seventh or eighth month and the infant may be delivered before full term, if necessary by operation. These methods have been shown to produce the best chance for the baby.

After delivery it is common for the diabetic condition to be temporarily improved and the dose of insulin must again be watched carefully. The babies of diabetic women are usually big and tend to lose a lot of weight in the first week. This is usual and need not worry the mother. Feeding of the infant is likely to be normal.

Anemia

In the United States most women take an adequate diet and, when not pregnant, they are not anemic. In other countries where the diet does not contain so much protein or iron, anemia is often a problem with women in the child-bearing age groups. It is not uncommon to meet women starting a pregnancy with their blood at 50 per cent of strength. This should be rigorously treated by iron medicines, tablets and injections.

In pregnancy the demands of the baby and the natural dilution of the blood cause most women to drop the iron content of the blood to about 80 per cent of their normal level. A few, living on poorer diets, drop even more than this.

Treatment. The best means of treating this anemia is to prevent it, and this is achieved by taking a good mixed diet with plenty of meat and green vegetables. Many prenatal clinics supplement this by prescribing extra iron in the form of tablets to all pregnant women. These tablets often produce associated constipation and sometimes nausea. If this occurs, the patient should tell the doctor at her next visit and the type of tablet can be changed. Among the forms of iron in common medical use are ferrous sulphate, ferrous gluconate, ferrous succinate and ferrous fumarate.

Occasionally, despite these treatments and without any bleeding to account for it, a woman progresses through pregnancy with a low blood iron level or it might fall in the later weeks. It would be dangerous to allow a patient to go into labor in an anemic condition and so, in the later weeks of pregnancy, more intensive preparations of iron are given. This may take the form of intramuscular or intravenous injections, and if they are of no avail, blood transfusions may be required to ensure that the woman goes into labor in a fit state.

A few forms of anemia do not respond to treatment with iron by itself. These can be diagnosed by laboratory tests and may require other medicaments, e.g. folic acid, in addition to iron.

BLOOD TESTS. It is usual for every woman who has prenatal care to have her blood checked at her first visit to a clinic. The blood which is then taken from a vein is tested for its iron content (hemoglobin level), and for the mother's blood group (O, A, AB, or B) and Rhesus group (positive or negative) (see Physiology, p. 240; a routine test for the reaction to syphilis (Wassermann test) is often done as well. After this most women have their hemoglobin rechecked at about thirty to thirty-six weeks and this is the final test unless there is something to make the doctor think the patient is becoming anemic.

The best prevention of anemia in pregnancy is a sensible diet and the taking of a reasonable number of iron tablets.

Thyroid Diseases

Women who have hyperactive thyroid glands are in the same age-group as those who become pregnant and so the two conditions are found to overlap. Pregnancy usually makes the condition worse, and more energetic treatment is necessary. If surgical treatment is indicated, there is no reason for the presence of the child to stop such treatment and in many cases, in the middle months of pregnancy, an operation can be the best therapy. The dosage of thyroid depressant drugs being taken by a pregnant young woman must be carefully watched because the dose may need to be increased and there is a slight risk that the drugs may affect the infant in the womb. For a similar reason, the radio-active treatment of hyperactive thyroid glands is not used in pregnancy.

Women with an underactive thyroid rarely become pregnant but they occasionally do so under good treatment. When this occurs their dosage of thyroid extract tablets may need careful supervision, but they, like the hyperactive patients, may look forward to a normal labor and a healthy infant.

Nervous Diseases

Epilepsy

Many women with epilepsy become pregnant. They are usually under sedative treatment before they become pregnant and this should be continued and carefully watched. A few epileptics improve in pregnancy only to relapse afterwards and the dosage of anti-epileptic drugs may need revision up to a year after the birth of the child. Labor is usually normal but, in regard to the infant, the hereditary nature of this condition should be remembered.

Disseminated Sclerosis

This condition is one that has natural periods of relapse and exacerbation and it is often hard to judge the effect of pregnancy, a condition lasting nine months, on a disease whose natural cyclical process may take many years. If pregnancy occurs in a period of remission from the disseminated sclerosis it is likely to be uneventful and to have no effect on the development of the nervous disease. Should the pregnancy come, however, when a relapse is occurring, the effect on the mother may be adverse. In such cases, it may be wiser to terminate the pregnancy if the risk of serious deterioration to the mother is great.

Acroparesthesia
(*Tingling in the Fingers*)

In late pregnancy, patients often get a tingling of the fingers of one or both hands, especially affecting the first and second fingers. This tingling may become more severe, increasing to a throbbing or burning sensation. It is due to compression of one of the hand nerves on the inside of the wrist. The sensation can always be relieved by raising the arm on pillows or a cushion, and sometimes a high sling is effective. Complete recovery always takes place after delivery.

Cramps

Pregnant women often suffer from muscular cramps of the calves, feet and thighs. These usually occur in the later months and are worse when the patient is in bed and relaxed. The cramps can always be dispersed by moving and rubbing the affected muscles, and sometimes calcium tablets, 30 grains daily, are helpful. This condition also always ends after pregnancy.

Alimentary Disorders

Excessive Salivation

This condition is fairly rare but distressing because such large volumes of saliva may be produced that the patient cannot swallow at all. Usually it starts about the second month but always stops by the fourth or fifth month. Astringent mouth washes may be prescribed and belladonna sometimes relieves the excessive secretion.

Dental Decay

During pregnancy a great demand on calcium is made by the growing fetus. If there is any small breach in the enamel covering the mother's teeth, then the tooth substance underneath will rapidly be eroded by decay. All cavities should be carefully filled.

Dental decay can be postponed by a high calcium diet, regular cleaning of teeth and twice-yearly visits to the dentist. If teeth have to be extracted during pregnancy, then either local injection anesthesia or a good general anesthetic carefully given may be used with safety to mother and child.

Heartburn

This is a common complaint of the later months of pregnancy and is due to the enlarging uterus pushing up on the stomach and forcing some of the acid stomach contents into the gullet, whose sensitive lining is irritated by the acid. The heartburn is often worse after meals and at night when the patient lies flat.

Treatment is usually with antacids (magnesium trisilicate, and by improving the posture at night with a 'throne' of pillows, so that the patient sleeps propped upright. When the pregnancy is over, the condition ceases.

Abdominal Pain

During the course of pregnancy many women experience vague transient pains in the stomach. Some of these are due to stretching of the walls of the uterus and its associated ligaments. Others may be due to pressure of the enlarging organ on other structures. However, if the pain lasts more than an hour or so, and if it is accompanied by vomiting, then the patient should consult a doctor. One of the more serious conditions such as appendicitis may occur and these diseases require urgent and prompt treatment in order to save not only the health of the mother but the life of the baby.

Constipation

This is a common accompaniment of pregnancy and often begins in the first month. It may be accompanied by flatulent dyspepsia and piles, and probably is due to a reflex inhibition of the intestine.

Prevention is the best treatment and this may be done by ensuring a good diet containing plenty of roughage, and drinking plenty of fluid especially in warm weather. If the condition is established, bland laxatives such as liver salts should be used at first and then, if necessary, senna, or cascara. It is wise to avoid mineral oil in pregnancy, as well as castor oil and other violent purgatives.

Hemorrhoids

In pregnancy, especially if the patient is constipated, piles are common. Local cleanliness must be practiced after every bowel action and if any piles are protruding they should be replaced by pressure with a small pad of raw cotton. Usually no injection or operation is used during pregnancy for much natural improvement occurs after delivery. If, however, there is excessive pain, a pile may have thrombosed and this is best treated by a small operation under local anesthesia.

Skin Diseases

Psoriasis

This unfortunate disease involves chronic scaling of the skin of the chest, back, elbows and knees and is fairly common in young women and often occurs in the pregnant. It tends to get better during the pregnancy itself but unfortunately recurs afterwards in its former degree.

Urticaria

This is an allergic skin rash which appears suddenly after an irritant substance has been in contact with a sensitive person. This irritant could be food, dust, or even the pollen of some flowers. In pregnancy, urticaria occurs very frequently and often in a more severe form.

It is best treated with antihistamines, both as an ointment to apply to the area and also as tablets to be taken by mouth.

Pruritus Vulae

This is an itching of the external genitals. It is usually due to a discharge from the vagina. During pregnancy the patient must ensure that she is scrupulously clean and, if daily baths are impossible, she should have an 'all-over wash.'

The discharge may be an increase in the normal secretions due to the increased blood supply to the genital organs in pregnancy; or it may be due to a mild infection with *Trichomonas* or monilia (see Diseases of Women, p. 489). The infections can be treated by specific therapy but the patient can help herself by taking a bath each day into which a handful of kitchen salt has been dissolved. Her doctor will advise her of other treatments for the vaginal discharge.

Fibroids

Many women, often those past thirty-five, have fibroids in the walls of the uterus. These masses of fibrous tissue are not cancers but smooth irregularities. Commonly they are multiple and small (like a group of marbles) and when like this they do not affect the pregnancy but, in some cases, large ones occur and may cause symptoms.

Their presence in the uterus sometimes makes conception less likely and the risk of miscarrying is increased. This, however, depends on the site of the fibroid tumor.

Later on in the fourth or fifth month a fibroid may outgrow its blood supply and undergo degeneration in the middle. This produces pain and, provided the diagnosis can be made confidently, the treatment is non-operative, but this is often difficult and an operation may be required to exclude appendicitis or a piece of twisted tissue.

The fibroid itself if close to the surface may twist and shut off the blood vessels. Further, the fibroid may become infected. Still later in pregnancy, a fibroid may cause a malpresentation of the baby so that a breech or part of the trunk may present (Fig. 1).

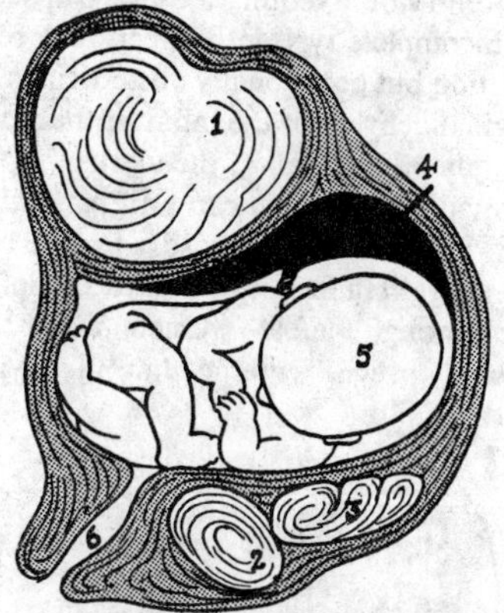

Fig. 1. *FIBROIDS IN THE UTERINE WALL causing the baby to lie in the transverse position.* 1, 2, 3. *Tough fibroids in the uterine wall hamper its elasticity and prevent the infant from moving into the normal (head down) position for birth.* 4. *Placenta.* 5. *Infant's head.* 6. *Neck of uterus.*

Once labor starts, most fibroids give little trouble in themselves and tend to be pulled up above the baby as it is born. Occasionally they do not allow the uterus muscle to contract properly, leading to long labor, while poor contraction after delivery may allow the uterus to remain relaxed, and bleeding could occur.

The above complications with fibroids are all very rare and, provided the patient is in the capable hands of an obstetrician, the potential troubles can be circumvented.

Ovarian Cysts

Many women have small cysts on one or both ovaries. If one of these enlarges it may be felt at a prenatal examination. Usually they cause no trouble in pregnancy or labor but one of them may twist on its stem and this causes pain and may require an operation. Often quite large ovarian cysts found in pregnancy disappear after delivery.

Cervical Erosion

The neck of the uterus, in common with the rest of that organ, becomes very vascular in pregnancy and sometimes a small erosion occurs. This causes an increased clear discharge from the vagina and occasionally the erosion bleeds so that a little bright red or brown discharge occurs. This is not serious but should be reported to the doctor who may then exclude other, more serious conditions (see pp. 490 and 496). After delivery the erosion usually gets smaller but may require a light electrical cautery.

Varicose Veins

Dilated surface veins of the external genitals or legs may occur for the first time during pregnancy. They cause aching and look unsightly and are due to the bulk of the baby and uterus pressing on the veins in the abdomen that drain the lower extremities. The varicosities get worse as pregnancy progresses, but after delivery, although they may not go away completely, they get very much better. During the pregnancy it is better not to operate, and if the leg veins are uncomfortable, an elastic stocking may be worn.

BLEEDING IN EARLY PREGNANCY

Usually for the nine months she is carrying and for two or three months afterwards, a woman has no vaginal bleeding and no monthly menstrual periods. Indeed, this lack of bleeding is used as an indicator of pregnancy, and the patient's doctor uses it to calculate the duration of pregnancy. Hence should any pregnant woman bleed vaginally, she should report this to her doctor for, although it may not be serious, there are a few conditions that must be ruled out.

Vaginal bleeding in pregnancy may be best considered in two groups, (a) early bleeding before five months, and (b) bleeding after this time.

Continuation of Periods

A few patients do have a little spotting of blood at the time when they would have expected their periods, i.e. at 4, 8, and even at 12 weeks. This is considered to be due to the maturing embryo not completely filling up the cavity of the uterus. It is not a serious condition and has no effect on the health of mother or baby.

Abortion

The word 'abortion' is synonymous with the word 'miscarriage,' and is used medically to cover all expulsions of the embryo baby before it is viable. While lay people tend to use 'miscarriage' for the natural event, they tend to keep the word 'abortion' for the induced or criminal expulsion. This does not apply to the doctor, who uses the word 'abortion' to cover both situations.

The abortion is the expulsion of the embryo before the baby is considered mature enough to survive on its own. Infants are usually thought to be capable of survival after the twenty-eighth week of pregnancy, but, in spite of this definition, infants delivered before that time have occasionally survived. Probably an abortion is the commonest accident of pregnancy and, although it is not usually attended by any special dangers, each patient should have medical care since infections or other troubles may occur and urgent aid be required.

It is hard to get accurate figures of the incidence of this risk, but probably about one pregnancy (with early bleeding) in five ends in an abortion, and the majority of these women go on to normal pregnancies, if they wish, later in life.

Causes. The causes of an abortion are usually not known and, excluding gross disease in the mother, it is postulated that there is something wrong with the embryo. This would be nature's way of keeping the species fit, and many an embryo that is aborted in early pregnancy would never have lived into childhood.

Usually the first symptom of abortion a patient has is a little bleeding, in the eighth to tenth week, of bright red blood. This may occur once in the day and is painless. If ignored, a little more bleeding may occur the following day, and a heavier bleed after this, possibly accompanied by lower abdominal cramps. If still untreated, some time after this the embryo will be expelled in a minute labor with small labor pains.

Threatened Abortion. The patient has a little bleeding, but no pain. Should she rest in bed and take things quietly, then no more may happen and the embryo will not have been dislodged. The woman can go on to a perfectly normal labor at the end of her pregnancy, and have a normal infant.

Inevitable Abortion. Pains accompany the bleeding from an early stage and, since the neck of the uterus is open, abortion will certainly follow.

Complete Abortion. The patient expels the embryo, its sac of membranes and the developing placenta completely, and the uterus is empty. This occurs in later abortions after the fourteenth to sixteenth weeks.

Incomplete Abortion. When the patient has expelled most of the uterine contents herself but a small piece of membrane or placenta remains attached to the wall of the uterus, the abortion is incomplete. This is usual in abortions before fourteen weeks. Bleeding continues from the cavity and the uterus cannot contract down properly. It is wise therefore to remove these fragments by a small operation of curettage which must be performed in hospital under an anesthetic.

Legal Abortion. A number of states in the United States have recently passed abortion acts. The laws vary and abortion should be performed in compliance with the law.

Criminal Abortion. When a pregnancy is terminated by other than natural means, or than under the legal conditions specified above, this is a criminal act. 'Back door' abortions are very dangerous and foolish. Countless thousands of women end up with pelvic infection and ill health for the rest of their lives.

Missed Abortion. Should the embryo die in the uterus and not be passed within a day or so, the tissues are slowly absorbed and the size of the uterine bulk shrinks. Often such patients retain the mass of tissue for some weeks or months and difficulty may be experienced in hastening the expulsion. It is a trying time for a patient, and many doctors try to speed up the process by any means at their disposal that is safe for the patient. When this is over the mother may go on to have normal babies afterwards.

NOTE. If properly looked after, a woman will be perfectly well after an abortion and can usually, under medical advice, go on to have a normal family later.

Ectopic Pregnancy

Occasionally the fertilized ovum settles outside the uterine cavity. The commonest of these outside sites is the Fallopian tube (Fig. 2). When this happens, the egg grows for a few weeks and erodes the wall of the tube. Eventually it bursts, usually into the abdominal cavity.

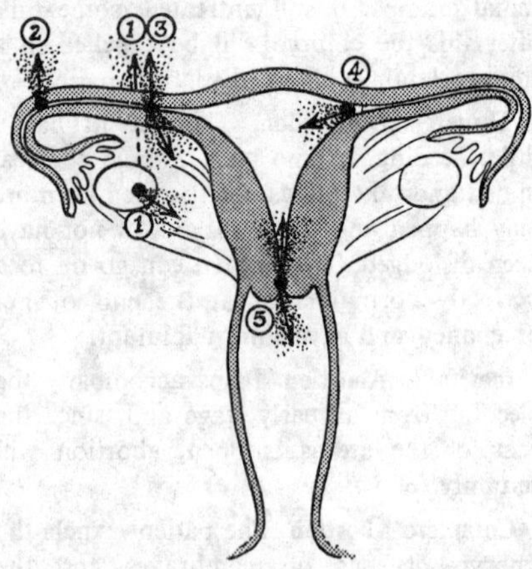

Fig. 2. *SITES OF ECTOPIC PREGNANCY. A diagrammatic illustration showing the various places, other than the uterus, at which a fertilized egg may settle and attempt to develop. 1. In the ovary—it may burst into the abdominal cavity or bury into the broad ligament. 2. In the outer end of the Fallopian tube—it may burst into the abdominal cavity. 3. In the inner end of the Fallopian tube—it may burst into the broad ligament or into the abdominal cavity. 4. In the angle of the uterus adjoining the Fallopian tube—it usually bursts into the uterus. 5. In the cervix—it usually bursts into the vagina, but may go into the uterine cavity.*

The patient usually feels acute pain in the lower abdomen. She may have missed a period or the rupture can occur before four weeks have passed, but this is not always so. Often the woman is shocked and collapsed from loss of blood internally. The condition requires blood transfusions and urgent operation to save the woman's life.

It occurs more commonly in the tropics.

Vesicular Mole

A rare cause of bleeding in early pregnancy is the vesicular mole. The patient bleeds and passes a lot of material like small grapes. This indicates a breakdown of the placenta, and the patient needs the uterus emptied and scraped. A patient with this condition is watched carefully by the doctor to avoid late complications.

Bleeding from Outside the Uterus

Examination of the diagram of the female genital tract shows that the bleeding can come from several sites not connected with the developing baby; the cervix, walls of the vagina or entrance may be involved and the blood can even come from the rectum and be mistaken for vaginal bleeding (Fig. 3).

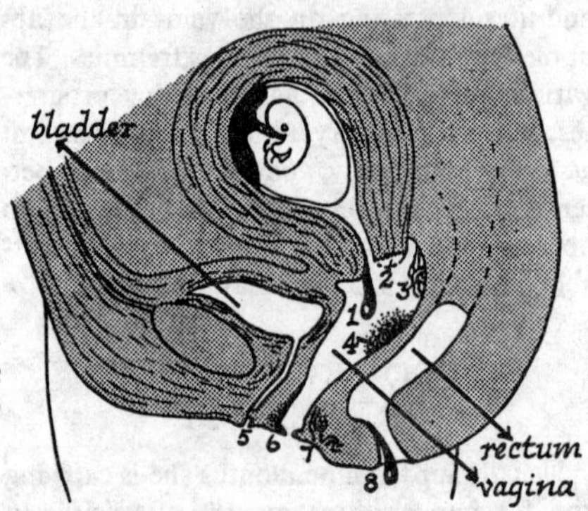

Fig. 3. *PREGNANCY BLEEDING (indirect). During pregnancy there may be bleeding from the vagina or rectum which is not directly associated with the presence of the developing fetus. One or more of the following disorders may be the cause of this bleeding. 1. Polyp of cervix. 2. Erosion of cervix. 3. Varicose veins of vagina. 4. Inflammation of vagina (vaginitis). 5. Wart of caruncle at entrance to the urethra. 6. Inflammation of the vaginal entrance (vulvitis). 7. Varicosities of the vulva. 8. Hemorrhoids of the anus.*

BLEEDING IN LATE PREGNANCY

Late Bleeding

After twenty-eight weeks of pregnancy, a different set of factors come into play, and most commonly bleeding is associated with some separation of the placenta. A few patients may bleed from some trouble of the cervix or vagina (see above) but this is rare. It should be remembered that labor sometimes starts with a show of blood rather than of mucus. Some women start labor earlier than they expect, and their bleeding may be a normal event.

Placenta Previa

Normally the placenta, or afterbirth, is implanted at the upper end of the uterus (Fig. 4). After the baby is born, the uterus becomes smaller by contraction of its walls and the placenta is sheared off and passed without trouble. Occasionally, however, the placenta is implanted below the baby in the lower part of the uterine cavity and this may make it dangerous for the baby to be born by the normal method.

The patient at first feels well and pregnancy progresses in a normal fashion. Some time in the last three months, there is a slight show of bright red blood. This is painless and often repeated each day. Still no pain is felt. If neglected the bleeding will increase in severity until a large hemorrhage will drive the patient to hospital.

Treatment. Should a woman have such bleeding, she should report to her doctor immediately. It is possible he will want her to go into hospital and there she will probably be rested in bed completely. By doing this the bleeding is eased and the baby given a chance to grow bigger.

When the doctors think the infant is large enough to stand a good chance, the patient is examined to ascertain which type of placenta previa is present. The marginal type would be compatible with a vaginal delivery while that completely covering the neck of the womb would require a caesarean section. The incomplete type in between may require operation but occasionally obstetricians allow a vaginal delivery of the infant if the placenta is mainly on one wall of the uterus.

Provided the patient can wait patiently and 'bide with her medical advisors for the boring time of waiting in hospital until the infant is large enough, most women who had a placenta previa emerge happily with a healthy child.

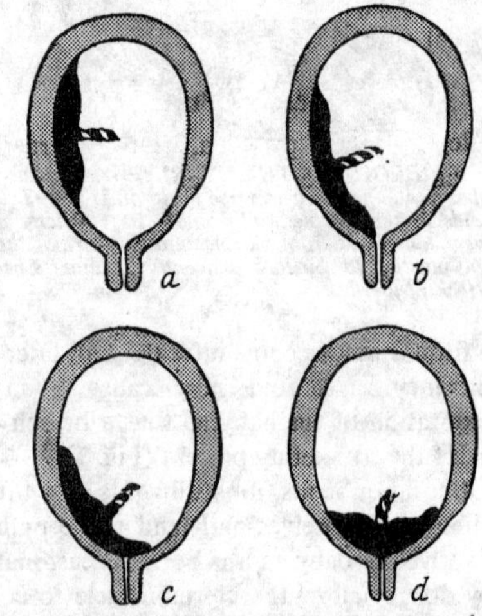

Fig. 4. *PLACENTA PREVIA. Location of the placenta on the wall of the uterus. a. Normal at upper end of the uterus. b. Marginal site encroaching on the neck of uterus. c. An incomplete placenta previa partially covering the undilated neck of the uterus. d. A complete cover of the neck of the uterus.*

Accidental Hemorrhage

Earlier reference was made to pre-eclampsia, that specific disease of pregnancy during which the blood pressure could rise. An occasional complication of this is that some bleeding occurs between the placenta and the wall of the uterus. This cuts off some of the baby's blood supply and is a serious risk to the child.

Different amounts of bleeding occur and infants and mothers differ in their response but usually the mother first notices a pain in the abdomen alongside the enlarged uterus and then some hours later has a trickle of dark blood from the vagina. She should seek medical advice at once.

Treatment depends on the state of the mother and baby, and may consist of blood transfusion and bed rest or, if the baby's condition warrants, caesarean section.

It is to exclude this sort of complication that patients attend prenatal clinics regularly and have constant checks on their health.

CAESAREAN SECTION

This operation's name is derived from the Lex Caesare (or Emperor's Law) which concerned the birth of a child by cutting the mother's abdomen. It is nothing to do with Julius Caesar who, as far as we know, was delivered normally. With better and more comfortable anesthetic facilities available now, it is a safe operation for the mother and, in certain circumstances, the only way of ensuring the delivery of a live baby.

In many cases the obstetrician will have to decide to deliver a certain patient by this route before labor starts. This is an elective operation (advantageous to the patient but not necessary to save life) and can usually be planned in advance. The mother is told well beforehand and is usually taken into hospital for rest before the operation.

The operation would be performed if the pelvis of the mother were too small to allow the baby's head to pass through. It would be folly to try to squeeze the child through, and a safer route is by operation through the mother's abdomen. Similarly, if a very big infant is expected, as happens with diabetic mothers, a caesarean section is often safer for both the baby and the mother. Should the infant be lying in an unusual position and the risks of a vaginal delivery be too great, a section is safer.

When the mother has had a caesarean section in a previous delivery, care is always taken to watch for complications. It by no means follows that the patient is bound to be delivered by operation a second time. Many women have normal pregnancies and deliveries after a previous operative delivery.

DISEASES OF YOUNG CHILDREN

Causes of Ill Health in Children

Ill health in children may be due to a variety of causes.

1. **Heredity,** from inborn weakness or disease of the parents or grandparents.

2. **Infection.** Infectious illnesses are common in infancy and early childhood and they may be followed by complications. The recuperative powers of children, however, are considerable, and once an infection has been overcome, convalescence is usually rapid. The chief source of entry of infection into the body is the throat and the back of the nose, and in all cases of feverish illness the throat and ears should be examined.

3. **Psychological Influences.** Nervousness in children is frequently inherited from parents who are themselves highly strung and neurotic. More often, however, it results from improper management, and the nervous mother or nurse is likely to mismanage the infant in various ways. In such cases the infant may acquire a nervous condition by suggestion which is subtly and unconsciously transmitted from the grown-up persons in control. The child has little knowledge of itself, and is able to see itself only through its mother's eyes, so that it tends to become whatever is thought of it, whatever is said of it and whatever is feared for it. This is more likely to occur in the case of the only child in a community of adults. The dismay and agitation which is excited in them by any abnormality of health or conduct on the part of the child cannot be hidden from him, and may turn what would otherwise have been a trivial disturbance into something formidable and difficult to treat.

4. **Improper Feeding.** This can lead to many troubles, especially in children under two years of age. Causative factors include gross lack of vitamins (especially A, D and C) and, in infants under three months of age, underfeeding and mismanagement.

The adequate feeding of infants and children and the essentials for a balanced diet are dealt with fully in Baby Care, pp. 99-113, and in Food and Nutrition, pp. 65-75.

5. **Poor Hygienic Conditions,** with lack of sunshine, warmth, fresh air and exercise. These are now not such a problem in the United States.

Babies and children should have as much fresh air and sunshine as possible but this can be overdone in winter by over-conscientious mothers. Living in overheated rooms may make a small child more susceptible to colds: about 21° C (70° F) is the best temperature for the family living room. Bedrooms should never be stuffy, even in winter.

Inadequate domestic hygiene, too, can contribute to ill health. Badly washed feeding bottles may lead to thrush and diarrhea; shared family handkerchiefs spread germs around; and cooked food exposed carelessly to flies may cause avoidable infections.

SOME COMMON RASHES

Illness	*Type of Rash*	*Other Symptoms*
Measles	Starts as small pink spots behind the ears and round the mouth. Spreads rapidly. Becomes blotchy. Fades in 3 to 5 days.	Fever. Cough. Running eyes and nose. Small white spots surrounded by redness inside mouth (Koplik's spots) a pear before the rash.
German Measles (Rubella)	Diffuse pink-red rash. Fades rapidly.	Slight fever. Running nose. Glands in back of neck enlarged.
Chickenpox	Red spots which become blistery, scab over, and fade. If scratched leave a scar. Appears in crops. Starts on face and body, later to limbs.	Fever. Slightly 'out of sorts.'
Scarlet Fever	Red rash on body and limbs. Peeling of skin after 7 to 10 days.	Sore throat. Fever. Vomiting. Whiteness around mouth. 'Strawberry' tongue.
Nettlerash (*Urticaria*)	Itchy red raised spots. May be blistery.	
Heat Rash	Raised red spots. May itch.	Sweating, as child is usually over-clothed.
Eczema	Itching blistery areas. When scratched they burst and 'weep.' Crusts form. May become infected.	If itching severe, child very upset.

Symptoms of Ill Health in Children

Unlike an adult, a child who is ill is often unable to describe his symptoms. Particular attention must therefore be paid to a departure from his usual behavior. Slight ailments often make the child unwilling to run about, while an acute illness quickly lessens his normal vitality and destroys his natural interest in toys. The appetite is usually reduced, vomiting is common, and dark rings may appear round the eyes. Especial attention should be paid to any suggestion of earache or of discharge from the ear, since it may give rise to serious consequences.

Nervous children are particularly apt to suffer from restlessness, irritability, disturbances of sleep, bad dreams, and nightmares. Thumb sucking, nail biting, squinting, stammering, attacks of faintness and early muscular fatigue are also common in children of a nervous temperament.

The Examination of Children

Children are easily frightened, and much patience may have to be exercised by anyone who undertakes their examination. The first thing is to determine if the child has any fever, and if the pulse rate is increased.

1. **Fever.** In younger children, the temperature may be taken in the groin, armpit, or in the rectum. The rectal temperature is the most accurate, and special thermometers which are safe from the danger of breaking may be used for this purpose. In older children, the temperature may be taken in the usual way, under the tongue. It must not always be concluded that, because the child may have a little temperature, he is ill. The younger the child, the more likely is he to develop a temperature from slight causes, and many children who are in perfectly normal health will show a rise of temperature to 100° F or more after exercise, which, however, quickly returns to normal on resting.

2. **Increase of Pulse Rate.** At birth the normal pulse rate is 120–140 beats per minute. At the age of one year it is 100–110, at five years 100, and at twelve to fifteen years it settles down to the normal adult rate of 72 beats per minute.

Disturbing factors such as excitement, exercise, fever, and pain, will easily produce a rate of 120, 140, or 160 beats per minute. A variation of the pulse rate with the phases of breathing is common in children and is of no significance.

3. **Increase of Respiration.** The rate of respiration in children varies with the age:

Age	*Rate per Minute*
Birth	30–40
1 year	25
5 years	20
10–15 years	18 (normal adult rate)

Many normal children breathe quite irregularly, often with short bouts of rapid shallow respiration interspersed with periods of normal rhythm. An increase in the respiration rate is common in pneumonia and other diseases affecting the lungs.

4. **Rashes.** If a child is feverish, look for a rash as he may be starting an infectious illness (see p. 511).

5. **Throat.** Any child who is found to have fever should also have the throat examined. This should never be omitted, even though the child may not complain of a sore throat. If this is not done, cases of tonsillitis, etc. may be missed.

6. **Ears.** Any child who complains of earache, tenderness near the ear or discharge from the ear passage should if possible have the ear drum examined by a doctor. Neglect of an inflamed ear drum may lead to the development of mastoid infection, and may possibly lead to deafness in later life.

7. **Urine and Stools.** The urine should be examined for evidence of infection, and the stools for looseness, blood, mucus, and threadworms.

8. **Hair and Scalp.** The hair and scalp should be examined for parasites, eczema, etc.

General Treatment of Sick Children

Preventive Treatment. Taking the whole range of childhood, from birth to school leaving, all children who are in good health should be protected against smallpox (by vaccination), and by inoculation against whooping-cough, diphtheria, and tetanus. Protection against poliomyelitis is usually given by mouth. For inoculation details, see Fevers and Infectious Diseases, pp.265 - 266 .

Treatment of Acute Illness. The most important measures are nursing, a suitable diet, and plenty of fluid. Treatment by drugs plays only a minor part. See also Home Nursing, pp. 45-53.

FLUID. An ample supply of fluid is very important, especially in the case of infants who are ill. Unlike adults, they cannot ask for a drink, and water must be offered at frequent intervals. It is not uncommon for a well-nourished infant, weighing say 15 lbs, to lose 8 oz. in the first twenty-four hours of an attack of acute diarrhea, the loss of weight being accounted for almost entirely by the loss of fluid from the blood and tissues. There is practically no disease, except acute surgical conditions of the abdomen such as appendicitis, in which unlimited fluids should not be given.

GLUCOSE. In nearly all conditions glucose is also of great value and may be given in water and fruit juice at intervals during the day. In older children the dose may be three teaspoonfuls or more at a time.

DRUGS. In cases where drugs are necessary, the dosage must be modified according to age, the usual formula being:

$$\text{Adult dose} \times \frac{\text{age of child}}{\text{age} + 12}$$

A useful sedative prescribed by doctors for young children is phenobarbital (see Treatment of Convulsions, p. 519). Aspirin (junior dose) is also efficacious.

DISORDERS OF THE HEART AND BLOOD

Hemolytic Disease of the Newborn

(*Erythroblastosis Fetalis*)

This blood disorder occurs at birth or within the first two or three days of life.

Causes. It is due to destruction of the infant's red blood cells by antigens which pass via the placenta from the mother's blood. It usually occurs when the infant is of the Rhesus-positive blood type (inherited in these cases from the father) and the mother is Rhesus-negative (see p.240). There is always the risk in this kind of pregnancy that the Rhesus-positive factor in the fetal blood may pass into the mother's circulation. The mother's blood resists the factor by forming antibodies to protect her, but, unhappily, the antibodies or antigens are most harmful to the infant's blood cells. It is rare for a first child to be affected, but the risk increases with subsequent pregnancies in which Rhesus-positive fetuses are carried; the risk is about one in twenty-two.

Symptoms. The newborn child is very pale or becomes so during the first twenty-four hours (three days in mild cases). The spleen is enlarged, and jaundice and edema may be present in severe cases. Laboratory examination of the blood shows a reduction in the number of red cells and an increase in the white.

Treatment. PRENATAL ASSESSMENT is essential. The blood of all pregnant women should be tested for Rhesus antibodies in the Rhesus-negative mothers. This is done at about the thirty-second week of pregnancy. If the mother's blood is highly sensitized, it is often advisable to promote an early delivery to save the infant.

EXCHANGE TRANSFUSION: Immediately after birth in severely affected infants, Rhesus-negative blood is injected through the umbilical vein while the damaged blood is removed at about the same rate. This usually takes about two hours. Occasionally, transfusion is done prenatally, via the mother.

MILD CASES. In mild cases a simple blood transfusion may be all that is required to increase the number of red cells, and some infants do not even need that assistance. Regular checking of the condition of the blood, however, is necessary for six weeks.

Congenital Heart Defects

A congenital heart defect may or may not be associated with cyanosis (blueness). An infant with cyanosis is known as a 'blue baby.' Defects that occur include holes in the heart (ventricular or atrial septal defects), patent ductus arteriosus, pulmonary or aortic stenosis, and so on. Single or multiple defects may be present.

In severe cases, the baby may be cyanosed from birth and may not live. Mild cases may be without symptoms.

Causes. In some cases there is a hereditary tendency, but in others the defects may be due to the mother having had rubella in early pregnancy.

Treatment. If there is only a slight limitation of the child's energy and activity, he should be allowed to develop his own powers as fully as he can.

In many cases, however, the patient is severely disabled from birth owing to the defective circulation. Such children require careful nursing and feeding, together with abundant fresh air and sunshine. They need to be protected as far as possible from cold, dampness and all the forms of fevers and diseases which are especially common in childhood. Surgical treatment is possible in some cases and is especially successful in simple single defects. New techniques are continually being devised.

DISORDERS OF THE JOINTS AND BONES

Congenital Dislocation of the Hip

This is a condition which occurs before birth but only becomes evident some weeks or months after birth. It may be on one or both sides and affects the fit of the head of the femur (hip bone) into its socket in the pelvis. It is important that the condition should be recognized early because prompt treatment leads to good results whereas neglect may cause a permanent limp and later gross osteoarthritic changes in the hip or hips.

In congenital dislocation the head of the femur is not well developed and the roof of the socket is too shallow so that the femoral head slides in and out. This does not matter too much while the infant is young but once he starts to crawl and some weight is transmitted through the hip, the femoral head is thrust further out all the time and the ligaments and capsule of the joint become more and more stretched.

Diagnosis should be made if possible before the stage of weight-bearing. If the dislocation is one-sided there is asymmetry of the limbs. The leg looks too short and the creases are different in the two sides. The mother may notice difficulty in putting on diapers because

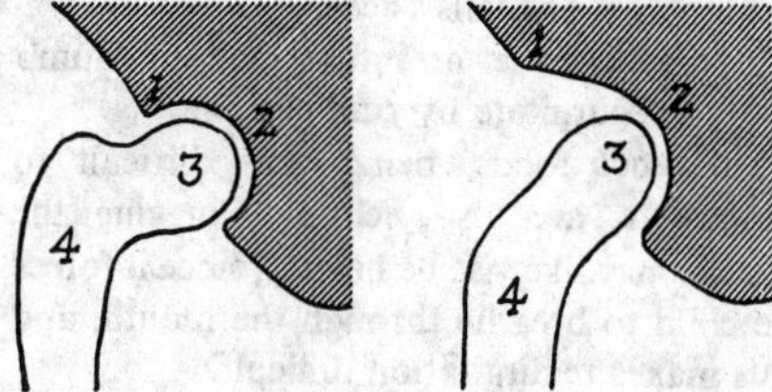

Fig. 1. *CONGENITALLY DISLOCATED HIP. Diagrams to show the normal relationship of the hip socket to the head of the hip-bone (femur) in a very young infant; and the inadequately shaped socket and femur head of a congenitally imperfect hip.*

the affected leg cannot swing out and she may further notice a click on such movement. The infant, if allowed to grow older before the diagnosis is made, may be a late walker and when he starts will have a painless limp, dipping if there is a one-sided dislocation and waddling if it affects both sides.

The diagnosis is made by the doctor examining the child and confirmed by X-ray photographs of the joint.

Treatment. This depends upon the stage at which the condition is seen. If the infant is examined and the diagnosis made in the first six months of life, a simple harness or plaster may be used to hold the limbs out to allow the femoral head to grow into the pelvic socket, thus enlarging and deepening it. Although the position of the infant looks uncomfortable, this is not so and the child is usually very happy in the plaster after the first day, treatment usually being continued for three to six months.

Should the child be first seen at one or two years, once weight-bearing has begun, the outlook is less good but still treatment may be successful by means of a traction frame which pulls the head out of its false position to allow it to return to its true place slowly; this is a slow treatment taking many months. If necessary an open operation may be necessary to make the socket deeper and increase the shelf of bone above.

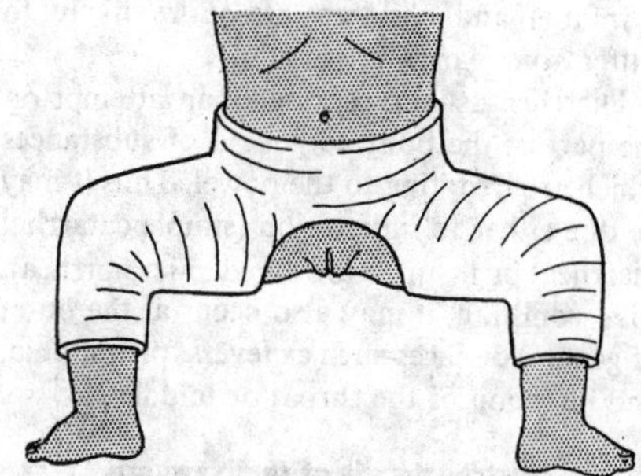

Fig. 2. *PLASTER SUPPORT to hold out widely the hips and legs of an infant with congenital dislocated hip so that the femoral head of the thigh bone will grow properly into position in the pelvic socket, and at the same time enlarge and deepen it.*

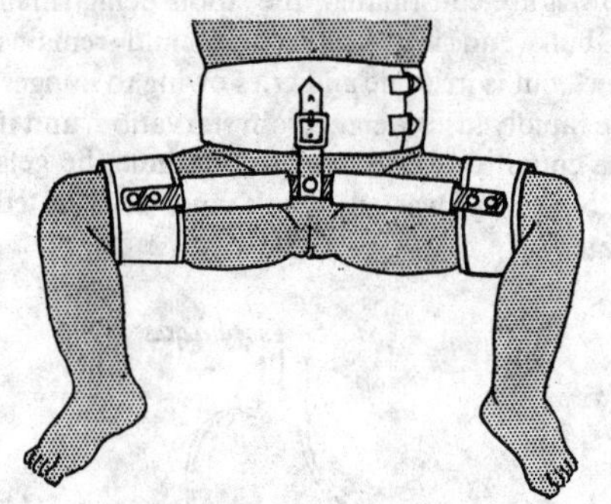

Fig. 3. *DENIS-BROWNE HARNESS for a case of congenital dislocated hip. It serves the same purpose as the plaster support in Fig. 2.*

If the patient is brought after the age of seven, the above treatments are no good and further surgery is required to make the best of a deformed hip.

All infants should be examined at birth and again in a few months by their doctors in order to pick up this fairly rare but potentially disabling condition, since treatment given early is very successful.

DISORDERS OF THE TEETH

Teething

Symptoms. Teeth-cutting generally begins between the ages of 5 and 7 months. There may be no unusual symptoms, but it is common to get some of the following temporary disturbances:

pain; the child puts his fingers in his mouth and screams when attempts are made to look at his teeth;

incessant flow of saliva;

increased movements of the bowels (diarrhea);

bronchitis;

fretfulness, and loss of sleep.

Diagnosis. The most important conditions which may be confused with teething are early pneumonia and inflammation in the ears. It is particularly important therefore that the child's chest and ears should be examined by a doctor if there is any considerable constitutional disturbance.

Treatment. A most effective remedy is 100 milligrams of soluble aspirin given every four to six hours.

Defective Dental Development

Delayed dentition of the milk teeth and subsequent defects of development are usually due to improper feeding during the first three years of life. A deficiency of vitamins A and D and of vitamin C is a common cause of this condition. Sufficient vitamin A is necessary for the normal formation of the enamel, vitamin C for the normal formation of the dentine, and vitamin D for the process of calcification or hardening.

Defective development and decay of the temporary teeth commonly cause derangement of their permanent successors. It is therefore very important that the temporary teeth should be properly preserved until they are shed in the usual way.

Caries or Decay of the Teeth

Dental caries always begins in the spaces in and around the teeth where food is liable to collect. When the food contains a large amount of sticky sweet carbohydrates, consisting largely of starch and sugar, it tends to adhere to the teeth and leads to excessive bacterial fermentation with the production of acids. The enamel is destroyed by the acid, and calcium is dissolved out of the dentine. The remaining tissues in the teeth are then softened, leading to the formation of a cavity. The pulp of the tooth is thus exposed to infection, and suppuration may ensue, leading to an abscess. The abscess may perforate the bone of the jaw and form the familiar 'gum boil,' or it may affect the cheek or neck.

The general health of the child may thus be affected by poisons which pass into the blood stream. The removal of septic teeth often leads to an improvement in nutrition so that the child begins to put on weight.

Prevention. Diet and mouth hygiene are important factors.

DIET. The importance of breast feeding for the development of good teeth cannot be too strongly insisted upon. If this is not possible, a properly balanced artificial diet, supplemented with cod-liver oil and orange juice, and later egg yolk, fresh fruit and vegetable juices will provide the necessary factors.

In older children it is important to limit the consumption of soft and sugary food which does not require much mastication and clings to the teeth. Too much white bread, and too many sticky sweets such as toffee are harmful. Chocolate and sweets may be allowed after meals before the teeth are cleaned.

The diet should contain sufficient milk, with a good supply of hard and fibrous substances such as brown bread, rusks, toast, vegetables and fresh fruit, particularly apples. When such foods are eaten, the act of chewing cleans the teeth.

MOUTH HYGIENE. Cleansing of the teeth by means of a toothbrush night and morning, and if possible after meals, is to be encouraged as a habit early in childhood. It should be started never later than the age of three years. A soft brush should be used, care being taken not to injure the gums. It should not be brushed across the teeth, but always from the gums towards the biting surface, No food should be taken after the evening cleansing, which should therefore be done just before going to bed. Simple rinsing of the mouth with water after each meal is to be encouraged.

DENTAL INSPECTION. The teeth should be inspected regularly by a dentist every six months from the age of three.

See also p. 117 and p.356.

DISORDERS OF THE DIGESTIVE SYSTEM

Disorders of digestion are probably the most common of illnesses in infancy and early childhood, and the chief symptoms of such disorders are vomiting, colic and diarrhea.

Vomiting in Infancy

Regurgitation

Sometimes there is a return of an excess of food directly at the end of feeding. It often occurs in breast-fed babies, with a scanty vomit of milk hardly altered in character, since it has not yet been subjected to digestion in the stomach. The vomiting is not forcible, and is unattended by discomfort or colic. The stools are quite normal, and there is no loss of weight, or failure to gain in the normal way. It usually occurs if the child is moved' about too much after a feed but, apart from attention to this point, it may be disregarded.

Dyspeptic Vomiting

It is important to recognize that there is an easy transition from regurgitation to an actual dyspeptic type of vomiting, in which there may be a considerable loss of food so that the infant fails to thrive. In such cases there is an interval between the meal and the vomiting and the vomited matter is sour, having undergone partial digestion in the stomach.

It may be that the child is placed flat on its back immediately after the feeding and in his efforts to bring up swallowed air also brings up mouthsful of food. Another fault is feeding through too small a nipple.

To prevent regurgitations, the baby should be given a rest half way through the feeding and held upright over the shoulder and patted on the back in order to allow him to expel any wind. After the feeding he should again be placed in an upright position and the 'wind' brought up.

Obstructive Vomiting
(Pyloric Stenosis)

This is a special type of vomiting caused by thickening of the muscle at the outlet of the stomach. It causes an obstruction to the passage of food from the stomach to the duodenum. It is much more common in boys than in girls, and often occurs in the first-born in a family. It is rare, however, for more than one child in a family to be affected. Breast-fed and bottle-fed babies are equally predisposed to the condition.

Symptoms. The most prominent symptom is vomiting, the feedings being readily taken, but not retained. It commonly begins between the third and fourth weeks, and is characteristically forcible or projectile in character, the food being shot out several feet. Vomiting may occur after each feeding or at less frequent intervals, in which case more than one feeding is returned when it occurs, the previous formula having remained in the stomach. The bowels are constipated, the stools being small in bulk and infrequent. The child remains alert, but is irritable and cries owing to hunger. He rapidly loses weight from starvation, and if the condition is allowed to continue, he gets into a very wasted, weak and dehydrated state.

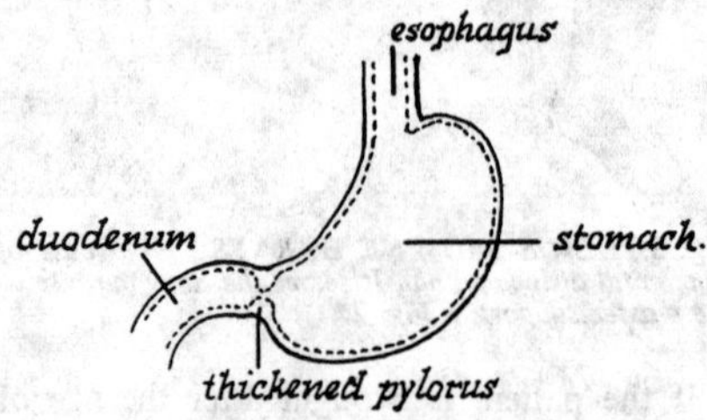

Fig. 4. *PYLORIC STENOSIS. In very young infants suffering from this disorder, the pylorus muscle, ringing the end of the stomach, is unusually thick so that the food cannot pass through into the duodenum. The condition can be remedied by operation.*

Treatment. This is usually by operation. The child must be under constant medical attention.

Nervous and Habitual Vomiting

When each one of the above-mentioned types of vomiting has been excluded, there remains a group which may be called habitual or nervous vomiting. It may be projectile in type. This type of vomiting does not usually affect the baby, who continues to thrive. He usually grows out of it by six to nine months of age.

Rumination

In addition to vomiting, the nervous type of infant may develop the habit known as rumination: it seldom occurs in breast-fed babies. It never begins before the fourth month, and is seldom well developed before the sixth month.

Symptoms. After taking the meal in the ordinary way, the child is quiet for a time. It then begins to perform certain movements by which the muscles of the abdomen are thrown into a series of violent contractions, the head being held back and the mouth kept open. After a period of persistent effort, a successful contraction forces up a considerable quantity of milk into the mouth. The infant lies with an expression of the greatest satisfaction on its face, and subjects the milk to innumerable chewing and sucking movements before swallowing it again.

Rumination is characteristically a secret habit. Only when the child is alone in a drowsy vacant state does it indulge in the act, and if it is openly watched it immediately stops. Ruminating infants tend to lose weight. Once the habit is acquired it tends to persist for several months, and it may be very difficult to eliminate.

Treatment. Rest and quiet are essential, together with very careful management of the child by an experienced nurse. The meals should be given in a quiet place and must not be hurried. Probably the best results are obtained by interesting the child in his surroundings, and every effort must be made by the mother or nurse to distract the child's attention until he falls asleep.

It is better to let an infant suck his thumb than to regurgitate by rumination.

Thickened foods, being very difficult to regurgitate, are also helpful. Plugging the nostrils may likewise be helpful, since it forces the child to breathe through the mouth, and thus makes regurgitation difficult.

Colic

Colic is a form of painful cramp in the bowels which causes the baby to draw up its legs and scream. It is usually felt in the region of the navel. It is most frequent during the early months, and is more common in bottle-fed than in breast-fed babies.

Causes. AIR SWALLOWING. The breast-fed child is apt to swallow air if left sucking too long on an empty breast, or if suction is difficult, either because of a scanty flow of milk or because the mother's nipples are poorly formed. The bottle-fed child is apt to swallow air if the bottle is held incorrectly, if the nipple hole is too small, or if he is not 'burped' properly after his feed.

COLD FOODS. Foods which are given too cold readily cause colic in very young infants. Hence the necessity of warming foods to the proper temperature.

Symptoms. The child screams violently from abdominal pain, and continues until the paroxysm is relieved either by the passage of wind from the stomach or bowel, or after a bowel movement. The legs are drawn up and the abdomen is distended and held rigid.

Treatment of the Cause. The method of feeding must be inquired into and the stools should be examined. Any errors of feeding must be corrected (see Baby Care, p. 103 105).

NOTE. *If an attack of colic occurs suddenly* in an infant who is usually quite well, it is best to call in a doctor, since in some cases it may be due to obstruction of the bowels. *On no account should castor oil or any strong laxative be given without direction from a doctor.*

Diarrhea

Infants and children are more likely to suffer from diarrhea than adults.

Diarrhea usually represents an attempt on the part of the body to get rid of substances which are irritating to the bowel. Thus it may be due either to indigestion (simple catarrhal diarrhea) or to infection (epidemic diarrhea). Like vomiting, it may also occur at the onset of general diseases such as fevers, pneumonia, and infection of the throat or middle ear.

Gastroenteritis of the Newborn
(Epidemic Diarrhea of the Newborn)

This infectious diarrhea and vomiting which occurs during the first month of life is believed to be due to a virus; in some cases where epidemics have broken out in maternity units the bacteria *Escherichia coli* has been the cause of the illness. The onset is usually sudden and both breast-fed and bottle-fed infants are affected equally.

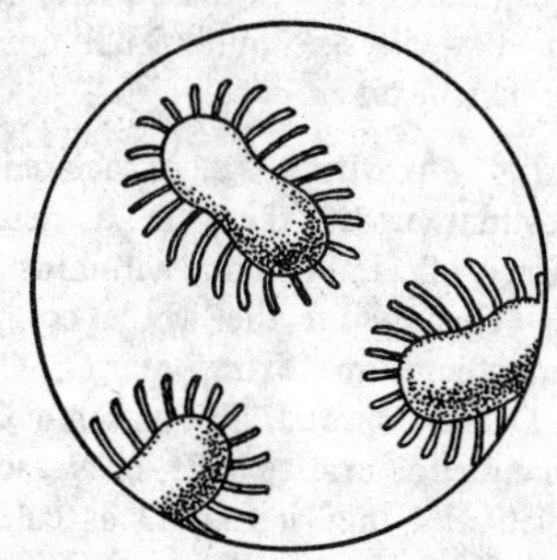

Fig. 5. *ESCHERICHIA COLI. This type of bacterium is commonly found in the human colon (large intestine) where it appears to do little harm. Certain strains, however, are more virulent and sometimes cause gastroenteritis in the newborn.*

Symptoms. The infant refuses to suck, is fretful and passes explosive watery stools. Vomiting is usual, but in mild cases it may be absent. The eyes appear slightly shrunken, though bright. The tongue is dry and the lips often bright red. Within two or three days the infant loses weight.

Treatment. The doctor must be called in promptly and he will decide whether the infant is to be nursed at home (mild cases) or will require hospital care. Milk foods must not be given for twenty-four hours. Water containing salt (sodium chloride) in the strength of 1 teaspoonful to 4 pints of water is given in small quantities every one to two hours during the day, and every four hours at night. Sometimes glucose is prescribed in the saline solution. As the diarrhea lessens, milk may be reintroduced diluted in the feedings.

Drugs are not usually necessary in mild cases but, in more severe cases, antibiotics and sulphonamides are prescribed according to the type of organism which is found to be causing the infection. Castor oil or other purgatives must not be used.

Diarrhea in the Breast-fed Child

Green stools may sometimes occur in breast-fed babies when there is no obvious error with regard to the quantity or quality of the milk. If the child is putting on weight and otherwise thriving, no notice need be taken of it.

Diarrhea in the Bottle-fed Child

This may follow the addition of too much sugar (sugar indigestion), or it may indicate that the child's tolerance for has has been overstepped (fat indigestion). Protein indigestion, on the other hand, is usually associated with constipation.

Infective Diarrhea

(Summer Diarrhea of Infants; Infant Cholera)

Infants and young children are especially liable to attacks of severe diarrhea during long spells of hot weather with the increase of dust and flies. This type of diarrhea is especially common in hot climates where the greatest hygienic precautions should be taken to guard against it.

Infantile diarrhea, however, is not confined to the summer months. Overcrowded homes and faulty feeding which lower the baby's resistance to bacteria also play a part in causing an outbreak. By far the greatest number of cases occur in bottle-fed babies.

Symptoms. The complaint usually begins suddenly with vomiting and fever. Soon the stools become frequent, green and watery, with the appearance of chopped spinach. In severe cases the child may be rapidly and gravely debilitated from loss of tissue fluids.

Treatment. In every case of severe diarrhea in an infant, a doctor should be called in at once.

HYGIENE. Since the complaint is usually infectious, all soiled diapers should be disinfected by soaking in 1 in 40 carbolic solution, and then by boiling. Disposable diapers are useful because they can be burned. The greatest care must be taken to clean all feeding utensils and to protect them from flies. All milk should be boiled before it is given to the infant.

IMMEDIATE TREATMENT. It is important that the child should be kept warm and, if possible, isolated from other children.

All milk food must be stopped for twelve to forty-eight hours, until the acute diarrhea has subsided. Instead of the usual bottle of milk, give the same amount of warm boiled water at the usual time, or smaller quantities more frequently.

Sulphonamides and antibiotics are often given to counteract secondary infection and recovery is quicker than when they are withheld. Castor oil should never be given.

LATER TREATMENT. When feeding is resumed after the preliminary period of starvation, it should be done very cautiously. Feedings are given at first in very weak form and in small quantities, and any additions must be made very slowly, their effect on the stools, temperature and general condition of the child being carefully noted.

Diarrhea in Older Children

This will be treated much as for adults. See Diarrhea, p. 369.

Constipation in Infancy and Early Childhood

A constipated stool is a hard formed stool. It cannot be said to exist if the child merely has infrequent movements, say once every two days, provided the stool is normal in consistency, and the child is getting on well. In such cases no treatment is required, except to make sure that the child is having sufficient water in addition to its food.

Causes

ERRORS OF DIET. Constipation is more common in breast-fed than in bottle-fed infants, and the most usual cause is insufficient food or fluid. It is particularly common in the later months of breast feeding, when it usually indicates that the child is not getting sufficient breast milk, or water, or both.

In bottle-fed infants constipation may also be caused by insufficient food or water. It may be due to over-dilution of the milk, which then becomes deficient in fat or sugar. During the second year, too much milk and insufficient fruit and cereals may give rise to constipation.

FAULTY HABITS are often due to lack of proper training; the toddler has not been taught to expect an action of the bowels at about a given time of the day.

SPASM OR TIGHTENING OF THE ANUS. This is usually due to fissure or crack in the anus.

WEAKENED ABDOMINAL MUSCLES, as in rickets. In such cases the child is pale and irritable, and fails to gain weight.

OBSTRUCTION OF THE STOMACH OR INTESTINES. In such cases vomiting is a prominent feature, and there is considerable loss of weight, the stools being small, dry and dark in color. In such cases, pyloric stenosis is likely to be the cause (see p. 514).

Symptoms. Constipation may exist without any symptoms of disturbed health. Often the only symptom is pain, due to intestinal colic.

Treatment

EXTRA WATER. For infants, 30 to 120 milliters (1 to 4 ounces) of warm boiled water should be given an hour before the evening feed.

ADJUSTMENT OF DIET. (*a*) *Milk.* Milk mixtures often need readjustment, and it may be necessary to reduce the protein and modify the sugar. Brown sugar is more laxative than white.

(*b*) *Fruit.* This should be given in the form of fruit juice, or fruit or vegetable puree.

Other Additions to Diet. Give constipated babies over the age of four months extra cereal foods and add finely chopped vegetables to the diet.

DRUGS. Laxative drugs should only be given to infants and young children as a last resort, since they may start a bad habit which is only got rid of with great difficulty. In any case, they should only be used as a temporary measure while the diet is being adjusted.

Pure olive oil is a useful and natural lubricant which may be given by mouth, or mineral oil two or three times daily.

ANAL SPASM. In cases which are due to spasm of the anus, the bowel movements should be kept soft by prune puree or mineral oil. Such cases are often relieved by stretching the anus with the finger well greased and with nail cut short.

For constipation in older children, see pp. 367 to 368.

Thrush

This is a fungus infection which may occur in the mouth of bottle-fed babies. See section on Skin, p. 471.

Kwashiorkor

The deficiency disease of kwashiorkor results from a mixed deficit of protein and vitamins in the diet. It occurs in Africa, the West Indies, India and parts of the Far East, and derives its name from the African Ga language, signifying 'red boy.'

Usually children below the age of four are affected and they appear as undernourished infants with pot-bellies, swollen legs, sores around the mouth, and pale skin and hair. The hair acquires a gray-red tinge (hence the name of the disease) and loses its natural curl. The infants often have diarrhea, passing loose, pale, fatty stools. Parents usually notice the ill child to be apathetic and rarely actually crying or screaming, but often whimpering and listless. Indeed, those who have seen much of this illness say that when the child smiles he is well on the road to recovery.

The liver is often affected by fatty disease and this is one of the most important aspects of the illness to be corrected.

This illness is found mainly in children after weaning, in poor areas, for their diet of cereals, cassava, plantains, yams and maize is poor in protein; people in these areas do not get much milk and meat, the main providers of protein in the human diet.

Treatment. The essence of treatment is feeding. The child requires protein in a form that he can take. Often a very ill baby will be anemic as well and will have to have blood transfusions, which will in themselves start the protein treatment. Older children can usually begin to take protein by mouth in the form of cows' milk, and high-protein meat extracts can be added if tolerated. This regime should be continued until the child has no more diarrhea and then gradual weaning to a full diet with vitamin extracts is undertaken.

Intussusception

By intussusception is meant the invagination of one part of the intestine into another, like the finger of a glove. It occurs usually in infancy between the ages of four and eighteen months, affecting as a rule fat and well-nourished boy babies. It never occurs in wasted infants. It accounts for three-quarters of all cases of intestinal obstruction in young children. (See p. 372.)

Symptoms. There are three main symptoms:

ABDOMINAL PAIN, of sudden onset and colicky in nature. The pain is spasmodic and severe while it lasts, and it occurs at intervals for twenty-four to thirty-six hours.

VOMITING. This is severe and repeated, and occurs just after the pain.

PASSAGE OF BLOOD AND MUCUS BY THE RECTUM. This appears at some interval after the onset of the pain and vomiting. Intussusception leads to paralysis of the bowel. When this occurs the child becomes drowsy and collapsed and the spasms stop.

Treatment. Treatment is by operation, and the earlier this is performed the better the outlook.

Celiac Disease

Celiac disease is a chronic digestive disorder occurring in infants and young children who show no signs of any organic disease of the abdominal organs. It is due to an idiosyncrasy to the gluten in wheat, giving rise to a failure of the intestines to absorb the fat of the food. The disease is commoner in girls than in boys, and its onset is usually between the seventh and twenty-fourth months.

Symptoms. The onset is usually gradual, with loss of appetite, vomiting, looseness of the bowels and nervous symptoms, the child becoming introspective and irritable. There is no disease in which loss of appetite is so constant or so pronounced. The three main features are large pale stools, enlarged abdomen and retarded growth.

The stools are typically unformed, and may be passed two or three times in the twenty-four hours. They are bulky and porridge-like in appearance, and their consistency may vary from that of putty to one of diarrhea. They are pale in color, and are particularly offensive. These characteristics are due to the abnormal amount of fat present in them.

Enlargement of the abdomen is caused by weakness of the muscles of the abdominal wall and by flatulent distension of the intestines. The abdomen has a doughy feel to the touch.

There is loss of weight with wasting of the muscles and retarded development (infantilism). The buttocks are noticeably small in size and contrast strikingly with the enlarged abdomen. The face is pale. Rickets is often present.

Treatment is essentially a matter of a gluten-free diet. When the child first comes under the doctor's care, the listless lack of appetite needs to be dealt with gently.

SLOW TRANSITION. It is best to make the transition by getting the child to take two pints of skimmed milk daily. This should help to improve the diarrhea and also lessen the irritability which is so trying to parents and siblings alike. Ripe mashed banana may then be given, and calves' foot jelly. A month or two later cornflakes, rice pudding, and stewed apple can be tried.

Gradually a normal diet for the child's age can be attained with the strict proviso that foods containing wheat-flour or rye-flour are *never* eaten by the patient.

GLUTEN CONTENT. Gluten-free wheat-flour makes a very crumbly loaf, many bakers will bake gluten-free loaves to order. Cornflour, oat-flour and rice do not contain gluten, but the following do—ordinary bread, biscuits, custard powder, all-bran, shredded wheat, grape-nuts, semolina, macaroni, ice-cream, malted milk, and puddings made from wheat-flour.

Foods suitable are—all meats, fish, eggs, cheese, vegetables such as tomatoes, peas, beans, and cabbage, potato in small quantities, bananas and other fruits, cornflour, cornflakes (maize flour in these), rice, honey, jam, boiled sweets, and milk. Small amounts of butter may be taken.

VITAMINS AND MINERALS. Associated with the intestinal upset there is a defective absorption of important vitamins and minerals. Throughout the whole course of treatment, therefore, extra vitamin C and vitamin D are required. The vitamin C can be taken either as orange juice, or as ascorbic acid tablets and the vitamin D as calciferol tablets or Calcium with Vitamin D Tablets. The attendant anemia should be remedied by the administration of ferrous sulphate 60 to 120 milligrams thrice daily.

DISORDERS OF METABOLISM

Acidosis

By acidosis is meant an acid condition of the blood caused by certain abnormal products of oxidation, the chief of which is acetone.

The energy which is expended on muscular activity and on emotional activity is derived from the stores of carbohydrate in the body. Normally, there is only a small reserve. In some children, and especially in those of an eager excitable temperament, the carbohydrate reserves are very easily exhausted by fatigue, excitement or feverish illnesses; with insufficient carbohydrate, the child is forced to consume the body fat which is the second main store of energy. When the body is short of carbohydrate, however, the fats are incompletely broken down to the normal end products of combustion, namely, water and oxygen, the process stopping halfway with the production of what are known as ketone bodies, the chief of which is acetone. This acetone circulates in the blood and is eliminated from the system partly in the breath, partly in the urine.

Acidosis is thus a symptom and not a disease in itself, and it may occur in a number of different disorders, all of which, however, are associated with carbohydrate starvation. Thus it occurs during periods of starvation, feverish illnesses, and in association with disorders of digestion, as during the change from breast feeding to bottle feeding. It is well known that when young children take a journey, they are often 'out of sorts' on the second day. This is usually due to acidosis resulting from disturbances of digestion. The chief cause of carbohydrate starvation, however, is vomiting. Thus, it occurs in cases of vomiting with diarrhea in vomiting after anesthetics, and in the condition known as cyclical vomiting (see p. 417).

Acidosis is commonest during the first seven years of life. Young children who are subject to the complaint usually outgrow it within a few years.

Cyclical Vomiting

Cyclical vomiting is a condition allied to acidosis in which severe attacks of vomiting, often lasting from one to four days, occur at intervals of a few weeks.

The attacks first appear between the ages of two and seven, and attain their maximum at about four years of age.

The attacks take place more often in winter than in summer and tend to disappear spontaneously, usually either at the beginning of the permanent dentition (i.e. the cutting of the permanent teeth at the age of six years, or at puberty).

The subjects of this disorder often suffer from infantile eczema, and may later develop migraine or some form of allergy.

Symptoms. The attack begins suddenly after a few hours of lassitude. Dark rings appear under the eyes and vomiting sets in. There is intense thirst, but even water is rejected by the stomach. The bowels are usually constipated, and the vomiting is often accompanied by fever and abdominal pain. The attack may easily be confused with that in appendicitis or intussusception. It usually lasts for one, two or three days, and a child of four years may lose as much as seven pounds in weight during this period.

Treatment of an Attack. The child should be put to bed in a quiet darkened room. A clinical examination should be made to exclude any surgical condition.

GLUCOSE should be given, if possible by mouth, 3 teaspoonsful in a glass of water, flavored with fruit juice, such as orange or lemon juice. This should be repeated as often as the child can take it, and at least every two hours. If big drinks are returned, only sips from a spoon should be given at frequent intervals. If the vomiting makes it impossible for the child to keep down the glucose drinks, a solution of glucose may have to be given by the rectum (two teaspoonsful of glucose in eight ounces of water as an enema every two hours). It is not necessary to use medicinal glucose, the commercial product known as liquid glucose being quite as efficacious. It can be obtained at any large grocery store. Glucose is simply carbohydrate in a form which requires no digestion. It is absorbed very quickly from the stomach.

Six hours after vomiting has stopped, diluted milk, or weak sweetened tea or oatmeal may be given. Recovery is usually rapid, and the diet can be quickly increased.

Prevention of Attacks. The most important part of treatment is prevention.

MANAGEMENT. With children who are subject to attacks of vomiting, wise understanding and considerate control are of the greatest importance. Physical exercises, gymnastics, and dancing are of great value.

The bowels should be kept regular.

DIET. *Limitation of Fat.* A moderate limitation of fat may be advised. Milk should be given in the usual quantities.

Increase of Carbohydrate. A free provision of carbohydrate is as necessary as a moderate limitation of the fat. Glucose, being the most easily assimilated form of carbohydrate, is of particular value. It should be given regularly over a period in doses of three teaspoonsful in a glass of orangeade or other fruit drink on rising in the morning, at 11 a.m. and at bedtime.

Extra carbohydrate may also be given in the form of honey, barley sugar, or cane sugar after meals. Chocolate and toffee contain a good deal of fat and should be limited. All kinds of fruit and vegetables are allowed.

Alkalosis and Tetany

Alkalosis. By alkalosis is meant an increase in the alkaline reaction of the blood. It may occur in cases of gastric disorder associated with much vomiting, or after the prolonged administration by mouth of alkalis such as bicarbonate of soda. Any severe case of alkalosis is likely to be complicated by the condition known as tetany.

Tetany (*Spasmophilia*). Tetany is a condition of over-irritability of the nervous system with an abnormal excitability of the muscles, resulting in spasms of the muscles of the hands and feet and of the larynx, and often giving rise to convulsions. It may occur as a result of alkalosis (usually after prolonged attacks of diarrhea and vomiting), and in any condition in which there is a deficiency of calcium in the blood. Thus it is most commonly seen in cases of active rickets. It is commonest between the age of six months and two years, and in the late spring months when the child's supply of vitamin D in the system is at its lowest. In older children it may occur with celiac disease (p.416).

It should not be confused with tetanus (lockjaw), a disease caused by an organism which infects a cut or wound.

Symptoms. The most important are:

CARPO-PEDAL SPASMS (spasms of the muscles of the arms and legs). The arms are usually first affected; they are bent at the elbow and held against the chest. The wrists are also bent and the hand is held in what is called the 'accoucheur's position.' Occasionally the muscles of the face are affected, giving rise to the so-called 'carp mouth' in which the lips are protruded like those of a fish.

SPASM OF THE GLOTTIS (spasm of the muscles of the larynx). This gives rise to a sudden shutting of the glottis or passage to the windpipe which creates a feeling of strangulation and difficulty in breathing so that when the child takes a deep breath he emits a peculiar crowing sound (laryngismus stridulus) which may be repeated several times. The disease is sometimes mistaken for whooping-cough.

Laryngismus stridulus is commonest between the ages of 6 and 15 months, and is usually brought on by fright, annoyance, cold air, etc. Thus, it may result from a sudden severe frost which comes on during the night and causes a rapid lowering of the bedroom temperature.

CONVULSIONS. Convulsions may follow any slight disturbance. They may be difficult to distinguish from epileptic convulsions (see p. 436).

Treatment. To raise the blood calcium level, 300 mg to 1 gram of calcium chloride should be given in water or milk every four hours. Calcium gluconate may also be given by mouth or by injection.

For further treatment of convulsions, see p. 519.

Prevention of Tetany. This consists mainly in the prevention and treatment of the underlying disease such as rickets (p.392), or celiac disease (see p. 416).

Cod-liver oil should be administered regularly, but if this cannot be tolerated, capsules of the oil should be given. Plenty of sunlight is necessary, and if this is not available ultraviolet irradiation should be arranged for. Both of these measures assist the absorption of calcium into the system.

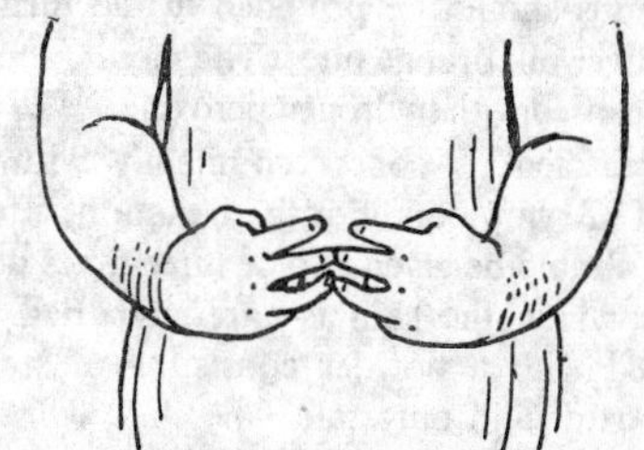

Fig. 6. *SPASM OF THE WRIST AND HAND MUSCLES IN TETANY.* (See text.)

Pink Disease

(*Acrodynia*)

This disease affects young children between the ages of 4 months and 2½ years, and is slightly commoner in males than females. The cause is obscure. Inadequate vitamins may aggravate the condition.

Symptoms. The disease starts as a mild feverish illness with a cold in the head and symptoms of slight bronchitis. After the fever there may be a quiescent period lasting from two to four weeks, but it is followed by loss of appetite, and severe sleeplessness, the child becoming very miserable and depressed. The hands and feet become cold and begin to swell. They are bright red in color resembling raw beef, or looking as if they had been dipped in boiling water. There is cold clammy perspiration and a scattered rash like a sweat rash on the trunk and limbs. The mouth becomes very sore, and the teeth may drop out, although they appear to be perfectly healthy. The nails may also become loose and drop off, and the hair comes out, leaving bald patches. Hypersensitivity to light is a feature.

The disease may be complicated by bronchopneumonia, diarrhea or infection of the middle ear.

Course. The complaint may last for three to nine months, during which time incessant care and vigilance may have to be exercised. In the absence of complications, however, complete recovery occurs and there are no recurrences.

Treatment. Where possible, the child should live in healthy surroundings in the country and in good weather he may be kept in a crib out of doors. Careful nursing is essential. Light clothing only should be worn, so that there is a minimum of sweating. It should be of silk or cotton, which is far less irritating than wool or flannel. The eyes should be protected from bright light. Careful feeding is essential, in order to overcome the very poor appetite. Children with pink disease, however, are able to digest a moderately full diet if they are carefully fed by spoon. Plenty of cold fluids should be given in small quantities at frequent intervals, and ice-cream is of particular value. Extra vitamins should be provided in the form of cod-liver oil, orange juice. The mouth should be cleansed with hydrogen peroxide.

Treatment is concerned mainly with the relief of symptoms. For the irritation, a tepid bath should be given two or three times daily, after which the skin is carefully dried and dusted with a powder consisting of starch, zinc oxide and pure talc. The child will then often fall off to sleep naturally for two or three hours. A calamine and zinc oxide lotion may also be used to relieve the irritation.

The hands and feet should be protected with cotton gloves and socks to prevent them from being scratched and, if necessary, the arms may have to be splinted. When there is much irritation of the hands and feet, allow the child to hold them from time to time in cold water. If insomnia is persistent, a mild sedative may be prescribed by a doctor.

DISORDERS OF THE SKIN

Sore Buttocks

Sore buttocks are usually due to irritation caused by a diaper which has been soiled by acid urine or stools, as in diarrhea. Occasionally it is caused by a diaper which has been washed with harsh detergents or those containing soda, and then insufficiently rinsed.

The rash is distributed as a blotchy eruption on the convex surfaces of the buttocks, thighs and abdomen.

Treatment. The diapers should be of soft material, and should be frequently changed. They should be washed with any soap which does not contain an excess of soda, or with a mild detergent. After washing, all traces of soap or detergent must be carefully removed by thorough rinsing. Soaking the diapers in a solution of benzalkonium chloride (use strength as given on the label) after rinsing will help to prevent a rash. Disposable diapers are recommended if the rash is severe. They should be changed often.

The buttocks should be washed regularly at each change of diaper, and kept as dry as possible. If a rash develops, the buttocks may be wiped with warm olive oil each time the diaper is changed, followed by the free application of a simple cream consisting of equal parts of castor oil and zinc ointment. Do not use waterproof pants while the child has a rash. Such material holds in all the moisture and causes water-logging of the child's skin.

For resistant rashes, a few applications of 1 per cent picric acid lotion will often clear up the last traces.

Heat Spots
(Prickly Heat)

This is one of the commonest skin affections occurring in infants and young children, and nearly all infants have it in some degree at some time or other. The spots are seen usually between the ages of six months and three years, and they are commonest in the summer months.

They appear as a rule in the evening, and consist of oval or irregular red blotches up to half an inch in diameter. They are generally situated on the lower part of the back and round the waist, but they may occur on the limbs as well. They are intensely irritating until the child scratches the top off them, when they cease to itch, but start to ooze serum which then dries into small crusts.

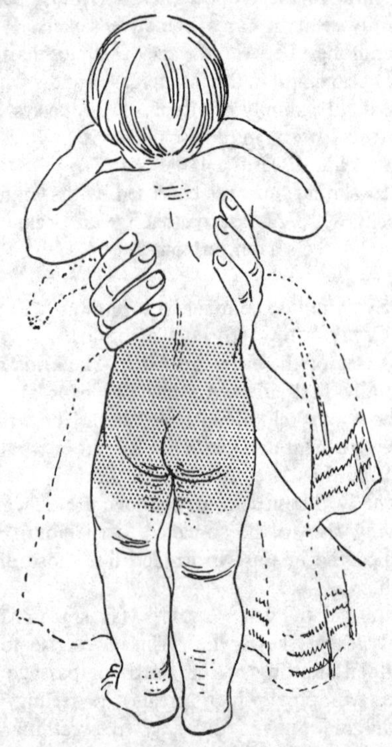

Fig. 7. *AREA AFFECTED BY PRICKLY HEAT indicated by shading.*

Treatment. The child should be kept cool and not overclothed; the bowels should be regulated to act every day. There should be no excess of starchy food, sugar and sweets in the diet.

The irritation may be allayed by the external application of a lotion containing 2 per cent of phenol in calamine lotion. In obstinate cases it may be necessary to send the child to stay in a different house, or with relatives. When this is done, it is often found disappears spontaneously.

Infantile Eczema

Infantile eczema is the most distressing skin complaint of young children.

Cause. Eczema is not a disease in itself but the inflammatory reactions of the skin to external irritation; it only occurs in highly sensitive predisposed infants. A baby's skin is so sensitive that it is easily irritated by external contacts, and the infant's face, being exposed, is the part which is most liable to be affected. Among such external irritants are washing with strong soaps or hard water, imperfect drying in cold weather, and exposure to sudden changes of temperature such as to cold winds or hot fires. A combination of two or more of these irritants causes the skin of the cheek or forehead to become flushed, and further irritation gives rise to eczema.

Symptoms. Most infants with eczema are plump and overfed. In babies under two years of age the eczema usually begins on the forehead or cheek as a redness and roughness of the skin. As a result of rubbing and scratching a raw weeping surface is produced and the discharge dries into crusts. When fully developed the eruption has a characteristic mask-like distribution over the forehead, cheeks, chin, and often the scalp, leaving free the eyelids, nose and mouth. Itching is generally worse at night, so that sleep is interfered with and the child may become nervous and difficult to manage. In cases which persist beyond the second year the eruption may also be present in patches on the limbs and trunk. It is likely to persist at the bends of the elbows and at the back of the knees.

Course. The disorder varies from time to time, having a great tendency to relapse when nearly cured. In spite of careful treatment it may last for several weeks, or even for several months, but even without treatment it almost always clears up, at least on the face and scalp by the age of two years.

Treatment. It is a disease which calls for much care and patience on the part of the mother and nurse, and babies who suffer from eczema should be under the supervision of a doctor. The secret of successful treatment is to keep the parts protected from every form of external irritation and from scratching.

The child should be protected from cold winds, and shaded from direct sunlight. He should not be allowed to get overheated, either from exposure to hot fires or from over-clothing. Clothing is a matter of considerable importance, and only silk or cotton, or a mixture of both should be allowed to come in contact with the skin. Wool acts as an irritant, and warm garments should only be put on over the silk or cotton underclothes. Blankets should be faced with linen, so that no wool comes in contact with the baby's face or body. Nylon shirts and dresses are best avoided since they do not allow a free enough circulation of air around the skin.

Water and soap are irritants, and should not be used for washing until the normal condition of the skin has been regained. Warm olive oil or mineral oil should be used for cleansing purposes.

It is important to prevent the child from rubbing and scratching, and it may be necessary to put the arms into splints, a roll of cardboard being tied round the arm from the shoulder to the wrist.

LOCAL APPLICATIONS. Some form of hydrocortisone cream or ointment is used in most cases of eczema. It is applied in small quantities three times a day. In severe cases, tar preparations are often used.

It may often be necessary to continue the treatment for some weeks or months, but if a wasting is noticed in the napkin area, steroid ointment must be stopped for several weeks.

DIET. The diet should be adjusted to the age of the child. If the baby is being fed on the breast it is best to continue. If artificially fed, it may be wise to reduce the amount of sugar in the diet.

For eczema related to food allergies, see section on Allergy, p.482.

Narrowing of the Foreskin, and Circumcision

The foreskin or prepuce acts as a protective covering for the sensitive mushroom-like end of the penis. It should be free, and capable of being pulled back completely so that the whole glans is exposed. In very young babies the foreskin is often narrow and cannot be retracted so as to expose the glans completely. This condition will usually correct itself in a few weeks.

In some infants, the foreskin is adherent to the glans, and its opening may be so narrow that it impedes the passage of the urine. When this is the case a doctor should be informed, in order that a little operation may be done to break down the adhesions and dilate the opening by stretching it with forceps. This can be done without an anesthetic for children under the age of one year. The after-treatment is important, and consists in pushing back the foreskin twice daily for a week, once daily for a second week, and after that once every other day for a week. In all cases great care must be taken to see that the foreskin is pulled forward again. At the end of three weeks, it usually remains free from adhesions and sufficiently dilated so that it does not need to be touched any more.

Circumcision. The operation of circumcision is probably often done unnecessarily. It should be reserved for cases where the foreskin is very long or inflamed. If it has to be done, the earlier it is done the better. Between the ages of two and six years, little boys often suffer from fears of losing or damaging the penis, and circumcision at such a stage can do psychological harm.

DISORDERS OF THE NERVOUS SYSTEM

Convulsions in Infancy and Early Childhood

A convulsion is probably the commonest medical emergency in childhood. The tendency to convulsions is greater in infancy than at any other age, and steadily diminishes as the child grows older. This susceptibility in infancy is explained by the immature state of the nervous system at birth. So long as this immaturity exists the baby is disposed to sudden attacks of uncontrolled diffusion of nervous energy from relatively minor disturbances. Irritations which might cause a baby to have a convulsion do not have the same effect on a child of five or older.

Causes. When a convulsion occurs in an infant or young child, it should be regarded as a symptom of some underlying disorder, and not as a disease in itself.

FEVERS. Convulsions are particularly apt to occur at the onset of an acute feverish illness with a sudden rise of temperature, such as whooping-cough, pneumonia, measles, scarlet fever or chicken pox. Acute inflammation of the middle ear may sometimes cause convulsions in predisposed children. Convulsions due to fever are usually transitory and do not leave any tendency to repeated fits unless there are complications in infection of the middle ear.

RICKETS. A common predisposing cause of convulsions is tetany, which is associated with a diminished amount of calcium in the blood. This occurs in rickets (see Deficiency Diseases, p. 398, which is due to a shortage of vitamin D in the system. In such conditions the nervous excitability of the infant, which is naturally high, becomes aggravated on account of the shortage of calcium in the blood, so that minor irritations are liable to give rise to a fit. It is therefore unwise to attribute a convulsion to such a minor condition as teething without looking for an underlying cause such as rickets. Convulsions associated with rickets are more common in the second half of infancy and in artificially fed children. The attacks usually cease at the end of the second year.

BIRTH INJURY AND BRAIN HEMORRHAGE may precipitate convulsions in the newborn infant; other associated symptoms are usually cyanosis, inability to suck, and fever.

EPILEPSY. In cases where there is a family history of epilepsy, infantile convulsions may be epileptic, since it has been estimated that at least one-eighth of all cases of epilepsy begin during the first three years of life. In such cases the convulsions are often periodic in their occurrence, and may recur over periods of weeks or months.

BREATH-HOLDING. These attacks occur in spoiled children but, if treated lightly, they may lead to convulsions. Firm handling of the small child and calm treatment are important.

Symptoms. Fits may occur in a great variety of forms. In the mildest type, the baby may simply become stiff and pale, rolling up his eyes, and appearing to be unconscious for a few seconds. Sometimes this may be associated with a twitching of a single muscle, or with a few jerking movements of the limbs.

A more severe type of convulsion has much in common with a major epileptic seizure in an older patient.

Such attacks begin suddenly and unexpectedly. The face grows pale, the eyes are rolled upwards, so that the pupils are hidden behind the upper lids, and in a moment or two continuous twitchings begin in the limbs or face, and rapidly spread to involve the whole body. The child may be incontinent. After a time, which may vary from a minute or so to half an hour or more, the spasms gradually cease, leaving the child prostrated, and generally unconscious or extremely drowsy.

Treatment of the Convulsion. Whatever is done should be done immediately, and a doctor should be sent for at once, as the fit may be a sign of some impending illness.

DRUGS. Chloral hydrate and potassium bromide may be safely given for infantile convulsions. The doctor may prescribe a small dose of phenobarbital as a sedative between convulsions.

Treatment of Underlying Causes. These must be carefully sought for and treated. Thus any tendency to rickets should be corrected (p. 398). The treatment should be continued for several months, to prevent relapse.

Acute inflammation of the middle ear should be looked for and, in cases due to this cause, prompt medical care is essential. For teething with convulsions, 100 milligrams of aspirin may be given every 6 hours for 2 or 3 days to a baby of six months.

Convulsions which recur over periods of weeks or months are probably epileptic in nature, and may be treated on a doctor's advice with phenobarbital in doses of 30 milligrams twice daily for a child of two or three years. See epilepsy, pp.436-438.

Brain Disorders and Mental Deficiency

There is great variation in the degrees of incapacity, both mental and physical, of infants born with inadequate brains, inborn errors of metabolism, or inherited degenerations, as well as those whose brains are permanently affected by birth injury or by early illness such as meningitis. Each case needs assessing separately as the incapacity can be alleviated in some cases and little can be done for others from the medical point of view.

Mongolism (*Down's Syndrome*). About one in four of idiots suffer from this inborn genetic fault—an extra chromosome in their cells. With patience the higher grade mongol babies can be trained to walk, feed themselves and sometimes to be independent in toilet habits although at a much slower pace than a normal child. No known drugs are of use for this condition.

Cerebral Palsy. These children suffer from varying degrees of spasticity (muscle tenseness and rigidity) owing to damage in the muscle-controlling brain cortex and the basal ganglia, probably at birth. Some suffer only from a mild difficulty in walking whereas others can scarcely walk at all and find speech difficult.

The brain lesions are irreversible but in many cases the intellectual functions are not damaged, so these children may go to a special school for education and training.

Inborn Errors of Metabolism. If the disorder in the baby is recognized early and the appropriate drugs regularly given, the child is likely to grow up into a fairly normal adult, though he will always need to take the vital drug. This is particularly so in cretins if given thyroid treatment right from babyhood (see Diseases of Metabolism, p. 395).

Headache

Headache in childhood is extremely common, although it may be difficult to recognize. It may occur in many disorders, the most common cause being some intestinal disturbance such as constipation or indigestion.

It is often present with fever, and a child with acute tonsillitis or acute infection of the ear may make no other complaint than that of headache. It is usually an early symptom of infectious disease such as measles, pneumonia, or scarlet fever.

Nervous children of the restless, rapidly exhausted type are very subject to headache, and it is particularly common in rheumatic children. It is also a symptom of bilious attacks from acidosis and of attacks of cyclical vomiting. Another form of nervous headache in children is due to migraine, when it may be also associated with fever and vomiting.

Head Rolling

This habit is sometimes met with in infancy. It is characterized by forcible rubbing of the back of the head from side to side against the pillow, so that the hair at the back of the scalp is completely rubbed off. One explanation is that the head sweats, so that contact with a hot and moist pillow gives rise to itching which is relieved by friction.

It is sometimes caused by inflammation in the ear.

Treatment. A bran pillow with a slight depression in the center should be provided. Inflammation of the ear, or rickets, if present, should be appropriately dealt with.

Head Banging

It is difficult to assign a cause to this curious condition. It may result from pain in the head or ears, but in most cases no explanation can be found, and it is remarkable with what force a child will continue to bang his head against the sides of his cot without apparently experiencing any pain. Such habits are practically harmless unless they are allowed to become fixed, in which case they may aggravate an existing nervous condition. It is important to make sure that the general management of the child is satisfactory.

DISORDERS ASSOCIATED WITH THE RESPIRATORY SYSTEM

Infants and young children are very vulnerable to infections passed on via the breath (droplet infection) of those handling them, and, in fact, diseases of the respiratory system form the largest single cause of death in the first few months of life.

Colds

In all young infants, colds in the head, with running nose and redness of the pharynx, should never be regarded lightly.

Treatment. Leave the infant in his crib out of a draft and with the room temperature 17·5° C (just below 65° F). Give as much fluid —fruit juice and water, boiled water, or thin barley water—as the child will take. Dilute the milk if there is feverishness. Clear the nasal passages before feeding time, perhaps by instilling a few dilute ephedrine drops into each nostril while the child's head is held slightly back.

Prevention. All persons with head colds should refrain from handling an infant. If the mother herself has a cold, it is advisable for her to wash her hands before attending to the infant and wear a mask over her nose and mouth when feeding or tending him. The masks must be boiled after use, or disposable ones burned.

Pneumonia

In newly born infants unable to clear their respiratory passages by coughing or unable to move from the position they are placed in, pneumonia is an extremely dangerous disease. Inhalation of amniotic fluid or vomitus is often a predisposing cause. Respiration is often irregular but may be rapid. The infant fails to suck and appears collapsed, and there may be diarrhea.

Treatment. The infant must be placed with head low so that fluid can drain from the lungs, and his position should be changed often. An antibiotic is given. In severe cases the infant may need the aid of oxygen.

Bronchitis and Pneumonia

In small children it is often difficult to differentiate these two illnesses. Infection is usually spread from the nose and throat to the lower part of the lung.

Treatment. Although in the feverish stage the child should be as little disturbed as possible, his position must be changed regularly so as to drain away fluid and excess mucus, and to prevent bedsores. Plenty of boiled (partly cooled) water, and fruit juices are necessary for the patient, and milk is less important for the first few days. Antibiotics will be prescribed by the doctor according to the micro-organisms causing the pneumonia.

The bronchitic child may be the 'father' of the bronchitic man for the child does not easily grow out of it.

Cough

A cough is a symptom of an infection or disorder affecting the throat and respiratory organs. To remedy the cough the underlying cause must be dealt with. Common causal conditions are:

- Infected tonsils and adenoids
- Sore throat, inflammation of the throat
- Bronchitis, bronchopneumonia
- Measles
- Nervousness and indigestion
- Whooping-cough; this cough comes in paroxysms and is worse at night.

Young children are rarely able to expectorate adequately and the sputum is usually swallowed. This can lead to further infection unless the underlying cause is put right. The bowels should be kept in good order, too.

Suppressive Treatment. To suppress a troublesome cough, particularly in bronchitis, an infant of about six months may be given a cough medicine containing codeine under a doctor's direction. To assist sleep, 200 milligrams of chloral hydrate may be given.

Steam medication, using a special kettle with a long funnel, often brings relief. To the water in the kettle 1 to 2 teaspoonsful of compound benzoin tincture is added, and the steam flows into a homemade tent made by placing a sheet over the crib (leaving the foot end open for the entry of the steam).

Deformities of the Chest

Deformities of the chest wall may occur with surprising rapidity in early childhood as a result of faulty breathing associated with disease. The commonest deformities are pigeon chest and funnel-shaped chest.

Pigeon Chest. In this the thorax comes to a point in front, and the lower ribs are drawn inwards owing to deficient entry of air into the chest and a consequent diminu-

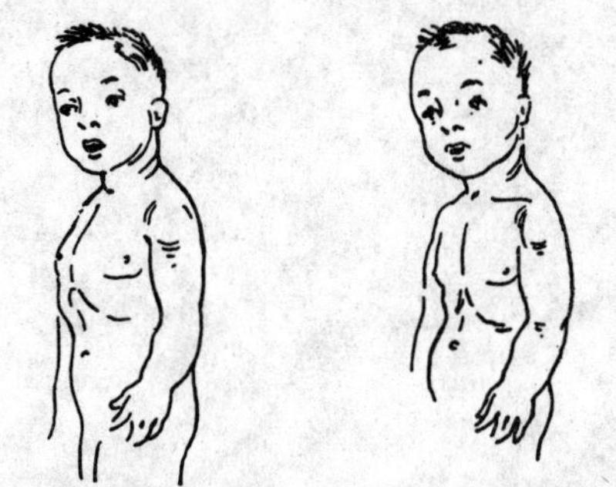

Fig. 8. *PIGEON CHEST* and *FUNNEL-SHAPED CHEST in young children.*

tion of its natural movements. This may occur in obstruction of the throat and nose by enlarged tonsils and adenoids, in whooping-cough, and after recurrent attacks of bronchitis.

The Funnel-shaped Chest, in which the breast-bone is depressed and drawn inwards towards the spine, is seen in weakly children.

As growth and development proceed in conjunction with improved health, most children with chest deformities tend to improve. Drill, gymnastic exercises and breathing exercises are of the greatest importance in helping to correct the deformity.

Breathing Exercises. They should be carried out in the open or in a room with widely open windows. The clothing should be light. The exercises should be practiced for ten minutes three times a day for about two months. Then the time may be reduced to five minutes morning and evening as a regular habit for at least twelve months.

Before beginning the exercises, the nose should be blown vigorously on a handkerchief to clear the nostrils. Inhalation through the nose should then be practiced with the teeth clenched and the mouth firmly closed.

In order to secure concentration on the proper movements of the diaphragm, it is usually helpful to start the course with the child lying down, with the knees drawn up, arms loosely at the sides, and shoulders kept well down. When breathing in, the child should learn to keep the upper part of the chest still, so that the breathing is performed mainly by the diaphragm. When breathing out, the abdominal wall should contract, sinking in towards the spine.

The diaphragmatic breathing may be followed by blowing exercises in the standing position. Small balls of paper or ping-pong balls should be blown across a table. There must be one long blow, not many short ones.

Enlargement of the Neck Glands

Enlargement of the lymphatic glands of the neck is extremely common, and may be found at any age. They are in fact more often enlarged than any other set of glands, but in all cases the glands of the elbow region, armpits and groins should be examined as well. The enlargement may be acute or chronic.

Acute Enlargement. This is generally an indication of septic absorption from some focus of inflammation in the surrounding area.

TONSILS AND ADENOIDS. In the case of infected tonsils and adenoids the first glands to be involved are those below and behind the angle of the lower jaw.

THE FACE AND SCALP. In cases of inflammation of the lower lip, chin or lower jaw, e.g. impetigo, the glands beneath the lower jaw are found to be enlarged. Inflammation of the scalp causes enlargement of the glands at the back of the neck.

German measles often causes enlargement of the glands at the back of the neck.

Treatment should in all cases be directed to eliminating the cause.

Chronic Tuberculous Enlargement is due, as a rule, to infection taking place through the tonsils. It is generally an entirely localized condition, with no evidence of tuberculosis elsewhere in the body, and it seldom leads to generalized infection of the system.

It usually affects children between the ages of two and four. At first the infected glands are separate and painless, but softening may occur later with reddening of the overlying skin.

Treatment. If the enlargement is extensive and the general condition of the child is poor, a general tuberculosis routine is essential, with complete rest, good feeding with extra vitamins, cod-liver oil, etc., open air and sunshine.

Ear Infections

Throat infections in small children may spread along the course of the Eustachian tube to the inner ear causing otitis media and also leading to mastoiditis. This is dealt with in the section on Diseases of the Ear, Nose and Throat, p. 330.

DISEASES OF OLD AGE

THE CHANGES OCCURRING IN ADVANCED LIFE

Growth, maturity and decline are the three main phases of our life as human beings. During the period of growth or development the constructive processes of the body are more active than are those of a destructive nature due to wear and tear. In old age a reversal of these processes becomes apparent, and the body organs and tissues fail to carry out their functions as efficiently; they gradually become less active and produce less energy and, unless some illness or disability intervenes, there is a slowly progressive decline in recuperative powers and capacity for action or effort.

In old age the inevitable and progressive loss of vitality may be accelerated by factors such as ill health, illness or an unfavorable mode of life or habits.

For most people a gradual adjustment to a life within their capacities must be made as age increases, but many persons cannot merely resign themselves to tedious inactivity and must find new interests and pursuits which make less demand upon their energies. It is indeed greatly to their advantage and contentment that they should do so, since satisfactory diversions of mind and body will often prevent undue introspection and preoccupation with minor disabilities. The general health should receive care and attention, with avoidance of worry, strain, excesses, or exposure to infection.

The Aging Process

The aging process continues throughout the lifespan of each individual. All the processes which are involved are not yet fully understood—nor why some people 'age' quicker than others. Wide individual differences have been found during investigations of aging, and certainly the slow failing of the controlling endocrine glands and their hormone secretions, as well as of the delicate tissues of the nervous system, play an important part in the gradual breakdown of regulatory mechanisms.

Most, but not all, physiological processes show progressive changes with age. The blood sugar and the osmotic pressure of the blood, for example, remain the same throughout the life of a normal person. On the other hand the actual amount of blood pumped through the heart is diminished, and the kidneys become less efficient at excreting waste products. The blood pressure and the pulse rate recover more slowly after exercise as a person grows older.

Why is this? It has been found that there is an actual gradual loss of active cells in various organs, especially in the cardiovascular and genito-urinary systems. Moreover it is probable that the cells remaining in old tissues are less able to do their work.

DISEASES IN OLD AGE

In many persons the effects of past illnesses or injuries only become apparent in later life and are the causes of various disabilities in old age; they may play as big a part in causing senility as factors of heredity.

The following diseases are only considered in so far as they relate to old age. Fuller details of the diseases and their treatment will be found in the respective sections dealing with the heart, the chest, the digestive system, etc.

Cardiovascular Diseases

High Blood Pressure (*Hypertension*). Gradual changes in the walls of the blood vessels, with hardening and loss of elasticity (arteriosclerosis), bring about circulatory impairment in the various systems of the body. About 23 per cent of persons over fifty years of age die from the effects of high blood pressure, nevertheless fairly high systolic pressures, at about 200 millimeters of mercury, may persist for a number of years without causing an undue degree of heart failure or other ill effects, providing the arterial walls are not markedly diseased. When gross arteriosclerosis is present, the blood vessels of the brain, heart, kidney or eye may be affected. Possible complications include strokes, heart failure, coronary thrombosis, and deterioration of vision.

TREATMENT depends on the severity of the high blood pressure. If there are no symptoms then no specific treatment is advised. Otherwise, general management includes reduction of weight in the obese, modification of physical (and mental) activities, rest, and salt restriction. Drugs to reduce the blood pressure (hypotensive drugs) may be used. These drugs fall into three main groups: centrally acting drugs of the rauwolfia group, ganglion blocking drugs, and peripherally acting drugs (see also p. 307). These drugs must be used with care in the aged as mental confusion or cerebral thrombosis can result when the blood pressure is unwisely lowered.

Heart Disease. As age advances the heart may be affected in a number of ways. There may be valvular disease or muscle impairment, the blood vessels supplying the heart may be diseased or the heart affected as a result of respiratory disease (cor pulmonale). The heart tires more easily in these cases and is less capable of sudden strain or prolonged effort.

When heart failure sets in there are warning symptoms of breathlessness on exertion, swelling of the ankles or legs, cough, and sometimes blueness of the lips. When coronary artery disease is present, angina pectoris or coronary thrombosis may develop. Cardiac asthma is a characteristic condition associated with heart failure and usually high blood pressure in old persons.

TREATMENT of heart failure includes rest, diet, and restriction of the use of salt in foods and drinks, with the administration of digitalis and, maybe, diuretics.

Patients with coronary thrombosis are often treated in hospital, especially if the attack is severe. Anticoagulant drugs are not generally used after the age of 65 as the resulting diminished blood coagulation may give rise to cerebral hemorrhage or other disorders.

Cardiac asthma may be very distressing and then requires immediate treatment with morphine, aminophylline, and oxygen.

Respiratory Diseases

Bronchitis. Many old people suffer from chronic bronchitis.

CAUSES. Factors which play an important part in causing this distressing condition are smoking, irritant substances in dust, smoke or fumes, and damp and cold. In some cases the bronchitis follows a severe respiratory infection. The condition is always worse in winter when further bronchial irritation occurs. Especially dangerous is smog. The high humidity reduces dispersal of the polluted air which is inhaled into the bronchi and causes excessive secretion of mucus. Other dangers to the bronchitic in winter are cold air and ice-cold bedrooms, especially if the sufferer has been breathing in well-warmed air in a warm room during the day. The contrast is a shock to the lung tissues.

TREATMENT aims, in the first place, at reducing bronchial irritation. A move to a dry, warm, clean climate is seldom possible, but avoidance of adverse weather conditions, and living in a warm house are essential. Doors and windows should be sealed during fog. Much benefit is obtained by giving up smoking.

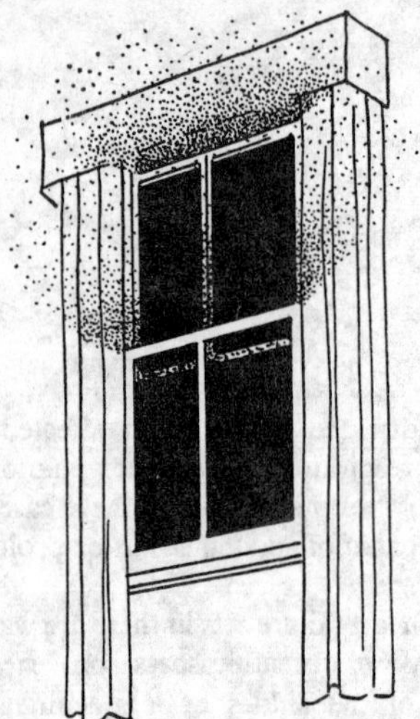

Fig. 1. *SMOG is devastating to those who suffer from bronchitis. It will creep through every crack and cranny. Shut windows closely on foggy smoke-polluted days.*

Antibiotics are used during attacks of acute bronchitis due to infection. In some people acute infections are so frequent that continuous antibiotic treatment (usually tetracycline) is advised. Other drugs used include bronchodilators (e.g. ephedrine) to control wheezing, and cough mixtures.

Pneumonia. This is more common in older persons and is especially prone to develop after operations, fractures, or other illnesses necessitating prolonged rest in bed. For this reason the elderly patient should not be kept in bed for longer than is absolutely necessary. The mortality rate from pneumonia is much higher in old people than in younger subjects, the heart being unable to endure the period of strain or the toxemia (see pp. 272-74).

Prompt recognition of the condition, and treatment with modern antibiotics have reduced the danger to a certain extent, but there are some types of pneumonia in the elderly debilitated patient where antibiotics are less effective, and in these cases skilled nursing is of the utmost value.

Alimentary Canal Diseases

Dyspepsia, flatulence, constipation and other digestive disorders are common in old age, but should not be ignored.

Cancer. In dyspepsia with loss of appetite, cancer of the stomach may be present and an investigation by a doctor should be made. The passage of blood in the feces with loss of weight, alternating constipation and diarrhea, and perhaps colic, suggest cancer of the bowel.

Constipation. The weakness of the various muscles around the back passage in an elderly person predisposes to constipation. If ignored, constipation can cause a lot of distress in this age group, and a stage may be reached where the feces become impacted in the lower bowel and will necessitate manual removal.

TREATMENT. Drastic purgation is harmful. Suitable exercises to try and improve the musculature may be of benefit. A high roughage diet is advisable; this will include plenty of green vegetables, carrots, parsnips, peas and wholemeal bread. The all bran cereal is a useful source of roughage—and the person should be advised to drink plenty of water. If the doctor prescribes a laxative, his instructions concerning the dose must be carefully adhered to. The distasteful enema which used to be a routine treatment in cases of severe chronic constipation has been replaced, to some extent, by suppositories These are a valuable form of treatment and have made life more pleasant for many elderly persons.

The *Lactobacillus* in yoghurt is often helpful in maintaining a less constipated condition of the bowel in old people.

Hemorrhoids *(piles)* are very common and are worse in a constipated person. They may cause considerable discomfort and pain. Piles are occasionally caused by disease in the intestine, e.g. cancer of the rectum, and should therefore be seen by a doctor.

Kidney and Bladder Diseases

The kidneys usually function less well in the general arteriosclerosis which affects persons with arterial disease. There is a tendency to ascending bladder and kidney infection in old people. This type of infection is apt to be chronic or recurrent and, although it may be comparatively symptomless or may only give rise to discomfort such as scalding or frequency of micturition, and aching of the back

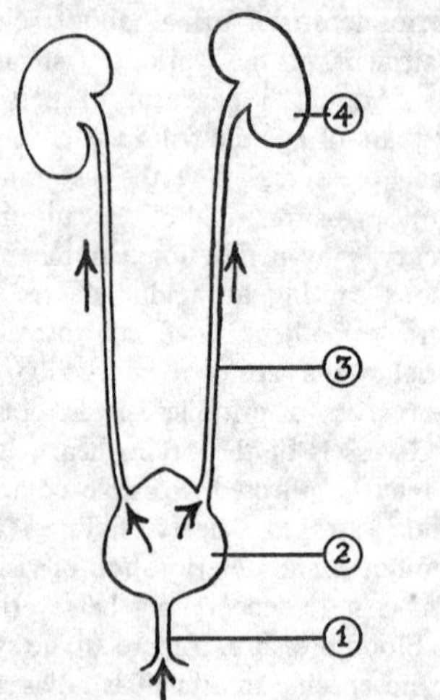

Fig. 2. *ASCENDING KIDNEY INFECTION. A mild infection of the urethra, if neglected, especially in older people, can cause infection of the bladder (cystitis) which, in turn, if untreated, may spread upwards to the kidneys.*

or bladder, it will nevertheless (if not treated) cause kidney changes which interfere with the excretion of waste products.

In men, enlargement of the prostate gland is generally present in about 50 per cent of those over seventy years of age. Prostatic stone or bladder stone is also commoner in old people (see Diseases of the Urinary System, p. 415).

Central Nervous System Diseases

Strokes. The elderly person with a high blood pressure and degenerative disease of the blood vessels of the brain is especially liable to suffer a stroke. Apoplexy may have a sudden onset with loss of consciousness passing to deep coma, or it may come on gradually, frequently during sleep. The commonest type of stroke is a cerebral thrombosis. Other types include cerebral hemorrhage and embolism.

The results of a stroke depend on the portion of the brain involved. Some cases, where a large portion of the brain is affected, are fatal within a few hours or days of the onset. Some result in paralysis of one side of the body which may be temporary or permanent. Other possible sequels include slurred speech, paralysis of one side of the face, loss of speech, and incontinence of urine. (See pp. 430-31).

TREATMENT. Management and nursing are the essentials of treatment. While the patient is unconscious special attention should be paid to keeping the air passages clear (false teeth out), moving him from side to side to avoid lung congestion, and preventing bedsores. Penicillin may be advised to prevent pneumonia.

When consciousness is regained the encouraging outlook of relatives and medical staff is most important. Modern physiotherapy methods and various ingenious mechanical aids are capable of rehabilitating a large percentage of patients who have suffered from a stroke.

Senile Dementia. This is the condition commonly known as second childhood. It is due to degenerative disease of brain blood vessels. The patient is forgetful, querulous, irritable and perhaps suspicious, or he may be disinterested, simple-minded and apparently oblivious of current events, or helpless in regard to personal care and hygiene. Simple senile degeneration is generally associated with changes in character and intelligence, especially in comprehension and powers of memory.

Senile delirium is accompanied by hallucinations and fear, and may develop after injuries or operations. It may be of short duration, but in chronic cases death may follow from exhaustion. Increased sexual excitability is often noted, and sleeplessness at night is often distressing. The patient is generally self-centered, with delusions; he may be avaricious, malicious, and develop untidy or dirty habits. Finally there may be complete childishness, loss of memory, and indifference to friends, events, or personal care.

Paralysis Agitans. When cerebral atheroma affects a certain part of the brain (the basal ganglia) paralysis agitans (Parkinsonism) results. The features of this condition are a mask-like face, tremor of the eyelids, jaw and limbs, muscle rigidity, dribbling of saliva and a shuffling gait (p. 433).

The rigidity and dribbling may be controlled to a certain degree by drugs.

Skin Diseases

The dry and impoverished condition of the skin in old age predisposes to various complaints such as bedsores, parasitic disorders, eczema, varicose ulcers or varicose eczema, pruritus and prurigo, warts, and ecthyma. Scrupulous cleanliness will prevent many of these disorders, and a thorough toilet should be performed daily.

Pigmentation is also a common occurrence in elderly persons; it may be most conspicuous on the exposed parts such as the face, neck and hands, or may develop in patches over the trunk and limbs.

Cancer of the skin (epithelioma) and rodent ulcer are sometimes seen in persons of advanced years. A rodent ulcer is usually situated on the face, and is now treated by irradiation with good prospects of cure (see Diseases of the Skin, p. 478).

Bone and Joint Diseases

Fractures. The bones become rarefied and brittle in old age, and thus fractures are common results of falls or injuries. Union of the bone fragments is apt to be slow and convalescence tedious. In the case of fractures of the leg it is unwise to keep the patient in bed for a prolonged period of time as pneumonia, encouraged by static position, is a common sequel. It should be emphasized that even a slight trip-up is enough to cause

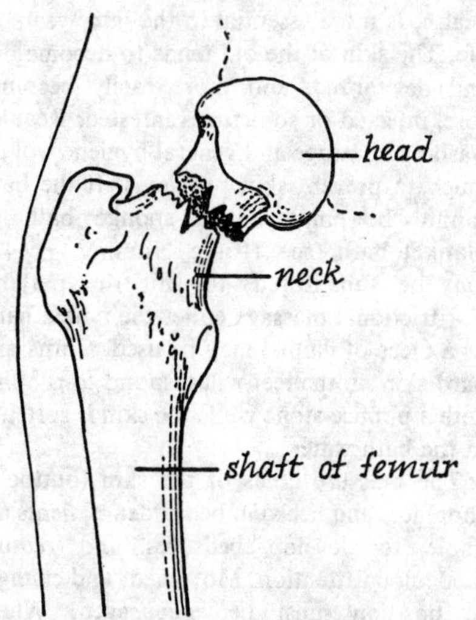

Fig. 3. *FRACTURE OF NECK OF FEMUR. One of the more common fractures occurring in old people who fall.*

a fracture of the upper part of the leg (neck of femur) in an elderly person. This type of fracture is sometimes overlooked, especially where the patient is stubborn and does not want the doctor called. Delayed treatment often results in a permanent disability.

Arthritis. Arthritis, especially osteoarthritis, is very prevalent in old people; the hip, knees and spine are the sites generally affected, and the pain and stiffness are indeed an affliction, and often severely limit the patient's activities. Deformities of the finger joints (Heberden's nodes) are a common but less painful occurrence, the pain often disappearing in earlier years while the swelling persists (pp. 529 and 531).

TREATMENT. Physiotherapy and mechanical aids can help the patient a great deal. Physiotherapy at home is ideal in severe cases, as many elderly persons dislike having to be taken to the hospital several times a week.

Cancer

Although cancer commonly develops after the age of forty or forty-five, it increases in frequency in persons up to about eighty-five years; the incidence of this disease then declines. In old people cancer is often only slowly progressive owing to the low state of vitality of the body.

TREATMENT. The treatment of a particular cancer will depend on its site and on how far it has already progressed. Because of its slow growth in the older person a bright outlook of permanent cure can be held in many cases.

The forms of treatment include surgical operation and/or irradiation (radiotherapy with X-rays, beta particles, and radioactive isotopes). Sex hormones may be used in the treatment of cancer of the prostate and the breast.

MEDICAL TREATMENT OF THE OLD

A good relationship between the patient and his doctor is of the greatest importance in geriatric practice. When choosing a new doctor for an old person a sympathetic physician who has time and patience are the qualities to look for.

Although little is known about the influence of old age on drug action, certain factors should be borne in mind when medicines are required for old people.

SMALLER DOSES. The torpid condition of the system in old age often necessitates smaller doses of medicine.

FLUID MEDICINES. Pills and powders sometimes pass through the stomach and bowels in the same state in which they are swallowed. Fluids are more readily effective, especially when the more active medicinal ingredient is mixed with wine, or some stimulating tincture, or aromatic water.

MEDICINE BY RECTUM. It is sometimes necessary to administer drugs via the rectum, in cases where the patient cannot swallow.

Suitable Medicines for the Old

The potential dangers of anticoagulants and hypotensive drugs in the elderly have already been mentioned. A similar risk of coronary or cerebral thrombosis exists if over-zealous administration of antidiabetic drugs gives rise to hypoglycemia.

The **corticosteroids,** too, must be used with caution because of their side-action on the skeleton, which is already brittle in the elderly.

All metallic medicines must be given sparingly, and with caution. Iodine and potassium iodide are not very well tolerated by old people.

Narcotics must sometimes be used but habitual use of sedatives should be avoided when possible. Routine use of a sedative drug is sometimes necessary to induce sleep.

Bromides and **barbiturates** have a tendency to accumulate in the old and may give rise to confusion and restlessness. The danger of accidental overdosage with barbiturates is increased where the old person is absent-minded or confused, and these drugs are toxic in the presence of alcohol.

The barbiturate group of drugs can be useful, however, if the above facts are borne in mind.

Tranquilizers. The tranquilizer drugs are of great value in the geriatric field: chlorpromazine is especially effective in senile confusion; phenelzine and imipramine are used in depressive states *(but they are very dangerous if taken together).* Where morning stimulation is necessary, dexamphetamine is useful.

Vitamins. Some cases of senile confusion, where undernutrition and/or alcoholism are prominent features, will respond well to vitamin injections in massive doses.

Tonics. Various tonics, bitters and carminatives may be of value to an elderly person who feels he is deriving benefit from them.

Surgical Operations

The spectacular advances in modern anesthesia in recent years has meant that age itself is no longer a contraindication to surgery, whether of a minor or major nature.

If the general health of the patient is such that a general anesthetic is inadvisable then local anesthesia may be used (see p. 597).

GENERAL CARE

Habits

Old persons often lose the power of adapting themselves to change. The discontinuance of the moderate habitual use of alcohol or tobacco by an old person, although the use of either has an acknowledged harmful tendency, will frequently prove distressing or even fatal. It is generally better that moderately indulgent habits of the aged should be allowed to remain unless some intercurrent illness requires them to be modified.

The various social services available to the elderly, and the ways in which emotional difficulties can be avoided, especially in 'rejected' old people, are fully dealt with in the section 'Grandparents and the Elderly,' pp. 153–59.

Diet

The diet of old people should be easy to digest. It should contain sufficient vitamins, milk, protein and cereals, but rich foods and much fat are better avoided. Small, light and frequent meals are generally best for persons of advanced years. They should never eat to excess or repletion, but should eat slowly and chew their food very thoroughly.

Fats. There is evidence to suggest that unsaturated fatty acids contained in animal fat play a part in the causation of arteriosclerosis (hardening of the arteries). Medical opinion is divided on this matter, but it is reasonable to suggest that butter and fatty meat should be restricted, and vegetable oil should be used in cooking.

Milk is a nutritious food for most old persons; it may be citrated to make it more digestible. Yoghurt, and peptonized milk are very easily digested by infants or by old persons. Various types of baby foods are useful during times of illness when a light diet is advised, or in old people who are not able to chew their food. They are of special value when a busy housewife has little time to prepare this type of diet.

Vegetables and Fruits. Potatoes, beets, carrots, parsnips and asparagus are generally suitable vegetables; peas, beans, cabbages, etc., should not be eaten in cases of dyspepsia for fear of causing mechanical irritation and providing too much roughage.

Ripe fruits taken in moderation are refreshing. Among these, ripe apples, pears, peaches, bananas, apricots and grapes are useful sources of vitamin C, and their consumption should be encouraged.

Wine and alcohol in moderation should not be withheld if the elderly person wants it, except in certain conditions such as digestive disturbances. Indeed, drinking a glass of beer can be of real value during convalescence and

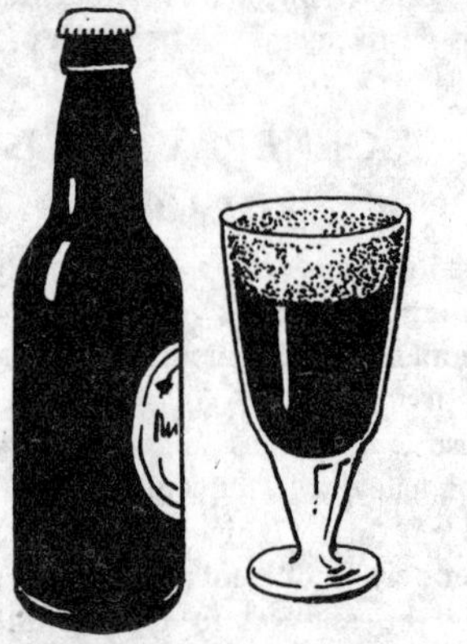

Fig. 4. *A GLASS OF BEER provides a pleasant and nourishing 'pick-me-up' for old people.*

in debility. Beer has a high calorie and carbohydrate content and the live yeast it contains is a rich source of vitamin B.

It must be remembered, however, that alcohol should not be given to a person who is taking barbiturates.

Nutritional Deficiencies in Older People

These arise from a continually faulty or insufficient diet which, in old people living alone, sometimes becomes either generally poor in quantity, or in variety, or both. Poverty, ignorance, incapacity, inability to go shopping or plan meals, debility and dislike of cooking appetizing dishes may all play a part in causing a state of subnutrition or malnutrition in old and lonely people. A diet that is reduced in quantity is very often also poor in the quality of the essential items required for adequate nourishment. It is not always very easy to detect mild subnutrition or lack of certain food factors, but loss in weight or flabbiness of skin are indicative, and there may be signs of vitamin deficiencies.

The commonest fault is probably the preponderance in the diet of the cheaper carbohydrate articles (cereals, bread, biscuits, and other starchy foods), with lack of the more expensive protein items (meat, fish, eggs, cheese and milk) and of vegetables and fresh fruit.

The 'Meals on Wheels' scheme, run in many areas by volunteers for bringing appetizing, ready-prepared hot meals to old people who live alone, is a great advance in the prevention of nutritional deficiencies. These welfare facilities help to guard the health of the less robust or perhaps slightly incapacitated elderly person who, by this service, can continue to live in his own home, where he is usually happier than in hospital or in an institution.

Old people who prepare food for themselves should not rely too much on pots of tea and bread and butter or margarine; stewed fruit, grated or cream cheese should be substituted for jam sometimes. Eggs are easily cooked in a variety of ways. Fruit purees, lettuce, cress, tomatoes, and other digestible salads are appetizing and help to guard against constipation. Vegetable soups also provide a variety of flavor and, with added milk, whole barley, or thickened with oat, pea, or wholemeal flour, are suitable for evening suppers. Milk puddings (blancmange or custard) or milk and cereals are easily digested; jellies may be eaten with sponge cake or oaten biscuits.

Milk drinks may be varied by flavoring with cocoa, or other proprietary milk foods. These are easily prepared and are especially useful at bedtime as they help to overcome sleeplessness.

When nutrition has been neglected and the patient comes under medical care, food concentrates containing concentrated protein, vitamins and minerals are frequently advised.

In severe cases, hospital admission may be necessary for the purpose of general care and urgent nutritional restoration. Treatment usually includes the administration of vitamins and iron by injection.

Sleep

Aged people should have sufficient rest and sleep. They should retire at a reasonable hour and often require more sleep than persons in middle life. Eight or ten hours in the twenty-four is not too much in most cases. An afternoon rest is also often refreshing.

Many old people get up very early; they disturb a household (sometimes because they are deaf or have to potter about in the half-dark without their glasses) by making early breakfast, and so on. This early rising is often just a bad habit, although early morning insomnia in the aged is a well recognized phenomenon. A later bedtime may solve the problem.

Sleeplessness. Although the old require a good deal of rest, it is unfortunate that many can only sleep for short periods. A large number of persons advanced in life complain of inability to sleep. Many old people deceive themselves and really sleep much more than they are aware, but they often insist that they cannot sleep at all, night after night.

Narcotics and sedatives should be avoided if possible, but it is sometimes necessary to resort to them, in which case they should be prescribed by a doctor. Sleep may sometimes be encouraged by taking an earlier or a lighter supper, or by gentle exercise in the open air. Occasionally a glass of wine, or a little dilute whisky taken just before retiring will induce somnolence. Light reading in bed may also be of help.

Care of the Skin

Attention to the skin, always important to health, is more essential in the later years of life. The skin of the old tends to become dry and devitalized, and more easily becomes sore, infected or sometimes infested. Regular washing, massage and general hygiene will do much to prevent skin problems. If the bath cannot be employed, a sponge bath or blanket bath (see Home Nursing, p. 47) may be substituted, to suit the patient. For frictional massage either the naked hand or a piece of flannel may be used. Corns and hard skin on the feet will respond to rubbing with a pumice-stone while the skin is softened in the bath water.

The pressure areas of the skin (buttocks, shoulders and heels) in bedridden patients are liable to develop bedsores and require meticulous attention. Movement and changes in position must be encouraged. Where normal turning of the body is impracticable, an alternating air pressure mattress is of great value. Alcohol rubs, regularly carried out, are also useful in preventing bedsores. See also Home Nursing, p. 47.

Exercise

Always important during all periods of life, moderate exercise is also often beneficial in old age, but the aged should always exercise with discretion, and not immediately after a meal has been taken. Walking and light work in the garden are suitable when they can be undertaken, bearing in mind that undue fatigue is injurious.

Susceptibility to Cold

Aged people sometimes suffer very much from cold hands and feet and, indeed, from poor circulation and low temperature generally. This is mainly due to hardening of the arteries. The clothing of old people should be loose, and warmer than that of younger people. Wool, or wool and silk, may be worn next to the skin; woolen clothes are generally required in cold weather, being poor conductors of heat. Unless they are obese, old people seldom suffer discomfort from heat.

During winter nights, the old, especially those who are prone to attacks of angina pectoris, are apt to suffer very much from cold. On going to bed, therefore, they should be warm; and on cold nights they should have a hot-water bottle or an electric blanket. A window can be kept partially open if desired. However, in industrial atmospheres open windows will do more harm than good in winter.

It is not generally realized that, apart from winter illness, the effect of very low environmental temperature itself can have extremely dangerous consequences to the elderly. Due to inadequate provision of warmth from hot-water bottles, warm bedding, enough food, etc., the very old may develop the condition of accidental hypothermia, a grave state of affairs which may prove fatal.

DISEASES OF THE JOINTS AND MUSCLES

AFFECTIONS OF THE JOINTS

Arthritis

A joint consists of the ends of the bones forming the joint, together with their ligaments, joint capsule, the cartilage covering the bone surfaces, and the joint membrane called the synovial membrane. Any of these different parts may be affected in arthritis, according to the form of disease present, while in synovitis the synovial membrane is mainly involved.

Arthritis is the name given to certain diseases of the joints; they may be of an inflammatory nature, as in tuberculosis, or may be due to wear and tear, causing damage of the joint as in osteo-arthritis, or may be due to the involvement of the tissues of the joint in a general bodily stress reaction as in acute rheumatism.

Arthritis may be due to many causes, some of which are recognized and others remain doubtful.

1. **Arthritis arising from Known Causes.**

(a) From injury which often becomes chronic.

(b) From infections due to gonococcal, dysenteric, or pneumococcal organisms, or tuberculosis, or associated with specific diseases such as scarlet fever, enteric fevers, syphilis and septicemia.

(c) From gout.

(d) From nervous disorders.

(e) From blood disease such as hemophilia and purpura.

(f) From deficiency diseases such as rickets or scurvy.

2. **Arthritis due to Obscure Causes.**

(a) To acute rheumatism.

(b) To infective forms of unknown or non-specific origin.

Some of these diseases begin in the cartilage, some develop in the synovial membrane, and others in the heads of the bones, but they do not necessarily remain confined to the original structure, and one form merges into another, so that arthritis may be accompanied by synovitis, etc.

Effusion, or the secretion of fluid into the joint cavity, is a common sign of irritation and causes swelling, usually with some pain. It may not always be easy to diagnose the cause or extent of joint affections at the beginning, and in most cases an X-ray investigation is advisable in all but simple sprains. Even if the acute condition subsides there may be residual loss of movement, stability or strength, or a tendency to chronic arthritis, and much depends on correct treatment in the early stages.

Infective Arthritis

Tuberculous Joint Disease

This begins in the synovial membrane, or in the periosteum, or in the bone end; it is commonest in children or young adults. The hip or knee is most frequently affected, and the early symptoms are pain, limitation of movement, and wasting of the muscles round the joint, with perhaps a hot skin, and some fluid in the cavity. Later, swelling and sharp pain at night occur. If untreated, abscesses and fever will follow.

The disease tends to be very chronic, and the treatment requires complete rest and immobilization of the joint by splints or plaster, with sanatorium or general tuberculous treatment. The outlook is favorable if the disease is treated early (see pp. 352-3).

Gonococcal Arthritis

This condition is not very common, and vigorous penicillin treatment produces excellent improvement. (See also Venereal Diseases, p. 291.)

Pneumococcal, Typhoid and Pyemic Arthritis

These forms require specialized treatment, related to the original disease. Antibiotics may be used in the early stages, but arthritic joints are treated as for chronic rheumatic diseases in general (see below).

Rheumatic Diseases in General

Rheumatic diseases, both of the acute and chronic types, are unfortunately very prevalent in countries with temperate climates, and are a serious source of ill health.

COLLAGEN DISEASES. Rheumatic fever, rheumatoid arthritis, polyarteritis nodosa, systemic lupus erythematosus and associated diseases form a group which are sometimes called collagen diseases. Collagen fibers are part of the loosely structured connective tissue (see Fig. 3 in Anatomy, p. 218) which is found all over the body; it gives support to various organs, carries blood vessels from one part to another, and forms a supporting framework for the lining of blood vessels and the lining of the synovial sacs in joints. When there is degeneration of collagen fibers the connective tissue may collapse. What causes this degeneration is not yet known but it is suggested that some allergic process may account for it.

RHEUMATOID ARTHRITIS generally runs a chronic course for many years, but it is never too late for some hope of improvement. In severe cases, unless treated, the disease progresses intermittently, with increasing joint deformity and disability. Only about 10 per cent of cases are seriously crippled, and the outlook depends on early remedial treatment.

Sedimentation tests of the blood should be carried out at regular intervals, and any underlying disorder or predisposing causes of the rheumatic condition must be attended to. Local infection (as from decayed teeth or infected tonsils), an unhygienic environment, poor general constitution, unsuitable occupation, recent illnesses, grief, and so forth may all play a part in favoring the onset of rheumatoid arthritis.

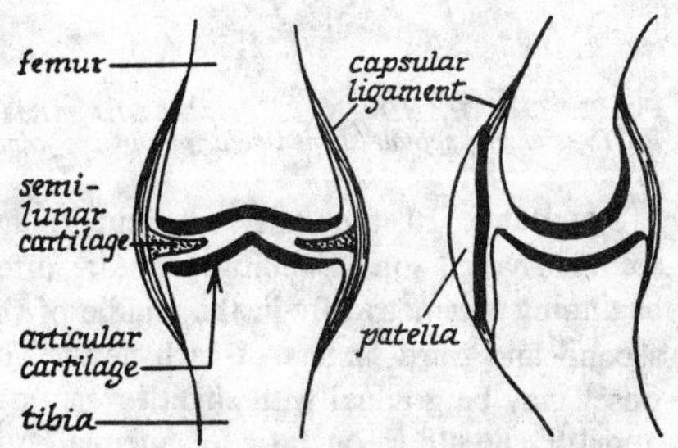

Fig. 1. *KNEE JOINT (front and side views). Despite its simplification, the diagram shows how vulnerable is the joint, with its complexity of tissues, to infection, inflammation, damage, and strains.*

Often a fairly long course of treatment is required, and must be conscientiously persevered in, since no sudden or dramatic results or benefits can be expected.

Chronic arthritis is not confined only to elderly people, and in fact rheumatoid arthritis typically affects women (in the proportion of 3 women to 1 man) in their forties.

OSTEO-ARTHRITIS occurs rather later in life, generally after the age of forty years. This disease is really a degenerative condition of the joints, often as a result of wear and tear, although there may be a constitutional tendency underlying the aging process of the joint structures.

It is increasingly believed that minor congenital abnormalities of the joints can lead to the development of osteo-arthritis. Falls or occupational injuries which affect the joints can also accelerate the degeneration process, e.g. agricultural workers are often affected in the hips and spine.

Rheumatoid Arthritis

Causes. The causes of this disease are still uncertain, and are probably multiple; cases are divided into an infective or toxic type, and a non-infective variety which is probably due to glandular or constitutional disturbances. Rheumatoid arthritis is often familial; poor feeding, damp or ill-ventilated houses are contributory factors, and influenza, shock, or anxiety may precede an attack. Rarely, gonorrhea may be responsible. The complexion often becomes sallow, and the appetite and body weight diminish, while numb and cold extremities, irregular menstruation, and digestive disorders are common.

A menopausal form of rheumatoid arthritis is also recognized, developing during or after the climacteric.

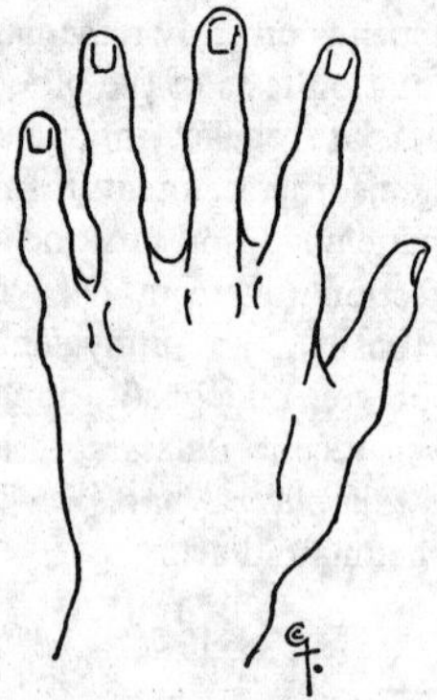

Fig. 2. *THE HAND IN RHEUMATOID ARTHRITIS, showing spindle-shaped deformity of the joints.*

Symptoms. In the early or acute stage spindle-shaped joint swellings appear, often beginning symmetrically in the middle of the second and third fingers of each hand. The onset may be gradual with slight fever, poor appetite, lassitude or fatigue, anemia, and loss of weight; the hand muscles undergo

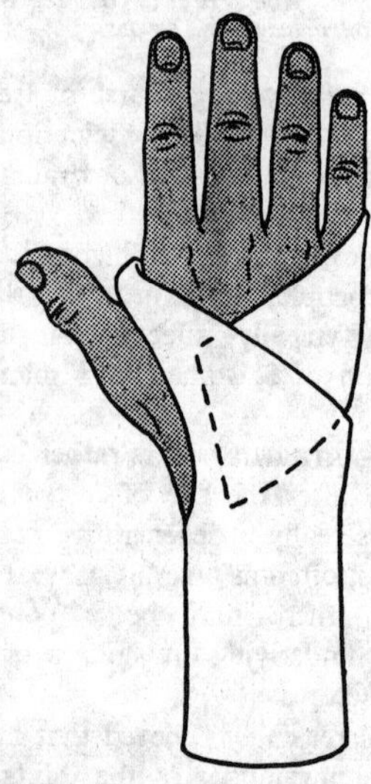

Fig. 3. *PLASTER SPLINT for the hand of a patient with acute rheumatoid arthritis. In the early stages of the disease, complete immobilization of the swollen joints is essential.*

wasting and the fingers become bent. Soon the wrists and elbows may be involved, and less frequently the knees; pain is considerable and may interfere with proper sleep. The disease often abates during pregnancy, but later on reappears with added severity.

In rheumatoid arthritis (as opposed to osteo-arthritis and intermediate forms) the soft tissues around the joint are first affected, the inflammation then spreading to the cartilages which may adhere together and cause permanent stiffness. Anemia may occur, with pallor and an accompanying rapid pulse, and perhaps slight breathlessness. The acute stage may subside in six months or longer in older persons, but the chronic form of the disease often persists.

Treatment

Treatment varies according to the stage of the disease developed in the patient when he comes under medical care. In early acute cases, treatment is directed towards relief of symptoms, improvement of general health, and in the use of the affected joints.

General Measures in Acute Conditions. When several joints are swollen and there is general malaise with fever and anemia, complete rest in bed is necessary for several weeks or months, during which time careful nursing is required. Patients are sometimes nursed on lamb's skin to protect pressure points. A firm mattress, open texture blankets, and footrests with footcages to support the bedclothes are used to prevent foot deformities, and maintenance exercises are given for general health. The rest from use and weight-bearing helps relieve the pain and spasm.

Diet should be ample, with plenty of protein, eggs, milk and fruit—vitamin C is important for stimulation of the metabolism of collagen tissue.

Acutely swollen joints are immobilized in plaster of Paris splints for one to two weeks since rest is better than passive movements in the early stages. When the swelling and pain have subsided the splints can be removed, and active exercises are given several times a day to prevent permanent stiffness; heat is also beneficial. When the fever drops the patient is allowed up for increasing periods, and physiotherapy is given, with wax baths for the hands and feet, faradic footbaths, radiant heat, infra-red rays or short-wave diathermy. (See Physiotherapy, p.176.)

In Chronic Cases physiotherapeutic measures are still needed. Hydrotherapy (see p. 177) is particularly beneficial. Active movement, exercise, and massage under the guidance of a skilled physiotherapist will prevent worsening of deformities and enable once-bedridden patients to become gently ambulant.

For those with fixed deformities, especially of the hips and other joints, plaster casts are most valuable in taking the strain from the muscles. Crutches and walking cylinders should, if possible, be used only as interim aids until the patient's muscles are re-educated.

Occupational therapy, e.g. weaving, basket making, or leather work, is very useful in restoring hand movements. Vocational training schemes now exist for the rehabilitation of suitable cases (see Occupational Therapy, p.181).

Drug Treatment in Acute Conditions. ASPIRIN or calcium aspirin is still the most useful drug, 4 to 8 grams daily. CODEINE tablets, two or three times daily may be used for severe pain.

PHENYLBUTAZONE (Butazolidin) also relieves pain and is sometimes prescribed when response to aspirin is unsatisfactory, but in up to 40 per cent of patients nausea, vomiting, rashes, edema, vomiting of blood, blood in the urine, anemia, etc. develop.

HYPNOTICS, e.g. barbiturates, for sleepless ness, and IRON PREPARATIONS when anemia is present are often useful.

GOLD SALTS, are given by intramuscular injection in selected cases under careful medical supervision, but toxic reactions may occur, with rashes, purpura, albumin in the urine, jaundice, diarrhea, or soreness of the mouth. Such symptoms must be reported by the patient at once.

CORTISONE, HYDROCORTISONE, AND THE SYNTHETIC STEROIDS. After more than ten years of controlled trials it was concluded that cortisone and hydrocortisone in favor of the tolerable doses was not more effective than aspirin after one, two or three years. Cortisone causes complications such as acne, growth of hair on the face, increased blood pressure, glycosuria, nervousness and depression, and in some cases peptic ulcer, tendency to fractures, psychotic disorders, or revival of dormant tuberculosis.

On sudden withdrawal of the hormone, the arthritis might become worse, with great weakness, loss of appetite and weight, depression and general muscular pains and stiffness. These results have led to discontinuation of cortisone and hydrocortisone in favor of the synthetic steroid compounds such as prednisolone, triamcinolone, and dexamethasone. These are more powerful, and control symptoms in smaller doses. They cannot be given if the patient has a peptic ulcer, high blood pressure, or decalcification of the bones. Any patient using steroids should carry a card naming the preparation, dose, and doctor in charge.

CORTICOTROPHIN (ACTH: a hormone from the anterior pituitary gland) is given to stimulate the patient's own adrenal glands. Long-acting preparations are used, injections being given once daily, but they may cause edema and high blood pressure, although gastric effects are much less common. Good results are obtained in up to 75 per cent of cases.

IBUPROFEN is a useful non-steroid antirheumatic agent. It reduces stiffness and so improves joint movement. It is well tolerated by patients.

HYDROCORTISONE FOR LOCAL USE. The injection of a hydrocortisone or of a steroid compound into a joint reduces the pain and swelling for a few days up to three weeks in about 50 per cent of cases.

Chronic Menopausal Arthritis

This form develops in women during the

'change of life' or menopause, usually affecting the obese type of woman. The knees are most often involved, but the hands may also show arthritic changes. The joints are swollen and painful, and finally the condition resembles osteo-arthritis.

Treatment aims at reduction in weight when this is above the normal, and patients need to train themselves to live on a reduced diet. Thyroid gland extract may be prescribed, and occasionally Lugol's iodine is prescribed. Heat treatment and hydrotherapy are used, and the joints must be rested, with little walking for some weeks. Crepe or adhesive bandages may be used to support the knees. Spa therapy is highly recommended.

Table Showing Features of Joint Diseases

	Acute Rheumatism	*Rheumatoid Arthritis*	*Osteo-arthritis*	*Gout*
Age	Young adults	Persons over 25 years of age	Middle-aged and old persons	Middle age and later life
Sex	Either sex	Generally women	Either sex	Generally older men
Cause	Unknown. Possibly due to infection	Often due to reaction to general bodily infection	Injuries, old age, wear and tear	Uric acid in the blood
Joints	Generally affects the larger joints, often in succession	The small joints of the hands and feet are especially affected but others may suffer also	One large joint is generally affected such as the hip, knee, or part of the spine	Several joints such as the big toes, fingers, elbows, or knees
Fever	At the beginning	During the early stages	None	May occur
Deformities	None	Joints like spindles; often much swelling and deformity	Slight	Chalky lumps over the joints and on the ears
Heart	Sometimes affected	Not involved	Not involved	May be disease of the blood vessels
Treatment	Aspirin and similar drugs	Heat treatment locally; hydrotherapy; gold injections; cortisone group of drugs. Liniments, general measures	Similar to measures for rheumatoid arthritis, especially local heat	Diet. Colchicine. Allopurinol. Local treatment

Osteo-arthritis

(*Osteoarthrosis*)

Osteo-arthritis differs from the preceding in attacking first the joint cartilages and then the bone beneath, especially in the large weight-bearing joints such as the hips, spine, and knees; it also occurs later in middle life in individuals of sturdy build, usually men.

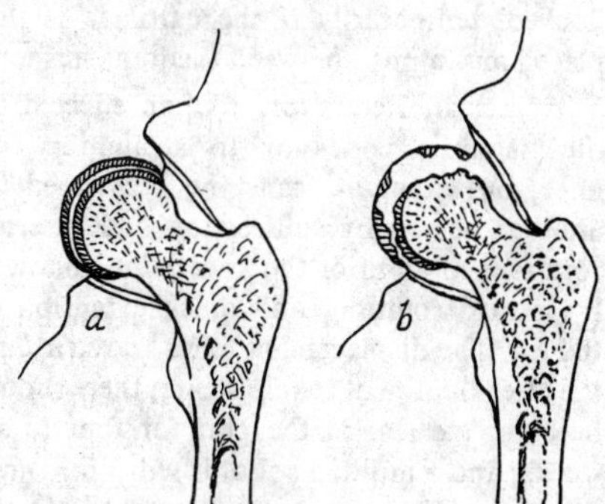

Fig. 4. *BONE CHANGES IN OSTEO-ARTHRITIS.* a. *Normal head of bone, covered with firm cartilage and smooth synovial membrane, can move freely in the socket.* b. *An arthritic head of bone with eroded and pitted cartilage and general degenerative changes which cause pain when the patient moves about or puts his weight on the joint.*

Causes. Heredity, advancing age, repeated injuries or strains, and strenuous occupations are the predisposing causes, rather than infection as in rheumatoid arthritis; it is not a simple disease but a progressive destruction of the joint surfaces. Intermediate forms between this disease and rheumatoid arthritis also occur, the commonest affecting women during the menopause.

Symptoms. The onset is gradual, and does not affect the general health; slight aching and stiffness are felt round the joint after exertion, and these gradually become worse, while creaking may be noticed. The bone ends become 'mushroom' in shape and, as the cartilages disappear, the bones rub together, giving rise to pain of varying severity, usually worse at night or in damp weather. There may be associated senile changes of high blood pressure, impaired kidney function, and arteriosclerosis.

Certain trades show distinctive joint involvements, such as blacksmith's elbow, laborer's spine, and foot-arch trouble in standing occupations. The affected joint becomes stiff and painful on rotation, although there is less pain on bending; in the hip the pain is often referred to the knee, and as the weight is shifted to the other leg, spinal curvature develops.

Although probably incurable, osteo-arthritis can be so far checked that symptoms diminish, and the outlook is fair if the disease is attended to in the early stages, but much less so as it advances. The relief of muscular spasm alone considerably reduces the pain.

Treatment. Avoidance of exposure to cold, wet, or excessive heat, with adequate periods of rest especially after middle age, choice of suitable occupation, and avoidance of damp clothes will reduce the tendency to osteo-arthritic disease of the joints.

When symptoms develop, an X-ray examination is advisable to show the extent of bone destruction. Plenty of rest is essential to allow all possible repair, and the diet must be limited to reduce the weight (see Obesity, p. 394), avoiding rich food, eggs, liver, and alcohol or a too liberal use of salt. Light diet, with fruit, vegetables, cheese, and 3 to 4 pints of fluids daily, usually causes both swelling and pain to abate.

Drugs are useful only to relieve pain, but aspirin or paracetamol three times a day may be tried under medical advice.

External applications of Scott's dressing or methyl salicylate ointment are of comfort. Hydrotherapy and short wave therapy are most important to relieve pain and encourage movement; for fat patients with several arthritic joints, spa medication is advised. Later, manipulation, and possibly an appliance for hip or knee-joint cases, may enable the patient to get about more comfortably. In some cases surgical treatment is used to fix the joint so that it cannot be bent, and so relieve the pain.

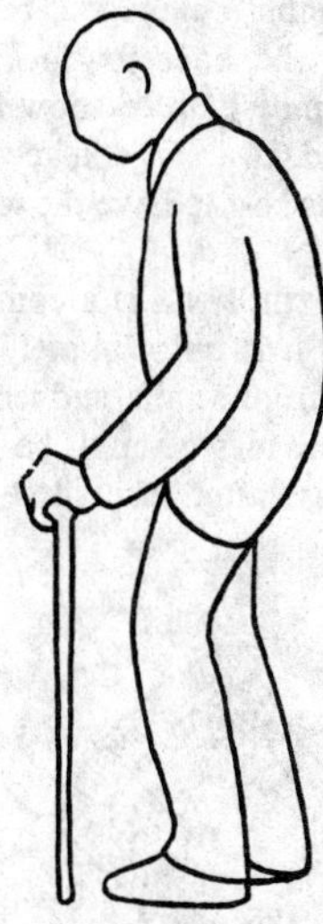

Fig. 5. *LABORER'S SPINE. After years of constant stooping and weight lifting, the affected spinal joints gradually become fixed in this characteristic position.*

Acute Synovitis

Acute synovitis, or inflammation of the joint membrane with the formation of fluid in the joint cavity, may follow an injury such as a sprain; the fluid may be clear or may become infected by bacteria so that pus is formed.

Sometimes acute synovitis may occur in association with acute fevers such as scarlet fever, rheumatic fever, gout, or gonorrhea.

Symptoms. Injury leads to the sudden formation of fluid in the joint, which may also contain blood. An injury of this type is liable to cause stiffness from adhesions, and if the sprain is severe there is often chronic thickening of torn ligaments, with some weakness of the joint. At the time of the injury there is often severe pain, followed by a dull aching pain as the fluid forms.

Treatment. When the joint is swollen it is necessary to rest the limb, keeping the leg raised on a bed or couch if the lower limb is affected. Cold compresses and firm bandages may be applied as a counter-irritant for twenty-four hours (after which time the skin will be reddened) to help the absorption of the fluid. Massage and gentle movements should be given when the fluid disappears and the pain is less. A firm supporting crêpe bandage or elastic support should then be worn as normal movements are again allowed. Great care should be taken not to strain the joint again by sudden movements or twists.

In the case of the knee joint the cartilages sometimes become damaged, being partially torn, causing the knee to 'lock.' An X-ray examination may help to show the extent of the injury and, if a surgeon recommends an operation, it is best to have the torn cartilages removed.

WATER ON THE KNEE is a common type of synovitis and it is unfortunately often recurrent. Any form of strain, sudden twisting, or strenuous activities should be avoided for some months after the first attack has subsided.

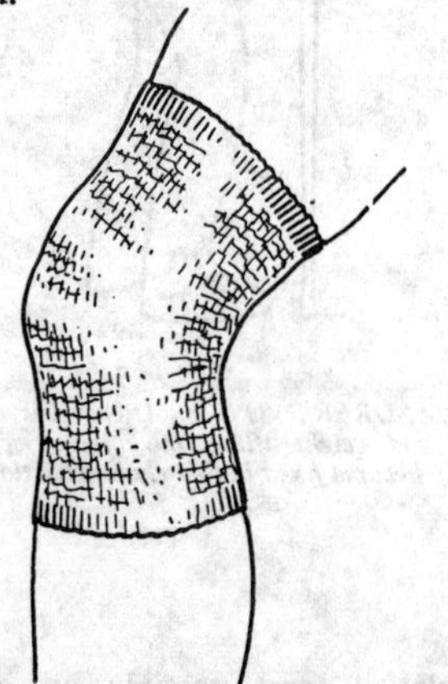

Fig. 6. *AN ELASTIC KNEE-CAP gives support to the weakened knee once the swelling of synovitis has been reduced. A cap may need to be worn for months or years.*

INFECTED SYNOVITIS. Complete rest of the joint is necessary, with hot compresses; sometimes a doctor will draw off the fluid to reduce the swelling and ease the strain on the ligaments, and the joint may be washed through with sterile saline solution.

Acute Suppurative Synovitis

Suppurative synovitis may follow injuries which penetrate the joint, or infections such as pneumonia, typhoid fever, gonorrhea, pyemia, or extension of infection from adjoining parts. It is likely to develop into acute arthritis and affect the bones of the joint.

Symptoms. The joint is very swollen, red and hot, and is usually kept in a somewhat bent position. The fluid in the joint may form a fluctuating swelling, and movement of the part is extremely painful.

Treatment. When pus forms, the purulent fluid may, if the case is seen early, be drawn off by a syringe with a sterile needle introduced into the joint by a surgeon.

In late cases drainage is secured by surgical incisions, with irrigation. In both cases movements must be carried out as soon as possible to prevent final stiffness of the joint. Antibiotics are now often used early in such cases, to reduce the risk of infection and pus formation.

Loose Bodies in Joints

Different types of 'loose bodies' are sometimes present in joint cavities; they are generally the result of chronic synovitis, injury, or tuberculosis. They lead to symptoms of sudden pain and locking if they get caught between the joint surfaces of the bones, and fluid is likely to be formed in the joint. The knee and elbow are the joints generally affected.

The joint should be opened by a surgeon and the loose body removed.

Gout

Although this disorder affects joints, it has an origin entirely different from rheumatism. It is due to disturbance of the purine metabolism of the body, and is dealt with in the section on Diseases of Metabolism, p. 391.

Ankylosing Spondylitis

This is a fusing arthritis of the spine occurring in young males. Its exact cause is unknown but it is probably part of a general body response to a specific infection.

Symptoms. The onset is slow and, after repeated attacks of 'lumbago,' the spine becomes stiff and poker-like. Twists may occur and eventually the whole spine and possibly the hips become immobile.

Treatment. The best treatment is radiotherapy, and this may arrest the process for years. Phenylbutazone may be effective for those patients who are radio-resistant.

Fixation of a Joint

(*Stiff Joint: Ankylosis*)

A joint may become fixed and stiff as a result of injury or disease. The fixation may be *false*, when it is the result of the formation of scar tissue in the skin or muscles around the joint, as may often occur after burns or wounds; this type of stiffness is also seen with deformities or untreated dislocation of joints.

ANKYLOSIS may be incomplete when it follows gonococcal or rheumatoid arthritis, chronic synovitis with adhesions, or tuberculous arthritis with scar tissue. In complete, or BONY ANKYLOSIS, the ends or surfaces of the bones become joined together so that the movements of the joint are lost. This may occur in suppurative arthritis, osteo-arthritis, or syphilitic disease of joints.

Torn Cartilage

A torn cartilage is a common injury of the knee joint, and consists of a tear of the cartilage (usually the internal semi-lunar cartilage) from its attachment to the tibia. The injury occurs from sudden twists of the knee when it is bent, as in football or other sports. There is violent pain, and the knee is 'locked' temporarily if the cartilage is displaced and nipped between the joint surfaces.

Treatment. Reduction is often effected by the patient's endeavor to straighten the knee, but otherwise must be performed by another person by full flexion and external rotation, rotation of the knee joint, followed by inward rotation, and quick extension of the leg. The displacement tends to recur, and the after-treatment requires care; there should be complete rest of the part for four to six weeks, and a molded splint is worn for three months. Operation for removal of the cartilage is often advisable, since healing of cartilage is always poor and recurrent attacks of synovitis are common.

Injuries of Joints: Dislocations

See Fractures and Dislocations, pp. 543-56.

Treatment depends largely on the cause. In fibrous fixation with few adhesions, manipulation, massage and radiant heat may give good results. Manipulation under an anesthetic (except in tuberculous cases) may also be tried. Surgical treatment is often valuable, a new joint being formed, but this cannot be done in tuberculosis of joints as it is likely to excite recurrence of the disease.

AFFECTIONS OF THE MUSCLES

Fibrositis

(*Muscular Rheumatism: Myositis: Myalgia: Non-articular Rheumatism*)

Fibrositis is a common painful condition

of muscles and sometimes of fibrous tissues. It is usually sudden in onset, with stiffness as a characteristic feature. The neck, back, shoulders, upper arm, chest and buttocks are mainly affected. In some cases the disorder may involve the joint capsule, nerve sheaths, tendons, bursae and the synovial membrane of the joints. Lumbago is a common form of fibrositis.

Chronic fatigue, gout, hypersensitivity of the skin to cold, and occupational strains—especially when they are associated with damp or chills—may be responsible. It may also follow injuries, influenza, tonsillitis or other acute infection, certain glandular deficiencies, or the menopause in women. Worry, mental conflict, or excessive muscular tension in anxiety states is increasingly thought to be one of the causes of an attack of fibrositis. This tension may give rise to aching and fatigue in certain muscles. Such cases of a psychogenic nature must be carefully distinguished from those arising from physical causes. The chronic condition is often seen in older people, especially in those who suffer from gout.

The affected muscle is very tender to touch and nodular lumps may be felt which tend to shift their position, this being caused by contraction of part of the muscle. Pain may be very intense in the early stage and complete rest in bed may be necessary. Acutely tender areas known as 'trigger spots' may develop. An attack of fibrositis may last only for a few days but, especially in cold weather, it may continue for some weeks. If neglected it may become a chronic condition.

Faulty posture may cause persistent aching pain particularly in the neck, back or lumbar region, either in obese people or the thin type with spinal kyphosis or lordosis (see p. 541). Flat foot may also cause low backache. See also Neuritis, pp. 423.

Treatment. GENERAL MEASURES IN ACUTE CASES. The part affected should be rested as much as possible and the patient kept warm and well away from draughts. Heat in the form of poultices, hot-water bottles or an electric blanket gives relief of pain and shortens the attack.

A light but nourishing diet is allowed, and 6 to 8 glasses of water should be drunk daily; Vichy or other alkaline waters are very suitable.

Free sweating should be encouraged and may be induced by hot baths, but care must be taken when the patient is elderly not to cause exhaustion.

For the treatment of the highly painful 'trigger spots,' the doctor has first to locate them by pressing over the whole tender area and then injects a local anesthetic solution into them. It may be necessary to repeat the injection once or twice. The procedure gives great relief immediately. A week's course of heat, massage and active exercises should follow. If neglected, the pain will often lead the sufferer to seek comfort by walking or sitting badly, thus causing imperfect muscle balance which in turn creates further strain and recurrence.

IN CHRONIC CASES hot-air baths, hydrotherapy, diathermy, exercises, and massage are very effective. The out-patient clinics of many hospitals provide these therapies.

Infiltration of painful 'trigger spots' is as important in chronic as in acute cases.

There is no need for special diets.

Drug Treatment. Aspirin, calcium or soluble aspirin taken three times a day help to relieve the pain.

Colchicine should be used for those with fibrositis linked with gout.

An effervescent saline preparation may be effective in acute cases.

Spa Treatment combines the psychological benefit of a holiday with absence from the worries associated with work or home, as well as regular medication together with massage and hydrotherapy.

In obese patients the most important factor in treatment is adequate reduction in weight.

Occasionally a change of occupation may be advisable to avoid further risks of chills, strain or excessive fatigue.

Lumbago

Pain in the lumbar region may arise from many causes, but in most cases the condition is due to lumbago, or fibrositis in the muscles of the back, aggravated by sudden cold from sitting in a draught, or by wet feet or other exposure.

Great pain is felt in the loins, the onset often being very sudden, and the pain is much worse when stooping or rising is attempted.

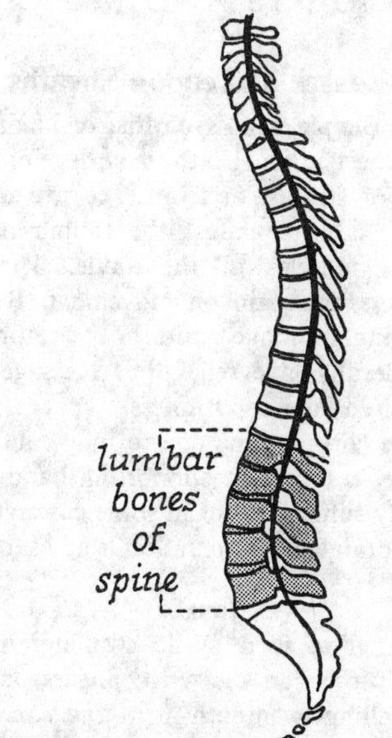

Fig. 7. *LUMBAGO is fibrositis of the lumbar area of the spine* (*shaded*).

In more chronic cases a careful examination should be made, since pain in the lumbar region is usually due to degenerative changes in one or more of the gristle-like discs between the spinal bones. In women, persistent backache may be due to some pelvic disorder, and should be investigated.

Faulty posture in obesity, flat feet, or strain of the back muscles in certain occupations may also lead to lumbar pain. These postural defects should be corrected by remedial exercises.

Treatment. The general measures used in fibrositis may also be adopted in lumbago, such as heat in the form of hot-water bottles, or an infra-red heat pad applied to the part. Diathermy, radiant heat, and massage are also used. See above.

In very chronic cases with tenderness in the lumbar muscles, injection of a local anesthetic, combined with heat treatment, massage and exercise, often gives considerable relief.

In other cases where general measures do not appear to improve the condition, or in cases of sacro-iliac strain, manipulation of the spine under a general anesthetic by a surgeon is advised. See also above).

Wasting of Muscles

(*Muscular Atrophy*)

Wasting of muscles is a fairly common condition which may be due to many different causes. It may affect one muscle or group of muscles only, or all the muscles of the body may participate.

General Wasting is often due to chronic exhausting disorders such as tuberculosis, cancer, typhoid fever, general malnutrition, or other prolonged illnesses.

Disuse Atrophy is seen when some part of the body is kept at rest for a long time, as when a fractured limb is kept in a plaster cast.

Local Wasting develops as a result of diseases of the nerves supplying that part, so that nutrition is disturbed; this is seen in poliomyelitis, or after injuries to nerves or to the spinal cord, as in bullet wounds or other accidents which damage a nerve. Local wasting also occurs as a result of disuse of muscles, as after fractures.

Certain Muscle Diseases such as progressive muscular atrophy, myasthenia gravis, and other hereditary muscle disorders (*dystrophies*) also produce severe and extensive wasting.

Treatment. Physiotherapy may often prevent or improve wasting of muscles when the nerves are not affected. Massage and exercises, electrical treatment, and various forms of heat treatment are the chief means employed.

Muscular Cramps and Spasms

Muscular cramps of a severe type occur in general diseases such as tetanus (lockjaw), and tetany, which are described under these headings on p. 275 and p. 402. Polyneuritis may also give rise to cramp.

Periodic Cramp and Nocturnal Cramp. Periodic cramps often occur in normal persons; these painful contractions may come on during a resting period, or as a result of cold or fatigue. Warmth, and rubbing or exercising the part generally relieves the pain. In cold weather or in cases of poor circulation sturdy shoes and warm stockings should be worn.

Cramp at night, or nocturnal cramp, is sometimes distressing; cold, restlessness and fatigue during the daytime should be avoided. Aspirin, 600 milligram doses, before retiring is sometimes effective, and tolazoline hydrochloride, 25 milligrams two or three times a day, is sometimes given.

Arteriosclerosis. In old people suffering from arterial disease and poor circulation of the blood, cramp in the calves of the legs is a fairly common symptom; it usually comes on during walking, and may be severe. This form of cramp is sometimes relieved by a course of hormone treatment under a doctor's supervision.

Pregnancy. Cramps are fairly common in pregnancy, and may be a sign of a lack of calcium in the mother's blood. Calcium in the form of calcium lactate tablets, Calcinate, or else iron, calcium and vitamin D tablets may be taken regularly from the third to the eighth months of pregnancy.

Nocturnal Jumps. Some people find that when they are just falling asleep they are roused by sudden starts or 'jumps' of the legs. These may be due to temporary anemia of the brain, and the sufferer should sleep with the head low, or the foot of the bed may be slightly raised.

Injuries of Muscles

Bruising

Bruising of muscles causes pain on movement similar to that produced by a sprain.

The condition is generally relieved by rest for a few days, cold compresses and gentle massage. In very severe cases, with considerable injury or laceration of the muscles, contraction and deformity may follow.

Rupture of Muscle

Rupture of a muscle sometimes occurs on sudden strain or exertion; the parts usually affected are the thigh, calf (in 'tennis leg'), inner side of the thigh (rider's strain), the neck muscles of an infant during labor, 'tennis elbow,' the biceps muscle of the arm, the Achilles tendon of the heel, and the tendon of the knee-cap. Sudden pain and inability to move the muscle are followed by swelling and discoloration; sometimes the separation of the muscle can be felt.

Treatment consists in complete rest for at least three weeks, with relaxation and firm support of the limb. In a few cases, surgical treatment is preferable. Massage is generally advised, with a gentle return to movement, and care in after-use of the part, with careful avoidance of further strain.

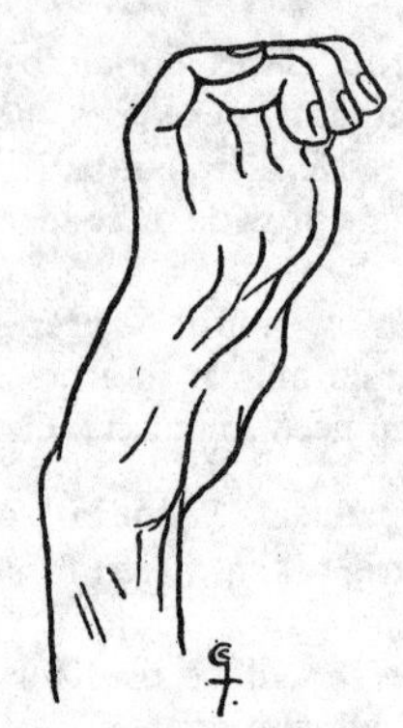

Fig. 8. *VOLKMANN'S ISCHEMIC CONTRACTURE OF THE RIGHT HAND*

Contractures

Contractures of muscles sometimes follow injuries such as severe bruises or lacerations, when the circulation to the part has been affected, especially when tight bandages or unsuitable splints have been used. Contractures of the hand and forearm are liable to follow injuries or fractures of the elbow-joint, with wasting of the forearm (see Fig. 8).

Tumors

Tumors of muscles are rare, except in cases secondary to growths elsewhere in the body. Fibromas and lipomas are benign growths which may be removed surgically. A fibroma rarely undergoes malignant changes and becomes carcinomatous.

OTHER AFFECTIONS OF THE JOINTS AND MUSCLES

Diseases of Tendon Sheaths

Acute Simple Teno-synovitis, or inflammation of the tendon sheath, may develop after sprains or strains, or from excessive use. It is most liable to affect the thumb or the peroneal muscles of the ankle. There is tenderness and pain on movement. Rest, a supporting bandage, and hot compresses will generally give relief, but massage may be required later for stiffness.

In the chronic type due to long-continued over-use, rest with a supporting bandage is generally sufficient, but in some cases aspiration or drainage by operation is advisable.

Ganglia

A ganglion is a cystic swelling, and is generally seen on the wrist, fingers or foot. The swelling is smooth, firm and somewhat movable without causing much pain; it contains mucoid fluid. In most cases surgical excision is recommended, but occasionally the contents may be removed by aspiration. Ganglia often recur in the same individual.

A compound ganglion of the palm of the hand is a more serious condition as it is usually due to tuberculosis of the tendons of the wrist, and may lead to permanent stiffness.

Bursitis

A bursa is a small sac which forms near a joint, usually in a site exposed to pressure. When such a sac becomes inflamed the condition is called bursitis; it may be acute or chronic, and may develop either as simple inflammation with effusion, or as a suppurative condition.

Gouty bursitis commonly develops behind the elbow joint. Other common sites of bursitis are around the knee joint; in front of the knee-cap; below the knee-cap; behind the Achilles tendon of the heel; near the hip joint; below the tuberosity of the haunch bone; and behind the deltoid muscle on the outer side of the upper part of the arm.

Acute Simple Bursitis is often due to strain, especially in gouty or rheumatic persons; it causes pain, tenderness and heat of the part. Complete rest of the part and hot compresses usually effect a cure, but occasionally removal of the bursal sac is indicated. Suppuration should be treated surgically like an abscess, with incision and drainage.

Chronic Bursitis may follow the acute type or may develop more insidiously, as in 'housemaid's knee.' Fluid forms within the bursa, causing adhesions and tenderness, with much thickening of the part. In many cases removal of the sac is the best course, but rest and the application of counter-irritants, or painting with iodine, may be successful in giving relief. In some cases, hydrocortisone injected into the bursa, followed by exercises and heat treatment, will give much improvement.

Small loose bodies known as 'melon seed' bodies sometimes form in the bursa, from coagulated lymph.

Deformities

Torticollis

Torticollis, or wry-neck, causes turning of the head to the affected side as a result of spasm or contraction of the neck muscles. It may be a congenital condition, as in infants when it occurs after labor with difficulty in delivering the child. When it occurs later in life it is caused by rheumatism or exposure to cold, or from scarring in severe burns, or reflex spasm from irritation due to inflamed glands or cellulitis of the neck; epileptiform spasm, or occasionally syphilis (by the formation of gummata in the muscle) may cause torticollis; hysterical cases sometimes occur, or wry-neck may develop after poliomyelitis.

Treatment consists in ascertaining the cause, and the use of massage and appropriate manipulation. The infantile type should be treated early and, if properly managed, an operation may be avoided.

In the rheumatic type, aspirin, and oil of wintergreen liniment soon help to give relief from pain; any decayed teeth should be attended to. Sometimes surgical division of the muscle or tendon, with stretching, may be necessary in the congenital type of case.

Dupuytren's Contracture

In this condition there is a slowly progressive contraction of the fourth and fifth fingers of one or both hands, so that the fingers are gradually drawn into the palm, and cannot be straightened. The disease is often hereditary and is most commonly seen in middle-aged persons. Operative treatment is the only means of improving the movements of the fingers, but a permanent cure cannot be promised.

Hammer-toe

This is a contraction of one of the toes, so that it is permanently bent. The second toe is most often affected. The condition may be hereditary, or associated with deformity of the foot, or may be caused by wearing short shoes.

Excision of the joint, or amputation of the toe, gives satisfactory results.

Flat Foot

This is an affection of one or both feet and is associated with dropping of the arches and turning out of the foot in varying degrees (Figs. 9 and 10). The condition may be congenital or acquired; causes of the latter include rachitic tendencies, weakness or paralysis, inflammatory conditions, injuries (especially after Pott's fracture), and prolonged strain from standing or carrying heavy weights.

To obtain the strength necessary to enable the weight of the body to be carried in a light, graceful and easy manner, the foot is not placed entirely flat on the ground, but a long arch passing from the heel to the ball of the foot is formed by the bones of the foot; these are normally supported by muscles and ligaments. A shorter transverse arch is also normally present between the ball of the big toe and the base of the little toe.

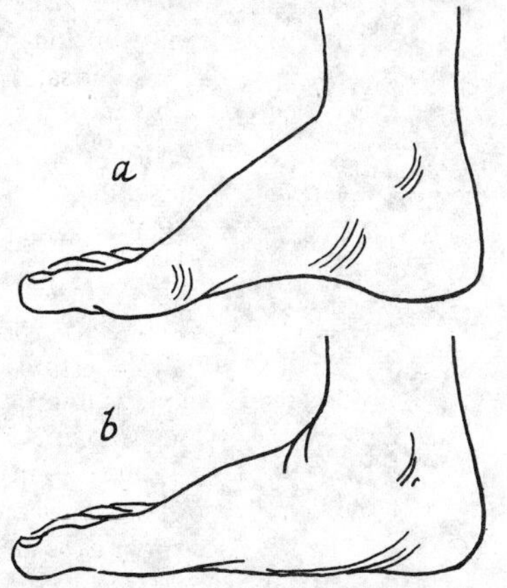

Fig. 9. *ARCH OF RIGHT FOOT.* a. *Normal arch* b. *Dropped arch resulting in flat foot.*

The presence of flat foot may be determined by wetting the sole of the foot and placing it on a dry board. In flat foot the imprint will show an unusually large part of the surface of the bottom of the foot; if there is no degree of flat foot the imprint will show only the toes, ball, and heel of the foot, and the outer edge, the whole resembling a crescent; the raised part of the arch in normal feet, as in Figs 9a and 10a, does not touch the board.

Symptoms. The symptoms felt during the development of flat foot are persistent pain and weakness at the site of the weakness in the foot; great discomfort or even pain is felt if standing is continued over long periods. Sometimes the pain is most severe in the muscles behind the external malleolus of the ankle, especially in the early stages.

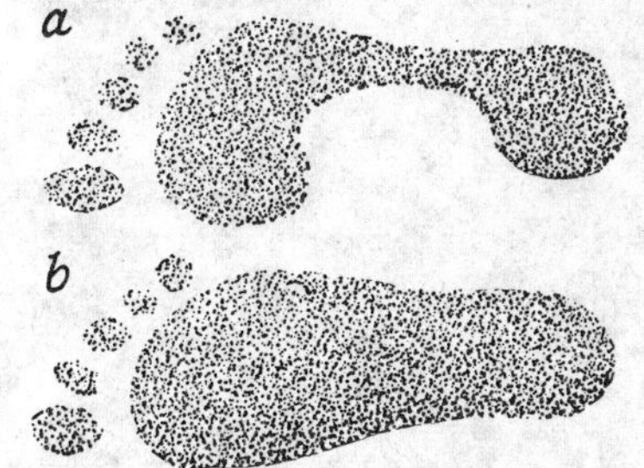

Fig. 10. *IMPRINT OF SOLE OF FOOT indicates the condition of the arch.* a. *Normal arch.* b. *Flat foot.*

There are four degrees of this disability, which may involve the transverse arch as well as the longitudinal.

1. The muscles and ligaments on the inner side and the sole of the foot are stretched and weakened, but the flattening of the arch can be corrected by voluntary effort.
2. The muscles are further weakened, and there is spasm of the muscles behind the ankles; the flattening of the arch is more pronounced, but the patient can still stand on tiptoe without aid.
3. Adhesions form, and the condition is less painful, owing to chronic stretching of the ligaments.
4. There is deformity of the foot, and some degree of arthritis of the joints. At this stage no amount of rest or massage will correct the flattening.

In the early stages pain may be quite severe, but as the condition grows worse and the ligaments become permanently stretched, there is less discomfort and pain, although the buoyancy of the gait is lost.

Treatment. In the early stages complete rest, with massage, electrical treatment and exercises are given, and shoes properly fitted. Later, prolonged standing must be avoided, and specially made arch supports may be useful in preventing further descent of the sole, but they must be made to the individual requirements. The shoes should also be modified by thickening the sole on the inner sides and building the heel forward to carry the weight on the outer side.

In late cases active treatment is generally of little use, but modified shoes and arch supports improve the gait. Occasionally surgical treatment is given.

Dropped Metatarsal Arch

A dropped transverse metatarsal arch from the ball of the foot to the little toe may also occur with flatfoot; hardened skin or calluses are formed, causing aching and discomfort. An elastic band may be used to support the foot, with a pad under the sole behind the ends of the metatarsal bones to help raise the transverse arch.

Metatarsalgia

In this condition there is a sharp neuralgic pain below the ends of the metatarsal bones of the foot, especially between the fourth and fifth toes. In many cases the pain is due to pressure on the nerves between the toes, owing to dropping of the transverse arch, and there may also be calluses on the sole of the foot. Occasionally the pain is due to gout or rheumatism.

Treatment consists in rest and massage; it is advisable that a shoe with a low heel should be worn, and that a bar be fixed on to the sole of the shoe behind the heads of the metatarsal bones. This will relieve the pressure on the nerves between the toes. In long-standing or severe cases surgical treatment with removal of the head of the bone may be adopted to give relief.

Bunion

This is a deformity of the inner side of the first joint of the big toe, and the toe often appears to be partially out of joint. The swelling and projection of the joint exposes it to irritation from the shoe, and to repeated attacks of inflammation, while the deformity makes it difficult for the sufferer to wear ordinary shoes.

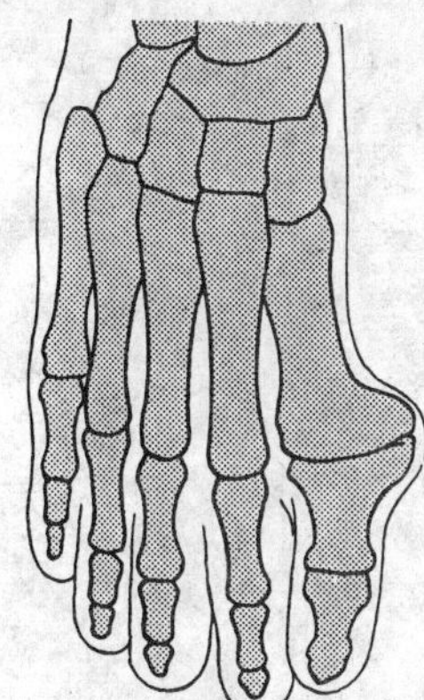

Fig. 11. *BONES OF THE FOOT SHOWING A BUNION, i.e. deformity of the inner side of the first joint of the big toe.*

Treatment. Remove the pressure from the part by wearing a suitable shoe; when there is any inflammation, keep the foot rested and elevated upon a chair, applying heat, compresses, etc. Well-fitting boots or shoes with a straight inner border should be worn, or a toe-post between the big and second toe also helps to keep the big toe in correct position; by this means the pressure against the side of the toe is removed. An operation for the removal of the bunion and of the enlarged joint may be performed, and usually gives good results.

DISEASES OF THE BONES AND SPINE

The bones that make up the skeletal support of the body are the toughest tissues that a human being possesses, but they are not inanimate. They are supplied with blood vessels and nerves as well as special cells in the marrow which make the blood corpuscles; they live and grow like other parts of the body, and they may also become diseased.

The main diseases are inflammatory and infective conditions (including necrosis, rarefaction, thickening, osteomyelitis and periostitis), which may be acute or chronic; new growths and cysts, both benign and malignant; and the general diseases of rickets, scurvy, osteomalacia, Paget's disease, acromegaly, and other rarer affections.

NON-SURGICAL DISEASES OF BONE

Non-surgical diseases of bones include various common conditions, and those which are less frequently seen.

Clubbing of the Fingers or Toes

'Clubbing,' or swelling of the end phalanges, is met with in cases of congenital heart diseases, in some lung diseases, and other chronic diseases. There is seldom much pain and only slight stiffness, but the condition is somewhat unsightly. The finger tips are red and swollen, and the nails are brittle and ridged. There may also be some swelling and arthritis of the ends of the long bones of the limbs, or of other bones. In some cases the clubbing disappears when the original disease is cured, but more often it persists.

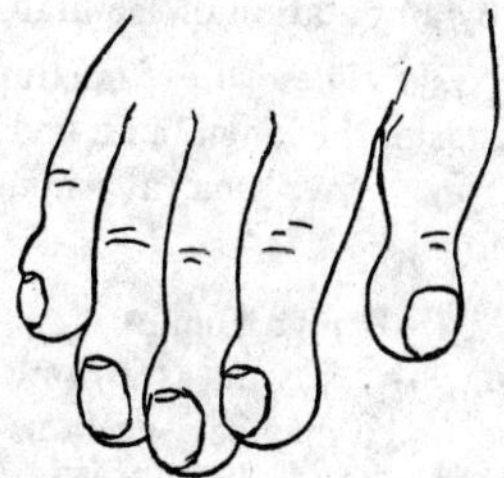

Fig. 1. *CLUBBED FINGERS. This rounding of the finger ends occurs in persons suffering from congenital heart diseases or certain lung diseases. It seldom causes pain.*

Treatment must be given to the primary lung or heart disease, the local treatment of the bones being directed towards relieving symptoms as they develop, as in other cases of arthritis.

Paget's Disease
(*Osteitis Deformans*)

This is an uncommon condition, and consists in rarefaction of various bones such as the skull, limbs, spine, pelvis and ribs. The bones become thickened and deformed, the skull enlarging and the limb bones becoming bent. The disease generally occurs in persons over forty years of age, giving rise to pains in the affected bones, but the general health otherwise remains good. The condition is slowly progressive, and occasionally sarcoma (cancer) or cysts develop in the bones.

Treatment. The general health must be watched, and occasionally supporting spinal apparatus may be required. No known treatment has much effect on the course of the disease but calcium, parathyroid extract and vitamin D are often given. Aspirin is also used, under medical direction, as an alternative.

Fragilitas Ossium

Fragilitas ossium, or 'brittle bones,' is a rare condition of newborn infants; it may cause numerous fractures of the bones and then generally proves fatal; if the child lives, various deformities may develop.

Rarely, the condition develops for the first time in the adolescent. When this happens the outlook is not so serious.

Osteomalacia
(*Adult Rickets*)

This is a chronic disease mainly affecting women who live confined lives in the poorest quarters of industrial cities in the East, and who are inadequately fed and have many pregnancies.

The bones become soft and bend easily, and the condition may not be recognized until it is well advanced. Pain is generally felt early, and later deformity or fractures may draw attention to the condition of the bones. The course of the disease may be rapid or may extend over a number of years.

Treatment. A very nourishing diet is required, with plenty of milk, eggs, fish and meat. Phosphorus, calcium, and cod-liver oil and vitamin D may be ordered by a physician; sunlight and ultraviolet irradiation are also beneficial.

Achondroplasia

This is a comparatively uncommon condition. Subjects with the disease are the typical stunted dwarfs sometimes seen in circus troupes; these persons have large heads, normal-sized bodies, but very short legs and arms; in consequence they appear to be stunted. The general health is generally good, and intelligence is normal. The condition often occurs in several members of one family, and may be hereditary. There is no known means of cure or alleviation. Many infants with achondroplasia are still-born or die shortly after birth; an achondroplasic woman will probably require Caesarean section if she becomes pregnant.

SURGICAL DISEASES OF BONE

Osteitis

Inflammation of a bone, or osteitis, may be acute or chronic; it may be the result of an injury, or may be due to blood-borne infection. The bacteria which are generally responsible for the infection of bone are the common pus-producing germs, the bacillus of tuberculosis, and the spirochete of syphilis.

Symptoms and Signs. The common signs of inflammation of a bone develop, to a greater or lesser extent, according to the severity and cause of the infection. Pain is usually severe in acute cases, and is worse at night or when pressure is applied to the part. In some cases of bone infection there are grave constitutional symptoms, and the diagnosis is then often difficult, especially when there are no apparent injuries or wounds; in the early stages such a case may be mistaken for some acute general fever such as scarlet fever, or for erysipelas or cellulitis.

Types. Inflammation in the long bone of a limb can take three forms:

1. The periosteum, or the membrane covering the bone, may be first involved, causing *periostitis*.
2. The marrow-cavity may be mainly involved, as in *osteomyelitis*.
3. In *epiphysitis* the end of the bone is affected.

Course. Inflammation of a bone always begins in the parts supplied by blood vessels, but is likely to be followed by changes in the dense parts composed of mineral substance.

The formation of fluid exudate which occurs in the bony canals during inflammation causes an increase of pressure which reduces the blood supply; this may be followed by destruction or death of the surrounding bone.

When a part of a bone dies, or undergoes *necrosis*, the dead fragment is called a *sequestrum*. Such a fragment may have to be removed by a surgical operation, or it may be gradually pushed towards the surface of the body, and be discharged through the skin, through an opening known as a sinus. A sinus is often slow in healing, owing to the discharge of pus which continues after the bone fragment has been extruded.

In less severe cases absorption of bone occurs, leading to rarefaction, or *caries*; in other cases condensation, or *sclerosis*, of the bone follows.

Periostitis

Periostitis is the inflammation of the membrane covering the bone, and may be acute or chronic. Deeper inflammation involves the bone and marrow, and is known as osteomyelitis (see below), which is generally a serious disease with acute onset.

Acute periostitis alone generally follows specific fevers, pyemia, blows or injuries, exposure to X-rays, gout or extension from local infection; while the chronic type may be due to syphilis, tuberculosis, gangrene, or suppuration.

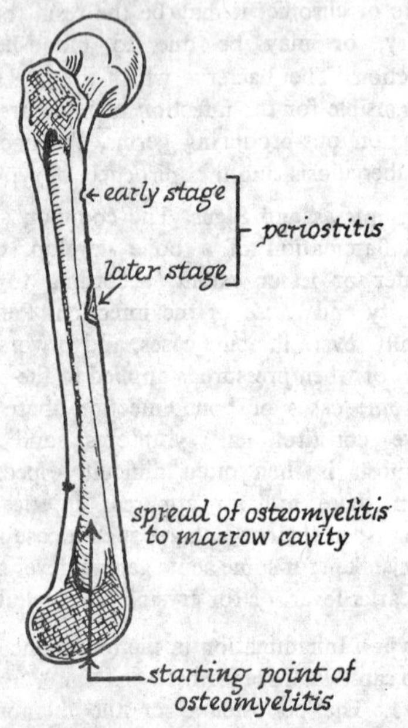

Fig. 2. *INFLAMMATION OF BONE (osteitis), due to infection brought via the blood vessels, may affect the outer membrane causing periostitis, or may spread deeply into the bone and marrow cavity causing osteomyelitis.*

Symptoms. There is severe pain, and there may be swelling or redness if the disease is near the surface. If an abscess forms it may break through the skin and small dead fragments of bone may be discharged from time to time (see also Osteitis).

Treatment. It is essential to have absolute rest and elevation of the part at first, and the application of heat. If pus is suspected, surgical drainage is often required to prevent deep infection of the bone.

Osteomyelitis

Osteomyelitis is a deep inflammation of the bone and marrow. It occurs more often in children and may follow a slight injury or abrasion; it is sometimes precipitated by compound fractures, acute fevers, or pyemia, but in other cases there may be no apparent predisposing cause.

Acute Osteomyelitis

Symptoms. There is sudden onset of pain of a boring character, swelling and redness if the affected part is near the surface, limitation of movement, with tenderness along the bone, fever, chills, malaise, vomiting and toxemia. The disease often starts near a joint, especially the lower end of the femur of the thigh or the radius of the forearm, and the upper end of the tibia or shin-bone, and of the humerus or arm-bone, and spreads rapidly through the marrow cavity. Infected particles may enter the blood stream and give rise to pyemia.

Early diagnosis is extremely important to prevent severe destruction of the bone.

Treatment. The use of antibiotics in the early stages of osteomyelitis has revolutionized the treatment and course of the disease, so that in many cases surgical treatment may be avoided.

Surgical treatment is often indicated to drain out pus; the wound is left open and lightly packed, later being irrigated daily with sterile saline solution. Amputation is occasionally necessary to save life.

Chronic Osteomyelitis

Chronic osteomyelitis, often in association with chronic periostitis, sometimes occurs after injuries, or typhoid fever or other infections such as rheumatism. In some cases a local abscess, may develop, especially in the leg bones; an open operation is usually necessary, since the diseased part seldom heals of its own accord.

Tuberculosis of Bones

Tuberculosis of the bones generally develops in young people, often being a sequel to tuberculous infection in the chest or the abdomen. Abscesses form in the bone substance or in the marrow cavity, while the surrounding bone slowly becomes absorbed (*caries*) or it may become dense (*sclerosis*). Small fragments of dead bone (*sequestra*), often become separated off and discharged through the skin. These dead pieces of bone are soft, and break easily; they are somewhat like cheese in appearance, and of a yellowish color.

The ribs, sternum (breastbone) and spinal column are often the site of tuberculous periostitis, while tuberculous osteomyelitis affects the fingers, the bones of the foot, and the long bones; children are liable to develop tuberculosis of the finger bones after acute fevers.

Treatment consists in measures to assist the general health, with complete rest and immobilization of the diseased part for a long period. This may mean staying in hospital for many months, and even years, to allow proper healing. Antituberculous drugs such as streptomycin are given, and surgical treatment may be required to deal with sinuses or diseased fragments of bone. See p. 353.

See also Pott's Disease, p. 540.

Syphilis of Bones

Syphilis affects the bones as a chronic affection, attacking the periosteum and the bone substance itself. The condition usually appears in the late stages of the disease and is manifest by thickening and pain in the long bones and shin.

Occasionally, babies born of mothers with untreated syphilis may be affected, but this could be prevented by prompt treatment of the mother during pregnancy.

See also Venereal Diseases, p. 289.

Tumors of Bone

Cysts

Fibrocystic Disease of Bone. In this condition single cysts develop in the shafts of the long bones, especially the humerus and the femur. The disease is most common in young people, and may give rise to fractures, owing to thinning of the bone substance, with loss of strength.

Hydatid Cysts. In the form of a hydatid cyst, the larval form of the sheep-dog tapeworm may sometimes invade the lungs and liver of man, and occasionally the long bones or pelvis (see also p. 387). There may be thickening of the bone around the cyst, or later a fracture may follow.

Cysts within a long bone can only be removed by amputation of the limb.

Blood Cysts. These are sometimes found near the ends of the long bones, and probably develop from a myeloma, a benign form of bone tumor.

Benign Tumors

Osteoma. An osteoma is a tumor derived from bone, and it may be cancellous (spongy), or composed of dense ivory bone.

A Cancellous Osteoma grows near the ends of the long bones, especially the radius of the forearm and the femur of the thigh. It is hard and usually painless unless it presses on nerves, in which case it may be removed by an operation.

An Ivory Osteoma consists of very hard bone, and is generally seen in the orbit of the eye, the bony passage of the ear, the frontal sinus, the mastoid bone, or the jaw.

Exostosis. This small projection of bone may sometimes follow inflammation of the part. It may involve a tendon at the point of its attachment, as at the heel, and another common site is below the nail of the great toe, causing the nail to become raised up. These small tumors should be removed by a surgeon.

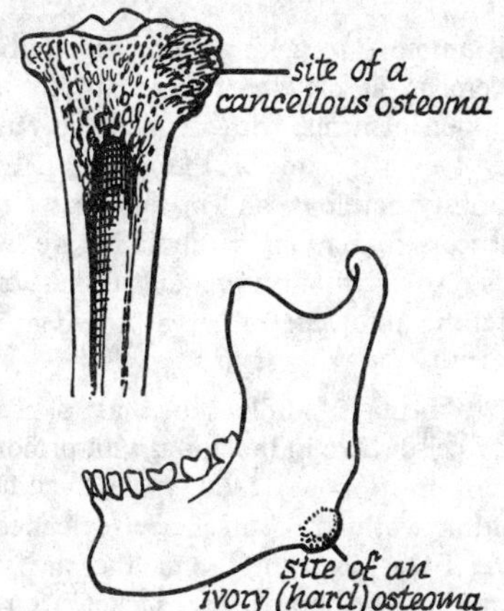

Fig. 3. *OSTEOMA. Two forms of a benign type of tumor of the bone.*

Chondroma. A chondroma is a tumor originally formed of cartilage, but later it may become converted into bone. In a long bone such a tumor is of slow growth, while in the bones of the hand there are often many small tumors which cause the bones to become expanded.

Myeloma. This is a rare tumor occurring in young adults before the age of thirty, in the ends of the long bones, especially the femur and the tibia, and also in the jaw, ribs, spine, and the bones of the wrist and foot. It may be caused by injury, and later fractures may follow. The early symptoms are vague, with pain, or sudden fracture of a bone; on X-ray examination punched-out areas are seen in the bones.

Malignant Tumors

Sarcoma. This is a very malignant type of tumor which affects young people, often between the ages of ten and twenty years. The leg is generally the site of the growth, the femur commonly being involved. Severe boring pain is felt which is worse at night, and soon a visible swelling appears. The condition may be confirmed by X-ray examination, and no time should be lost in procuring treatment, since secondary growths usually develop extremely quickly. The whole limb is usually removed by operation but results are often disappointing, and the average period of survival is seldom longer than about two years.

Cancer of Bone. Secondary cancerous deposits in bones are fairly common when cancer develops in some other organ of the body. These deposits are most often seen in cases of cancer of the lungs, the prostate gland, the testicles, or the breast. Cancer of the adrenal glands often gives rise to secondary growths in the skull, while cancer of the thyroid gland is sometimes associated with secondary tumors of the skull, the vertebrae, and the long bones of the limbs.

Sometimes the primary or original growth is not discovered during the patient's lifetime. The first sign of secondary cancer of bone is usually a sudden fracture in a long bone. An X-ray examination in these cases shows a rarefied area in the shaft of the affected bone; the growth may not progress very rapidly and sometimes the fracture will become reunited.

Occasionally X-ray treatment relieves the pain and diminishes the rate of growth of the malignant deposit.

RICKETS

Rickets generally begins in the first two years of life, and is one of the deficiency diseases (see p. 398). Rickets is due to deficiency of vitamin D in the diet, lack of sunlight, and deficiency of calcium and phosphorus.

In the early stages the infant is pale and suffers from gastro-intestinal disturbances; there are general flabbiness of the muscles, perspiration of the head at night, and sometimes convulsions; 'crowing' of the larynx is often characteristic. The bones become tender, and the ends of the long bones of the limbs and the ribs are thickened. The head and forehead have a typical square appearance, the fontanelles of the skull remaining open after the usual time for closure. Sometimes the child is pigeon-chested, and there may be curvature of the spine, 'knock-knees' and bow legs. The bones may finally become permanently deformed, if not attended to at an early stage.

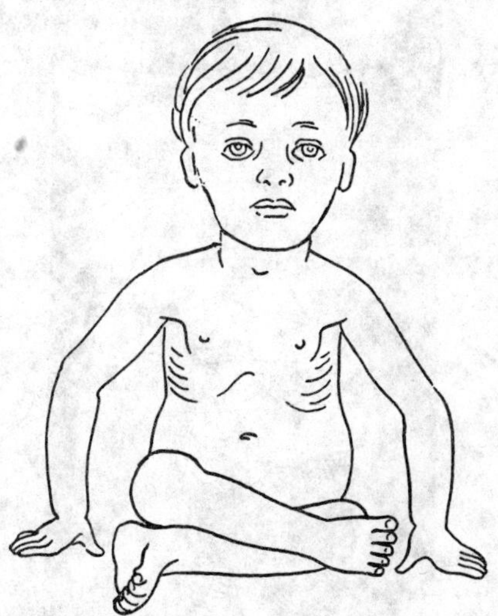

Fig. 4. *RICKETS. A characteristic posture of a rachitic child.*

Treatment consists in adequate and varied diet, particularly with cows' milk, limewater, eggs and cream. Vitamin D with fresh air and sunshine are essential. Prevention of deformity can be obtained by manipulation, with rest and recumbency and, if necessary, the use of supporting splints. Surgical treatment of bones is occasionally necessary.

Adolescent Rickets. See Osteomalacia, p.357.

DEFORMITIES

Knock-knee

In knock-knee the legs are bent outwards from the knee; the condition may be present on one or both sides, and often occurs in conjunction with flat foot and spinal curvature (scoliosis). Knock-knee occurs in young children with rickets, and in young adolescents who are growing rapidly and whose work entails weight carrying or long hours of standing. It may also follow injuries or fractures near the knee.

At some stage in early walking many children go through a phase of knock-knee. This is not a serious condition but is merely due to incoordination of the immature walking muscles. It usually resolves itself within a few months, but often worries the child's parents while it lasts.

Treatment. In rickety children the general condition must be dealt with, and anti-rachitic treatment given for a long period. Rest in bed, massage, and the use of splints firmly applied to the outer sides of the legs and thighs, will often be successful in correcting the deformity. In adolescents, rest, massage, and the use of a walking caliper, splint and boot are advised. Some cases require surgical treatment.

Bow Legs

Bow legs are found in rickety children who have been allowed to run about during acute rickets; the legs are curved outward and forward. Anti-rachitic treatment must be adopted and carried out for a prolonged period, and manipulation or surgical operation may also be needed. See also Rickets, p.398.

Club Foot

Club foot is a deformity in which the foot is bent and deformed so that the patient does not stand on the sole of the foot when he puts his weight on that leg. There are different types of the deformity; in the commonest form the heel is drawn up and the sufferer walks on the outer edge of the foot. In other cases he may walk on his heel, or the foot may be turned inward or outwards. Club foot is usually hereditary and present from birth, or it may develop later as a result of poliomyelitis, nerve injuries, or nerve diseases, scarring with contraction after injuries or infection, shortening of the leg, or irregular growth of the leg bones as in osteomyelitis.

Treatment. Massage, manipulation, and bandaging with malleable splints may be sufficient in early cases; when the deformity is severe, however, an operation is necessary.

Cervical Rib

This is a condition in which there is an overgrowth of the sixth or seventh vertebrae in the neck, so that a fibrous cord or a complete rib is developed. This may press on the subclavian artery or on the nerves to the arm, causing neuralgia on the inner side of the arm and forearm, with weakness of the thumb, and some wasting of the muscles of the hand.

The rib may be present on one or both sides, and is generally found in young women.

Treatment consists in removing the rib by a surgical operation.

Webbed Fingers and Toes

This is a condition sometimes seen in newborn infants, which can be corrected by a surgical operation.

Polydactylism

Occasionally children are born with more than five digits on a hand or foot, but these can easily be removed by a surgeon.

DISEASES AND INJURIES OF THE SPINE

Spina Bifida

This is a condition sometimes seen in newborn infants; some part of the back wall of the spinal canal is deficient, and there may be protrusion of the cord. In some cases the child may be stillborn, or may only live for a few days. In other cases surgical treatment is possible, occasionally giving very good results. The ultimate prognosis depends, however, on whether or not the child subsequently develops hydrocephalus (water on the brain).

Fractures and Dislocations

These are dealt with in detail in the section on Fractures, pp. 543-56.

Sprains and Injuries

Sprains are caused by sudden severe bending or twisting of the spinal column so that the spinal muscles and ligaments are torn. Such injuries are common in riding, diving, or railway accidents. The pain varies according to the severity of the sprain and, when very severe, causes rigidity, with inability to move. Absolute rest is required, with massage when the pain becomes easier. Six to eight weeks in bed may be necessary.

Sacro-iliac strain, due to strain of the joint between the sacrum and pelvic bones, is common in women, especially after confinements; a supporting corset gives relief if properly fitted.

Injuries to the spinal column may cause spinal concussion, spinal shock, compression of the spinal cord, or injury or destruction of the cord. The effects of the injury, as from blows, bullet wounds, or falls on the head or directly on the back, depend on the site involved. In cases of injury to the neck death may be instantaneous, but in the lower parts of the column paralysis may develop if the cord is injured, or there is pressure from hemorrhage.

Treatment is mainly surgical, with prevention of sepsis in open injuries or penetrating wounds. In spinal shock, without gross injury to the cord, the paralysis often passes off within a few weeks.

Slipped Discs

Under muscular stress or strain, usually due to an accident, the fibrocartilage discs between the vertebrae may become displaced and the pulpy center partly extruded into the spinal canal, thus pressing on nerve roots. This is known as prolapsed or slipped discs. In the lumbar region it may cause sciatica.

The sequence of treatment is (1) rest in bed; (2) wearing a supporting plaster jacket for a short period only; (3) lumbo-sacral support; (4) spinal manipulation to restore muscle function; and (5) exercises for the extensor muscles of the spine.

Prevention of this condition may be helped by proper use of the back in lifting heavy objects. The back should always be kept straight, the body being lowered by bending at hips, knees, and ankles.

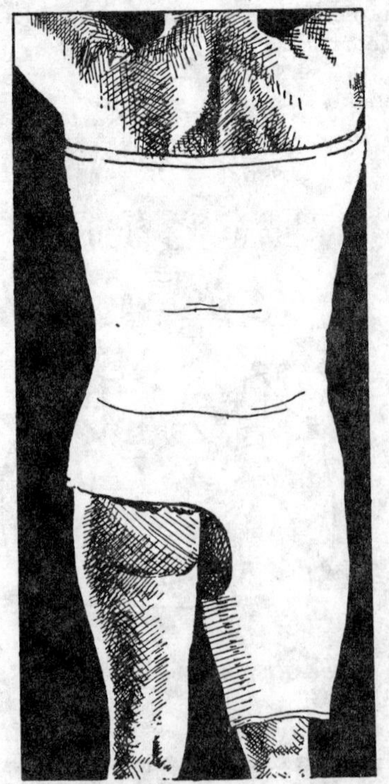

Fig. 5. *PLASTER SUPPORT for a sciatic patient with prolapsed disc in the lumbar region.*

Pott's Disease

Tuberculosis of the spine, or Pott's disease, generally occurs in children under ten years of age, but occasionally young adults develop the disease after accidents or injuries to the spine. It is the cause of the deformity known as hunch-back. Softening of the bodies of the affected vertebrae occurs, followed by collapse from the weight of the trunk, with backward deformity, and often angular curvature.

Symptoms are aching pain, especially on movement. It may be referred to the legs, abdomen or arms, with rigidity and tenderness over the site of the disease. Later, deformity develops, and in some cases there is abscess formation; paralysis is rare. Most cases recover with fixation and stiffness of the vertebrae involved, and a varying degree of deformity.

Treatment is similar to that of tuberculosis elsewhere in the body, with prolonged immobilization and rest in a recumbent position with the spine over-extended to correct the deformity, and the use of a supporting apparatus or jacket. Surgical treatment is often used to shorten the rest period by providing support to the spine with bone grafts, or by evacuating abscesses and dead bone.

Arthritis

Osteo-arthritis and other forms of chronic arthritis of the spine are fairly common. Such conditions cause much pain and stiffness and occasionally produce deformity, especially in old persons who have done much heavy manual labor. (See Diseases of the Joints, p. 531 for treatment.)

Coccydynia

This is a fairly common condition with pain over the coccyx or tail-bone. It may follow childbirth or injuries, but there may be no apparent cause. Sometimes removal of the coccyx is carried out to give relief.

Spinal Meningitis

This may follow injuries or wounds; paralysis develops and, except in cases which can be treated by antibiotics, the spinal cord may be destroyed, with a fatal termination.

DEFORMITIES OF THE SPINE

There are several varieties of curvature of the spine, the main types of deformity being:

SCOLIOSIS, or lateral curvature, with some twisting and rotation of the vertebrae, in the dorsal and lumbar parts of the spine.

KYPHOSIS, or backward curvature, generally in the center dorsal portion of the spine between the ribs.

LORDOSIS, or forward curvature of the lumbar spine below the ribs.

These types may be combined in the same person.

Scoliosis

Scoliosis occurs in young adolescents, especially anemic girls. It may be secondary as a compensating posture in hip disease or other deformities of the legs or feet, or may follow diseases of the chest or spine such as rickets, caries of the spine, empyema or lung disease. Scoliosis occasionally develops after poliomyelitis, or may be congenital.

Symptoms. At first there is a projection of one collar-bone, or one side of the chest (on the side of the convexity of the curve), or one shoulder is elevated and is thought to be 'growing out,' the shoulder blade being higher and more prominent than its fellow. On examination, one shoulder and side of the chest will be found to be rounded (convex) and lifted up with the ribs widely separated, while the other is sunken and concave, with the ribs crowded together. The opposite hip bone protrudes and the spinal column has a curve, as in Fig. 6. Generally the primary curve is to the right in the dorsal region, with a second curve to the left in the lumbar region.

Causes. The condition is often caused by weakness, strain, habit, posture or occupations which keep the body in a laterally distorted position. It develops in quickly growing children with bad habits in sitting and standing, or in young people fatigued through prolonged standing. The muscles may also become so weakened in young girls or women of sedentary habits that they cannot maintain the spine in the normal upright position. In severe or long-standing cases the patient is listless; there may be indigestion from displacement of the abdominal organs.

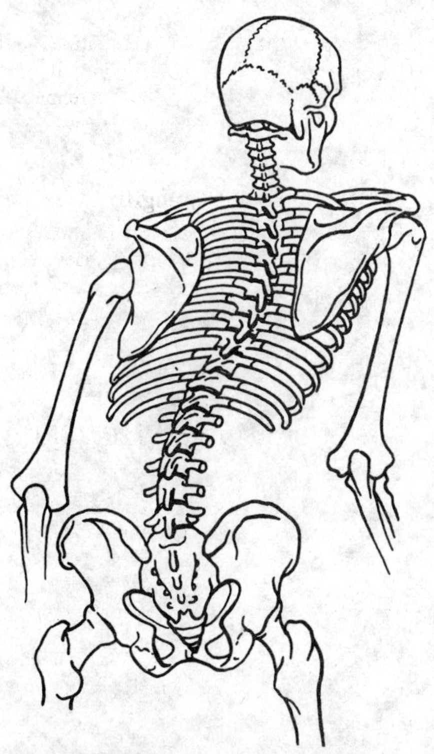

Fig. 6. *LATERAL CURVATURE OF THE SPINE.*

Examination. The patient should be stripped for examination and the spinous processes of the vertebrae are marked with a colored pencil. The pelvis may be seen to be tilted or 'oblique,' and flat foot or knock-knee may also be noted. If the curve disappears when the patient stands as erect as possible, or when he hangs by the hands from a bar the curvature is curable. If it only partly disappears a complete cure may not be possible, although treatment may arrest the trouble. A large single curve is worse than a double curve.

In some cases deafness in one ear, or poor eyesight is present. Regular examination of schoolchildren and gymnastic training in cases of poor or faulty posture greatly help in preventing postural types of curvature where no structural disease is present.

Treatment. The first thing is to find what particular habit of posture of the body has given rise to the deformity.

The cause must always be treated, and deformities of the leg or foot must be corrected or compensated. The general health must be given every attention as regards fresh air, nourishing food and regular meals. Massage, cold bathing and daily remedial exercises for some months, with avoidance of fatigue, and sometimes manipulation, are required. Rest in the lying-down position on a flat inclined board is necessary for two hours daily. Spinal supports should be used only in severe cases. A plaster jacket is used with success in some cases, being applied to correct the deformity, but its use should be restricted to those who are under skilled medical care.

Kyphosis

Kyphosis sometimes occurs in rickety infants and is then generally only temporary, although severe cases may lead to permanent deformity. Adolescent 'round shoulders' are very common, due to weakness, short-sightedness, anemia, and certain occupations involving close work. The child looks listless, the head is poked forwards, the shoulders droop, the chest is flat, and the abdomen probably protrudes. This type of deformity also develops in shoemakers and porters and others whose occupation involves constant bending. In old persons senile kyphosis is very common, and it sometimes follows injuries or diseases of the spine.

Treatment includes remedy of the cause where possible, correction of faulty posture, with massage, electrical treatment and remedial exercises taught by a physiotherapist or skilled person, with avoidance of fatigue and care of the general health.

Lordosis

In lordosis the deformity is in the lumbar region and there is generally some other form of spinal curvature or deformity present also. It occurs as a compensating posture in pregnancy, obesity, and large abdominal tumors.

BACKACHE

Backache may be due to a variety of disorders, so the spine must be carefully examined for tender areas, and the pelvis and abdominal organs must also be examined. An X-ray photograph of the spine should be taken, and a careful test made of the urine.

Due to Affections of Spinal Bone or Joints. Injuries of the head, or the back of the pelvis, are often a source of backache afterwards. An X-ray examination may show some bony injury or displacement. Bony injuries which are most likely to lead to backache are minor fractures which may not be diagnosed at the time of the injury. Of the minor types of fractures causing backache, the two most common are compression fractures and fractures of the transverse processes of the lumbar vertebrae. The first should be treated by fixation or immobilization in a plaster case and by the use of a spinal support afterwards, while the second may be treated by strapping and exercise. In long-standing cases surgical treatment for fusion of the vertebrae will bring permanent relief.

Locked Joint. Locking of the joints between the vertebrae is an occasional cause of pain, and occurs after sudden strains. It may affect any part of the spine from the neck to the lumbar spine, or the lumbo-sacral joint. Manipulation is often useful in these cases to relieve pain, and to increase mobility.

Strain of the Ligaments. Any factor which leads to an alteration in the weight-bearing axis of the spine or lower limbs, or distorts the normal curves of the spine, or stretches the joints, may lead to persistent pain as a result of strain of the ligaments. These conditions may arise from injuries, such as sudden falls, from childbirth, or from faulty postures or muscular weakness.

Sacro-iliac Strain may follow various injuries, especially childbirth; there is severe pain in the lower part of the back which is worse after sitting or on bending. Manipulation under an anesthetic often relieves the pain, and massage and exercises are then given for a month afterwards. A supporting corset is also used by many women who find the specially fitted belt relieves the condition.

Lumbo-sacral Strain gives rise to pain and stiffness when the patient bends forwards, or when the back is turned round while the patient is sitting down. This pain is felt just above the sacrum. Manipulation is seldom effective, more benefit being gained from skilled massage and infra-red irradiation. Physical exercises are also used when the posture is faulty. If the pain is made worse by driving a car the seat should be raised up and drawn forward to prevent complete extension of the legs in using the control pedals.

Postural pain may follow conditions which affect the weight-bearing ligaments of the spine. Thus flat foot, corns, high heels, sedentary occupations, or fatiguing work, obesity and many other conditions may lead to changes of stress in the spinal ligaments. The cause should be discovered and, as far as possible, removed.

Vertebral Disease. Tuberculosis, osteo-arthritis, and secondary cancer in the spine are other causes of pain in the back.

TUBERCULOSIS, or caries of the spine, may be diagnosed in the early stages by pain and stiffness during movement, muscular rigidity, and X-ray examination. The treatment is described on p.538.

OSTEO-ARTHRITIS of the spine is often relieved by careful manipulative treatment, combined with radiant heat or diathermy, and with massage.

CANCER deposits may settle in the spine from any primary source but the commonest are the growths of the breast in women and the prostate gland in men.

Due to Muscular Affections. Chill, exposure to damp, or heavy sweating and congestion of the muscles when the clothes are not quickly changed are common causes of acute backache, especially in gouty or rheumatic individuals. A very hot bath, a thorough rub down and 600 milligrams of aspirin often relieves this type of pain. Infra-red irradiation, diathermy, or brisk massage are also useful. Massage with oil of wintergreen is also useful; kaolin compresses will provide heat to the affected part.

Sometimes painful nodules persist, which may be treated by injections of local anesthetics. See p. 533.

Due to Nervous Causes. This type of backache may be due to pressure upon the spinal nerves, or to disease of the nerves themselves. In other cases where there is no apparent cause for the pain, as after injuries without actual structural damage, an 'anxiety state' may be present, which should be treated by psychological methods in conjunction with massage, and other physiotherapeutic means.

Due to Referred Pain. In all obscure cases of backache a thorough examination should be made to exclude septic conditions of the teeth, tonsils, sinuses, urine and pelvis, etc. Diseases of the internal organs may give rise to pain in the back, for example aneurysm, lung diseases or growths, gastric disease, affections the of gall-bladder or liver, or diseases of the kidneys, pancreas, or pelvic organs (such as chronic infection of the cervix).

FRACTURES AND DISLOCATIONS

A fracture is a break, either partial or total, in a bone, which is usually produced by injury or violence. Fractures, however, may be the result of old age, or of diseases such as paralysis, or of bone diseases such as tuberculosis or cancer; the fracture is then said to be 'spontaneous.'

Causes. Fractures may be caused by:

1. direct violence, when the bone breaks at the site of the blow.

2. indirect violence, when the bone is broken at some distance from the point of impact; in long bones the fracture is then often oblique or spiral.

3. muscular action, which causes fractures of some small bones such as the knee-cap (patella), or the olecranon of the humerus at the elbow joint.

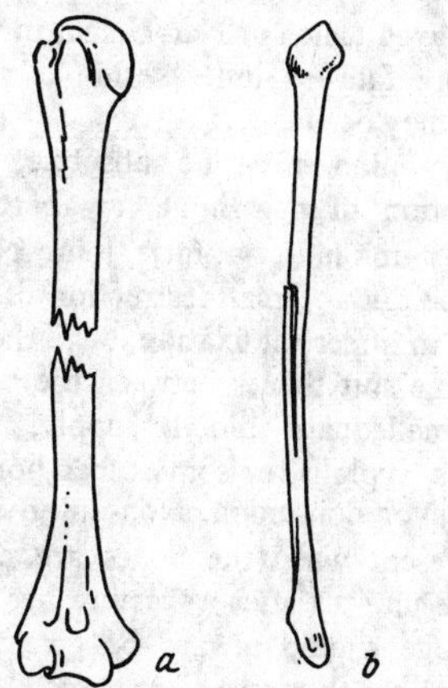

Fig. 1. *SIMPLE FRACTURE.* a. *Fracture of humerus.* b. *Greenstick fracture of fibula in a young child.*

Types of Fractures

A Simple Fracture is one in which the bone is broken without much injury to the surrounding parts, and without any wound of the flesh. This is also called a 'closed fracture.' A complete fracture may be T-shaped, transverse, oblique, longitudinal, or spiral.

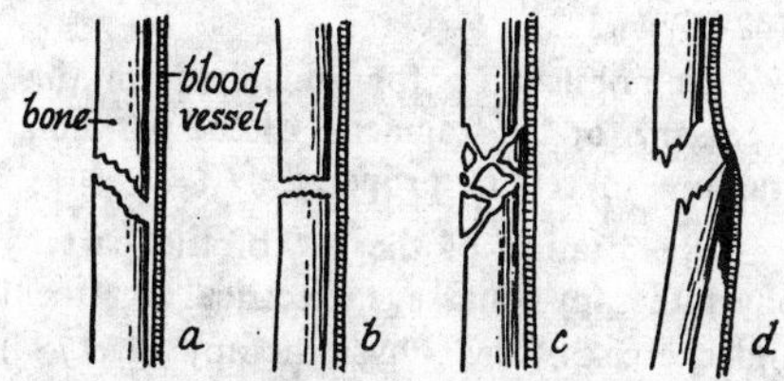

Fig. 2. *FOUR VARIETIES OF FRACTURES.* a. *A simple oblique fracture.* b. *A simple transverse fracture.* c. *A comminuted fracture, with fragmentation of the bone.* d. *A complicated fracture showing injury to blood vessel from sharp splinter of bone.*

Greenstick Fractures occur in children when the bone bends, and only partially breaks, owing to its soft immature structure (Fig. 1, b).

A Comminuted Fracture is one in which the bone is broken or splintered into several pieces, necessitating great care in handling (Fig. 2, c).

A Compound Fracture consists of a fracture in continuity with an external wound; an end of the broken bone may protrude through the flesh and skin, or the wound may communicate with the bone below, as in a bullet wound. The fracture may be transverse, oblique, spiral, or longitudinal.

A Complicated Fracture is one in which, besides the breaking of the bone, there is dislocation of a joint, injury of blood vessels or nerves, the extensive tearing of the soft parts, or injuries of the bowels, lungs, or some other internal organ. The fracture itself may be transverse, oblique, spiral, or longitudinal.

Fractures of the skull may be stellate, fissured, depressed, etc. (See p. 545.)

Diagnosis

A fracture can generally be diagnosed by the patient's symptoms, by the signs of appearance of the part, and the history of the accident or injury. When characteristic signs are absent, the diagnosis may be made from a history of sudden severe pain, followed by deformity and local tenderness on pressure; the fracture must be confirmed by X-ray examination. When the injured part is examined, great care must be used so that further damage or pain is not caused; the part should be compared with the corresponding region on the opposite side of the body.

History. The patient's own account may provide some clues as to the likely extent of the injury. Severe crush injuries often cause fractures, and sometimes the bone may have been heard to snap at the time of the accident.

Symptoms. The chief symptom of a fracture is generally pain at or near the site of the injury, with tenderness on pressure. There is also disability of movement or use of the part, with pain on attempted movement. Swelling and deformity may be seen, but are not necessarily present in all fractures. In some cases swelling may mask the deformity, especially at the ankle.

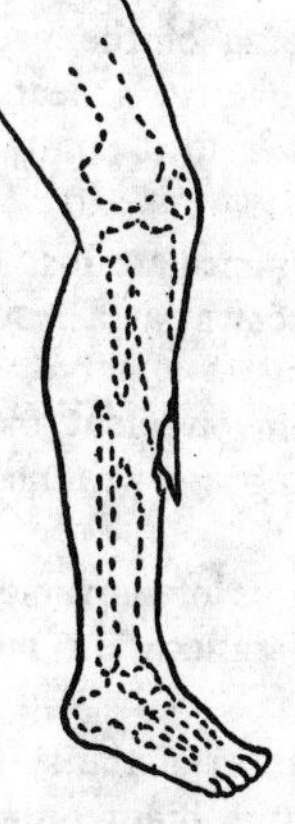

Fig. 3. *COMPOUND FRACTURE OF SHIN-BONE, with the upper part of the bone projecting through the flesh and skin.*

The limb or part may be misshapen or held in an unnatural position, or there may be obvious shortening. If the fractured bone is near the surface of the skin it may be seen to be irregular in outline or shape.

Grating of the bony fragments (crepitus) may be heard when the bone is moved slightly or is examined, but this should *never* be tested for except by a doctor, since a compound fracture or further damage may be produced by unskilled handling.

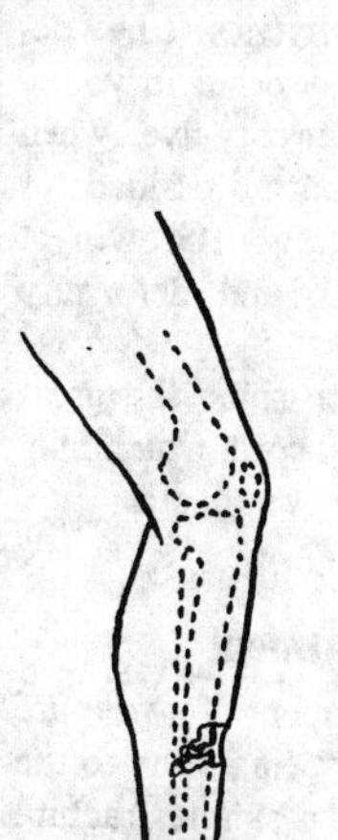

Fig. 4. *COMPOUND FRACTURE OF SHIN-BONE, with the open wound penetrating among the broken fragments of the bone.*

X-ray Examination. When there is any doubt, the case should be treated as a fracture until an X-ray examination has been made or the patient has been seen by a doctor.

Transport. When the patient is unconscious or when there are signs of injury to the head or spine, especial care must be taken in moving or transporting him.

Associated Disorders due to Fractures

A fracture, apart from the local injury, usually also results in shock; in some cases there may be hemorrhage, or later there may be reactionary fever, delirium tremens in alcoholic subjects, and other systemic disturbances.

Shock. For an account of shock, its causes, effects on body tissues, and treatment, see Wounds and Their Care, p. 557. For the first-aid treatment of shock, see First Aid, p. 21.

Complications. A fracture may also cause injury to surrounding tissues, organs, or other parts of the body immediately after injury, in the course of healing, or as a result of unsatisfactory healing.

ARTERIES. Hemorrhage, gangrene, or aneurysm may follow a fracture causing damage to a main artery.

VEINS. Clotting, or swelling of the part, may be caused by injury of a vein near a fracture. This may lead later to a contracture of the muscles.

NERVES. There may be immediate loss of sensation or power of movement as a result of a fracture causing injury to a nerve, or later symptoms of nerve involvement may follow, such as tingling, numbness, weakness, or even paralysis.

JOINTS. Adhesions and loss of movement may lead to arthritis, or dislocation may occur.

OTHER ORGANS. In fractures of the skull, pelvis or ribs, injuries to the brain or abdominal organs or lungs may be severe.

AN IMPACTED FRACTURE is one in which the broken ends of the bone are driven into one another.

SEPARATION OF AN EPIPHYSIS (the developing end of a bone) may occur in young persons under the age of twenty-five, when the parts of the bone are not all ossified (or joined together by bony tissue). Growth of the bone may be affected, and deformity produced.

SPINE. In fractures of the spine the great danger is injury to the spinal cord, which may be followed by paralysis or even death.

First-aid Treatment

The aim of first-aid treatment of a fracture is to prevent further injury being done to the part, especially to prevent a simple fracture from becoming compound or complicated, or a compound fracture from becoming infected or complicated.

1. **Promptness.** As a general rule the patient should be attended to on the spot, since careless or inexpert handling in moving him might increase the effects of the injury. Often a provisional stretcher, splint, sling or other support can quickly be found and applied, as when someone is injured in a busy street, or when it is necessary to take a patient to hospital. Unless the patient is in danger from hemorrhage or some other form of risk, therefore, always render the part immovable by some splint or support, before removing him.

2. **Hemorrhage.** When bleeding occurs it must be attended to at once. Place the patient in a comfortable or suitable position, expose the injury and apply pressure by means of the fingers and thumb on the appropriate pressure point (see First Aid, p. 24). Then use a sterile pad and bandage to control the bleeding (p. 25).

3. **Support** the injured part, placing it with great care in as natural a position as possible.

4. **Splints, Bandages and Slings** should be used as required in individual cases.

Splints should be firm, and sufficiently long to support the joints above and below the fracture. They should be light and strong, and at least as wide as the limb. Wooden or light metal splints are generally used, but sticks, strong cardboard, brooms or umbrellas etc. may be used as temporary emergency substitutes. Whatever form of support is used should be well padded on the surface next to the limb with raw cotton or other soft material. When no splint is available for first aid, an injured arm may be very carefully bound to the body; a fractured leg should always be tied to its fellow for additional support, with wide bandages round the thighs, above and below the knees, at the ankles and around the feet (p. 34).

Great care must be used when applying the splints and bandages so that the injured part is kept well supported and the bones are not further displaced. Bandages must be applied firmly but not too tightly, to hold the splints in position. The upper bandage should always be applied first. (For diagrams of bandages and slings, see First Aid, pp. 26-30.)

A Stretcher may be improvised in an emergency by using a shutter, door, or broad piece of wood covered with rugs, coats or straw; over these is laid a piece of sacking, a rug or blanket which is useful for lifting the patient off the stretcher.

An alternative method is to pass two poles through the sleeves of two or three coats turned inside out. The coats are buttoned up. Strips of wood bound to the ends of the poles complete the stretcher.

A stretcher of some sort must be obtained as soon as possible and should be covered with padding, blankets or garments; the stretcher should be gently slid beneath, and the patient laid on it by a sufficient number of people to raise him easily from the ground. The stretcher should then be carried by four people, two at each end, moving steadily with great care, and keeping exact step with each other. If these persons take hold of the ends of two poles fixed under the stretcher, they will find they can carry it much more easily. (See illustrations, pp. 20-21).

Union of Fractures

The union of fractured bones is slower than that of severed skin or muscle. If the ends or parts of the bone are kept steadily in position together, they soon become surrounded by a blood clot called 'primary callus' which gradually becomes converted into bone.

Callus is formed between the bone and the outer covering membrane or periosteum (external callus), in the marrow cavity (internal callus), and between the bone ends (permanent callus). An internal or external callus gradually disappears after union of the bone fragments. Callus takes from two to three weeks to form, and is converted into bone in about six or eight weeks in favorable cases. In old persons, union of the broken bone fragments may, however, be delayed for weeks or months, or there may be fibrous union, or non-union.

Time Required for Union. Fractures of the ribs and collar-bones normally unite with comparative firmness in about a month; fractures of the arm unite in six weeks and those of the thigh and leg in eight weeks. A broken bone will unite much sooner in a robust and healthy person than in a debilitated patient, and sooner in young than in old people.

The time required for the splint or plaster case to be worn varies with the part injured, the severity of the injury, the health of the patient and any associated complications.

Massage is generally required and should be started as soon as possible; this must be given by a skilled exponent.

Delayed Union or Non-Union, in which the fracture fails to unite within a reasonable time, may occur.

Non-union may be absolute, with no formation of new bone, or there may be fibrous union, or a false join. Non-union may be due to great destruction of part of a bone, to imperfect fixation, or to the pressure of some soft tissues between the bone ends. An inadequate blood supply, old age, rickets, syphilis, or some other bone disease also favor non-union. Non-union is said to be present when the bones are not united twelve months after a fracture has occurred. Massage should always be given, and the general health must be improved.

Surgical treatment by bone-grafting, wiring, or other methods may be required to assist the union of the bone fragments.

GENERAL TREATMENT OF FRACTURES

There are three essential aims in the treatment of fractures.

1. Early reduction of the fracture, and correction of the displacement of the bone fragments.

2. Immobilization for the length of time necessary for the fragments of the particular fracture to reunite properly.

3. Restoration of the use of the part by physiotherapy—massage, electrical treatment and exercises. (See Physiotherapy, p. 175.)

Compound Fractures. Because there is an associated break in the skin or an exposed wound in compound fractures, treatment involves additional measures to eliminate the added danger from infection. See pp. 553 and 557

Reduction

Reduction can generally be accomplished by a surgeon by manipulative methods. General or local anesthesia is usually required to overcome the spasm and pain in the part, in order to allow relaxation of the muscles. Often some form of continuous extension is required, such as the use of weights which are attached to the limb by various devices.

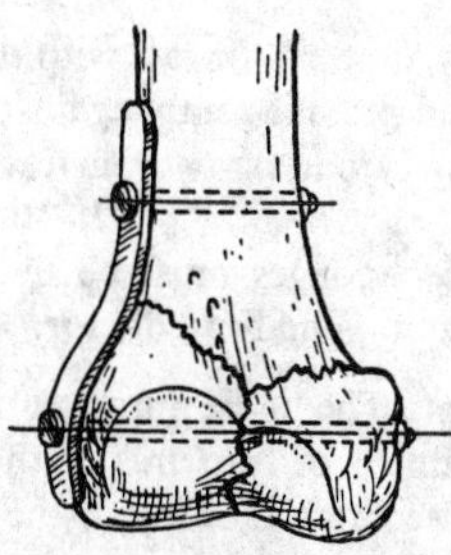

Fig. 5. *SURGICAL REPAIR OF FRAGMENTED BONE with a steel plate screwed to lower end of femur.*

Reduction lessens the displacement, bringing the fragments of the broken bone together and adjusting them to each other so that they regain their natural position. This is achieved by what surgeons call manipulation, extension, counter-extension and coaptation. An X-ray examination is usually made before manipulation to show the position of the fractured parts and the extent of the displacement. When a fracture has been set, it may be X-rayed again to confirm the satisfactory position of the bone fragments.

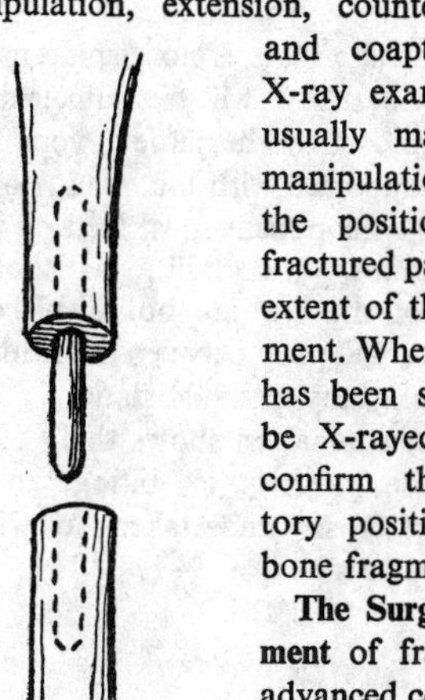

Fig. 6. *BONE PEG used to repair and fix long bone fractures. Sometimes a wire peg is used.*

The Surgical Treatment of fractures has advanced considerably during the last quarter of a century and technique has improved. Open operation is now advocated in order to reduce a fracture if closed reduction is impossible (as occurs with some thumb fractures), or is not accurate enough (some ankle fractures). It is also used when it is necessary to fix the fragments of bone by silver wire, screws, nails, pegs of bone, or metal plates. Such aids are employed with good results and permit earlier use of the limb.

There is, however, a grave danger of introducing infection, and strict asepsis must be used to get good results.

Immobilization

To maintain the ends or fragments of the broken bone steadily in contact in the correct position, so that union can occur by the natural process of callus formation, the part or limb must be made immovable. Immobilization of the limbs is generally achieved by the use of splints which may be made of leather, metal (gutter splints), plaster of Paris, plastics or celluloid. The splints should be broader than the limb and must always be well padded. For some hours after a limb is broken the surrounding parts continue to swell, and if the limb is bound up immediately with splints or plaster of Paris, these may require watching and possible readjustment. The lowest part of the limb should be kept under observation for signs of blueness, coldness, or numbness, which show that the splint is too tightly applied and is preventing proper circulation of the blood, and must be readjusted.

Skeleton splints, such as Thomas's knee splints are used to maintain fixation with traction. Caliper splints are used to allow the patient to move about, when he has sustained some injury to the bones of the leg, and weight-bearing must be prevented. The weight of the body is transferred from the pelvis through the side supports of the caliper, instead of being borne by the injured leg (see Fig. 30, p. 551).

Other parts, such as the clavicle, or ribs, may be supported by strapping or bandages properly applied.

Massage and Exercise

Massage and exercises under skilled supervision are required in most fractures and should generally be started early. (See also Physiotherapy, pp. 175 and 177.)

Slings. In fractures of the shoulder or arm, a sling is generally used. This, if well made and properly applied, supports the part and allows the patient to move about and go out-of-doors while union takes place.

Plaster of Paris Bandages

In many simple fractures, as for instance a fracture in the shaft of the lower part of the leg, and in certain cases of fractures at the ankle joint, plaster of Paris and a caliper enable the patient to move about with the use of crutches, whereas if splints were used it would not be advisable to allow him to move about until the bone had united.

Plaster of Paris bandages may be bought prepared for use and are ready for application after being entirely covered by warm water until the bubbles of air cease to rise. Temporary splints which may have been used for support are removed, and a layer of raw cotton or circular stockinet may be applied round the limb. Over this the prepared plaster bandages are firmly and evenly rolled. These should be smoothed over and the limb held in proper position until the plaster is quite set, which usually takes from fifteen to twenty minutes, depending on the temperature of the water used for wetting the bandage. Plaster casts may be left on from two to eight weeks if they do not become loose or broken; the cast may be split by cutting down lengthwise from top to bottom with a sharp knife or shears, care being taken not to go through the plaster suddenly and thus injure the skin.

SPECIAL FRACTURES

Fractures of the Skull

These are always dangerous, owing to the associated brain injury; in all cases of fracture of the skull some degree of concussion is present, and this may be severe. In some cases considerable laceration or bruising of the brain may occur. A fracture of the base of the skull is generally more dangerous than fracture of the vault; both may exist simultaneously. Fractures of the vault are often caused by a direct blow, while those of the base are caused by indirect violence as from a fall.

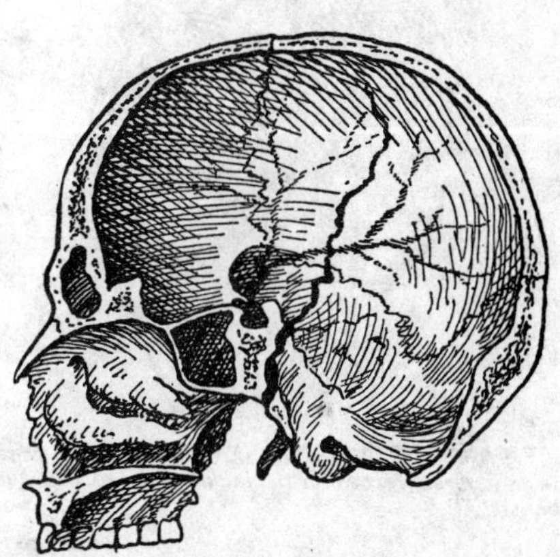

Fig. 7. *FISSURED FRACTURE OF SIDE OF THE SKULL. The fracture crosses the middle meningeal artery.*

Fractures of the Vault may be fissured by extension from the base, star-shaped or depressed, and they are always compound except in the case of 'pond' fractures in infants from birth injuries. In every case there is some degree of concussion and bruising of the brain. In depressed fractures, or when there is bleeding within the skull, compression of the brain also occurs.

Depressed fractures of the vault, causing pressure on the brain, usually require surgical treatment.

A Fracture of the Base may be longitudinal or transverse, and may involve the anterior, middle, or posterior compartments of the skull.

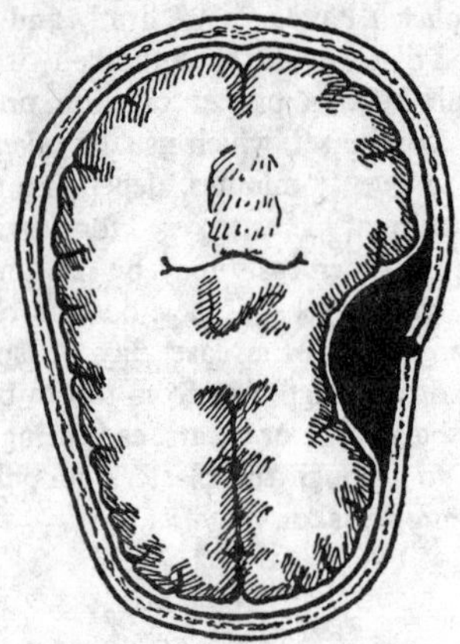

Fig. 8. *BLOOD CLOT AFTER SKULL FRACTURE. An extensive blood clot, due to breaking of blood vessels as in Fig. 7, causes compression of the brain.*

Symptoms. The symptoms vary with the severity of the injury and the type and site of fracture produced. They include unconsciousness (which may be immediate or delayed), vomiting, unequal pupils, and paralysis. A swelling may be visible on the skull, or there may be a visible wound through which a

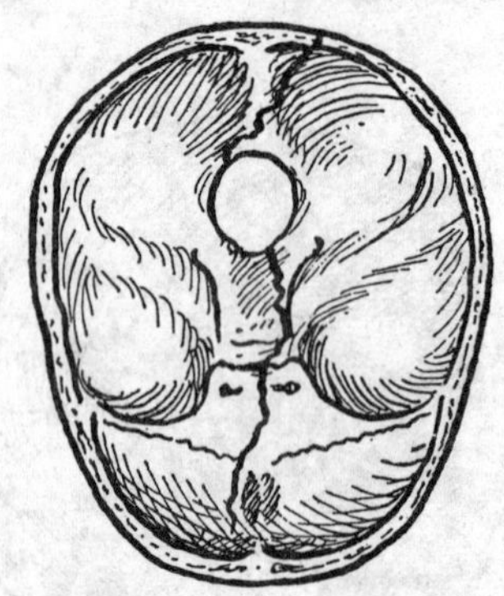

Fig. 9. *FRACTURE OF BASE OF SKULL. A transverse fissured fracture in the middle fossa of the skull base.*

fracture of the vault may be felt with a sterile probe.

In fractures of the base the patient is often unconscious, but not invariably so; he may be temporarily stunned, and then regain consciousness; afterwards he may again lapse into unconsciousness owing to pressure on the brain as a result of bleeding within the skull. There may be protrusion of an eye, with nose-bleeding, bleeding from either ear, or escape of cerebral fluid from nose or ear. Sometimes blood is swallowed and later this may be vomited.

Immediate Treatment. A clean sterile dressing is applied to any scalp wound or injury, if present. Remove any false teeth, and look for any other injuries.

Keep the patient lying flat and, if he is unconscious, watch his breathing to see that it is not obstructed by blood or vomit in the throat, or by the tongue falling backward. Unconscious patients are best treated by gently turning them on their side so that the airway is kept clear.

Ice may be applied to the head by means of an ice bag. If the patient cannot swallow, intravenous feeding may be necessary.

The pulse must be carefully watched by the nurse, and the bladder may require to be emptied by means of a catheter.

Stimulants must *not* be given. (See also First Aid, p. 31.)

A fluid or soft diet is usually given for several days.

General Treatment consists of rest in bed for some weeks while the patient is under a surgeon's care.

If there is an open wound associated with a localized depressed fracture of the vault, the wound edges are excised by a surgeon, together with any fragments of bone. If the surrounding bone is much depressed, it is then elevated, and the scalp wound sutured.

In fissured fractures of the base, no special treatment is indicated regarding the position of the bone fragments. When the fracture is open, or compound, through the ear, nose or pharynx, infection must be guarded against by the use of the correct antibiotics while the wounds are kept sterile by dressings.

Restlessness and irritability may need to be allayed by sedatives. Incontinence sometimes follows head injuries.

In all cases the patient must be carefully watched for signs of compression of the brain, which may be delayed in appearing, and which may render a surgical operation necessary.

Prolonged mental rest is necessary in after-treatment.

Fractures of the Bones of the Nose

The nose is often broken by a direct blow, with displacement of the fragments, causing swelling, deformity, and nose-bleeding. The nasal septum may also be injured.

Treatment. Injuries of this kind may generally be corrected under a general anesthetic by passing guarded forceps up the nostril, and adjusting the bones into their natural position, at the same time using pressure by the fingers on the outside of the nose. If the septum is displaced, rubber tubing is used to correct the deviation. A splint should then be molded to fit over the nose, and is worn for seven to ten days; prophylactic antibiotics may be prescribed. If infection of the nose follows the fracture, both internal and external splints must be removed.

Fractures of the Lower Jaw

Fracture of the lower jaw usually occurs near the chin, but may also take place near the angles of the jaw. It may be simple or compound into the mouth, and may be diagnosed by the pain, bleeding from the gums, swelling, inability to move the jaw or to speak properly, the irregularity, indentation, or swelling felt by the finger, the irregularity of the teeth, and the crepitus or grating sensation. If the fracture occurs at the upper part near the joint, the jaw is displaced towards the fractured side. The patient should not try to speak.

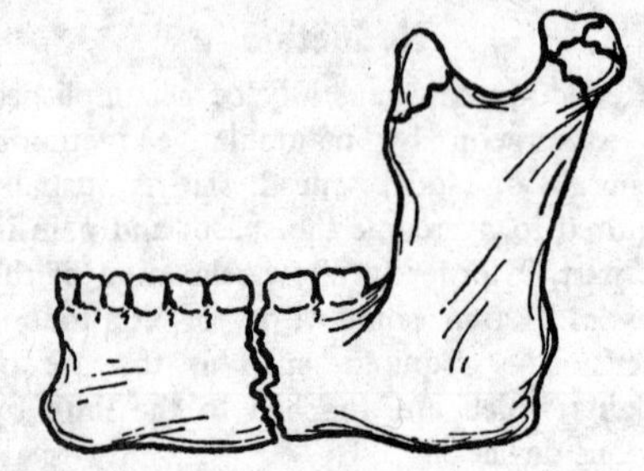

Fig. 10. *LOWER JAW. A fracture of the mandible, or lower jaw.*

First Aid. Support the jaw with the palm of the hand and press it gently against the upper jaw, and apply one or two narrow bandages as illustrated on p. 31. If the patient vomits, the bandages must be removed and reapplied later. Send for a doctor.

Treatment. The most important principle in the treatment of fractures of the jaw is to ensure the accurate meeting of the teeth with their opposite teeth. A dental surgeon should be consulted if necessary.

If there is much displacement, the fragments can be easily replaced in position while the patient is under an anesthetic, and a dental model is taken; an internal wire dental splint is then used. In other cases a suitable molded external splint is used if there is much oral sepsis, or absence of teeth precludes a wire splint; this will ensure a perfect fit of the teeth.

In cases where there is no displacement, a simple jaw bandage will be sufficient; this must be removed if the patient vomits, the jaw being supported with the hand. For four to five weeks the patient must feed on fluids, such as soups, and milk, so that the fragments of the jaw are not displaced by chewing. A small prop between the teeth used during feeding may be of assistance.

If X-ray examination shows that the teeth do not close properly on biting, an open operation may be undertaken to wire or plate the fragments.

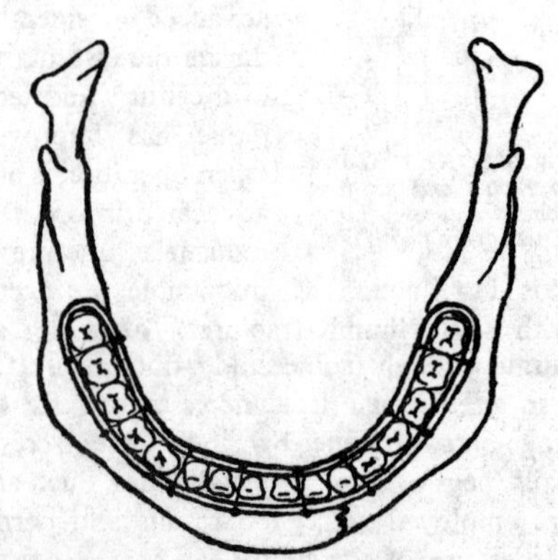

Fig. 11. *DENTAL SPLINT. A wire dental splint is often used on a fractured lower jaw to ensure proper alignment of teeth with those of the top jaw.*

If the fracture is compound, osteomyelitis, septic pneumonia or pyemia may develop as a result of infection of the bone. The infection can usually be cleared with antibiotics.

Fracture of the Collar-bone

This accident usually occurs near the middle of the bone, and is often caused by falls on the arm and shoulder; the outer end, however, is sometimes broken. Fractures of the collar-bone (clavicle) are common in children.

Symptoms. Pain and tenderness are felt at the place of the injury, and there is inability to lift the arm. A small prominence may be noted at the point of the fracture, and the distance from the point of the shoulder to the breast-bone is shorter than on the other side; the shoulder drops downwards, forwards, and inwards. The patient often supports the elbow with the opposite hand to relieve the tension on the fracture. To examine a case of suspected fracture of the collar-bone, compare the two bones and see whether the shoulders have the same shape

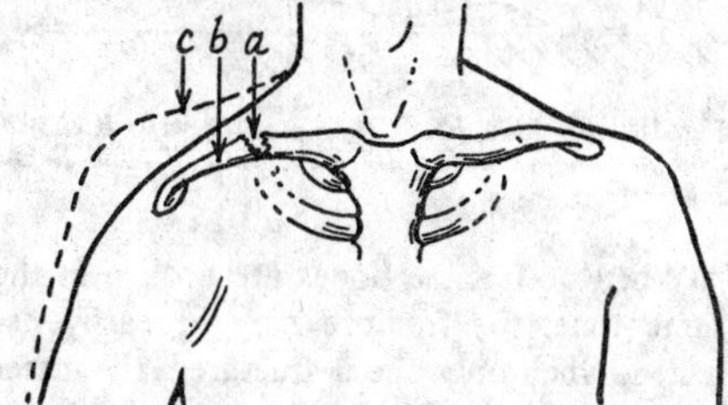

Fig. 12. *COLLAR-BONE FRACTURE. Fracture of the right collar-bone at this site is fairly common. Note the depression of the shoulder.* a. *Site of the fracture.* b. *Collar-bone.* c. *Outline of shoulder before injury.*

of outline. Fractures of the collar-bone seldom cause any final disability, and union nearly always occurs, although there is often a slight deformity over the fracture.

Treatment. Remove the coat and other upper clothing.

For Fractures of the Shaft. For first-aid treatment use a sling, with a pad about four inches wide and two inches thick under the armpit; gentle massage, and movement of the hand are allowed from the onset. The arm is kept at rest by a broad bandage or second sling applied round the elbow and passed round the body, being tied on the opposite side. Test the pulse at the wrist, and if necessary relax the bandage slightly. (See Fig. 57, p.33 .)

A simple way of retaining the fragments in position so that a good result is secured is to place the patient in bed with a narrow pillow behind the shoulders, and the elbow supported; the shoulder then falls backward of its own accord. In cases in which it is especially important to prevent deformity for cosmetic reasons, this method of treatment is the best. The recumbent position should be maintained for three weeks, the arm afterward being kept in a sling and gently exercised.

The figure of eight is useful if both collar-bones are broken. A handkerchief or triangular bandage is folded over a thin roll of bandage, tied round each shoulder, with a reef knot behind. A pad is placed in the middle of the back and the free ends of the two bandages are tied over the pad to draw the shoulders backwards. The arm or arms are then supported in a sling. When only one collar-bone is injured the sling is worn over the sound shoulder. A third bandage, which binds the arm to the chest, may also be worn by day, and this bandage should always be used in bed at night.

The shoulder supports may be dispensed with in about two weeks, and the sling is used for three to four weeks. Manual work may be resumed in six to eight weeks.

For Fractures of the Acromial (Outer) End of the collar-bone there is usually little displacement, but the outer fragment may slip downwards.

When there is no displacement, a sling

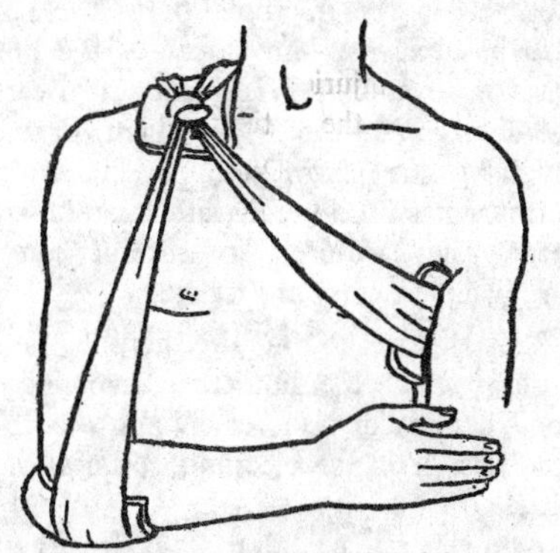

Fig. 13. *FRACTURE OF OUTER END OF COLLAR-BONE. Since there is seldom much displacement in a fracture of the outer end of the collar-bone, this method of fixation is usually adequate.*

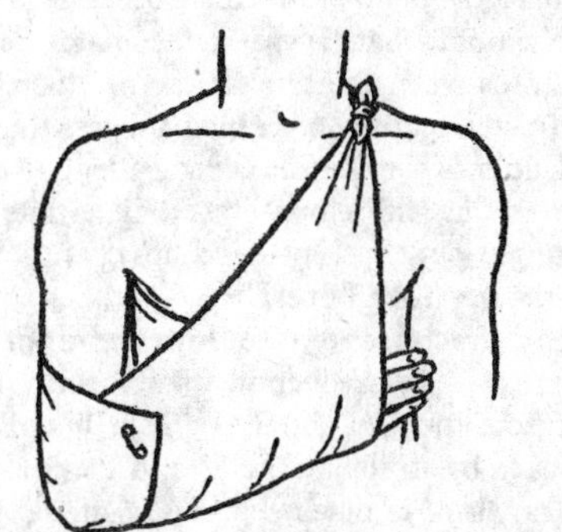

Fig. 14. *SLING FOR A FRACTURED COLLAR-BONE where there is no displacement.*

worn to support the arm is sufficient, keeping the elbow raised.

Fracture of the Shoulder Blade

When this uncommon accident happens, the body of the bone is generally broken across by some great direct violence. In a few cases the acromial end next to the collar-bone is broken.

Symptoms. Great pain is felt on moving the shoulder, and a grating sensation may be felt by the surgeon when placing one hand on the upper end of the bone, and moving the lower portion with the other. There is usually not much displacement in fractures of the body of the bone, the fragments being held in position by the muscles attached to the scapula.

Treatment. For first-aid treatment a broad bandage is applied at its center to the armpit on the injured side and taken round the chest; the ends are crossed over the uninjured shoulder, and tied in the armpit below. The arm on the injured side is supported by a sling. Reduction of the fragments into position is not required. The patient should rest in bed for a few days; this position of the arm should be maintained for four weeks and the arm must be gently exercised after a few days. Good function generally results, even though the fragments are not in perfect position. Heavy work must not be attempted for six to eight weeks.

A second method of immobilizing the part is to use supporting strapping applied to the chest when the patient has breathed out as fully as he can; the strapping encircles two-thirds of the circumference of the chest and is then covered with a flannel bandage.

Fracture of the Acromion

Fracture of the acromion, or the end of the scapula which unites with the collar-bone, may be shown by the flattening of the shoulder; the broken part is drawn down by the action of the deltoid muscle, and the arm is helpless.

Treatment. The injured part must be supported in the same way as a fracture of the outer end of the collar-bone; the elbow must be raised, and the arm fixed to the side of the chest. This position is kept for three to four weeks. No pad should be put in the armpit for this would push the broken fragment outward. Gentle movements of the arm may be begun about the fourth week, with return to work after about eight weeks.

Fractures of the Humerus

The bone of the upper arm is most frequently broken near the center of the shaft although it may be fractured near the shoulder or elbow; in the latter case there is often also a dislocation. (See Figs. 1a, 15, 16, 17.)

A fracture of the shaft causes grating of the broken ends against each other which may be either heard or felt by a surgeon. The arm may also be misshapen, shortened and helpless; if the ends of the shaft of the bone overlap each other, it will be shortened.

First Aid. If the fracture is at the upper end of the humerus, the arm must be supported by a sling; a bandage is passed round the chest and over the arm to bind the arm to the body; tie under the opposite armpit.

If the middle or lower end of the bone is

broken, bend the forearm across the chest with the elbow at a right angle.

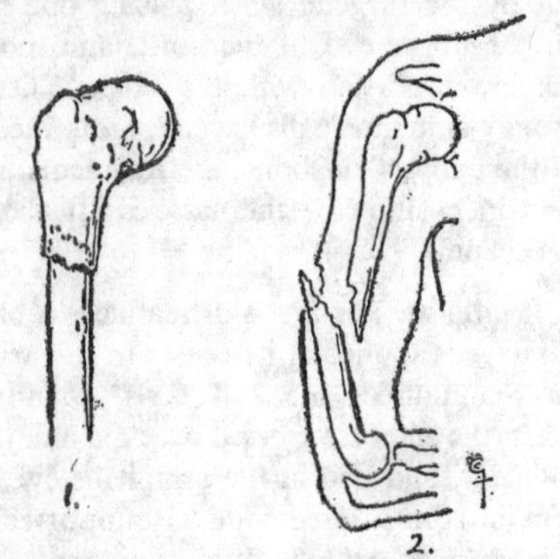

Fig. 15. *FRACTURES OF THE HUMERUS.* 1. *An impacted fracture.* 2. *A compound fracture with an external wound.*

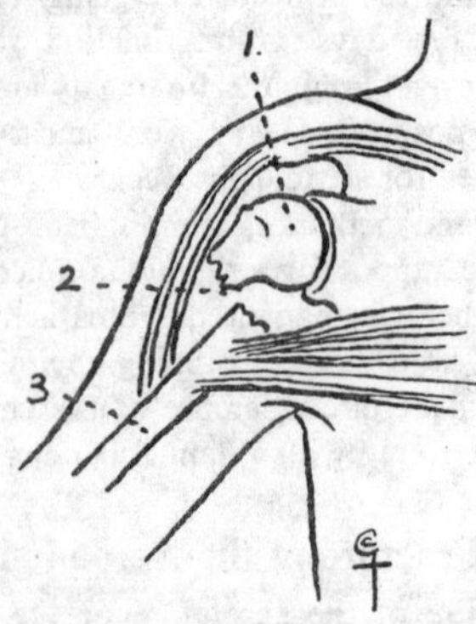

Fig. 16. *FRACTURE OF HUMERUS WITH DISPLACEMENT.* 1. *Head of humerus in shoulder joint.* 2. *Site of fracture.* 3. *Shaft of humerus displaced by pull of the muscle from the chest.*

Treatment. An X-ray photograph should be taken to show the displacement. If there is an associated dislocation of the shoulder or elbow joint, this must be reduced before the fracture is set.

In impacted fractures of the neck of the humerus a sling is worn for four weeks, with gentle movements after one week. Massage should be continued for six weeks.

Fractures of the upper end of the bone, or fractures of the neck with displacement, may be treated on an abduction shoulder splint. Open operation may be necessary in some cases when there is much displacement.

Fractures of the shaft of the bone may be oblique, transverse, spiral or comminuted. They rarely require manipulation, and may be immobilized in plaster of Paris with the arm in a sling. Non-union is not uncommon. Massage should be given from the first, and movements of the shoulder may generally be started after two weeks. Splints may usually be discarded after one to two weeks, the sling being kept for one week longer.

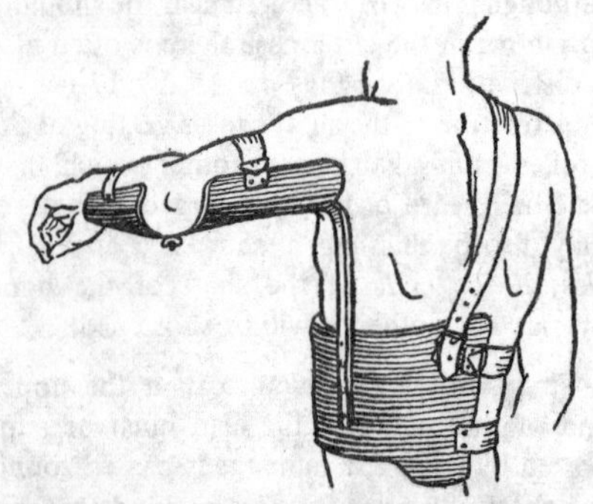

Fig. 17. *SHOULDER ABDUCTION SPLINT for fracture of the glenoid fossa of the scapula and of the surgical neck of the humerus.*

For Fractures of the Lower End, if there is no displacement after reduction, the arm may be kept flexed in a sling, with the forearm in supination.

In most cases fixation for three to six weeks is sufficient; meanwhile massage and movements may be commenced, a sling still being worn. On rare occasions an open operation is required where there is much deformity. Fractures involving either the elbow or the shoulder joint often cause permanent stiffness, even after careful treatment.

Fractures of the Elbow

This may be shown by the patient being unable to move the arm without pain, and by crepitus, and also by the swelling and severe pain felt in the fractured part. There may also be abnormal movement of the bones. An X-ray examination is essential to ascertain the damage and the displacement. Fractures involving the elbow joint often result in permanent stiffness, even after careful treatment. They require very careful handling during any attempt at first aid.

Treatment. The fracture may be at the lower end of the humerus, involving one condyle only, or transversely above both the condyles, or in the olecranon process of the ulna.

As a general rule, all cases of fracture and dislocation occurring about the elbow joint, *excepting* a fracture of the olecranon process of the ulna, are treated with the elbow fully flexed (or bent) with the forearm in full supination, that is with the palm facing upwards when the arm lies across the chest. In fractures of the olecranon process the arm is held in a sling in the older patient so as to prevent a stiff elbow resulting, while the younger patient may have an operation to fix the fractured bones.

For fractures of the lower end of the humerus, after reduction of deformity by a surgeon, the arm should be kept flexed in a sling or by strapping the arm to the forearm, unless there is much separation of the fragments, in which case an operation may be necessary.

Early gentle massage is given from the outset, and gentle movements of the hand are allowed; assisted active elbow movements should be begun after two weeks; the wrist is then gradually lowered every two or three days.

For fractures in this region it is important to watch the initial swelling of the joint when the arm is flexed, or there may be obstruction of the blood supply to the forearm, as shown by swelling and blueness of the fingers, and a poor pulse at the wrist. These signs require immediate straightening of the forearm and loosening of the bandages; an urgent operation is required if the color of the fingers does not immediately improve, otherwise there may follow loss of power in the arm (Volkmann's contracture) or gangrene.

Fractures of the Forearm

The lower part of the arm between the elbow and wrist (forearm) has two bones: the ulna extends from the inner side of the elbow to the wrist at the root of the little finger and the shorter radius lies on the outer or thumb side.

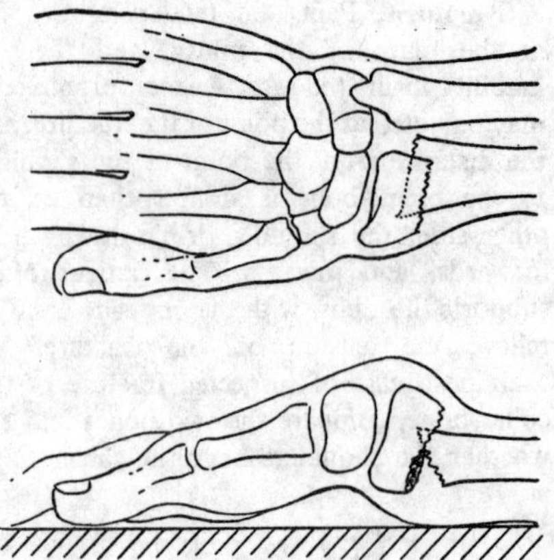

Fig. 18. *COLLES' FRACTURE of the wrist is known, as a 'dinner-fork' deformity. Top, back of hand Below side view.*

When both these bones are broken at the same time, the fracture may be easily detected; when only one is fractured, the intact bone keeps the other in place and the injury is not so apparent. A transverse fracture of the radius within an inch of the lower articular surface is known as Colles' fracture; it is one of the commonest injuries, and is generally due to a fall upon the hand with the wrist extended.

First Aid. For fractures of the forearm when one or both bones are involved, raise the forearm so that it lies across the chest, with the arm bent at a right angle at the elbow, and the palm of the hand against the body. Support the forearm and elbow in a large sling.

Treatment

1. **Fracture of the Ulna.** Fractures of the upper end involving the olecranon process of the elbow joint often require fixing by surgical operation, but if this cannot be undertaken, the arm is immobilized in a sling. This position is maintained for three weeks, during which time graduated exercises are started by a trained physiotherapist.

Fractures of the shaft are easily detected; the deformity must be reduced and the forearm kept in plaster of Paris in semi-pronation, that is, with the thumb pointing directly upwards when the arm is bent across the chest for support in a sling. The plaster should be worn for four to six weeks.

2. **Fractures of the Shaft of the Radius.**

These cause pain, deformity, crepitus and abnormal mobility. The deformity is reduced by manipulation as far as possible. If there is no displacement, the elbow is bent to a right angle, and the forearm put up in the supinated position, with the palm facing upwards when the arm lies across the chest, or in the semi-pronated position (as above) according to the site of the fracture; the latter position is used for fractures of the lower part of the bone. A plaster of Paris slab is applied to the back of the forearm. If there is some displacement, this must be reduced and the arm is fixed with the elbow joint extended, and the fore-arm supinated; plaster of Paris is then applied to the forearm and arm and worn for two weeks. the elbow being bent and the arm supported in a sling in supination. Open operation, with pegging or plating, may also be necessary to correct the displacement.

COLLES' FRACTURE. Fracture of the lower end of the radius just above the wrist, with impaction of the fragments, is known as a Colles' fracture; this is a very common injury especially in old persons, and is caused by falling on the outstretched arm. It produces a typical 'dinner-fork' deformity, with abduction of the hand and backward displacement of the lower fragment and hand. The fracture is about an inch above the wrist, and somewhat oblique, and the fragments are usually impacted. Union generally occurs readily, but some degree of deformity with adhesions, and weakness of grip are common sequels. Reduction of the deformity is essential, and requires slight traction with pressure between the surgeon's hands over the fragments, and manipulation into place. In some cases the deformity tends to recur. The forearm is then put in a split plaster cast and massage must be started at once, with movements of the fingers. Active movements of the wrist are permitted after about two weeks.

3. **Fractures of Radius and Ulna.** When both bones are broken there is usually some overlapping of both bones; the elbow must be kept fixed to prevent cross-union of all four fragments of the shafts. If the displacement cannot be reduced as shown by X-ray examination, an open operation is required, or traction must be applied for a long period by special apparatus.

Fractures of the Wrist, Hand, and Fingers

Any of the bones of the wrist or hand may be broken either by direct injury or by a fall upon the hand. In many cases the diagnosis can only be made by an X-ray photograph. Suspicion of the presence of the fracture arises from the existence of localized pain and tenderness with stiffness and loss of movement.

Fracture of the Carpus (Wrist). Fracture of the scaphoid bone is the most common injury to the carpal bones of the wrist. This is an injury of young people. It is often difficult to diagnose even with X-rays, but when found it must be treated by plaster of Paris immobilization often for months to get a good result.

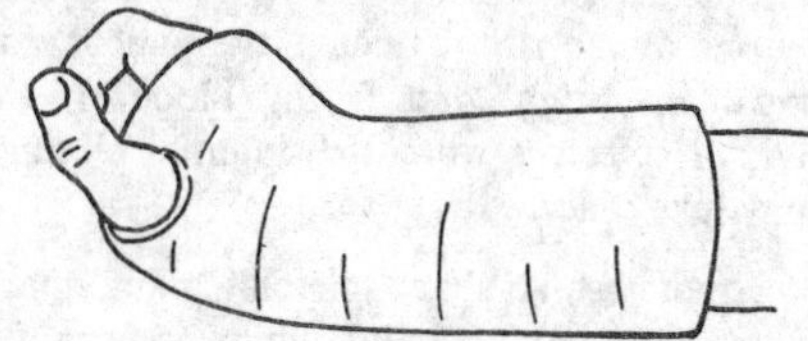

Fig. 19. *PLASTER OF PARIS COCK-UP SPLINT for various fractures of the wrist.*

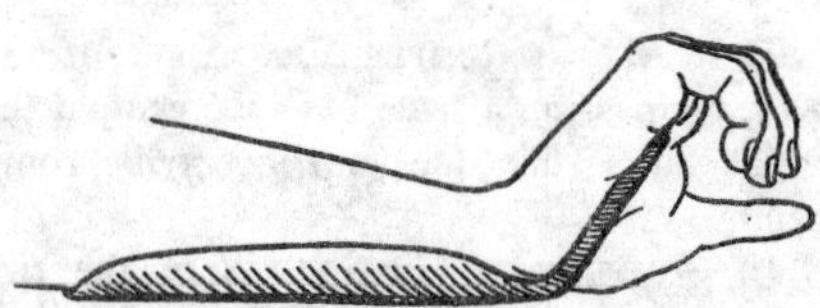

Fig. 20. *METAL COCK-UP SPLINT for the wrist.*

In fractures of the other carpal bones the wrist should be supported in splints or a plaster cast, the hand being slightly bent upwards (dorsiflexed). One or both fragments may be removed if there is much pain or stiffness.

In Fracture of the Metacarpals (hand bones) there is usually no displacement of the fragments. For first aid, a padded splint is applied to the front of the hand, reaching from the tips of the fingers to the middle of the forearm. This is kept in place with a figure of eight bandage round the hand, and a bandage round the forearm. Occasionally extension on a wire frame is required if overlapping of the fragments is present.

For fractures of the fingers, narrow splints may be used, and the hand must be rested. In all the above cases a sling should be used, but massage and exercises must be given. Bennett's fracture is an oblique fracture of the metacarpal bone of the thumb, and must be treated by prolonged extension.

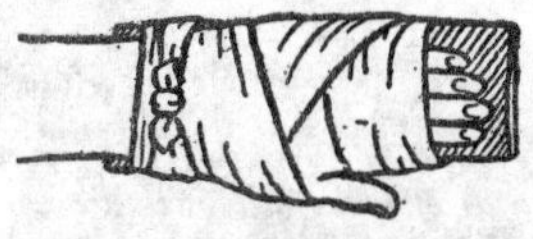

Fig. 21. *FIRST-AID SPLINT AND BANDAGE for fractures of the metacarpal bones of the hand.*

Fractures of the Spine

The spine may be broken by *direct force*, as when a heavy weight falls on the back; or by *indirect violence*, as when a paratrooper lands heavily on his heels.

COMPLETE FRACTURES. When the back is broken the fragments of the vertebrae are liable to become displaced and may injure the spinal cord, causing paralysis or loss of sensation in those parts of the body below the site of the fracture; common sites of complete fracture of the spine are between the neck and upper part of the dorsal region, and at the lower end of the dorsal and upper lumbar regions.

INCOMPLETE FRACTURES. In less severe cases, one of the transverse or spinous bony processes of vertebra may be broken from its attachment to the body of the vertebra, causing severe pain on movement or other symptoms of pressure on a nerve. Incomplete fractures are generally caused by direct violence and may be accompanied by injury to the spinal cord, or spinal concussion.

A COMPRESSION FRACTURE, which is always due to indirect violence, occurs when the spongy body of the bone is crushed. One or more vertebrae may be involved, causing pain, angular deformity, tenderness and rigidity. Concussion of the spinal cord also occurs in these types of injuries.

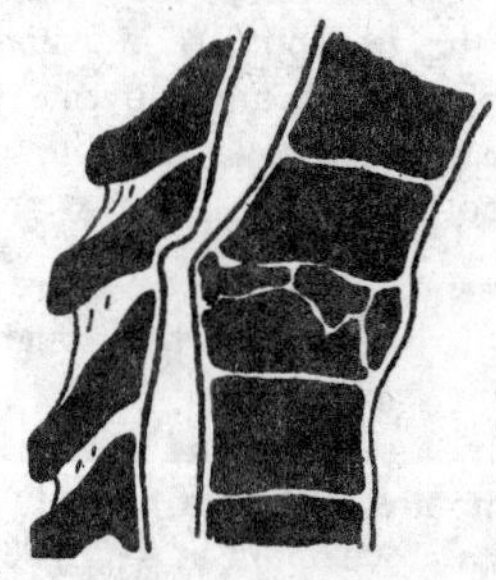

Fig. 22. *COMPRESSION FRACTURE OF SPINE involving the body of a vertebra and giving rise to compression of the spinal cord.*

First Aid for Spinal Injuries

1. Insist on the patient lying completely still, since any handling or movement may involve the spinal cord and increase the injury or even cause death.

2. With great care place the legs together, and then tie a bandage in a figure of eight round the feet and ankles, the knot being arranged to lie under the soles of the feet. Then apply broad bandages round the knees and highs, to keep the limbs steady.

3. In the meantime send for a doctor and treat the patient for shock (see p. 21), with warmth and hot drinks if the patient can swallow. If he is unconscious be sure to watch that the tongue does not fall backwards in the throat, and cause suffocation; it may be grasped with a handkerchief and kept forwards.

TRANSPORT is a procedure only to be undertaken with great caution. It must first be decided in which position the patient should be moved.

1. *If he is unconscious*, or if the site of the injury is uncertain, the patient should be carried face upwards. He is also carried in this way when the injury to the spine is in the region of the neck, that is, when he is conscious but cannot move his arms or legs, and has no sensation in them. If the neck

is injured, firm pads about 4 inches thick are very carefully placed one on either side of the neck.

2. *If the patient is conscious,* but cannot move either of his legs, and has no sensation in them although he can move his arms, a fracture may be present in the thoracic or lumbar parts of the spine and the patient should be carried face downwards, lifting him by slings placed under the upper part of the thighs and pelvis in order to keep his spine extended.

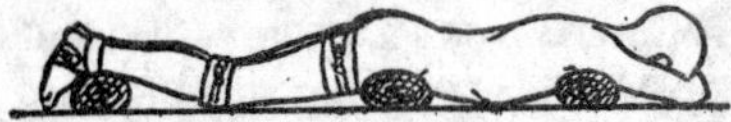

Fig. 23. *FIRST AID IN FRACTURE OF THE SPINE. The patient who is conscious and has an injury or suspected fracture in the dorsal or lumbar region of the spine should be placed face downwards (prone) on a stretcher with firm pillow (or rolled cloth) supports under the shoulders, pelvis, and ankles.*

NOTE. Only skilled first aiders should attempt the transport of a patient with a spinal injury, and any movement must be carried out with great caution, gentleness, and support.

Treatment. In compression fractures, flexion or bending of the spine must be *absolutely* avoided. A plaster jacket is applied by a surgeon and must be worn for several months, although the patient may be allowed to move about at a fairly early stage. Later a spinal brace may be required.

Fracture-Dislocations of the Spine

Fracture-dislocations generally occur in the lower neck or upper part of the spine; the upper segment is usually dislocated forwards, becoming impacted. The spinal cord may be compressed or entirely ruptured. Even if the bony injury is corrected the damage sustained by the cord is permanent. There may be paralysis, deformity, swelling, crepitus and tenderness, with considerable shock. Cystitis, incontinence or retention of urine, and bed-sores are common sequels.

Complete fracture-dislocations above the fourth vertebra are immediately fatal. In other cases the higher the injury, and the greater the damage, the greater is the danger to life.

Treatment. In cases which survive, absolute rest is essential. Surgical treatment may be given later, and careful nursing to prevent bedsores is of the greatest importance.

Fractures of the Ribs

This accident may result from blows, crush injuries of the chest, or even from violent coughing especially in the pregnant and in the old. One, two, or more ribs may be broken at a time, according to the extent of the injury. Fracture of the ribs is more common in middle-aged and old persons on account of the loss of elasticity of the bones as age advances.

The sixth, seventh, eighth, and ninth ribs are those most often fractured, the break usually occurring midway between the spine and the breast bone. If the lungs are injured by one of the rib fragments, the patient may cough up bright and frothy blood. If the liver or spleen is wounded, internal bleeding may take place.

Symptoms. A sharp piercing pain, made worse by breathing, coughing or other movements, is present. The breathing is short and shallow and there is a grating sensation when the patient takes a long breath if the hand is laid upon the injured part.

First Aid. IN SIMPLE FRACTURES of the ribs, try passing a wide bandage around the chest, but if this does not give relief soon, remove it.

IN COMPLICATED FRACTURES of the ribs (when some internal organ is injured) do *not* apply supporting bandages. Let the patient lie down and support him so that the body is inclined to the injured side. Loosen the clothing and treat as for internal hemorrhage and shock; support the arm on the injured side in a large sling.

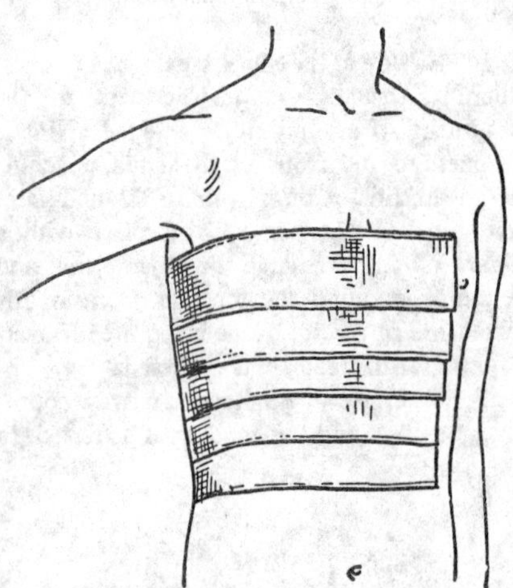

Fig. 24. *SUPPORT FOR RIB FRACTURES. Overlapping strips of adhesive plaster are applied to the affected side of the chest.*

Treatment. The patient should be kept in bed. The injured side is strapped with overlapping strips of non-stretch adhesive plaster applied around the chest when the patient has let out his breath as much as possible; this controls the movements of respiration on that side and gives as much rest to the part as possible. Complications should be treated according to their nature. When a rib is fractured by direct violence the chest may be supported by sandbags instead of by strapping.

Fracture of the Breast-bone

Symptoms. The injured breast-bone (sternum) may be depressed, causing difficulty in breathing, with cough, spitting of blood, pain, inability to lie on the back, and a grating noise caused by breathing. The fracture is usually due to direct violence such as a kick in the chest.

Treatment. Undo all tight clothing. The patient should rest in bed, with a pillow between the shoulders. Should the broken part be displaced downwards, it must be replaced by manipulation or operation.

Occasionally, when much violence occurs to the front of the chest, as in head-on collisions in motor-car accidents, the whole sternum and the ribs attached to it are stove in. It is then an urgent matter to fix these multiple fractures in order that breathing can occur, and traction to the whole chest wall may be required.

Fractures of the Pelvis

These fractures are dangerous, often being associated with some other injury, such as rupture of the bladder, urethra, or bowel, or injury to the great veins or arteries. Fortunately, however, they are only caused by severe injury, and do not often occur.

They may be complete, as from crush injuries, or incomplete, as when the true pelvis escapes injury and only some peripheral part is damaged.

First Aid. See p. 33.

Treatment. Place the patient in the easiest possible position, and keep him entirely at rest in bed. Generally a catheter should be kept in the bladder, so that the urine may be passed easily. Damage to the bladder or bowel has to be treated by open operation.

Complete rest on a firm bed must be ordered for six weeks or two months, and weight-bearing is forbidden for at least three months. Pressure sores must be avoided by careful nursing.

If the extreme lower end of the sacrum, the coccyx (see Anatomy, p. 221), be broken, there is pain on walking, defecation or straining. The separated portion may if necessary be replaced by introducing the finger into the rectum. The bowels must be kept gently opened by mineral oil or laxatives. The patient should rest in bed until firm union has occurred. A fracture of the coccyx may give rise to persistent pain (*coccydynia*), for the relief of which excision of the coccyx may be necessary.

Fractures of the Thigh-bone

The points where the thigh-bone (femur) is liable to be broken are at its upper end or neck, the center part of the shaft, or the lower end near the knee-joint.

FRACTURE OF THE NECK OF THE FEMUR is especially likely in elderly persons who accidentally fall, owing to the brittle state of the bones in old age. Union of the fracture is also often delayed or defective in these cases unless surgical treatment for fixation is given. The shaft of the femur, on the other hand, is strong and is usually only broken by severe violence as in motor-cycle accidents.

Fracture of the neck of the femur causes the thigh to be turned outwards, and there is shortening of the leg.

FRACTURE OF THE SHAFT. The deformity and displacement vary according to the site and direction of the fracture.

A fracture in the shaft may be straight

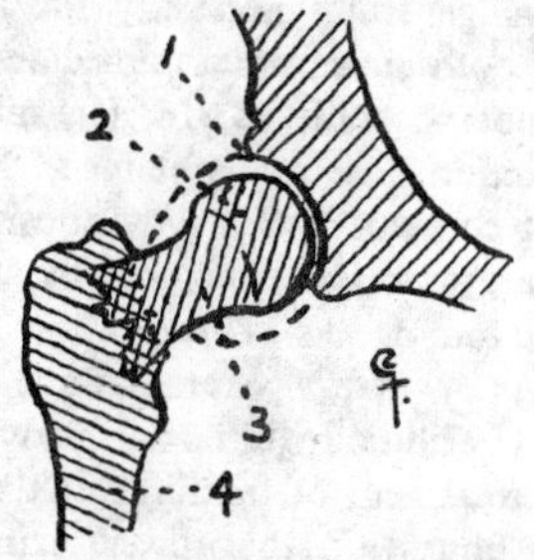

Fig. 25. *FRACTURE OF NECK OF THE FEMUR OUTSIDE THE JOINT CAPSULE, WITH IMPACTION* (*Extracapsular fracture.*) 1. *Capsule of hip joint*. 2. *Head of femur*. 3. *Neck of femur*. 4. *Shaft of femur*.

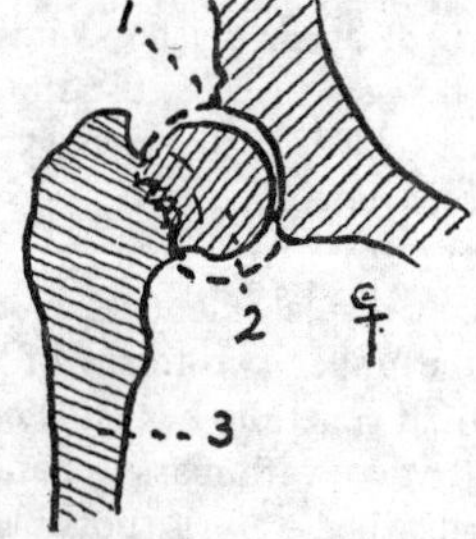

Fig. 26. *FRACTURE OF NECK OF THE FEMUR, INSIDE THE JOINT CAPSULE.* (*Intracapsular fracture.*) 1. *Capsule of hip joint*. 2. *Head of femur*. 3. *Shaft of femur*.

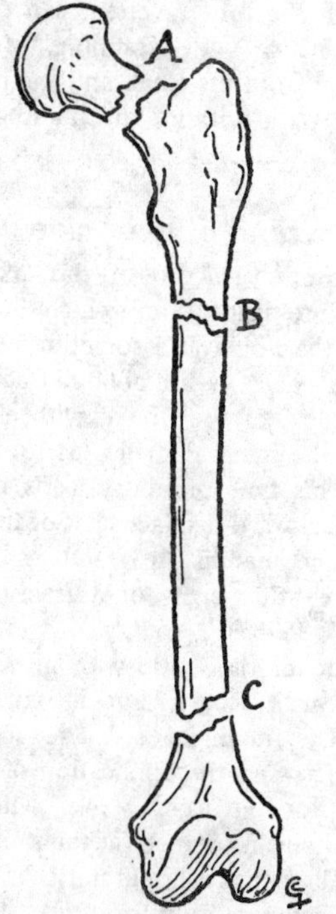

Fig. 27. *VARIOUS FRACTURES OF FEMUR.* A. *Fracture of the neck of the femur, within the capsule.* B. *Fracture below the trochanters.* C. *Fracture at lower end of shaft.*

across the bone or oblique; when oblique, the point of one of the fragments may penetrate one of the large muscles or blood vessels of the thigh.

When the break occurs in the upper third of the shaft, the upper fragment is flexed and turned outwards. The lower part is drawn up and displaced with rotation. In the middle part there is less displacement, but there may be considerable overlapping. In the lower third, the lower fragment may be displaced backwards, injuring the blood vessels.

Symptoms. A fracture in the neck of the femur may be difficult to diagnose before an X-ray examination is made, but as a general rule the patient is unable to lift the heel from the ground while he is lying on his back. A fracture in the middle of the bone, if it is transverse, may be shown by swelling, or some irregularity may be felt by the hand; if it is oblique, the ends of the bone will overlap each other and the limb will be shortened, sometimes to the extent of three inches. The foot will also lie on the outer side.

First Aid should only be performed by those trained in the specialized techniques (see First Aid, p. 34). If no trained help is available, and the injured person must be moved, tie the legs together.

Treatment. The treatment depends on the site of the fracture and on the age of the patient. In old persons setting of the limb may be postponed until the initial shock has

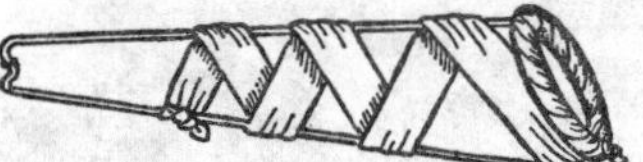

Fig. 28. *THOMAS'S HIP SPLINT. The frame, interlaced with bandages, makes a trough for support of the leg.*

subsided. The patient should be put to bed and given stimulants, and a Thomas's hip splint applied to the injured limb to prevent movement of the leg. Alternatively, immobilization can be achieved with sandbags.

FOR FRACTURES OF THE SHAFT, the deformity should be reduced by traction under anesthesia, an extension splint applied and suitable weights added. Extension is maintained either through a metal pin in the shin bone, or plaster on the skin. Where the deformity cannot be reduced by extension, an open operation is sometimes essential, so that the interposing muscle fragments can be removed, and apposition and alignment secured. Extension is then maintained as above.

FOR CHILDREN, extension with skin traction is used from four years onwards. Below this age the gallows splint gives excellent results. This comprises vertical extension of the limb, with the child in bed, both legs being suspended by strapping to a cross-bar supported on vertical poles. A weight of 3 to 6 lbs. is usually sufficient to raise the buttocks slightly from the bed.

The Thomas's knee splint combined with traction can be used for a large number of

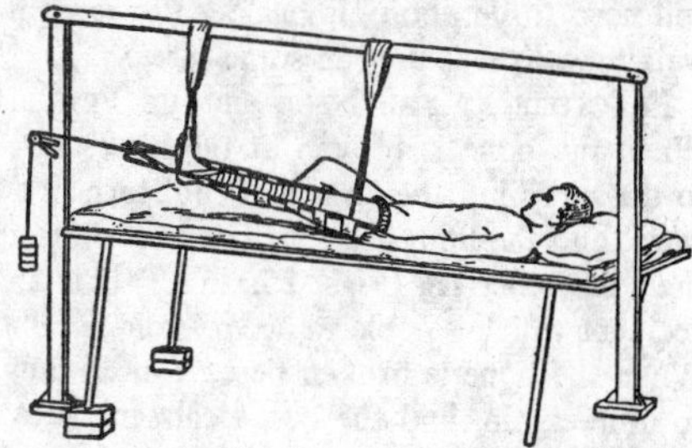

Fig. 29. *THOMAS'S KNEE SPLINT with weight and pulley traction for a fracture of the middle of the thigh-bone (femur).*

fractures of the thigh and leg; extension is easily obtained by weight or body traction. When a fracture of the thigh-bone has been reduced and fixed upon the splint it should invariably be X-rayed, to ascertain that the

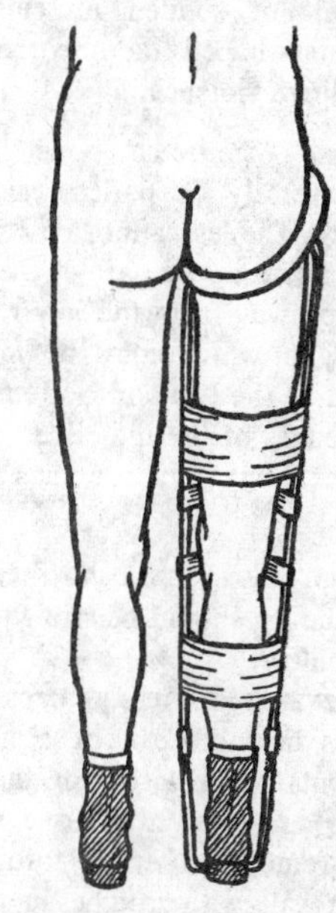

Fig. 30. *A CALIPER SPLINT. This splint is used for walking and prevents the weight of the body being borne on the leg-bones.*

position is as perfect as possible. X-ray examination can be made with the splint in position without disturbing the limb.

Eight to ten weeks will be required for the bones to unite, during which time the patient

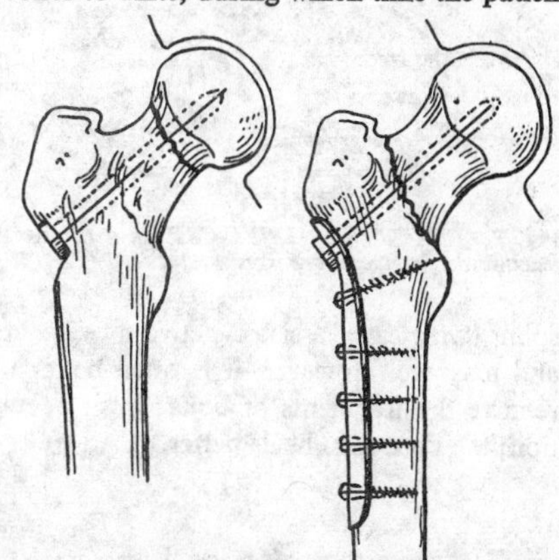

Fig. 31. *PIN AND PLATE REPAIR OF FRACTURE* Left, *a simple pin is used where the fracture is close to the head of the femur and there is enough 'bite' on the rest of the neck.* Right, *a pin and plate are used where there is not enough bone on the near side of the fracture to give sufficient grip.*

will need to lie upon his back. Afterwards a walking caliper is used in some cases.

FRACTURE AT THE NECK OF THE FEMUR. When the bone is broken at the neck close to the hip joint, the knee and foot turn outward, and the limb is an inch or two shorter than the other leg (Figs. 25, 26). This is an accident which is liable to occur in old people When the bone is broken here, it often fails to unite again, and the best treatment is by operation to insert a nail into the neck of the femur with or without a plate added. By this means, old people can be got moving from bed very soon.

Fractures of the Knee-cap

The knee-cap (patella) may be broken transversely across or in the form of a star; the first fracture is the most common, and is the result of sudden muscular strain. Stellate or star-shaped fractures are generally caused by direct violence.

Symptoms. When the bone is broken across transversely the patient cannot stand upon the leg. The leg cannot be straightened at the knee. The upper part of the knee-cap is drawn up away from the lower fragment, leaving a gap which may be felt by the fingers, and at the top and bottom of which the rough edges of the movable bones may be felt. The joint becomes distended with blood.

Treatment. For first aid see p. 34; basically, the leg should be straight, with the heel on a pillow.

IN TRANSVERSE FRACTURES across the bone, operation is the only means of securing union, the fragments being wired together. Passive movements are allowed in one week, and active movements after a fortnight. The patient can walk with crutches in about three or four weeks, and union is firm in about six weeks.

IN STELLATE FRACTURES caused by a direct blow the fragments are not separated widely, but pain and bruising are apparent. Treatment consists in resting the leg on a back

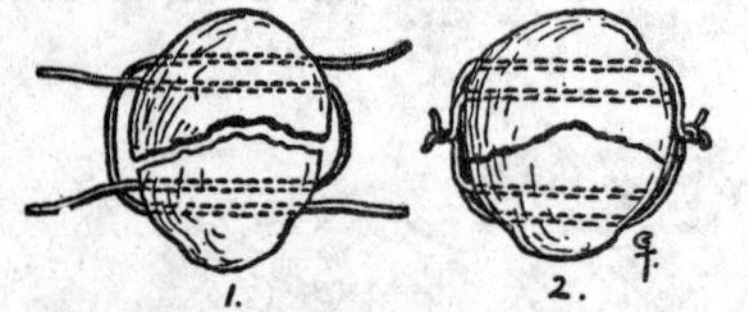

Fig. 32. *FRACTURED KNEE-CAP. In a transverse fracture the fragments are fixed with wire.*

splint, with early assisted active movements and massage. However, it is often better to remove the fragments of bone by an operation; the knee then heals better.

Fractures of the Leg

The leg is that part of the lower limb between the knee and ankle, and has two bones. The smaller bone on the outer side is the fibula; the larger bone on the inner side is the tibia, or shin-bone. When only one bone is broken the deformity may not be apparent. A fracture of the fibula about three inches from the ankle may be mistaken for a sprain or a dislocation. If both bones are broken, it is impossible to stand upon the limb.

FRACTURES OF THE TIBIA AND FIBULA

In cases of direct violence, as from blows, both bones are broken at about the same level, the fractures being transverse, and usually causing little displacement. *In indirect violence* the tibia breaks between the middle and lower thirds, and the fibula breaks slightly higher up. The fractures may be oblique or spiral. The lower fragment is drawn upwards, and the upper fragment may penetrate the skin causing a compound fracture.

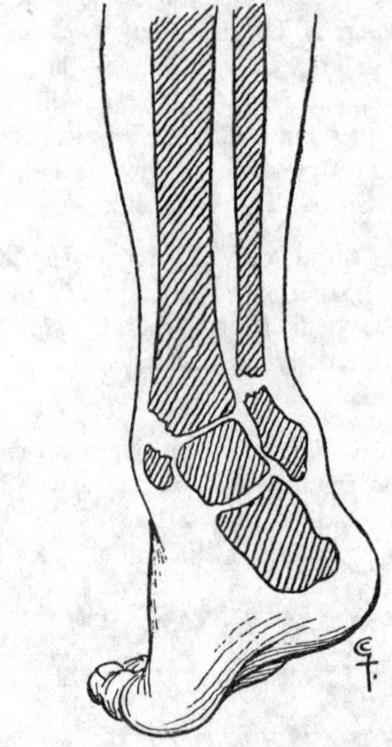

Fig. 33. *POTT'S FRACTURE OF THE ANKLE*

When only one bone is fractured, the fracture may involve the upper or lower end of the tibia or its shaft, or the fibula alone may be fractured, the so-called Pott's fracture of the lower end just above the ankle being a common injury. (See Figs. 33, 34, 35, 37.)

FRACTURE-DISLOCATIONS OF THE ANKLE are common injuries, usually caused by twisting the foot, or tripping. Displacement of the foot is commonly outwards and backwards, and in severe cases upwards also (Pott's fracture) or occasionally it may be inwards, or even absent.

First Aid. Support the limb by holding the ankle and foot in the natural position.

Treatment. Reduction must be achieved by manipulation, extension, or operation. The exact position of the fragments must be determined by X-ray examination, which will assist very greatly in reduction.

FRACTURES OF THE SHAFT OF THE TIBIA. These commonly occur below the middle third of the bone, and there is often some angular deformity without much shortening of the limb. The displacement is reduced and the parts are then kept in position by means of a plaster cast to the leg above the knee, with the foot at right angles. The cast is worn for six weeks (or four weeks in children) but is split at three weeks so that massage may be given. After six weeks a lighter walking cast is substituted.

FRACTURES OF BOTH TIBIA AND FIBULA. Lateral displacement is not usually great, but overlapping is always present. In some cases prompt extension under a general anesthetic allows the deformity to be corrected so that a plaster cast may be applied.

A Thomas's splint with extension and traction is generally necessary for fracture involving both bones when immediate reduction cannot be achieved. In determining if full correction has been obtained, the limb should be compared with the opposite limb. This apparatus may be replaced by a plaster cast after four weeks. The position may be confirmed by X-ray examination. Six to eight weeks will be required for recovery.

In the treatment of fractures of the shafts of both bones of the lower extremities, which are common, three conditions should be fulfilled; first, extension, then apposition and fixation of the fragments, and third, support and immobilization. Using the method of fixation in plaster, with traction, the patient being allowed to use the leg while union takes place, still gives very good results in transverse fractures.

FRACTURES OF THE FIBULA. There is seldom much displacement when the break occurs in the upper two-thirds of the bone. The leg should generally be rested completely for a week or two, with massage, and walking is permitted when this is possible without pain.

In the lower third of the shaft there is little displacement as a rule, and fixation of the leg, with the foot inverted, can usually be made effective with strapping. Massage may be given from the start, and the patient can usually walk without much discomfort after a week.

Fractures of the Ankle

The commonest fracture of the ankle is a Pott's fracture-dislocation, which involves the end of the fibula and sometimes the tip of the tibia. There is an oblique fracture in the lower third of the fibula, with either a fracture of the internal malleolus, or a torn ligament. This type of injury leads to outward and backward displacement of the foot, with pain and inability to stand, associated with all the other signs of a fracture (see Figs. 33, 34, 35, 37).

A fracture of the ankle with inward displacement also occurs, but is much less common. The treatment is full reduction of the deformity, and the application of a split plaster cast for four to six weeks, with massage and passive movement at the third week onwards. The patient should not bear his full weight on the ankle joint for at least two full months. The heel of the boot or shoe is often raised on the inner side for six months, and an ankle-strap may be worn by the patient.

DIFFERENT TYPES OF FRACTURES OF THE ANKLE

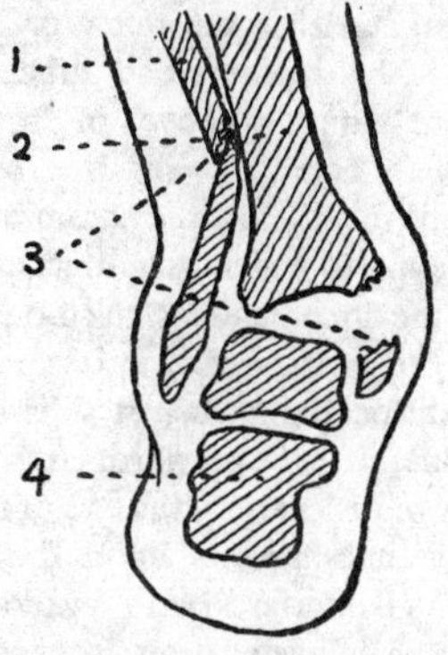

Fig. 34. *POTT'S FRACTURE OF THE ANKLE, WITH OUTWARD DISPLACEMENT OF THE FOOT (a common type). 1. Shaft of fibula. Shaft of tibia. 3. Site of fracture. 4. Os calcis of heel.*

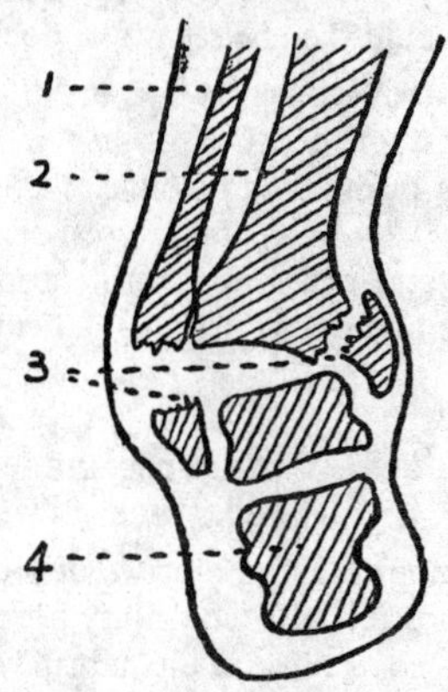

Fig. 35. *POTT'S FRACTURE OF THE ANKLE, WITH INWARD DISPLACEMENT OF THE FOOT (an uncommon type). 1. Shaft of fibula. 2. Shaft of tibia. 3. Site of fracture. 4. Os calcis of heel.*

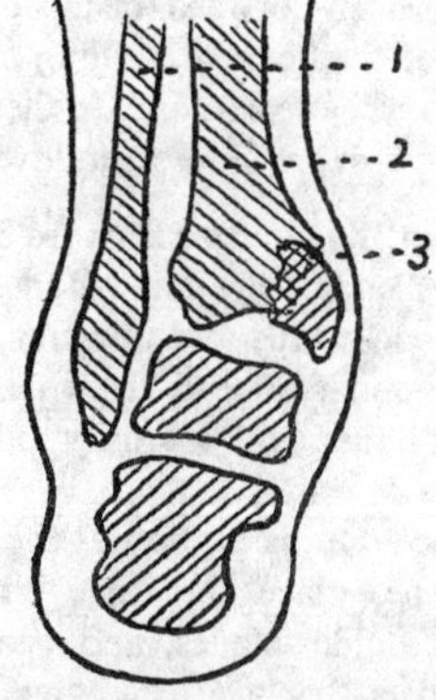

Fig. 36. *DUPUYTREN'S FRACTURE OF THE LOWER END OF THE TIBIA. 1. Shaft of fibula. 2. Shaft of tibia. 3. Site of fracture.*

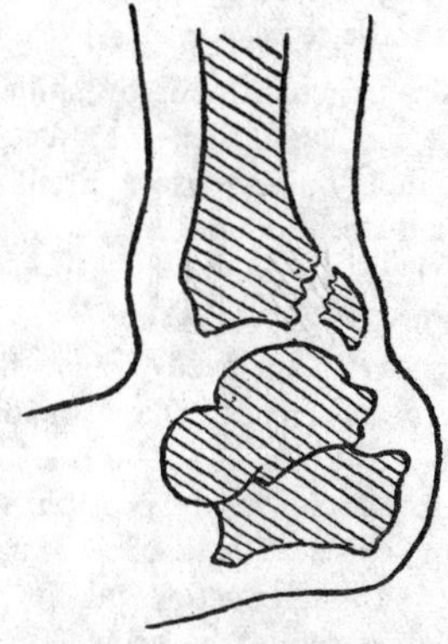

Fig. 37. *A POTT'S FRACTURE OF THE ANKLE, with backward displacement of the heel.*

Fractures of the Bones of the Feet

The actual nature of the injury must be determined by X-ray examination; there are often other injuries of the muscles or ligaments, since the fracture is often caused by a crush injury.

First Aid. The shoe and stocking are carefully removed, and a padded splint is applied to the sole of the foot from the heel to the toes; this is kept in place with a figure eight bandage applied around the foot and ankle. The foot may then be kept supported in a slightly raised position on a firm cushion. (See First Aid, p. 34.)

Treatment. A fracture of the metatarsal bones is likely to cause some damage to the transverse metatarsal arch of the foot. This should be borne in mind, and the foot should be inverted and immobilized with adhesive strapping or plaster of Paris, with a pad placed in the arch. The body weight should not be borne on the foot for about two months after the injury.

A useful and simple expedient that may be used in all fractures of the lower extremities is some form of cradle to prevent the bedclothes coming in contact with the injured parts. (See illustrations in Home Nursing, p. 46.)

FRACTURES OF THE HEEL-BONE often require surgical treatment, with reduction by weight extension through a transfixion pin in the bone, combined with squeezing in a special vice, and prolonged immobilization in plaster, with subsequent use of an arch support to prevent flat foot, which is a common sequel to foot injuries.

In fractures of the astragalus the fragments sometimes need to be removed surgically.

COMPOUND FRACTURES

When an external wound of the skin communicates with the broken ends of the bone, the injury is called a compound fracture. The wound is often caused by one of the ends of the bone penetrating or protruding through the muscles and skin. But, however caused, a compound fracture is of a much more serious nature than a simple one, and it is particularly dangerous when a joint is involved, owing to the danger of infection.

Treatment. (See also Wounds and Their Care, pp. 557-60.) The first thing after the injury is to shield the wound against further infection and to induce it to heal by first intention, that is without suppuration. To do this, the wound must be rendered as clean and free from dirt, bacteria, and devitalized tissue as possible. Surgical toilet must be carried out under a general anesthetic. The skin is carefully cleansed with some disinfectant such as alcohol, ether, or tincture of iodine. The wound is cleansed; tags of skin or flesh are removed and the skin edges are excised, to form a new healing surface. When the fracture has been manipulated into position, the edges are then approximated with nylon stitches. Sterile dressings and appropriate plaster of Paris are applied, and antibiotics given.

It will be necessary to keep the weight of the bedclothes off the limb by a bed-cradle.

Should the wound heal by first intention, treatment may be the same as for a simple fracture; but this unfortunately does not always occur.

Complications which may arise later on are pneumonia, bedsores, gangrene, ossification of the muscles, Volkmann's contracture, and crutch palsy from pressure of the crutch in the axilla. These can generally be prevented when the case is in the hands of a surgeon.

Late complications may be the formation of *sequestra* (dead fragments of bone), which are pushed up to the surface and cause discharging sinuses which may fail to heal unless the fragments are removed. The question of amputation must be decided by a surgeon when the process of recovery seems likely to be endangered by complications.

DISLOCATIONS

The bones of the skeleton are connected with each other by joints or articulations. The surfaces of bones which are adjacent within a joint and where movement may take place are called articular surfaces. Movable joint surfaces are normally covered by cartilage to enable them to move smoothly upon each other.

In most cases the bones within joints are bound together by cartilage and ligaments; by the aid of these the joint movements are supported and controlled.

There are three main types of joints, which vary in their range of movement.

1. In sutures there is no joint cavity and the joint is immovable. Such a joint occurs in the bones of the dome of the skull.

2. Other joints have limited movement, such as the joints between the vertebrae of the spine, and the joint between the pubic bones of the pelvis.

3. Joints with free movements, such as are found in the limbs.

These freely moveable joints are divided into various kinds: (1) the ball-and-socket type, which has a rotary motion, as the shoulder and hip: (2) the angular, hinge or pump-handle type, as the elbow, ankle, and knee: (3) the gliding joints, as between the collar-bone and breast-bone, and the joints of the wrist and knee.

The ball-and-socket joints have the greatest range of movement and are most liable to become dislocated.

For illustrations of the types of joints, see Anatomy, pp. 222-23.

Types of Dislocation

A dislocation is a displacement of one or more of the bones forming a joint. The joints which are most commonly dislocated are those of the lower jaw, shoulder, elbow, thumb, and fingers. Dislocation is often the result of some injury by external force, whereby the ends of the bones forming the joint became separated. The joint is moved beyond its normal range, and if the bones form a ball-and-socket joint, the head of one bone is dislodged from the socket, and tears the joint capsule.

SIMPLE. A dislocation is simple when there is no wound penetrating the synovial membrane, or joint cavity.

COMPOUND. It is compound, or open, when associated with a wound.

COMPLETE. A dislocation is complete when the articular surfaces are entirely separated.

INCOMPLETE. Dislocation is incomplete when the separation is only partial (subluxation).

Recent dislocations are usually reduced without great difficulty by a surgeon. Old dislocations are often difficult to reduce, especially in the larger joints, and sometimes cannot be reduced at all without a surgical operation.

A fracture-dislocation denotes a fracture near the dislocated end of one of the bones.

Congenital dislocations are those with which a child is born, even though diagnosis is delayed for some months. A common example is the hip joint (see p. 512).

Dislocations due to injury are the form commonly seen.

Pathological dislocation occurs in certain diseases which may affect the joint cavities, or the supporting structures.

Symptoms of Dislocation

The symptoms of dislocation are pain and inability to use the joint, and the head of the bone may be felt to be in an unnatural place. The limb is shortened, lengthened, or deformed, and the joint may be misshapen; in recent cases there are also severe pain, bruising and swelling.

First Aid for Dislocations

A first-aid helper should not attempt to reduce a dislocation.

If the accident occurs when the patient is out-of-doors the part should be supported in a comfortable position with pads of cotton or some folded pieces of soft cloth; slings, splints and bandages are used as required to steady the part and prevent jolting. The patient should then be seen by a doctor.

If the accident occurs indoors the patient should rest on a couch or bed in as comfortable a position as possible. The pain can be relieved by cold compresses or, if these cease to give relief, use warm applications instead until a doctor sees the patient.

Reduction and Treatment of Dislocations

It is important to reduce a dislocation as soon as possible after the injury because later considerable swelling of the part may obscure the diagnosis. The displacement may cause injury to the surrounding parts by pressure, and it is much more difficult to reduce a dislocation after some lapse of time.

An anesthetic is usually required to permit sufficient relaxation of the muscles to enable the bones to be replaced.

Reduction is carried out by skilled manipulation according to the joint affected. After reduction daily massage is required.

When a dislocation and a fracture occur at the same time, the dislocation must receive attention first.

Reduction is achieved when the limb regains its natural length, shape and direction, and is able to perform the normal range of movements which are not possible while the dislocation exists. The pain is immediately diminished upon reduction taking place. In cases where it cannot be achieved by manipulation, an open operation is sometimes necessary.

SPECIAL DISLOCATIONS

Dislocation of the Lower Jaw

Yawning or gaping very wide is the usual cause of this dislocation. One or both sides of the jaw may be disjointed.

Symptoms. If one side is dislocated, the chin is displaced towards the normal side, the normal range of movement is lost, and the jaws are partially open. If both sides are dislocated at once, the mouth is kept opened, the chin projects, with a hollow in front of each ear, and there is great pain, inability to speak, and dribbling of saliva from the mouth.

Treatment. To effect reduction, stand in front of the patient, insert the thumbs inside the patient's mouth, and press firmly downwards on the lower jaw at the angles, either beside or behind the back teeth, at the same time lifting the chin with the fingers.

Reduction occurs with a snap, and the thumbs must be kept away from the teeth.

After the jaw is set, it should be kept bandaged for a few days. No solid food which requires chewing should be taken for a short time.

Dislocation of the Collar-bone

Dislocation of the collar-bone (clavicle) may occur at either the inner or the outer end, that is, by the inner end attached to the breast-bone slipping above, in front of, or behind that bone; or by the outer end slipping above or below the acromion process of the scapula to which it is attached.

When the inner end of the bone slips in front of the breast-bone, it is said to be a forward dislocation; when it slips under the breast-bone, it is backward. In the backward type of dislocation, the end of the collar-bone sometimes presses upon the gullet or trachea, and interferes with swallowing and breathing. The dislocation is generally the result of a direct blow.

Dislocation of the outer end may be upwards or downwards, and is usually caused by a blow or a fall. Upward dislocation of the inner end is rare.

Symptoms. In forward dislocation of the inner end of the bone, a swelling may be felt at the top of the breast-bone. In the backward dislocation, a depression or hollow is seen.

Treatment. To reduce a forward dislocation of the inner end of the collar-bone, draw the shoulders backwards and upwards, by which means the collar-bone is drawn away from the breast-bone, and is easily pushed into place.

To reduce the dislocation at the outer end of the bone, place the knee between the patient's shoulder-blades, and steadily draw his shoulders backwards. After reduction apply a figure of eight bandage over both shoulders and stress the components together every day for a fortnight. Some undue mobility and prominence of the clavicle usually remains.

Dislocation of the Shoulder Joint

This is the commonest dislocation seen in adults. The head of the long bone of the arm (humerus) may be displaced in four different directions: (1) downwards into the armpit (axilla), which is the commonest type; (2) forwards, under the muscles of the breast; (3) backwards, upon the back of the shoulder blade; and rarely (4) upwards, if the acromion and coracoid processes of the shoulder blade are fractured

Symptoms and Signs. Dislocation is recognized by the shoulder losing its rounded shape and becoming flattened, by the lengthening of the arm, and by severe pain and loss of mobility. The elbow is displaced from the side and the head of the bone is felt in an abnormal position.

Treatment. When the head of the humerus is displaced from the joint, and the direction of the shaft of the bone does not correspond with the displacement present (indicating an associated fracture), an X-ray photograph should be taken before reduction treatment is carried out. It is also advisable to have an

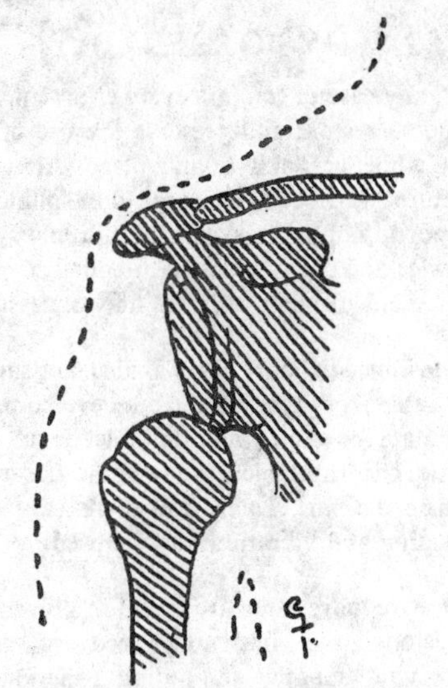

Fig. 38. *DISLOCATION OF SHOULDER JOINT with downward displacement of the humerus.*

X-ray photograph taken of every dislocation after reduction.

To effect the reduction in the first two forms of displacement, (1) Kocher's method of manipulation often succeeds, and is the only one required in certain forms of shoulder dislocation. Take the arm on the patient's injured side, bend the elbow at right angles and place it close to the side of the body, and while pressing the elbow steadily downwards, rotate the forearm outwards as far as possible; then carry the elbow, still flexed, inwards and upwards across the chest, and then flick the hand to the opposite shoulder. The head of the humerus often slips back into place with ease. (2) A surgeon may attempt reduction by extension, that is putting pressure in the armpit against the head of the bone. Then, taking hold of the arm above the elbow or at the wrist, he pulls steadily. If reduction cannot be effected, the muscles may be relaxed under anesthesia. Extension, however, is best avoided.

After the reduction, a sling will be required, and three weeks' or a month's rest. Massage should be begun at once, with assisted active movements after about a week.

Recurrent dislocation of the shoulder joint is not uncommon and may require operation.

Dislocation of the Elbow Joint

Of this there are six varieties. In the first and most common type, both bones of the forearm (radius and ulna) are dislocated backwards; in the second both are displaced forwards; in the third or lateral, both are dislocated (usually incompletely) to one or other side; in the fourth, the ulna alone is forced backwards; in the fifth the radius is forced forwards, and in the sixth the radius is thrown backwards. Partial dislocation, or 'pulled elbow,' is fairly common in young children, being caused by pulling the child along by the forearm.

In general, these dislocations are often complicated by a fracture; the displacement is then apt to recur and requires an operation.

Treatment. In the first three types of case the surgeon's knee is placed in the bend of the elbow and the forearm slightly extended and then bent upon it, the surgeon grasping the upper arm with one hand and the forearm with the other. In the last two varieties the elbow is bent at a right angle, and with traction and pressure over the head of the radius, reduction follows.

If there is no fracture the arm should be kept flexed in a sling and cold compresses applied. Careful massage may be begun in twenty-four hours; assisted active movements are started in five days. In three to four weeks the sling may be dispensed with.

These types of dislocation may be followed by damage to the nerves of the forearm and hand.

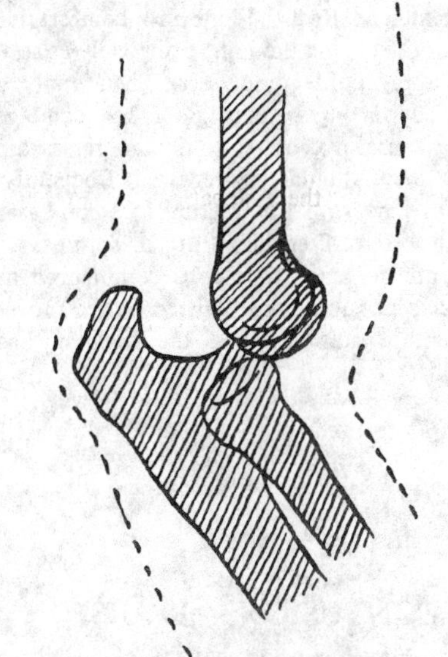

Fig. 39. *DISLOCATION OF THE ELBOW JOINT with backward displacement of the ulna.*

Dislocations of the Wrist

These are uncommon and are caused by falls upon the hand. Both the radius and ulna may be displaced backwards or forwards upon the wrist, causing a projection either in front or behind. The dislocation is reduced by extension of the hand from the forearm, with manipulation. An X-ray examination is required, since these dislocations may be combined with fracture.

Treatment. Put a straight splint on the front, and another on the back of the forearm and hand, with compresses on both sides of the wrist, and a bandage over the whole. Support the forearm in a sling and reduce the swelling by cold compresses, cooling lotions, etc.

Dislocations of the Bones of the Hand

Rarely, one of the carpal bones may be pushed out of its place so as to form a projection on the hand. To replace the bone, anesthetize the patient, then steadily press upon it, apply cold compresses on the front and back of the wrist, with straight splints to support the joint, and bandage these in place. Put the forearm in a sling. If reduction cannot be accomplished the bone sometimes has to be removed surgically.

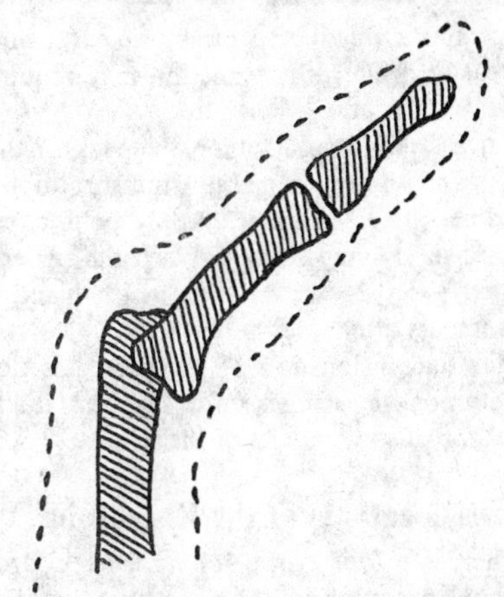

Fig. 40. *DISLOCATION OF A FINGER JOINT, with forward displacement of the second phalanx.*

Dislocations of the finger joints may generally be corrected, extension being combined with flexion of the displaced phalanx over the head of the bone from which it has been dislocated backwards. Sometimes dislocation of the thumb is difficult to reduce, and requires an operation because in many cases the dislocation is accompanied by a small fracture.

Dislocations of the Hip Joint

There are four types: backwards and downwards, forwards and downwards, backwards and upwards, and forwards and upwards. Dislocations of this joint are rare and may be confused with fracture of the neck of the thigh-bone; a fracture may be distinguished from dislocation of the hip joint by X-ray examination. Dislocation may be congenital with shallow deformity of the socket, and these cases are often bilateral.

The backward and upward displacement is the most common type.

Treatment. For replacing the bone, the anesthetized patient lies on his back upon a table or on the floor. The surgeon, standing on the injured side, directs gradual flexion and adduction, with final circumduction and bringing the leg down straight; this replaces the head of the bone in the socket of the hip. An X-ray examination should be made to ascertain that the bone is not injured.

The patient is kept in bed for seven to ten days, with his knees tied together by bandages and a broad belt round his hips. Movements may then be started, but standing and walking are not permitted for three weeks. The displacement is liable to recur.

Dislocations of the Knee-cap

The patella, or knee-cap, may be displaced

outwards, causing a projection on the outer side of the knee, and inability to bend the knee; or it may be dislocated inwards, causing similar inability to bend the knee, and deformity on the inner side.

Treatment. To restore the bone to its place, extend the leg and flex the thigh, then manipulate the bone into place. Vertical dislocations are due to direct violence, and are easily dealt with; reduction may require an anesthetic.

Put a straight splint upon the back of the limb, and make moderate pressure upon the knee by a bandage. Apply cold compresses or cooling lotions. Keep the patient in bed for two weeks, with assisted active movements after seven to ten days.

Habitual dislocation of the patella is not uncommon in women, and the best treatment for this is removal of the patella.

Dislocations of the Knee Joint

There are four types: forward, backward, inward and outward; the dislocation may be complete or incomplete. These injuries may be due to severe violence or to disease of the knee joint.

They are corrected by extension and counter-extension from the ankle and thigh, and pressure upon the head of the displaced bone.

Treatment. When the dislocation is the result of injury, the knee, after reduction, must be immobilized for several weeks. Usually the cartilages within the knee joint become torn, with severe pain and locking of the knee. Manipulation under an anesthetic enables the cartilage to be replaced, but displacement is liable to recur.

Loose bodies, consisting of cartilage fragments or joint membrane, sometimes develop in the joint, and should be removed surgically if they cause pain, swelling or locking.

Dislocations of the Ankle

These may occur in a forward, backward, outward (commonest), or inward direction. (Figs. 34, 35, 36, 37.) Dislocation is often associated with a Pott's fracture (p. 552).

Treatment. For fracture-dislocations of the ankle, which are comparatively common, manipulation under general anesthesia by a surgeon is required. The leg and foot are then put in a plaster of Paris support. The patient may attempt to use the limb at an early stage. In other cases the plaster cast is split, and massage is given after about two weeks. Later the inner side of the shoe is raised by a leather wedge on the sole.

Other forms of dislocation of the ankle generally require surgical treatment.

SPRAINS

A sprain is a forcible wrenching and twisting of a joint to such a degree as to stretch and tear the ligaments of the part and sometimes to injure a tendon. The symptoms are severe pain, tenderness, swelling, and bruising of the parts, with stiffness and partial inability to move the part. In elderly persons the effects of sprains may be very persistent and disabling, causing pain and stiffness for many weeks or even months.

Treatment. Rest the limb in a comfortable position, keeping the joint completely at rest, and apply cold compresses. Then apply a firm supporting bandage, a crêpe bandage being a useful type. If cold compresses are used they should be renewed frequently. X-rays may reveal a fracture in some cases which were at first thought to be sprains.

Gentle massage should be commenced as soon as possible, and assisted active movements are started when the swelling has subsided.

CONTUSIONS—BRUISES

When the soft parts of the body sustain an injury from a blow or sudden violent contact with a hard object, without breaking the skin, the injury received is called a bruise. This accident generally ruptures a number of the smallest blood vessels or capillaries which leak blood under the skin, producing a black and blue patch, or livid spots (ecchymosis). A black eye is an example of a severe bruise.

Treatment. Apply cold applications at first to prevent bleeding from the small vessels under the skin. Gentle massage and rest in bed for elderly persons is often required when there is much pain on movement, or where there is bruising of the muscles below.

PHYSIOTHERAPY

In any case of fracture every effort must be made to restore and preserve the use of the part while union is taking place. After the fracture has been set, and the splints or supporting apparatus have been applied, the muscles and joints must be attended to so as to prevent ultimate stiffness and uselessness.

Massage. In most cases skilled massage is advisable from the outset, to relieve pain and stimulate the circulation; this must be smooth, gentle, and rhythmical, and should not cause pain in the part. Later, deeper massage with kneading and vibration may be used.

Passive movements are useful in preventing adhesions and hastening recovery while preserving muscle and joint function In these movements there is complete relaxation by the patient, the movement of the part being carried out by the physiotherapist. The movement is quite involuntary and there should be no opposing spasm, so that the movement is quite painless. 'Forced' movements in the early stages are injurious, and must be avoided. They may, however, be occasionally employed later on to overcome adhesions.

Active movements should be allowed and encouraged directly they can be achieved without causing pain. In joints not immediately affected by the fracture, such as the fingers in fractures of the forearm, such movements may be used early.

Active movements are extremely important to recovery of the use of limb or part. From simple to more complex movements, the patient goes through a progressive range of activity relying less and less on assistance from the physiotherapist until he can perform movements unaided.

Exercises are employed to strengthen the muscles and joints when union is sufficiently firm to stand the strain or the weight of the body.

Electrical treatment is employed to restore the tone and use of the muscles by inducing them to contract. This is particularly useful after a limb has been immobilized for a long period and the muscles have become weak from disuse.

WOUNDS AND THEIR CARE

A wound is a breach in the continuity of the skin or tissues. It may be due to accident, surgery, or disease.

Accidental Wounds. The variety is endless, and the resulting wound may be a simple breach of skin, or complicated by the presence of a foreign body or by further damage such as severed nerves, arteries, tendons or muscle, or fractured bone.

ABRASIONS are superficial wounds with loss of skin, such as may follow a fall causing grazing.

INCISED WOUNDS are clean cuts produced by sharp instruments such as a knife or razor. These wounds usually gape and bleed freely. A blunt object wounding the scalp may produce a wound that looks like a clean cut.

PUNCTURED (PENETRATING) WOUNDS may appear trivial but can penetrate deeply, damaging internal organs or tissues. This type of wound can be caused by daggers, knives, nails, toy arrows, darts and shotgun pellets. These wounds are especially dangerous as the damage to internal structures may not give rise to any symptoms until several hours after the injury. Furthermore, foreign bodies may be lodged far in.

LACERATED WOUNDS are torn wounds with irregular edges, and may not bleed much. They are especially liable to infection. Blunt objects, machinery, animals' claws or crushing injuries will cause lacerations.

Surgical Wounds are produced during operations. Most surgery begins with an incision and ends with closure of the wound with stitches. Healing is usually simple.

Disease causing Wounds. Examples of wounds due to disease include the varicose ulcer and frostbite.

HEALING OF WOUNDS

A knowledge of the healing process is helpful in understanding the whys and wherefores of wound treatment. Whatever the mode of healing the final result is a fibrous scar. No known method of treatment can restore the tissues exactly as they were before injury.

Healing by first intention is the aim of wound treatment. This means the direct union of the two well-matching edges of the wound by agglutination. In order to achieve this result certain prerequisites are necessary: the wound must be clean, the edges must be close together, and the blood supply must be adequate. There must also be a sufficiency of certain nutrients, especially vitamin C, and the affected part must be rested. The stages involved in first intention healing are:

1. exudation of serum at the wound edges to bind them together;
2. capillary budding from either side to bridge the gap;
3. laying down of layers of collagen fibrils;
4. invasion of the fibrils by scar-forming cells (fibroblasts); and
5. formation of the scar (fibrous tissue).

Healing by granulation occurs if the edges of a wound are not close together (as in large open wounds), in infected wounds, or in the presence of a foreign body. Granulations in the wound appear as small, rounded, pink, fleshy masses. The granulations gradually contract to reduce the size of the wound. A granulated wound may be very tender. The healing is usually associated with some degree of sloughing.

Healing by blood clot takes place in clean wounds filled with blood clot. It is similar to healing by granulation, the whole blood clot being replaced by scar tissue.

Healing under a scab is common in clean surface wounds. The scab protects the part while union proceeds.

Scars

Scars may sometimes give rise to trouble when healing is complete. Deformity may result from excessive shrinkage and the resultant disability may be simply cosmetic or involve loss of function such as the restriction of movement. A scar may be especially liable to ulceration (varicose ulcer) and an injured scar is difficult to heal again.

Keloid is a complication occurring particularly after burns. Tumors invade the scar making it smooth, enlarged and maybe claw-like. The tendency to keloid formation is inherited and is commoner in tuberculous and negroid families.

Treatment of keloid consists of X-ray or radium therapy either directly on the enlarged scar or after it has been reduced surgically.

LOCAL TREATMENT OF WOUNDS

Prevention of Infection

Prevention of infection is of prime importance. Only a clean wound can heal by first intention with the minimum of scar tissue and a speedy return to normal function. Surgical repair and grafting are only successful if infection has been prevented. Furthermore, secondary bleeding from the wound is prevented.

At the time of injury the wound may become contaminated from the clothes and skin of the injured person. Other sources are external dirt, foreign bodies, weapons used, etc. Later, germs may be introduced while the wound is being dressed—the germs may come from the attendant, from the dressings themselves, from the air, and from the patient.

Tetanus (Lockjaw). There are two methods of guarding against tetanus—active and passive immunization. The most satisfactory way is the routine giving of tetanus vaccine to babies (usually in conjunction with diphtheria and whooping-cough vaccine) by three spaced injections (active immunization). Others who should be immunized are special-risk people such as agricultural workers and soldiers. Reinforcing doses should be given five and ten years after the original course, and at the time of injury.

Persons who have not been actively immunized can be temporarily protected at the time of injury by an injection of tetanus antitoxin (passive immunization). Even a minor wound may be a possible source of entry for tetanus micro-organisms, especially those contaminated by dirt from the road, stables, or field.

The Minor Wound

The minor wound should be cleaned with soap and water. The best way is under running warm tap water. The person dressing the wound must have freshly washed hands and the dressings should be as sterile as possible. After the wound is cleaned, dry gauze and a plaster or bandage, are applied. No antiseptics are necessary for a trivial wound. Indeed, some are considered harmful because as well as killing germs they may damage tissue cells and thus delay healing.

The Major Wound

At the Scene of the Accident. The wound should be covered with some type of dressing —sterile gauze if possible, if not, a clean handkerchief, towel, or the cleanest material available. This should be bandaged over firmly but not tightly, and left until medical aid is obtained.

If bleeding is present a pressure bandage should be added. Arrest of bleeding by the application of pressure is the safest method. If the hemorrhage is severe, then a tourniquet may have to be applied. This must be done properly, and preferably by a doctor or trained First Aider. The tourniquet must be tight enough to obstruct the artery as well as the vein. (The commonest mistake is to have the tourniquet too loose, thus making the bleeding more profuse.) The wider the tourniquet the better. The time of application must be noted in writing. The tourniquet should be released after half an hour and may be reapplied if necessary.

At the Hospital. The wound will now have to be exposed for inspection. Germs can enter it from the hands, nose, throat or clothing of the nurse or doctor. To minimize this risk the attendant should wash and dry his hands, and he should wear a mask. The old dressings are taken off with forceps, the wound examined and further action decided on.

X-rays may be needed to detect broken bones. Other injuries, such as internal injuries, must be excluded, and the extent of any nerve or tendon injury must be assessed by clinical examination. Blood transfusion is given where necessary, and shock (see below) is treated.

If it is decided that repair or exploration of the wound is necessary (as is the case in most major wounds) then the patient is moved to the operating room, where the room itself, the instruments and the dressings are all as sterile as possible. The operating staff is gowned, masked and 'scrubbed up.' These precautions are very important as a number of germs found in hospital have become resistant to many of the available antibiotics (bacterial resistance).

Either general or local anesthesia is used (see Anesthetics, pp. 596-97).

The wound is first cleansed thoroughly, as well as a wide area of skin around it. Superficial wounds may be actually scrubbed with a scrubbing brush. The inside of the wound is washed out with water or saline.

A simple incised wound is then stitched and dressed.

A more complicated wound may now have to be opened up to show the full extent of the damage. This applies particularly to penetrating wounds. Bleeding blood vessels are tied off. Bits of metal or gravel, bullets, etc. are then removed and the wound cleaned out again. Any dead tissue is cut away.

Repair of deeper structures, such as bone plating or nailing, stitching of blood vessels, and repair of tendons is then carried out. This is followed by stitching the wound layer by layer, if this is indicated, and finally skin stitching (p. 559.). Occasionally drainage of the wound is desirable.

Dressing. The wound is then dressed with gauze, and then bandaged (all sterile), and put at rest. The arm may be placed in a sling and a serious limb wound may need a plaster of Paris protection. The dressing is left in place for between five and ten days without being disturbed, unless there is a rise in the patient's temperature, or pain, when the wound is inspected earlier.

GENERAL TREATMENT

Antibiotics

Penicillin, by injection as a rule, is usually given as a routine in the prevention of infection in major wounds. It is given at first in large doses and as soon as possible after the injury. The antibiotic treatment is carried on for five to seven days. Wounds which are thought to be contaminated with penicillin-resistant germs (for example, wounds near the buttock, or those exposed to 'hospital germs') are protected by giving the patient an alternative antibiotic, usually tetracycline.

Shock

Signs and Symptoms. The patient is pale. In a severe case, he may be blue (cyanosed), especially in the finger tips, lips and ears. He is cold and clammy and may be frankly sweating. He feels faint, giddy and nauseated, and may vomit. On the other hand, he may be unconscious, or he may be anxious and garrulous. The pulse may be slow at first, then quickly becomes very rapid and feeble. The blood pressure is lowered (although it may be raised at first). The breathing is shallow and rapid.

The above picture is modified according to the severity of the state of shock. A transient fainting attack may be the only sign in a mild case.

Causes. Traumatic shock is usually associated with loss of blood or plasma. Psychological and neurogenic shock are not necessarily associated with such loss.

Psychological causes are apprehension, terror or fear—a nervous person may suffer from severe primary shock as a result of a trivial injury such as a cut finger. The sight of the blood (rather than the amount lost) is the causative factor. Conversely, a person who suffers an injury while his mind is engrossed, such as a soldier in the heat of battle, may be oblivious of his injury, though his wound is serious.

Neurogenic causes are stimuli affecting sensitive nerve centers, such as a blow on the solar plexus or on the testicle. Neurogenic shock may also be associated with multiple injuries.

Traumatic shock develops within a few minutes to a few hours after injury. It is the result of severe injury, bleeding, or burns where there is blood or plasma loss.

Physiology of Shock. The body in shock is not in a state of useless failure. On the contrary, there is a defensive mechanism at work. The nervous and chemical systems are fighting to keep the circulation going and the blood pressure up.

One way in which this is done is by closing off, to a large extent, the blood circulation to the skin and gastro-intestinal tract, and directing the available blood to the organs where it is most needed—the brain and the heart. It is this process which brings about the pale, cold, sweating skin. When the fight is over, then true collapse sets in.

The body goes through the following phases in the production of shock.

The Alarm Reaction

1. Neurogenic phase. This consists of general stimulation of the autonomic nervous system. If the person is particularly sensitive to vagal stimuli, i.e. faints easily, then the parasympathetic system is predominant, producing a slow pulse, pallor and lower blood pressure.

One of three events may then take place: (a) immediate recovery, e.g. after fainting at seeing a mouse; (b) immediate death (rare, but can occur if the stimulus is sufficient and subject highly responsive); or (c) the sympathetic system becomes predominant, releasing adrenaline which produces a faster pulse, raised blood pressure and diversion of the circulation to heart and brain. People not especially of the 'vagal type' will not go through the stage of parasympathetic stimulation but will immediately show signs of sympathetic stimulation.

2. Humoral phase. The released adrenaline stimulates the anterior pituitary gland to release corticotrophin (A.C.T.H.). This hormone acts on the cortex of the adrenal glands, causing them to produce the steroid hormones, cortisone and hydrocortisone.

The Resistance Stage. This is reached when shock is established and the body is fighting a defensive battle. The raised heart rate is maintained and vasoconstriction fully established. The blood pressure falls as shock progresses. If the stimulus is removed and treatment instituted, gradual recovery takes place. If the stimulus is overwhelming then death may take place at this stage. Otherwise the third stage is reached.

Failure of Resistance. This is characterized by a severe fall in blood pressure, generalized vasodilatation, deep coma and death.

Treatment at Scene of Accident. Reassurance of the shocked patient is very important; an attitude of cheerful confidence counteracts the natural fears of an injured person and is not only humane, but a valuable therapeutic measure.

The clothing should be loosened and the patient placed in the horizontal position. He should be turned to one side if unconscious. Hemorrhage is controlled, and the wound dressed as already described. A bad fracture is immobilized and the patient removed to hospital as soon as possible.

Hot-water Bottles. These should not be applied. It has been explained that the cold skin is a defensive mechanism. If heat is applied to the body, the skin blood vessels dilate and the blood, which is being directed to the brain and heart, returns to the skin.

HOT TEA, ETC. The only time this is useful is in psychogenic shock (brandy is better). Otherwise nothing should be given by mouth. This is because an anesthetic may be necessary, and food or fluid in the stomach may cause vomiting and choking. Furthermore, the blood vessels to the stomach are constricted so any fluid given would not be easily absorbed. If the patient complains of thirst his mouth may be rinsed out.

Treatment at the Hospital. The most important single factor in shock production is fluid loss. The doctor will assess whether immediate transfusion is necessary—for this can be a life-saving procedure. The transfusion will consist of whole blood, plasma, or a plasma substitute. Blood is taken for cross matching as soon as possible.

APPLICATION OF ARTERIAL LIMB TOURNIQUETS is a useful procedure in cases of extreme severe shock. This excludes the limbs temporarily from the circulation, allowing the blood to reach the essential organs.

Morphine has no place in the treatment of shock unless pain is the sole cause.

CONSEQUENCES OF WOUND INFECTION

If a wound is neglected or becomes contaminated during treatment then it will become infected. The effects of infection are first seen locally and then, if the infection is severe and treatment fails or is delayed, general effects are noted.

Local Effects

Inflammation is the first manifestation and it is characterized by redness, pain, heat, swelling, and loss of function (not all necessarily present in any one case). If the inflammation is superficial then cellulitis of varying extent occurs. If the inflammation is deep in a wound then the swelling occurs deep down so that the stitches seem to be under tension. There is tenderness, and then hardness of the part follows.

The acute inflammation may subside in a few days or may progress to suppuration, ulceration, sloughing, and even gangrene in certain cases.

Suppuration. If this occurs then pus is seen in the superficial wound. In the deep wound an abscess may form and may burst to the outside, sometimes discharging a stitch with the pus.

Ulceration and **sloughing** of an infected wound are more likely in an old or debilitated patient, and in diabetics. The surface tissue cells are slowly destroyed and an open 'sore' is formed. There are three recognized stages in ulceration.

EXTENSION. The floor of the ulcer is covered with slough, exudate, and persistent discharge.

TRANSITION. The ulcer is preparing for healing. The floor becomes cleaner, sloughs separate and discharge becomes less. Granulation tissue then covers the ulcer bed.

HEALING. The granulation tissue is gradually replaced by fibrous tissue which eventually contracts to form a scar.

Gangrene is the death of large portions of tissue with putrefaction. There is cessation of blood circulation to the part, loss of heat, sensation, and function, as well as swelling and discoloration. A line of demarcation forms which separates the gangrenous mass from healthy tissue. Gangrene may follow as a direct result of crushing injuries, or indirectly as a result of severe injury to blood vessels at some distance from the site of gangrene.

GAS GANGRENE. Certain micro-organisms, e.g. *Clostridium welchii*, are capable of producing gas in dying tissues. They are thought to be introduced into the wound via infected clothing. The infection can spread rapidly. It is recognized by tenseness, swelling and crepitus (crackling) at the site of the wound, and by a severe generalized toxemia. Cases in which gas gangrene is likely should be given gas-gangrene antitoxin and penicillin prophylactically.

General Effects

Toxemia. Toxins are poisonous substances liberated in infection by micro-organisms, and if a sufficient amount is absorbed into the circulation then toxemia results. This is characterized by fever, a rise in pulse rate, sweating and loss of appetite. In severe cases the temperature may be subnormal.

Septicemia and **Bacteremia** (blood poisoning). These conditions are due to the actual presence of micro-organisms in the bloodstream. In septicemia the bacteria multiply in the blood. Clinically the condition is often heralded by chills (severe uncontrollable shivering). The temperature is then intermittent and chills may continue. The patient feels very ill. Sweating, diarrhea, anemia, hemorrhage, and jaundice may be features.

Pyemia. This is caused by pus-making particles in the bloodstream. Such a particle (embolus) enters the circulation and then lodges in a blood vessel too small for it to pass through, forming a secondary abscess. These may occur in the lungs, liver, skin, joints, etc.

Pyemia gives rise to chills, high intermittent fever and profuse sweating. The pulse is weak and rapid, appetite is lost and delirium may follow. Jaundice may develop. Multiple abscesses may form a week or so after the onset of the disease.

Systemic Treatment. In all but minor forms of wound infection and its sequelae, antibiotics will be given. Before the course is started a swab should be taken from the wound for culture of the organisms in it so as to determine which antibiotics they will respond to (sensitivity). Where blood poisoning is suspected, blood culture tests should be made. Penicillin is usually the antibiotic of choice, but where strains of bacteria resistant to it are suspected (or found) another antibiotic is given.

If anemia is present it must be treated promptly and effectively. A nutritious diet is ordered and pain is relieved.

Local Treatment. The part is rested. If there is pus under tension, it is let out by incision (lancing). In certain cases antibiotics in powders or in creams are applied locally.

If the stage of ulceration is reached the ulcer is cleansed and may be enclosed in an elastic adhesive dressing extending well beyond the ulcer's limits. This is left on for a week or longer to allow healing to proceed.

Gangrene is treated by keeping the part dry, as moisture encourages further infection. Antibiotic powder is applied. If a limb is affected then raising it helps the return of blood from the part. Where gangrene has followed a crushing injury, amputation may be necessary.

Stitching of Wounds. The object of stitching a wound is to bring together damaged structures and to appose the skin edges so that healing can take place by first intention. The choice of stitching material depends to some extent on the surgeon.

CATGUT and chromic catgut (catgut sterilized in chromic acid) are absorbed by the body. The former ceases to be effective after about seven days, the latter after fourteen days. Catgut is usually employed for stitching structures under the skin, such as muscle.

Other materials used for stitching include thread, many kinds of silk, kangaroo tendon, fine stainless steel wire (single or braided), horse hair, human hair and synthetic substances such as nylon.

NEEDLES. The needle may be curved or straight and of varying sizes according to the thickness that must be stitched.

An atraumatic needle has no hole, the thread is welded on. It is used for stitching delicate structures such as intestine.

A round-bodied needle is used for tissues under the skin such as muscle and other soft structures.

A cutting needle is used for tough tissues such as skin and fascia.

METAL CLIPS. These are spiked U-shaped pieces of metal which are used instead of stitches to appose skin edges, particularly thin loose skin such as on the neck.

All materials used for stitching are thoroughly sterilized before use to prevent infection.

STITCHES. The actual stitching up may consist of a continuous suture (as in domestic sewing) or of individual unconnected stitches known as interrupted sutures. The advantage of continuous suture is that it is quicker and the disadvantage that if one part breaks down then the whole suture is vulnerable. It is more often used for deep structures (intestines, membranes, etc.). Interrupted stitches are used for skin and muscle, particularly where strength of the suture is important.

Simple Stitch. In at one edge, out at the other and tied in a reef knot.

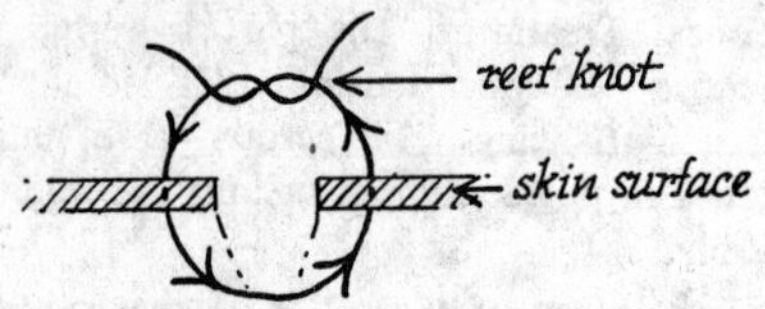

Fig. 1. *SIMPLE STITCH*

Mattress Stitch. Used where extra support is necessary.

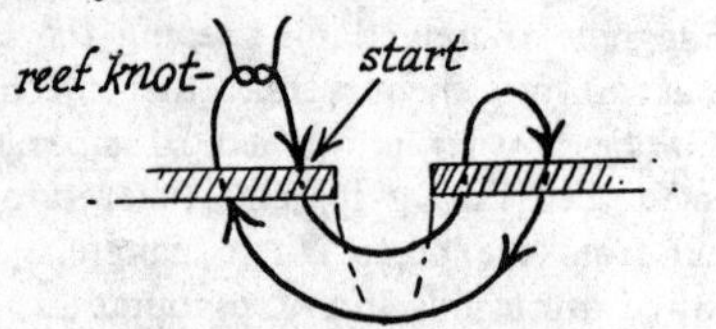

Fig. 2. *MATTRESS STITCH*

Figure of Eight Stitch. Often used for tendons.

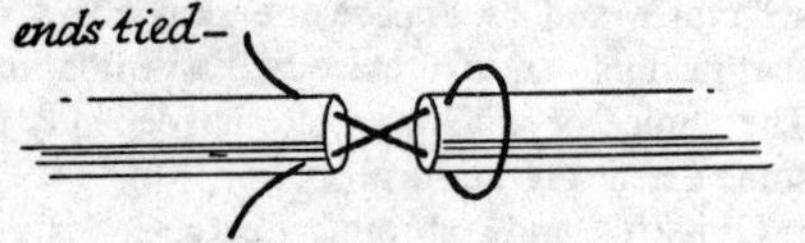

Fig. 3. *FIGURE OF EIGHT STITCH*

Tension Stitch. Used to reinforce simple stitching where there is much gaping.

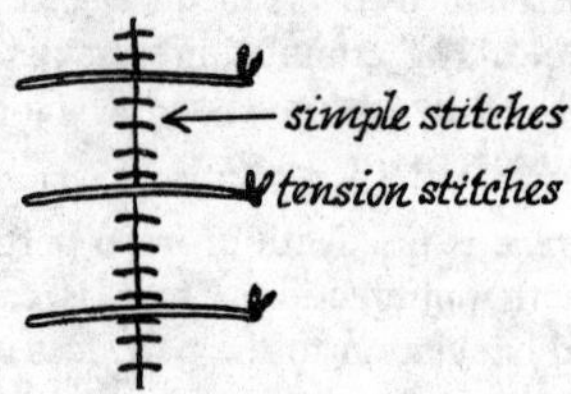

Fig. 4. *TENSION STITCH*

It is interesting to note that stitching and clips are not the only ways in which wound skin edges can be brought together. In parts of the body where the skin is supple, even long gaping superficial wounds can heal satisfactorily if the edges are apposed with *'butterfly' adhesive bandages* and the part adequately rested.

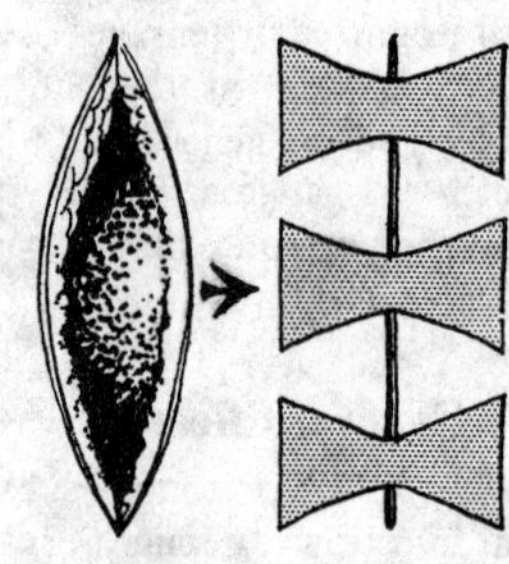

Fig. 5. *'BUTTERFLY' ADHESIVE BANDAGES*

SKIN GRAFTING

This useful procedure hastens the healing of large wounds deprived of skin, and of ulcers. The skin is usually taken from a healthy part of the patient's own body. The skin from another person will be 'rejected'—the exception to this being in the case of identical twins. The bare surface must be clear from infection, and if granulation has taken place it is scraped away before grafting. Various methods of skin grafting are available. Either split skin or whole skin is used.

Fragments of skin are taken, usually from the front of the thigh, with a razor or special instrument known as a dermatome. The electric dermatome is useful in difficult cases. The grafts are transferred to the prepared area, each being placed in contact with the other, and a dressing is applied.

The scar produced is thin, and the skin may die if a successful blood supply has not developed from beneath the graft. One knows whether the graft has taken within a week of the procedure.

Pedicle Grafting. Whole skin is used in pedicle grafting. Here a flap of skin is left partly attached at its source and the rest swung over on to the area to be grafted. When the graft has taken the pedicle is divided.

The hand, face and scalp most often require these full thickness grafts.

DISORDERS DUE TO PHYSICAL AGENTS

EFFECTS OF SUN AND HEAT

Sunburn

Individuals vary in their reaction to exposure to the sun. When the skin is exposed to 'strong' sunlight without previous acclimatization, it will become sunburned. The reaction appears not less than two hours after exposure and may go on developing for up to twelve hours.

The reaction varies from redness and soreness to swelling of the skin, extreme discomfort and erythema, and blisters which may contain blood. As the redness fades, so a transitory browning develops. This pigmentation is soon lost as the skin peels profusely. A more lasting tan begins in the next week and fades in about two months. Extensive sunburn, quite apart from heat stroke, may be accompanied by generalized symptoms of headache, nausea, lassitude and even fever.

Cause. The burn is due to radiation in the invisible part of the light spectrum, which is well reflected by water, snow and ice and excluded by window glass. It is absorbed by atmospheric smoke.

Prevention. Graduated exposure to the sun builds up the horny layer in the skin which prevents excessive sunburn reaction.

Various substances which are commercially available are produced in the form of creams, sprays and lotions. They are said to filter off the harmful radiation, but gradual acclimatization is the most sensible method of protection.

Treatment. Mild cases are treated by the application of calamine lotion to the sunburned areas. In severe cases, the patient requires bed rest as well. Alcohol must be avoided. Pain-relieving drugs may be necessary.

Prickly Heat

This is an acute heat rash associated with excessive sweating and is common in the tropics. It may affect any part of the body. A pricking burning sensation and itching are present. The lesions may become infected as a result of scratching. (See also p. 468.)

Prevention. The clothing should be loose and the rooms air-conditioned. Previous suntan prevents prickly heat.

Treatment. A warm bath and application of a soothing solution. But the only cure in chronic cases is removal of the sufferer to a different climate.

Heat Exhaustion

This is most commonly seen in persons exposed to shade temperatures of 110° F (43° C), especially when this is continued for several days. Exertion increases the risk. Hot damp climates are more dangerous than hot dry climates, and people of over forty are more susceptible than younger persons. Men working in extreme artificial heat, such as furnacemen, ships' firemen and glass workers, may also suffer from heat exhaustion.

Symptoms. The symptoms are weakness, faintness, giddiness, nausea and sweating. The skin is cold and clammy, the temperature normal or subnormal, and in some cases the pupils are dilated.

Cause. In addition to salt loss through sweat and urine, it is thought that there is a direct heat action on the brain.

Treatment. Recovery is usually rapid with treatment though fatalities occasionally occur. The patient should be laid on his back in a cool place, and his clothing loosened. A warm bath may be helpful. Salt drinks are given, and the patient kept under observation. In severe cases saline may have to be given via a vein (intravenously).

Heat Cramps

Agonizing cramps, starting in the calves and moving to the arms and abdominal muscles, are especially liable to occur in workers in very hot atmospheres who are in a poor general condition. It usually comes on if water has been drunk copiously after sweating. Abdominal colic and vomiting are common symptoms if the intestine is affected.

Cause. Heat cramps are due to loss of salt largely via the sweat and urine. The sufferer has a lowered level of sodium in his blood serum.

Treatment. Men working under conditions which involve much sweating should take extra salt routinely. This can be taken in the form of effervescent flavored tablets.

Morphine by injection may be necessary if the cramps are severe. The lost salt is replaced by mouth, or intravenously where there is vomiting.

Heat Stroke

Heat stroke (sunstroke; heat hyperpyrexia) usually comes on gradually with confusion, irritability, headache, drowsiness and pyrexia which, if untreated, proceeds to a sudden rise in temperature (maybe up to 43° C, or 110° F) with delirium, convulsions, and death.

Occasionally the onset is sudden and dramatic, with fits and coma. In other cases there is gastro-intestinal upset with nausea and vomiting (and maybe diarrhea), followed three to four days later by a sudden onset of high fever.

Cause. Heat stroke is due to a failure of the heat controlling mechanism of the brain.

Prevention. Hard work and exercise in hot climates should be restricted to the morning and evening. The diet must include plenty of salt and water, and additional salt in the form of tablets should be taken. Alcohol should not be drunk during the day. The clothing must be light and loose, and the head and neck protected.

Treatment. The patient is laid on a bed with a porous mattress and freely circulating air around him. If this is not available he is placed in a bath of cold water up to the neck, and massaged. The rectal temperature is taken every minute and when 39·5° C (103° F) is reached, the patient is wrapped up and ice packs applied to his head and neck. The salt loss is replaced. If fits are present, then blood letting, lumbar puncture, or anethesia may be necessary.

When the acute condition has been overcome, the patient is kept under observation for three weeks or so, and sedatives may be necessary. A move to a more temperate climate is advised in severe cases.

ELECTRICAL INJURIES

Electrical injuries may be due to lightning, or to contact with charged wires or rails. Household electrical appliances which have been wired without care, or open electric fires in bathrooms are two avoidable danger spots in the home.

The resulting injuries depend on the voltage of the current, the length and completeness of contact, the degree of insulation, the moisture of the skin, and the general bodily health. Alternating current is usually more dangerous than direct current. Currents of over 500 volts often produce fatal injuries, although death may follow shock from much lower voltages. If the hands are wet, the grip cannot be relaxed when a person is grasping a wire charged with over 50 volts.

STROKE FROM LIGHTNING. The head is struck and the body may show various types of burns. The brain is injured mainly by disruption, but also by the heat produced by the current. The muscles contract violently, and are in spasm for a short time.

As the person is struck, he usually falls unconscious. He is pale and pulseless, and breathing ceases. Death may take place or this state of 'apparent death' ends either on its own or after artificial respiration has been applied. The subject is then drowsy, and complains of headache and (fortunately) cannot remember what happened. Recovery may take several days but there may be immediate after-effects such as pains in the body and limbs, giddiness, cramps, disturbances of sight and hearing, and the effects of burns.

Permanent defects of memory, speech and gait may be observed. Eye cataract is another possible sequel.

In Electrical Injuries a mild shock causes a violent tingling, and the person may feel faint. These symptoms abate as contact with the 'live' object is broken.

In severe shock, spasm involving the whole body is followed by loss of consciousness with cyanosis, and death may result. The symptoms are similar to those caused by lightning. There may be subsequent hysteria from the severe shock and burn.

The resulting burns may produce a black and dry appearance. They seldom suppurate but heal very slowly. There may be gangrene of the surrounding parts.

Prevention. During severe thunderstorms, especially in the tropics, it is safest to be indoors with doors and windows shut, and away from the chimney. Out of doors it is best to shelter in a ditch or closed car, etc., trees and wire fences being avoided.

In industry, electrical apparatus must be made absolutely safe and it should be checked periodically. In the home, plugs must always be carefully wired. Electric blankets should be serviced regularly. Avoid using electrical tools and kitchen appliances when you are tired and keep them out of children's way.

Treatment. Switch off the current. If this is impossible care must be taken by the rescuer to avoid receiving an electric shock himself. He should stand on some dry insulating (non-conducting) and non-metallic surface such as linoleum, a rubber mat, or glass, and should cover his hands with rubber gloves, newspaper, felt hat or dry rain coat. If these are not available the subject may be pulled away by a dry crooked walking stick, a dry broom or a dry rope. An umbrella should not be used as the metal ribs may conduct the current. Never use bare hands, and do not touch the patient's skin, shoes, or wet clothes.

After rescue, and if the patient's breathing has stopped, the ideal method of resuscitation is as follows. Lay the patient flat on his back with a cushion or pillow under the neck to extend the head. Then perform external cardiac massage, 10 strokes, followed by one good mouth-to-mouth, or mouth-to-nose respiration (see p. 22) — then repeat these procedures aiming to do so six times in one minute (i.e. 60 strokes of cardiac massage and 6 respirations). This should be continued until breathing is resumed, or until medical help arrives, or until the attendant is exhausted.

External Cardiac Massage. The principle of this procedure is to squeeze the heart between the spine and the anterior rib cage. The casualty must be lying flat on his back on a hard surface, e.g. the floor, not on the bed.

The attendant squats across the casualty's abdomen. He places the fist of the left hand at the bottom of the sternum and slightly to the casualty's left side. The right palm is placed on top of the left fist. The fist is sharply pushed by the right hand, hard down towards the vertebral column. This is followed by complete release. The procedure is repeated approximately 60 to 80 times per minute. The force used should be sufficient to tire the attendant severely in ten minutes.

These methods should only be attempted by a rescuer who has practiced them or seen demonstrations. Older methods of artificial respiration (p. 22) should be employed by the completely untrained person.

The patient should also be treated for shock (p. 21) and must rest afterwards under medical observation. Burns must receive appropriate treatment (p. 468). Painful cramps, which may occur when the casualty is conscious, may be treated by massage.

MOTION SICKNESS

Travel by sea, air, train and car can produce motion sickness, as can other forms of repetitive irregular motion such as a swing, a lift, or a roundabout. It is caused by the unusual stimulation of the eye, the vestibular apparatus in the inner ear, and the postural sensory system of the muscles and joints. Psychological factors, such as apprehension, play a part, and the liability is accentuated by cold, unpleasant odors and dyspepsia. The disability is commoner in people who have migraine.

Symptoms. The characteristic symptoms are giddiness, double or disturbed vision, nausea and vomiting, pallor and prostration. Very young infants are immune, and old people are less apt to develop motion sickness. Toleration may sometimes be developed by habitual travel, but some persons appear never to lose the tendency.

Seasickness is the most disabling form. The first symptoms are salivation and yawning with severe nausea. Retching and violent vomiting follow, with giddiness, headache and depression. In prolonged seasickness, exhaustion and lassitude may be followed by collapse. The symptoms quickly subside when the motion stops. On long voyages the passenger's condition generally improves after a few days, and his appetite returns.

Prevention. Before traveling, a susceptible person should take moderate exercise, avoid alcohol and have a light meal two hours before embarking. On board he should keep warm and lie down. The most favorable position on a ship is in the center. In an airplane the head should be rested back on the head rest.

Half an hour before the journey, the traveler may take one or two tablets of hyoscine (for short journeys), or an antihistamine. The latter are suitable for longer journeys.

Dimenhydrinate is also a valuable prophylactic, but apt to produce drowsiness (as are the other antihistamines to a lesser extent).

Treatment. During an attack the sufferer should be kept warm and quiet and should lie down. Hyoscine or cyclizine tablets may be given. If vomiting is severe, dimenhydrinate may be given by injection. Small dry meals should be taken, e.g. biscuits, toast, sponge cake, or cold chicken. Sodium bicarbonate, glucose or alcohol may also give relief.

See also Diseases of the Digestive System, pp. 362.

DECOMPRESSION SICKNESS

This is also known as caisson disease, compressed air illness, and diver's paralysis. Decompression sickness arises under the following circumstances.

1. When workers in compressed air are decompressed too quickly. Such workers include those excavating underwater, in pressurized caisson chambers, for deep foundations for bridges, tunnels, etc.

2. When deep-sea divers or men escaping from submarines come up too quickly to the surface.

3. When airmen or air passengers in unpressurized cabins climb too rapidly to high altitudes.

Cause. The condition is due to the liberation of a mixture of gas bubbles (82 per cent nitrogen, 16 per cent carbon dioxide, and 2 per cent oxygen) in the blood and tissues. The bubbles are especially released into fat-rich structures such as the spinal cord. The oxygen and carbon dioxide rapidly diffuse away. The nitrogen cannot do so.

Apart from gas-bubble release, decompression can affect certain cavities in the body which enclose air, e.g. the ears, the sinuses, and the intestine.

Symptoms which may arise include ear discomfort, sinus pain, and abdominal distension and pain. The symptoms due to decompression sickness include the following: dull, shifting pain in the joints, bones and muscles, known as the 'bends' (because the arms become fixed in a bent position); redness and pruritis of the skin, known as the 'itch;' coughing and an odd sensation behind the sternum, known as the 'chokes;' and giddiness, known as the 'staggers.'

There may also be nausea, vomiting, and ringing in the ears. If the spinal cord is affected various types of paralysis and other nervous system manifestations may result.

Delayed complications after repeated attacks most commonly occur in the bones and joints. They may not become evident until six months or more later, and may eventually lead to osteo-arthritis.

Prevention. Divers, caisson workers and others exposed to the risk of decompression sickness should be carefully chosen. The age (20 to 40 years is most suitable), the general health, and the stature (obese men are bad risks) must all be considered. If acute infection of the upper respiratory tract is present, the man should not work until it has cleared up.

The time of exposure to the high pressure must be limited. A diver going down to a compression of more than 50 lbs per square inch should do so only for a few minutes.

If the return to normal atmospheric pressure is slow enough, the condition never occurs. Divers are brought up in stages, waiting at certain depths for increasing lengths of time. Caisson workers pass through a series of chambers in which the air pressure is gradually lowered and where they wait in a similar way.

Nowadays aircraft are provided with pressurized cabins for passengers and crew. Thus decompression sickness does not occur in modern aviation except perhaps in air crashes.

Treatment. Once the condition has occurred symptoms are relieved if the affected person is returned to the high pressure. This is done in a recompression chamber and the subject is then decompressed very slowly, for at least five hours.

SPACE FLIGHTS

To adjust to the sudden change caused by acceleration when a space capsule is launched and to adapt their heart and breathing systems to the environment within the capsule, astronauts have to be specially prepared. For three hours before the launch they breathe 100 per cent oxygen to remove nitrogen from the body tissues (see Decompression Sickness).

The space capsule is, of course, fully pressurized—as is the space suit which the astronaut wears—so that the astronaut is still subjected to pressure similar to that at the earth's surface.

ALTITUDE SICKNESS

The pressure of oxygen in the atmosphere at altitudes over 10,000 feet is sufficiently reduced to cause some oxygen lack in the blood and tissues. The susceptibility to the resulting altitude sickness varies in different people. The elderly and those with heart or lung disease will succumb, whereas the young and healthy can stand up to it well.

Symptoms. The first symptoms are slurred speech, blunting of the mental faculties, and inco-ordinated movements. Then come headache and weakness. If the degree of under-oxygenation is increased then coma and fits occur, and finally death.

Acclimatization can be produced by increased respiration, by an increase in the number of red cells in the blood (polycythemia), and by an increase in the lung blood vessels.

High mountain climbers avoid altitude disorders by carrying and using oxygen.

RADIATION HAZARDS

Apart from natural radiation, to which all human beings are subjected and adapted, the man-made radiations include medical X-rays, industrial X-rays, radiotherapy, atomic bomb fall-out, atomic energy, and luminosity from watches. The subject is dealt with on p. 191.

MEDICAL AND TECHNICAL PROCEDURES

The following procedures are processes used in medicine (a) for treatment of a disorder or disease (therapeutic use), or (b) as a means of investigating what is wrong with the patient (diagnostic use), or (c) as a preparatory stage to further treatment. They are presented in alphabetical order.

Acupuncture

This is a Chinese traditional surgical procedure, practiced in China many centuries before the Christian era. In recent years it has been introduced into western cultures.

Purpose. Acupuncture therapy is supposed to relieve internal congestion and restore the equilibrium of body functions. It is used for the treatment of arthritis, headache, convulsions, lethargy and colic. There is no known physiological basis for acupuncture. However, a large part of the benefit from its use may be psychosomatic. How it works is not known.

Method. There are 365 specified acupuncture sites on the human trunk, extremities and head. Needles made of a variety of metals and of various shapes and sizes are inserted into these spots.

Adequate anesthesia for major surgery has been achieved by use of manipulated or electrically stimulated needles.

The Artificial Kidney

This is a device which temporarily takes over the functions of the kidneys, to remove waste products from the blood.

Purpose. The artificial kidney is most useful in acute renal failure, which occurs in such conditions as crush injuries, burns, poisoning, and obstetrical hemorrhage. Its use in chronic renal failure is now being perfected.

The blood is 'washed' by the artificial kidney. Metabolites, e.g. urea, accumulate in the blood as a result of faulty kidneys and, in excessive quantities, are injurious to the body. Urea is removed in the 'washing,' and other substances that can be removed are ingested poisons such as aspirin, barbiturates, and antifreeze fluid (ethylene glycol).

Method. The artificial kidney works on the principle of osmosis (see Physiology, p. 237). Blood is pumped from the patient into a long 'sausage' of semipermeable cellophane wound around and around. The coil is in a bath of fluid, isotonic with blood, but containing no urea. The urea (or other poison) diffuses out and the 'purified' blood is returned to the patient. See p. 411.

The 'kidney' is usually run for about six hours at one time. The procedure can be repeated until the cleansing function of the kidney has been restored. Constant blood-checks are made during this dialysis, and the length of running time is determined by the result.

Some hundreds of small machines are now in use in patients' homes today as well as the large machines in big hospitals.

Barium Meal

The whole of the gastro-intestinal tract can be shown up by X-rays if it contains barium sulphate. The barium sulphate powder is made into a liquid and drunk. X-ray pictures taken at intervals then show any distortions or faults in the tract.

Purpose. Diseases of the alimentary tract which may require investigation include difficulty in swallowing, dyspepsia, and pain in the abdomen. If a peptic ulcer or growth is present, it will be shown up on the X-ray plate.

Methods. A Barium Swallow is used to investigate the esophagus. The patient is given a mouthful of barium sulphate paste and holds it in his mouth until he is told to swallow it. The descent of the barium, as it outlines the esophagus, is then watched on the X-ray screen.

Barium Meal. No medicines which would show up on X-ray plates, e.g. alkali mixtures or iron tablets, should be taken for a week before the meal. Nothing is taken by mouth for six hours before the meal and, if a follow-through is being done, food and drink should not be taken for another six hours.

Barium sulphate is swallowed and a series of films are taken 1, 3, 6, and 24 hours later (for a follow-through).

Barium Enema. The patient is first given a soap and water enema two hours before the examination. The barium enema is given with the subject lying on the X-ray table. The passage of the barium through the lower bowel is observed by the radiologist on the X-ray screen. Permanent X-ray pictures are also taken.

Blood Transfusion

Blood from a human donor is given via a tube into the vein of a recipient with a compatible blood group (see Physiology, p. 239-40).

Purpose. Blood transfusions are given for acute hemorrhage due to injury or surgery, and for severe gastro-intestinal hemorrhage from the stomach (hematemesis), or from the large bowel (melena). Severe nose bleeding and bleeding from the womb may sometimes necessitate blood transfusion. It is also given in chronic anemia not responding to other therapy, before operations, and during convalescence. It is often required for hemophiliacs (congenital bleeders).

Method. The recipient's blood is first tested to find its group and cross-matched against the donor's blood. The blood used is usually stored blood. In special cases fresh blood or concentrated red blood cells are given.

The transfusion is usually given through a vein in the forearm, and the arm splinted to keep it still. Tubing is kept in place with adhesive tape, and the bottle suspended from a stand. The rate of flow of the blood is carefully adjusted by the medical attendant.

If an arm vein is not available it may be necessary to use a vein in the ankle.

Bronchoscopy

Bronchoscopy is the passage of an illuminated tube into the trachea and bronchi.

Purpose. Diagnostic. Conditions such as lung abscess, pneumonia that is not responding to treatment, and unexplained hemoptysis (coughing up of blood) should be examined to exclude cancer of the lung. A biopsy (tiny sample of tissue) of any suspicious material is taken. Other conditions investigated include tracheobronchial tuberculosis and lung collapse.

Therapeutic. Bronchoscopy is used for removal of foreign bodies, aspiration of secretions and mucus, and relief of lung collapse.

In Anesthesia. When a patient is to be given an anesthetic before surgery, endobronchial tubes and blockers are positioned via a bronchoscope.

Method. The examination is made while the patient is anesthetized. Atropine is usually given beforehand, with or without morphine. The tube is passed through the open mouth and glottis into the trachea, and then into either main bronchus.

Local anesthesia is used when the risk of a general anesthetic is too great. Many operators use a local anesthetic from choice: this method requires the patient's full co-operation.

Hoarseness of the voice and sore throat may be a temporary after-effect of bronchoscopy. See illustration, p. 342

Cardiac Catheterization

Blood samples are obtained from the great veins and the right side of the heart by the introduction of a catheter.

Purpose. This procedure is used in the study of some types of heart disease, such as hole in the heart and pulmonary stenosis.

Method. The patient is given sedatives and prophylactic penicillin.

A fine, flexible, plastic catheter is introduced into the arm vein and gently pushed up the vein through the thoracic inlet and into the right side of the heart. The procedure is controlled by X-ray screening. Blood samples are taken at intervals and the pressure in the heart chambers and veins recorded.

Catheterization of the Bladder

A rubber tube (catheter) is passed through the urethra into the bladder, in order to draw off urine.

Purpose. Bladder catheterization is done in the following cases:

1. to obtain urine from women for a bacteriological examination of the urine;
2. to relieve urinary retention due to an enlarged prostate, urethral stricture, after labor, or after surgical operations;
3. to obtain a specimen of urine from an unconscious person, e.g. in diabetic coma;
4. to make sure the bladder is empty before surgical operations.

Method. Catheterization must be carried out under strict aseptic conditions because of the danger of introducing infection into the bladder. All instruments, towels, etc., including the catheter, are sterilized. The attendant wears a mask and scrubs up. The patient lies on his back, on sterile towels, with the receiving vessel between the legs.

CATHETERIZATION OF WOMEN. The vulva and labia are swabbed with cetrimide. The catheter is lubricated and gently inserted into the urethral opening below the clitoris. It is carefully pushed upwards for 2 to 3 inches until the urine flows through the catheter.

CATHETERIZATION OF MEN. The penis is cleansed with cetrimide, the foreskin being pushed back if necessary. The penis is held up with the left hand and the lubricated catheter gently passed through the urethra into the bladder, without using force. If any difficulty is experienced a local anesthetic is injected up the urethra—this takes some 15 minutes to become effective.

In cases of retention with severe bladder distension, the bladder should not be entirely emptied at once; the catheter may be left in place, closed with a small cork, and the urine let out gradually.

SUPRAPUBIC CATHETERIZATION. Where catheterization from below has failed, e.g. in severe urethral stricture, the patient is given a general or local anesthetic and a cut is made through the skin above the pubis so that the front of the distended bladder is exposed. A catheter is inserted by means of an introducer. The wound is closed and the end of the catheter attached to a dripper to allow the urine to flow out slowly.

Dialysis

Dialysis is a process whereby metabolites in a strong solution diffuse through a membrane into a weaker solution. It is the principle upon which the artificial kidney works (see p. 565) and the procedure is called *hemodialysis* or *extracorporeal dialysis.*

There is another related procedure known as *peritoneal dialysis*. For this, a nylon catheter inserted into the peritoneum by paracentesis (see p. 568) is connected to two bottles (2 liters) containing a solution suitably prepared to diffuse out the harmful metabolites within the body. This solution, the dialysate, is run into the peritoneal cavity, remains there for 20 to 30 minutes, and is then drained away. The process is continued for 24 to 48 hours.

Peritoneal dialysis is employed when an artificial kidney is not available or when the build-up of urea or other metabolites in the blood is relatively slow.

Ear Syringing

This consists in the injection of fluid into the ear under pressure.

Purposes. When hard wax accumulates in the outer ear, impinging on the ear drum, impaired hearing results. Wax is removed by ear syringing.

Syringing is also used to remove profuse discharge and debris in cases of otitis externa, after careful drying of the ear. More harm than good can come of the process if performed by an inexperienced operator.

Method for Wax Removal. Before treatment, the hard wax is softened by the instillation of sodium bicarbonate ear-drops three times a day for two to three days.

The patient sits in a chair with a towel around the shoulders and an emesis tray held below the ear to receive the water. The ear is syringed with warm water under pressure. As soon as the main mass of wax has been removed the patient can usually hear much more clearly. Slight giddiness may be experienced after the syringing. This is to be expected and it wears off after a few minutes.

Electroencephalography

This is a graphic recording of the electrical currents developed in the cortex of the brain. It is used for investigating neurological disorders such as epilepsy.

Encephalography

This is a process by which air is introduced into the subarachnoid space after lumbar puncture. The air rises to the brain ventricles. X-ray pictures then taken will show the size and shape of the ventricles. This procedure is especially useful in investigating some brain tumors.

Enemas

An enema is fluid introduced into the rectum via the anus. The fluid may be water or oil, and it may be medicated.

Purposes. 1. To empty the bowel of feces, as in fecal impaction in the elderly, intractable constipation, or at the beginning of labor.

2. To empty the bowel of gas.

3. To cleanse the bowel before colonic operations.

4. For therapeutic purposes such as replenishing of body fluids in mild dehydration with water or with glucose saline; giving of drugs such as opium and paraldehyde; reducing cerebral edema by giving a 25 per cent magnesium sulphate solution rectally; and giving corticosteroids rectally in the treatment of ulcerative colitis.

5. To induce anesthesia with thiopentone. Rectal thiopentone is especially useful in the induction of anesthesia in children.

Method. The patient lies on the edge of the bed on his left side, with the knees drawn up. A rubber sheet and towel are arranged for protection. The enema nozzle is lubricated and carefully inserted up to 3 to 4 inches. The fluid is then run in slowly under pressure from a funnel or douche bag until the required amount has been introduced. A greater pressure is obtained by raising the level of the funnel and the foot of the bed. This sends the fluid far around the colon—a high enema. A small quantity of fluid and less pressure reaches the rectum and lower colon—a low enema.

For an evacuant enema the fluid is retained as long as the patient can manage. He should lie quite still and then empty the bowel when he can hold the fluid no longer.

SIMPLE ENEMA: 2 to 4 pints of warm water and soap are used (for ordinary bowel evacuation).

TURPENTINE ENEMA: 30 milliliters of turpentine oil made up to 600 milliliters with Simple (soap) Enema; for gross flatus.

OLIVE OIL ENEMA: 180 ml of warm olive oil are run in slowly. An hour later a soap and water enema is given (useful in fecal impaction).

COLONIC WASHOUT: Before operations on the colon and for instrumental examinations (sigmoidoscopy) 3.5 to 4 liters of fluid is run in slowly, 250 to 500 ml at a time, and siphoned back.

DISPOSABLE ENEMA: This is a small-volume enema containing sodium phosphate and diphosphate in solution (approx. 100 milliliters). The container consists of a polythene bag with an adjustable plastic nozzle. The nozzle is inserted into the back passage and the container squeezed. The whole process takes only 10 minutes or so.

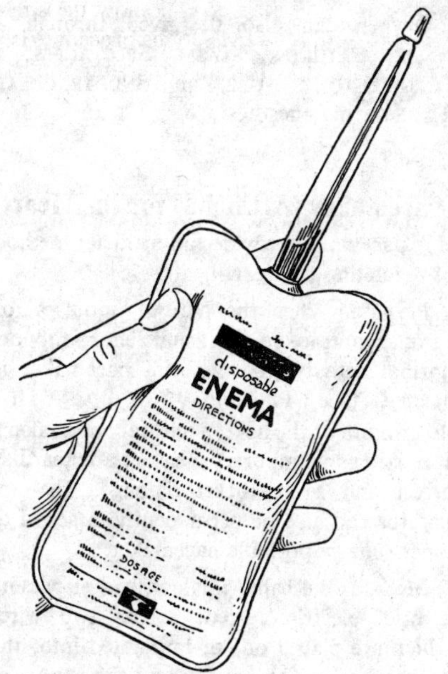

Fig. 1. *DISPOSABLE ENEMA. The contents of the plastic tube are squeezed through the long nozzle into the rectum of the constipated patient.*

This type of enema is of great value in home nursing, and for old people. One of its advantages is the fact that the patient can administer it himself.

Gastric Intubation

This is the passage of a soft rubber tube through the nose or mouth, down the esophagus and into the stomach.

Purpose. DIAGNOSTIC. The stomach contents are aspirated (brought up) through the tube and can be examined. This is useful in cases of suspected cancer of the stomach, peptic ulcer, and in pernicious anemia.

THERAPEUTIC. *Tube Feeding.* Food can be introduced into the stomach through a stomach tube. Patients who are unconscious but not vomiting can be fed in this way, as can those who cannot swallow, e.g. in fractured jaw. Some patients with peptic ulcer are prescribed a continuous drip of milk and alkali through the tube. Tube feeding is also used to nourish persons on hunger strike, or psychotic patients who refuse to eat. A tube is forcibly passed into the stomach.

Gastric Aspiration. Continuous vomiting causes discomfort and exhaustion which can be prevented by bringing up the stomach contents. Continuous suction can be effected by using an electrically-driven pump.

Method. If the tube is passed for diagnosis, the patient has nothing to eat or drink after 8.0 p.m. on the evening before the test. Retching can be avoided during the passage of the tube if the patient breathes deeply and evenly.

The tube is lubricated. The patient sits upright supported by pillows at the back The tube is passed through either the nose or the mouth.

NASAL ROUTE. The best nostril is chosen and the surface membrane of the nose anesthetized. The tube is pushed through the nostril to the back of the throat and the patient told to swallow. As he swallows the tube is pushed down through the esophagus and into the stomach. The patient is asked not to swallow his saliva during a diagnostic test but to spit into a basin.

ORAL ROUTE. The mouth is opened and the tube passed to the back of the tongue. The lips are then closed and the patient swallows while the tube is pushed gently down. If the pharynx is very sensitive it may be anesthetized.

Gastric Lavage
(Stomach Washout)

Purpose. The washing is done to remove swallowed poisons, to aid treatment of patients in diabetic coma, in pyloric stenosis, in acute gastric dilatation, and prior to operations on the stomach. The procedure is also performed when intestinal tuberculosis is suspected, the stomach washings being searched for tubercle bacilli.

Method. See p. 39 and illustration.

Injections (Parenteral)

An injection is the administration, by means of a needle and syringe, of substances into the body, other than via the alimentary canal. (see also p. 585.)

Purpose. Drugs and nutrients are given by injection for the following reasons:

1. when rapid action of a drug is necessary;
2. when it is desired to administer a drug which has no effect if given by mouth, e.g. insulin and adrenaline;
3. for delayed absorption, e.g. intramuscular iron;
4. for a local action of a drug, e.g. injection into a joint to ease its movement;
5. for local anesthesia;
6. for diagnosis, e.g. to test the patient's reaction to possible allergens.

Method. For any hypodermic injection the needle and syringe must be sterilized before use. The attendant washes his hands. The syringe is carefully filled with the solution according to the required dose. The syringe is inverted and emptied of air.

The skin is swabbed with alcohol and the needle inserted quickly to the required depth. Before injecting the solution, the plunger is drawn out gently to ensure that a vein has not been pierced. Puncture of a vein is only used for intravenous injections. The correct dose is injected, the needle withdrawn and the puncture swabbed with alcohol.

INTRADERMAL INJECTIONS are used for some skin sensitivity tests. A fine small needle is used to enter the skin but not to pierce below it.

SUBCUTANEOUS INJECTIONS are used for giving small amounts of non-irritating substances. The rate of action of the drug is slowest when given at this site. The most suitable areas are the outer surface of the upper arm or thigh. The needle pierces through the skin but does not enter muscle.

INTRAMUSCULAR INJECTIONS are used for giving large volumes of solutions, or for viscid or irritating substances. The action of a drug is more rapid when given into the muscle. A longer needle is used, and for giving viscid solutions it should have a wide bore.

The site for the injection is chosen to avoid piercing nerves or arteries. The outer part of the upper half of the thigh and the upper outer quadrant of the buttock (to avoid the sciatic nerve) are commonly used. Small amounts may be injected into the outer part of the upper arm.

INTRAVENOUS INJECTIONS. When rapid action of a drug is required, or if the substance, e.g. aminophylline, digoxin, and calcium gluconate, is too irritating to be given by other routes, the injection is made into a vein—usually the vein in the crook of the arm or on the back of the hand. A tourniquet is placed around the arm, the vein is punctured, the tourniquet released, and the substance injected slowly.

INTRACARDIAC INJECTIONS. Drugs can be injected directly into the heart as a lifesaving measure, e.g. adrenaline in cardiac arrest.

EPIDURAL INJECTIONS are sometimes used for anesthesia, and in orthopedic treatment to break down adhesions. Severe headache after lumbar puncture can be relieved by the epidural injection of saline. The solution is injected outside the outer membrane surrounding the cerebrospinal fluid which bathes the spinal cord.

NERVE BLOCKS are used for regional anesthesia and for tooth extraction. Injection into a nerve is used in the treatment of such conditions as trigeminal neuralgia of the face.

JOINT INJECTIONS. Hydrocortisone is injected into the joint in some joint disorders, e.g. rheumatoid arthritis.

SINUS INJECTIONS. Antibiotics are injected directly into the sinuses in some cases of sinusitis.

Intravenous Infusions

These infusions are given into a vein to replace loss of water and electrolytes (charged particles of important salts in solution in the body's fluids).

Purpose. In many conditions, water and electrolytes are lost in excess by the body and unless they are replaced serious consequences result (see Physiology, p. 239). Water depletion occurs in coma, shipwreck, or difficulty in swallowing. Salt depletion arises after excessive sweating. Salt and water depletion is a consequence of kidney diseases, extensive burns, diabetic coma, and vomiting. Depletion of potassium as well as of salt (sodium chloride) often follows diarrhea and vomiting, and some cases of nephritis.

These substances can be replaced by various routes—through the back passage, under the skin, and through a vein. Replacement into a vein is used when the loss is severe, when the patient (possibly unconscious) cannot take enough by mouth, when vomiting is present, and when circulatory collapse has occurred.

Method. The drip set used is essentially similar to a blood transfusion set. The rate of drip will depend on the condition of the patient. The most commonly used solutions are glucose solution, and glucose saline solution, with added potassium when necessary. Biochemical checks of the blood are made to judge the amount and type of replacement necessary.

Ionization

This is the introduction, by means of an electric current, of ions (electrically charged particles) into the tissues of the body for therapeutic purposes.

Purpose. The main use of ionization is in the treatment of the 'sensitive' areas of the nose of patients who suffer from hay fever. The aim is to give the mucosa immunity against the irritant producing the attack. It is also useful in other types of rhinorrhea. Excellent results are occasionally obtained in children.

Method. The nose is packed with gauze or cotton which has been soaked in 1 per cent zinc sulphate solution. An electric current is passed through the nose. At the first application the current is passed for a short time only as some patients may react very strongly to the treatment. Three applications, at weekly intervals, are usually sufficient; the third may last about 20 minutes.

Lumbar Puncture

Lumbar puncture consists in the insertion of a hollow needle into the subarachnoid space (containing cerebrospinal fluid) below the end of the spinal cord.

Purposes. 1. A lumbar puncture is performed as a diagnostic measure when meningitis, subarachnoid hemorrhage, etc., is suspected. Cerebrospinal fluid is obtained and sent for pathological examination.

2. The measurement of the pressure of the fluid is useful in the investigation of some neurological conditions.

3. If air or radio-opaque substances are introduced into the subarachnoid space, X-ray photographs will show up irregularities in the structures.

4. Local anesthetics and antibiotics can be injected into the subarachnoid space through a lumbar puncture.

Method. If the patient is nervous or restless a sedative is given. Children over one year are always sedated, and occasionally a general anesthetic is required.

The patient lies on his left side with a pillow under his head. His knees are bent up to the chin and his hands clasped beneath his knees. The purpose of this posture is to bend the spine, making the procedure easier. If the position is found difficult an assistant helps by placing one hand behind the neck and the other behind the knees, and drawing them together.

The operator scrubs up and wears a gown, mask and gloves. Every precaution is taken to prevent infection. The patient's skin is painted with antiseptic and a local anesthetic is injected, infiltrating deep into the tissues. The fine lumbar puncture needle, with the stilette in place, is then inserted carefully through the anesthetized area until it impinges on the ligament over the spine. There is a 'give' as the needle pierces it and enters the subarachnoid space. The stilette is withdrawn and the cerebrospinal fluid drips through the needle.

The pressure of the fluid is measured with a manometer. The patient is asked to relax at this point—if he is too tense a false reading is obtained.

The fluid is then collected into small bottles for examination. The needle is taken out and the skin puncture sealed with raw cotton soaked in collodion.

Headache may develop a few hours after lumbar puncture and is relieved by analgesics and salt drinks by mouth.

Oxygen Therapy

Extra oxygen is needed for:

1. The relief of anoxia (oxygen lack in the blood), in respiratory obstruction, severe pneumonia, emphysema, severe asthma, and coal gas poisoning.
2. Cancer radiotherapy (some forms) because oxygen increases tumor sensitivity.
3. The relief of headache after air encephalography.
4. The relief of gaseous bowel distension.
5. Certain forms of anesthesia.

Method. Oxygen is usually supplied in cylinders of varying sizes. As oxygen burns well, precautions must be taken to avoid fire; attendants must not smoke.

OXYGEN TENT. This is made of airtight transparent material with loose aprons to tuck in with the bedclothes. It must be carefully set up to obtain a sufficient oxygen concentration. Part of the oxygen supply is passed through ice to cool the gas. The patient's movements in the tent are unrestricted and the tent is especially useful for long-term oxygen therapy. The main disadvantage is that the tent has to be taken down for examination of the patient.

INCUBATOR. This is a special type of oxygen tent for nursing premature or ill babies.

FACE MASKS. The mask may be either nasal, leaving the mouth free, or oronasal, covering the mouth and nose, when the patient is a mouth breather. (p.273).

Oxygen can also be given through a NASAL CATHETER, NASAL SPECTACLES, a TRACHEOSTOMY TUBE, an ENDOTRACHEAL TUBE during anesthesia.

Pacemaker (Artificial) for the Heart

A pacemaker provides an artificial method of regulating the heart beat.

Purpose. When the natural impulses for cardiac contraction are insufficient to support normal activity, the artificial pacemaker is needed (see Physiology, p. 242, for description of the heart's natural pacemaker). It is used as a temporary measure after cardiac arrest and severe heart damage. The apparatus can also be permanently attached to a person as a portable pacemaker.

Method. Basically, this consists of passing a brief electric current across two wires which are placed on, or implanted into, the heart muscle. The battery and the source of contact breaking are outside the body and can be worn on the lapel of a coat.

Paracentesis of the Abdomen

Paracentesis is the surgical puncture of a body cavity.

Purpose. To remove excessive fluid from the peritoneal cavity in the condition known as ascites, which may occur in cirrhosis of the liver, tuberculous peritonitis, secondary cancer in the peritoneum, etc. The fluid gives rise to discomfort and breathlessness.

Method. Sedatives are given if necessary. The bladder must be empty, otherwise it may be punctured inadvertently—a catheter is therefore passed just before the procedure. The patient lies flat on his back with a many-tailed bandage under him (see Fig. 26, p.382).

The procedure is done under aseptic conditions. The skin is prepared and the area to be punctured is infiltrated with a local anesthetic.

The site chosen is usually the right or left side below the umbilicus.

A small cut is made in the skin and through this opening a trochar and cannula are introduced until a 'give' is felt as the peritoneum is penetrated. The inside of the trochar is removed and the fluid emerges. This should not be released too quickly. The end of the cannula is attached to rubber tubing and a clip controls the rate of flow.

The bandage is wrapped around the abdomen and tightened as the swelling goes down.

Paracentesis of the Pericardium

Purpose. Where fluid has accumulated around the heart, some is removed for examination to determine whether the condition is due to tuberculosis, infection, or cancer.

Method. The heart is usually approached from just below the sternum but a route through the chest wall may be necessary. Preparation of the skin and local anesthesia are followed by the actual aspiration of fluid from around the heart.

Paracentesis of the Ear
(*Myringotomy*)

Purpose. In otitis media, myringotomy is indicated where

1. despite antibiotics and other measures there is excessive pain;
2. there is fluid in the middle ear causing a hearing defect;
3. pus in the middle ear is causing bulging of the drum and spontaneous perforation seems inevitable.

Method. A good light is essential. The patient is anethetized. The external ear is cleaned and a reversed J-shaped incision made with a special knife in the posterior part of the ear drum. Pus or fluid then discharges. A gauze wick is inserted into the ear to help drainage.

Tracheostomy
(*Tracheotomy*)

This consists in the creation of a hole in the trachea affording communication between the trachea and the atmosphere.

Purposes. 1. To relieve difficulty in breathing owing to an obstruction above the site of tracheostomy, as in diphtheria, cancer of the larynx, and acute laryngotracheobronchitis (severe croup), or the presence of a foreign body.

2. To increase the effective ventilation of the lung, as in severe emphysema.

3. For sucking out secretions in the absence of effective cough, as in some forms of pneumonia.

4. For prolonged artificial ventilation with an automatic ventilator, as in tetanus and poliomyelitis.

5. For extensive operations on the larynx.

The tracheostomy may be either temporary or permanent—the latter in cancer of the larynx and after laryngectomy.

Method. Either a local or a general anesthetic is used. In very urgent cases where there is immediate danger of asphyxia, the procedure can be done without anesthesia.

The head is held far back (hyper-extended). The skin is incised and the muscles in front of the trachea divided. A window is cut through the second, third, or fourth tracheal cartilage and a sterilized tracheostomy tube inserted (see Fig. 13 in Fevers, p. 269). The tube needs to be changed at frequent intervals.

The presence of a tracheostomy does not mean that the patient cannot talk, for if he places a finger over the opening of the tube, natural phonation can result.

Venepuncture

Venepuncture is the taking of blood from a person, via a vein.

Purposes. 1. To obtain a blood sample for analysis;

2. to withdraw blood to use for a blood transfusion, or to relieve high blood pressure.

Method. The procedure is relatively painless. Any vein which is palpable and well supported may be used—usually in the crook of the arm, on the back of the hand, or at the wrist.

The needles and syringe are sterilized before use. The patient should lie down and if blood is taken from an elbow vein the elbow should be kept fully extended. A tourniquet is applied at the top of the arm. The skin is cleaned. The patient may be asked to clench and unclench his fist in order to distend the vein. The needle is then introduced through the skin and into the vein and the blood drawn off.

When enough has been obtained the tourniquet is released and the needle withdrawn. A swab is held firmly over the puncture for a few minutes.

CAPILLARY BLOOD. When a very small amount of blood only is required, capillary blood is obtained by pricking the lobe of the ear or the finger, or the heel in infants. The selected site must be warm to ensure a free flow of blood.

SOCIAL SECURITY AND MEDICARE

THE BASIC IDEA

The basic idea of social security is a simple one. During working years employees, their employers, and self-employed people pay social security contributions which are pooled in special trust funds. When earnings stop or are reduced because the worker retires, dies, or becomes disabled, monthly cash benefits are paid to replace part of the earnings the family has lost.

Part of the contributions made go into a separate hospital insurance trust fund so that when workers and their dependents reach 65 they will have help in paying their hospital bills. Voluntary medical insurance, also available to people 65 or over, helps pay doctors' bills and other medical expenses. This program is financed out of premiums shared half-and-half by the older people who sign up and by the federal government.

Nine out of ten working people in the United States are now building protection for themselves and their families under the social security program.

MONTHLY CASH BENEFITS

To get monthly cash payments for yourself and your family, or for your survivors to get payments in case of your death, you must first have credit for a certain amount of work under social security. This credit may have been earned at any time after 1936.

Most employees get credit for ¼ year of work if they are paid $50 or more in covered wages in a 3-month calendar quarter. Four quarters are counted for any full year in which a person has $400 or more in self-employment income. A worker who receives farm wages gets credit for ¼ year of work for each $100 of covered wages he has in a year up to $400.

You can be either fully or currently insured, depending on the total amount of credit you have for work under social security and the amount you have in the last 3 years. The table on page 000 shows which kinds of cash benefits may be paid if you are fully insured and which kinds may be paid if you are currently insured.

If you stop working under social security before you have earned enough credit to be insured, no cash benefits will be payable to you. The earnings already credited to you will remain on your social security record; if you later return to covered work, regardless of your age, all your covered earnings will be considered.

Fully Insured. Just how much credit you must have to be fully insured depends upon the year you reach 65 if you are a man, or 62 if you are a woman, or upon the date of your death or disability.

The amount of credit you will need is measured in quarter-year units of work called quarters of coverage; but for convenience, the following table is given in years. The people in your social security office will be glad to give you further details if you have questions.

You are fully insured if you have credit for at least as many years as shown on the appropriate line of the following chart.

If you reach 65 (62 if a woman) or die or become disabled	*You will be fully insured if you have credit for this much work*
In 1965	3½ years
1967	4
1969	4½
1971	5
1975	6
1979	7
1983	8
1987	9
1991 or later	10

If you become disabled or die before reaching 65 (62 for a woman), you are fully insured if you have credit for ¼ year of work for each year after 1950 and up to the year of your disability or death. In counting the number of years after 1950, omit years before you were 22.

No one is fully insured with credit for less than 1½ years of work and no one needs more than 10 years of work to be fully insured. Having a fully insured status, however, means only that certain kinds of cash benefits may be payable—it does not determine the amount. The amount will depend on your average earnings.

Currently Insured. You will be currently insured if you have social security credit for at least 1½ years of work within 3 years before you die or become entitled to retirement benefits.

Amounts of Monthly Payments

The amount of your montly retirement or disability benefit is based on your average earnings under social security over a period of years. The amount of the monthly payments to your dependents or to your survivors in case of your death also depends on the amount of your average earnings.

The exact amount of your benefit cannot be figured until there is an application for benefits. This is because all of your earnings up to the time of the application may be considered in figuring your benefit. The Social Security Administration will, of course, figure your exact benefit at that time.

You can estimate the amount of the worker's benefit, however, by following the steps given below.

1. Count the number of years to be used in figuring your average earnings as follows:
   - If you were born before 1930, start with 1956;
   - If you were born after 1929, start with the year you reached 27.

   Count your starting year and each year up until (but not including):
   - The year you reach 65, if you are a man;
   - The year you reach 62, if you are a woman;
   - The year the worker becomes disabled or dies, for disability or death benefits.

   (Note: At least 5 years of earnings must be used to figure retirement benefits and at least 2 years to figure disability or survivor benefits.)
2. List the amount of the worker's earnings for all years beginning with 1951. (Include earnings in the year of death or the year disability began.) Do not count *more than* $3,600 for each year 1951 through 1954; $4,200 for each year 1955 through 1958; $4,800 for each year 1959 through 1965; $6,600 for 1966 and 1967; and $7,800 for 1968 and after.
3. Cross off your list the years of lowest earnings until the number remaining is the same as your answer to step 1. (It may be necessary to leave years in which you had no earnings on your list.)
4. Add up the earnings for the years left on your list, and divide by the number of years you used (your answer to step 1).

The result is your average yearly earnings covered by social security over this period.

Look in the table entitled 'Examples of Monthly Cash Payments' and estimate your benefit from the examples given there.

Increasing Payments by Additional Work. If you work after you start getting benefits and your added earnings will result in higher benefits, your benefit will be automatically refigured after the additional earnings are credited to your record.

Special Payments. Special payments of $46 a month ($69 for a couple) can be made under the social security program to certain people 72 and over who are not eligible for social security benefits. These payments are intended to assure some regular income for older people who had little or no opportunity to earn social security protection during their working years.

People who reached 72 in 1968 or later need credit for some work under social security to be eligible for special payments. Those who reached 72 in 1968 need credit for ¾ year of work under social security. The amount of work credit needed increases gradually each year for people reaching 72 after 1968, until it is the same as that required for retirement benefits. (This will be in 1972 for men and 1970 for women.)

The special payments are not made for any month for which the person receives payments under a federally-aided public assistance program. The special payments are reduced by the amount of any other governmental pension, retirement benefit, or annuity.

Payments to people who have credit for less than ¾ of a year of work covered by social security are made from general revenues, not from social security trust funds.

EXAMPLES OF MONTHLY CASH PAYMENTS

Average yearly earnings after 1950 [1]	$923 or less	$1800	$3000	$4200	$5400	$6600	$7800
Retired worker—65 or older / Disabled worker—under 65	64.00	101.70	132.30	161.50	189.80	218.40	250.70
Wife 65 or older	32.00	50.90	66.20	80.80	94.90	109.20	125.40
Retired worker at 62	51.20	81.40	105.90	129.20	151.90	174.80	200.60
Wife at 62, no child	24.00	38.20	49.70	60.60	71.20	81.90	94.10
Widow at 62 or older	64.00	84.00	109.20	133.30	156.60	180.20	206.90
Widow at 60, no child	55.50	72.80	94.70	115.60	135.80	156.20	179.40
Disabled widow at 50, no child	38.90	51.00	66.30	80.90	95.00	109.30	125.50
Wife under 65 and one child	32.00	51.00	70.20	119.40	164.60	177.20	183.80
Widow under 62 and one child	96.00	152.60	198.60	242.40	284.80	327.60	376.20
Widow under 62 and two children	96.00	152.60	202.40	280.80	354.40	395.70	434.40
One child of retired or disabled worker	32.00	50.90	66.20	80.80	94.90	109.20	125.40
One surviving child	64.00	76.30	99.30	121.20	142.40	163.80	188.10
Maximum family payment	96.00	152.60	202.40	280.80	354.40	395.60	434.40

[1]Generally, average earnings are figured over the period from 1950 until the worker reaches retirement age, becomes disabled, or dies. Up to 5 years of low earnings or no earnings can be excluded. The maximum earnings creditable for social security are $3,600 for 1951-1954; $4,200 for 1955-1958; $4,800 for 1959-1965; and $6,600 for 1966-67. The maximum creditable in 1968 and after is $7,800, but average earnings cannot reach this amount until later. Because of this, the benefits shown in the last column on the right generally will not be payable until later. When a person is entitled to more than one benefit, the amount actually payable is limited to the larger of the benefits.

DISABILITY PAYMENTS

The risk of disability hangs over all of us. When disability occurs, it may affect a family's financial security more than the retirement or even the death of a worker.

Protection against the loss of earnings because of disability became a part of social security in 1954. In the years since, this disability protection has been expanded and improved several times.

The disabled people who get monthly benefits come from all walks of life: the 40-year-old salesman who has had a heart attach; the 23-year-old secretary sidelined for more than a year by an auto accident; the 53-year-old widow who is crippled with advanced arthritis; the retired worker's 32-year-old son who has been mentally retarded from birth.

Each person who applies for disability benefits is considered for services by the vocational rehabilitation agency in his state.

This section tells you what you need to know about the social security disability provisions—how they affect you and your family, now or in the future.

Who Can Get Benefits Because of Disability?

The social security program provides disability protection in three different situations. Monthly benefits can be paid to:

- Disabled workers under 65 and their their families. (See below.)
- Persons disabled in childhood (before 18) who continue to be disabled. These benefits are payable as early as 18 when a parent receives social security retirement or disability benefits, or when an insured parent dies. (See page 573.)
- Disabled widows, disabled dependent widowers, and (under certain conditions) disabled surviving divorced wives of workers who were insured at death. These benefits are payable as early as 50. (See page 573.)

The Disabled Worker

A Disabled Worker Needs Some Work Credits. If you are a worker and become severely disabled, you will be eligible for monthly benefits if you have worked under social security long enough and recently enough. The amount of work you will need depends on your age when you become disabled:

- *31 or older:* If you become disabled before 1972, you need credit for 5 years of work out of the 10 years ending when you become disabled. The years need not be continuous or in units of full years.
- *24 through 30:* You need credit for having worked half the time between 21 and the time you become disabled.
- *Before 24:* You need credit for 1½ years of work in the 3-year period ending when your disability begins.

When Is A Worker Disabled? A worker is considered disabled under the social security law if he has a physical or mental condition which:

- Prevents him from doing any substantial gainful work, and
- Is expected to last (or has lasted) for at least 12 months, or is expected to result in death.

(Payments may be made to a person who meets these conditions even if he is expected to recover from his disability.)

The medical evidence from your physician or other sources will show the severity of your condition and the extent to which it prevents you from doing substantial gainful work. Your age, education, training, and work experience also may be considered in deciding whether you are able to work.

If you can't do your regular work but can do other substantial gainful work you will not be considered disabled. (For an exception involving blind workers, see below.)

Special Provisions for the Blind. A person whose vision is no better than 20/200 even with glasses (or who has a limited visual field of 20 degrees or less) is considered "blind" under the social security law.

If a person who meets this test of blindness has worked long enough and recently enough under social security, he is eligible for a disability "freeze" even if he is actually working. Under the "freeze," years in which he has low earnings (or no earnings) because of disability will not reduce the amount of his future benefits, which are figured from his average earnings.

A person 55 to 65 who meets this test of blindness and who has worked long enough and recently enough under social security can get cash disability benefits if he is unable to perform work requiring skills or abilities comparable to those required by the work he did regularly before he reached 55 or became blind, whichever is later. (Benefits will not be paid, however, for any month in which he *actually performs substantial gainful work.*)

A blind worker under 55 can become entitled to cash benefits only if he is unable to engage in *any* substantial gainful work.

Dependents of Disabled Workers. While you are receiving benefits as a disabled worker, payments can also be made to certain members of your family. These family members include:

- Your unmarried children under 18.
- Your children 18 through 21 if they are unmarried and attending school full time.
- Your unmarried children 18 or older who were disabled before reaching 18 and continue to be disabled.

(*Note:* Stepchildren and adopted children also may qualify for benefits on your record.)

- Your wife at any age if she has in her care a child who is getting benefits based on your social security record because he is under 18 or because he has been disabled since before 18.
- Your wife 62 or older even if there are no children entitled to benefits.
- Your dependent husband 62 or older.

If You Also Receive Workmen's Compensation. If you are a disabled worker under 62 and are entitled to both social security disability benefits and workmen's compensation, the total monthly payments to you and your family may not exceed 80 percent of your average monthly earnings before you became disabled. (A worker's *full* earnings, including any amounts above the maximum creditable for social security, may be considered when his average earnings are figured for this purpose.) Social security benefits must be reduced if combined benefits from social security and workmen's compensation would otherwise be over this limit.

The Person Disabled Since Childhood

If you have an unmarried son or daughter 18 or older who became disabled before 18 and is still disabled, he or she may start receiving childhood disability benefits:

- When you begin to receive social security retirement or disability insurance benefits, or
- At your death if you had enough social security work credits for the payment of benefits to your survivors.

A person disabled before 18 needs no social security work credits to get benefits. His payments, based on the earnings of his parent, may start as early as 18 and continue for as long as he is disabled. The decision whether a person has been disabled since childhood is made in the same way as the decision whether a worker is disabled. (See page 572.)

If a child with a severe medical condition is now receiving child's insurance benefits which are scheduled to stop when he reaches 18, he or someone in his family should get in touch with the social security office a few months before he reaches 18 to see about continuing the benefits past 18 on the basis of disability.

The mother of a disabled son or daughter who is entitled to childhood disability benefits may also qualify for benefits *regardless of her age* if she has the son or daughter in her care.

The Disabled Widow or Widower

Before a 1967 change in the social security law, a widow could not get monthly benefits until she reached 60 unless she had in her care a child entitled to benefits based on her husband's earnings. A dependent widower could not, under any circumstances, get payments based on his deceased wife's earnings before he reached 62.

Now, if you are disabled and are the widow, dependent widower, or (under certain circumstances) the surviving divorced wife of a worker who worked long enough under social security, you may be able to get monthly benefits as early as 50. The benefits will be permanently reduced, with the amount of the reduction depending on the age at which benefits start (see the table on monthly cash benefits). You need no work credits of your own to get benefits based on the earnings of your deceased spouse.

A widow or widower may be considered disabled only if she or he has an impairment which is so severe that it would ordinarily prevent a person from working and which is expected to last at least 12 months. Vocational factors such as age, education, and previous work experience cannot be considered in deciding whether a widow or widower is disabled (as they may be for a disabled worker).

In general, you cannot get these benefits unless your disability starts before your spouse's death or within 7 years after the death. However, if you receive benefits as a widow with children, you can be eligible if you become disabled before those payments end or within 7 years after they end. (This 7-year period protects the widow until she has a chance to earn enough work credits for disability protection on her own social security record.)

A disabled widower can get benefits based on the earnings of his wife only if she was providing at least half his support at the time of her death. A disabled surviving divorced wife may get benefits based on the earnings of her former husband only if their marriage lasted 20 years or longer, and he was contributing to her support at the time of his death (or was under a court order to do so).

Disability Benefit Payments

When Benefits are Payable. Because the law provides a 6-month waiting period, payments to a disabled worker and his family or to a disabled widow or widower generally cannot begin until the 7th full month of disability. If you are disabled more than 7 months before you apply, back benefits may be payable (but not before the 7th month of disability). It is important to apply soon after the disability starts because back payments are limited to the 12 months preceding the date of application.

If you have recovered from a disability which lasted 12 months or more but have not yet applied for benefits, you may still be eligible for some back payments. But if you wait longer than 14 months after you recover to apply, you may not be eligible for any back benefits.

A person disabled in childhood may get benefits beginning with the month his parent starts receiving retirement or disability benefits or the month his insured parent dies. There is no 6-month waiting period.

Your benefit payments may continue as long as you remain unable to work. (In general, if someone marries while he is receiving benefits as a person disabled in childhood or as a disabled widow or widower, the benefits will stop. In some cases, however, they can be continued. You can get more information about these exceptions from your social security office.)

Amounts of Monthly Payments. The amounts of your monthly disability benefit is based on your average earnings under social security over a period of years. The amount of the monthly payments to your dependents also depends on the amount of your average earnings.

The exact amount of your benefit cannot be figured in advance. This is because all of your earnings in your social security record at the time of your application must be considered. The Social Security Administration will, of course, figure your exact benefit at that time.

You can estimate the amount of your benefit, however, by following these steps:

1. Count the number of years to be used in figuring your average earnings as follows:
   - If you were born before 1930, start with 1956;
   - If you were born after 1929, start with the year you reached 27.

   Count your starting year and each year up until (but not including) the year you become disabled.

   (*Note:* At least 2 years of earnings must be used to figure disability benefits.)
2. List the amount of your earnings for all years beginning with 1951. (Include earnings in the year disability began.) Do not count *more than* $3,600 for each year 1951 through 1954; $4,200 for each year 1955 through 1958; $4,800 for each year 1959 through 1965; $6,600 for 1966 and 1967; $7,800 for 1968 through 1971; and $9,000 for 1972 and after.
3. Cross off your list the years of lowest earnings until the number remaining is the

EXAMPLES OF MONTHLY CASH DISABILITY BENEFITS

	Average yearly earnings after 1950*						
	$923 or less	$1800	$3000	$4200	$5400	$6600	$7800
Disabled worker	70.40	111.90	145.60	177.70	208.80	240.30	275.80
Disabled worker and wife at 62	96.80	153.90	200.20	244.40	287.10	330.50	379.30
Disabled widow at 50	42.80	56.10	72.90	89.00	104.50	120.30	138.00
Disabled widow at 55	52.00	68.10	88.60	108.10	127.00	146.10	167.70
Disabled worker, wife under 65 and one child (maximum family payment)	105.60	167.90	222.70	308.90	389.90	435.20	482.70

*The maximum earnings creditable for social security are $3,600 for 1951-54; $4,200 for 1955-58; $4,800 for 1959-65; $6,600 for 1966-67; and $7,800 for 1968-71. The maximum creditable starting with 1972 will be $9,000, but average earnings usually cannot reach that amount until later; therefore, benefits based on average earnings of $9,000 will not be payable until later.

same as your answer to step 1. (It may be necessary to leave years in which you had no earnings on your list.)

4. Add up the earnings for the years left on your list, and divide by the number of years you used (your answer to step 1).

The result is your average yearly earnings covered by social security over this period.

Look in the table on monthly benefits and estimate your benefit from the examples given there.

Disability Benefits Are Not Paid in Addition to Other Social Security Benefits. Benefits because of disability are not paid in addition to other monthly social security benefits. If you become entitled to more than one monthly benefit at the same time, the amount you receive will ordinarily be equal to the larger of the benefits.

If you become disabled after you start receiving social security benefits (early retirement benefits, for example, or benefits as a wife or widow), it may be to your advantage to switch over to benefits based on disability. For instance, if you start receiving reduced retirement benefits at 62 and then become disabled at 63, your benefit may be higher if you change to disability payments.

If the benefit you were receiving before you became disabled was a reduced widow's benefit or a reduced retirement benefit, your disability benefits also will be reduced to take into account the number of months you received the other benefits. Even with this reduction, however, your disability benefits may be higher than the benefits you were receiving.

The people in your social security office can give you the amounts of the different benefits in this situation.

Effect of Work on Benefit Payments. If you receive benefits because of disability (as a worker, a person disabled from childhood, or a disabled widow or widower), you are subject to the general rule under which some benefits are withheld if you have substantial earnings. There are special rules, which include medical considerations, for determining the effect on your disability payments of any work you might do. See page 575 for further details.

If you are a disabled worker and one of your dependents (who is not disabled) works and earns more than $1,680 in a year, some of his benefits may be withheld. In general, $1 in benefits is withheld for each $2 he earns between $1,680 and $2,880; and $1 in benefits is withheld for each $1 earned over $2,880.

But no matter how much that person may earn in a year, he will get the full benefit for any month in which he neither earns over $140 as an employee nor renders substantial services as a self-employed person.

The Disability Decision

Evidence of Disability. If you are applying for benefits because of disability, you will be asked to provide medical evidence to support your claim. The evidence is usually a medical report from your doctor, hospital, clinic, or institution where you have been treated.

When you apply for benefits, the people at the social security office will assist you in requesting these reports and help you in every way possible to fill out your application and get the necessary evidence. (However, you are responsible for any charges made by the doctor or hospital for preparing the reports.)

On the medical report form, your doctor, hospital, institution, or agency is asked to give the medical history of your condition: what the doctors have found to be wrong with you, how severe it is, what the medical tests have shown, and what treatment you have received. They are not asked to decide whether or not you are "disabled" under the social security law.

When this medical evidence has been obtained, the social security office will send the complete record to an agency in your home state (usually the vocational rehabilitation agency). There the evidence is reviewed to see if you should be considered disabled under the law.

A team of trained people in the state agency—a physician and a disability evaluation specialist—will consider all the facts in your file. If additional information is needed, the state agency may ask you to get this evidence or to have a medical examination at government expense.

Decisions of Other Agencies. The rules in the social security law for deciding whether a person is disabled are different from rules in some other government and private disability programs. Some people receiving disability payments from another government agency or from a private company may be found not eligible for social security disability benefits. However, the report of any examination made for another agency, as well as the decision itself, may be considered in determining whether you are eligible under the social security program.

Examples of Disabling Conditions. Certain conditions which are ordinarily severe enough to be considered disabling under the law are described in the Social Security Regulations. Copies of these regulations are available in any social security office. Following are some examples of disabling conditions listed in the regulations:

1. Loss of major function of both arms, both legs, or a leg and an arm.
2. Progressive diseases which have resulted in the loss of a leg or which have caused it to become useless.
3. Severe arthritis which causes recurrent inflammation, pain, swelling, and deformity in major joints so that the ability to get about or use the hands has been severely limited.
4. Diseases of heart, lungs, or blood vessels which have resulted in serious loss of heart or lung reserve as shown by X-ray, electro-cardiogram, or other tests; and, in spite of medical treatment, there is breathlessness, pain, or fatigue.
5. Diseases of the digestive system which result in severe malnutrition, weakness, and anemia.
6. Serious loss of function of the kidneys.
7. Cancer which is progressive and has not been controlled or cured.
8. Damage to the brain or brain abnormality, which has resulted in severe loss of judgment, intellect, orientation, or memory.
9. Mental illness resulting in marked constriction of activities and interests, deterioration in personal habits, and seriously impaired ability to get along with other people.
10. Total inability to speak.

In the case of workers and persons disabled since childhood, conditions less severe than those listed in the regulations can be considered disabling. This is because age, education, training, and work experience can also be taken into account for these applicants.

You Will Be Notified Of The Decision In Your Case. After you have submitted the evidence needed for the decision on your disability application, you do not have to do anything more. You will receive a notice from the Social Security Administration as soon as a decision has been reached in your case.

If Your Application Is Denied. If you get a letter notifying you that you are not entitled to benefits, the letter will tell you the reason. The doctors and other experts who have studied your case may have found that your condition is not serious enough for you to be considered disabled under the law. Or the evidence may show that your condition is of a type which is not likely to continue for 12 months or more.

In some cases, a disabled worker's application under the disability provisions may be denied because he did not work long enough or recently enough (as explained on page 572).

A letter of denial for disability benefits does *not* mean that a decision has been made about your eligibility for any other type of social security benefits. It means only that you are not now eligible to receive social security disability benefits.

If your application is denied, you may, if you wish, present new evidence concerning your disability. Your social security office will be glad to see that any new evidence you may have is presented and that your case is reconsidered.

If you have no new evidence to offer but feel that the decision in your case is not correct, you still may ask your social security office to have your case reconsidered. If you believe that the results of this reconsideration are not correct, you may request a hearing before a hearing examiner of the Social Security Administration. There is no charge for reconsidering your claim or for a hearing.

If you have received notice of the hearing examiner's decision and believe the decision is not correct, you may ask for a review by the Appeals Council of the Social Security Administration in Washington, D.C.

If you believe the decision of the Appeals Council is not correct, you may take your case to the Federal Courts.

Vocational Rehabilitation And Special Employment Services

Whether or not you are found eligible to receive benefits because of disability, you may be offered help in improving your condition and in preparing for and finding work.

When you apply for social security disability benefits, you will be considered for vocational rehabilitation services by your state vocational rehabilitation agency. That agency provides counseling, training, and other services that you may need to help you get back to work. Information in your file is made available to help the people in that agency decide whether you can benefit from rehabilitation services and, if so, what kinds of services will be most useful to you.

Rehabilitation services generally are financed by state-federal funds. In some cases, however, social security pays the costs of rehabilitating those receiving disability benefits. Rehabilitating beneficiaries is expected to save social security money because, in the long run, the cost should be less than the expense of paying them benefits.

You may also get employment counseling and special placement services from your State Employment Service.

People who become entitled to benefits because of disability will not be paid those benefits if, without good cause, they refuse counseling, training, or other services offered to them by their state vocational rehabilitation agencies.

If You Recover Or Return To Work

If your claim for disability benefits is approved, you are required by law to inform the Social Security Administration if your condition improves or if you return to work. You may do this either by sending in the post-card form which will be given you for this purpose, by writing a letter, or by visiting your social security office.

If You Recover From Your Disability. If at any time medical evidence shows that your condition has improved so much that you are no longer disabled, you will still receive benefits for a 3-month period of adjustment. This period includes the month in which your condition improves and 2 additional months. Benefits will then be stopped.

Trial Work Period. If you are a disabled worker or a person disabled in childhood and you return to work in spite of a severe condition, your benefits may continue to be paid during a trial work period of up to 9 months (not necessarily consecutive months). This will give you a chance to test your ability to work. If after 9 months it is decided that you are able to do substantial gainful work, your benefits will be paid for an adjustment period of 3 additional months.

Thus, if you go to work in spite of your disability, you may continue to receive disability benefits for up to 12 months, even though the work is substantial gainful work. If it is decided that the work you are able to do is not substantial and gainful, you may continue to receive benefits. Of course, should your condition improve so that it becomes no longer disabling, your benefits would be stopped (after a 3-month adjustment period) even though your trial work period might not be over.

A disabled widow, disabled dependent widower, or disabled surviving divorced wife is not eligible for a trial work period. If she or he begins to do substantial gainful work, benefits will stop 3 months after the work begins.

If You Again Become Disabled

If you become disabled a second time within 5 years after your disabled worker's benefits were stopped because you returned to work or recovered (within 7 years if you are a disabled widow, disabled dependent widower, or disabled surviving divorced wife), your benefits can begin with the first full month in which you are disabled. Another 6-month waiting period is not required. You are not eligible for a trial work period.

If you reapply for benefits as a disabled worker, you will need to meet the disability work requirements at the time of your new application (see page 572).

FAMILY PAYMENTS

Monthly payments can be made to certain dependents:

- When the worker gets retirement or disability benefits;
- When the worker dies.

These dependents are —

- Unmarried children under 18, or between 18 and 22 if they are full-time students;
- Unmarried children 18 or over who were severely disabled before they reached 18 and who continue to be disabled;
- A wife or widow, regardless of her age, if she is caring for a child under 18 or disabled and the child gets payments based on the worker's record;
- A wife 62 or widow 60 or older, even if there are no children entitled to payments;
- A widow 50 or older (or dependent widower 50 or older) who becomes disabled not later than 7 years after the death of the worker or, in the case of a widow, not later than 7 years after the end of her entitlement to benefits as a widow with a child in her care;
- A dependent husband or widower 62 or over;
- Dependent parents 62 or over after a worker dies.

In addition to monthly benefits, a lump-sum payment may be made after the worker's death.

Under the law in effect before February 1968, there were circumstances in which benefits could be paid to children of a woman worker only if she had worked 1½ out of the last 3 years before she retired, became disabled, or died, or if she had actually provided most of the child's support. This provision, which prevented payment of benefits in some cases, has been removed. Now children are considered dependent on both their mothers and their fathers, and they may become eligible for benefits when either parent becomes entitled to retirement or disability benefits or dies.

Payments may also be made under certain conditions to a divorced wife at 62 or a surviving divorced wife at 60 (or a disabled surviving divorced wife 50 or older). To qualify for benefits, a divorced wife must have been married to the worker for 20 years and also meet certain support requirements. Benefits also can be paid a dependent surviving divorced wife at any age if she is caring for her deceased former husband's child under 18 or disabled who is entitled to benefits. For more information about this provision, get in touch with your social security office.

Monthly payments to the wife or dependent husband of a person entitled to retirement or disability payments generally cannot be made until the marriage has been in effect at least 1 year unless the couple are parents of a child. Payments can be made to the widow, stepchild, or dependent widower of a deceased worker if the marriage lasted 9 months or longer; or in the case of death in line of duty in the uniformed services, and in the case of accidental death if the marriage lasted for 3 months, under special circumstances.

Amount of Your Family's Benefits. Cash benefits to your dependents, and to your survivors in case of your death, are figured from the amount of your retirement or disability benefit.

Permanently reduced benefits are received by:

- Workers and their wives who choose to start receiving retirement benefits while they are between 62 and 65;
- Widows who choose to start receiving benefits between 60 and 62; and
- Disabled widows and disabled dependent widowers 50 or older who receive benefits before they reach 62.

The amount of the reduction depends on the number of months they receive benefits before they reach 65 (62 for widows and disabled dependent widowers). On the average, people who choose to get benefits early will collect about the same value in total benefits over the years, but in smaller installments to take account of the longer period during which they will be paid.

If a person could be entitled to monthly benefits based on the social security records of two or more workers, he will receive no more than the largest of the benefits.

The lump-sum payment at a worker's death is ordinarily three times the amount of his monthly retirement benefit at 65, or $225, whichever is less.

Benefits Not Taxable. Social security benefits you receive are not subject to federal income tax.

An Application Is Necessary

Before payments can start, an application must be filed.

When you are nearing 65 or if you become disabled, get in touch with your social security office.

It is important for you to inquire at your social security office 2 or 3 months before you reach 65, not only for the possibility of retirement benefits, but also for Medicare benefits, which are available whether or not you retire. If you wait until the month you reach 65 to apply for the medical insurance part of Medicare, you will lose at least one month of protection. It is always to your advantage to apply before you reach 65, even if you do not plan to retire. If you have high earnings which would increase the amount of your benefit in the year you are 65 or later, your benefit amount will be refigured. You will always be sure of receiving benefits at the highest possible rate.

When a person who has worked under the social security law dies, some member of his family should get in touch with the social security office.

If you cannot come to the social security office—perhaps because you are housebound or hospitalized—write or telephone. A social security representative can arrange to visit you.

Long delay in filing an application can cause loss of some benefits, since back payments for monthly cash benefits can be made for no more than 12 months.

An application for a lump-sum death payment must usually be made within 2 years of the worker's death.

Proofs Needed. When you apply for social security benefits, take your own social security card or a record of your number; and if your claim is based on the earnings of another person, his card or a record of the number.

You will need proof of your age. If you have a birth certificate or a baptismal certificate made at or shortly after your birth, take it with you when you apply. If you are applying for wife's or widow's benefits, take your marriage certificate; if your children are eligible, their birth certificates.

Take your Form W-2, Wage and Tax Statement, for the previous year; if you are self-employed, a copy of your last federal income tax return.

Proof that the applicant was being supported by the insured person is required before benefits can be paid to a parent after the death of a working son or daughter, or to a husband or widower whose working wife has retired, become disabled, or died. Generally, this proof must be furnished within 2 years after the worker dies, or in the case of husband's benefits, within 2 years after his wife applies for cash benefits.

Do not delay applying because you do not have all of these proofs. When you apply, the people in your social security office can tell you about other proofs that may be used.

If you apply for retirement or survivor payments and supply all of the necessary information and then 4 to 6 weeks go by after the time you thought your benefits should start and you do not hear about

TYPES OF CASH BENEFITS

This table shows the principal types of payments and the insured status needed for each.

Retirement	
Monthly payment to—	*If you are—*
* You as a retired worker and your wife and child	Fully insured.
Your dependent husband 62 or over	Fully insured.
Survivors	
Monthly payments to your—	*If at death you are—*
* Widow 60 or over or disabled widow 50-59	Fully insured.
* Widow (regardless of age) if caring for your child who is under 18 or disabled and is entitled to benefits	Either fully or currently insured.
Dependent child	Either fully or currently insured.
Dependent widower 62 or over and disabled dependent widower 50-61	Fully insured.
Dependent parent at 62	Fully insured.
Lump-sum death payment	Either fully or currently insured.
Disability	
Monthly payments to—	*If you are—*
You and your dependents if you are disabled	Fully insured and if you meet work requirements explained on page 14.

* *Under certain conditions, payments can also be made to your divorced wife or surviving divorced wife.*

your claim, get in touch with your social security office. There are special procedures for speeding payments in these cases and your social security office will be glad to do everything possible to prevent delays in your payments.

Information Is Confidential. Under the law and regulations, social security records are confidential. Information from your record may not be disclosed without proper authorization.

If You Work After Payments Start

When you apply for retirement or survivors insurance benefits, your social security office will explain how any future earnings you may have will affect your payments and when and how to report your later earnings to the Social Security Administration. The explanation that follows is intended to give a general idea of the conditions under which benefits are paid to people who are still working.

For taxable years ending after 1967, the following rules apply:

If you earn $1,680 or less in a year, you get all the benefits.

If you earn more than $1,680 in a year while you are under 72, the general rule is that $1 in benefits to you (and your family) will be withheld for each $2 you earn from $1,680 to $2,880. In addition, $1 in benefits will be withheld for each $1 of earnings over $2,880.

Exception to the general rule: Regardless of total earnings in a year, benefits are payable for any month in which you neither earn wages of more than $140 nor perform substantial services in self-employment.

The decision as to whether you are performing substantial services in self-employment depends on the time you devote to your business, the kind of services you perform, how your services compare with those you performed in past years, and other circumstances of your particular case.

Benefits are also payable for all months in which you are 72 or older, regardless of the amount of your earnings in months after you reach 72.

Your earnings as a retired worker may affect your own and your dependents' right to benefits. If you get payments as a dependent or survivor, your earnings will affect only your benefit and not those of other members of the family.

Earnings which must be counted ——

Earnings from work of any kind must be counted, whether or not the work is covered by social security. (There is one exception tips amounting to less than $20 a month with any one employer are not counted.) Total wages (not just take-home pay) and all net earnings from self-employment must be added together in figuring your earnings for the year. However, income from savings, investments, pensions, insurance, or royalties you receive after 65 because of copyrights or patents you obtained before 65 does not affect your benefits and should not be counted in your earnings for this purpose.

In the year in which your benefits start and the year your benefits end, your earnings for the entire year are counted in determining the amount of benefits that can be paid.

Earnings after you reach 72 will not cause any deductions from your benefits for months in which you are 72 or over. However, earnings for the entire year in which you reach 72 count in figuring what benefits are due you for months before you are 72.

For more information about how working after you apply for benefits will affect your retirement or survivors payments, inquire at your social security office.

Beneficiaries Outside the United States. Special rules affect the payment of benefits to people outside the United States. If you intend to go outside the United States for 30 days or more while you are receiving benefits, ask your social security office for Leaflet No. SSA-609.

If you are not a citizen or national of the United States, your absence from this country may affect your right to benefits. The people in your social security office will be glad to explain these provisions to you.

Reasons Why Payments Stop

When monthly payments are started, they continue until they must be stopped for one of the reasons given below. If any of these occurs, it must always be promptly reported to the Social Security Administration.

Marriage—Benefits for a child, an aged dependent parent, a disabled dependent widower, a divorced wife, a disabled widow, or widow receiving mother's benefits generally stop when the beneficiary marries a person who is not also getting social security dependent's or survivor's benefits.

There is an exception for the widow who remarries after reaching age 60. If she could have qualified for benefits on her deceased husband's record, she may still get benefits on that record. She would qualify for ½ of her deceased husband's retirement beneit, or (at 62) for the amount of the wife's benefit on her later husband's record, whichever is larger. A similar provision applies to widowers who remarry after 62.

Divorce—Payments to a wife or a dependent husband generally end if a divorce is granted. However, if a wife 62 or older and her husband are divorced, benefits to the wife may continue if the marriage lasted at least 20 continuous years before the divorce. (If a wife under 65 and her husband are divorced after 20 continuous years of marriage, she may receive benefits at 62 or later provided certain conditions are met. For more information, get in touch with any social security office.)

No child "in her care"—Payment to a wife under 62 or to a widow or surviving divorced wife under 60 will generally stop when she no longer has in her care a child under 18 or disabled. A widow or surviving divorced wife who is 50 or over and is severely disabled should get in touch with her social security office for information about any benefits that may be payable.

Child reaches 18—When a child reaches age 18, his payments stop unless he is—

- Disabled (if so, he and his mother may be eligible for benefits for as long as he is disabled), or
- A full-time, unmarried student (if so, he may be eligible for benefits until he reaches 22).

Adoption—When a child is adopted, his payments end unless he is adopted by his stepparent, grandparent, aunt, uncle, brother, or sister after the death of the person on whose record he is receiving benefits.

Death—When any person receiving monthly benefits dies, his or her payments end.

Disability benefits—When the benefits payable to a person stop because he is no longer disabled, the benefits payable to his dependents also stop.

If payments end because of any of these reasons, the last check due is the one for the month before the event.

MEDICARE

HEALTH INSURANCE FOR PEOPLE 65 AND OVER

Nearly all people 65 and over are eligible for health insurance protection under Medicare, including some people who do not have enough credit for work covered by social security to qualify for monthly cash benefits.

There are two parts to Medicare: hospital insurance, and for those who choose, medical insurance.

Eligibility for Hospital Insurance. If you are 65 or over and are entitled to social security or railroad retirement benefits, you are automatically eligible for hospital insurance; if you are not entitled to either of these benefits, you should ask about hospital insurance and medical insurance at your social security office.

Nearly everyone who reached 65 before 1968 is eligible for hospital insurance, including people not eligible for cash social security benefits.

If you reached 65 in 1968 or later and are not eligible for cash benefits, you will need some work credit to qualify for hospital insurance benefits. The amount of credit required depends on the year of your 65th birthday. Eventually the amount of work required for hospital insurance will be the same as for social security cash benefits.

After you establish your eligibility, you receive a health insurance card, which shows that you have hospital insurance, medical insurance, or both.

Your Hospital Insurance

Your hospital insurance will pay the cost of covered services for the following care:

- Up to 90 days of inpatient care in any participating hospital in each benefit period. For the first 60 days, it pays for all covered services except for the first $60 ($52 until January 1, 1971). For the 61st through the 90th day, it pays for all covered services except for $15 a day ($13 a day until January 1, 1971). (For care in a psychiatric hospital, there is a lifetime limit of 190 hospital benefit days.)

A "benefit period" begins the first time you enter a hospital after your hospital insurance starts. It ends after you have not been an inpatient for 60 days in a row in any hospital or in any facility that mainly provides skilled nursing care.

- A "lifetime" reserve of 60 additional hospital days. You can use these extra days if you ever need more than 90 days of hospital care in any benefit period. Each lifetime reserve day you use permanently reduces the total number of reserve days you have left. For each of these additional days you use, hospital insurance pays for all covered services except for $30 a day ($26 a day until January 1, 1971).
- Up to 100 days of care in each benefit period in a participating extended care facility, a specially qualified facility which is staffed and equipped to furnish skilled nursing care and many related health services. Hospital insurance pays for all covered services for the first 20 days and all but $7.50 a day ($6.50 a day until January 1, 1971) for up to 80 more days, *but only if:*
  —You are admitted because you need additional care for a condition treated while you were in a hospital;
  —You need continuing skilled nursing care, not just help with such things as bathing, eating, dressing, walking and taking medicine at the right time;
  —You are admitted within 14 days after your discharge from a hospital where you were an inpationt for at least 3 days in a row;
  —You are in an extended care facility which is approved for Medicare payments.
- Up to 100 home health "visits" by nurses, physical therapists, speech therapists, or other health workers *but only if:*
  —Your condition is such that you need skilled nursing care on an intermittent basis or physical or speech therapy;
  —The services are ordered by a doctor and are furnished by a home health agency which takes part in Medicare;
  —A plan for your care is established by a doctor within 14 days of your discharge from the hospital or extended care facility;
  —Your care is for further treatment of a condition for which you were treated in the hospital or extended care facility;
  —The visits are made within 12 months after a qualifying stay of at least 3 consecutive days in a hospital or after your discharge from an extended care facility.

If you sign up for medical insurance, you will also be eligible for the other home health visits described below.

Enrolling For Medical Insurance

The medical insurance part of Medicare is voluntary and no one is covered automatically.

You will receive this protection only if you sign up for it within a specified period.

You will have protection at the earliest possible time if you enroll during the 3-month period just before the month you reach 65. You may also enroll the month you reach 65 and during the 3 following months, but your protection will not start until 1 to 3 months after you enroll.

If you do not enroll during your first enrollment perod, you will have another opportunity during the first 3 months of each year, provided this period begins within 3 years after you had your first chance to enroll. However, if you wait to enroll, you may have to pay a higher premium for the same protection; and your coverage will not begin until 3 to 6 months after you enroll.

Medical insurance is financed with monthly premiums paid by people 65 and over who have signed up for this insurance. The government matches these premiums dollar for dollar. The medical insurance premium is $5.30 per month for the 12-month period ending June 30, 1971.

Once you enroll for medical insurance, you do not have to do anything to keep your protection. It continues from year to year without any action.

If you wish to drop your medical insurance, you may give notice to do so at any time. Your medical insurance protection will stop at the end of the calendar quarter following the quarter you give notice.

Your Medical Insurance

Generally, your medical insurance will pay 80 percent of the reasonable charges for the following services after the first $50 in each calendar year:

- Physicians' and surgeons' services, no matter where you receive the services—in the doctor's office, in a clinic, in a hospital, or at home.
  (You do not have to meet the $50 deductible before your medical insurance will pay physician charges for X-ray or clinical laboratory services when you are a bed patient in a hospital. The full reasonable charge will be paid, instead of 80 percent.)
- Home health services ordered by your doctor even if you have not been in a hospital—up to 100 visits during a calendar year.
- A number of other medical and health services, such as diagnostic tests, surgical dressings and splints, and rental or purchase of durable medical equipment.
- Outpatient physical therapy services—whether or not you are homebound—furnished under supervision of participating hospitals, extended care facilities, home health agencies and approved clinics, rehabilitation agencies, or public health agencies.
- All outpatient services of participating hospitals, including diagnostic tests or treatment.
- Certain services by podiatrists (but not routine foot care or treatment of flat feet or partial dislocations of the feet).

For More Medicare Information. For more information on the health insurance programs, get in touch with your social security office and ask for a copy of Leaflet No. 43.

FINANCING THE PROGRAMS

Federal retirement, survivors, and disability benefits, and hospital insurance benefits are paid for by contributions based on earnings covered under social security.

If you are employed, you and your employer share the responsibility of paying contributions. If you are self-employed, you pay contributions for retirement, survivors, and disability insurance at a slightly lower rate than the combined rate for an employee and his employer. However, the hospital insurance contribution rate is the same for the employer, the employee, and the self-employed person.

As long as you have earnings that are covered by the law, you continue to pay contributions regardless of your age and even if you are receiving social security benefits.

How Contributions are Paid. If you are employed, your contribution is deducted from your wages each payday. Your employer sends it, with an equal amount as his own share of the contribution, to the Internal Revenue Service.

If you are self-employed and your net earnings are $400 or more in a year, you must report your earnings and pay your self-employment contribution each year when you file your individual income tax return. This is true even if you owe no income tax.

Your wages and self-employment income are entered on your individual record by the Social Security Administration. This record of your earnings will be used to determine your eligibility for benefits and the amount of cash benefits you will receive.

The maximum amount of earnings that can count for social security and on which you pay social security contributions is shown in the following table:

Year	*Amount*
1937-50	$3,000
1951-54	3,600
1955-58	4,200
1959-65	4,800
1966-67	6,600
1968 and after	7,800

Earnings over the maximums may have been reported to your social security record and may appear on your earnings statement, but cannot be used to figure your benefit rate.

When you work for more than one employer in a year and pay social security contributions on wages over $7,800 for 1968 and after, you may claim a refund of the excess contributions on your income tax return for that year. If you work for only one employer and he deducts too much in contributions, you should apply to the employer for a refund.

A refund is made only when more than the required amount of contributions has been paid.

Questions about contributions or refunds should be directed to the Internal Revenue Service.

This table shows the schedule of contribution rates now in the law:

CONTRIBUTION RATE SCHEDULE FOR EMPLOYEES AND EMPLOYERS (EACH)

Years	Percent of Covered Earnings		
	For Retirement, Survivors, and Disability Insurance	For Hospital Insurance	TOTAL
1968	3.8	0.6	4.4
1969-70	4.2	.6	4.8
1971-72	4.6	.6	5.2
1973-75	5.0	.65	5.65
1976-79	5.0	.7	5.7
1980-86	5.0	.8	5.8
1987 and after	5.0	.9	5.9

CONTRIBUTION RATE SCHEDULE FOR SELF-EMPLOYED PEOPLE

Years	Percent of Covered Earnings		
	For Retirement, Survivors, and Disability Insurance	For Hospital Insurance	TOTAL
1968	5.8	0.6	6.4
1969-70	6.3	.6	6.9
1971-72	6.9	.6	7.5
1973-75	7.0	.65	7.65
1976-79	7.0	.7	7.7
1980-86	7.0	.8	7.8
1987 and after	7.0	.9	7.9

The Trust Funds

Social security contributions for retirement, survivors, and disability insurance go into the Federal Old-Age and Survivors Insurance Trust Fund and the Federal Disability Insurance Trust Fund. They are used to pay the benefits and administrative expenses of these programs and may be used for no other purpose.

There are two other trust funds—a Federal Hospital Insurance Trust Fund, into which hospital insurance contributions are placed, and out of which hospital insurance benefits and administrative expenses are paid; and a Federal Supplementary Medical Insurance Trust Fund, into which the enrollees' premiums, along with the Government's matching contributions, are placed, and out of which the benefits and administrative costs of the medical insurance program are paid.

Funds not required for current benefit payments and expenses are invested in interest-bearing U.S. Government securities.

Certain costs, however, are financed from general funds of the U.S. Treasury, including the cost of hospital insurance benefits for people who are uninsured for cash social security benefits; the Government's share of the cost for supplementary medical insurance; and cash payments for certain uninsured people 72 and over.

Kinds of Work Covered

Almost every kind of employment and self-employment is covered by social security. Some occupations, however, are covered only if certain conditions are met.

Farming. You receive social security credit as a farm operator or rancher if your net earnings from self-employment are $400 or more in a year. You must report your net earnings from self-employment as a part of your income tax return.

If your gross earnings from farming in a year are between $600 and $2,400, you may report two-thirds of your gross earnings, instead of your net earnings, for social security purposes. If your gross earnings from farming are more than $2,400 and your net earnings are less than $1,600, you may report $1,600 for social security purposes.

If you rent your farm land to someone else, you receive social security credits, for your rental income if you "materially participate" in the actual production of the farm commodities or the management of production.

Ministers and Members of Religious Orders. Before 1968 income from the ministry received by a clergyman (ordained, commissioned, or licensed ministers, Christian Science practitioners, and members of religious orders who have not taken a vow of poverty) was not covered by social security unless the clergyman signed a form stating that he wanted it to be covered.

For taxable years ending after December 1967, earnings from services as a clergyman will automatically be covered unless the clergyman files an application to have it excluded, stating that he is conscientiously opposed, or opposed by reason of religious principles, to receiving social security benefits based on services as a clergyman.

A clergyman who qualifies to be excluded from coverage may complete Form 4361 and file it with the Internal Revenue Service. This form may be secured at any social security office or at any Internal Revenue Service office. Once this form is filed it cannot be withdrawn.

Clergymen who elected coverage for any year before 1968 will not be affected by the new provisions. They will continue to be covered.

A clergyman reports his income and makes his tax contributions as if he were self-employed, even though he may be working as an employee.

In general, a clergyman who entered the ministry in 1968 or earlier had until April 15, 1970, to file the form.

Members of religious orders who have taken a vow of poverty are not covered by social security.

For more information about social security coverage for clergymen, ask for a copy of Leaflet No. 9 at your social security office.

Family Employment. Work done by a parent as an employee of his son or daughter in the course of the son's or daughter's trade or business is covered by the law. Domestic work in the household of a son or daughter is not covered unless special conditions are met.

Work for a parent by a daughter or son (also a stepchild, adopted, or foster child) under 21 is not covered.

Also not covered is any work performed by a wife for her husband or by a husband for his wife.

Household Workers. A domestic worker's cash wages (including transportation expenses if paid in cash) for work in a private household are covered by the law if they amount to $50 or more from one employer in a calendar quarter.

If you employ a household worker who will come under the law and you are not receiving the forms for making the earnings reports, ask your social security office or your Internal Revenue Service office for a copy of Leaflet No. 21. This leaflet explains how to get the forms and make the reports.

Employees Who Receive Tips. Cash tips amounting to $20 or more in a month with one employer are covered by social security.

You must give your employer a written report of the amount of your tips within 10 days after the month in which you receive them. Your employer will collect your contributions due on these tips from other wages he owes you or from funds you turn over to him for that purpose. Otherwise, your contribution must be paid by you to the Internal Revenue Service.

If your report is late or incomplete, you will be liable for your social security contribution on tips not reported, and you may also be subject to a penalty in an amount equal to ½ of that contribution.

Your employer includes your tips reported to him along with your other wages in his social security wage reports and on Form W-2, but he does not have to match your social security contribution on the tips.

If you receive tips, you can get further information at your social security office.

Employees of Non-profit Organizations. Employees of non-profit organizations operated exclusively for religious, charitable, scientific, literary, educational, or humane purposes, or for testing for public safety, may be covered by the social security law if—

- The organization waives its exemption from the payment of social security contributions by filing a certificate (Form SS-15) with the Internal Revenue Service, and
- Those employees who wish to be covered indicate their desire to participate by signing the Form SS-15a that goes with the certificate.

Employees who sign the form and employees who are hired or rehired after the calendar quarter in which the waiver certificate is filed are covered. If any employee of a non-profit organization earns wages of less than $50 in a quarter, his wages for that quarter are not covered.

Employees of State and Local Governments. State and local government employees may be covered by social security under voluntary agreements between the individual state and the Federal Government.

Farm Employees. When you work for a farmer, a ranch operator, or a farm labor crew leader, you earn social security credits:

- If the employer pays you $150 or more in cash during the year for farm work, or
- If you do farm work for the employer on 20 or more days during a year for cash wages figured on a time basis (rather than on a piece-rate basis).

For more information about farm labor crews and the conditions under which the farmer or the crew leader is the employer, get Leaflet No. 15 from your social security office.

Household workers employed on a farm or ranch operated for profit are covered under the same rules as other farm employees.

Federal Employment. Most employees of the Federal Government not covered by their own staff retirement system are covered by social security.

Military Service. Active duty or active duty for training you perform as a member of the uniformed services of the United States after 1956 counts toward social security protection for you and your family. From 1957 through 1967 your basic pay was credited to your social security record.

For active duty after 1967, your credits for each month of active duty will generally amount to your basic pay plus $100. No additional deductions will be made from your pay for the extra $100 credits. You cannot, however, get social security credit for more than $7,800 in any year, including the extra credits.

For Active Duty After September 15, 1940, and Before 1957—

Social security credits of $160 a month are given to most veterans who served during this period. When credits are given, they county the same as wages in civilian employment. These credits are not actually listed on your record, but if they would affect your benefit, the people in the social security office will ask for proof of your military service when an application is filed on your record.

Railroad Employment. Earnings from railroad work are reported to the Railroad Retirement Board and not to the Social Security administration. Your social security record will not include any work you may have done for a railroad.

Benefits based on work for a railroad are ordinarily paid by the Railroad Retirement Board. However, if you have less than 120 months (10 years) of railroad service when you retire or become disabled, your earnings for railroad work after 1936 are considered in figuring your disability or retirement payments under the social security law.

A retired worker who has at least 120 months of railroad service and who has also done enough work under social security to qualify for social security benefits may receive retirement benefits under both railroad retirement and social security.

Survivors of a worker can be entitled under one system only, either railroad retirement or social security, even though the worker may have been entitled during his lifetime under both. Regardless of which program will pay the benefits, records of the deceased worker's railroad earnings after 1936 and his earnings under social security will be combined to determine payments to survivors.

American Citizens Working Abroad. U.S. citizens employed by American employers in foreign countries or aboard vessels or aircraft of foreign registry are covered by social security. Seamen and airmen employed on American vessels or aircraft are usually covered regardless of citizenship.

U.S. citizens working abroad for a foreign subsidiary of an American corporation may be covered if the parent firm makes an agreement with the Secretary of the Treasury to see that social security contributions are paid for all U.S. citizens employed abroad by the foreign subsidiary.

Foreign Agricultural Workers. Agricultural work performed by foreign workers admitted to the United States on a temporary basis to do agricultural work is not covered.

Foreign Exchange Visitors. Work performed by foreign nationals temporarily in the United States to study, teach, conduct research, etc. under a foreign exchange program is not covered under social security if it is performed to carry out the purpose for which they were admitted to the country.

Social Security Cards

You must have a social security number if your work is covered by the social security law or if you receive certain kinds of taxable income. Your social security number is also used for income tax purposes. Show your card to each of your employers when you start to work. Upon request, show it to anyone who pays you income that must be reported.

You can get a social security card at any social security office. The number on your card is used to keep a record of your earnings and of any benefits to which you and your dependents become entitled.

You need only one social security number during your lifetime. Notify your social security office if you ever get more than one number.

If you change your name, or if you lose your social security card, go to a social security office to get a card showing your new name or a duplicate of the card you lost.

Checking Your Record. Each employer is required to give you receipts for the social security contributions he deducts from your pay. He does this at the end of each year and also when you stop working for him. These receipts, such as Form W-2, will help you check on your social security record. They show the amount of your wages that counts for social security. For most kinds of work, your wages paid in forms other than cash—for instance, the value of meals or living quarters—must be included. For domestic work in a private household or for farm work, only cash wages count.

You should keep a record of the amount of self-employment income you have reported.

You should check your record from time to time to make sure your earnings have been correctly reported. This is especially important if you have frequently changed jobs. Simply ask your social security office for a postcard form to use in requesting a copy of your record, complete sign, and mail it.

If Your Records Do Not Agree. If your records of your earnings do not agree with the amounts shown on the statement you get from the Social Security Administration, get in touch with your social security office promptly. If you write, give your social security number, the periods of work in question, your pay in each period, and your employer's name and address. If the earnings in question were from self-employment, include the date your tax return was filed and the address of the Internal Revenue Service office to which the return was sent.

Right of Appeal

If you feel that a decision made on your claim is not correct, you may ask the Social Security Administration to reconsider it. If, after this reconsideration, you are not satisfied the decision is correct, you may ask for a hearing by a hearing examiner of the Bureau of Hearings and Appeals. And, if you are not satisfied that the decision of the hearing examiner is correct, you may request a review by the Appeals Council. The Social Security Administration makes no charge for any of these appeals. You may, however, choose to be represented by a person of your own choice, and he may charge you a fee. The amount of such a fee is limited and must be approved by the Social Security Administration.

Someone in your social security office will explain how you may appeal and will help you get your claim reconsidered, or request a hearing.

If you are still not satisfied, you may take your case to the Federal courts.

Social Security Offices

The Social Security Administration has over 800 offices conveniently located throughout the country. These offices have representatives who regularly visit neighboring communities.

If any of your questions about monthly social security benefits or Medicare are not answered in this booklet, call, write or visit your social security office. The people who work there will be glad to answer questions and to explain your rights. They will also assist groups and organizations in informing their members about social security through talks, films, and other planned activities.

For the address of your social security office, look in the telephone directory under Social Security Administration, or ask at the post office.

PHARMACY

Pharmacy is a science which may be defined as the collection, preparation, and compounding of medicinal substances, and its history is part of the history of medicine.

Early Origins. There were compounders of medicine in Babylonia and the word *pasisu*, which described a compounder of ointments and cosmetics, is equal to our word *pharmacist*. The latter word derives from the Greek *pharmakon*, a drug or poison, and is probably Egyptian in origin.

Although magic played a great part in the treatment of disease in early times, a knowledge of the values of many drugs was gradually accumulated, and the later Assyrians (1100 to 600 B.C.) became skillful in the preparation of medicines. Dioscorides, who lived in Greece in the first century A.D., described 500 medicinal plants as well as 90 earths and metals and drugs of animal origin. Many of these were still included in the pharmacopoeias of the years 1900-10. His treatise on Materia Medica was the authority for nearly fifteen centuries.

The ancient Romans were slower than the Greeks in establishing medicine as a rational science and often resorted to magical rites when their few remedies failed. So the distinction between drug sellers and poisoners and sorcerers gradually blurred, and the whole *pharmacopoloi* gained sinister reputations.

By about 160 A.D. the well-known classical physician, Galen, had raised the status both of pharmacy and of medicine, and his name is remembered in the term 'galenical' which is still used for such preparations as infusions, tinctures, and decoctions.

In medieval England, the compounding of medicines was the job of the apothecary who supplied the remedies prescribed by the physician. Later, the apothecaries began to do their own prescribing and called in the aid of the chemists who prepared mineral compounds chiefly for medicinal use. Early in the eighteenth century they joined with the dealers in herbs, known as druggists, and the title 'chemist and druggist' came into being.

Pharmacopoeias and Formularies

Information on the substances that have been found useful in curing diseases and on the best methods of preparing and combining them has always been much sought after. This information has been collected and published in books from earliest times by many authorities.

Early pharmacopoeias were essentially lists of medicinal substances and preparations, with information as to the source, nature and properties of the substances and directions for making the preparations. Modern pharmacopoeias, in contrast to this, concentrate principally on the identity, quality, and purity of the drugs.

Prescriptions

The prescription is the written document by means of which a doctor gives the pharmacist instructions for preparing medicine for a particular patient. From the specimen given below it will be seen that prescriptions can be separated into several parts.

1. All prescriptions begin with the symbol ℞, an abbreviation of the Latin word 'recipe,' meaning 'take thou.'

2. The list of ingredients follows, and the quantities of each. These are usually written in abbreviated English or Latin. The quantities are given in the metric system of weights or measures though older doctors sometimes use old formulae.

3. Then come the doctor's directions to the pharmacist regarding such things as the way the ingredients are to be compounded and the total quantity to be sent. Unless the doctor wants some unusual medicine made up, the pharmacist will follow an appropriate formula, or supply officially recognized ready-made tablets, ointments, etc., named by the doctor.

4. Lastly, the prescription indicates the directions that the doctor wants to appear on the label. This is called the 'signature,' from the Latin 'signetur' (let it be labelled). These directions are usually written in abbreviated Latin; the commoner ones appear below.

Recording the Prescription. A prescription will bear the name and address of the patient for whom it is made, as well as the signature of the doctor and the date. Prescriptions for children are often marked 'pro inf.' (for a child and also state the age of the child.

A specimen prescription is given below with its translation.

℞
Tab. Acid. Acetylsal. 300 mg.
Mitte 100
Sig. 2 (or ii) tab. every four hours

TRANSLATION
Take thou:
Acetylsalicylic Acid Tablets 300 milligrams
Send 100
Label them: Two tablets to be taken every four hours

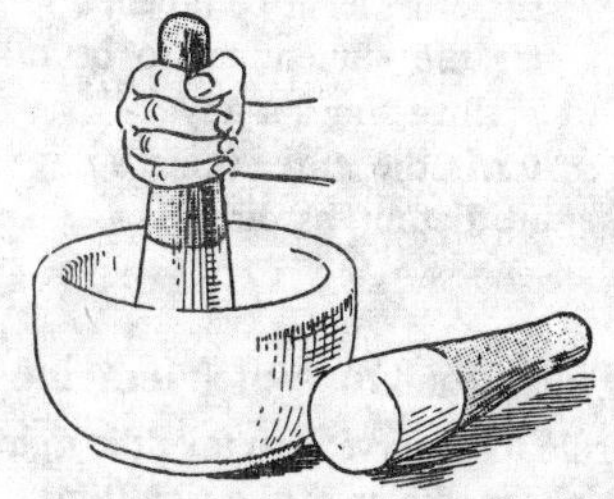

Fig. 1. *MORTAR AND PESTLE. Crystals, powders, or dried herbs are placed in the bowl of the mortar and pounded finely with the pestle. This age-old method of preparing medicines is being superseded by large-scale manufacturing processes.*

The Signs and Abbreviations on a prescription constitute a useful form of shorthand. They are derived from Latin phrases, since all medical communications were originally carried on in Latin. The more generally used terms are given below with their full Latin forms and the English meanings.

ʒ	drachma, a drachm (60 grains); or a fluid drachm (60 minims)
℥	uncia, an apothecaries' ounce (480 grains) or a fluid ounce (480 minims)
ss	semis, half (used in conjunction with the above signs, thus: ℥ss half an ounce)
a.c.	ante cibum, before meals
aa.	of each
ad	to, or up to
ad lib.	ad libitum, freely
aq. bull.	aqua bulliens, boiling water
aq. dest.	aqua destillata, distilled water
aq. gel.	aqua gelida, cold water
b.d.	bis die } twice a day
b.i.d.	bis in die } twice a day
c̄.	cum, with
cap.	capiatur, let it be taken
coch.	cochleare, spoonful
d.d.	de die, daily
dil.	dilutus, diluted
ex. aq.	ex aqua, in water
ft.	fiat, let it be made
ft. mist.	fiat mistura, let a mixture be made
h.s.	hora somni, at bedtime
in d.	in dies, daily
in p. aeq.	in partes aequales, in equal parts
m.d.	more dicto, as directed
mitt.	mitte, send
n.	nocte, at night
o.m.	omni mane, every morning
p.a.a.	parti affectae applicandus, to be applied to the affected part

p.r.n. pro re nata, when required, occasionally
p.c. post cibum, after food
q.d. quater die, four times a day
q.q.h. quarta quaque hora, every four hours
q.s. quantum sufficiat, sufficient
s.a. secundem artem, according to the art
s.o.s. si opus sit, if necessary
sig. signetur, let it be labelled
t.d.s. ter die sumendus, to be taken three times a day
t.i.d. ter in die, three times a day
ut dict. ut dictum, as directed

Taking a Dose of Medicine

The rule to observe is to take the right dose of the right medicine at the right time.

The Right Dose. Modern medicines are powerful remedies and their introduction has usually been preceded by much hard work to find out the most suitable doses. The doctor acts on this information in prescribing the medicine and judges the dose for each patient. He also decides how often this dose should be taken, and all the information is given to the patient or written briefly on the label. *It is important that these instructions are carefully followed if the greatest benefit is to be obtained* from the medicine and also because the doctor will then be in a better position to assess the results of the treatment than he would if the medicine were taken carelessly.

Measuring the Dose. Liquid medicines which are to be taken by mouth are sometimes ordered to be given by the tablespoonful, the dessertspoonful, or the teaspoonful. Although convenient for the patient, these measures are not really satisfactory because one teaspoonful varies from 3·5 to 5 milliliters and one tablespoonful from 14 to 20 milliliters.

Liquid medicines are now reformulated to give a standard dosage either as a 5 ml or 10 ml dose. This means that the patient receives a consistent dose. It is important, therefore, that every medicine chest should be equipped with a metric measuring glass and a 5-ml spoon.

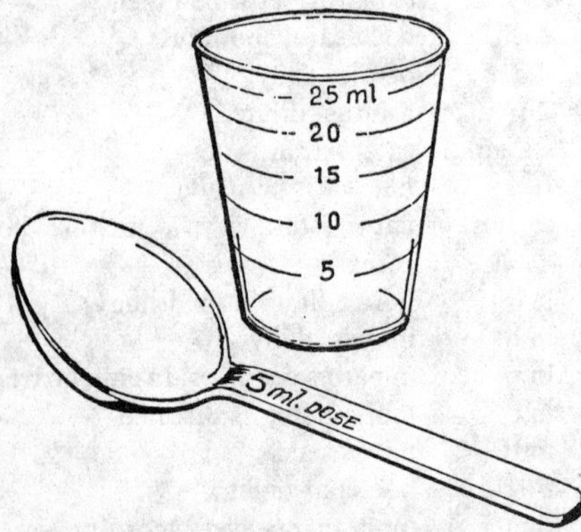

Fig. 2. *FOR MEASURING LIQUID MEDICINES. A milliliter measure for a dose with water and a 5–ml spoon.*

Measuring glasses or plastic medicine measures are particularly suitable for medicines which have to be taken with water, such as many mixtures. They should be prescribed in unit doses of 10 milliliters. This is easily measured in the glass and 'topped up' with the same or double the amount of water.

It is not important to measure the precise amount of water but the whole of any diluted medicine must be taken otherwise the benefit will be lost.

For powders, it is best to weigh the dose if suitable scales are at hand, otherwise remember that a teaspoonful means a level teaspoonful.

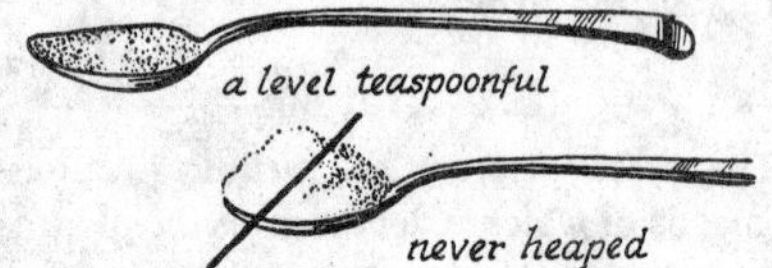

Fig. 3. *A TEASPOONFUL. For simple home use, a 'teaspoonful' is a level one, never heaped.*

The Intervals of time between doses should be carefully watched. The commonest instructions are that the medicine should be taken three times a day and it is usually intended that the three doses should be evenly spread over the normal waking day. With medicines such as antibiotics and sulphonamides, however, the instructions are often that the doses should be taken every six or eight hours and this usually means that a dose should be given at the stated interval throughout the twenty-four hours, including doses during the night. The purpose of this is to keep the amount of drug in the bloodstream up to a certain level all the time until treatment is finished. The body is constantly trying to get rid of the drug and if the dose is not taken at the right time the amount of drug in the blood will fall below the level required to combat the disease. It is obviously unwise therefore to fail to give a night dose because the patient is asleep. It is even more unwise to give a double dose last thing at night to avoid having to wake up during the night. A double dose could be an overdose and it is also unusual for it to keep up its effect for twice the period of a single dose. If there is any doubt as to the time at which the medicine should be taken the doctor or the pharmacist should be consulted.

PHARMACEUTICAL PREPARATIONS

The berries and roots, the clays, minerals, and molds with healing properties, the chemicals which destroy bacteria have all to be selected and prepared with the greatest care and precision for the making of medicines, and in this lies the art of pharmacy. Some drugs are only effective if given in the form of injections, others in tablets or capsules, and some are only suitable for external use in lotions or ointments. Some chemicals will not dissolve in water but will do so in oils. Two substances which may each be highly valuable medicinally will antagonize each other if mixed together.

The pharmacist, whether he works in a large factory producing medicinal preparations by the ton or dispensing prescriptions at the back of his shop, needs to know how the various substances he uses interact with one another and the most suitable forms in which they can be prepared for the patients.

The following accounts of the different types of preparations in common use are arranged for convenience in alphabetical order.

Balsams are resins, or mixtures of oils and resins, but today the name is often applied to cough mixtures, many of which contain aromatic oils and resins.

Capsules are containers for drugs and are swallowed with the contents. They are of two kinds—hard and flexible.

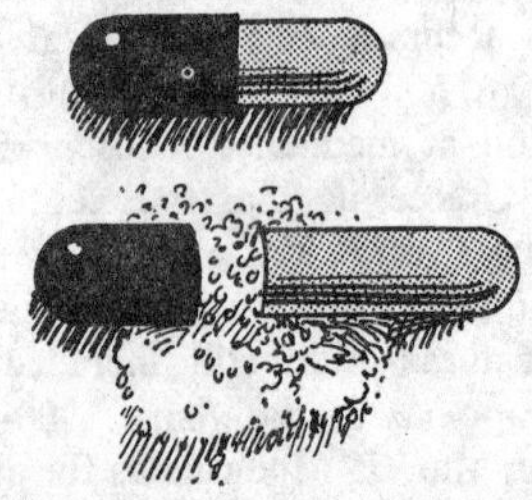

Fig. 4. *HARD GELATIN CAPSULES. When the capsule has been dissolved by the gastric juices, the powdery contents are more rapidly absorbed than tablets would be.*

Hard Capsules are made from hard gelatin containing glycerin. They consist of two parts. The drug is filled into the lower section and the tightly-fitting top is slipped over it. These capsules may be clear or distinctively colored. They are widely employed for hypnotic medicaments such as the barbiturates, and for certain types of time-release preparations, such as granules of amphetamine. They are also used for some antibiotics. The powdery contents of hard capsules are more easily absorbed by the body than swallowed uncrushed tablets.

By soaking hard capsules in formaldehyde they may be made resistant to gastric secretions and dissolve only when they reach the intestines. Such capsules are called 'enteric-coated.'

Flexible Capsules are made of soft gelatin and are mainly used for oily liquids such as halibut-liver oil; they are also used for some powdered drugs such as antibiotics.

Collodions are liquid preparations for painting on the skin. When dry, a flexible cellulose film is left over the wound. Collodions contain imflammable matter and should be stored in their small fluted containers in a cool place.

Creams, in pharmacy, are semi-solid emulsions containing medicaments and are for external use only.

Drops is a term used to refer to medicaments which are either taken internally in drop doses, or which are used for dropping into the eyes, ears, or nose.

NASAL DROPS are medicated watery or oily solutions which are put into the nose by means of a dropper.

EYE-DROPS are sterile solutions of medicaments in water (usually with a bactericidal substance to prevent contamination), or in oil.

EAR-DROPS are prepared by dissolving the medicament in water, glycerin, or weak spirit.

Dusting-powders are mixtures of powders intended for application to the skin. They are usually made of starch, purified talc, or kaolin, and may contain medicaments such as zinc oxide, salicylic acid, boric acid, etc. They should be sparingly applied and not used on broken skin.

Elixirs are strong or nauseous medicaments in a clear pleasantly flavored solution, often containing alcohol or glycerin as well as sugars. Fruit syrups are often added for children.

Emulsions. When two liquids which will not mix together, for example oil and water, are prescribed in the same mixture, the chemist uses an emulsifying substance which has the effect of keeping one of the liquids dispersed in the form of tiny droplets throughout the other. The resulting preparations are thick, usually white liquids called emulsions. The term is sometimes used for emulsified lotions intended for external use, such as liniments.

Before use, an emulsion should be well shaken. If it has been kept for a long time it may separate into two layers, the top one being watery. Such emulsions are 'cracked' and should be thrown away.

Enemas are liquid preparations which are injected into the rectum. They are used to wash out the lower bowel, especially before operations, to relieve impacted feces, or to adminster medicinal substances directly into the bowel. They are given by means of an enema syringe (see p. 566).

Enemas are packed in colored, fluted, glass bottles and labeled 'not to be taken by mouth.' Some are available in disposable packs (see p. 567) which are especially convenient for a busy nurse.

Extracts are made from vegetable substances. The root, whole plant, berries or stem is put whole or cut up into a solvent such as water, alcohol, or ether. By various processes such as infusion, maceration, percolation, and evaporation, the valuable medicinal substance is freed and made into a liquid or a soft or a dry extract. These are seldom prescribed now but are used for making mixtures.

Gargles are solutions of medicinal substances in water and they are used for the prevention and treatment of throat infections. Common salt, a teaspoonful to a pint of water makes a useful gargle. Aspirin gargle, two or three tablets crushed and stirred in warm water, is often of benefit in cases of sore throat.

Gels are semi-solid jellies made from a non-fatty substance such as gelatin or tragacanth and into which a medicament is incorporated during preparation.

Inhalations are liquid preparations containing volatile substances which are vaporized and inhaled so as to bring the medicaments into contact with the lining of the respiratory tract. When the substances are volatile at ordinary temperatures the preparation is sprinkled on a piece of material and inhaled directly, e.g. eucalyptus oil on a handkerchief, but the usual method is to add the inhalation, e.g. compound tincture of benzoin to hot but not boiling water and breathe in the vapor for five or ten minutes. The head and the bowl or jug should be covered with a towel to prevent the vapors from escaping too quickly.

Injections are sterile solutions or suspensions of medicaments which are injected through the skin, i.e. parenterally. They are used when a rapid action is required, or when the medicine cannot be effectively given by mouth. Injections are also used to obtain a localized action as when a dentist injects local anesthetics near a tooth which is to be drilled or removed. Injections require great care in administration and are usually given by doctors and nurses.

Intradermal, or intracutaneous, injections are injected into the skin. Subcutaneous, or hypodermic, injections are put just a little deeper, under the skin. Intramuscular injections are administered deep into a muscle, usually the thigh or buttock. Intravenous injections are given directly into the bloodstream by inserting the needle into a vein; large volumes of solutions given in this way are called intravenous infusions and perfusions. Intrathecal, intracisternal, or peridural injections are given into parts of the spinal cord and the brain. (See also p. 567.)

Injections must contain no living microorganisms which, if introduced into the body with the injection, might cause infection. To ensure that injections are not contaminated they are prepared under very strict conditions of cleanliness. To keep injections bacteria-free, special containers are used. Ampules are small, single-dose, all-glass containers made with a tapering neck. After the sterile injection is put into the ampule, the open end of the neck is sealed by melting in a flame. When the doctor is ready to give the injection, he draws a small file across a special constriction above the shoulder of the ampule and withdraws the correct dose, measuring it by marks on the syringe. The

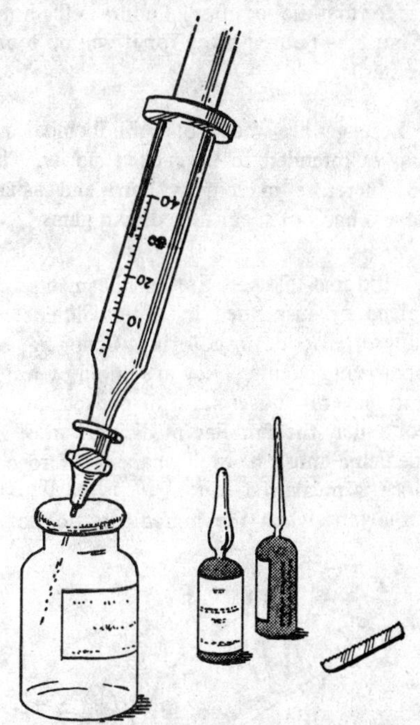

Fig. 5. *VIAL AND AMPULES. Certain medicaments for injection are supplied in vials (small bottles) covered with a special top through which the sharp point of the syringe needle can pierce, and a dose of the injection fluid is withdrawn; these vials contain many doses. Other injections are best supplied in single doses which are sealed in small glass ampules of varying shapes but each has a constriction on the neck to provide a suitable breaking point.*

other type of container is a glass phial or vial which contains several doses and is closed with a rubber cap. Strict cleanliness must be observed in withdrawing each dose. The screw top protecting the rubber cap is removed and the top of the rubber washed with a piece of raw cotton moistened with alcohol. The needle of the syringe is then forced through the rubber and the correct dose withdrawn. Insulin injections are put up in such containers.

Liniments are liquid or semi-liquid preparations used on the skin to soothe and relieve pain, or to stimulate. They should not be applied to broken skin as they often contain poisonous ingredients (and so are supplied in plainly marked bottles).

Lotions are for use upon the skin. The medicaments are usually dissolved or suspended in water but when a cooling effect is desired alcohol is used. Lotions are either dabbed on to the skin with raw cotton, or applied on cloth or raw cotton and covered with a piece of waterproof material. Lotions which are to be used to wash out body cavities are warmed gently and used with special syringes or douches.

Calamine lotion is a useful soothing lotion for many skin conditions.

EYE LOTIONS are sterilised solutions of medicaments in water which are used undiluted for first-aid or home treatment. They are usually dispensed in coloured fluted bottles with plastics screwcaps and a breakable seal. If any of the solution is left after use for first-aid, or after 24 hours in the home, it must be poured away for it will no longer be sterile.

Lozenges are small, solid, mildly medicated masses intended to be sucked slowly. They are therefore made very hard and usually have a basis of sugar mixed with gums.

Mixtures. These are medicaments dissolved or suspended in watery liquids and they often contain coloring, flavoring, and preserving agents. They are taken by mouth and several doses are dispensed in one container, the familiar medicine bottle. The medicine must be well shaken before each dose is measured out. This is particularly important when the ingredients do not all

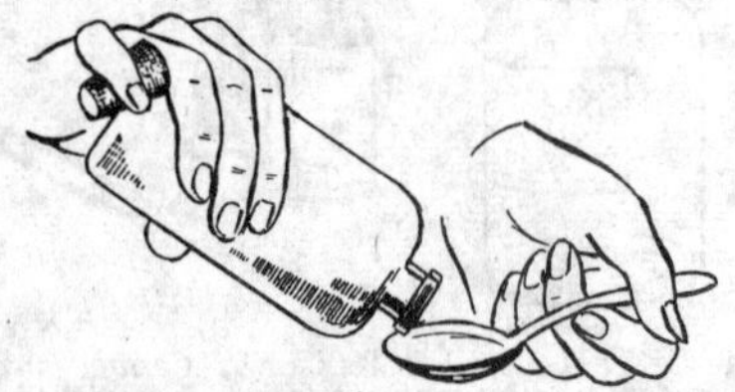

Fig. 6. *THE CORK. When measuring out a dose of liquid medicine hold the cork as shown to prevent its getting dirty or contaminated.*

dissolve. When the label on the bottle states that the mixture is to be taken in water, a volume of water equal to the dose of the mixture is usually sufficient. Greater amounts of water should be avoided, otherwise the patient has to swallow a large quantity of what is usually an unpleasant liquid.

For adults, the dose of a mixture is usually 10 milliliters although this varies according to the prescription. For children, smaller doses, one 5 ml-spoonful, are often prescribed. Mixtures are generally preferable to tablets or capsules for children, because mixtures are more easily taken and can be pleasantly flavored.

Mouth-washes are antiseptic, astringent, or deodorant preparations which are usually made in concentrated form to be mixed with warm water before use. If it is in tablet form, dissolve one tablet in a wineglassful of warm water.

Ointments are semi-solid preparations made mainly with greasy substances in which a medicament is incorporated. There are three classes of ointments.

1. Those used for their protective value on the outer skin are non-absorbent and are usually made with an oily base. They often contain antiseptic and counter-irritant medicaments.

2. Those with a softening and absorbent action are made of lard, soap, or non-fatty bases.

3. Those which are intended to be absorbed through the skin and allow the penetration of the medicament to deeper layers always contain wool fat (lanolin).

Ointments in small quantity are made on a marble or porcelain slab, the ingredients being rubbed down with a spatula until they are thoroughly mixed. Powdered substances are sifted and incorporated with a little of the basis until the mixture is quite smooth; semi-solid and liquid ingredients are then added and the rest of the basis gradually worked in.

Ointments are usually dispensed in collapsible tubes and screw-capped jars.

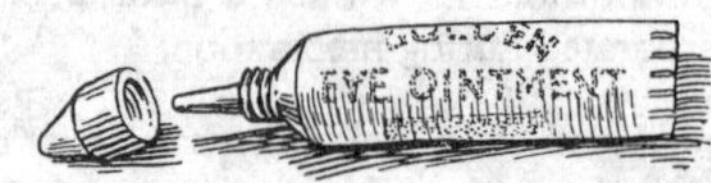

Fig. 7. *EYE OINTMENTS are usually packed in small collapsible tubes fitted with narrow-bore nozzles to permit the extrusion of a fine thread of the ointment which can be applied directly to the eye or the lid.*

Paints. These medicated liquids are applied to the skin or mucous surfaces. Skin paints evaporate quickly leaving a film of the drug on the skin.

Pastes are medicated preparations which are spread on cloth and applied to the skin. They usually contain glycerin or paraffins as their bases and a large proportion of powder is incorporated, this powder constituting the chief difference between a paste and an ointment.

Pessaries are used to introduce medicinal substances into the vagina. They are usually made from theobroma oil (cocoa butter). The basis is gently warmed until melted and the medicament mixed in. It is then cooled in specially shaped molds. Some pessaries are made in the form of tablets, and they should be inserted as they are.

Pills are usually spherical in shape, although occasionally ovoid. They were once a very popular form of giving medicine but their use has greatly diminished since the introduction of tablets.

Plasters. These are strips of elastic or non-elastic materials, coated with rubber or synthetic rubber, which are used for holding the edges of wounds together or to protect cuts from getting dirty.

Poultices are used to apply heat to different parts of the body. They are soft pastes which should be spread hot upon cloth, placed on the body, covered with waterproof material, and topped with a thick cloth to keep in the heat.

Starch poultice is made by boiling one part of starch with ten parts of water until a thick paste is formed. Kaolin poultice is one of the most efficient poultices: it is made from powdered kaolin and glycerin, and medicated with boric acid, peppermint, thymol, and wintergreen.

Powder. This word is used in two different senses in regard to dispensed medicines. It either refers to a bulk powder, or to a single dose wrapped flat in a paper and usually packed in a box with several other similar packets each containing a dose. Powders in individually wrapped doses were very much used before tablets displaced them.

Bulk powders often contain several ingredients and may be taken for the treatment of indigestion, or as laxatives, e.g., compound licorice powder. The best way of giving the powder is to stir it into a sugary water and make it into a drink.

Powder for dusting upon the skin is described on p. 585.

Salts. These are mainly mixtures of chemical salts, often in crystals, which when dissolved in water give a preparation similar to naturally occurring spa mineral waters. The name 'salts' is often applied to smelling bottles (smelling salts) although they do not always contain chemical salts, and to crystalline bath salts.

Solutions. In pharmacy a solution or liquor is the term used for a limited number of preparations which are simple solutions of chemicals in water. A few solutions are made by allowing two chemical substances to react in water. The pharmacist often keeps ready strong stock solutions of poisons or powerful drugs from which he can make mixtures as required.

Sterile solutions in water are intended for applying to cut surfaces and for washing out the bladder and the peritoneum.

SOLUTION-TABLETS, as their name implies, are intended to be dissolved in water to provide a solution for external use. They are usually larger than the tablets which are taken by mouth.

Spirits are mainly solutions of volatile oils in alcohol. They are made either by dissolving the oil in alcohol, or by distillation. Some spirits are compound preparations and contain medicaments other than volatile oils. Spirits are generally used as ingredients of mixtures, but may be taken by sprinkling a few drops on a lump of sugar.

Sprays are liquid preparations applied to the nose, throat, or other parts of the body by means of an apparatus which produces a fine mist. The main use of sprays is for the relief of symptoms in chronic respiratory conditions such as asthma, bronchitis, and hay fever.

Substances used medicinally in sprays are adrenaline (for asthma), ephedrine (for nasal congestion), and antihistamines.

Suppositories are medicated solid preparations suitably shaped for easy insertion into the rectum.

Glycerin suppositories contain no other medicament and are used as a safe effective laxative for the lower bowel. They are made in various sizes—one gram for infants, two grams for children, and four grams for adults.

Suppositories should be carefully inserted into the rectum; they do not require warming or moistening before use.

Syrups are strong solutions of sugar in water to which medicinal substances and, in many cases, flavoring agents are added.

Tablets are a comparatively modern method of administering medicines, having replaced the pills which were in use even in very early times.

Most solid drugs can be made into tablets and the modern machines can turn them out by the million. Most tablets are intended to be swallowed with a drink of water, but not all. Some should be dissolved in water before being taken, for example potassium chloride tablets. Effervescent tablets are also dissolved in water before use; they produce copious effervescence which makes a more pleasant drink. Hypodermic tablets, which are used to prepare solutions for injection, must be made under aseptic conditions. Certain types of tablets are heavily compressed to make them very hard. They are meant to be sucked slowly and resemble lozenges; they often contain antiseptic substances for the treatment of infections of the mouth and throat.

Tablets have become the most widely used of all dosage forms because they have a number of advantages over mixtures, and powders. They provide a convenient method of taking an accurate dose of medicine. They can be carried about easily and kept readily available for the next dose. No measure is necessary and the patient is not likely to get doses varying in quantity. If the medicines are bitter or nauseous the tablets can be coated, and this also helps to keep the medicine in good condition. The small size of tablets means that they can be easily dispensed by the pharmacist and that they occupy very little room.

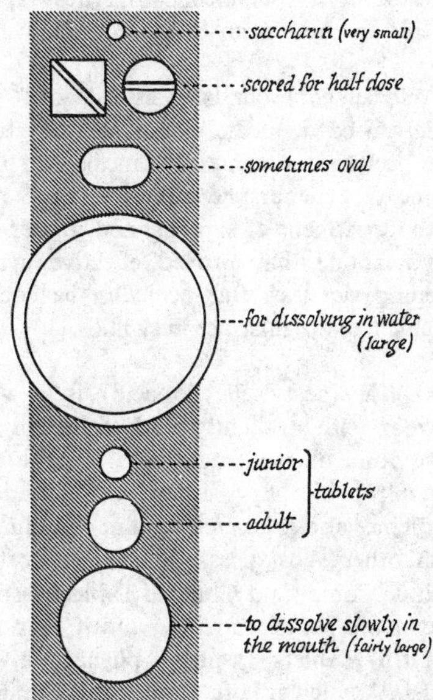

Fig. 8. *TABLETS are of many colors, thicknesses, shapes, and sizes. Large tablets are usually intended for dissolving in water.*

Tablets are made by compressing the ingredients in a die between two punches on a tablet machine. Some preliminary treatment is necessary to ensure that the tablets will disintegrate properly in the body, and yet will withstand handling.

Tablets must contain an accurate dose of the medicament and although they must be hard enough to withstand shaking while being carried about, they must not be so hard that they will not disintegrate in the stomach or intestines. They must be smooth and uniformly colored and should not chip or split during normal handling.

Coating Tablets. There are several reasons for putting an outer covering on compressed tablets. (1) Unpleasant tastes can be effectively disguised with a sugar coating; (2) certain tablets containing substances which can decompose under the action of moisture in the air can be protected by a layer of varnish; (3) some drugs, required for treatment of the bowels, are destroyed in the acid juices of the stomach but when the tablets are given an enteric-coating they will pass through the stomach untouched but break up in the intestines.

Sugar coatings are applied by tumbling the tablets in revolving coating-pans containing syrup until they are covered with a thin layer and then allowing them to dry: this process is repeated several times. Dyes are frequently added to the final layer to provide a distinctive color. Another modern process consists in compressing the coating on to the tablet.

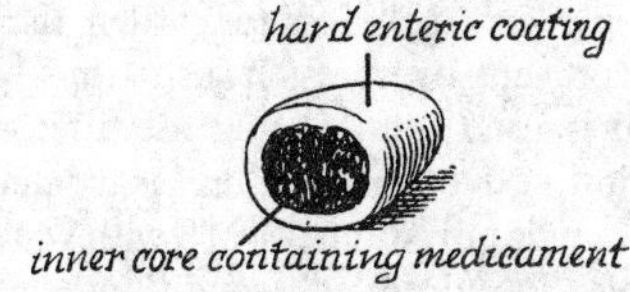

Fig. 9. *ENTERIC-COATED TABLETS. The medicament in these tablets is only effective if it reaches the intestines. In order to prevent the acid secretions of the stomach affecting it as it passes through, the tablet is given a special hard coating which can only be dissolved by the alkaline secretions of the intestines.*

Identification. Most tablets are circular in shape with flat or curved surfaces, and some have a deep groove across the middle so that they can easily be broken into halves. Others are heart-shaped, oval, or nearly spherical. Many are colored. Some makers mark their tablets with the name of the substance in a code number. It is, however, unwise for a patient to depend only on the appearance because many tablets are very similar in color and shape. Some manufacturers stamp the initials of the firm on their tablets and thus the same letters appear on widely differing tablets so that no attempt should be made to use these letters as a guide. Similarly, tablets which are made of the same drug or chemical may bear different initial letters because they have been made by a different firm. If a patient receives a second batch of tablets bearing different initials from those he was given previously, he should not conclude that the wrong tablets have been supplied.

Tinctures are fairly dilute solutions, usually in alcohol, of the active principles of vegetable drugs. Three processes are used in making tinctures: simple solution, maceration, and percolation. The last two are based on extraction of the active principle of a crude drug by means of a solvent, usually alcohol. Tinctures may be simple, that is made from one drug, or compound, made from more than one drug.

DRUGS AND MEDICAMENTS

A

Acacia (gum arabic; senega gum) comes from a small tree, *Acacia senegal*, which grows in the forests of Northern Africa near Ethiopia. The Ark of the Bible is said to have been made from acacia wood.

The gum is obtained by making cuts in the bark of the tree and allowing the thick sap to exude. The drops or 'tears' are allowed to harden and are either powdered or dissolved in water to form acacia mucilage. Powdered acacia is employed in the preparation of tablets and lozenges as a binding agent, and the powder or mucilage is used in the preparation of emulsions and to suspend insoluble powders in mixtures. A useful gum can be easily made by quickly rinsing 40 grams of acacia tears with water to remove dust and then dissolving them in 60 milliliters of water. For medicinal use a little chloroform is usually added to the mucilage as a preservative.

Acetic Acid is a clear colorless liquid with a strong sour taste and an agreeable smell. Three strengths are commonly used. The pure acid, glacial acetic acid, which sets to a glass-like mass when cooled, is applied with a camel-hair brush to destroy corns and warts, but is caustic if left too long on the skin. A 33 per cent solution of the acid is used in liniments. Dilute acetic acid, made by mixing one part of the 33 per cent acid with four parts of water, is used as an ingredient of mixtures for its diaphoretic and expectorant action.

Acetylsalicylic Acid. See under Aspirin.

Acriflavine. See under Proflavine.

Adrenaline is a hormone obtained from the adrenal (suprarenal) glands of sheep and other animals. When injected into the body it causes a great increase in the blood pressure. Since small doses injected locally constrict blood vessels, adrenaline is included in injections of local anesthetics to check bleeding. Adrenaline injection, which contains the equivalent of 1 in 1,000 of adrenaline, is useful for urticaria, asthma and hay fever, and when given into a vein it stimulates the heart beat in cases of sudden failure.

Adrenaline solution, which also contains the equivalent of 1 in 1,000 of adrenaline, is applied externally to stop bleeding from small wounds. It is also incorporated in nasal sprays for the treatment of hay fever, coryza and bleeding from the nose.

Agar. This substance is prepared by drying out into strips a mucilage made from various species of an alga called *Gelidium*. The thin grayish white strips or flakes swell into a stiff gelatinous mass in cold water. The best 'gels' are obtained from Japanese and Australian agar.

Crushed like bran and added to moist food, it has no nutritive value and passes through the intestines unchanged but in passing it absorbs moisture, increases the bulk of the feces, and promotes peristalsis—a useful quality for constipation.

Alcohol (ethyl alcohol; ethanol) is the product of fermentation of the juices of many vegetable materials. When these fermented liquors are distilled a mixture containing approximately 95 per cent of pure alcohol is obtained. Pure alcohol (absolute alcohol; dehydrated alcohol) is prepared from this by removal of the water. Weaker strengths are made by adding water.

Alcohol is used to extract the active principles from animal and vegetable drugs, as in the preparation of tinctures and extracts. 70 per cent alcohol is a good antiseptic and is used to keep sterilized hypodermic syringes in. When applied locally, alcohol has a cooling effect on the skin. When taken internally, in the form of wines and spirits, it has a depressing effect on the brain. It increases the flow of saliva and gastric juice and so is an aid to digestion. Because of its action in dilating the blood vessels in the skin it produces a sensation of warmth but it should not be taken before going out in the cold.

INDUSTRIAL METHYLATED ALCOHOL is alcohol (95 per cent) mixed with wood naphtha to make it undrinkable. It is free of duty and is therefore used instead of pure alcohol in many preparations for external use. Surgical alcohol is a mixture of industrial methylated alcohol, castor oil, and other substances and is applied to the skin to prevent bedsores. It is also used to sterilize the skin before an injection. Both of these spirits are colorless liquids and should be distinguished from the purple mineralized methylated alcohol which is commonly known as methylated alcohol. The latter is not suitable for treating bedsores. Wood naphtha contains methyl alcohol which causes blindness when it is drunk; it is therefore very dangerous to drink any form of methylated or surgical alcohol.

Almond (*Prunus communis*) is a tree growing in Asia and southern Europe; two varieties, sweet and bitter, are known. Almond oil, a fixed oil, is obtained from the seeds of both trees. It is demulcent and laxative. Rubbed into the skin it prevents chafing, and is used in the preparation of cold cream and other toilet articles.

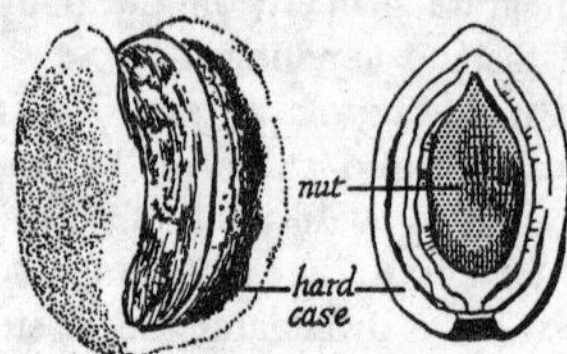

Fig. 10. *ALMOND. The dull green, soft, outer case splits to release the hard pitted shell containing the edible nut. The nuts are crushed and pressed to release the oil.*

Aloes is the dried juice of the leaves of several species of *Aloë* which grow in East and South Africa as well as in Europe, the West Indies and America.

The use of aloes in medicine goes back to ancient times. It is a cathartic which acts mainly in the lower bowel about eight to twelve hours after being taken. Griping pain sometimes results from its action and, because of its irritant effect, it should not be used in inflammatory conditions of the intestines. It is more irritating than cascara, rhubarb, or senna. Aloes is a useful purgative in some cases of chronic constipation, but should not be taken by pregnant women. Extract of aloes is the dried aqueous extractive.

Alum is either potassium aluminium sulphate (potash alum) or ammonium aluminium sulphate (ammonia alum). Both forms are colorless crystals or a white powder with a sweetish astringent taste.

Alum is astringent, and is used externally as a 1 per cent solution to harden the skin and so prevent bedsores. It also stops bleeding and is used for this purpose after tooth extraction. Glycerin of alum is sometimes used as a paint or, diluted 1 in 8 with water, as a gargle in ulcerated conditions of the throat, but continuous use should be avoided because alum has a deleterious effect on the teeth. A mixture of 15 parts of alum and 85 parts of talc is used as a foot powder for hardening the skin of the feet.

Aluminum is a soft silvery white metal. Powdered aluminum is applied, as a paste with zinc oxide, to the skin around colostomies and ileostomies to protect it from irritation.

Aluminum hydroxide gel, a thick white suspension usually flavored with peppermint, is used as an antacid in the treatment of peptic ulcers, 1 to 2 5-ml spoonfuls being taken 2- to 4-hourly. The dried gel is used to prepare tablets, usually flavored with peppermint; they should be chewed and not swallowed whole. Many proprietary antacid preparations contain aluminum hydroxide gel, often with other antacids such as magnesium hydroxide.

Ammonia is a colorless gas with a very pungent unpleasant odor. In various forms and mixed with other medicaments it is used in medicine both internally and externally.

It is also used in certain fluids as a cleansing agent for general domestic purposes. Dilute ammonia solution (ammonia water) is often an ingredient of diaphoretic and stimulant mixtures. Aromatic spirit of ammonia (sal volatile) is prepared by dissolving ammonium bicarbonate in a strong solution of ammonia with alcohol and water flavored with lemon and nutmeg; doses of 1 to 4-milliliters in water are taken as a stimulant in fainting.

AMMONIUM BICARBONATE and AMMONIUM CHLORIDE are used as ingredients of expectorant cough mixtures. The chloride is also given in large doses to make the urine acid before giving certain diuretic drugs which increase the flow of urine. The bicarbonate has a carminative action and has been used for dyspepsia.

Amyl Nitrite is a clear golden inflammable liquid with a pleasant sharp smell. When inhaled it causes a fall in blood pressure lasting for two or three minutes; flushing of the face and perspiration usually accompany its use.

Antidepressants. Two types of drugs are used to treat depression—those such as amphetamine which stimulate the central nervous system directly, and those such as phenelzine which act by interfering with certain body chemical reactors (monoamine oxidases) to produce accumulation of natural brain stimulators, e.g. serotonin and noradrenaline. Certain antidepressants such as tranylcypromine have both qualities.

For use in psychiatric disorders see p462.

Antihistamines. See p. 482.

Arrowroot (maranta) is the starch from the rhizome of *Maranta arundinacea*, and a mucilage prepared from it is a useful article of diet for the sick and convalescent. It is easily digested and has demulcent properties of special benefit to those with bowel complaints.

Arsenic compounds were at one time widely used in medicine but are very toxic. The related organic arsenicals—arsphenamine and neoarsphenamine—are of value in the treatment of syphilis, and a later one, tryparsamide, has proved effective against sleeping sickness. But penicillin has ousted arsenic from regular use in syphilis.

Aspirin (acetylsalicylic acid) is a white powder with a slightly acid taste and is a compound of acetic acid with salicylic acid.

Aspirin is the basis of most headache medicines and it is often used in combination with other substances. Official preparations include Compound Codeine Tablets (aspirin, phenacetin, and codeine) and Compound Aspirin Tablets (aspirin, phenacetin, and caffeine) which are often called A.P.C. tablets.

Some persons have an idiosyncrasy for aspirin and since it is likely to upset them or make them ill, they should be familiar with alternative names by which it is known.

Aspirin relieves pain and reduces fever. The normal dose for an adult is 300 to 600 milligrams. 4 to 8 grams administered once to four times a day, is used for acute rheumatism, but this treatment should only be followed under medical supervision.

Aspirin tablets are usually made in 300-milligram strength; and double strength tablets may also be obtained, as well as smaller tablets for children. The tablets should preferably be crushed and swallowed with a drink of water or milk. Aspirin is also prescribed in mixtures. A gargle of aspirin is often effective in sore throat and can be made from the tablets, using one tablet, finely crushed, to each tablespoonful of warm water, and shaking well.

If large quantities of aspirin and other analgesics are taken, the kidneys are overloaded in excreting them and harmed.

Atropine. See under Belladonna.

B

Balsam of Peru. This is a dark brown viscous balsam which exudes from the trunk of the tree, *Myroxylon perirae*, after it has been beaten and scorched. The trees grow in forests in central America. The balsam is antiseptic and has been used, generally as an ointment, for skin diseases, bedsores, and chilblains.

Balsam of Tolu is a soft tenacious pale brown substance produced by incising the trunks of the tree *Myroxylon balsamum* which grows in South America. The balsam is used as a flavoring agent, especially in cough medicines and lozenges. It is an ingredient of compound benzoin tincture.

Barbiturates. The barbiturates are a group of drugs which have a hypnotic action, that is, they induce sleep. They do this by depressing the central nervous system. There is great variation in individual response to these drugs and the dose required to induce sleep in one person may be twice that needed by a second person and perhaps a half of that required by a third. On average, a dose of 100 milligrams of a barbitrate drug, taken before going to bed, will produce a satisfactory night's sleep for those suffering from insomnia.

Phenobarbital is used in the treatment of epilepsy, being given in small repeated doses to maintain a state of mild sedation.

Thiopentone is given by intravenous injection as an anesthetic for short operations; occasionally it is given alone but more usually in combination with more powerful anesthetics (see p. 597).

Barbiturates do not relieve pain but, when analgesia is required as well as sedation, they are given with a pain-relieving drug such as aspirin or phenacetin.

It is *dangerous to take alcohol* during treatment with barbiturates because the combined effect on the brain may cause severe and dangerous depression of the central nervous system. A dose of barbiturate which when given alone would produce normal sleep may, if taken with alcohol, result in prolonged coma or dangerously shallow breathing.

It is unwise to keep a supply of barbiturates at the bedside, because a patient may repeat his dose several times during the night while too drowsy to realize what he is doing.

POISONING by barbiturates, with its shallow breathing and coma, is treated by giving oxygen, washing out the stomach by means of a stomach tube, and injecting drugs which stimulate the central nervous system. See also p. 41.

Belladonna (deadly nightshade) is a tall perennial plant (*Atropa belladonna*) which grows wild in England and other parts of Europe; it prefers shady sites and rubbish heaps and produces yellow and purple flowers which are followed by dark purple and black berries. These berries have an attractive appearance but are *extremely poisonous* because they contain the alkaloid ATROPINE. One of the effects of atropine on the human body is to dilate the pupil of the eye, making it appear lustrous. The juice of the plant was used for this purpose in the Middle Ages by Italian women and received the name 'bella donna' (beautiful lady).

All parts of the belladonna plant contain atropine. The aerial parts (stem, leaves, flowers and fruits) constitute Belladonna Herb and this is used in the preparation of the dry extract and the tincture.

Belladonna Root is used in the preparation of the liquid extract, which was formerly employed in making belladonna plasters.

Belladonna is now mainly used, in combination with antacids, for the relief of spasm in gastric and intestinal conditions.

Benzoic Acid is a light, white, feathery substance which has a mild antiseptic action and prevents the growth of molds. Compound ointment of benzoic acid is applied to the scalp, body and nails in the treatment of ringworm. Benzoic acid is also used as a preservative in pharmaceutical preparations. SODIUM BENZOATE has a similar action. An anti-rust solution for surgical instruments contains sodium benzoate, 1·5 grams, and chlorocresol, 0·2 gram, in 100 milliliters of water.

Benzoin (gum benzoin; gum benjamin) is a brittle, brownish-red resin which is formed when the trunks of the *Styrax* trees are cut. Compound tincture of benzoin is used as an inhalation for the relief of nose and throat congestion, one teaspoonful being added to a pint of very hot water and the steam inhaled. It can also be applied undiluted to small cuts as an antiseptic and to stop bleeding.

Bismuth and its salts are effective in the treatment of syphilis and are injected intramuscularly for this purpose. The metal itself is used in a very finely divided form (precipitated bismuth) suspended in a solution of dextrose. The salts of bismuth used are the sodium tartrate, the oxychloride and the salicylate.

Other salts, principally the carbonate, have been widely used as antacids but their popularity for this purpose is declining.

Applied externally, bismuth salts have a protective action, and ointments and dusting-powders containing the carbonate, the subgallate or the nitrate are used. Suppositories of the subgallate are used in the treatment of hemorrhoids (piles).

Borax (sodium borate) occurs naturally and is made by boiling native calcium borates with sodium carbonate. It is a transparent crystalline substance with a sweetish saline taste and is soluble in water. Solutions are used for their mild antiseptic action as gargles (one teaspoonful in half a pint of warm water) and mouth-washes. A mixture of equal parts of borax, sodium bicarbonate, sugar and salt makes a nasal spray, a tablespoon being dissolved in a pint of warm water.

Boric Acid (boracic acid) occurs as colorless crystals or a white powder and has a bitter taste. It is poisonous and can be absorbed through the mucous membranes and broken skin. For these reasons it is not given internally, and it should be used with caution as douches, lotions, dusting-powders and ointments. It has been extensively used as an antiseptic in surgical dressings; boracic dressings used to contain about 40 per cent of boric acid but this has now been reduced to 5 per cent because of the dangers of absorption. Borated talc (boric acid, 1 part, starch, 1 part, and talc, 8 parts) is a useful dusting-powder but for babies it is better to use powders which do not contain boric acid. A solution of the crystals (two level teaspoonsful in a pint of warm water) is a soothing eye-lotion, skin lotion, and mouthwash. A starch compress containing about 5 per cent of boric acid is used for softening and removing crusts in eczema and other skin conditions.

C

Caffeine is an alkaloid obtained from various plants, including tea, coffee and cola. It occurs as a white powder or as white shining needle-like crystals. It has a bitter taste. Caffeine stimulates the nervous, muscular, and respiratory systems and the heart. It also increases the flow of urine. When taken in caffeine-containing drinks such as tea and coffee it helps to ward off fatigue, and combined with aspirin or phenacetin in tablets it is useful in the treatment of migraine. Caffeine is used to stimulate the heart and kidneys in heart failure, chronic nephritis, and dropsy. Caffeine citrate, 125 to 300 milligrams taken before retiring and again during the night, will sometimes bring relief to adult sufferers from bronchial asthma.

In some persons, especially those with weak hearts, normal medicinal doses may cause side-effects such as headache, restlessness, nausea, vomiting, palpitations and insomnia.

Calamine is a basic zinc carbonate which is colored by incorporating ferric oxide. It is a pink to reddish brown powder. Since it has a mild astringent action on the skin, it is used in dusting-powders, lotions and ointments to relieve the irritation of skin rashes and dermatitis. Calamine lotion is a useful cooling application for sunburn. An oily lotion is used in eczema.

Camomile Flower (anthemis; Roman camamile). The camomile plant *(Anthemis nobilis)* grows wild in the northern parts of Europe. The flowers have yellow central discs with white petals radiating from them. They contain a volatile oil (camomile oil) which is blue when freshly extracted but gradually changes to greenish-yellow. The flowers act as a bitter; in large doses they have an emetic action. Camomile tea is a domestic remedy for indigestion. It is made by infusing 1 ounce of the dried flowers with a pint of boiling water: dose 2 to 8 tablespoonsful. The flowers are also used as a poultice. Powdered camomile is an ingredient of some hair shampoos.

Camphor (gum camphor) is a colorless, transparent crystalline substance with a very characteristic, aromatic odor and a pungent taste which is followed by a feeling of coldness. It is obtained from the wood of an evergreen tree (*Cinnamomum camphora*) which grows in Japan, China, and Taiwan. The wood is cut into small pieces and heated in a current of steam which blows the camphor into a condensing apparatus. On cooling, the camphor solidifies and is purified by sublimation. This gives the powdery form known as 'flowers of camphor,' which is often compressed to produce 'blocks' and 'tablets.' Synthetic camphor is manufactured from oil of turpentine.

INTERNAL USE. When taken by mouth camphor is carminative and irritant and is used in the treatment of coughs as camphorated opium tincture (paregoric).

EXTERNAL USE. When applied to the skin, camphor dilates the blood capillaries and causes a sensation of tingling and warmth followed by slight numbness. It is used in liniments and lotions for neuralgia, lumbago, fibrositis, etc. A mixture of camphor and hard and soft paraffins (camphor ice) is an emollient application to chilblains.

Cannabis (=Bhang, Hashish, Indian Hemp, 'Pot,' Marihuana) is a plant whose leaves and flowers are smoked as Reefer cigarettes and its extracts swallowed. It produces effects similar to those of alcohol. It is a depressant, causing a loosening of brain control: the smoker feels emotional excitement, his laughter becomes uncontrolled, his sense of time inaccurate, and he has hallucinations and illusions.

The habit of taking cannabis is readily formed since the taker is almost invariably a person who desires to escape from reality. Prolonged habitual use causes mental, moral, and physical deterioration and often insanity. Cannabis has no known therapeutic value.

Capsicum (cayenne pepper; red pepper) is the dried ripe fruit from various kinds of capsicum plants. The fruits of some varieties are known as 'chillies' and 'paprika.'

Capsicum is a powerful irritant and rubefacient. When taken internally it is carminative and also stimulates gastric secretions. Capsicum tincture is prepared by percolating the powdered fruits with alcohol (60 per cent).

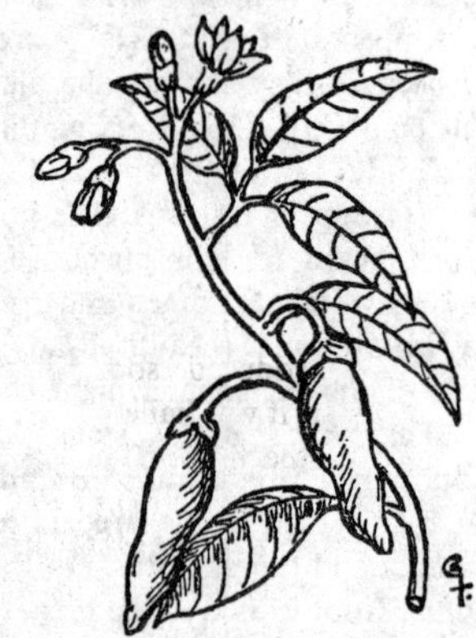

Fig. 11. *CAPSICUM or Red Pepper. The longish red berries and the seeds inside them are ground to a fine powder which tastes intensely hot; it also has a warm stimulating effect upon the skin.*

Caraway (*Carum carvi*) is a biennial herb, native to Europe and Asia; the seeds ripen in August of the second year and the dried ripe seeds are employed in medicinal preparations. Caraway is a mild stomachic and carminative. It is of value in flatulence and colic, and as a flavoring agent in medicines and cooking.

Cardamom (*Elettaria cardamomum*) is a perennial herb native to southern India and also cultivated in Ceylon. The seeds contain a volatile oil which is carminative and is used as an aromatic flavoring agent. The seeds are retained in the capsular fruits until required in order to retain as much as possible of the volatile oil.

Cascara is a shrub (*Rhamnus purshiana*) which grows in British Columbia, California, and other parts of North America. The name cascara sagrada means 'sacred bark' and it is the dried bark which is valuable in medicine. It is collected and dried at least one year before being used. Cascara has a mild purgative action and is valuable in chronic constipation. Its mild action and the fact that the dosage need not be increased with prolonged use make it a useful laxative for habitual constipation during pregnancy and for persons with piles. Cascara is best given at night, a soft stool being evacuated eight to twelve hours afterwards. Preparations containing cascara include an elixir and liquid extract, both of which are taken in a dose of 2 to 5 milliliters.

Castor Oil (oleum ricini) is a fixed oil obtained by expression from the seeds of *Ricinus communis* a tall shrub native to India but cultivated in all warmer regions of the world. Castor oil produces marked irritation of the intestinal mucosa, causing purging but without much griping. Copious watery stools are produced. Children require a comparatively larger dose than adults: dose 1 to 6 5-ml spoonfuls (5 to 30 millilters). The disagreeable taste and character of castor oil may be disguised by giving it floating on orange juice or water flavored with essence of cinnamon or peppermint, or by boiling it for a few minutes with a little sweetened milk and flavoring it with cinnamon or peppermint. It may also be taken in capsules.

EXTERNAL USE. Castor oil is used for its bland emollient action. Zinc and castor oil cream is a soothing application especially for young children. Castor oil is also used as an ingredient of eye preparations.

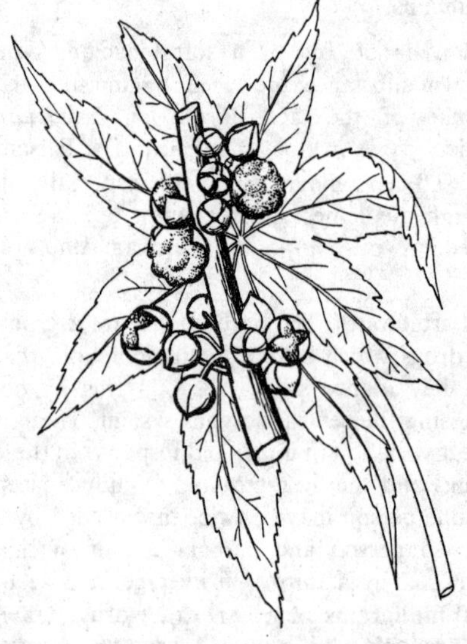

Fig. 12. *CASTOR OIL PLANT. The brown mottled seeds which lie in the pods are the size of small plump almonds. They are crushed to produce the oil.*

Chalk for medicinal use is purified by a washing process. It is a white powder almost insoluble in water. It is used as an absorbent and antacid, mainly in mixtures.

In the treatment of diarrhea, chalk is often combined with opium, or mixed with aromatics. In the treatment of acidity chalk is usually mixed with magnesium carbonate, bismuth carbonate and sodium bicarbonate. Externally, it is sometimes used, with calamine or zinc oxide, as a dusting-powder.

Chlorpromazine was one of the first tranquilizing drugs, and is still very widely used in the treatment of major psychiatric disorders, including schizophrenia and manic-depression. It is valuable for calming aggressive and hostile patients in mental hospitals, making them more cooperative. it can be given by mouth or by injection. It produces a calming effect without clouding the patient's consciousness or impairing his judgment.

Chlorpromazine does not itself relieve pain but when it is given with pain-reducing drugs it has the effect of intensifying their action, so that they can be given in much lower dosage than usual. Because of this, chlorpromazine is given with morphine in the treatment of severe pain such as that of cancer.

Chlorpromazine is also used before operations in order to make the patient calmer and more easily anesthetized.

A number of side-effects may occur during treatment with chlorpromazine, and they include skin rashes, drowsiness, dryness of the mouth, constipation and an increased pulse rate. A more serious effect, which occurs only occasionally, is jaundice, but it disappears when treatment is stopped.

Cinchona Bark (Peruvian bark) is the source of quinine, quinidine, and many other similar alkaloids of great value in medicine. The trees originally grew on the western slopes of the Andes in South America and the bark was brought to Europe in the early seventeenth century by the Jesuits who had discovered its value in the treatment of malaria. The drug was given the name Cinchona by the Swedish botanist Linnaeus, in memory of the Spanish Countess of Chinchon, who is said to have been cured of malaria in Peru in the seventeenth century.

When its curative properties were first discovered, the bark was taken in powder form, a teaspoonful in a glass of wine. Now the chief use of cinchona bark is for the extraction of its alkaloids, and these and similar synthetic drugs have replaced cinchona itself for the treatment of malaria.

Colchicum (autumn crocus; meadow saffron) is a perennial plant native to the temperate parts of Europe; it also grows in northern Africa. The flowers, which are pale purple, appear in the early autumn. The underground part of the plant is a corm and this, as well as the seeds, are used medicinally in Great Britain; in France the flowers are also used. There is no difference in the action of the various parts because in all of them it is due to the presence of the alkaloid colchicine.

Colchicum is a specific for gout and is given as a dry or liquid extract or as a tincture; colchicine is also used, being extracted from the plant by complex processes and made into tablets. Colchicine and all parts and preparations of the plant are *highly poisonous*. The dose of colchicine is 0·5 to 1 milligram, and of the tincture 0·5 to 1·5 milliliters; repeated doses are taken at intervals of a few hours until the pain is relieved or until vomiting or diarrhea occurs, when further treatment must be stopped. It is more effective in the treatment of acute than of chronic gout.

Cortisone and the Corticosteroids. Cortisone and the closely related hydrocortisone are natural hormones secreted by the cortex or outer part of the adrenal gland. The corticosteroids are mainly synthetic compounds very similar to the natural hormones. These substances have no effect on bacteria.

After many trials all over the world the cortisone group of drugs has proved of value for three forms of treatment.

1. When the body's natural supply of hormones from the adrenal cortex is defective, as in Addison's disease or after surgery on the gland, the corticosteroids are used for replacement.

2. When the adrenal gland is overactive and produces too much of the natural hormones, administration of the steroids 'damps down' the overactivity.

3. The corticosteroids have an excellent effect in reducing inflammation, and it is this quality that makes them so helpful in rheumatism, and in eye and skin inflammation.

Use in Rheumatoid Arthritis. When cortisone was introduced soon after the Second World War, it was hailed as a wonder drug which would be the long-awaited cure for rheumatic complaints. By reducing inflammation it relieved the pain and reduced the stiffness of rheumatoid arthritis, thereby allowing greater movement of the affected joints, so that it appeared to be curing the disease. Unfortunately it was found that although cortisone can suppress the symptoms, it cannot cure rheumatoid arthritis or even check its progress. In large-scale trials there proved to be very little difference between patients treated only with cortisone and those treated only with aspirin.

Nevertheless, corticosteroids are sometimes valuable in rheumatoid arthritis to suppress inflammation while other forms of treatment are being carried out. They are usually given by mouth as tablets, although sometimes hydrocortisone and prednisolone are given by injection directly into an affected joint such as the knee. Cortisone is sometimes given by intramuscular injection. Administration of these drugs must be under close medical supervision and, to ensure this, patients are usually treated in hospital.

Side-effects often occur, and may include edema, rounding of the face, congestive heart failure, peptic ulceration and delayed wound healing. At the end of a course of treatment the drug must be withdrawn gradually; if it is suddenly stopped there may be very serious symptoms.

Corticosteroids are seldom given to people suffering from active tuberculosis, diabetes, congestive heart failure, or chronic kidney disease, and great care must be taken if they are given to the elderly.

Use in Eye Inflammations. The corticosteroids are often used to relieve inflammatory conditions of the eye, such as allergic conjunctivitis and keratitis. Hydrocortisone and prednisolone are very frequently used for this purpose, being applied in eye-drops or eye ointments.

Use in Skin Diseases. Skin diseases, such as eczema and pruritus, which are associated with allergy or hypersensitivity, are treated by the application of lotions, creams or ointments containing hydrocortisone, prednisolone, fludrocortisone, dexamethasone, or betamethasone. These preparations are usually effective in relieving pain and irritation, but the relief does not persist after treatment has been stopped.

The Corticosteroids all have the same basic actions, but these vary in degree, and the various compounds each have special indications.

Betamethasone is used for skin complaints, but it has been used too for rheumatoid arthritis, for which it is given in tablets.

Cortisone is used mainly for replacement therapy after adrenalectomy and in Addison's disease, for the control of overactivity of the adrenal gland, and for the treatment of rheumatoid arthritis.

Deoxycortone is used as an adjunct to cortisone in the treatment of Addison's disease and after adrenalectomy.

Dexamethasone is used mainly for rheumatic complaints. It is very potent.

Fludrocortisone is used mainly in skin preparations to relieve inflammation.

Hydrocortisone is used for external application in eye and skin preparations, for injection into inflamed joints in rheumatoid arthritis, and in a retention enema for the treatment of ulcerative colitis.

Prednisolone and Prednisone are used for rheumatic diseases; they are potent so smaller doses are required.

D

Dandelion is a perennial herb (*Taraxacum officinale*) native to Europe. The young tender leaves are used as a food and the rhizome and roots are used medicinally, given as a liquid extract and as a juice from the fresh root. Dandelion is a bitter and is mildly laxative. Herbalists use the roots to prepare dandelion 'coffee'.

Digitalis (foxglove; fairy bells; ladies' glove) is a biennial plant, *Digitalis purpurea*, growing widely in the United States and other temperate countries. It is now cultivated in many parts of the world for its valuable medicinal properties. The leaves are the part used in medicine and these are collected either from the first year plants, or from those of the second year. After collection they must be dried as quickly as possible at about 60° C.

Digitalis improves the force of the heart beat and will therefore increase the flow of urine in patients with dropsy.

Digitalis is usually administered as tablets containing 60 milligrams of Prepared Digitalis, i.e. standardized powdered leaf. The tincture is prepared by percolating the dried leaves with alcohol.

An alternative method of using digitalis is to extract from the leaves the substances which produce the medicinal effect. These glycosides include the following:

DIGITALIN: a mixture of the glycosides obtained from the foxglove seeds and which must be carefully distinguished from

DIGITOXIN: one of the most powerful glycosides obtained from foxglove leaves; it is also known as DIGITALINE CRYSTALLISÉE. It is given as small pills (granules) or by injection.

Wooly foxglove leaf (Austrian foxglove) comes from the plant *Digitalis lanata*, which is a native of Austria and the Balkans. From it is obtained another foxglove glycoside called DIGOXIN, which is also used in the treatment of heart diseases either as tablets or by injection.

Foxglove leaves and all the preparations and substances obtained from them are *highly poisonous* and powerful medicines, and must only be used on the advice of a doctor.

E

Ergot. This is a minute fungus that grows on the grains of growing rye. Epidemics of ergotism (severe muscle pains, cold skin, dry skin gangrene, nausea, diarrhea, leg weakness) have occurred after ingestion of ergotized rye bread. Medieval midwives used crude ergot for abortions as it stimulates uterine muscle. It is now used, in capsules or tablets, to check hemorrhage after delivery.

Eucalyptus Oil is a volatile oil obtained from the leaves of eucalyptus trees, of which the blue gum-tree or Australian fever tree (*Eucalyptus globulus*) is one of the best known. These trees, which are mostly evergreen, grow in Australia and Malaya. The oil is antiseptic and deodorant. It is used with other ingredients as an inhalation in the treatment of colds and other respiratory infections, either sprinkled on a handkerchief or added to boiling water and the steam inhaled. When mixed with an equal quantity of olive oil it is a useful rub in rheumatism.

EUCALYPTOL (cineole) is the principal constituent of eucalyptus oil. It is less irritating to the mucous lining of the nose and throat than the oil itself and is given in lozenges which usually also contain menthol.

G

Gentian (gentian root) is the plant *Gentiana lutea*, the dried roots and rhizome being the parts used medicinally. The plant grows in the mountainous regions of Europe and Asia Minor. Gentian root has been used for centuries and its name is said to have been derived from Gentius, King of Illyria.

It is a bitter, stimulating the gastric juices and improving the appetite. It may be used in gastric dyspepsia and anorexia and is used in tonics for debility and during recovery from exhausting illnesses. Preparations used are the compound infusions and the compound tincture, which are flavored with orange and lemon peel and cardamom seeds.

Ginger is a perennial plant (*Zingiber officinale*) native to tropical Asia and now cultivated in many tropical countries. The dried and scraped rhizome is used in medicine as a powder and as a tincture and syrup. The syrup is made by mixing one part of strong ginger tincture with enough simple syrup to produce twenty parts.

Ginger is a stimulant and carminative which is valuable in acute flatulence or colic. It is sometimes given with purgatives to prevent griping. The syrup has been used in some medicines to disguise their nauseous taste. As a homely remedy a hot infusion known as 'ginger tea' has been used as a diaphoretic in colds: a pint of boiling water is added to half an ounce (15 grams) of the powdered or bruised root: dose 2 to 4 tablespoonsful.

Griseofulvin. See under Antibiotics, p. 598.

Gum. See under Acacia and Tragacanth, or under Benzoin.

H

Hydrocortisone. See under Cortisone.

Hyoscyamus (henbane; poison tobacco) is a native of Great Britain and other parts of Europe. It was introduced into America where it grows in the north-eastern states. There are many varieties, both annual and biennial. The drug is usually collected from *Hyoscyamus niger* and consists of the leaves and flowers. These contain the alkaloids hyoscyamine and hyoscine (scopolamine) which are extremely poisonous. Hyoscyamus is used as a liquid extract, a dry extract, or a tincture to relieve griping pains such as those caused by some purgatives. For this reason it is often included in laxative pills.

Hyoscyamus preparations are *poisonous*. They should only be taken under medical supervision.

EGYPTIAN HENBANE is a herbaceous perennial (*Hyoscyamus muticus*) which grows in the desert area between Egypt and India. It is collected chiefly in Egypt and is used for extracting the alkaloid hyoscyamine.

I

Imipramine is used to alleviate mental depression and can be given by mouth or by injection. It may occasionally cause blurred vision, sweating, or dryness of the mouth. (Dangerous if used with certain other drugs.) It is not suitable for epileptics and schizophrenics. See also Tranquilizers, p. 596.

Iodine is a heavy, bluish-black metallic substance with a strong characteristic odor. Taken internally in the form of a solution or as the iodides it is used in the treatment of diseases of the thyroid gland. Lugol's solution (aqueous iodine solution), which contains iodine 5 per cent and potassium iodide 10 per cent, is often administered. Iodine is a powerful antiseptic. Weak iodine solution (tincture of iodine) is painted on small cuts and wounds as a first-aid treatment but continued application inflames the skin and may lead to blistering. Colorless tincture of Iodine ointment and non-staining iodine ointment are used as counter-irritants for chilblains.

Ipecacuanha (*Cephaëlis ipecacuanha*) is a low straggling shrub growing in Brazil and Colombia. The dried rhizome and roots are used in medicine.

It is mainly used in the form of a liquid extract or tincture. Large doses have an emetic action; smaller doses are diaphoretic and expectorant. As a diaphoretic, sometimes combined with opium it is useful in feverish conditions and to abort colds in their early stages. Its expectorant action is of value in acute bronchitis. Children tolerate it well. The dose of the tincture is 0.25 to 1 milliliter as an expectorant, or 5 to 20 milliliter as an emetic.

L

Licorice is a perennial herb (*Glycyrrhiza glabra*) indigenous to southern Europe and Asia. The powdered root is used in the preparation of pills and to dilute some powdered extracts. The extract and liquid extract are often included in cough preparations for their demulcent and expectorant properties. The liquid extract is a useful flavoring agent for mixtures. Licorice preparations will not mix well with acids since the active principle is precipitated. Compound licorice powder, made by mixing senna and licorice powder, of each two parts, fennel and sublimed sulphur, of each one part, and sugar, six and a half parts, was a popular domestic remedy for constipation, especially for children; it is effective without causing purging: dose, one teaspoonful.

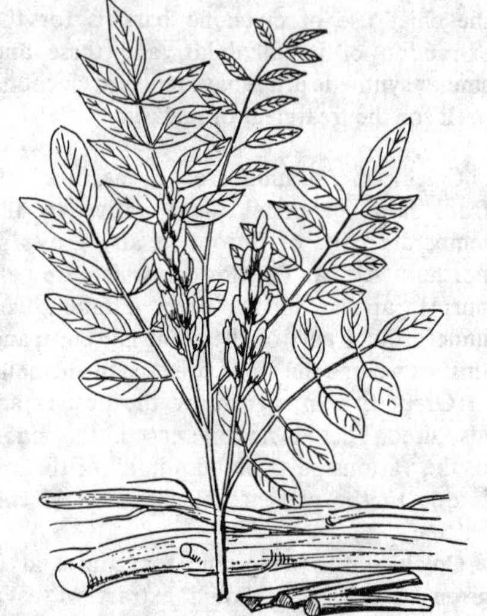

Fig. 13. *LICORICE. The* Glycyrrhiza *plant grows in Europe and has spikes of blue pea-like flowers. The dried fibrous roots are used for the making of licorice extract, or licorice powder.*

Linseed (flaxseed) is the dried ripe seed of flax (*Linum usitatissimum*), an annual plant which is widely cultivated. It bears blue flowers in June and July and the seeds ripen in August. Medicinally, linseed has both demulcent and emollient actions due to the mucilage and oil which it contains. Poultices made by mixing the ground linseed meal with hot water are of value in inflammatory conditions such as boils.

BOILED LINSEED OIL, which is used for furniture polishing, etc., is prepared with toxic substances such as lead, and should never be taken or used medicinally.

LSD (lysergic acid diethylamide) is synthesized from ergot, a fungus on rye. Minute amounts, taken by mouth, produce hallucinations of time, form, color, and space, the taker feels he is observing himself from a distance and reveals what is deeply in his unconscious (this is the reaction which is useful in psychiatry). He also becomes restless, dizzy, he feels nausea, sweats, his temperature rises, blood pressure falls, breathing quickens, he has prickling sensations, his pupils dilate, and his mouth is dry. No treatment is known.

M

Magnesium Oxide (magnesia) occurs in light and heavy forms and is used as a laxative and antacid, particularly for children. The light powder is preferable for mixtures and the heavy for powders and tablets.

Magnesium Carbonate occurs in two forms—light and heavy. Both are antacid and laxative. The light form can be taken as a powder or mixed in milk; it is also used as a suspending agent for volatile oils in inhalations. Heavy magnesium carbonate, mixed with other antacids such as kaolin, bismuth carbonate and magnesium trisilicate, is used in powders. Compound rhubarb powder contains both light and heavy magnesium carbonates, rhubarb, and ginger (dose 0·6 to 4 grams). Fluid magnesia (magnesium bicarbonate solution) is a mild laxative and antacid for children; it has a slightly bitter taste and should be sweetened.

Magnesium Sulphate (Epsom salts) is an odorless colorless crystalline substance with a bitter saline taste. Taken in doses of ½ to 4 teaspoonsful in a glassful of water, it acts as a powerful purgative in about one to two hours. If only a little water is taken the action may be delayed for about twelve hours. Dried and powdered magnesium sulphate may be mixed into a thick paste with glycerin and a little phenol and applied to boils and carbuncles on absorbent cotton.

Male Fern (aspidium) is used in the eradication of tapeworms. The plant (*Dryopteris filix-mas*) is widely distributed in the northern hemisphere, and the part used in medicine is the underground stem (rhizome), which must be collected late in the autumn and carefully dried so that the internal part remains green. The rhizome is extracted with ether and the extract mixed, after removal of the ether, with peanut oil.

Male fern does not kill the tapeworm but paralyzes it, so that its hold becomes loosened and the worm can then be washed out with a purge. The extract is best taken as a liquid, the required dose, usually 3 to 6 milliliters, being well mixed with powdered acacia and enough water to make about 45 milliliters. This is swallowed on an empty stomach and a purge is then given; saline purges are better than castor oil. Male fern extract is also given in hard gelatin capsules. This disguises the taste, but the capsules are not so reliable in action and the liquid is preferable.

Meprobamate is of value in the treatment of anxiety and mental tension but is of less value for persons who are depressed. It has been used to relieve the unpleasant symptoms which arise during treatment for alcoholism and drug addiction. See also Tranquilizers, p. 596.

Mercury (hydrargyrum; quicksilver) is a shiny silvery-white liquid metal, familiar as the liquid in a thermometer. It was known to the Greeks and has had considerable use in medicine ever since. It is used as a purgative and in the treatment of syphilis. For its purgative effect, it is given in the form of mercury pill (blue pill) or pill of mercury with rhubarb.

In the treatment of syphilis, mercury was for centuries the only known remedy. It was given by mouth in pills, or by injection, and also as ointments because mercury is absorbed through the skin. Mercury combines with many metals to form amalgams and some of these are used as dental fillings.

ANTISEPTIC USE. A number of mercury salts and organic compounds are used as antiseptics and some are effective against parasites and fungous infections. Complex mercury compounds, such as mersalyl and meralluride, when injected into the body have the property of increasing the flow of the urine. They have been widely used for this purpose but are now being replaced by newer substances which have the advantage that they can be taken by mouth.

Compounds of mercury which are used as antiseptics include yellow mercuric oxide, which is chiefly used in an eye ointment for conjunctivitis, and mercuric chloride (corrosive sublimate). The latter is made up into solution-tablets colored blue; one tablet gives a pint of a 1 in 1,000 solution which is satisfactory for general disinfectant purposes and as a skin antiseptic. Weaker solutions (1 in 5,00 to 1 in 10,000) should be used for cleaning wounds.

Organic compounds of mercury are often stronger antiseptics and are less irritating and poisonous. Phenylmercuric nitrate and phenylmercuric acetate are commonly used. A 1 in 1,500 solution is suitable for application to the unbroken skin, but for cleansing wounds it should be diluted to 1 in 20,000. Both salts are effective as 0·05 to 1 per cent ointments in the treatment of fungus infections of the skin. They are also spermicidal and are used in some contraceptive creams.

AS A PURGATIVE. Mercurous chloride (calomel) is a heavy white tasteless powder. It is a purgative and is best taken at night in a dose of 30 to 120 milligrams and followed next morning by a saline purgative.

Monoamine Oxidase Inhibitors. These drugs, commonly termed MAO, are a type of antidepressant (see p. 588) used mainly to treat patients suffering from agitated depression. They elevate the mood. But at the same time they produce in susceptible patients a number of severe reactions such as jaundice, dizziness, agitation, constipation, impotence, and defects of vision. If taken with other drugs, or even with other types of antidepressants or some wines and alcohol, the patient usually develops a violent headache, there is a rise in blood pressure which may lead to intracranial hemorrhage or acute heart failure.

These drugs are usually administered as tablets, sometimes as injections.

Morphine. See under Opium.

Mustard (*Sinapis alba*), white or yellow mustard, is native to Europe. The ripe seeds are used medicinally as a rubefacient, generally in the form of a poultice commonly, though incorrectly, termed 'mustard plaster.' The mustard should be mixed with some substance such as flour before wetting since it is too strong to use undiluted. Liquids such as alcohol, glycerin or vinegar should not be added as they have a weakening effect upon the mustard mixture. It will cause blistering if allowed to remain on the skin for too long. Mustard is a fast-acting emetic, particularly useful in cases of narcotic poisoning. As a condiment it stimulates the mucous membrane of the stomach and aids digestion. Obstinate hiccup may sometimes be relieved by mustard.

O

Opium is the dried juice obtained from the unripe capsules of the opium poppy (*Papaver somniferum*). This annual plant grows up to four feet in height and is native to Asia but is cultivated in other parts of the world. After the petals of the flowers have fallen and the capsule is becoming mature, several cuts are made into it. From these cuts a white juice oozes on to the outside of the capsule.

It is left to dry for twenty-four hours and is then scraped off.

Opium is used in the treatment of diarrhea, for the relief of colic and mild insomnia, and as a diaphoretic. Aromatic chalk mixture with opium is useful for intestinal treatment. Paregoric is prepared from opium tincture (laudanum), camphor, benzoic acid, anise oil, and alcohol. It contains 0.05 per cent of morphine and the most usual dose given is one to two 5-ml spoonsful.

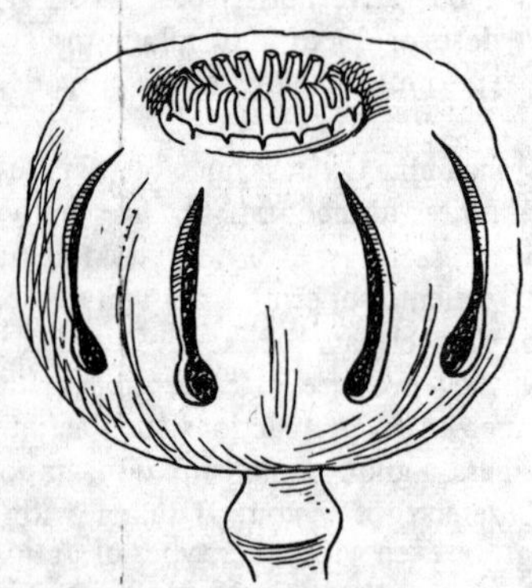

Fig. 14. *OPIUM POPPY CAPSULE. The capsule, or seed pod, is pierced to allow the sticky juice to ooze out. This gummy substance is scraped off and pressed into lumps. The minute seeds inside contain no opium.*

The narcotic action of opium is chiefly due to the presence of morphine (usually about 10 per cent), but other important alkaloids contribute. These include codeine and noscapine, which are also important in medicine.

OIL. The seeds in the capsule of the opium poppy do not contain morphine or other narcotic substances and are used for food. They are known as maw seed and are expressed to obtain poppy seed oil (maw oil) which has a pleasant almond taste and is used as a substitute for olive oil, which it greatly resembles in properties. By treating poppy-seed oil with hydriodic acid, an iodinated oil is obtained, preparations of which are used to show up the bronchial tract for X-ray examination (see p. 342).

P, Q, R

Penicillins. See under Antibiotics, p. 598.

Peppermint (*Mentha piperita*) is a perennial herb native to Europe. It was cultivated by the ancient Egyptians and today it is widely grown for commerce throughout the world. The active principle is a volatile oil similar to menthol which is distilled from the fresh overground parts of the flowering plant. It is aromatic and stimulant. Peppermint water is used in stomach medicines intended to relieve spasmodic pains and flatulence and to allay nausea. The strong taste is useful for covering the unpleasant flavor of other ingredients in medicines, and the addition of peppermint to some purgatives reduces their griping effect. Peppermint oil is taken in lozenges, or 1 to 3 drops may be taken on a lump of sugar or in sweetened water. It is also taken in the form of peppermint spirit (dose: 0·3 to 2 milliliters) with sweetened water. Peppermint water is widely used as the vehicle in mixtures and mouth-washes.

Perphenazine is chemically related to chlorpromazine. It has a depressant action on the brain so it is used in the treatment of schizophrenia and acute manic states. It has a tranquilizing effect without producing sleep (hypnosis). It can be given by mouth or by injection. During treatment with perphenazine certain other unwanted effects—tremor, blurred vision and excessive salivation—may be observed in the patient. See also Tranquilizers, p. 596.

Phenacetin is a white crystalline odorless substance which is used to reduce the temperature and to relieve pain. The dose is 300 to 600 milligrams and the drug is administered in tablets each containing 300 milligrams. It is also used as tablets with other pain-relieving drugs such as aspirin and codeine. It is an ingredient of aspirin, phenacetin and caffeine tablets (A.P.C. tablets). Some authorities advise that phenacetin should not be taken for long periods at a time.

Podophyllum (mandrake; May apple) is the dried rhizome and roots of *Podophyllum peltatum*, a perennial herb native to America.

Podophyllum is a cathartic. When taken internally, it produces watery stools and often causes much griping. In small doses, it is used, combined with aloes or cascara, in chronic constipation. Its purging action is reduced by a small quantity of belladonna or hyoscyamus extract. It is usually employed as podophyllum resin, a light brownish powder. Large quantities of the resin must be handled carefully because of its intensely irritant properties which can cause conjunctivitis.

Potassium (kalium) is one of the so-called alkali metals. It is an essential constituent of the body, and its compounds are used in medicine for many purposes.

POTASSIUM HYDROXIDE (caustic potash) is a powerful caustic which has been used to remove warts. A 5 per cent solution in water is used as a cuticle solvent. Burns on the skin caused by potassium hydroxide should be flooded with water and then with dilute acetic acid or vinegar.

POTASSIUM BICARBONATE is taken in a dose of 1 to 2 grams in water as an antacid. It is included in mixtures with expectorants to loosen the phlegm.

POTASSIUM BROMIDE is a white crystalline substance with a salty taste. It is widely given, usually with other ingredients, as a sedative. A draught of chloral hydrate and potassium bromide before retiring induces sleep. 'Three bromides mixture' contains the bromides of ammonium, potassium and sodium dissolved in water with flavoring and coloring added. Continued administration of bromides may bring on skin rashes which usually clear on stopping the medicine. Potassium bromide is sometimes prescribed as tablets, usually containing 300 milligrams. They are dissolved in water and not swallowed whole because they break up very slowly in the stomach and may cause pain.

POTASSIUM CHLORATE is a mild astringent used as a gargle, tablet or lozenge to alleviate some disorders of the mouth. The tablets each contain 300 milligrams and should be sucked slowly. Potassium chlorate should not be given to children. The gargle is made by dissolving 6 grams in 300 ml of water and mixing with an equal quantity of warm water before use. *All chlorates are explosive.* Do not carry the tablets loose in the pocket or in a paper bag, and keep them out of contact with matches. Potassium chlorate must not be confused with potassium chloride.

POTASSIUM CHLORIDE, a white crystalline substance, is the form of potassium employed to maintain an adequate supply of potassium in the blood when the level of this essential ingredient is reduced after vomiting, diarrhea or heavy urine loss. Potassium loss may also follow the use of diuretics, which increase the amount of urine and potassium discharged from the body. The unpleasant taste may be partly disguised with lemon juice. Injections of potassium chloride are given in very dilute solution as an intravenous drip, usually with sodium chloride and calcium chloride (Ringer's solution). A similar solution called Hartmann's solution or Ringer-lactate solution contains sodium lactate as well.

POTASSIUM CITRATE is made up into mixtures, sometimes with hyoscyamus, which are given in inflammation of the bladder. The citrate makes the urine alkaline.

POTASSIUM IODIDE is an expectorant and is also used as a means of introducing iodine into the body, especially before operations for goiter. In some districts where simple goiter is common because the water supply is deficient in iodine, potassium iodide in small doses will prevent the disease.

POTASSIUM NITRATE (niter; saltpeter) is used in gargles with potassium chlorate for the relief of sore throat.

POTASSIUM PERMANGANATE occurs as dark purple crystals with a greenish metallic luster. 1 in 1,000 to 1 in 5,000 solutions are used for their antiseptic action as gargles, and for vaginal and urethral irrigation. They can be readily prepared from solution-tablets. One of these solution-tablets when dissolved in a pint of water gives a 1 in 1,000 solution, or in 5 pints of water a 1 in 5,000 solution. A strong solution, 1 in 20, is a powerful styptic. The crystals are reputed to act as an antidote to snake poisoning. A 1 in 500 solution in water is used to wash out the stomach in the treatment of poisoning by opium or morphine. Potassium permanganate stains the skin brown; the stain may be removed by washing with weak solutions of oxalic or sulphurous acid.

POTASSIUM ACID TARTRATE (cream of

tartar) is a pleasant tasting substance which can be used as a non-irritating laxative.

Prednisolone and **Prednisone.** See under Cortisone.

Prochlorperazine has an action similar to that of chlorpromazine (p. 590). In small doses it is given for the treatment of mild emotional disturbances, giddiness and migraine, and larger doses are used for schizophrenia, mania, and psychoses. See also Tranquilizers, p. 596.

Proflavine, acriflavine, aminacrine, and euflavine are crystalline powders used in dilute solution as local antiseptics. Their action is not affected by body fluids or pus and they are suitable for cleaning wounds, usually as a solution containing one part of the substance in 1,000 parts of water or normal saline. Acriflavine is also used in the treatment of burns and is incorporated in wound dressings.

Stains on the skin caused by these substances may be removed with very weak solutions of hydrochloric acid.

Quinine. See under Cinchona.

Radio-isotopes. See p. 192.

Reserpine is obtained from a plant, rauwolfia, which grows in India and Africa. It is used in the treatment of high blood pressure (hypertension), producing a gradual relaxation of mental tension and a reduction in blood pressure. It is also used in the treatment of schizophrenia and anxiety states. During treatment the patients sometimes have peculiar dreams, skin rashes and gastric upsets but these cease when the drug is stopped. See also Tranquilizers, p. 596.

S

Sodium (natrium) is a soft white alkali metal. It is an essential constituent of the body and is used in many forms for medicinal purposes. The most important of its salts and compounds are described below.

SODIUM BICARBONATE is taken by mouth, about 1 gram in water, to relieve flatulence and heartburn, but it is better taken with other antacids such as magnesium carbonate or magnesium trisilicate. It may be sucked as a tablet for the same purpose. Compound sodium bicarbonate tablets (soda mints) contain 300 milligrams, with peppermint oil. Taken half-an-hour before meals with a bitter such as gentian, it promotes appetite. Sodium bicarbonate dissolves mucus so it is used as a mouth-wash or gargle (1 to 4 per cent in water). A teaspoonful each of sodium bicarbonate and borax in half a pint of water makes a solution which can be mixed with an equal amount of warm water for a nasal wash. A weak solution (half a teaspoonful in half a pint of water) relieves irritation in urticarial rashes. Sodium bicarbonate is also used as an eye lotion to wash out the eyes after splashes with acid substances. It is available as a sterile solution containing 3·5 per cent of sodium bicarbonate. It is used undiluted; any not used within 24 hours must be discarded.

SODIUM CARBONATE (common soda) is an alkali used as a 1 in 200 solution in water to soften encrustations on the skin in eczema. Five ounces in 30 gallons of water makes an alkaline bath. Moistened and rubbed on the bite, it relieves wasp stings. A special form, crystal soda, is used in bath salts.

SODIUM CHLORIDE (common salt) is one of the most important salts in medicine. A 0·9 per cent solution in water (normal saline; physiological saline) has some of the properties of blood and is given by intravenous injection and per rectum to patients who cannot take fluids by mouth. Dextrose is often added to the solution to provide the patient with nourishment.

Sodium chloride is taken by mouth to replace that excreted by the body. The normal daily intake is between 5 and 15 grams and this is usually provided in the diet. When an excessive amount is excreted, for example because of excessive sweating in hot climates, a 0·5 per cent solution may be taken. Sodium chloride tablets, which usually contain 300 milligrams, should be dissolved in water or sucked. A strong solution in water is a useful emetic in the treatment of poisoning.

SODIUM CITRATE prevents the formation, by the rennet of the stomach, of large curds from milk. It is therefore given to invalids and infants to make milk more digestible. For this purpose, it is supplied as tablets each of 125 milligrams of sodium citrate. The tablets should be crushed and dissolved in a little water and the solution added to the milk. For invalids, 60 to 180 milligrams is needed for 40 milliliters of milk. For infants, one tablet dissolved in a teaspoonful of water is added to each feed.

Sodium citrate also prevents stored blood from clotting.

SODIUM HYDROXIDE (caustic soda) is a powerful caustic. A 1 in 40 solution in glycerin is used as a cuticle remover. If the skin is burned, it should be flooded with water and then with dilute acetic acid or vinegar.

SODIUM SALICYLATE is used in the treatment of acute rheumatism, a dose of 1.5 grams being given every three or four hours. It may produce headache, noises in the ear, sweating and skin eruptions, but these effects pass off when the drug is stopped. It tends to irritate the stomach, and sodium bicarbonate is therefore given at the same time. If tablets are prescribed, they should be dissolved in water; the taste may be disguised with orange tincture or clove infusion.

Squill (*Urginea maritima*) is a perennial plant growing from a bulb. It grows in sandy soil along the Mediterranean coast. The bulbs are collected in the autumn and the fleshy inner parts are sliced and dried for medicinal use. Squill has an irritant effect on the stomach and if given in large doses causes nausea and vomiting, while in smaller doses it acts as an expectorant. It is mainly used for coughs, especially in combination with other expectorants such as ipecacuanha and ammonium bicarbonate. It has been used as a diuretic and as an emetic.

Stilbestrol is a white tasteless powder often prescribed as a substitute for the natural female sex hormones or estrogens. It is used for alleviating menopausal symptoms, for suppressing lactation, and in cancer of the breast and prostate. It is given by mouth as tablets but sometimes by injection.

Sulphonamides. Sulphanilamide and similar compounds became widely used during the Second World War, under the name 'M and B,' for the treatment of infections and for the dressing of wounds.

The sulphonamides halt bacteria by taking the place of essential vitamins upon which the bacteria are dependent. They are effective in the treatment of pneumonia, dysentery, meningitis, and infections caused by hemolytic streptococci. They are usually taken by mouth as tablets or mixtures, although they may be given by injection in severe infections.

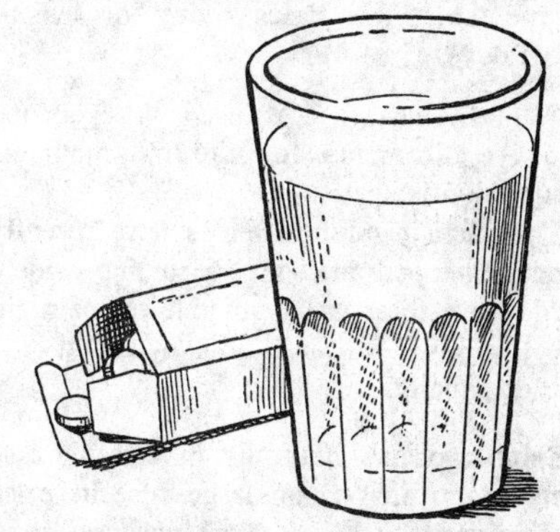

Fig. 15. SULPHONAMIDE DRUGS. *Because sulphonamide drugs tend to form crystals in the kidneys and thereby upset the urinary flow, patients taking these medicaments should always drink plenty of water or other fluids.*

Resistance to the sulphonamides develops comparatively rapidly, and so courses of treatment do not as a rule last for more than a week or ten days. It is important that treatment should be begun as soon as possible after the onset of an infection. A large first dose is given in order to produce a high concentration of the drug in the bloodstream and this concentration is maintained by giving smaller doses at regular intervals.

The commonest danger associated with sulphonamide treatment is the formation of crystals of the drug in the urine, which may result in damage to the kidneys. To prevent this crystallization, the patient is given plenty of fluids during the period of treatment.

Although the various forms of sulphonamide have saved countless lives, many doctors are giving up their use owing to the toxic effects they have. All sulphonamide drugs depress bone marrow, affecting the blood-cell-forming ability; they sensitize the patient, producing connective tissue disorders; they cause serious skin rashes; and many strains of micro-organisms in the world are now quite resistant to them—particularly the organism causing gonorrhea.

Antibiotics are as effective as sulphonamides for all bacterial infections in man and are immeasurably safer.

SULPHADIMIDINE This is probably the most active and widely used sulphonamide, and is effective in the treatment of a variety of infections. It is given by mouth as tablets containing 0.5 gram and as mixtures; six-hourly dosage is necessary to maintain an effective concentration in the bloodstream. It rarely causes side-effects.

SULPHAFURAZOLE is used in the treatment of infections of the urinary tract.

SULPHAMETHIZOLE is given in tablets containing 0.1 gram, also for urinary tract infections. The usual course of treatment is one tablet five times a day for five to seven days.

SULPHACETAMIDE is used in eyedrops and eye ointments for the treatment of conjunctivitis.

Long-acting sulphonamides have recently been developed and are becoming widely used. With these, it is possible to maintain effective blood concentrations by giving only one dose daily.

Sulphur occurs naturally in volcanic districts (Italy, Sicily) and large deposits exist in Louisiana. For medicinal purposes it is purified by the process known as sublimation. Precipitated sulphur is given as a laxative in confections and lozenges, or it may be mixed with milk, syrup, honey or molasses. Sublimed sulphur is included for its laxative action in compound licorice powder.

In the treatment of scabies, sulphur is applied to the skin, as an ointment containing 10 per cent of precipitated sulphur, or as compound sulphur lotion.

SULPHURATED POTASH is also used in the treatment of scabies, acne and other skin affections, either as a medicated bath (8 ounces in 30 gallons of water) or as a lotion.

T

Tranquilizers. The group of drugs known as the tranquilizers comprises a large number of compounds, of varying chemical composition, which have the ability to stimulate or depress the central nervous system. They are very valuable for the relief of the anxiety, tension and agitation which are frequently associated with emotional disturbance and mental illness (p. 461).

Tranquilizers should be taken only under medical supervision, as their use can be habit-forming and can even lead to addiction. Like many other drugs, they are of great value when administered wisely and when really required, but they are harmful if taken indiscriminately without an understanding of their possible dangers.

There are many drugs which have a tranquilizing effect; the more commonly used are: chlorpromazine (p. 590), perphenazine (p. 594), prochlorperazine (p. 595), trifluoperazine (below), imipramine (p. 592), meprobamate (p. 593), and reserpine (p. 595).

Trifluoperazine is given, by mouth or by injection, to control patients who are in acute psychotic states. In smaller doses it is used for the treatment of mild mental and emotional disturbances, as well as for nausea and vomiting. See also Tranquilizers, above.

U–Z

Wintergreen (*Gaultheria procumbens*) is a small woody evergreen plant native to North America. The leaves have been used in medicine but their properties are due entirely to the oil which they yield. Oil of wintergreen has largely been replaced by methyl salicylate.

Witch Hazel (*Hamamelis virginiana*) is a shrub or small tree indigenous to the United States and Canada. The dried leaves and bark are used in medicine for their astringent and hemostatic properties. It is applied to bruises, minor wounds and sprains, as either the tincture or the liquid extract, diluted with water. The dried extract is used in suppositories containing 200 milligrams for treatment of piles. An ointment is used as an astringent application for the same purpose.

Zinc Oxide. A white tasteless powder which is used for its mild astringent effect on the skin. It is usually applied in creams and ointments, often with castor oil or arachis oil, and sometimes with an added medicament. It is often included in dusting-powders with talc and starch. Zinc and castor oil ointment is widely used to prevent napkin rash and to soothe inflamed skin conditions.

ZINC COMPOUNDS. Other zinc salts are also used externally. Zinc carbonate and its variant CALAMINE are both useful in lotions and ointment. ZINC UNDECENOATE in an ointment or dusting-powder is used for athlete's foot.

ANESTHETICS

Anesthetics are agents (gases or liquids) which, when the vapor is taken into the body, eliminate body sensation. The loss of sensation may be partial and confined to a small area of the body while the patient still remains fully conscious. This happens with local anesthetics such as cocaine. With other anesthetics, the patient may lose consciousness and be completely insensitive to pain. This happens after administration of a general anesthetic such as ether.

General Anesthetics

Premedication. It is important that before a patient is anesthetized for an operation he should be in a calm and relaxed state, so that the anesthetic will take effect rapidly. As most people are tense and nervous at the thought of an operation, they are given hypnotic and muscle-relaxing drugs beforehand to relieve their apprehension. If the muscles are made to relax, less anesthetic is required. The premedication also reduces the likelihood of shock and lowers the blood pressure, thus preventing constriction of blood capillaries and reducing bleeding at the site of the operation. Salivary and respiratory secretions are also reduced. The drugs used for this pre-operative medication are barbiturates, morphine, hyoscine, and atropine.

Administration. General anesthetics are given by inhalation. They are either gases (nitrous oxide, cyclopropane) or volatile liquids (ether, chloroform, trilene, halothane) which, when inhaled, cause loss of consciousness. There are three methods of giving an inhalation anesthetic.

1. OPEN METHOD. The anesthetic, usually ether or chloroform, is dropped directly on to a pad placed over the patient's nose and mouth. This rather crude method is only suitable for producing very short periods of anesthesia.

2. SEMI-CLOSED METHOD. This uses an apparatus by means of which the anesthetic passes from a storage cylinder into a rubber bag, from which it is inhaled by the patient through a gas-tight face mask or a tube inserted in his trachea. It is exhaled through a valve into the room. By this method it is possible to include more than one cylinder of gas in the circuit, so that two or more anesthetics can be used at once. Oxygen is usually given at the same time. The flow of each gas from its cylinder is regulated by taps.

3. CLOSED METHOD. The apparatus used is similar to that described above, except that the exhaled air does not go into the room. Instead it is breathed back into the circuit, the carbon dioxide being absorbed by a container of soda lime which is included in the circuit between the mask and the rubber bag.

Stages of Anesthesia. There are four main states of anesthesia.

1. INDUCTION. As administration of the anesthetic begins, the patient begins to feel giddy and sleepy, although he is still conscious and able to talk.

2. EXCITEMENT. He begins to lose consciousness. His breathing becomes irregular, his pulse is rapid and strong, and his pupils are dilated.

3. SURGICAL ANESTHESIA. Excitement disappears. The pupils constrict and the reflexes begin to disappear, the first to go being those which control the voluntary muscles, and then the centers controlling coughing, vom-

iting and blinking are paralyzed. This stage can be subdivided into four planes.

(a) The eyes rove about and respiration is deep and regular. Operations other than abdominal can be performed at this stage.

(b) The eyes become still, and breathing becomes weaker and less regular. Operations on the lower abdomen are possible.

(c) There is only abdominal respiration. The upper abdomen can be operated on.

(d) Very deep anesthesia, passing on to stage 4.

4. Paralysis of the Medulla. If too much anesthetic is given, the medulla (the portion of the brain adjacent to the spinal cord: it controls breathing and heart action) becomes paralyzed. Breathing becomes very shallow and irregular, the pulse is rapid, the blood pressure falls and the pupils dilate. Death will probably occur from respiratory failure.

It will be seen from this that dilatation of the pupil and irregular breathing and pulse rate may mean that anesthesia is either too deep (stage 4) or too shallow (stage 2). The anesthetist is able to distinguish between these two stages by the muscular tone of the patient and by the depth of his respiration. An electroencephalogram shows significant changes with each stage of anesthesia.

Principal Inhalation Anesthetics

Chloroform, a volatile non-inflammable liquid, is more potent than ether and is less irritant to mucous membranes, so that it causes less nausea and vomiting. It is, however, more dangerous than ether; it may cause serious respiratory depression or a sudden fall in blood pressure. For this reason, chloroform is not given to patients with respiratory or heart disease.

Cyclopropane is a safe anesthetic gas which has a rapid action and which can be used to maintain anesthesia for comparatively long periods. It is used for all types of surgical operation and is particularly useful in chest surgery and obstetrics.

Ether is a safe volatile anesthetic which is very widely used, both alone and in conjunction with other inhalation anesthetics. It is, however, irritant to mucous membranes, and stimulation of the salivary glands and the gastric mucous membrane leads to post-operative nausea and vomiting. This effect on mucous membranes means that ether cannot be used for chest surgery, or given to patients with damage to the trachea, bronchi, or lungs.

Halothane is a very potent volatile anesthetic which is effective in very low concentrations and has a rapid action. Anesthesia can be maintained for long periods and recovery is rapid.

Nitrous Oxide (laughing gas) is a very safe anesthetic which has a very rapid action. It is used alone for short operations, such as dental extractions, and to induce anesthesia prior to maintenance with longer-acting anesthetics such as ether. It can be used in conjunction with oxygen to maintain anesthesia for longer operations.

Trichloroethylene is slightly less potent than chloroform, but is less toxic. It is used alone for induction of anesthesia and for short operations and, in conjunction with other longer-acting anesthetics, for longer procedures. It does not irritate mucous membranes.

Local Anesthetics

These are drugs which, when applied to the skin or given by injection, produce a loss of sensation in the area of their application. This is brought about because the numbed nerve endings in the skin or mucous surface are temporarily unable to send pain and other impulses to the brain.

The original local anesthetic was cocaine, but as it produces addiction it is seldom used nowadays except for application to the eye. There are three ways of using local anesthetics.

1. Surface Anesthesia. This is produced by applying a local anesthetic to a body surface, where it blocks the sensory nerve endings. Drops containing cocaine or amethocaine are used to deaden pain in the eye while the surgeon removes foreign bodies which have become embedded in the cornea. Lozenges containing a local anesthetic, usually benzocaine, are given to block the nerve endings of the throat and larynx before inserting a stomach tube or a bronchoscope. Benzocaine is also incorporated in ointments used for the relief of pruritus, and in suppositories to relieve the pain of piles.

2. Infiltration Anesthesia. This is the method used in such minor operations as dental extractions and the stitching of small wounds. The local anesthetic is injected into and around the field of operation, usually in conjunction with adrenaline which constricts the blood capillaries in the area, thus preventing the anesthetic from spreading too far. Loss of sensation quickly results, and lasts for an hour or longer. The two drugs which are usually used for infiltration anesthesia are lignocaine and procaine.

3. Spinal Anesthesia. This is a method of general anesthesia which is used in major operations when inhalation methods cannot be used, for example in some types of chest surgery. A local anesthetic is injected into the subarachnoid space of the spinal canal, causing paralysis of the spinal nerves. This method of anesthesia has the advantages of producing complete muscular relaxation, and of causing little or no post-operative shock.

Anesthetics in Dentistry

The most usual method of obtaining anesthesia before dental procedures is to inject a local anesthetic, usually lignocaine or procaine, into the gum beside the tooth which is to be extracted or drilled. The area around the tooth quickly becomes numb, the effect lasting for about an hour before it begins to wear off.

Less widely used now, but at one time very important in dentistry, is nitrous oxide (laughing gas) which is given by inhalation. It produces a short period of unconsciousness, long enough for most dental procedures, and it very rarely has any unpleasant after-effects.

Twilight Sleep

In obstetrics, an alternative procedure to anesthesia is sometimes used. It is known as 'twilight sleep.' The pain of childbirth is reduced by treating the mother with morphine and hyoscine. The effect is said to be due to amnesia (loss of memory), which means that the patient feels pain at the time, but forgets about it, so that the final result is just the same as if there had been no pain at all.

This procedure increases the risk to the infant.

ANTIBIOTICS

The antibiotics are a group of complex chemicals which are produced during the growth of certain micro-organisms. These chemicals have the power of preventing the growth of many species of bacteria other than the one which has produced them. Some antibiotics are very effective against a large number of bacteria causing disease in human beings but others are only useful against a few.

The first antibiotic to be discovered was penicillin, which was isolated from a mold growth by Sir Alexander Fleming in 1928. A great deal of work was done subsequently by Sir Howard Florey and others, and by 1940 penicillin was being manufactured on a large scale. Many other antibiotics have since been isolated, and their contribution to medicine is a very large one. Most of them are prepared from cultures of molds or bacteria, although some can be manufactured synthetically.

Antibiotics fight diseases by preventing or inhibiting the growth of the organisms which cause the disease; they do not necessarily kill the invading organisms but prevent their multiplication. They vary in their activity. Some antibiotics, such as penicillin and streptomycin, are effective against a small range of bacteria and are termed 'narrow-spectrum' antibiotics. Others, such as the tetracyclines, are effective against a wide range of bacteria, and also against some viruses, fungi and rickettsias; they are described as 'broad-spectrum' antibiotics.

The introduction of antibiotics revolutionized the treatment of many infectious diseases, including tuberculosis, typhoid fever, meningitis and syphilis, which at one time were often fatal but which are now curable by antibiotics.

Generally speaking, the antibiotics are very safe and rarely cause toxic effects. A few people may become sensitized to a particular

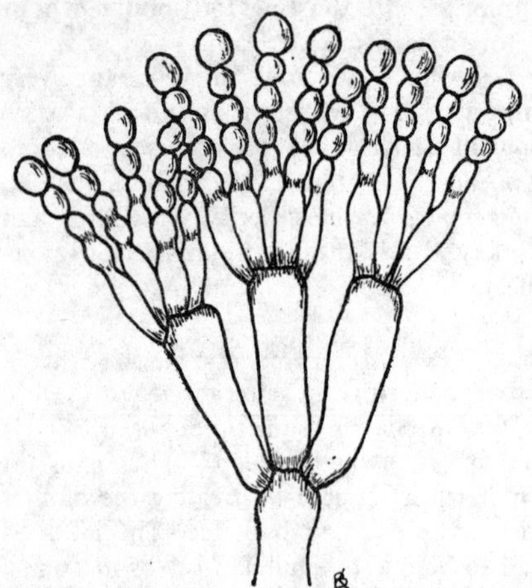

Fig. 16. *PENICILLIUM NOTATUM (magnified). The spore heads of the mold from which penicillin is derived.*

antibiotic so that it makes them ill, but such people are usually able to tolerate a different type of antibiotic instead. Another danger is that strains of bacteria which are at first sensitive to an antibiotic may gradually develop resistance to it, so that it is no longer effective against them. Because of this, most antibiotics are available only on a doctor's prescription and are reserved for the treatment of diseases for which they are really necessary.

Some of the more important antibiotics are discussed below.

The Penicillins are particularly effective against infections caused by the streptococcal bacteria. They are used in the treatment of infected wounds, boils, carbuncles and abscesses, acute tonsillitis, scarlet fever, rheumatic fever, some types of meningitis and of pneumonia, acute osteomyelitis, gonorrhea, syphilis, and yaws. They are given by mouth in tablets or mixtures, or by injection. Penicillin used to be widely used in ointments, eye-drops, ear-drops and lozenges, but external application is now discouraged because too casual and frequent use of penicillin may lead the bacteria to develop a strong resistance. The patient invaded by such resistant bacteria will then find that penicillin is valueless to him.

The early penicillin preparations had to be given by injection frequently, but synthetic penicillins are now made which have a more prolonged and steady action, and which are effective by mouth as well as by injection.

Benzylpenicillin or **penicillin G** is the most widely used antibiotic in the world. It is usually given by injection intramuscularly and only by mouth in mild infections. Fairly frequent dosage, at intervals of two to six hours, is necessary because the drug is rapidly excreted by the body.

Phenoxymethylpenicillin or **penicillin V** is given by mouth, as tablets, capsules, and flavored mixtures. It is excreted more slowly than benzylpenicillin and therefore remains longer in the bloodstream; the dosage is usually every four to eight hours.

Ampicillin is a penicillin which destroys upper respiratory bacteria and is taking the place of tetracycline for that infection. It is also useful in the treatment of urinary infections.

Methicillin is an expensive penicillin which has been found to be effective against some bacteria which are resistant to all other penicillins. It is only effective when given by injection, and used in hospitals for severely ill patients who cannot be cured by other penicillins.

Cloxacillin. For patients only moderately ill this is a useful synthetic penicillin similar to methicillin but it is given by mouth.

The Tetracyclines are a group of broad-spectrum antibiotics which are very similar both in their chemical structure and in their action. The most important members of the group are **chlortetracycline oxytetracycline** and **tetracycline.** They are used in the treatment of a wide variety of infections, including those mentioned above under The Penicillins.

Unlike the penicillins, the tetracyclines are effective against some virus infections, such as psittacosis and Q fever. They are often used in the treatment of infections of the urinary tract, such as amebic dysentery.

The tetracyclines are given by mouth in capsules, tablets, and flavored mixtures. They are also given by injection. Unlike penicillin, they are very effective when applied externally in the treatment of infections of the skin, eyes and ears. Many preparations are available for this purpose, including eye-drops, eye ointments, ear-drops, skin lotions, creams, and ointments.

Streptomycin is a broad-spectrum antibiotic which is very effective against the bacteria which cause tuberculosis. It is given by injection and is of particular value in tuberculous meningitis. It has the disadvantage that resistance to it develops quickly. This can be counteracted by giving it at the same time as other antituberculosis drugs, such as isoniazid and para-aminosalicylic acid. The two latter drugs are usually given by mouth in capsules.

Toxic effects occur more often with streptomycin than with the penicillins or the tetracyclines. The hearing nerves are often affected, and permanent deafness may occur if the treatment is not stopped. Skin rashes often occur.

Chloramphenicol, the first antibiotic to be manufactured synthetically, has been shown to cause serious toxic effects and it is now confined to the treatment of typhoid fever for which it is very effective.

Erythromycin is effective against the same range of bacteria as penicillin but, as it is more toxic, it is reserved for the treatment of penicillin-resistant infections. It is given by mouth in tablets, capsules and mixtures.

Griseofulvin is an antibiotic which, when taken by mouth, has the ability to reach the horny layers of the skin and the hair follicles. When these are infected with ringworm or other fungous skin infections, the griseofulvin halts the infection. It usually takes about four weeks before the hair is replaced on the scalp but sometimes as long as six months before infected nails have regrown healthily. Griseofulvin is usually prescribed as tablets in a dose of up to 1 gram daily.

Neomycin is sometimes used to treat intestinal infections, but it is usually applied externally in creams for skin infections, and in eye-drops for eye infections.

Nystatin is active against fungi. It is used in the treatment of moniliasis, an infection due to a yeast-like fungus which affects the vagina and the intestine. It can be given by mouth, but for vaginal moniliasis it is usually used as pessaries.

Polymyxin B is used in the treatment of infections of the urinary tract.

New antibiotics are still being introduced. They are valuable for the treatment of infections which have become resistant to the better established antibiotics. Among them are cephaloridine for a variety of severe infections; carbenicillin for *Pseudomonas* infections; colistin for enteritis, burns infection, and meningitis; cycloserine for tuberculosis; gentamycin for *Pseudomonas* infection (but it may damage hearing).

VACCINES AND ANTISERA

Antisera

Antisera are preparations of serum, the fluid portion of blood, containing protective factors known as antibodies. To obtain antibodies virulent germs are grown in culture nutrients; the toxins (poisons) they produce, or the germs, are injected into animals (often horses) causing the animals to retaliate and make antibodies in their blood.

When a serum containing antibodies is injected into a patient at the beginning of his illness, the antibodies react against the germs. This is only an emergency remedy—passive immunity. Vaccines are needed for long-lasting active immunity.

Sera are administered by a physician.

Botulinum Antitoxin. For persons who have eaten tainted food but who are slow in showing signs of food poisoning (blurred vision, giddiness, vomiting, difficulty in swallowing) a dose of at least 10,000 units is given intramuscularly; large doses intravenously are given to those already showing signs of poisoning. Only of value early in the disease.

Diphtheria Antitoxin. A large dose of diphtheria antitoxin should be given at the earliest possible moment, whenever there is reason to suspect diphtheria; treatment may be repeated if necessary. May also be used to give passive immunity to contacts.

Scarlet Fever Antitoxin. Although almost entirely superseded by sulphonamides and antibiotics, it is of some value in severe cases.

Streptococcus Antiserum. For Puerperal Fever; Erysipelas; Ulcerative Colitis, etc. Superseded by antibiotics and sulphonamides.

Rabies Antiserum. Only in conjunction with the Vaccine, see below.

Venom Antiserum. Because of the varieties of poisonous snakes, each country has different antisera to counteract the poisons of the snakes which are native to it.

Gas Gangrene Antitoxin (3 types). Used in abdominal surgery for the treatment and prophylaxis of the toxemia of acute abdominal obstruction and peritonitis.

Staphylococcus Antitoxin. For boils, carbuncles, acne, acute periostitis.

Tetanus Antitoxin. The serum should be given in large doses in cases of wounds contaminated by dirt and at the earliest possible moment when tetanus develops. Injections are continued weekly until symptoms abate.

Human Immunoglobulin. This is the fraction of human blood which in normal adults contains the antibodies against disease micro-organisms. It is given by intramuscular injection to protect susceptible contacts of several infectious diseases.

Vaccines

Vaccines are standardized liquids containing killed germs or much weakened living bacteria or viruses or their toxins which retain the capacity to stimulate the production of antibodies in the recipient's blood—active immunity. They are usually given by subcutaneous or intramuscular injection.

Vaccines are administered by a physician. Very few are available commercially.

Catarrh or Cold Vaccines. As prophylactics against common colds.

Cholera Vaccine. For prophylactic use.

Diphtheria Vaccines. To immunize persons against diphtheria and preferably for children under one year old. Natural immunity after 10 years of age is first tested with Schick Test Toxin; reactors are given 1 of 4 forms of vaccine, 2 or 3 doses at 4-week intervals.

Influenza Vaccine. Immunity is short-lived.

Measles Vaccine. A recent product. Two types available—killed virus vaccine and a live attenuated type. They give short protection, the former for about a year, the latter for about 4 years.

Pertussis Vaccine (Whooping-cough Vaccine). Recommended to be given at age of 3 to 6 months to protect vulnerable young children. Three doses are given with intervals of 2 and of 6 months.

Plague Vaccine. For use in contacts.

Poliomyelitis Vaccines. For immunization against poliomyelitis, 3 doses with intervals of 2 and 6 months, starting age 3 months, are advised. This vaccine is given on sugar by mouth. The earlier injection vaccine is much less used now. See p. 107 and p. 266

Pollen Vaccines. For the prevention of Hay Fever.

Rabies Vaccine. For the prevention of rabies in persons bitten by a rabid dog (or other animal). A dose of the Antiserum should be given as quickly as possible, then 14 daily injections of the vaccine; size of dose depends on the severity of the bites.

Tetanus Vaccine. For prevention of tetanus, three well-spaced doses in normal persons will cause production of antibodies which will persist in the blood for a long time. For agricultural and demolition workers, and children. Given in a mixed vaccine (diphtheria, tetanus, and pertussis) to infants.

Tuberculin. Used for diagnostic purposes.

Typhoid-Paratyphoid Vaccine (T.A.B. Vaccine). A widely-used protective against typhoid and paratyphoid. Immunity lasts for 1 to 3 years.

Typhus Vaccine. This lessens the severity of the disease. During an epidemic reinforcing doses should be given every three months. Not commercially available.

Yellow Fever Vaccine. One subcutaneous dose protects against yellow fever for many years. Not for babies under 9 months. Not commercially available.

Mixed Vaccines. Certain simple vaccines may safely be given together in one injection. See p. 107 and p. 266.

OSTEOPATHY

A dictionary definition of osteopathy reads as follows: a system of healing based on the belief that the human body can effect its own cure with the aid of manipulative treatment of the spinal column. The American Osteopathic Association (AOA) carries that definition several steps further. The profession of osteopathic medicine is concerned with the prevention, diagnosis, and treatment of human illness, disease, and injury.

The Doctor of Osteopathy, D.O., is a fully trained physician who prescribes drugs, performs surgery, and selectively utilizes all that modern science offers to maintain and restore the health of his patients. In addition, the D.O. focuses special attention on the biological mechanisms by which the musculoskeletal system, through the nervous and circulatory systems, interacts with all body organs and systems in both health and disease.

The D.O. recognizes that the musculoskeletal system (the muscles, bones, and joints) make up over 60 percent of the total body mass. He or she also recognizes that all body systems, including the musculoskeletal system are interdependent. Because of this interdependency, a disturbance in any one system may cause altered function in other systems of the body. The interrelationship of body systems is effected through the nervous and circulatory systems. The emphasis on the relationship between body structure and organic functioning gives a broader base for the treatment of the patient as a unit.

Physicians and surgeons (D.O.s) use structural diagnosis and manipulative therapy along with all the other more traditional forms of diagnosis and treatment to care effectively for patients and to relieve their distress.

Osteopathic research and practice have shown that disorders of the musculoskeletal system do occur to some degree almost invariably whenever illness is present. At times these disorders are simply outward manifestations of internal distress. At other times they may set off a chain reaction that perpetuates disease and interferes with the body's natural ability to recover. At still other times the disorder itself may trigger the disease process.

The additional care offered through palpation and appropriately applied manipulation provides an added dimension of health care. When used with accepted diagnostic and therapeutic techniques, this becomes a comprehensive health care directed to the whole person.

The Founder of Osteopathy

Andrew Taylor Still was born in Virginia in 1828 and died in 1917. His father was a medical missionary on the western frontier and it was only natural that the young man should follow into the practice of medicine. Dr. Still, a licensed physician, practiced medicine in Kansas and served in the Union Army during the Civil War. He gradually became more and more dissatisfied with the practice of medicine as he found it at that time. Such things as bleeding, purging, and cupping were common attempts at cures at that time. Dr. Still noted that many times the patient was not helped by these crude methods.

Dr. Still did not originally set out to establish a new form of medicine. He simply turned to the study of human anatomy as a means of alleviating suffering. What he found was not well-received by the practicing doctors of his day.

The philosophy and science of osteopathic medicine were first described by Dr. Still in 1874. Dr. Still observed much crude therapy in the practice of medicine, as well as an overuse of drugs.

He felt that disease was the result of "anatomical abnormalities followed by physiological discord." He believed that ill health had a specific cause and that the cause had a location. Perhaps his strongest belief was that in a person's body there is a capacity for health rather than illness and that the body can usually manage to heal itself.

The medical profession of that day did not take kindly to Dr. Still's observations. He was branded by many as unrealistic, unproven, and unscientific. Despite his lack of approval from his peers, Dr. Still continued to practice medicine as he now saw it. He was considered by some patients to be a miracle healer, and he himself had great faith in his ideas. He continued to work in medicine.

In 1892 Dr. Still founded the American School of Osteopathy in Kirksville, Missouri. He states that the purpose was:

"To improve our present system of surgery, obstetrics, and treatment of disease generally, and place the same on a more rational basis and to impart information to the medical profession . . ."

Still's original concept of osteopathy was to exclude the use of most drugs. This was a reaction to an overuse of drugs at the time, which was hindering patient recovery. The early D.O.s used only those drugs that were needed for anesthetics and antiseptics in surgery.

Today the osteopathic doctor works on principles that were begun by Dr. Still. The most important aspect of this is that the body's tendency is toward health and not toward disease. The patient is treated with a combination of manipulation of the musculoskeletal system, drugs, and, if needed, surgery. But the continuing philosophy of the D.O. is that the body is its own best physician.

What is a D.O.?

There are two types of licensed physicians in the United States today. One is the D.O., the Doctor of Osteopathy. The other is the M.D., the Doctor of Medicine. Both of these doctors have taken the prescribed amount of premedical training. Both have usually graduated from an undergraduate college and received four years of training in a medical school. Both take at least one year's internship in a hospital with an approved intern-training program. If the doctor wishes to go into a medical specialty, he then undertakes a further residency program toward that end.

Whether one becomes a D.O. or an M.D., the road toward complete medical training is essentially the same. The difference is that the osteopathic physician receives an additional training in what the osteopathic profession considers a more comprehensive health care.

Eighty-six percent of D.O.s provide primary health care to individuals and families. The remaining 14 percent are specialists in such fields as surgery, radiology, and psychiatry. More than half of all D.O.s are general practitioners located in towns and cities having less than 50,000 people. In many rural communities D.O.s are the only physicians available.

Today osteopathic medicine has been recognized as a separate but equal branch of American medicine. Federal and state governments and private and public health agencies offer the same rights as well as the same professional obligations to the osteopathic physician as they do to the allopathic (M.D.) doctor. Osteopathic physicians are eligible and serving in all branches of the United States armed forces. They serve as medical officers in the Civil Service Commission, U.S. Public Health Service, and the Veterans Administration. They serve as public health officers, coroners, insurance examiners, and school team physicians.

The American Osteopathic Association contends that the osteopathic profession's continuing educational emphasis on general practice rather than on medical specialization best serves the true health care needs of the American public.

The D.O., like all allopathic doctors, must obtain a license to practice from a state licensing board. Each state board sets its own requirements and then issues the license to the physician for use in that state alone. All states in the United States allow osteopathic physicians to provide the same range of professional services as provided by the M.D.

The Training of a D.O.

Admission to a college of osteopathic medicine requires a minimum of three years of preprofessional education in a college or university accredited by a regional educational association. Over 97 percent of all students entering colleges of osteopathic medicine hold bachelor's degrees or higher. A few students are in programs that give a bachelor's degree after three years of undergraduate study plus one year of their professional education.

In addition to a broad cultural background on the undergraduate level, an entering osteopathic student must have completed a required number of hours in physics, biology, and inorganic and organic chemistry. All prospective students must take the Medical College Admissions Test, with scores sent to the osteopathic colleges they wish to attend.

The degree of Doctor of Osteopathy requires four academic years of study: two years devoted to anatomy, physiology, chemistry, pathology, bacteriology, immunology, and pharmacology; and two years devoted to clinical subjects. Inherent in all osteopathic study is the interrelationship of structure and function as a reciprocal factor in health and disease. Structural factors in disease processes are stressed, and students are trained in osteopathic manipulative therapy and in medical, therapeutic, and surgical procedures.

Integrated throughout the curriculum is special instruction in osteopathic principles dealing with the interrelationship of all body systems in health and disease, and special training in osteopathic palpatory diagnosis and manipulative therapy.

After graduation, almost all D.O.s serve a 12-month rotating internship, with primary emphasis on medicine, obstetrics/gynecology, and surgery. This is conducted in an osteopathic hospital approved for such training by the American Osteopathic Association.

D.O.s who wish to become specialists must serve an additional two to four years of residency or fellowship training. To be applicable for formal certification, such training must be approved by the AOA and the appropriate osteopathic specialty board.

All colleges of osteopathic medicine and their affiliated teaching hospitals receive federal and state financial assistance.

Because of the osteopathic profession's high standards, AOA accreditation means automatic participation in government programs such as Medicare and Medicaid.

All 50 states and the District of Columbia provide for the unlimited practice of medicine and surgery by osteopathic physicians.

Osteopathic Hospitals

Some 200 osteopathic hospitals located in 31 states provide more than 25,000 beds for treatment of the sick and injured.

An estimated 825,000 patients are admitted to osteopathic hospitals each year, resulting in some 6.3 million patient-care days of care. In addition, the hospitals' outpatient departments accept some 3.1 million patients each year for emergency and other ambulatory care.

The Federal Government has designated the American Osteopathic Association as the official accrediting agency for osteopathic hospitals participating in the Medicare and Medicaid programs. Those hospitals seeking accreditation must meet the minimum standards of the Medicare law as well as special standards established by AOA for distinctly osteopathic care not provided in other hospitals.

Summary

Osteopathic medicine focuses special attention on the biological mechanisms by which the musculoskeletal system, through the nervous and circulatory systems, interacts with all body organs and systems in both health and disease.

The emphasis is appropriate, since osteopathic research and practice have demonstrated that disorders of the musculoskeletal system, in some degree, almost invariably are present when illness occurs.

Sometimes these disorders are simply outward manifestations of internal distress. At other times they may have a neurologic chain reaction that perpetuates disease and interferes with the body's natural recuperative powers. At still other times the disorder itself may cause the disease.

The differences between the practice and theories of osteopathy and allopathic medicine are matters of differing emphasis rather than a dispute over scientific truth. Osteopathy holds no positions in opposition to established scientific data.

There is an added dimension to osteopathic medicine not always present in allopathic practice. It is the combination of the idea that the body is its own best healer plus the use of good diagnosis and thorough treatment, using all that modern science has to offer. This provides a comprehensive health care directed by the physician to the whole person.

THE FAMILY PET

To give a child the responsibility for the well-being of his own pet, with the consequent discipline of regular feeding and grooming, will implant early in life a sense of kindness and consideration which will be invaluable. The child should be old enough to carry out these duties without undue parental assistance. Rabbits or hamsters are comparatively simple animals to look after, and five- to six-year-olds can usually be entrusted with their care. The more complex and demanding attention needed by a dog is usually within a child's capacity by the age of eight or nine.

It is extremely cruel to keep any pet in unsuitable conditions. However much love is lavished on it, it will suffer if its needs are not properly attended to. Only the small breed of dog should be kept by city dwellers, unless a large garden is available. Neither dogs nor cats should be shut up in an apartment all day without some human companionship. Fish, tropical or cold water, and cage birds are the least demanding of pets and are ideal for apartments.

Whatever the choice, make suitable preparations before buying. Do not keep a bird in the cardboard box, or the fish in the small glass bowl, supplied by the dealer. All pets—mammals, birds, reptiles or fish—need plenty of space, suitable living quarters and regular feeding. Only then will your family enjoy the pleasure and companionship a pet can give.

MAMMALS

Mammals are the group of animals whose females suckle their young during infancy. Most mammals have a hair or fur growth on their bodies. Into this category come all the popular pets—dogs, cats, rabbits, hamsters, etc. They are the most companionable and entertaining of pets but, because of their more complicated natures, they require greater care and attention than the lower species such as birds and fish.

Dogs

An affectionate animal, the dog is easily the most popular domestic pet. There is a wide choice, with a breed suitable for every family whatever the circumstances.

There are two main types: sporting dogs, which by their size are more suitable for country families, and non-sporting dogs which can be divided again into working dogs and toy dogs.

Sporting dogs include terriers, hounds such as whippets used for racing, and gun-dogs like the setters and labradors.

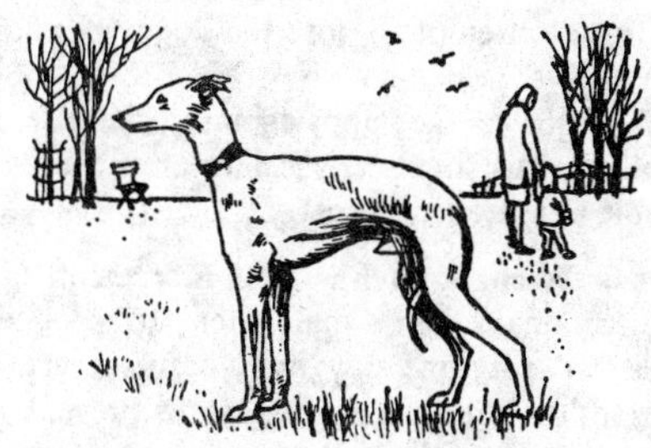

Fig. 1. *WHIPPET: a sporting dog.*

Working dogs include sheep-dogs, collies and the bull mastiff, an excellent watch dog. These are all lively, comparatively big animals and, if kept in cities, should have at least regular access to a park.

Toy dogs are the ideal pet for small houses and apartments. Pekinese, pomeranians, pugs, poodles and Welsh corgis are all excellent, but even they need regular exercise. A walk twice a day plus a game with a ball is often sufficient and is well within the scope of any owner.

Pedigrees. When paying a fair price for a dog which is claimed to be a thoroughbred, your guarantee is the Kennel Club registration certificate, which names the dog's parentage.

The Kennel. If your dog is to live out of doors, the kennel should be slanted and weatherproof, with a bed of clean straw. It should face, where possible, south-west in winter and north-east in summer, and should ideally be raised above ground level. The whole of a dog's run should be of concrete so that it can easily be kept clean. The door should be on the broad side. If the run cannot be enclosed with railings, there may be times when a chain is desirable. A dog must not, however, be kept habitually chained. To give a good measure of freedom a simply erected running chain may be installed (see Fig. 3).

A dog living indoors should have his own bed. A box or basket is best, so that the dog is shielded from drafts. The box may have a mat or cushion, which should be shaken every day. House manners can be easily taught with kindness, and the dog can be expected to go to its bed when told.

Feeding. Two meals a day are best for adult dogs, although many thrive on only one. If the animal is to be alert at night, give the main meal in the morning and only a small amount in the evening; otherwise the two meals can be equal. Keep to a regular time

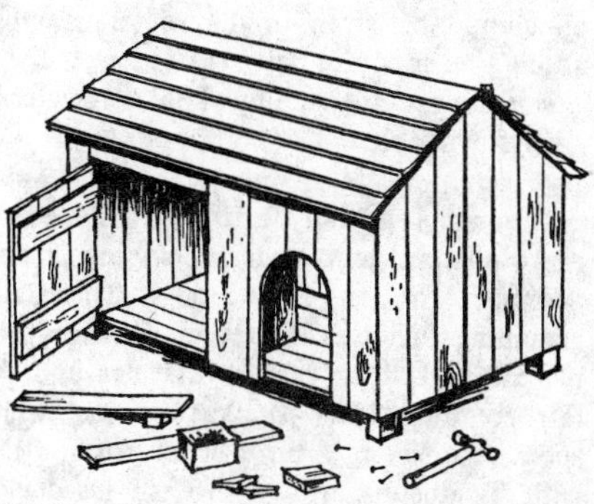

Fig. 2. *THE KENNEL should be raised above ground level to keep the floor dry.*

and on no account give snacks between meals or feed the dog tit-bits from your table, as this makes him a perpetual nuisance and endangers his health. It is important to realize that dogs do not masticate their food, nor does the saliva contain any digestive ferment to break up the starch. The teeth merely reduce food to a size that can be safely swallowed, and this is one reason why correct feeding is of great importance.

MEAT should constitute at least a quarter of the total diet. The remaining three-quarters can consist of household scraps and wholemeal biscuit or stale brown bread. Raw or lightly cooked liver is invaluable since it

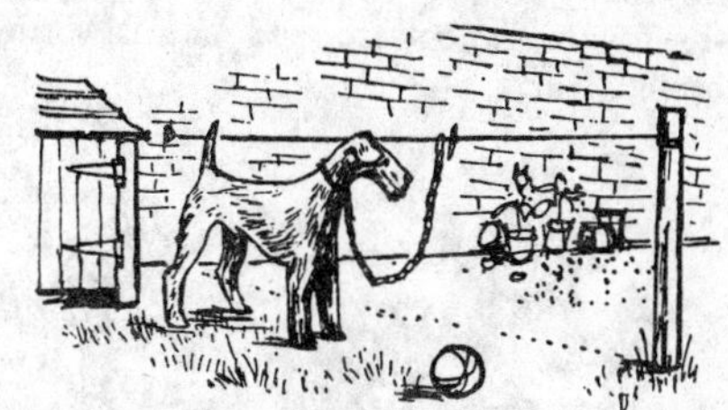

Fig. 3. *A RUNNING CHAIN. An Irish terrier on a running chain has a fair measure of freedom, though he should not be habitually chained.*

contains essential vitamins and minerals. When liver is unobtainable, and particularly during the winter, vitamins can be given in the form of a daily yeast tablet. Fish bones should never be given, neither should the bones of game, poultry or rabbit, which splinter and can cause serious abdominal injury. Oatmeal porridge can be substituted for bread and biscuit. A limited amount of potato cooked in the skin supplies starch and mineral salts.

VEGETABLES are not essential as the dog, unique among domestic pets, is able to manufacture vitamin C in its digestive organs. Nevertheless, such vegetables as cabbage and onions, and, if the dog shows a liking for them, apples and bananas, may be offered from time to time to provide variety.

WEANING. Puppies, for the first few weeks of weaning, require a larger proportion of raw or slightly cooked meat, cut in pieces. The rest of the puppy's diet can be cows' milk, cereal and bread-and-milk. Cod-liver oil should be given in the winter months, about a teaspoonful daily.

It is important that a bowl of fresh water is always available.

Grooming. A daily brushing will keep a dog's coat in good order. Combing is also necessary for long-haired dogs. This daily grooming will quickly reveal whether your pet has picked up vermin. The flea and the less common louse (look for ivory white specks the size of a pin's head) can be dealt with by dusting with a modern insecticide powder containing gammexane. Avoid powders containing dicophane (D.D.T.) as cases of poisoning can occur.

Kindness and human companionship are just as essential as correct feeding. A dog that is shut away from the society of human beings for long periods is always an unhappy dog. So play with your dog and encourage your children to do the same, bearing in mind that very young children sometimes hurt a dog unwittingly.

House training requires patience. The time it will take depends on the age of the dog. A young puppy treated with kindness will very soon understand what is wanted. He will become a perfect companion, always ready to do anything you wish. If a dog is badly treated and his mistakes are roughly punished, the animal's nerve will be destroyed and he will become a coward and untrustworthy through fear.

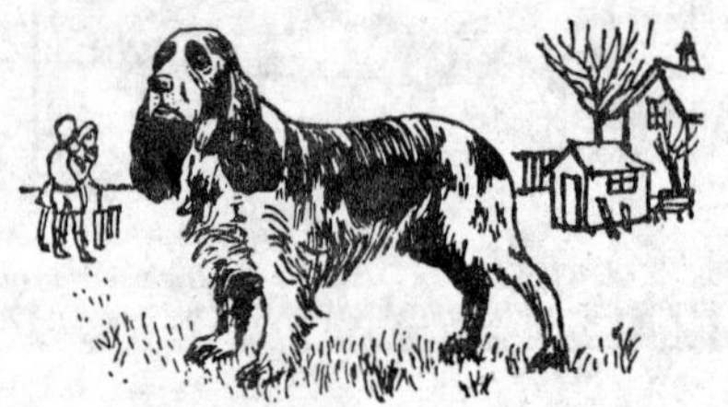

Fig. 4. *COCKER SPANIEL*

Training must be regular and should be given primarily by one member of the family. The aim should be to make the dog recognize and automatically obey certain short words and gestures such as 'Heel,' 'Drop,' 'Good Dog,' 'Bad Dog.' Obedience, especially at first, should be rewarded with pats or tit-bits.

Common Ailments. If a dog has an internal upset he will correct it by fasting for one or two meals. When food is continually refused, consult a veterinary surgeon. Avoid using condition powders: with a well-balanced diet they are superfluous.

Ear irritation should be dealt with by a veterinary surgeon, but a few drops of warm castor oil in the ear will alleviate the condition temporarily.

Signs of more serious illness are easily detected in a normally healthy animal. If he is listless, lacks appetite, vomits or has a distended stomach, call in a veterinary surgeon. Do not attempt to dose the dog with patent remedies.

To protect the puppy against distemper and other virus diseases, vaccines are now available at a moderate cost.

Breeding. A bitch is often more gentle and affectionate than a male. Her period of heat lasts twenty-one days and occurs every six months. The only sure ways to prevent her associating with dogs is to keep her indoors or in a kennel with a wired-in run. Should a mesalliance occur, an injection within 36 hours from a veterinary surgeon can prevent the pregnancy.

The gestation period is nine weeks. There may be any number of puppies in the litter, varying with the breed, but five is the average. It should be unnecessary to interfere with the birth, but a veterinary surgeon should be called in promptly if the bitch appears to be having difficulty.

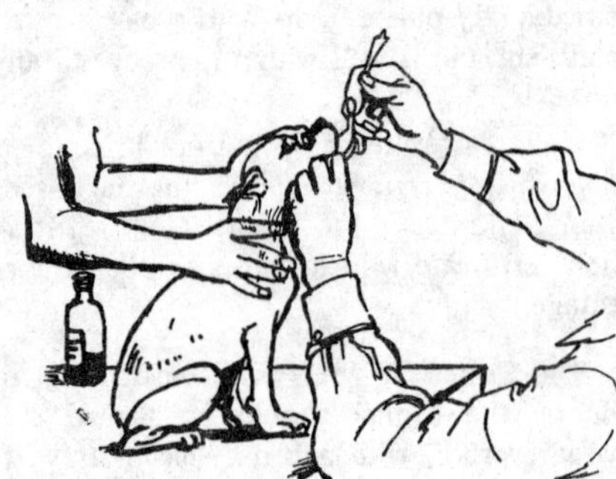

Fig. 5. *GIVING MEDICINE to a boxer puppy.*

Weaning should start after six weeks, when the puppy may be gradually introduced to a more varied diet. This may start with minced or scraped meat. The puppy will need three meals a day at this stage, and the addition of biscuit will help him with his teething. A few drops of halibut- or cod-liver oil and vitamin tablets should be given daily. Bones may be given from the age of six months.

Give the puppy its own basket and begin training it early. Do not over-exercise young puppies or let the children overtire them.

Do not dispose of surplus members of a litter before they are fully weaned, two months is the earliest.

The Law requires that every adult dog have the name and address of its owner on its collar. Neglect of this results in thousands of dogs being irretrievably lost. Should you lose your dog contact the police or the S.P.C.A. (Society for the Prevention of Cruelty to Animals), who find and care for many lost dogs.

A license must be taken out annually for dogs.

Cats

Unlike dogs, cats are nervous sensitive creatures which require especially gentle treatment. Properly looked after, they can be lovable and satisfying pets. It is unwise, however, to allow children to pull them about or squeeze them. They should never be lifted by the skin of the neck after the mother has ceased to carry them in this way.

In the country, cats often prefer to stay out at night, but most town-dwelling cats are safer kept at home and provided with a comfortable bed and a tray. They can roam the house and will keep it free from mice.

Never buy a kitten less than eight weeks old; it may cause permanent ill health to the kitten if it is taken from its mother too early. Watch for bright eyes, a firm body and liveliness. Signs of ill health are dullness, sneezing or coughing, and watery eyes.

A neighbor with unwanted kittens or a pet shop are good sources of supply, but if you contact the local S.P.C.A. they will often be glad to give you a kitten which has been brought in for destruction.

Bedding. A cat likes a warm clean bed. A large box or basket containing a cushion covered in washable material is suitable. The basket should be raised from the ground to avoid drafts.

Feeding. Kittens need three to four meals a day after they cease regular suckling, the amount of solid food being gradually increased. Feed adult cats twice a day with a quantity equal to 1 ounce for every pound of the cat's weight.

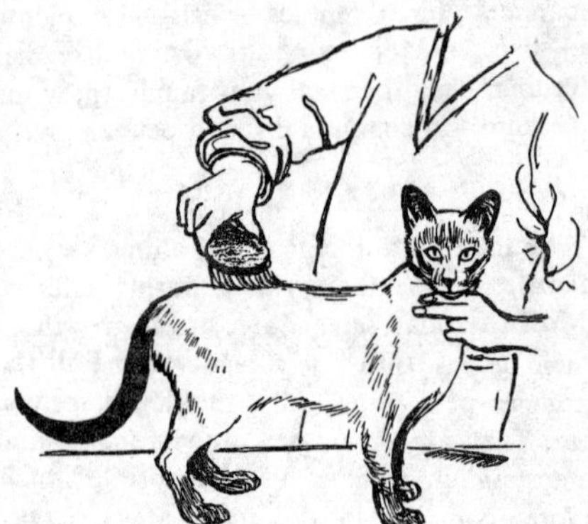

Fig. 6. *GROOMING a blue-point Siamese cat.*

Cooked meat and fish and a little minced raw meat or liver must be given, sometimes mixed with green vegetables. The diet should be varied; it is wrong to feed only with fish and may lead to chronic disease.

The bones of chicken, rabbit, and fish are dangerous as they may pierce the intestines and cause death.

Cats love milk and cream. Where only pasteurized milk is available, a few drops of halibut-liver oil should be added to kittens' food daily, to avoid rickets. Kittens also benefit by yeast.

Fresh water should always be available, especially in summer.

General Care. Although cats are extremely clean in their habits, regular brushing and combing are beneficial especially during molting time to prevent the formation of hairballs (the hairballs are an accumulation of the furry particles swallowed by the cat when grooming itself), a source of stomach upset. Should fleas or other skin parasites appear, gammexane dusting-powders are better than bathing. Dust the cat lightly all over, and repeat after a week. This applies also to the cat's bed. Brush out most of the powder two or three hours after treatment. Do not use D.D.T. powders.

Provide a box or tray filled with sand, dry earth or soft peat litter. The box, about eighteen inches square, should always stand in the same place and should be regularly cleaned, otherwise the cat will not use it. With a little patience the cat can be trained always to use this tray.

A cat's collar should be of half-inch wide elastic, never of leather or ribbon as the cat may be caught up and strangled.

Ailments. Never dose a cat with patent medicines except on veterinary advice. Ear irritation, with scratching and shaking of the head, is a common trouble caused by tiny mites inside the ear. Pour a few drops of warm olive or castor oil into the ear as a temporary relief before seeking expert help. Wax appearing on the surface of the ear may be wiped away, but do not poke around inside.

Never apply kerosene or gas to a cat's skin. It will prove poisonous owing to the cat's habit of licking off everything on its fur.

If the cat has a skin disease or watery eyes, vomits or shows other signs of ill health, consult a veterinary surgeon or an S.P.C.A. clinic.

Breeding. Cats have two or three litters per year with a gestation period of around 65 days. A cat about to have kittens should have a comfortable bed in a warm sheltered spot where she will be undisturbed. Unwanted kittens should be removed immediately, but it is advisable to leave one or two for the mother to bring up. It is easier to find homes for males than females. If all the kittens must be destroyed or are born dead, move the mother to a fresh bed in another room immediately and keep her from the place of birth for several days.

Drowning of unwanted kittens is not recommended. If possible, take them either to a veterinary surgeon or an S.P.C.A. free clinic for destruction.

'Doctoring' of males is best done by a veterinary surgeon when the kitten is three to four months' old. Females can be operated on quite painlessly at around five months.

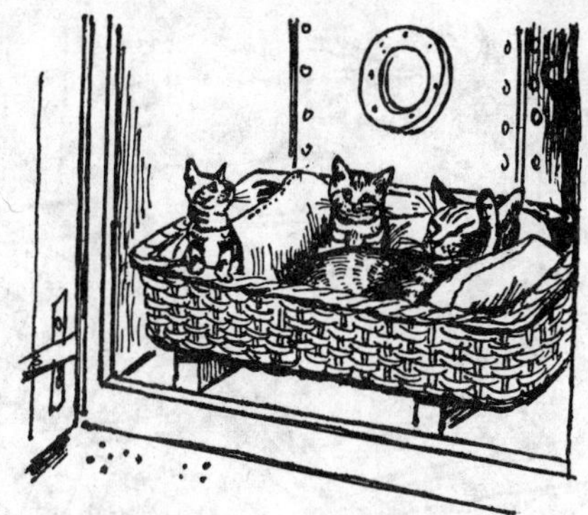

Fig. 7. *MOTHER CAT WITH KITTENS in a basket in a warm dry cupboard.*

Moving Home. Cats moved to a new home will occasionally return to old surroundings. To prevent this, the cat should be shut up in the new house for forty-eight hours, fed as usual, and provided with the earth tray. Let the cat roam about its new home but keep the windows closed. Allow it out for the first time about twenty minutes before feeding time; this ensures its return in almost every instance.

Guinea-pigs

(Cavies)

Breeds are generally divided into smooth- and rough-coated varieties. The long-haired Peruvian and the rosette-haired Abyssinian are most prized, but the coloring and breeds available increase each year.

A healthy guinea-pig is alert, bright-eyed and inquisitive, and has a firm compact body.

A suitable home should be provided before the animal is acquired. A box 2½ feet wide, 18 inches high and 18 inches from front to back is a good size for three guinea-pigs. Small-meshed wire netting should cover the front, with a door taking up a third of the width to make cleaning easy. Bedding may be hay or straw and should be changed weekly. Make sure the cage is rat-proof.

In summer, guinea-pigs benefit from being placed in a wire netting hutch on the lawn. The bottom should be covered with two-inch mesh wire netting to allow them to nibble the blades of grass.

Feeding. Guinea-pigs are voracious animals and should be fed a mixed diet two or three times a day. They will do well on bread and milk, with oats; warm milk is necessary in cold weather. Greenstuff such as watercress, and carrot tops and roots are essential. They should be put in a rack so that they do not become soiled. Rice, bran, barley or oatmeal can be given dry or mixed with a little water. Keep the dishes clean and remove unwanted food after the meal.

A plentiful supply of clean fresh water should always be available.

Breeding. It is usual to keep one male in a hutch with two females but at breeding time give the female a hutch to herself. The babies move at about three days old and should not leave their mother for a month.

General Care. Guinea-pigs are very timid and should not be handled often. Lift, when necessary, by holding just above the shoulder or by placing the thumb on one side, just under the forelegs, and the fingers on the other side.

Brush long-haired varieties with an ordinary hairbrush, every day. Do not use a comb. The guinea-pig should be trained to sit quietly on the palm while being groomed.

Golden Hamsters

White, piebald, cream and many other colors are now available through cross-breeding.

The ears of a young hamster should be covered with lots of fine silky hairs. As the animal ages, the ears become quite bare and shiny. When buying, look for a plump body covered with soft thick fur. The eyes should be examined for tumors.

A fully grown hamster is about five to six inches long. It should be without scars or sores of any kind. Choose a male for a young child; females are peevish when in season.

Housing. A cage should be at least 24 inches by 12 by 9 inches and made from hardwood at least five-eighths of an inch thick, as hamsters gnaw continually to keep their teeth in trim. No sleeping compartment is needed. The floor should be covered with sawdust and hay (not straw), changed frequently. Clean and odorless, the hamsters may be kept in the house or in a warm mouse-proof shed, but not in the open. When the weather is cold, they hibernate and look stiff and dead; leave them to awaken naturally. Hamsters must be kept in separate cages or they are likely to fight.

Feeding. The basic food is a puppy meal mash and table scraps (boneless meat or fish, egg, bacon rind, cheese, etc.). Oats or baked bread may be substituted. Leave dry food always at hand, and give about a tablespoonful of mash plus green food daily. Regular supplies of clean water or milk should be given in a small heavy pot.

Breeding. If kept warm, hamsters breed all the year round, coming into season every four or five days, but the main season is April to October. The gestation period is sixteen days, during which the female should not be moved or handled. The average number born is eight. The babies stay in the nest for eighteen to twenty-one days but begin to eat after five. Make sure the mother has ample nourishing food or she may eat her young. Sex the litters at about four weeks, and keep each sex group together in a cage until around eight weeks when they must be caged singly. Hamsters must be fourteen weeks' old before breeding.

Mice

Colors available include white, speckled grey, black, black-and-tan, brown, lilac, orange, and yellow. A healthy mouse has a thick glossy coat and bright eyes. Watch for and avoid any skin blemishes.

Housing. For three mice a cage must be not less than 18 inches long by 8 inches deep by 8 inches high; preferably it should be higher so that it can accommodate ladders and swings. Do not use revolving wheels. Hay bedding and sawdust must be changed at least once a week. Attach a nesting box for breeding. However clean the cage, there will inevitably be a slight 'mousey' odor.

Feeding. Feed morning and evening with a tablespoonful of oats or seed for each mouse. Dryish bread and milk is a good evening meal. Take away uneaten food, but leave a little green food such as watercress or dandelion, or some carrot. Give fresh water daily.

Breeding. Between six and twelve are born to a litter, nineteen to twenty-one days after mating. The young mice should be taken from the mother after three weeks and it is advisable to separate the sexes at this time as they might fight.

Never disturb the babies until they come out of the nest or the mother may kill them.

Do not breed from them until at least ten weeks old.

General Care. Handle the mice often to tame them. Lift by the root of the tail and put on your hand at once. A mouse will soon be content to stay on your hand if you stroke him lightly with one finger and groom his fur with a silk handkerchief.

Consult a veterinary surgeon for fungoid growths, lumps or tumors.

Rabbits

Gentle and easy to handle, the rabbit is an ideal pet for a child. Its average life is four to five years.

POPULAR TYPES OF RABBITS

For Food	*For Fur*	*To Show*
Flemish Giant	Champagne	Flemish Giant
Belgian Hare	Sitky	English
English	Angora	Dutch
Japanese	Chinchilla	Tan
Silver	Lilac	Silver
	Himalayan	Himalayan

Housing. Rabbit hutches should be large and have two compartments, the smaller one for sleeping. Cover the roof with tarred felt and let it project three to six inches over the front. If possible, the hutch should face south-west. Cover the floor with peat-moss litter, or with sawdust and straw, or wood chips. Clean regularly. Give the rabbits frequent excursions on a lawn in the summer.

Several does can be kept in one hutch. Bucks should be on their own since they tend to be unfriendly and do not make good pets.

Feeding. Feed rabbits twice daily. Grass, hay, greenstuffs and root crops are good. Bran mash can be fed, particularly in winter.

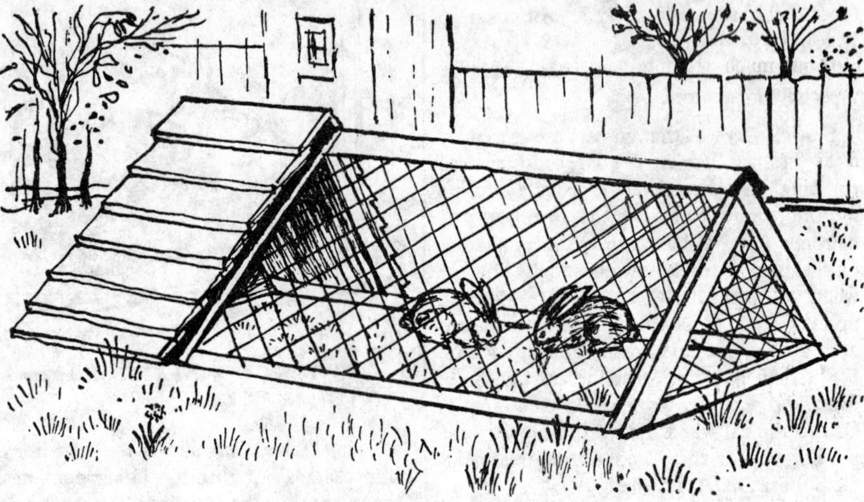

Fig. 8 *RABBITS IN A HUTCH. Excursions on the lawn in fine weather keep the rabbits fit and healthy.*

Never give frozen greenstuffs, raw green potatoes, rhubarb, foxglove, geranium, or any evergreen.

Remove all stale food and give fresh water in scrupulously clean bowls.

Breeding. Rabbits should not be bred from until nine months old. Mate young with old and put the buck and doe back in their own cages afterwards. The gestation period is around one month, and ten or more young may be born. They should, however, be reduced to eight at the most. Do not take them from the mother until they are at least six weeks old.

Hold a rabbit by the loose skin behind the head and support the body on the other hand.

Claws, if too long, should be trimmed with sharp pliers.

Flying Squirrels

Although expensive to buy, these unusual animals are easy and economical to keep.

They can be kept at room temperature in a parakeet breeding cage.

Feed on a little rolled oats, nuts, sunflower seed and greenstuff.

Flying squirrels breed readily in captivity and are easily tamed. They will swoop down on their owners from doors and picture rails with their wing-like membranes outstretched. They sleep by day, waking, as evening approaches, for food and exercise. Do not release the flying squirrel out of doors, although he appreciates an outing in the cage.

The mother has her young around February and should have a separate cage and plenty of nesting material. There are usually two to four to a litter and they must not be disturbed before they are four weeks old.

Chipmunks

The chipmunk, which originates in the Rocky Mountains, is about two inches in size and has a bushy tail and unbelievably bright eyes. He will be tame when you buy him and remains active throughout the year.

A pair will live in a two-foot square cage, with a sleeping box and an exercise wheel.

Feeding is extremely cheap— a few acorns, a small piece of raw meat twice weekly, and a few oats or sunflower seed daily. Occasionally give a small piece of fruit.

Rarely ill, chipmunks need no special attention.

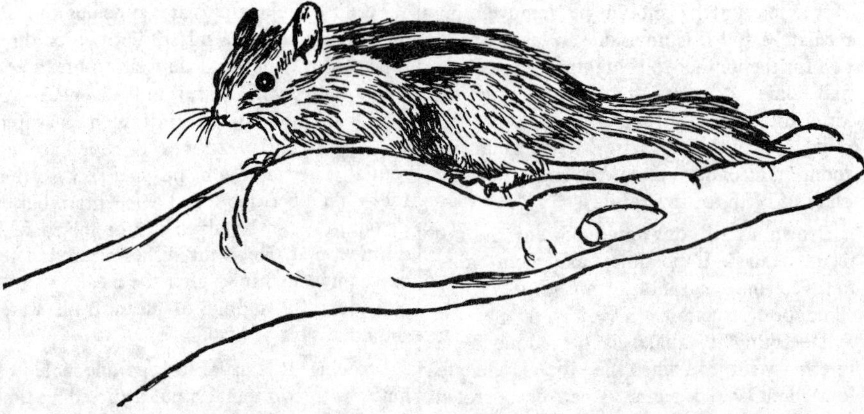

Fig. 9. *AN ADULT CHIPMUNK is only about two inches long, and is very tame.*

BIRDS

Wild birds should not be restricted to cage life, but much pleasure can be obtained by observing their habits in a natural environment and by providing them with food and a bath in your garden.

Cage birds can be divided into four groups.

1. Canaries.
2. Parakeets.
3. Foreign birds.
4. Native birds.

Canaries and parakeets are domesticated and make ideal pets, clean, entertaining and inexpensive both to buy and feed. Foreign birds such as the zebra finch and Java sparrow are also good family pets and are gaining in popularity.

Cage birds are naturally cheerful and sunloving creatures. It is not cruel to keep them in captivity. Canaries and parakeets have through generations become completely adjusted to cage life. If they escape, they are glad to return to the familiarity of their cage at the earliest opportunity.

Canaries

Canaries were brought from the Canary Islands between the thirteenth and fourteenth centuries and were the earliest domestic bird in the U.S.A. There are three varieties.

1. Type canaries, distinguished by certain shapes, e.g. the Yorkshire canary.

2. Singing canaries, the best known being the Roller, insignificant in appearance but with a superb song.

3. Color canaries. Yellow, blue, brown and white are basic, with infinite varieties.

Only the cock bird sings and it is therefore more expensive to buy than the hen. Unlike the parakeet, if kept alone a canary may cease its song.

The same type of cage or aviary described for a parakeet is also suitable for a canary. They adapt well to outdoor conditions providing they are not exposed to extreme cold. Canaries are particularly fond of bathing, so supply either a hanging pot or a saucer of water two or three times a week.

Feeding. Packaged canary seed can be purchased in pet stores.

Green food should be a regular item. Canaries will eat almost any type, particularly seeding grass and lettuce. Be sure it is fresh and uncontaminated with weedkiller, etc.

To digest their food, coarse sand or grit is needed, and a cuttle-fish bone provides essential minerals.

General Care. Accustom the bird to your voice and to your hand in the cage. It can then be brought out and allowed to fly round the room, returning to the cage when it is tired.

Ten years is the average lifetime of a canary.

Molting occurs in late summer or early autumn. Give a richer food mixture at this time and let the canaries bathe each day. If the canary seems off-color, isolate it, keep it warm and check the diet. Then call in expert advice.

Breeding takes place from April to July. If in condition, the cock will be in full song, while the hen is restless and flies back and forth calling. Put them in a roomy box-type breeding cage with a nest lined with felt. Put in a little nesting material, which can be bought in packets. Give the hen a little hard-boiled egg with crumbled biscuit each day.

The four or five eggs will be hatched within fourteen days. Do not disturb the nest or the hen may desert the eggs. After hatching, give soft food, or the hard-boiled egg mixture, or a proprietary egg food, two or three times a day. Remove uneaten food.

The cock will gradually take over the feeding of the young until the chicks are fledged at twenty-one days. The hen then begins to make another nest.

Parakeets

The most recently domesticated bird species is the parakeet. They have now ousted canaries as the most popular cage bird, and, for the beginner, they are the simplest to manage.

Almost every possible color is available. Among the best known are yellow, sky blue, violet, mauve, grey, dark and light green. The two main groups are blue and green, all other colorings being a variation or mutation produced by cross-breeding.

An adult bird's sex is easily identified by the color of the skin above the nostrils (the cere). The hen has a brown or cream cere whereas the cock's is bright blue. A young bird is more difficult to determine, but the male usually has a pinkish mauve cere.

One bird will live quite happily alone and will become more tame than a pair. A cock is a better pet than a hen.

Accommodation. The cage should be as large as possible and have two perches. An adequate breeding cage is at least 3 feet by 15 inches by 15 inches. An outdoor aviary is quite suitable, provided the sleeping quarters are dry and draft-free. The aviary should be made from half-inch wire mesh, the bottom of which should be buried about a foot below the soil to prevent rats from getting in. Make the perches from tree branches, excluding yew, laurel and privet which are harmful. Provide artificial heating in very severe weather.

Keep both the indoor cage and the aviary out of the direct rays of the sun and away from winds.

A swing can be put in the cage and a mirror or ping-pong ball, but an excess of toys tends to impede flight and harm the birds.

Feeding. Seeds, such as white millet and canary seed, plus greenstuff form the staple diet. These must be augmented by a cuttle-fish bone, grit placed in a small pot, and salt in the form of sea sand or rock salt mixed with the usual grain.

Lettuce leaves, cabbage, spinach and water-cress are liked by the parakeet and should be washed first. Do not give bruised or frosted leaves. Apple, carrot and orange pieces are all welcome additions.

Water must always be available and should be changed daily.

Taming. The process of taming requires gentleness and patience. Talk to your bird whenever you go near the cage and put your hand through the door, keeping quite still if he flutters and shows fear. Then softly stroke his head with the fingertip. After a while he will hop on your finger—a spray of millet seed on your hand may hasten the process. Talking continuously, withdraw your hand from the cage, avoiding any sudden movement. Before bringing the bird out of its cage, shut the doors and windows of the room. If the bird flies off, do not chase it. When it settles, approach gently and use the same technique to bring it on to your hand.

A parakeet kept on its own from babyhood will nearly always learn to talk, sometimes in a few weeks, sometimes at four to six months old. Repeat phrases constantly in a clear voice.

Breeding. With healthy stock, breeding is a simple matter. The season is from spring to late summer and two or three broods a year can be bred.

To tell whether the birds are in condition, look for firm plumage and increased activity. To be successful more than one pair of birds should be kept, in the same room if not in the same cage.

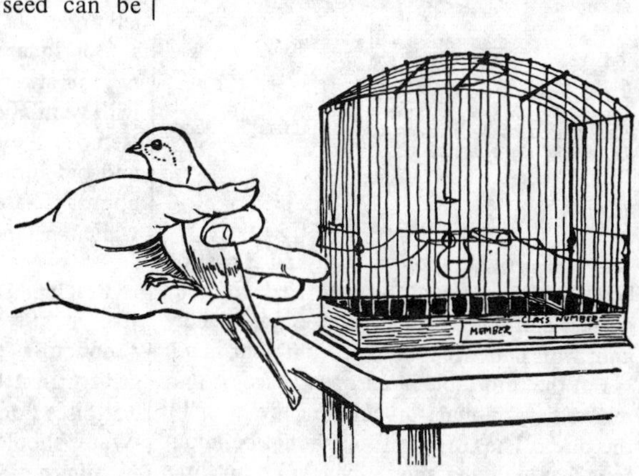

Fig. 10. *CANARY. A clear yellow canary: showing correct method of holding the bird.*

Supply a wooden nesting box, enclosed except for a circular hole. One side should be hinged or sliding to permit inspection. The base, removable for cleaning, must be concave so that the eggs do not roll. No nesting material is required. Supply two boxes, one for each pair, to prevent fighting. Five or six eggs, pure white in color, appear after a week or so of nesting. They are laid on alternate days and incubation commences after the first is laid and takes around seventeen days. The nesting box can be inspected without worrying the hen.

Plenty of fresh green stuff is important and cuttle-fish bone should always be available.

Four or five weeks will elapse before the birds are fully feathered and ready to leave the nest.

General Care. A saucer of tepid water can be put in shortly before the cage is cleaned as parakeets like to bathe.

Ruffled plumage, closed eyes, sleepiness, sneezing and coughing indicate a chill. Put the sufferer in a warm place on its own and keep the temperature constant. Give a teaspoonful of brandy or whisky in water.

A cold, causing running nostrils, can be treated by smearing menthol vaseline on the nostrils and by sprinkling the cage floor with eucalyptus. Again, isolate the bird.

Thinness and moulting can sometimes be corrected by giving sugar and rolled oats plus regular cod-liver oil.

But in all cases of ill health, take the bird to a veterinary surgeon.

Small Foreign Birds

Buy birds that are acclimatized to a temperate climate and they will be found hardy and cause very little trouble. Small finches and waxbills are especially suitable and may be kept safely in co-habitation.

Accommodation. Most foreign birds prefer a temperature of 45° F, but if there is a slight drop it will not worry them. A tubular electric heater will ensure a suitable heat during the winter months. Supply plenty of lukewarm water for bathing.

A standard bird cage, with narrow mesh for the smaller finch-type birds, is suitable. Many will live in an outdoor aviary if it is dry, draftproof, well lit and heated in extreme cold.

General Care. Indian millet and canary seed are basic foods, with white millet for the larger species. Green food is necessary, and some foreign birds are insectivorous. Grit and fresh water are just as necessary as for other birds.

Although most foreign birds can be released in a closed room, they are not as amenable to handling as parakeets and canaries and are more highly strung.

Most species will breed successfully under normal conditions.

The first treatment for a sick bird is warmth. It is advisable to consult a veterinary surgeon in cases of illness.

Parrots

Brilliantly colored, the parrot is also intelligent, an accomplished mimic and capable of becoming exceptionally tame. A drawback is the destructive beak, which precludes keeping a parrot in an aviary planted with shrubs or ornamental trees: it would tear the vegetation to shreds.

A strong spacious metal cage is essential, and the bird should be allowed out as often as possible. A spray should be used to bathe the parrot at least once a week.

A good seed mixture consists of sunflower and canary seeds with millet, hemp and peanuts added. The bird also needs fruit and greenstuff. Grit and plentiful water must always be provided.

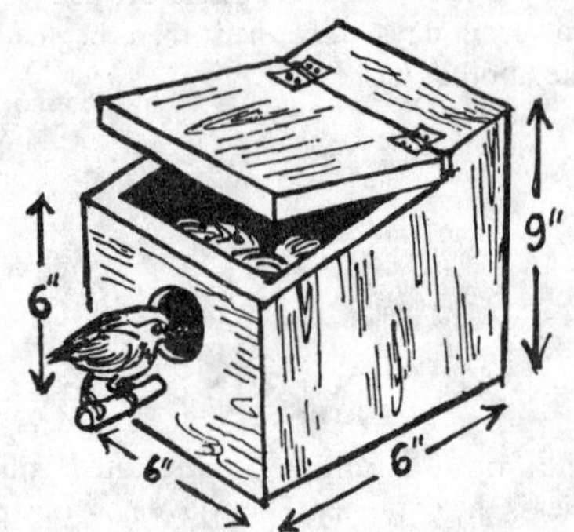

Fig. 11. *NESTING BOX for use in the garden.*

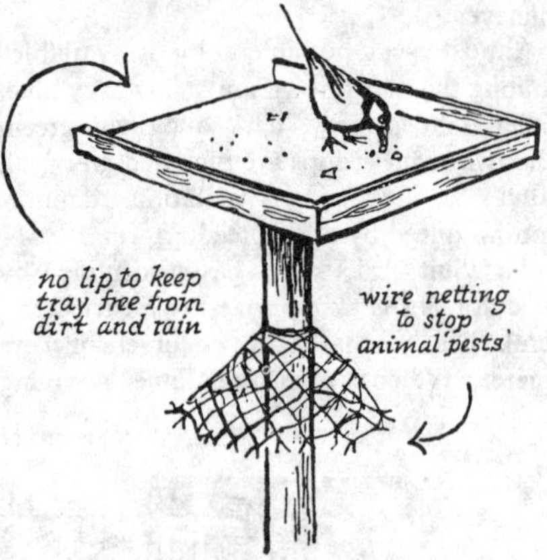

Fig. 12. *A BIRD TABLE should be about four feet above the level of the ground.*

Garden Friends

If you provide food, a bath and a nesting box, wild birds will be attracted to your garden and some will become quite friendly and, with patience, even eat from your hand.

Put the bird table in an open space so that marauding animals or children are seen by the birds. The tray for food should be about four feet high and should have a lip on three sides, the fourth being left open to allow stale food to be swept away.

Put out household scraps, grain and bread soaked in warm water in winter time. Pieces of suet and bacon rinds are appreciated by thrushes and blackbirds. Bones will be picked clean by insect eaters such as tits and robins.

At a distance from the table have a pole with horizontal perches on which you can place coconuts, millet sprays, nuts and swinging perches.

A simple wooden nest box will be used by almost all birds, but do not disturb them too much; birds like privacy. Fix the box not less than eight feet from the ground, facing north.

Place the bird bath away from food tables and have a dripping tap or fountain, if possible, for clean drinking water.

REPTILES

Reptiles are cold-blooded creatures which hibernate when living in cold climates. They are less responsive to human attention than mammals or birds, but many of them are a delight to keep by reason of their fascinating habits, coloring and movements.

Tortoises, lizards, chameleons, salamanders, alligators and other reptiles can be kept, and these more unusual kinds are growing more popular.

Tortoises

Land tortoises are the most common reptile kept as pets. They are imported from the Mediterranean shores and much suffering is caused to them on their journey when they are packed in layers in deep baskets. Buy a tortoise not later than July, as after this it will probably never become acclimatized and will die in the winter. The life span can be 100 years and more if the creature is well cared for.

If the eyes and mouth of a newly acquired tortoise are caked with mucus, bathe them in warm water so that the eyes open fully and the animal can eat and drink.

Housing. Tortoises must not be kept indoors. Provide a small cave or shelter in the garden during the summer months. Around October, when the tortoise becomes lethargic, place him in small box not less than a foot square. Fill the box with dry leaves, hay or straw, and cover with a lid pierced with ventilation holes. This will keep out rats. Remove the tortoise on a sunny spring day, and put him in a small bath of warm water about one-and-a-half inches deep, for a short while, keeping his head clear of the surface.

Feeding. Tortoises are vegetarians and will live happily on the greenstuff and weeds found in a garden. Protect precious plants with wire netting. Milk is not advisable, but tortoises do like brown bread soaked in jam. Water should always be provided.

Ailments. Ticks should be dusted with a gammexane insect powder and removed with tweezers after an hour. Do not use D.D.T.

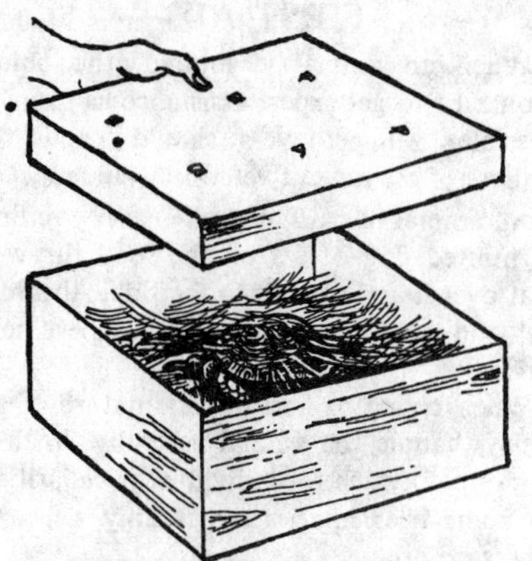

Fig. 13. *TORTOISE HIBERNATING for the winter in a box with dry leaves and hay. The box lid is pierced with ventilation holes.*

Dress cracks in the shell with flavine oil emulsion. Also rub it occasionally with olive oil, then clean with a dry cloth. Never pierce the shell in order to tie the tortoise to a lead.

If any other signs of illness appear, consult a veterinary surgeon.

Terrapins

These water tortoises have webbed hind feet and can be kept in a garden pond in summer. Put them in a heated tank or in a greenhouse in winter. They can be kept together with salamanders, newts, frogs or young alligators, but they will attack and kill fish.

They will eat almost anything. Aquatic vegetation and snails, fish and raw meat are suitable.

Terrapins do not breed in captivity.

Sunshine and clean water are necessary to health. Change the tank water three times a week. When handling, avoid their sharp mouths. Terrapins can be tamed with patience and by hand-feeding.

Other Reptiles

Lizards, salamanders, newts, chameleons, alligators and snakes are all reptiles which make interesting pets.

The slow-worm is the only variety of lizard to thrive in captivity. About a foot long, it can be distinguished from snakes by the fact that it has eyelids. Its body is scaled.

Keep slow-worms in a moist atmosphere and feed on spiders and earthworms. They hibernate in autumn until May when they breed. A large tank with moist sand, rocks and some plants makes a suitable home.

Newts and salamanders, which are amphibians, are best kept in an aquarium half filled with water, with rocks and plants projecting well above the surface. Cover the tank to lessen evaporation of the water, and also to prevent the amphibians escaping. Feed with small fish, earthworms or flies. If the creatures breed, transfer the newly hatched larvae to a separate tank and feed them on small water insects and pieces of earthworm. Newts and salamanders may die if handled too frequently.

Chameleons are hardy and easy to keep. The color changes happen very slowly and are due to their mood, health and the time of the day.

House them in a lidded tank in a warm spot. Put washed sand and a few plants in the bottom and keep the sand moist. Feed on small flies, moths and a little soft fruit from your hand, which will help to tame the chameleon.

Alligators are comparatively expensive to buy but cheap and interesting as pets. The vivarium should consist of a tank containing plants, rocks, and a pool about 4 inches deep. Control the water temperature at about 80°F. Supplement natural sunlight with an electric bulb to give a total of 12 hours a day.

Alligators will never outgrow their habitat. Put an eight-inch baby in a tank eighteen inches long and it will grow to eighteen inches. Transfer the alligator to a larger tank, and it will begin to grow again.

Feed on raw fresh meat, fish, worms and frogs.

If handled frequently—hold just behind the head so that he cannot turn and bite—your alligator will become tame and friendly.

Snakes, such as the grass and water snakes, make reasonably good pets and can be kept in a garden terranium. The center should be mound-shaped and surrounded by a concrete ditch filled with water.

All snakes are carnivorous. Grass and water snakes will only take young frogs. Four-lined snakes, imported from South Europe and West Asia, eat frogs and small mice, as does the dark green snake.

Snakes breed in springtime and the eggs should be kept buried in moist sand at a temperature of about 75°F, not in direct sunlight.

Most snakes hibernate in winter. They should not be fed frequently at this time unless kept in an artificially heated atmosphere. Several times a year the snake sheds its skin. A moist atmosphere will help, but do not attempt to assist this entirely natural process.

FISH

Fish, particularly the cold water varieties, are amusing and less trouble to keep than birds or mammals. The more common varieties are cheap to buy and, once installed in their tank, cost very little indeed in upkeep.

Goldfish

Goldfish originated in the fresh waters of eastern Asia.

The color may be white, orange, red or black, or a combination. Fancy goldfish are more delicate and should not be kept outdoors in winter. The normal goldfish is very hardy, however, and suffers no harm even should the pond water freeze. Barring accidents, goldfish live for six or seven years.

Housing. Do not keep goldfish in a round bowl. A rectangular indoor tank should have one gallon of water for each pair of fish. Plant weeds in sand on the bottom and clean the tank by siphoning the water into a bucket every week. Once a balance is established between the fish and plants, a complete change of water is unnecessary. Provided the deposit on the bottom is cleared out regularly, the water should stay quite clear.

Wait until sand and weeds have settled before introducing the fish. Place the aquarium out of direct sunlight and avoid sudden temperature changes.

In a garden pond little extra care is needed once the pool is established with a plentiful growth of water plants. These aerate the water, harbor food and provide the fish with shelter.

Apart from the aggressive stickleback, all other cold water fish may be kept safely with goldfish. Small water snails are useful as they act as scavengers.

Feeding. Prepared fish food is quite adequate but, if the fish are in an aquarium, offer them fresh food such as earthworms, bread crumbs, water fleas and insects. In an outdoor pond the fish will find their own fresh food, but if you give them small earthworms regularly they will become tame.

Breeding. Spawning takes place from May to August. The eggs, which are attached to plants, will hatch within a week and it is advisable to remove the eggs, with the plant, to a separate aquarium. Goldfish are cannibals and the parents will probably eat their eggs if they are left together.

The young fish will find their own food in a pond. In an aquarium, give them green water from a flower vase, supplemented by a little sieved egg yolk. After a month they can be fed with daphnia (water fleas).

Diseases

FUNGUS, a white spongy appearance on the skin, is highly infectious, so segregate the fish immediately. It is usually caused by insufficient cleaning of the tank or by a sudden temperature change. Disinfect the whole tank with strong permanganate of potash solution.

HARD DROPPINGS. If the droppings cling to the fish, it is constipated. Sprinkle a minute quantity of epsom salts on the water and give some raw food such as earthworm.

BLADDER DISEASE is present when the fish loses its balance and finds swimming difficult. It is incurable but not infectious.

SLIGHT AILMENTS can often be cured by putting the fish in green water, but it is often kinder to destroy. Consult an expert before doing this.

Use a net to catch goldfish and do not handle them.

Tropical Fish

All tropical fish must be kept in specially heated tanks at about 75°F. A thermostat will ensure a constant temperature.

Be careful in selecting the fish. Some species will fight, and the male and females of some types will attack each other. Barbels, guppies, live bearers, mollies, sword-tails, angels and zebras will live in harmony. Tetras, jewel fish and fighting fish should be segregated.

Housing. With a thermostat heater and possibly an aerator, a tank of minimum size (about one and a half cubic feet) is expensive but it will last for many years.

Keep the correct temperature constant, do not overcrowd a tank, provide plenty of plants to ensure sufficient oxygen and regularly clean out the excreta and other deposits on the bottom.

Segregate any fish which shows signs of illness, in order to prevent contagion.

Never handle fish: use a net very gently.

Feeding. Most of the prepared foods on the market are suitable, but live food should be given in addition, daphnia, shrimp pieces and garden worms all being appreciated. As a tonic, a little green water, taken from a flower vase in which the vegetation has decayed, is excellent.

Breeding. Breeding tropical fish is not advised for beginners, for it is a complex undertaking. Three or more tanks, each with carefully regulated temperature, are necessary, as males and females will fight and the eggs must be removed to prevent the parents devouring them.

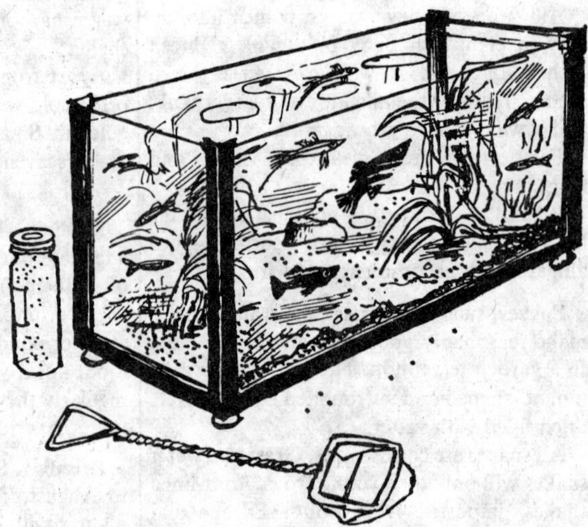

Fig. 14. *TROPICAL FISH IN TANK, containing black mollies, sword-tails and zebra fish. The net is to remove fish.*

VACATIONS

When you arrange to go away on vacation, do make adequate arrangements for your pet. It is not, as a rule, advisable to take a pet with you. In strange surroundings a dog or cat may be lost, or wander out on the sand and be cut off by the tide.

Animals, on the whole, are happier if left in capable hands at home even though they may pine at first. Hotel facilities are often unsuitable, even if the contrary is stated on the booking form, and it may be impossible to obtain the correct food.

Arrange with neighbors to leave the animal with them, giving all necessary instructions for feeding, cleaning and exercise. It is usually better to ask the neighbor to put out food in your own home for cats, as they will not adapt to a new home and the sudden absence of their owners, and may stray. Alternatively, there are special animal homes for cats and kennels for dogs where, for a reasonable fee, pets are properly looked after.

FIRST AID

When an animal is injured, the object should be to get expert assistance as soon as possible. All pet-lovers should know the address of the nearest veterinary surgeon.

An animal in pain may bite, so if you find an injured dog or cat on the road throw a coat over it and carry it to the side. Absolute rest and quiet are needed until expert help arrives.

When trying to find out the nature of an injury, handle the animal carefully. With a dog or cat, watch for individual peculiarities, for some bear injuries remarkably well and others do not.

Never be too hasty in assuming the animal is dead. It is better to treat a dead body than to neglect a live one.

Attend a severe hemorrhage first whatever other injuries there are. First get the animal in a restful position. You will then be able to handle it better with less chance of further injury.

Allow the animal plenty of space and air, keep it warm and be as speedy as possible. Massaging limbs restores circulation and should be employed where possible.

With burns or scalds, put the animal under restraint and apply strong cold tea.

A sting to a small bird or animal can be serious. A bee leaves its sting in the victim and it must be removed with a fingernail or blunt knife. If possible pinch up the affected area between finger and thumb for several minutes. Apply vinegar and, in case of shock, give adrenaline which is obtainable from chemists.

In cases of choking, skilled help is essential. Small objects can sometimes be extracted from the throat with the finger or a small pair of pliers, and lubrication with olive oil may be helpful.

Always wash your hands in disinfectant before touching wounds and be sure that anything you use in the course of giving first aid is scrupulously clean.

Fix bandages with adhesive tape. Cats and dogs will always attempt to pull a dressing or bandage off.

GLOSSARY

Abdomen. The belly.

Abdominal cavity. The cavity inside the belly.

Abduction. Drawn away from the mid-line of the body.

Abductor. A muscle which causes abduction.

Abortive. Not fully developed. Tending to induce abortion.

Abscess. A collection of pus.

Acetabulum. The socket of the hip joint.

Acidosis. Abnormal accumulation of acids in the body tissues and blood, with reduction of the alkali reserve.

Acromion. The projection of the shoulder blade which unites with the collar-bone.

Acute. Sudden. Of short duration. Sharp.

Adam's apple. The prominent thyroid cartilage in an adult male.

Adduction. Drawn toward the mid-line of the body.

Adductor. A muscle which causes adduction.

Adenoid. Overgrowth of glandular tissue at the back of the nose.

After-birth. The fleshy mass or placenta expelled from the womb after childbirth.

Ague. Malaria.

Albumin. A protein substance present in the blood, and in egg-white.

Alimentary tract. The digestive tract, from mouth to anus.

Allergy. Abnormal sensitivity, usually in relation to proteins.

Alopecia. Baldness.

Alveolar. Relating to (1) the teeth sockets; (2) the air-vesicles of the lungs.

Amenorrhea. Absence of menstruation.

Amnesia. Loss of memory.

Amniotic fluid. The fluid surrounding the fetus in the womb.

Amorphous. Without definite form.

Ampoule. Small glass phial containing a drug ready for use.

Anemia. Defect of blood (red cells). Deficiency of iron or red blood corpuscles in the blood; or presence of abnormal red cells.

Anesthesia. Lack of sensation, or lack of consciousness.

Aneurysm. A sac-like swelling formed by the dilatation of an artery, as a result of stretching of the wall.

Angina. Pain. Angina pectoris denotes pain in the region of the heart with sensation of suffocation. Vincent's angina is an inflammatory affection of the mouth or throat.

Ankylosis. A stiff joint. Fixation of a joint.

Anodyne. A medicament which relieves pain.

Anorexia. Loss of appetite.

Antacid. A substance which counteracts an acid.

Anthelmintic. A medicament which expels worms (helminths) from the bowel.

Antidote. A substance which counteracts the effects of a poison.

Antiscorbutic. A substance which prevents or cures scurvy.

Antisepsis. Prevention or counteraction of sepsis or infection.

Antispasmodic. A prevention of spasm.

Antisyphilitic. A preventive or a therapeutic measure for syphilis.

Antitoxin. A substance which counteracts a toxin.

Antrum. A hollow cavity, especially in a bone.

Anuria. Suppression of urine.

Anus. The extreme termination of the large intestine below the rectum.

Aperient. A laxative, or substance which opens the bowels.

Aphonia. Loss of voice.

Aphrodisiac. A substance which stimulates sexual excitement.

Aponeurosis. A whitish membranous investment of a muscle or tendon.

Apoplexy. Cerebral hemorrhage, or stroke.

Areola. A colored ring; the circle around the nipple.

Aromatic. Having a spicy smell or pungent taste.

Arrhythmia. Irregularity or absence of rhythm, usually of the heart beat.

Arteriole. A small artery.

Arteriosclerosis. Hardening of the arteries.

Artery. A blood vessel.

Arthritis. Inflammation of a joint, or degenerative changes in the articular surfaces or in the joint cartilages.

Articular. Pertaining to a joint.

Ascites. Fluid within the abdominal cavity.

Asepsis. Free from sepsis or infection.

Asphyxia. Suspension of breathing. Suffocation.

Aspiration. Withdrawal of fluid from a cavity, joint or ganglion.

Asthenic. Debilitated. Spare or slight physique.

Asthma. Paroxysms of difficulty in breathing, especially in expiration, with wheezing and constriction or spasm of the air passages.

Astragalus. Ankle bone.

Astringent. A substance with a drying-up, constricting or binding action. A medicine which induces constipation.

Ataxia. Irregularity of voluntary muscular action, with unsteadiness.

Athetosis. Purposeless movements of hands or feet; usually due to a brain lesion.

Atrophy. Shrinkage or wasting of a part of the body.

Auricle. The external ear; or an upper chamber of the heart.

Auscultation. The detection of physical signs in health and disease by listening to the breath sounds, or heart sounds, etc.

Autopsy. A post-mortem examination.

Axilla. The armpit.

Bacillus. A rod-shaped microbe.

Bacteria. Microbes or germs.

Bacteriophage. A biological agent which destroys and dissolves bacteria.

Bile. The fluid formed by the liver, with a yellow color in man, and a bitter taste.

Bladder. The gall-bladder is a pear-shaped bag on the under surface of the liver: it stores bile. The urinary bladder is a muscular bag in the lower pelvis: it is a reservoir for urine.

Boil. An inflamed swelling or abscess in the hair follicles or glands of the skin. A furuncle.

Bradycardia. Slow pulsation of the heart.

Bronchi. The air passages in the lungs.

Bubo. An inflammatory swelling in the lymphatic glands, usually in the groin or armpit.

Bulla. A large water blister.

Bunion. A deformity with swelling of the joint of the big toe.

Bursa. A sac or pouch, below a tendon, and often near a joint.

Bursitis. Inflammation of a bursa.

Calculus. A solid body or 'stone,' a concretion formed in certain parts of the body such as the kidneys or bladder.

Callosity. Local thickening of the skin.

Callus. The supporting tissue formed during the healing of a fractured bone.

Calorie. A unit for measuring heat. One calorie raises the temperature of one cubic centimeter of water by 1°C.

Cancellous. Resembling lattice work.

Capillary. As fine as a hair. A very small blood vessel.

Capsule. A membranous sac surrounding an organ or a part, as in a joint. Gelatinous container for drugs.

Carbuncle. An abscess involving several hair follicles of the skin and underlying tissues, common in diabetes and states of debility.

Carcinoma. Cancer.

Cardiac. Belonging to the heart.

Caries. Decay of a bone, or tooth.

Carminative. A medicine which relieves flatulence and pain in the bowels.

Carpal. Belonging to the wrist.

Cartilage. A firm white elastic substance covering the joint surfaces, and found in the larynx, trachea, etc. Gristle.

Caruncle. A small red fleshy growth, often at the urethral entrance.

Catamenia. The menstrual flow in women.

Catarrh. Inflammation of mucous membrane, with excess secretion of mucus.

Cathartic. Purgative.

Catheter. A tube for drawing off urine, mucus, etc.

Cell. A minute mass of protoplasm, enclosed in a membrane and containing a nucleus. The tissues of the bodies of animals and plants are composed of cells.

Cellular. Composed of cells.

Cerebellum. The hind and lower part of the brain.

Cerebral. Belonging to the brain.

Cerebrum. The main part of the brain, or forebrain.

Cervical. Pertaining to the neck, or the neck of the womb.

Chalybeate. Containing iron.

Chancre. A syphilitic ulcer, or 'primary sore' of syphilis.

Chemosis. Swelling of the conjunctiva of the eye. In severe cases the cornea appears to lie in a pit.

Chlorosis. A form of anemia seen in young women, causing a greenish pallor.

Cholagogue. A medicine which stimulates the flow of bile.

Cholecystitis. Inflammation of the gall-bladder.

Chordee. Painful erection of the penis in gonorrhea.

Chyle. The liquid products of digestion (mainly emulsified fats) in the intestines.

Chyme. The digested food pulp in the stomach.

Clavicle. The collar-bone.

Clonic. Alternating contraction and relaxation of spasm in a muscle.

Colic. Severe griping pain in the bowels, ureters, etc.

Colon. The large intestine.

Colostomy. A surgical opening from the colon through the abdominal wall to act as an artificial anus.

Colostrum. The early secretion before the milk in a nursing mother.

Coma. Insensibility, or profound stupor or unconsciousness.

Condyle. A protuberance at the end of a bone.

Confluent. Running together.

Congenital. Existing at or dating from birth.

Congestion. An abnormal accumulation of blood in a part.

Conjunctiva. The membrane lining the eyelids and covering the eyeballs.

Contagion. Spread of disease by direct contact with the body or discharges of the patient.

Contra-indicated. Not indicated.

Contusion. A bruise.

Convulsions. A fit; or involuntary contractions of the muscles of the body causing a seizure, sometimes with insensibility.

Cord, spinal. The column of nerves within the spine.

Cord, umbilical. The navel cord attached to the umbilicus and connecting the child to the mother's womb.

Cordate. Heart-shaped.

Cornea. The transparent layer covering the front of the eye.

Coronary. Encircling, as by a blood vessel.

Corrosive. Destructive, or eating away (a term used for certain poisons such as strong acids and alkalis, and corrosive sublimate).

Coryza. A cold in the head; nasal catarrh.

Costive. Constipated.

Counter-irritation. Irritation of one part which relieves congestion or pain in another part.

Crisis. The turning-point in the course of a disease.

Croup. Laryngitis in children, with spasm and hoarse cough.

Cutaneous. Belonging to the skin.

Cuticle. The outer skin.

Cutis. The true skin.

Cyst. A sac containing fluid or 'jelly,' or other soft matter

Cystitis. Inflammation of the bladder.

D.N.A. Desoxyribonucleic acid; the basic molecule of the cell nucleus.

Dandruff. Scurf.

Debility. General weakness.

Defecation. The act of evacuation of the bowels.

Deficiency disease. A disease resulting from lack of an essential substance, usually a vitamin.

Delirium. Mental excitement with restlessness, hallucinations, illusions or delusions. Seen in fevers, alcoholism, drug addiction, etc.

Delusion. Hallucination. Erroneous belief.

Dementia. Loss of the powers of mind.

Demulcent. A soothing soft substance used to alleviate inflamed mucous surfaces.

Dermis. The true skin.

Desquamation. Peeling or scaling of the outer layers of the skin.

Detergent. Cleaning; cleansing agent.

Diagnosis. Recognition of a disease by its characteristic symptoms or signs.

Diaphoretic. A medicine or treatment which induces sweating.

Diathesis. A particular disposition or state or habit, good or bad.

Diffusion. Spreading of a liquid or a gas through a membrane, or other medium.

Dilatation. Expansion. Distension of a hollow organ or structure.

Diluent. Watery drinks, which increase the fluidity of the blood or make the body fluids less viscid.

Diplopia. Double vision.

Dipsomania. A craving for alcoholic drinks.

Discrete. Separate.

Disinfectant. A substance which prevents or arrests infection by germs.

Disinfection. Destruction of germs.

Dislocation. Displacement of the bones of a joint.

Dissemination. Scattering over a wide area.

Diuresis. A profuse flow of urine.

Diuretic. A medicine or treatment which causes a copious flow of urine.

Diverticulitis. Inflammation of a pouch formed in the large bowel.

Dura Mater. The membrane lining the skull and spinal column, and forming the outer covering of the brain and spinal cord.

Dysarthria. Difficulty in speaking.

Dysmenorrhea. Difficult or painful menstruation.

Dyspepsia. Disorder of the digestive processes.

Dysphagia. Difficulty in swallowing.

Dyspnea. Difficulty in breathing.

Dysuria. Difficulty or pain in passing urine.

E.C.T. Electroconvulsive therapy.

E.E.G. Electroencephalogram.

E.N.T. Ear, nose and throat.

E.S.R. Erythrocyte sedimentation rate.

Eclampsia. Toxemic convulsions in pregnancy or the puerperium.

Ectopic. In an abnormal position. In ectopic pregnancy the fetus lies outside the womb.

Edema. Dropsy. Swelling due to serous effusion in a part of the body.

Emaciation. A wasted condition. Extreme leanness.

Embolism. The blockage of an artery by a clot, or by air or other foreign substance.

Emetic. A substance which induces vomiting.

Emmenagogue. A medicine used to stimulate the flow of the menses.

Emollient. A substance which softens or relaxes the tissues, when applied externally.

Emphysema. Distension of the tissues by air (especially the lungs).

Encephalitis. Inflammation of the brain.

Endemic. Prevailing or found regularly in a district or community.

Enuresis. Incontinence of urine.

Epidemic. Prevalent. Affecting a district or community at a certain time. A widespread outbreak of disease.

Epispastic. A substance which inflames the skin and raises a blister.

Epistaxis. Bleeding from the nose.

Epithelial. Belonging to the epithelium or outer layer of the skin or mucous membrane.

Eructation. Belching of wind or small amounts of fluid from the stomach.

Erythema. Redness of the skin, as in slight burns, or various rashes.

Escharotic. A substance which burns or destroys the tissues, and forms an eschar or slough.

Esophagus. Gullet or food-pipe.

Exacerbation. An increase in the severity of a disease or symptoms.

Exfoliation. The shedding of scales or flakes of skin.

Expectorant. A medicament which promotes or assists the coughing up of phlegm or sputum.

Extension. The act of straightening a part of the body such as a limb, or the spine.

Exudate. A discharge of fluid such as pus, sweat, serum, or muco-pus, through the tissues or a wound.

Farinaceous. Starchy.

Fauces. The pharynx, or back of the mouth, at the upper end of the throat.

Febrifuge. A medicine which allays or diminishes fever.

Febrile. Feverish.

Feces. The stools.

Fermentation. Chemical decomposition due to the action of germs, yeasts, etc.

Fetid. Foul-smelling.

Fibrosis. The formation of fibrous or scar tissue.

Fibrositis. Inflammation of connective tissue, such as joint capsules or muscles.

Fibrous. Composed of dense connective or scar tissue.

Filtration. The process of separation of solids from liquids by the use of a filter. Straining.

Fissure. A cleft or crack. It may be normal, as in the brain, or abnormal, as in anal fissure.

Fistula. An unnatural communication between two different structures.

Flaccid. Loose or flabby. Relaxed.

Flatulence. Distension of the stomach or bowels by gas or air.

Flatus. Air or gas in the stomach or bowels, or expelled from the stomach or rectum.

Flexion. The bending of a part, such as a limb.

Follicle. A gland, such as a hair follicle; a little bag or sac.

Fomentation. A hot, wet application to the surface of the body.

Fomites. Porous substances which may transmit contagion, e.g. clothing, toys, books.

Foramen. A small hole or opening.

Formication. A sensation like the creeping of ants.

Fulminating. Developing quickly and with rapid fatal termination.

Functional. Affecting the function or use, without change of structure in a part.

Furuncle. A boil or inflammatory swelling.

Furunculosis. A crop of small boils (especially of the ear passage).

Galenical. A drug of vegetable origin.

Ganglion. (1) A swelling in nerve tissue; (2) a cystic swelling arising from a tendon sheath or joint capsule.

Gangrene. Death of tissues or loss of vitality in a part, especially due to interference with the circulation.

Gastric. Pertaining to the stomach.

Gastritis. Inflammation of the stomach.

Genital. Pertaining to generation or reproduction.

Geriatrics. The branch of medicine dealing with the aging process and the diseases of old age.

Gestation. The period of pregnancy.

Gleet. A slimy discharge (generally gonorrheal) from a mucous surface.

Glossal. Pertaining to the tongue.

Glottis. The opening of the larynx, protected by the epiglottis.

Glycosuria. The presence of sugar in the urine.

Goiter. A tumor or swelling of the thyroid gland.

Gullet. The throat.

Granulation. A small red mass of new tissue containing blood vessels, formed in the repair of wounds, ulcers, burns, etc.

Hallucinations. Abnormal sense impressions or perceptions (such as apparitions or sounds) with no outward cause. Delusions, common in insanity.

Heartburn. A burning or acrid sensation in the stomach.

Hematemesis. Vomiting of darkish red blood, often with food particles. It indicates disease of the stomach or upper intestine.

Hematocele. A tumor containing blood.

Hematothorax. An effusion of blood into the pleural cavity.

Hematuria. The passage of blood in the urine.

Hemiplegia. Paralysis of one side of the body.

Hemoptysis. Expectoration of bright red frothy blood, often with sputum. It indicates lung injury or disease.

Hemorrhage. A flow of blood.

Hemorrhoids. Piles, or dilated veins of the anus or rectum.

Hepatic. Belonging to the liver.

Heredity. The transmission of qualities from ancestors or parents to the offspring.

Hernia. Rupture, or protrusion through an abnormal opening in the body.

Herpes. Small blebs or vesicles on the skin or lips due to virus infection. Herpes zoster is popularly called Shingles.

Hirsute. Hairy.

Hives. Nettlerash. Urticaria.

Hormone. A secretion from a ductless or endocrine gland.

Housemaid's Knee. Inflammation of the bursa in front of the knee-cap, with swelling.

Hydrocele. A swelling containing serous fluid in the scrotum or the spermatic cord.

Hydrocephalus. A collection of serous fluid within the skull or brain; 'water on the brain.'

Hydrotherapy. Treatment by the use of water, or medicated waters, either internally or externally.

Hydrothorax. Dropsy or fluid in the chest (thorax).

Hypermetropia. Long-sightedness.

Hypertrophy. Abnormal overgrowth, or dilatation of parts or organs, without change of structure.

Hypnotic. A substance or procedure which induces sleep.

Hypochondria. A nervous disorder often associated with indigestion, characterized by imaginary fears or ailments.

Hypodermic. Beneath the skin.

Hypotonic. With less tone than usual. A more dilute salt solution than the blood plasma.

Hysterectomy. An operation for removal of the uterus, or womb.

Hysteria. A nervous disturbance or disorder, often with paroxysms of crying, laughing or screaming, or a choking sensation in the throat. Counterfeit of some organic disease.

Idiosyncrasy. An individual peculiarity of constitution or temperament.

Immobilize. To render immobile. In surgery, the use of splints to hold immovable a normally mobile part, or the fragments of a fracture.

Impotence. Without sexual power.

Incontinence. Loss of control of the passage of urine or feces.

Incoordination. Failure of muscles or parts to work or move in harmony.

Incubation. The period between exposure to a specific infection and the onset of symptoms.

Indolent. Slow to heal, e.g. of an ulcer.

Infantilism. Delayed or imperfect development of mind or body.

Infection. The invasion of the body by germs or viruses which cause disease.

Infiltration. The spread of some abnormal substance in the tissues, such as a local anesthetic, or a malignant growth.

Inflammation. The changes occurring in tissues after infection, irritation or injury.

Inoculation. Vaccination, or the controlled introduction of the germ or toxin of a disease into a healthy person by injection or other methods to induce immunity.

Insidious. Advancing imperceptibly.

Insomnia. Sleeplessness.

Intercostal. Between the ribs.

Intestines. The bowels.

Intracranial. Within the cranium or skull.

Intramuscular. Within a muscle.

Intrathecal. Within the covering membranes of the spinal cord.

Intravenous. Within a vein.

Inunction. The application of drugs or medicated substances in the form of ointments.

Isotonic. Having the same strength of concentration as the blood plasma.

Itch. Scabies.

Jugular. Pertaining to the throat.

Kyphosis. A form of curvature of the upper part of the spine; hunchback.

Lachrymal. Pertaining to tears or secretion of tears.

Laryngitis. Inflammation of the larynx.

Larynx. The voice-box, in the upper part of the windpipe.

Latent. Concealed or dormant.

Laxatives. Medicines which induce relaxation of the bowels.

Lesion. Damage to tissues by an injury or disease.

Leucocytosis. An increase in the number of white corpuscles in the blood.

Leucorrhea. A whitish discharge from the vagina. 'Whites.'

Ligature. A cord or thread, or other strand for tying.

Lipoma. A benign fatty tumor.

Lochia. The discharge from the womb after childbirth.

Lumbago. Pain or fibrositis in the muscles of the lower part of the back.

Luxation. Dislocation.

Lymph. The alkaline fluid in the lymphatic vessels.

Lymphatic vessel. A vessel which conveys lymph.

Lysis. Gradual fall of a high temperature to normal.

Maceration. Softening by soaking.

Macula. A flat red or discolored spot on the skin.

Malaise. A vague or general feeling of ill-health.

Malaria. A fever conveyed by the bite of a mosquito infected with a malarial parasite.

Malignant. Generally cancerous. Malignant hypertension: progressive high blood pressure. Malignant endocarditis: a virulent and often fatal form of bacterial infection of the lining of the heart.

Mammary. Belonging to the breast.

Mandible. The lower jaw.

Mania. A mental disorder, or form of insanity, with great excitement and restlessness, and hallucinations or delusions.

Mastication. The act of chewing.

Mastitis. Inflammation of the breast.

Mastoiditis. Inflammation of the mastoid, or bony process, behind the ear.

Masturbation. Onanism. Abnormal sexual stimulation or gratification by the individual.

Meatus. An opening or mouth.

Melancholia. A mental disorder with depression and reduced activity of body and mind.

Melanoma. A black or pigmented tumor, usually cancerous.

Menorrhagia. Excessive menstrual flow.

Menses. The menstrual flow.

Mesentery. A membrane in the cavity of the abdomen which supports the intestines.

Metabolism. The chemical and physical processes in the body concerned in the assimilation of food, and in the growth, maintenance and repair of tissues.

Metacarpus. The five bones of the hand between the wrist and fingers.

Metatarsus. The five bones of the foot between the instep and toes.

Metastasis. Transmission from one part to another, as in a disease such as cancer.

Metritis. Inflammation of the womb.

Metrorrhagia. Bleeding from the womb between the periods, or after the menopause.

Micturition. The act of passing urine.

Monoplegia. Paralysis of one limb, or one side of the face.

Mucocele. An abnormally dilated cavity in the body due to the accumulation of mucus.

Mucus. The slimy secretion of the mucous membranes as of the nose, vagina, intestines, etc.

Murmur. An abnormal heart sound.

Myelitis. Inflammation of the spinal cord, or of the bone-marrow.

Myocarditis. Inflammation of the heart muscle.

Myopia. Short-sightedness.

Myxedema. A disease of adults (usually women), due to lack of thyroid gland secretion, with thickening of the tissues, especially the face, dullness of the mental faculties, and slowness of movement.

Narcotic. A medicine which relieves pain and induces sleep.

Nausea. A desire to vomit.

Necrosis. Death of a limited part of tissue, such as bone, muscle or brain, etc.

Neoplasm. A new growth, or tumor.

Nephritis. Inflammation of the kidney.

Nephrosis. A condition resembling chronic nephritis, of obscure origin.

Nettlerash. Allergic skin eruption attended by great irritation. Urticaria.

Neuralgia. Pain in a nerve.

Neuritis. Inflammation in a nerve.

Neurosis. A functional disorder of the nervous system, often with symptoms resembling organic disease.

Nevus. A birth mark, such as a pigmented mole (gray, brown, or almost black) or the so-called 'spider' and 'strawberry' nevus or port-wine stain, rich in blood vessels.

Nit. The egg of a louse.

Nucleus. The central dense zone in a cell, which controls the life processes of the cell.

Nutrient. Sustaining or nourishing.

Obstetrics. The science dealing with care of the pregnant woman and management of childbirth. The science of childbirth.

Occult. Obscure. Hidden.

Omentum. A fatty part of the peritoneum attached to the stomach.

Ophthalmia. Inflammation of the eyes, usually with discharge.

Ophthalmic. Belonging or pertaining to the eyes.

Opisthotonus. Extreme arching or extension of the back so that the body may rest on the heels and back of the head. Occurs in meningitis.

Oral. Pertaining to the mouth.

Orchitis. Inflammation of a testicle.

Orthopedics. Correction and treatment of deformities, and joint and muscular disorders.

Osmosis. Diffusion of liquids through a membrane.

Ossification. The formation of hard bone.

Osteoarthritis. Degenerative changes in a joint.

Osteomyelitis. Inflammation of a bone and its marrow.

Ovum. An egg.

Pain, Referred. Pain situated in a part of the body which is more or less remote from the cause of the pain.

Palliative. An agent which relieves symptoms but does not cure.

Papilla. A small raised point on the tongue, skin, or mucous membrane.

Papilloma. A wart; or small tumor of the skin or mucous surfaces.

Paracentesis. A procedure in which the abdomen, chest, ear drum, the pericardium, or a joint capsule is punctured and fluid is released.

Paralysis. Loss of power in a muscle or group of muscles or part.

Paraplegia. Paralysis affecting both sides of the body, usually both the legs, and part of the trunk.

Parasite. A living organism which feeds upon another living body.

Paroxysm. Occurring in sudden bouts. A sudden or acute attack.

Parturition. The act of childbirth.

Patent. Open. Not closed.

Pediatrics. The branch of medicine dealing with the diseases of childhood.

Pediculi. Lice.

Pelvis. The bony girdle below the abdomen, encircling the bladder, womb, rectum, etc.

Pemphigus. A skin eruption with watery blebs.

Pericarditis. Inflammation of the membranous sac surrounding the heart.

Perineum. The skin and tissues between the anus and sexual parts.

Periostitis. Inflammation of the membrane covering a bone.

Peripheral. Away from the center of the body.

Peristalsis. Muscular movements of the walls of the stomach and intestines which propel the contents.

Peritoneum. The membrane lining the abdomen, and covering many of the abdominal organs.

Peritonitis. Inflammation of the peritoneum.

Permeability. Porosity.

Pernio. Chilblain.

Petechiae. Very small dark red or purple spots, due to small hemorrhages into the skin or mucous membrane.

Phantom tumor. A tumor or swelling of the abdomen falsely suggesting or mistaken for pregnancy.

Pharynx. The upper part of the throat at the back of the mouth.

Phlebitis. Inflammation of a vein.

Phobia. A fear or apprehension without reasonable cause.

Photophobia. Aversion to light.

Phrenic. Pertaining to the diaphragm or the nerve to the diaphragm.

Pleura. The membrane lining the thorax and covering the lungs.

Pleurisy. Inflammation of the pleura.

Pneumothorax. Air in the cavity of the chest, outside the lungs.

Polyuria. Increased secretion of urine.

Pox. Syphilis.

Precordial. In front of the heart.

Prenatal. During pregnancy, before childbirth.

Priapism. Persistent painful erection of the penis.

Prognosis. The outlook in disease, or forecast of the probable course and outcome of any disorders.

Prolapse. Descent, or falling down, as of the womb or vagina.

Prophylactic. Preventive.

Protoplasm. The vital jelly-like substance of the cells of animals, plants, molds, bacteria, etc.

Pruritus. Itching of the skin.

Ptosis. Drooping of the upper eyelid, with inability to raise it.

Ptyalism. Increased salivation.

Puberty. The age at which the sexual organs begin to be fully active.

Puerperium. The lying-in period after childbirth, up to about three weeks.

Pyelitis. Inflammation of the upper end of the ureter within the pelvis of the kidney.

Pyemia. Pus in the blood.

Pyrexia. Fever.

Refraction. A change of direction made by rays of light when they pass obliquely through media of different density, as through air and water, or glass and air.

Remission. A reduction or disappearance of the symptoms of a disease.

Resolution. Dispersal of inflammation.

Respiration. The act of breathing.

Retroversion. Backward displacement, usually of the womb.

Rhinitis. Inflammation of the nasal membrane.

Rigor. A shivering attack; rigidity.

Rubefacient. An application which stimulates and reddens the skin.

Rupture. The breaking through or bursting through of an organ or part from the cavity in which it normally lies. Hernia. Breaking of a muscle or tendon, or bursting of an organ such as the spleen, bladder, kidney, etc.

St. Vitus's Dance. An earlier name for a form of chorea, a nervous disorder with irregular twitchings of the facial muscles and extremities.

Saline. Salt solution. 'Normal' saline has the same salt content as the blood plasma.

Sciatica. Pain in the sciatic nerve.

Sclerosis. Hardening of a tissue.

Scoliosis. Lateral curvature of the spine.

Scorbutic. Pertaining to scurvy.

Scrotum. The bag which contains the testes.

Scurvy. A deficiency disease due to lack of vitamin C.

Scybala. Hard masses of feces.

Sensory. Pertaining to sensation.

Sepsis. Infection by germs.

Sequestra. Dead fragments of bone.

Serous. Pertaining to serum.

Serum. The thin yellowish fluid which separates from the blood during clotting.

Shingles. See Herpes.

Slough. A dead portion of tissue which may separate from the living part.

Sordes. Offensive brown material which forms round the lips and mouth during severe fevers.

Spastic. Rigid or stiff. In spasm.

Speculum. An instrument used for examining the ear or vagina, etc.

Sphincter. A ring of muscle which serves as a valve at an opening, such as the anus, vagina, or mouth, etc.

Sphygmomanometer. An instrument for measuring blood pressure.

Sputum. Expectorated material.

Stasis. Stagnation.

Stenosis. Narrowing of a passage or opening, causing obstruction.

Sterilization. (1) Destruction of germs by disinfection; (2) the production of sterility or barrenness.

Stertor. Snoring or noisy breathing.

Stimulant. A preparation which increases activity, mental or physical.

Stomatitis. Inflammation of the mouth.

Strabismus. Squint.

Strangury. Pain and inability to pass urine except in small quantities.

Stricture. Narrowing or constriction, as of the gullet, urethra or rectum.

Stupor. A state of partial insensibility.

Styptic. A preparation which constricts the blood vessels when applied externally, and which helps to stop bleeding.

Subcutaneous. Beneath the skin.

Sudorific. A medicine which causes a profuse flow of perspiration. Diaphoretic.

Suppository. A medical preparation in the form of a small cone or cylinder, for use in the rectum in constipation, hemorrhoids, stricture, etc.

Suppuration. The formation of pus.

Syncope. Heart failure. Fainting. Circulatory failure.

Synovitis. Inflammation of the synovial membrane of a joint.

Tachycardia. Rapid action of the heart.

Talipes. Club-foot.

Tenesmus. A painful bearing down in the lower part of the bowel, with straining in attempts at defecation, even when the rectum is empty of feces.

Thrombosis. Clotting of blood in the arteries, veins or heart cavity.

Thrush. A fungous infection of the mucous membrane, especially of the mouth in babies.

Tinnitus. Noises in the ears.

Tissue. A part of the body composed of similar cells, e.g. muscle, skin, bone, fat, glandular tissue, etc.

Tone. A state of tension.

Torticollis. Wry-neck.

Tourniquet. An apparatus for reducing or arresting hemorrhage from a wound.

Toxic. Poisonous.

Transfusion. The passage of blood, saline or other fluids into the circulation of a recipient.

Trauma. Physical injury, as from a blow pressure, burn, or extreme cold. Mental injury.

Tumor. A swelling.

Ureter. The tube from each kidney which passes down to the bladder.

Urethra. The water passage from the bladder.

Vaccination. See Inoculation.

Vagina. The tubular front passage in women leading to the womb.

Vascular. Pertaining to blood vessels.

Venereal diseases. Syphilis, gonorrhea and 'soft sore.' They are propagated by sexual intercourse.

Venesection. The withdrawal of blood from a vein.

Vermifuge. An agent which expels worms.

Vertigo. Giddiness or dizziness.

Vesication. Blistering.

Virulent. Very potent or harmful.

Virus. A very minute ultra-microscopic living particle (smaller than bacteria) which can give rise to disease.

Viscera. Plural of viscus.

Viscous. Thick and sticky (of a fluid).

Viscus. An organ of the body such as the liver, stomach, heart, etc., contained in one of the body cavities.

Volatile. Capable of evaporating at a low temperature.

Wassermann Test. A test used in the diagnosis of syphilis.

INDEX

I

J

K

L

M

Q

R

S

Use the following pages to record medical information such as inoculations, diseases, operations, allergies, etc. for each member of the family